The Routledge Handbook of Social Work and Addictive Behaviors

The Routledge Handbook of Social Work and Addictive Behaviors is a definitive resource about addictive behaviors, emphasizing substance misuse, gambling, and problematic technology use. Contents address their prevalence in various communities and populations globally, theories related to their origins and etiology, and what is currently known about effective intervention strategies, education, and research. Social work's biopsychosocial, lifespan, and person-in-environment perspectives underpin the book contents which are applicable to a wide range of professional and social science disciplines. Contents are divided into five sections:

- The scope and nature of addictive behavior and related problems
- Addictive behavior across the lifespan and specific populations
- Interventions to prevent and address addictive behavior and related problems
- Issues frequently co-occurring with addictive behavior
- Moving forward

This handbook provides students, practitioners, and scholars with a strong focus on cutting-edge high-quality research. With contributions from a global interdisciplinary team of leading scholars, this handbook is relevant to readers from social work, public health, psychology, education, sociology, criminal justice, medicine, nursing, human services, and health professions.

Audrey L. Begun, MSW, PhD, Professor in the College of Social Work at The Ohio State University. For more information visit https://csw.osu.edu/about/faculty-staff/faculty-directory/begun-audrey-ph-d/.

Margaret M. Murray, MSW, PhD, retired as Director, Global Alcohol Research Program, National Institute on Alcohol Abuse and Alcoholism (NIAAA) at the National Institutes of Health (NIH).

The Routledge Handbook of Social Work and Addictive Behaviors

Edited by
Audrey L. Begun and Margaret M. Murray

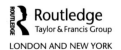

LONDON AND NEW YORK

First published 2020
by Routledge
2 Park Square, Milton Park, Abingdon, Oxon OX14 4RN

and by Routledge
52 Vanderbilt Avenue, New York, NY 10017

Routledge is an imprint of the Taylor & Francis Group, an informa business

British Library Cataloguing-in-Publication Data
A catalogue record for this book is available from the British Library

Library of Congress Cataloging-in-Publication Data
Names: Begun, Audrey L., editor. | Murray, Margaret M., editor.
Title: The Routledge handbook of social work and addictive behaviors /
edited by Audrey L. Begun and Margaret M. Murray.
Description: New York: Routledge, 2020. | Series: Routledge
international handbooks | Includes bibliographical references and index.
Identifiers: LCCN 2019050744 (print) | LCCN 2019050745 (ebook) |
ISBN 9780367195540 (hardback) | ISBN 9780429203121 (ebook)
Subjects: LCSH: Substance abuse. | Compulsive behavior. |
Substance abuse—Treatment. | Social service.
Classification: LCC HV4998 .R688 2020 (print) | LCC HV4998 (ebook) |
DDC 362.29/153—dc23
LC record available at https://lccn.loc.gov/2019050744
LC ebook record available at https://lccn.loc.gov/2019050745

ISBN: 978-0-367-19554-0 (hbk)
ISBN: 978-0-429-20312-1 (ebk)

Typeset in Bembo
by codeMantra

Contents

List of contributors   *ix*
Acknowledgments   *xvii*

1 Introduction to *The Routledge Handbook of Social Work
   and Addictive Behaviors*   1
   Audrey L. Begun and Margaret M. Murray

INTRODUCTION TO SECTION I
**The scope and nature of addictive behaviors
and related problems**   **17**

2 Introduction to psychoactive substances   18
   Audrey L. Begun

3 Global alcohol epidemiology: focus on women of childbearing age   39
   Svetlana Popova, Jürgen Rehm and Kevin Shield

4 Overview of addiction and the brain   58
   Aaron M. White and George F. Koob

5 The role of genes and environments in shaping substance misuse   78
   Cristina B. Bares and Karen G. Chartier

6 Psychological models of addictive behavior   95
   Audrey L. Begun

7 Social environmental contexts of addictive behavior   110
   Audrey L. Begun, Cristina B. Bares and Karen G. Chartier

8 Gambling disorder: the first behavioral addiction   129
   Lia Nower, Devin Mills and Wen Li (Vivien) Anthony

Contents

9 Internet Gaming Disorder and problematic technology use   142
   Wen Li (Vivien) Anthony, Devin Mills and Lia Nower

INTRODUCTION TO SECTION II
Addictive behavior across the lifespan and specific populations   157

10 Neonatal abstinence syndrome: recognition, management,
    and prevention   158
    *Kristina M. Reber, Amy B. Schlegel, Erica F. Braswell
    and Edward G. Shepherd*

11 Fetal alcohol spectrum disorder: evidence, theory, and
    current insights   174
    Christine Loock, Elizabeth Elliott and Lori Vitale Cox

12 The lay of the land: fetal alcohol spectrum disorder (FASD) as a
    whole-body diagnosis   191
    Myles Himmelreich, C. J. Lutke and Emily Travis Hargrove

13 The adolescent brain: predictors and consequences of substance use   216
    Lindsay R. Meredith and Lindsay M. Squeglia

14 Addictive behaviors during emerging adulthood   232
    Eric Wagner, Christine Spadola and Jordan P. Davis

15 Older adults and substance misuse   247
    Paul Sacco, Alexis Kuerbis and Robin Harris

16 Understanding addictive behavior from a human diversity perspective   262
    Christina C. Tam, Katherine J. Karriker-Jaffe and Karen G. Chartier

17 Substance use across the lifespan of the LGBTQ+ population   282
    Jacob Goffnett and Jeremy Goldbach

INTRODUCTION TO SECTION III
**Interventions to prevent and address addictive behavior
and related problems   297**

18 Intervening around addictive behaviors   298
    Allen Zweben and Brooke S. West

19 Current and emerging pharmacotherapies for addiction treatment   321
    Jeanelle Portelli, Vikas Munjal and Lorenzo Leggio

20 Screening, brief intervention, and referral to treatment (SBIRT) in
the substance use system of care 343
Corey Campbell, Douglas Smith, Kelly Lynn Clary and Lori Egizio

21 Mindfulness practices in addictive behavior prevention, treatment,
and recovery 355
Marjorie N. Edguer and Leigh Taylor

22 Working with children whose parents engage in substance misuse 366
Shulamith Lala Ashenberg Straussner and Christine H. Fewell

23 All drugs aren't created equal: exploring the general and specific
effects of psychoactive substances to understand child maltreatment
risk by drug type 381
Nancy Jo Kepple and Bridget Freisthler

24 Working with families affected by a member's addictive behavior 397
Megan Petra and Toula Kourgiantakis

25 The impact of addictive behavior on grandfamilies 410
Nancy Mendoza, Christine Fruhauf and Bert Hayslip, Jr.

26 Planning health promotion programs to prevent substance use
disorders and their consequences 423
Sylvia Roozen, Gerjo Kok and Leopold Curfs

27 Integrated care: identifying and intervening with substance
misuse in primary healthcare 436
*Stacey Saunders-Adams, Catherine Hechmer, Adriane Peck
and Margaret M. Murray*

28 Drug treatment courts 453
Margaret Lloyd and Michael Fendrich

29 Roles for social work and other professions in support of
recovery-oriented addiction policies and services 469
Clifford Bersamira

30 Policy reforms to reduce harms associated with substance misuse 482
Sheila P. Vakharia and Jeannie Little

31 Decriminalization and medicalization of cannabis: implications of the
Caribbean experience for global social work practice 497
Barris Malcolm

Contents

32 Emerging policy and practice responses to substance use with
currently and formerly incarcerated women   513
   Susan J. Rose and Thomas P. LeBel

INTRODUCTION TO SECTION IV
Issues frequently co-occurring with addictive behaviors   **527**

33 Understanding addictive behaviors and co-occurring disorders   528
   Amanda R. Reedy

34 Substance misuse and intimate partner violence   545
   Cecilia Mengo and Kenneth Leonard

35 Substance-involved sexual assault   560
   *Kelly Cue Davis, Mitchell Kirwan, Elizabeth C. Neilson
   and Cynthia A. Stappenbeck*

INTRODUCTION TO SECTION V
Moving forward   **577**

36 Implementation of evidence-based substance misuse prevention and
treatment interventions   578
   Alicia Bunger, Jim Lange and Erica Magier

37 Core health professional education curriculum for risky substance use
and substance use disorder   590
   Lena Lundgren, Meredith Silverstein and Siv Nyström

38 Using GIS and spatial analysis to better integrate context into our
understanding of addictive behaviors   601
   Bridget Freisthler and Nancy Jo Kepple

39 Emerging priorities for practice and research   618
   Audrey L. Begun and Margaret M. Murray

*Appendix A: diagnostic criteria for alcohol use disorder (AUD)
and substance use disorders (SUD) in DSM-5® and ICD-11 protocols*   *625*
Index   *629*

Contributors

Wen Li (Vivien) Anthony, PhD, Assistant Professor in the Rutgers University School of Social Work and Research Affiliate in the Center for Gambling Studies. For more information visit https://socialwork.rutgers.edu/faculty-staff/wen-vivien-anthony

Cristina B. Bares, MSW, PhD, Associate Professor in the University of Michigan School of Social work. For more information visit https://ssw.umich.edu/faculty/profiles/tenure-track/cbb

Audrey L. Begun, MSW, PhD, Professor in the College of Social Work at The Ohio State University. For more information visit https://csw.osu.edu/about/faculty-staff/faculty-directory/begun-audrey-ph-d/

Clifford Bersamira, AM, PhD, Assistant Professor in the Myron B. Thompson School of Social Work at the University of Hawai'i at Mānoa. For more information visit https://www.hawaii.edu/sswork/faculty/bersamira-clifford/

Erica F. Braswell, MD, Medical Director, H7B Neonatal Intensive Care Unit at Nationwide Children's Hospital (Columbus, OH) and Assistant Professor of Pediatrics at The Ohio State University. erica.braswell@nationwidechildrens.org

Alicia Bunger, PhD, Associate Professor in The Ohio State University College of Social Work. For more information visit https://csw.osu.edu/about/faculty-staff/faculty-directory/bunger-alicia-ph-d/

Corey Campbell, LCSW, doctoral student in the University of Illinois at Urbana-Champaign School of Social Work. For more information visit https://socialwork.illinois.edu/academics/doctoral-program-ph-d/student_directory/

Karen G. Chartier, PhD, Associate Professor in the Virginia Commonwealth University Social Work and Affiliate Appointment with the Virginia Commonwealth University School of Medicine Department of Psychiatry. For more information visit https://socialwork.vcu.edu/about/our-team/karen-g-chartier-phd.html

Kelly Lynn Clary, MSW, doctoral candidate in the University of Illinois at Urbana-Champaign School of Social Work. For more information visit https://socialwork.illinois.edu/academics/doctoral-program-ph-d/student_directory/

Contributors

Lori Vitale Cox, PhD, Director of the Elsipogtog First Nation Eastern Door Centre of Excellence for Diagnosis, Intervention, Research, and Prevention of FASD and Related ND Disorders, and Adjunct Professor in the University of British Columbia Faculty of Medicine, Department of Pediatrics.

Leopold Curfs, PhD, Professor Maastricht University and director Governor Kremers Center, Maastricht University Medical Center. For more information visit https://gkcmaastricht.nl/

Jordan P. Davis, MSW, PhD, Assistant Professor at the University of Southern California (USC) Suzanne Dworak-Peck School of Social Work, Associate Director of the USC Center for Artificial Intelligence in Society, and Associate Director of Research in USC Center for Mindfulness Science. For more information visit https://dworakpeck.usc.edu/academics/faculty-directory/jordan-davis

Kelly Cue Davis, PhD, Associate Professor in the Edson College of Nursing and Health Innovation at Arizona State University. For more information visit https://isearch.asu.edu/profile/3175330

Marjorie N. Edguer, PhD, Assistant Professor in Jack, Joseph, and Morton Mandel School of Applied Social Sciences at Case Western University. For more information visit http://msass.case.edu/faculty/medguer/

Lori Egizio, DSW, LCSW, Adjunct Professor and Trainer in the University of Illinois at Urbana-Champaign School of Social Work. For more information visit https://www.linkedin.com/in/lori-egizio-b75a1335

Elizabeth Elliott, AM, MD, Professor in Paediatrics and Child Health at the University of Sydney, Consultant Paediatrician and Heath of the New South Wales FASD Assessment Service, Sydney Children's Hospitals Network, and National Health and Medical Research Council Practitioner Fellow. For more information visit http://sydney.edu.au/medicine/people/academics/profiles/elizabeth.elliott.php

Michael Fendrich, PhD, Professor and Associate Dean for Research at the University of Connecticut School of Social Work. For more information visit https://ssw.uconn.edu/person/michael-fendrich-phd/

Christine H. Fewell, LCSW, PhD, Adjunct Professor in the Silver School of Social Work at New York University. For more information visit https://socialwork.nyu.edu/our-faculty/adjunct.F.html

Bridget Freisthler, PhD, Professor and Associate Dean for Research in the College of Social Work, The Ohio State University. For more information visit https://csw.osu.edu/about/faculty-staff/faculty-directory/freisthler-bridget/

Christine Fruhauf, PhD, Professor and Director of Extension Programs and Initiatives, Coordinator of Gerontology Interdisciplinary Minor, Human Development and Family Studies at Colorado State University College of Health and Human Sciences. For more information visit http://www.hdfs.chhs.colostate.edu/faculty-staff/fruhauf.aspx

Jacob Goffnett, MSW, doctoral candidate in the University of Illinois at Urbana-Champaign School of Social Work. For more information visit https://socialwork.illinois.edu/academics/doctoral-program-ph-d/student_directory/

Jeremy Goldbach, MSSW, PhD, Associate Professor and Director of the LGBT Health Equity Initiative at the Suzanne Dworak-Peck School of Social Work, University of Southern California. For more information visit https://dworakpeck.usc.edu/academics/faculty-directory/jeremy-goldbach

Emily Travis Hargrove, Member of the Adult Leadership Committee of FASD Change Makers, Founding Member of Self-Advocates with FASD in Action (SAFA), and Member of the FASD Center for Excellence Expert Panel of the Substance Abuse and Mental Health Services Administration (SAMHSA). For more information visit https://thearc.org/wp-content/uploads/forchapters/ARC_FASD2.pdf

Robin Harris, LMSW, University of Maryland School Medical Center.

Bert Hayslip, Jr., PhD, Regents Professor Emeritus of Psychology, University of North Texas.

Catherine Hechmer, LISW-S, LICDC-CS, Interprofessional Education and Practice Field Coordinator in the College of Social Work at The Ohio State University. For more information visit https://csw.osu.edu/about/faculty-staff/staff-directory/hechmer-catherine/

Myles Himmelreich, Member of the Adult Leadership Committee of FASD Change Makers. For more information visit https://preventionconversation.org/2019/06/28/adults-who-have-fasd-leadership-committee-of-fasd-change-makers-survey-about-life-as-we-live-it-for-older-teens-and-adults-who-have-fasd-or-think-they-do/

Katherine J. Karriker-Jaffe, PhD, Senior Scientist at the Alcohol Research Group of the Public Health Institute (California). For more information visit http://arg.org/staff/katherine-karriker-jaffe/

Nancy Jo Kepple, PhD, Assistant Professor in the University of Kansas School of Social Welfare. For more information visit http://socwel.ku.edu/people/faculty/kepple-nancy-jo

Mitchell Kirwan, PhD, Postdoctoral Scholar in the Edson College of Nursing and Health Innovation at Arizona State University.

Gerjo Kok, PhD, Professor of Applied Psychology in the Department of Work and Social Psychology at Maastricht University, Netherlands. For more information visit https://www.maastrichtuniversity.nl/prof-dr-gerjo-kok

George F. Koob, PhD, Director of the National Institute on Alcohol Abuse and Alcoholism (NIAAA) at the National Institutes of Health (NIH). For more information visit https://www.niaaa.nih.gov/directors-page

Toula Kourgiantakis, PhD, Assistant Professor in the University of Toronto Factor-Inwentash Faculty of Social work. For more information visit https://socialwork.utoronto.ca/profiles/toula-kourgiantakis/

Alexis Kuerbis, LCSW, PhD, Associate Professor, Silberman School of Social Work at Hunter College, City University of New York. For more information visit http://sssw.hunter.cuny.edu/staff-members/kuerbis-alexis-m-s-w-ph-d/

Jim Lange, PhD, Executive Director of the Higher Education Center for Alcohol and Drug Misuse Prevention and Recovery (HECAOD) at The Ohio State University, and Coordinator of Alcohol and Other Drug Initiatives at San Diego State University. For more information visit https://hecaod.osu.edu/about/leadership/

Thomas P. LeBel, PhD, Associate Professor of Criminal Justice & Criminology in the University of Wisconsin-Milwaukee Helen Bader School of Social Welfare. For more information visit http://uwm.edu/socialwelfare/people/lebel-phd-thomas/

Lorenzo Leggio, MD, PhD, MSc, Senior Investigator and Chief of the Joint NIAAA-NIDA Section on Clinical Psychoneuroendocrinology and Neuropsychopharmacology (CPN) at the National Institutes of Health. For more information visit https://irp.nih.gov/pi/lorenzo-leggio

Kenneth Leonard, PhD, Senior Research Scientist and Director of the Clinical and Research Institute on Addictions (CRIA) at the University at Buffalo and Professor of Psychiatry in the Department of Psychiatry at the Jacobs School of Medicine and Biomedical Sciences, University at Buffalo. For more information visit https://www.buffalo.edu/ria/staff/scientists/kleonard.html

Jeannie Little, LCSW, Executive Director of The Center for Harm Reduction Therapy, California. For more information visit https://harmreductiontherapy.org/staff/jeannie-little-2/

Margaret Lloyd, PhD, Assistant Professor, University of Connecticut School of Social Work. For more information visit https://ssw.uconn.edu/person/margaret-lloyd-phd/

Christine Loock, MD, FRCPC, DABP, Developmental and Social Pediatrician, Medical Director, Cleft Palate Craniofacial Program, British Columbia Children's Hospital, Co-Founder and Specialist Director for Research, Social Pediatrics RICHER Program, Co-Founder of British Columbia FASD CDBC Provincial Assessment Programs, and Associate Professor, Department of Pediatrics, Faculty of Medicine, University of British Columbia. For more information visit https://www.bcchr.ca/cloock

Lena Lundgren, PhD, Executive Director, the Cross-National Behavioral Health Laboratory and Professor, Graduate School of Social Work, University of Denver. For more information visit https://socialwork.du.edu/about/gssw-directory/lena-lundgren

C. J. Lutke, Member of the Adult Leadership Committee of FASD Change Makers. For more information visit https://preventionconversation.org/2019/06/28/adults-who-have-fasd-leadership-committee-of-fasd-change-makers-survey-about-life-as-we-live-it-for-older-teens-and-adults-who-have-fasd-or-think-they-do/

Erica Magier, MSW, LSW, doctoral student in the College of Social Work at The Ohio State University. For more information visit https://csw.osu.edu/degrees-programs/phd/meet-our-doctoral-students/magier-erica/

Barris Malcolm, MSW, PhD, Emeritus Associate Professor, University of Connecticut School of Social Work and Adjunct Faculty in Social Work at Sacred Heart University (Connecticut).

Nancy Mendoza, MA, PhD, Assistant Professor in The Ohio State University College of Social Work. For more information visit https://csw.osu.edu/about/faculty-staff/faculty-directory/mendoza-nancy-ph-d/

Cecilia Mengo, PhD, Assistant Professor in the College of Social Work at The Ohio State University. For more information visit https://csw.osu.edu/about/faculty-staff/faculty-directory/mengo-cecilia-phd/

Lindsay R. Meredith, BA, doctoral student in Clinical Psychology at the University of California, Los Angeles. For more information visit https://addictions.psych.ucla.edu/wp-content/uploads/sites/160/2019/07/CV_Lindsay_Meredith_July19.pdf

Devin Mills, PhD., Assistant Professor in Community, Family, and Addiction Sciences at Texas Tech University. For more information visit https://scholar.google.com/citations?user=Iuk4LYYAAAAJ&hl=en

Vikas Munjal, BS, Post-Baccalaureate Fellow at the Joint NIAAA-NIDA Section on Clinical Psychoneuroendocrinology and Neuropsychopharmacology (CPN) at the National Institutes of Health.

Margaret M. Murray, MSW, PhD, retired as Director, Global Alcohol Research Program, National Institute on Alcohol Abuse and Alcoholism (NIAAA) at the National Institutes of Health (NIH).

Elizabeth C. Neilson, MSW, MPH, PhD, Assistant Professor of Psychology at Morehead State University. For more information visit https://www.moreheadstate.edu/College-of-Science/Psychology/Faculty-Staff/Elizabeth-Neilsen

Lia Nower, JD, PhD, Professor in the Rutgers University School of Social Work, Director of the Center for Gambling Studies, and Director Addiction Counselor Training Certificate (ACT) Program. For more information visit https://socialwork.rutgers.edu/faculty-staff/lia-nower

Siv Nyström, PhD, former National Research Program Manager for the Swedish National Board of Health and Welfare.

Adriane Peck, LISW, Adjunct Faculty in the College of Social Work, The Ohio State University.

Megan Petra, PhD, Assistant Professor of Social Work in the College of Health and Human Services at The University of Toledo. For more information visit http://www.utoledo.edu/hhs/facultystaff/PetraMegan.html

Svetlana Popova, MPH, MD, PHDs, Senior Scientist, Institute for Mental Health Policy Research and Campbell Family Mental Health Research Institute, Centre for Addiction and Mental Health (CAMH), Canada, Associate Professor, Epidemiology Division, Office of Global Public Health Education & Training, Dalla Lana School of Public Health, University of Toronto, and Factor-Inwentash Faculty of Social Work, University of Toronto, Graduate Faculty Full Member, Institute of Medical Science, University of Toronto. For more information visit https://www.camh.ca/en/science-and-research/science-and-research-staff-directory/svetlanapopova

Jeanelle Portelli, PhD, Visiting Scientist at the Joint NIAAA-NIDA Section on Clinical Psychoneuroendocrinology and Neuropsychopharmacology (CPN) at the National Institutes of Health. For more information visit https://ned.nih.gov/search/ViewDetails.aspx?NIHID=2002308090

Kristina M. Reber, MD, Associate Division Chief of the Neonatology Section at Nationwide Children's Hospital (Columbus, OH) and Professor of Pediatrics at The Ohio State University College of Medicine. For more information visit https://www.nationwide-childrens.org/find-a-doctor/profiles/kristina-m-reber

Amanda R. Reedy, MSW, PhD, Associate Professor, Eastern Washington University School of Social Work. For more information visit https://www.ewu.edu/css/social-work/social-work/contact-us/

Jürgen Rehm, PhD, Senior Scientist, Institute for Mental Health Policy Research and Campbell Family Mental Health Research Institute, Centre for Addiction and Mental Health (CAMH), Canada, Professor and Chair, Addiction Policy, Dalla Lana School of Public Health, University of Toronto, Canada, Professor, Department of Psychiatry, Faculty of Medicine, University of Toronto, Canada, Senior Scientist, Pan American Health Organization (PAHO)/ World Health Organization (WHO) Collaborating Centre for Addiction and Mental Health, Head, Epidemiological Research Unit, Technische Universität Dresden, Klinische Psychologie & Psychotherapie, Dresden, Germany, Professor, Department of International Health Projects, Institute for Leadership and Health Management, I.M. Sechenov First Moscow State Medical University, Moscow, Russian Federation, and Faculty member, Graduate Department of Community Health and Institute of Medical Science, University of Toronto. For more information visit https://www.camh.ca/en/science-and-research/science-and-research-staff-directory/jurgenrehm

Sylvia Roozen, PhD, Researcher and Faculty of Psychology and Neuroscience, Applied Social Psychology, Department of Work and Social Psychology, Maastricht University Medical Center—Governor Kremers Center (The Netherlands). For more information visit https://www.maastrichtuniversity.nl/sylvia.roozen

Susan J. Rose, MSW, PhD, Professor of Social Work in the University of Wisconsin-Milwaukee Helen Bader School of Social Welfare. For more information visit https://uwm.edu/socialwelfare/people/rose-phd-susan/

Paul Sacco, PhD, Associate Professor and Associate Dean for Research, University of Maryland School of Social Work. For more information visit http://www.ssw.umaryland.edu/academics/faculty/paul-sacco/

Stacey Saunders-Adams, PhD, Assistant Professor of Social Work at Ohio University, Chillicothe Campus. For more information visit https://www.ohio.edu/chillicothe/facilities/profiles.cfm?profile=6A1CE58F-5056-A81E-8DCD5E4D2F89D3AF

Amy B. Schlegel, MD, MS, Medical Director of C4C Neonatal Intensive Care Unit at Nationwide Children's Hospital (Columbus, OH) and Assistant Professor of Clinical Pediatrics at The Ohio State University College of Medicine. For more information visit https://www.nationwidechildrens.org/find-a-doctor/profiles/amy-brown-schlegel

Edward G. Shepherd, MD, Section Chief of Neonatology at Nationwide Children's Hospital (Columbus, OH) and Associate Professor of Clinical Pediatrics in The Ohio State University College of Medicine. For more information visit https://www.nationwidechildrens.org/find-a-doctor/profiles/edward-g-shepherd

Kevin Shield, PhD, Assistant Professor in the University of Toronto, Dalla Lana School of Public Health, Epidemiology Division, and Head of the World Health Organization (WHO)/Pan American Health Organization (PAHO) Collaborating Centre for Addiction and Mental Health (CAMH). For more information visit http://www.dlsph.utoronto.ca/faculty-profile/shield-kevin/

Meredith Silverstein, PhD, Senior Research Associate at the University of Denver Butler, Institute for Families in the Graduate School of Social Work. For more information visit https://www.thebutlerinstitute.org/team/meredith-silverstein

Douglas Smith, PhD, Associate Professor and Director of the Center for Prevention Research and Development in the University of Illinois at Urbana-Champaign School of Social Work. For more information visit http://socialwork.illinois.edu/faculty-staff/douglas-smith/

Christine Spadola, MS, PhD, Assistant Professor in Phyllis and Harvey Sandler School of Social Work at Florida Atlantic University. For more information visit http://cdsi.fau.edu/ssw/people/spadola/

Lindsay M. Squeglia, PhD, Associate Professor in Psychiatry and Behavioral Sciences, College of Medicine, at the Medical University of South Carolina (MUSC). For more information visit http://academicdepartments.musc.edu/facultydirectory/Squeglia-Lindsay

Cynthia A. Stappenbeck, PhD, Associate Professor in the Department of Psychiatry and Behavioral Sciences at the University of Washington. For more information visit https://sites.uw.edu/cshrb/our-people/faculty/cindy-stappenbeck/

Shulamith Lala Ashenberg Straussner, PhD, Professor in the Silver School of Social Work at New York University, visiting professor to NYU Shanghai, China, and University of Amsterdam, The Netherlands, distinguished visiting professor at Hebrew University, Jerusalem, Israel, Fulbright distinguished chair at Masaryk University, Czech Republic, Fulbright senior scholar at Ben Gurion University, Israel, and Kiev, Ukraine, and founding editor of the *Journal of Social Work Practice in the Addictions*. For more information visit https://socialwork.nyu.edu/our-faculty/full-time/shulamith-lala-ashenberg-straussner.html

Christina C. Tam, MSW, PhD, Associate Scientist at the Alcohol Research Group of the Public Health Institute (California). For more information visit http://arg.org/staff/christina-tam/

Leigh Taylor, PhD, Visiting Assistant Professor, Department of Social Work, Florida Gulf Coast University, and Contributing Faculty, College of Social and Behavioral Sciences, Solomon School of Social Work, Walden University. For more information visit https://www.fgcu.edu/mariebcollege/facultystaff/#DepartmentofSocialWork and https://www.waldenu.edu/about/faculty/meet-our-faculty/member-profile/leigh-taylor

Sheila P. Vakharia, PhD, MSW, Deputy Director, Department of Research and Academic Engagements, Drug Policy Alliance, New York City, NY. For more information visit http://www.drugpolicy.org/sheila-p-vakharia-phd

Eric Wagner, PhD, Professor in Stempel College of Public Health & Social Work, Florida International University, and Director of the Community-Based Research Institute (FIU-CBRI). For more information visit https://stempel.fiu.edu/faculty/eric-f-wagner/

Brooke S. West, PhD, Assistant Professor of Social Work at the Columbia University School of Social Work. For more information visit https://socialwork.columbia.edu/faculty-research/faculty/full-time/brooke-s-west/

Aaron M. White, PhD, Senior Scientific Advisor to the Director, Office of the Director, National Institute on Alcohol Abuse and Alcoholism (NIAAA) of the National Institutes of Health (NIH).

Allen Zweben, PhD, Professor in Columbia University School of Social Work. For more information visit https://socialwork.columbia.edu/faculty/full-time/allen-zweben/

Acknowledgments

As the project editors, we would like to acknowledge the following without which this book could not have emerged:

- the copious, efficient, and effective clerical assistance provided by Ms. Ambir Myers in the College of Social Work at The Ohio State University;
- donation of the cover art from Ms. Amy Grambeau;
- suggestions and recommendations offered by reviewers of the initial project proposal and each subsequent iteration;
- the mentoring and educations we have received from the many scholars, practitioners, educators, and colleagues in multiple nations and diverse disciplines with whom we have had the privilege of "rubbing elbows" over the course of our careers;
- all that we have learned from the many individuals experiencing or affected by others' experiences with addictive behavior and making change;
- the many social workers who have dedicated their careers to the addictive behaviors arena, in research, teaching, practice, and advocacy, despite the many challenges and barriers encountered;
- the patience our colleagues, students, spouses, son, daughters, grandchildren, sisters, and friends have shown over the past year, their willingness to listen to our frustrations, and celebrate our successes.

Introduction to *The Routledge Handbook of Social Work and Addictive Behaviors*

Audrey L. Begun and Margaret M. Murray

Background

Substance misuse and substance use disorders, as well as obsessive engagement in behaviors such as gambling and internet gaming, are associated with significant problems for individuals, families, communities, and nations. These addictive behaviors and their associated problems underlie serious global public health, mental health, legal, economic, and social concerns. Social workers and members of other professions have much to offer in response to addictive behaviors and associated problems. However, social workers are not uniformly prepared through pre-service and in-service training to recognize, understand, and effectively respond to addictive behaviors and their associated problems. For these reasons, the co-editors and collaborating authors of this *Routledge Handbook of Social Work and Addictive Behavior* joined together to create a much-needed resource for informing social work and other professions about addictive behaviors and how these professionals can work together to approach problems and issues associated with addictive behaviors. To be most beneficial, prevention and treatment of addictive behaviors and related problems must rely on multiple perspectives, theories, disciplines, systems, and levels; therefore, an integrative resource on this broad topic is particularly relevant.

In keeping with social work traditions, prevailing frameworks in this handbook include:

- adopting a multi-level/multi-system perspective of addictive behavior issues and change strategies;
- adopting a biopsychosocial emphasis;
- adopting a life course perspective;
- emphasizing human diversity and responsibility to work from a position of cultural awareness and responsiveness;
- integrating evidence, theory, and knowledge to inform change strategies and social work interventions; and
- appreciating the multi-, inter-, and trans-disciplinary nature of issues, evidence, and change strategies.

The editors believe that *The Routledge Handbook of Social Work and Addictive Behaviors* will be of tremendous relevance to global social work and allied health professional audiences. Addictive behaviors and related problems intersect with a vast number of additional significant social work issues, and affect populations in every sector where social workers practice: physical health, mental/behavioral health, child and family welfare, intimate partner violence, sexual assault, workplace/economic sufficiency, legal/criminal justice systems, education, community violence, human trafficking, housing/homelessness, community development, service delivery systems, policy, research, and more. Addictive behaviors intersect with many of the 12 Grand Challenges for Social Work identified by the American Association of Social Work and Social Welfare: ensuring healthy development for all youth; closing the health gap; ending family violence; advancing long and productive lives; ending homelessness; promoting smart decarceration; and building financial capacity for all, among others (see http://grandchallengesforsocialwork.org/grand-challenges-initiative/12-challenges/).

Addictive behaviors and their associated problems cross demographic, geographic, and geopolitical lines; they appear among or affect almost all population groups in the world. These problems cross disciplinary lines and influence how social workers interface with members of other professions, paraprofessionals, and non-professional community members, including peer support, family, and natural/indigenous helping systems. Scholars contributing to this resource represent various professional disciplines and orientations, including one chapter from a team of young adults prenatally exposed to alcohol, further extending its relevance.

The handbook's general organization

The primary aims of *The Routledge Handbook of Social Work and Addictive Behaviors* are:

- to assemble a practical source of knowledge about the origins and emergence of addictive behaviors;
- to note the prevalence of addictive behaviors in a variety of communities and populations globally; and
- most importantly, to present what is currently known about effective solutions to optimally inform practice, education, and research in social work and other professions.

On balance, the co-editors were pleased with the scope of topics included, the high caliber and applicability of the content presented, and the interdisciplinarity of the book's authors and contents. Topics selected for inclusion were based on quality of the available evidence, urgency of emerging issues, and the important roles for social work and other professions. The resulting contents are organized into five general sections, each being briefly introduced and followed by its component chapters:

- Section I: The Scope and Nature of Addictive Behavior and Related Problems
- Section II: Addictive Behavior Issues across the Lifespan and Specific Populations
- Section III: Interventions to Prevent and Address Addictive Behavior and Related Problems
- Section IV: Issues that Frequently Co-Occur with Addictive Behavior
- Section V: Moving Forward.

Global perspective

The Routledge Handbook of Social Work and Addictive Behaviors was commissioned to identify and address issues, evidence, and strategies from a global perspective. Scholars recruited as authors engage in research and change efforts in many parts of the world, bringing their diverse experiences and expertise to the project, enhancing the book's global relevance. The global need for training social work and other professionals about substance misuse and addictive behaviors is evidenced in the United Nations Sustainable Development Goals specifically targeting increased prevention and treatment of substance abuse (UN, 2015) in response to World Health Organization's global statistics on morbidity and mortality of substance use and its effects (WHO, 2018a).

The misuse of alcohol and other substances is a causal factor in over 200 disease and injury conditions (WHO, 2018b), causing harm to millions, including dependence on these substances and a multitude of other serious acute and chronic health problems (WHO, 2010). For example, over 3 million deaths annually around the world are attributed to the harmful use of alcohol, representing over 5% of all deaths (WHO, 2018b). This statistic is particularly concerning among young adults aged 20–39 years, where 13.5% of deaths are attributable to alcohol. Chapters in Sections I, II, and III relate greater detail concerning worldwide patterns of alcohol use, alcohol use disorders, and fetal alcohol exposure as significant causes for concern in many countries.

Global impact is even greater when other substances are included in analyses: drug use disorders (other than alcohol) affect an estimated 31 million persons globally (WHO, n.d.). Among the world's 10.6 million persons who inject drugs, over half experience hepatitis C and 12.5% live with HIV; over 280,000 deaths were indirectly attributable to drug misuse via factors such as HIV and hepatitis infection from injection use (UNODC, 2018). Furthermore, "amphetamines are one of the most worrying threats of drug use in East and South-East Asia" (UNODC, 2018, p. 13). Cocaine use is increasing, particularly in North and South America; 18.2 million people globally were estimated to have used cocaine during 2016 (UNODC, 2018). While the "opioid crisis" has become widely reported in the United States, non-prescribed use of opioid pain medication (e.g. tramadol) is "soaring in parts of Africa" and "expanding in Asia" (UNODC, 2018, p. 1). Other than alcohol, the greatest degree of harm globally is attributed to opioids being misused and redirected from prescribed purposes: where drug use was implicated in the cause of death, opioids were responsible 76% of the time (UNODC, 2018). In fact, overdose deaths were considered a significant cause of the observed decline in overall national life expectancy during 2015–2016 in the United States (UNODC, 2018). "Evidence suggests that Canada is also affected" (UNODC, 2018, p. 6). Non-fatal overdose events remain significant personal, social, and public health concerns, as does fetal exposure to opioids.

Not only are addictive behavior problems global in the sense that they affect individuals, families, communities, and service delivery systems in many nations, but global in that many nations and governments are intricately involved in supply (production, distribution, regulation, and taxation), demand, control, and other policy relationships. International policing continues to be challenged by drug trafficking networks using "darknet" or "deep web" mechanisms—estimated as an annual $170 million to $300 million economy (UNODC, 2018, p. 7). Organized crime and gang activity related to addictive behavior (substance use and gambling) have significant micro-, mezzo-, and macro-level implications around the world. Global evidence concerning addictive behavior and related problems are addressed throughout the five book sections.

Emphasis on substance misuse

Readers will find an emphasis on addictive behavior related to alcohol and other substances. This emphasis has a great deal to do with classification schemes for addictive behaviors that influence social work practice; it also concerns current available evidence. A variety of substance use disorders classified by symptom severity and type of drug (alcohol, cannabis, opioid, and others) are recognized in the current Diagnostic and Statistical Manual (DSM-5) and International Classification of Disease (ICD-10) used by many professionals globally for diagnosis, treatment planning and billing for services, as well as by researchers in categorizing individual study participants. The ICD-10 is being replaced by the ICD-11, initially adopted in May 2019 with full implementation intended by January 2022 (WHO, 2018c). Appendix A presents a table detailing diagnostic criteria related to substance use and other addictive behaviors according to the DSM-5 and ICD-11.

Regardless of classification scheme, delivery of evidence-supported intervention strategies and adoption of effective policies for addressing substance misuse, substance use disorders, and their associated health/mental health problems "fall short" of what is needed (UNODC, 2018, p. 1). Recognizing this, the book's chapters examine micro-, meso-, and macro-/policy-level aspects of substance-related addictive behaviors and their prevention.

Gambling and gaming

Gambling disorders are recognized in the current DSM-5 and ICD-11. A systematic review of post-2000 literature reported lifetime history of problematic gambling and gambling disorder prevalence rates of up to 6.5% across the global population (Calado & Griffiths, 2016). Gambling problems during the past year were reported among up to 5.8% of the population in North America, South America, Asia, Europe, and Oceania. There exists a high degree of co-occurrence between problem gambling among persons meeting criteria for a substance use disorder, as well (Rennert et al., 2014). Problem gambling reflects a globally relevant addictive behavior with significant health, economic, social relationship, family, workplace, mental health, suicide, and legal consequences; hence, this important public health topic is included in Section I.

Considerable debate appears in the literature as to whether sufficient evidence exists to include a parallel diagnosis for gaming disorder (unspecified, online or offline; WHO, 2018d). Internet gaming disorder is potentially a DSM diagnosis if further evidence supports its future inclusion (Saunders, 2017). Clearly, problematic gaming does exist, at least among a minority of gamers, and excessive gaming involves significant functional and psychological impairment (Király & Demetrovics, 2017). Hazardous or problematic gaming (online or offline) may pose significant barriers to engaging in healthy social relationships, successful work and school performance, and physical and mental health. The co-editors elected to err on the side of including problematic internet gaming in Section I, particularly because the problem exists in multiple regions of the world.

What else does and does not appear?

The addictive behaviors arena is complex and constantly (rapidly) evolving on a global stage, and the team was confined by feasibility in the length of book that could be produced. Evidence concerning many additional forms of problematic technology involvement, such as smartphone use, currently remains limited (Panova & Caronell, 2018). Similarly, evidence is unclear regarding several other behaviors that might or might not reflect behavioral addictions, such as hypersexuality and compulsively engaging in buying/shopping. The editors chose to rely on existing scientific evidence regarding formally recognized addictive behaviors and believe that evidence about these can inform practice regarding other forms of potentially addictive behavior not included in this handbook. Future published evidence and revised classification schemas, as they are adopted, may lead to their inclusion in forthcoming editions.

Other potential topics may have been omitted simply because the editors were not sufficiently aware of their significance, and for this they apologize. For example, while included chapters reflect aspects of human diversity (Section II) and different service delivery sectors (Section III), other important groups and service delivery systems do not appear, such as addictive behavior in the workplace and employee assistance programs (EAPs). Chapters addressing varied biopsychosocial theories of addictive behaviors/disorders were included (Section 1), but certainly not all theories were covered; emphasis was placed on those with intervention implications and a reasonably strong evidence base. Chapters discuss multiple social work (and other profession's) intervention approaches (Section IV) and emerging science and curricula (Section V), but they do not cover all possibilities. The editors, who were responsible for recruiting and selecting the contributing authors, apologize for the inability to include chapters on several important topics. Readers are strongly encouraged to pursue knowledge on topics mentioned below through other resources.

Trauma and trauma-informed care

Numerous chapters refer to the significant role of trauma in the development and maintenance of addictive behaviors, as well as the importance of engaging in trauma-informed care in work with affected individuals. The topic is important enough to warrant social workers' further development. Evidence from multiple studies of potentially problematic substance use among both survivors of and first responders to major catastrophic traumatic events (natural disasters and terrorism attacks) depicts meaningful associations between post-trauma responses (scores on indices of post-traumatic stress disorder, PTSD) and alcohol, as well as tobacco/nicotine use levels and risky or hazardous use of these substances. The effects were particularly strong among individuals already engaging in heavy use (Bailey & Stewart, 2014). Other kinds of traumatizing events are associated with increased vulnerability to developing problems with addictive behaviors: adverse childhood experiences (ACES), sexual trauma, intimate partner violence, race- or gender-/sexuality-based violence and micro-aggression experiences, and community violence (Shin, McDonald, & Conley, 2018).

Active military and military veterans

A trauma-related topic concerns the world's population of military members and veterans, since much of what is known about trauma, as well as about the etiology and treatment of alcohol and other drug use disorders, was learned through studies of military and veteran groups. Individuals exposed to combat who develop PTSD experience substance use disorders at rates far exceeding what is observed in the general population: 31–76% experience a substance use disorder (Bailey & Stewart, 2014). Global figures suggest that a great number of individuals are potentially exposed to active duty/combat experiences that can result in comorbid PTSD (or trauma responses not meeting clinical criteria for PTSD) and substance misuse or substance use disorders. Worldwide, over 27.5 million persons were occupied as armed forces personnel in 2016 (International Institute for Strategic Studies, 2016), though it is unclear how many were exposed to active combat stressors and traumatizing events.

The transition from active duty to civilian life appears to be a critical period for developing substance misuse problems: in one study, use of marijuana and "hard" drugs increased during the immediate post-separation months, while alcohol, cigarette, and prescription drug misuse remained at levels endorsed during active duty (Derefinko et al., 2018). Furthermore, instances of sexual assault experienced by members of the military are finally recognized as potentially traumatizing events associated with an increased vulnerability to substance misuse, particularly among women and sexual minority service members (Gilmore et al., 2016). Social norms associated with military culture and stress associated with re-entering civilian life are also important considerations related to addictive behaviors, as are issues related to physical injuries, chronic pain, and physical or mental disabilities resulting from active duty experiences.

Immigrant and refugee populations

Experiences among the world's immigrant and refugee populations in their countries-of-origin prior to emigrating, during the process of migration, and once relocated, are all potentially relevant to social workers' understanding of addictive behavior and effectively intervening with these groups. For example, in a national sample survey, extended duration of the refugee period was associated with an increased risk for alcohol use disorder compared to non-refugee immigrants to the United States ("New Americans"), although the risk of other substance use disorders was less (Salas-Wright & Vaughn, 2014). In a study of 90 refugee camps across 15 countries between 2009 and 2013, clinic visits for alcohol or substance-related problems averaged 1,965 per month among men and 426 per month among women; in addition, considerable discrepancies were noted by country (Kane et al., 2014).

Drugs, gangs, and transnational organized crime

A topic the editors very much wished to include relates to the intersectionality between drugs, gangs, and organized crime at individual, community, national, and international levels. The most violent countries in the world are in the Americas (El Salvador, Honduras, Guatemala, Mexico, and the United States), with many homicide deaths attributed to drug-related violence, gang activities, trafficking, and organized crime (Rosen & Kassab, 2019). Violence not only affects individuals engaged in drug-related activities, it has a profound effect on communities fighting these criminal activities, nearby youth and families, as well as national and international policy. Escaping their country's violence, death threats, kidnapping, and other crimes against persons is cited as a prime driver of massive numbers of individuals, families, and unaccompanied minors attempting migration and seeking refugee status in recent years. The micro-, meso-, and macro-level forces and implications of these transnational substance-related drug, gang, and organized crime problems are important for social workers to understand.

Housing

Homelessness is a problem of significant magnitude: "In the European Union, more than 400,000 individuals are homeless on any one night and more than 600,000 are homeless in the USA" (Fazel, Geddes, & Kushel, 2014, p. 1529). This is a multiply faceted topic when considered in conjunction with substance misuse and substance use disorders. On one hand, evidence leads to conclusions that homeless and vulnerably housed individuals and families experience relatively high rates of substance use disorders compared to the general population, at least in high-income nations: between 8 and 15% for alcohol (4–16% in general population), 5 and 54% for other drugs (2–6% in general population), and 58 and 65% dually diagnosed with psychiatric conditions (less than 1% in general population; Fazel et al., 2014). The causal nature of this relationship is complex: substance misuse may contribute to housing vulnerability, housing vulnerability may contribute to substance misuse, other factors (such as mental disorders or criminal justice system involvement) may exacerbate both substance misuse and housing vulnerability, and these forces may interact in iterative patterns over time. Regardless of causal pattern, substance misuse is "recognized as a significant barrier to exiting homelessness" (Palepu et al., 2013, p. 1).

On the other hand, housing options are an important consideration in supporting recovery from substance-related problems and substance use disorder. Recovery housing models typically provide an abstinence-supporting living environment and peer support; some formats also integrate substance recovery supports and treatment services, including treatment for other health problems (Paquette & Panella Winn, 2016). The nascent research concerning recovery housing demonstrates positive impact on multiple outcomes (relapse prevention, homelessness, family reunification, criminal justice system involvement, employment, reduced treatment costs, and others); however, not enough research has yet been systematically conducted or evaluated (Paquette & Panella Winn, 2016). Thus, housing vulnerability/stability and recovery housing are important topics for developing greater social work awareness and knowledge.

Intended audiences

At present, the topic of addictive behaviors is not systematically taught in social work programs in the United States (Wilkey, Lundgren, & Amodeo, 2013). What occurs in other countries is not always clear. Literature on social work education indicates a striking need for research-supported addictive behavior content to be included at all levels—stand-alone, specialized courses for achieving depth of understanding, as well as information infused into core courses required across the curriculum to promote generalized, integrated knowledge. Uneven attention to evidence-informed practices related to addictive behaviors around the world characterizes the current state of social work education and under-preparation of a professional workforce for addressing addictive behaviors and their associated problems.

The Routledge Handbook of Social Work and Addictive Behaviors is designed for MSW, PhD/DSW, post-doctoral, and in-service trainees, including research scholars and educators of future professionals. Ideally, social work practitioners in any area of specialization will find what they need to know about the problems of and associated with addictive behaviors—challenges that intersect and intrude on many areas of professional practice. The interdisciplinary nature of addictive behavior problems means this resource also is relevant for students, researchers, educators, and practitioners in a wide range of disciplines: social work, public health, psychology, education, sociology, criminal justice, medicine, nursing, and others. Educators in undergraduate programs may also find specific chapters or sections of the book useful as assigned and supplemental readings.

Key concepts and trending topics

The addictive behaviors arena is highly complex and constantly developing. Because the problems are so pervasive and exert such powerful influences on the lives of individuals, families, communities, and nations, topics are often argued intensely and passionately by practitioners, researchers, scholars, policy decision-makers, and the general public. Here we address the use of language and terminology encountered throughout the book, as well as current trending topics to help readers understand both what is presented in the book and how it is presented.

Use of language

Throughout the book, authors and editors endeavored to use terminology in a consistent manner. Careful attention has been paid to authors' use of language, with potentially stigmatizing or depersonalizing labels avoided wherever possible (e.g. avoiding terms like "addicts," "users," and "subjects") in favor of person-first or experience-/behavior-focused language (see Begun, 2016). These language-use practices are modeled for readers.

Defining addiction

Throughout the *Handbook of Social Work and Addictive Behaviors*, DSM and ICD definitions of alcohol use disorder (AUD), substance use disorder (SUD), and gambling disorders were applied (see Appendix A). However, there is more to defining addictive behavior than clinical diagnostic labels, a matter complicated by differences in perspective from around the globe. As a start, consider the American Society of Addiction Medicine policy statement defining addiction (ASAM, 2011):

> Addiction is a primary, chronic disease of brain reward, motivation, memory and related circuitry. Dysfunction in these circuits leads to characteristic biological, psychological, social and spiritual manifestations. This is reflected in an individual pathologically pursuing reward and/or relief by substance use and other behaviors. Addiction is characterized by inability to consistently abstain, impairment in behavioral control, craving, diminished recognition of significant problems with one's behavior and interpersonal relationships, and a dysfunctional emotional response. Like other chronic diseases, addiction often involves cycles of relapse and remission. Without treatment or engagement in recovery activities, addiction is progressive and can result in disability or premature death.
>
> *(p. 1)*

Important aspects of this definition include recognition of:

- the impact of addiction on biological, psychological/emotional, social, interpersonal, and spiritual aspects of life;
- the brain-behavior nexus in the development and maintenance of addictive behavior;
- the common experience of cyclical relapse and remission; and
- the potential for problem progression.

The ASAM definition reflects a "disease model" perspective—a model popular in the United States and many other areas, but not without controversy and critics, particularly in other parts of the world.

Original disease model of addiction

The original disease model of addiction emerged during the 1950s and 1960s regarding alcoholism, viewing addiction as a primary disease, not secondary to other psychological conditions (Hartje, 2009). The original disease model was hailed as an important, less stigmatizing alternative than the prevailing moral model of that placed blame on individuals for their addiction and deemed them deserving of its consequences and punishment (Thombs, 2009). Viewing addiction as a disease, instead, allowed the person to be seen as the "victim" of an illness, deserving of compassionate care and medically supervised treatment (Thombs, 2009). In this model, an individual's choice to initially engage in substance use was made freely; however, once initiated, the disease could take over: "intense cravings are triggered via physiological mechanisms, and these cravings lead to compulsive overuse. This mechanism is beyond the personal control of the addict" (Thombs, 2009, p. 561).

Research by E. Morton Jellinek was credited with providing early support for a disease model of addiction (Hartje, 2009). Based on a non-random sample of surveys completed by 98 men responding to an Alcoholics Anonymous newsletter, later expanded to include 2,000 histories, Jellinek (1952) identified four progressive phases of the disease: the prealcoholic symptomatic, prodromal, crucial, and chronic phases. The "Jellinek Curve" reflected how specific behaviors and experiences relate to the disease's progression and recovery—the curve's very design reflects the perception of a person "hitting bottom" before being able to recover from addiction (see https://www.in.gov/judiciary/ijlap/files/jellinek.pdf). Despite methodological weaknesses in the evidence, the original disease model became popular with many practitioners and Alcoholics Anonymous programs, introducing significant implications:

- alcoholism was viewed as a chronic, progressive, incurable disease;
- professional treatment was specified as necessary to control this incurable disease;
- abstinence was viewed as the only defense against recurrence and the only reasonable goal for a person with this disease; and
- substituting a different drug for alcohol was expected to manifest the same disease symptoms and progression (Hartje, 2009).

The original disease model and principles have greatly influenced assessment and treatment practices over the past 60–70 years. There exist several key points around which the original disease model of addiction has been challenged.

Heterogeneity challenge to original disease model

Longitudinal studies documenting the natural course of alcoholism demonstrated significant inconsistencies with a disease progression premise: multiple patterns were observed among men still alive 60 years after beginning the study, including continued alcohol abuse, stable abstinence, and return to asymptomatic/controlled drinking (Vaillant, 2003). Tremendous individual variation exists in patterns of addictive behaviors, as well as the severity of problems experienced by individuals at different points in time. Jellinek (1952) admitted that his was an "average trend" model in which individuals do not necessarily exhibit all of the symptoms associated with a phase, may differ in the sequencing of symptoms, and may differ in the duration of each phase; furthermore, "nonaddictive alcoholic" individuals may experience the identified negative consequences of alcoholism without experiencing a loss of control over drinking, and women may experience the disease differently.

This high degree of variability (heterogeneity) in expression called into question the perspective that alcoholism (or any addictive behavior disorder) represents a single disease. Emphasis on the addiction/dependence end of the continuum of substance misuse "has resulted in a myopic view of substance abuse problems that has characterized them as progressive, irreversible, and only resolved through treatment" (Sobell, 2007, p. 2). Observed heterogeneity has informed the diagnostic schedules' differentiations (see Appendix A): different substances and addictive behaviors (e.g. gambling) have distinct diagnostic codes. If "addiction" were a single, uniform event there would be no need for multiple diagnostic categories—or different intervention strategies.

Subtypes versus stages of disease

There exist marked differences in how addictive behaviors are expressed even within a single substance type. Challengin Jellinek's stage model of alcoholism, for example, is evidence of heterogeneity in "types" of alcoholism derived from a national sample (United States). The investigators based their typology on clinical characteristics of individuals meeting criteria for an alcohol dependence per the DSM-IV-R criteria that preceded the DSM-5 (Moss, Chen, & Yi, 2007). This analysis of U.S. National Epidemiological Survey on Alcohol and Related Conditions (NESARC) data led the authors to identify five "subtypes" of alcohol dependence, demonstrating clinical heterogeneity within the diagnostic classification. The subtypes they identified were based on how participants clustered on diagnostic criteria, age of onset, family history, and presence of other co-occurring disorders. The five statistically determined clusters were labeled young adult (31.5%), young antisocial (21.1%), functional (19.4%), intermediate familial (18.8%), and chronic severe (9.2%) subtypes. The groups demonstrated differences in their patterns of drinking, help-seeking, and response to intervention, as well. This study, based on a large, nationally representative sample reflected heterogeneity among persons engaged in a specific addictive behavior, and the wisdom of avoiding stereotypes about them—for instance, while the chronic severe subtype was the least common, it reflects a common stereotype of alcohol dependence.

Treatment and the disease model

Additional important challenges to the disease model of addiction appear in the literature. Asserting that formal treatment for addiction is necessary has been challenged by evidence that many individuals experience significant, long-lasting improvement without engaging in formal treatment—sometimes referred to as "natural recovery" or "self-change"—typically, persons whose alcohol misuse is not of the most severe dependent nature (Sobell, 2007). Little is known about natural recovery in other substance misuse, though some evidence for its existence appears in the literature (e.g. Chen, 2006; Erickson & Alexander, 1989; Price, Risk, & Spitznagel, 2001). Possibly, the necessity for engaging in formal treatment varies by individual, severity of the problem, and characteristics of the substances or addictive behaviors involved.

Abstinence only prescription based on disease model

Viewing abstinence from substance use as the only defense against "disease" recurrence and the only reasonable goal for a person experiencing a substance use disorder has been challenged. Complete abstinence from all psychoactive substances is at one end of a continuum in treatment strategies, commonly applied in U.S. medical practice (Glenn & Wu, 2009). A debated position is that the continuum of recovery includes controlled substance use, including the type of substance which a person previously used problematically. Between these positions is a question of whether psychoactive medications used to treat substance use disorders reflect recovery or are only a prelude to recovery not achieved until these medications are no longer needed. This question relates to an assertion that substituting one substance for another, despite its being safer, more controlled, or reducing harm, simply maintains the disease rather than offering a cure.

The word "sobriety" originally, historically implied temperate, moderated indulgence, not necessarily complete abstinence—an abstinence interpretation emerged during the 1900s (Glenn & Wu, 2009). Evidence since the 1970s indicates that some individuals achieve controlled drinking despite having previously engaged in an "out-of-control" drinking pattern, contrary to "the prevailing belief that any alcohol consumption causes an inevitable loss of control over one's alcohol use" (Klingemann, 2016, p. 436). The debate about "controlled drinking," "reduced-risk drinking," and "moderation management" continues, and it is unclear how the evidence for and against it might apply to other substances and addictive behaviors. On the issue of the use of pharmacotherapy to assist in controlled drinking, recent meta-analysis concluded that three medications showed controlled drinking outcomes superior to a placebo, but the effects were small and inconsistent across studies (Palpcuer et al., 2018). With or without medication, reduced-risk drinking (RRD) is seen in many Western European countries as one pathway out of addiction, and a legitimate treatment goal (Klingemann, 2016). As previously noted, the ability to engage in controlled use following a substance use disorder may vary by individual, severity of the problem, and characteristics of the substances or addictive behaviors involved.

Closely associated with the abstinence issue lies an additional point of contention with the original disease model of addiction: the expectation that substituting a different substance for the primary addictive behavior (e.g. misuse of alcohol, cannabis, or opioids) simply continues manifestation of the same disease of "addiction" where the symptoms persist, as does the pattern of disease progression. This stance contributes to the hesitancy expressed by some practitioners that medically assisted treatment (MAT) and the use of pharmacotherapies to treat substance use disorders maintains the (incurable) disease rather than treating it. Evidence of the effectiveness of these approaches for many persons, including eventual weaning from medication, contradicts this contention.

Loss of control concept

The original disease model of addiction expressed another point with which scholars and practitioners have taken issue: applying "loss of control" as a defining criterion. The prior moral model attributed individuals' use/misuse of alcohol, tobacco, or other drugs to moral failure or personality weakness, holding them "personally responsible for creating suffering for themselves and others" (Thombs, 2009, p. 561). The original disease model, as previously discussed, did not take a position on a person's initial decision to use a substance, but argued that the "disease" may take over, eventually rendering an individual helpless to control the behavior. Heather (2017) argued against the "compulsion" aspect of the disease model where addictive behavior "is said to be carried out against the will," and "marks the turning point from normal, recreational drug use to addictive drug use" (p. 15). His counter argument does not support a moral failure/blame stance toward addiction; instead, he emphasized the power of environmental, contextual, and reinforcement paradigms operating to influence behavioral choices related to continued engagement in substance misuse (or other addictive behaviors). One problem with the loss of control concept is that individuals may reframe it in terms of, "I can't help myself," excusing themselves from taking responsibility for the behavior or taking steps toward recovery.

Contemporary brain disease model and biopsychosocial perspective

As previously noted, recognition of the brain-behavior nexus in the development and maintenance of addictive behavior is important and necessary to understanding, intervening around, and recovery involving addictive behavior and related problems. Evidence concerning the neurobiology of substance use and mechanisms involved in the transition to substance use disorders has expanded in many directions over the past two decades, contributing to a widening variety of treatment and prevention intervention strategies (Volkow & Koob, 2015; Volkow, Koob, & McLellan, 2016).

Proponents of a contemporary brain disease model of addiction argue that:

> After centuries of efforts to reduce addiction and its related costs by punishing addictive behaviors failed to produce adequate results, recent basic and clinical research has provided clear evidence that addiction might be better considered and treated as an acquired disease of the brain.
>
> *(Volkow et al., 2016, p. 364)*

The U.S. National Institute on Drug Abuse applies the following definition of addiction:

> Addiction is defined as a chronic, relapsing disorder characterized by compulsive drug seeking and use despite adverse consequences. It is considered a brain disorder, because it involves functional changes to brain circuits involved in reward, stress, and self-control, and those changes may last a long time after a person has stopped taking drugs. Addiction is a lot like other diseases, such as heart disease. Both disrupt the normal, healthy functioning of an organ in the body, both have serious harmful effects, and both are, in many cases, preventable and treatable. If left untreated, they can last a lifetime and may lead to death.
>
> *(NIDA, 2018)*

Chronic, relapsing diseases like diabetes or high blood pressure often have a strong behavioral health component—just as substance use disorders. While these disease conditions may worsen over time, the outcome is not immutable—outcomes can be affected by behavioral health interventions, as well as self-directed changes in behavior and/or environment.

Biology and psychology intersect where substances altering the brain's reward and emotional circuits influence individuals' experiences, learning, memory, affect, executive function, decision-making, expectancies, withdrawal symptoms, and cravings, with profound implications for continued engagement in addictive behavior, as well as strategies for changing addictive behavior patterns. Understanding brain-behavior processes is necessary; however, this alone does not impart sufficient knowledge. Biological and psychological processes do not occur in a vacuum, but within complex, impactful social contexts and physical environments. For example, evidence that early exposure to alcohol and other substance misuse increases the odds of developing a substance use disorder later in life (Odgers et al., 2008) invokes mechanisms of multiple types: changes to the brain (biology); learning, social learning, and expectancies (psychology); social norms and access (social context/environment). Not only does recovery occur within social contexts (Heather et al., 2018), biological, psychological, and social interventions all may play a role. Furthermore, social and psychological interventions can influence neurobiological processes (Volkow et al., 2016); biology does not confer destiny but has a powerful iterative relationship with the other domains. Viewing addictive behaviors from an integrated biopsychosocial framework is required and reflected throughout this book.

Harm reduction

A somewhat contested topic related to addictive behavior and related problems is harm reduction. First appearing in the literature during the late 1980s and early 1990s, the term "harm reduction" was used to describe attempts to reduce adverse consequences associated with substance misuse, without necessarily eliminating substance use (Single, 1995). Two general levels of harm reduction effort emerged in the literature: clinical practice and policy interventions. Underlying harm reduction is recognition of the potential harms associated with engaging in addictive behavior (e.g. substance misuse or problem gambling), as well as knowing that some individuals will continue to engage in these behaviors, at least for an unknown length of time, despite the potential for harms to self and others. "The essence of the concept is to ameliorate adverse consequences of drug use while, at least in the short term, drug use continues" (Single, 1995, p. 287). Clean needle exchange programs, medically supervised injecting facilities, heroin-assisted treatment, distribution of fentanyl testing strips, and wide public distribution of opioid overdose reversal kits (Narcan) are examples of harm reduction strategies at the program/policy level that have at least some supporting evidence for reducing the risk of infectious disease transmission and drug overdose, among other potential harms (see Drucker et al., 2016). Examples of harm reduction practices at the clinical level include nicotine replacement therapy to reduce the harms of smoking tobacco products and medication-assisted treatment (MAT) involving opioid substitution drugs (e.g. methadone, buprenorphine) to reduce harms associated with the use of unregulated "street" drugs.

While harm reduction as a public health and social work strategy makes intuitive sense on the surface, controversy revolves around philosophy and implementation, led to some degree by a misunderstanding of harm reduction (Drucker et al., 2016). One argument against harm reduction strategies is that it may be mis-perceived as sanctioning the problematic behavior. The evidence on this is mixed, however. For example, while zero-tolerance/abstinence-based messaging was more effective in curbing college students' future drinking in several studies (Abar, Morgan, Small, & Maggs, 2012; LaBrie, Boyle, & Napper, 2015), in another, this was true only among students who currently consumed two or fewer drinks per week; harm reduction messaging outcomes were more favorable among students currently engaged in heavy drinking (Napper, 2019). Thus, the anti-harm reduction argument that it seems to sanction the behavior, thereby contributing to the problematic behavior, is only partially supported by evidence. An argument that harm reduction (reducing the negative consequences) interferes with motivation to seek treatment and/or quit engaging in the problematic behavior is also countered with the argument that, as a result of engaging in harm reduction programming, individuals may then become encouraged to engage in treatment to reduce or cease substance misuse (Drucker et al., 2016). An argument against nicotine or opioid replacement therapies is that the person continues to experience substance dependence. However, use of these therapies may allow the individual to gradually become weaned from dependence in a controlled manner, supported by behavioral therapies (see Chapters 18 and 19). While this argument is offered in support of e-cigarettes/vaping as a harm reduction tool, evidence is mounting that significant risks of harm are associated with these devices (including injury from malfunctions/battery problems, chemical exposure not being reduced as much as advertised, worsening of the nicotine dependence, and poisoning of children and pets from the liquid nicotine).

Conclusions

This chapter established that identification, prevention, and treatment of addictive behaviors and disorders are critical targets for global health. What is known about effective strategies to address these issues has grown as research findings from many countries, often as a result of international collaborative efforts, resulting in new concepts and definitions of "addiction." Scholars from many disciplines continue to open new doors and windows to the development and implementation of effective strategies; accompanying these advances, the number of trained practitioners who have the skills to apply them must be increased.

The specific perspectives of the social work conceptual framework are ideal in identifying, preventing, and treating addictive disorders. These include: adopting biopsychosocial, multi-level/multi-system, and lifespan perspectives of addictive behaviors; emphasizing human diversity awareness and responsiveness; working from a strengths perspective; and integrating multi-, inter-, and trans-disciplinary evidence, theory, and knowledge to inform change strategies and interventions. The principles on which each of these is based can be applied to many different professions.

Given the wide reach of addictive disorders both in type and in prevalence, the book could not include every area of problem addictive behaviors that exist today among diverse populations. As discussed in the chapter, feasibility, global, and evidence-supported perspectives were applied in the decisions made regarding what to include. Where controversy exists, attempts were made to present different prevailing viewpoints. The co-editors hope that this book is useful as a resource for the intended audiences. To have a significant impact on reducing the harms to individuals, communities, and societies derived from addictive behavior, it is essential to have the best information disseminated as widely as possible to those dedicating their careers and lives to the helping professions.

References

Abar, C. C., Morgan, N. R., Small, M. L., & Maggs, J. L. (2012). Investigating associations between perceived parental alcohol-related messages and college student drinking. *Journal of Studies on Alcohol and Drugs, 73*(1), 71–79. doi:10.15288/jsad.2012.73.71

American Society of Addiction Medicine (ASAM). (2011). Public policy statement: Definition of addiction. Retrieved from https://www.asam.org/docs/default-source/public-policy-statements/1definition_of_addiction_long_4-11.pdf?sfvrsn=a8f64512_4

Bailey, K. M., & Stewart, S. H. (2014). Relations among trauma, PTSD, and substance misuse: The scope of the problem. In P. Ouimette & J. P. Read (Eds.), *Trauma and substance abuse: Causes, consequences, and treatment of comorbid disorders* (2nd ed., pp. 11–34). doi:10.1037/14273-002

Begun, A. L. (2016). Considering the language we use: Well worth the effort. *Journal of Social Work Practice in the Addictions, 16*(3), 332–336. doi:10.1080/1533256X.2016.1201372

Calado, F., & Griffiths, M. D. (2016). Problem gambling worldwide: An update and systematic review of empirical research (2000–2015). *Journal of Behavioral Addictions, 5*(4), 592–613. doi:10.1556/2006.5.2016.073

Chen, G. (2006). Natural recovery from drug and alcohol addiction among Israeli prisoners. *Journal of Offender Rehabilitation, 43*(3), 1–17. doi:10.1300/J076v43n03_01

Derefinko, K. J., Hallsell, T. A., Isaacs, M. B., Salgado Garcia, F. I., Colvin, L. W., Bursac, Z., . . . Klesges, R. C. (2018). Substance use and psychological distress before and after the military to civilian transition. *Military Medicine, 18*(5–6), 258–265. doi:10.1093/milmed/usx082

Drucker, E., Anderson, K., Haemmig, R., Heimer, R., Small, D., Walley, A., . . . van Beek, I. (2016). Treating addictions: Harm reduction in clinical care and prevention. *Bioethical Inquiry, 13,* 239–249. doi:10.1007/s11673-016-9720-6

Erickson, P. G., & Alexander, B. K. (1989). Cocaine and addictive liability. *Social Pharmacology, 3,* 249–270.

Fazel, S., Geddes, J. R., & Kushel, M. (2014, October 25). The health of homeless people in high-income countries: Descriptive epidemiology, health consequences, and clinical and policy recommendations. *Lancet, 384,* 1529–1540. doi:10.1016/S0140-6736(14)61132-6

Gilmore, A. K., Brignone, E., Painter, J., Lehavot, K., Fargo, J., Suo, Y., . . . Gundlapalli, A. V. (2016). Military sexual trauma and co-occurring posttraumatic stress disorder, depressive disorders, and substance use disorders among returning Afghanistan and Iraq veterans. *Women's Health Issues, 26*(5), 546–554. doi:10.1016/j.whi.2016.07.001

Glenn, J. E., & Wu, Z. H. (2009). Sobriety. In G. L. Fisher & N. A. Roget (Eds.), *Encyclopedia of substance abuse prevention, treatment, & recovery* (Vol. 2, pp. 828–832). Los Angeles, CA: Sage.

Hartje, J. (2009). Disease concept. In G. L. Fisher & N. A. Roget (Eds.), *Encyclopedia of substance abuse prevention, treatment, & recovery* (Vol. 1, pp. 292–295). Los Angeles, CA: Sage.

Heather, N. (2017). Is the concept of compulsion useful in the explanation or description of addictive behaviour and experience? *Addictive Behaviors Reports, 6,* 15–38.

Heather, N., Best, D., Kawalek, A., Field, M., Lewis, M., Rotgers, F., . . . Heim, D. (2018). Challenging the brain disease model of addiction: European launch of the addiction theory network. *Addiction Research & Theory, 26*(4), 249–255.

International Institute for Strategic Studies (IISS). (2016). The military balance 2016. Retrieved from https://data.worldbank.org/indicator/MS.MIL.TOTL.P1.

Jellinek, E. M. (1952). Current notes: Phases of alcohol addiction. Retrieved from https://www.jsad.com/doi/pdf/10.15288/QJSA.1952.13.673.

Kane, J. C., Ventevogel, P., Spiegel, P., Bass, J. K., van Ommeren, M., & Tol, W. A. (2014). Mental, neurological, and substance use problems among refugees in primary health care: Analysis of the health information system in 90 refugee camps. *BMC Medicine, 12,* 228–238. doi:10.1186/s12916-014-0228-9

Király, O., & Demetrovics, Z. (2017). Inclusion of gaming disorder in ICD has more advantages than disadvantages. *Journal of Behavioral Addictions, 6*(3), 280–284. doi:10.1556/2006.6.2017.046

Klingemann, J. (2016). Acceptance of reduced-risk drinking as a therapeutic goal within the Polish alcohol treatment system. *Alcohol and Alcoholism, 51*(4), 436–441. doi:10.1093/alcalc/agv141

LaBrie, J. W., Boyle, S. C., & Napper, L. E. (2015). Alcohol abstinence or harm-reduction? Parental messages for college-bound light drinkers. *Addictive Behaviors, 46,* 10–13. doi:10.1016/j.addbeh.2015.02.019

Moss, H. B., Chen, C. M., & Yi, H. Y. (2007). Subtypes of alcohol dependence in a nationally representative sample. *Drug and Alcohol Dependence, 91*(2–3), 149–158. doi:10.1016/j.drugalcdep.2007.05.016

Napper, L. E. (2019). Harm-reduction and zero-tolerance maternal messages about college alcohol use. *Addictive Behaviors, 89,* 136–142. doi:10.1016/j.addbeh.2018.09.024

National Institute of Drug Abuse (NIDA). (2018). Drugs, brains, and behavior: The science of addiction. Retrieved from https://www.drugabuse.gov/publications/drugs-brains-behavior-science-addiction/drug-misuse-addiction

Odgers, C. L., Caspi, A., Nagin, D. S., Piquero, A. R., Slutske, W. S., Milne, B. J., . . . Moffitt, T. E. (2008). Is it important to prevent early exposure to drugs and alcohol among adolescents? *Psychological Science, 19*(10), 1037–1044. doi:10.1111/j.1467-9280.2008.02196.x

Palepu, A., Gadermann, A., Hubley, A. M., Farrell, S., Gogosis, E., Aubry, T., & Hwang, S. W. (2013). Substance use and access to health care and addiction treatment among homeless and vulnerably housed persons in three Canadian cities. *PLOS One, 8*(10), e75133. doi:10.1371/journal.pone.0075133

Palpcuer, C., Duprez, R., Huneau, A., Locher, C., Boussageon, R., Laviolle, B., & Naudet, F. (2018). Pharmacologically controlled drinking in the treatment of alcohol dependence or alcohol use disorders: A systematic review with direct and network meta-analysis on nalmefene, naltrexone, acamprosate, baclofen and topiramate. *Addiction, 113*(2), 220–237. doi:10.1111/add.13974

Panova, T., & Caronell, X. (2018). Is smartphone addiction really an addiction? *Journal of Behavioral Addictions, 7*(2), 252–259. doi:10.1556/2006.7.2018.49

Paquette, K., & Panella Winn, L. A. (2016). The role of recovery housing: Prioritizing choice in homeless services. *Journal of Dual Diagnosis, 12*(2), 153–162. doi:10.1080/15504263.2016.1175262

Price, R. K., Risk, N. K., & Spitznagel, E. L. (2001). Remission from drug abuse over a 25-year period: Patterns of remission and treatment use. *American Journal of Public Health, 91*(7), 1107–1113. doi:10.2105/AJPH.91.7.1107

Rennert, L., Denis, C., Peer, K, Lynch, K. G., Gelernter, J., & Kranzler, H. G. R. (2014). DSM-5 gambling disorder: Prevalence and characteristics in a substance use disorder sample. *Experimental and Clinical Psychopharmacology, 22*(1), 50–56. doi:10.1037/a0034518

Rosen, J. D., & Kassab, H. S. (2019). *Drugs, gangs, and violence.* Cham, Switzerland: Palgrave Macmillan. doi:10.1007/978-3-319-94451-7

Salas-Wright, C. P., & Vaughn, M. G. (2014). A "refugee paradox" for substance use disorders? *Drug and Alcohol Dependence, 142*, 345–349. doi:10.1016/j.drugalcdep.2014.06.008

Saunders, J. B. (2017). Substance use and addictive disorders in DSM-5 and ICD 10 and the draft ICD 11. *Current Opinion in Psychiatry, 30*(4), 227–237. doi:10.1097/YCO.0000000000000332

Single, E. (1995). Defining harm reduction. *Drug and Alcohol Review, 14*, 287–290. doi:10.1080/09595239500185371

Sobell, L. (2007). The phenomenon of self-change: Overview and key issues. In H. Klingemann & L. C. Sobell (Eds.), *Promoting self-change from addictive behaviors: Practical implications for policy, prevention, and treatment* (pp. 1–30). doi:10.1007/978-0-387-71287-1_1

Shin, S. H., McDonald, S. E., & Conley, D. (2018). Patterns of adverse childhood experiences and substance use among young adults: A latent class analysis. *Addictive Behaviors, 78*, 187–192. doi:10.1016/j.addbeh.2017.11.020

Thombs, D. L. (2009). Moral model. In G. L. Fisher & N. A. Roget (Eds.), *Encyclopedia of substance abuse prevention, treatment, & recovery* (Vol. 1, pp. 560–563). Los Angeles, CA: Sage.

United Nations (UN). (2015). *Transforming our world: The 2030 Agenda for sustainable development.* Retrieved from: https://sustainabledevelopment.un.org/post2015/transformingourworld/publication

United Nations Office on Drugs and Crime (UNODC). (2018). *World drug report 2018, volume 2: Global overview of drug demand and supply.* Vienna, Australia: United Nations Office on Drugs and Crime. Retrieved from https://www.unodc.org/wdr2018/prelaunch/WDR18_Booklet_2_GLOBAL.pdf

Vaillant, G. E. (2003). A 60-year follow-up of alcoholic men. *Addiction, 98*(8), 1043–1051. doi:10.1046/j.1360-0443.2003.00422.x

Volkow, N. D., & Koob, G. (2015). Brain disease model of addiction: Why is it so controversial? *The Lancet: Psychiatry, 2*(8), 677–679. doi:10.1016/S2215-0366(15)00236-9

Volkow, N. D., Koob, G., & McLellan, A. T. (2016). Neurobiologic advances from the brain disease model of addiction. *The New England Journal of Medicine, 374*(4), 363–371. doi:10.1056/NEJMra1511480

Wilkey, C., Lundgren, L., & Amodeo, M. (2013). Addiction training in social work schools: A nationwide analysis. *Journal of Social Work Practice in the Addictions, 13*(2), 192–210. doi:10.1080/1533256X.2013.785872

World Health Organization (WHO). (2010). *ATLAS 2010: First global report on substance use disorders launched.* Geneva, Switzerland: World Health Organization. Retrieved from https://www.who.int/substance_abuse/publications/Media/en/

World Health Organization (WHO). (2018a). *World health statistics 2018: Monitoring health for the SDGs, sustaining development goals.* Geneva, Switzerland: World Health Organization. Retrieved from http://apps.who.int/iris/bitstream/handle/10665/272596/9789241565585-eng.pdf

World Health Organization (WHO). (2018b, September 21). *Alcohol fact sheet.* Geneva, Switzerland: World Health Organization. Retrieved from https://www.who.int/news-room/fact-sheets/detail/alcohol

World Health Organization (WHO). (2018c, June). *WHO releases new international classification of diseases (ICD-11).* Geneva, Switzerland: World Health Organization. Retrieved from https://www.who.int/news-room/detail/18-06-2018-who-releases-new-international-classification-of-diseases-(icd-11)

World Health Organization (WHO). (2018d, December). *ICD-11 coding tool.* Geneva, Switzerland: World Health Organization. Retrieved from https://icd.who.int/ct11_2018/icd11_mms/en/release#/

World Health Organization (WHO). (n.d.). *Management of substance abuse: Facts and figures.* Geneva, Switzerland: World Health Organization. Retrieved from https://www.who.int/substance_abuse/facts/en/

Introduction to Section I

The scope and nature of addictive behaviors and related problems

Responding to complex problems like addictive behaviors requires a complex theoretical understanding: no single theory or model of addictive behavior suffices to explain all aspects of these problems. This first section of *The Routledge Handbook of Social Work and Addictive Behaviors* examines the biological, psychological, and social context domains involved, as well as how these domains interact in a true biopsychosocial manner. We recognize that distinctions between biological, psychological, and social factors are somewhat arbitrary: different scholars sort them in different ways and different theoretical models address different aspects of the addictive behavior conundrum. While we tease these apart in this section, a framework for bringing them back together in an integrative fashion is presented in the book's final concluding chapter.

The eight chapters of Section I present existing and emerging evidence, knowledge, and theories concerning the scope, nature, and etiology/origins of addictive behaviors and their associated problems, applying a biopsychosocial lens. The section opens with a description of common types of psychoactive substances, their effects, global scope of their use/misuse, and basic principles concerning classification of substances and psychopharmacology. This is followed by a chapter focused on the scope of alcohol use, misuse, and use disorders, with an emphasis on women and fetal alcohol exposure. Biological models of addictive behaviors and their supporting evidence are presented in two chapters: one examines neurobiology, the other genetics and gene × environment interactions. The next two chapters discuss psychological and social context models. While much of this book emphasizes theory, evidence, and intervention concerning substance misuse, the two final chapters in Section I emphasize theory and evidence concerning two additional addictive behaviors: gambling and internet gaming disorders. The Section I contents, together with the first introductory chapter, lay the groundwork for the book's subsequent sections.

2

Introduction to psychoactive substances

Audrey L. Begun

Background

Much of this book discusses substance misuse as an addictive behavior potentially leading to development of a substance use disorder (SUD) and/or associated health, mental health, legal, social, and other problems. This chapter provides a basic introduction to seven categories of psychoactive substances most frequently misused. First, psychoactive substances are defined, followed by discussion of how psychoactive substances might be classified and the significance of mode of substance administration. Next, several important principles of pharmacokinetics (how drugs work) and pharmacology (i.e. tolerance and withdrawal) are presented. Seven categories or classes of psychoactive substances are described in terms of their actions and effects on human experience, behavior, and health: alcohol, sedative–hypnotics and central nervous system depressants, cannabis, hallucinogens, stimulants, opioids, and inhalants; prescription drug misuse is addressed where relevant. The chapter's goal is to provide social workers and other professionals with an orientation to better understand the nature of substances discussed throughout this handbook, and they may encounter in their work with individuals, families, and communities.

Psychoactive substances and their classification

Manufactured drugs and many naturally occurring substances have specific (and sometimes general) effects on the human body and how organ systems function when ingested, inhaled, absorbed, or otherwise consumed. The term "psychoactive" refers to substances affecting the mind (perceptions, thoughts, and emotions/mood), and thus affecting behavior through their influence on the brain; sometimes the word "psychotropic" is applied (affecting a person's mental state). While many psychoactive substances have important medicinal or other intended purposes, they represent a subject of concern because of the potentially harmful consequences associated with their misuse and the potential for developing a related substance use disorder.

Different types of psychoactive substances have different intended and unintended effects, largely due to their chemical nature. Thus, they may be categorized or classified in terms of their effects. Other classification schemes relate to their legal status, such as being legal or "illicit" substances. This latter approach is potentially problematic because legal status is inconsistent geographically (e.g. cities, counties, states, or nations), across population groups (e.g. "underaged" youth), time (e.g. prohibition periods), and purpose (e.g. medical versus "recreational" use).

Controlled substances

In the United States, many substances are classified in terms of the Drug Enforcement Agency (DEA) schedule of controlled substances. This schedule system combines information concerning a substance's abuse potential with its status as an accepted medical treatment in the United States. The schedule defines levels of control imposed over each substance (and sometimes, ingredients used in its manufacture), as well as defining penalties associated with distribution outside of approved channels. For example, Schedule 1 drugs are the most strictly controlled and have the most severe associated punishment. Schedule 1 substances presumably have high potential for abuse and no accepted medical use in the United States: for example, lysergic acid diethylamide (LSD) and ecstasy. Schedule 5 drugs remain controlled substances but have the least severe punishment; their potential for abuse is deemed low and they have approved medical uses. Examples are cough or anti-diarrhea medicine formulations containing low amounts of narcotics. They are controlled through prescription systems. The DEA classification system can be confusing because some therapeutic drugs medically prescribed in other countries may not be approved (yet) for medical use in the United States (see Chapter 30 for more information on Scheduled Drug policy). Additionally, new medical uses are emerging even for Schedule 1 drugs (e.g. marijuana and LSD). Scheduling problems also arise as new substances appear on the scene and are not yet subject to control (e.g. when stimulants produced from khat were first introduced as "bath salts").

Prescription drug abuse

Many chemical formulations with psychoactive features are available without a prescription. These are called over-the-counter (OTC) substances. Others are more closely regulated with the intent of access and distribution being controlled through prescription requirements. The difference between OTC and prescription (R_x) drugs may be in their components, the concentration of certain components, or a country's regulatory policies. In the United States, it is illegal to distribute scheduled drugs outside of the regulated prescriber system. For example, while it is legal for individuals to have in their possession a drug prescribed to them by a licensed physical/mental health care provider and obtained through a pharmacy, it is illegal for them to give or sell that drug to another person (illegal distribution). Prescription drug abuse involves legal substances being used outside of legally prescribed parameters, referred to as nonmedical use of medications/drugs, and is one common prelude to use of illegal substances. For example, analysis of 2008–2010 data from the U.S. National Survey on Drug Use and Health demonstrated that among at least four out of five individuals (82.6%) using heroin in the past year, nonmedical use of opioids predated their heroin initiation (Jones, 2013). Prescription drug abuse occurs at individual, dyad, and community levels.

Individual level

Individuals may engage in prescription drug abuse by pursuing access to more than what is allowed by prescription. For example, they may seek additional pain medications, possibly from multiple physical/mental health care providers or by "faking" medical conditions. Pharmacy computerized networking systems and regulated prescriber practices are designed to reduce this type of prescription drug abuse.

Dyad level

Prescription drug abuse may occur between individuals when one (with good intentions) shares a prescribed medication with a friend or family member, or when someone steals another's medication. Not only is this prescription drug abuse problematic for the person using it without a prescription, but the providing person may also have their own medical/mental health condition un- or under-treated. "Drug Take Back Events" are intended to reduce individuals' access to unused prescription medications and public education efforts are designed to reduce illegal prescription drug sharing.

Community level

Trafficking in prescription medications is a community-level problem where individuals (illegally) acquire supplies of controlled substances and sell them to others. While pharmacy network and prescriber practices are designed as supply reduction strategies, untold volumes of drugs illegally pass across national borders from countries where they are legally or illegally produced for this purpose.

Classification by effects

This chapter relies on categories related to the effects of psychoactive substances rather than their legal standing. Important to note is the distinction between the effects of a particular substance and possible additives of which a person may be unaware. For example, individuals may be unaware that the heroin they have acquired is contaminated with fillers like talc, cornstarch, or rat poison to increase the volume sold—a relative weakening of the drug, introducing potentially harmful products. Or, heroin may be intensified with methamphetamine or other opiates, like fentanyl or carfentanil, which increases the risk of drug interactions and overdose. This is a potential problem with any unregulated drug manufacturing or distribution, not just heroin.

One consideration is the addictive potential of different substance types. For example, WHO (2016) reported that in 1990s U.S. data, cannabis dependence occurred among 9% of individuals who had ever used it, compared to 32% for nicotine, 23% for heroin, 17% for cocaine, 15% for alcohol, and 11% for stimulant drugs. An estimated 5.6% of the world population (275 million persons) used psychoactive drugs other than alcohol in 2016 (UNODC, 2018). Other factors and effects also warrant attention concerning the seven categories of substances discussed in this chapter.

Alcohol is the first substance discussed because, worldwide, it is the most commonly used psychoactive substance (see Chapter 2). Global estimates are that 1.4% of the population experience an alcohol use disorder (AUD); this figure does not include individuals who engage in risky or problematic drinking that does not meet criteria for an AUD (Ritchie & Roser, 2019). By comparison, 0.9% of the global population is estimated to experience a substance use disorder to drugs other than alcohol (Ritchie & Roser, 2019). In the United States, 5.3% of individuals aged 12 years and older were estimated to have experienced an AUD during the past year, 2.8% another substance use disorder (SUD), and 0.9% a substance use disorder involving both alcohol and another drug (NSDUH 2017 data, SAMHSA, 2018).

This effects-based classification strategy is not without problems, either. For example, some substances do not fit neatly into a single category, such as caffeinated alcoholic beverages—caffeine is a stimulant, alcohol a depressant. Sale of premixed caffeinated alcoholic beverages was banned in the United States in 2010 because of their potential for harm (though individuals may still combine them on their own); although several European countries have restricted the sale of caffeinated beverages of any type, these mixed beverages may remain on the market in others. Another example is some drugs that have both sedative and dissociative effects (club drugs like ketamine and Rohypnol), so they could be discussed in either the sedative/hypnotic or hallucinogen/dissociative drug sections. Or, a drug like ecstasy/MDMA—amphetamine derivative (Molly) that has both hallucinogenic and stimulant effects.

Basic pharmacokinetics and psychopharmacology processes

While each substance type has unique actions, mechanisms, and effects, basic pharmacokinetic and psychopharmacological principles apply across the board. Important concepts for social workers and other professionals to understand include: the pharmacokinetics of dosage and metabolism, drug interactions, tolerance, and withdrawal. The significance of mode of administration is also important to understand, as are polydrug use/drug interaction effects.

Pharmacokinetics

As alcohol and other substances are consumed the body begins metabolizing them (breaking them down). The net result is that the dose exposure circulating in the body is not constant over time. In other words, the drug's concentration decays over time. Different substances (and modes of administration) vary in terms of the rate at which they are metabolized. To some extent, individuals differ in the rate at which their bodies metabolize specific substances, as well—genetics, body composition, age, and other individual differences are involved.

The pharmacokinetic principle concerning a substance's average dose decay rate is measured in a drug's "half-life." This is a measure of how long it takes for the drug's concentration in the body to be cut in half (50%). That rate remains steady so that one half-life takes the concentration down to 50% of what it was at the initial dose; two half-lives take it down another 50%, to a 25% dose, three take it to 12.5%, and so forth. This curve is related to what is known to be the dose range at which effects are experiences—with medication, this is called the drug's therapeutic range. The aim is to find an initial dose large enough to help the person for the longest time possible while low enough to minimize unwanted side effects or overdose (see Figure 2.1). In this example, the peak circulating dose appeared two hours after the drug was administered (100%), well within the drug's therapeutic/effects range (above 40%)—just a little above this peak level the risk of overdose appears. The therapeutic/effects range lasted for about five hours. The first half-life (50%) occurred at four hours; the second at six hours. However, administering the same dose again at this point, when 25% is still circulating, runs the risk of bringing the new peak above the overdose threshold.

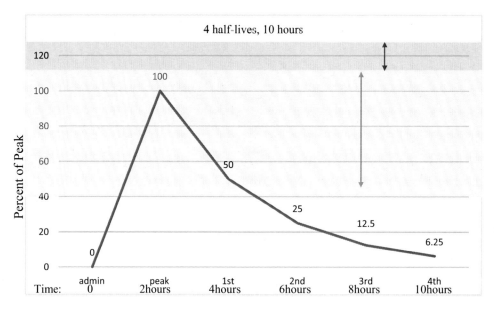

Figure 2.1 Hypothetical example of drug half-life and therapeutic range

Table 2.1 Home use urine drug tests may be positive for different substances (adapted from U.S. Federal Drug Administration, http://www.fda.gov/medical-devices/drugs-abuse-tests/drugs-abuse-home-use-test)

Drug Type	As Early as	For as Long as
Marijuana	1–3 hours	1–7 days
Cocaine	2–6 hours	2–3 days
Heroin/opiates	2–6 hours	1–3 days
Methamphetamine	4–6 hours	2–3 days

Why this matters

A "short acting" drug is metabolized quickly so that a person loses the effects sooner than for a "long acting" drug. This relates to the therapeutic range and timing of medications used in treating alcohol or other substance use disorders (see Chapter 19), as well as to substance misuse. One problem with drugs produced outside of controlled conditions (i.e. "street" drugs) is that the actual dose being administered is uncertain. Thus, the pharmacokinetic pattern may vary markedly from one use to the next. Another reason pharmacokinetics matter relates to detecting drugs in the body. Blood, urine, breath, and other measures can detect various substances either directly, as in blood alcohol levels (BAL) or concentrations (BAC), or indirectly in terms of known metabolites created as the drug is metabolized. Even though the original substance may disappear, the metabolites may take longer to clear the body. Average times that drugs continue to show up in urine drug tests, even though acute effects may have worn off, appear in Table 2.1.

Tolerance

Tolerance occurs when a person's brain and body begin adapting to repeated, chronic use of a substance such that effects diminish with the same dose levels over time; in other words, to achieve the same effect, increasingly greater doses of the substance are needed. For example, a person unused to drinking may experience alcohol's intoxicating effects (slurred speech, impaired balance and coordination) at a BAC of 0.08–0.15%, whereas a person experiencing a long-standing alcohol use disorder may not demonstrate these symptoms until a much higher level is reached—levels that would be incapacitating or even fatal for someone else (NIAAA, 1995). The tolerance phenomenon is often held accountable for contributing to overdose deaths among individuals experiencing a substance use disorder (e.g. opioids), unable to acquire the drugs over a significant time period (e.g. incarcerated or hospitalized), and return to using at the same level required when tolerance was high— these doses are no longer tolerated and can be fatal since the previously acquired tolerance diminished (Binswanger et al., 2012).

Note that tolerance may develop to an entire class of substance, not just to a specific drug in that group. Note also that tolerance to a substance, such as alcohol, is not protective for substance-related problems (NIAAA, 2016). The reason being that a person who does not feel the effects at one dose will consume higher levels until the desired effect is experienced. The higher dosing exposes the person to greater health risks.

Withdrawal

With sufficient chronic use of certain substances, the body begins to adapt the presence of the substance and becomes dependent on its presence for "normal" functioning; the body has become habituated to the drug's presence. When a person in this state of physical dependence significantly reduces or stops using that substance, the body goes through a withdrawal process. Withdrawal symptoms vary according to the type of substance and the previous level of exposure (amount and duration of use). Withdrawal from some substances (alcohol and benzodiazepines) carries a significant health risk and can be deadly if not medically supervised and managed. Thus, massive natural disasters (e.g. hurricane/typhoon/cyclone or tsunami) that interrupt individuals' access to these substances become significant public health and social work concerns (and for other reasons, too): individuals in affected areas may be susceptible to dangerous and potentially fatal withdrawal experiences.

Gradually reducing exposure, administering similar but safer/more controlled drugs (e.g. methadone or buprenorphine for opioid withdrawal), and medically managing symptoms of withdrawal from these drugs is preferable to abrupt cessation: this is known as a detoxification (detox) process. Withdrawal from substances carrying a moderate (heroin) or low risk (cannabis, nicotine, caffeine) can still be very unpleasant, and these symptoms often trigger relapse to use as a means of avoiding withdrawal. Longer-term withdrawal symptoms involving depression, anxiety, and sleep problems can be difficult to discriminate from primary mental health conditions.

Mode of administration

Not only is it important to understand the actions of different substances, but it is also important to recognize the influences of different modes of administration (e.g. ingesting, smoking/inhaling, injecting, absorption through the skin or under the tongue).

First, mode of administration determines the speed with which a substance begins to have its psychoactive effects. For example, substances consumed by ingestion (i.e. drinking or swallowing) take longer to begin circulating in the blood stream than substances consumed by more direct pathways such as injection directly into the circulatory system. Substances smoked or used as inhalants (i.e. "huffing") reach the brain rapidly as they are quickly absorbed from the lungs. Rapid psychoactive effects increase the addictive potential of using a substance as the reinforcement is experienced sooner and often more intensely.

Second, mode of administration may influence the substance's actual circulating dose and how long it lasts. For example, alcohol metabolism (breaking it down into its component chemical) begins in the digestive track, meaning that less circulates throughout the body compared to alcohol introduced directly into the blood stream. (This is an uncommon mode of alcohol administration outside of medical procedures.)

Third, different modes of administration are accompanied by differential health risks. For example, injection introduces higher risks of infection and infectious disease exposure than some other forms of administration. Smoking has long been recognized for its lung damage potential. Nasal inhalation ("snorting") of cocaine, methamphetamine, and opiates has an associated risk of damaging/destroying nasal passage architecture (Bakhshaee, Khadivi, Sadr, & Esmatinia, 2013; Greene, 2005). Ingestion of alcohol may affect digestive track cancer risk (Salaspuro, 2003).

Injection drug use has been studied as a public health concern at the global level, largely in conjunction with an emphasis on HIV transmission. Estimates of the percentage of persons who engage in injection use (sometimes called "persons who inject drugs" or PWID) were presented in the 2018 World Drug Report (UNODC, 2018). Globally, 0.17–0.30% of the population aged 15–64 years engaged in drug injection. Estimates are highest for Eastern and Southeastern Europe (0.82%), Central Asia and Transcaucasia (0.76%), North America (0.55%), and Oceania (0.53%).

Drug interactions

Taking more than one drug at a time can result in interactions that either increase or decrease their separate effects. One drug may amplify (potentiate) the effects of the other, having an additive effect, or the two drugs may interfere with each other's actions, cancelling some or all the effects. For example, consuming benzodiazepine and alcohol together potentiates their central nervous system depressant effects—increasing the risk of overdose symptoms like impaired breathing. Or, for example, combining alcohol and cocaine reduces the feelings of inebriation from the alcohol and increases the "high" produced by cocaine use; however, this combination is also more cardiotoxic (potentially damaging to the heart) than either substance alone (Pennings, Leccese, & Wolff, 2002). However, administering Narcan counters (cancels) many opioid effects making it a potentially life-saving intervention in opioid overdose situations. The problem of combined caffeinated (stimulant) alcoholic (depressant) beverages was previously introduced. Drug interaction effects are unpredictable, especially when the substances involved are of uncertain quality/quantity/dosage, making polydrug use (see Chapter 23) potentially riskier than use of one substance at a time.

This description of pharmacokinetic and psychopharmacology principles and the ways substances are often classified provides a foundation for learning about specific types of psychoactive substances. The next sections describe the seven types of psychoactive substances previously listed. Each description includes an explanation of what the substances are, their common effects, and statistics concerning their use/misuse. A useful resource for understanding more about different types of substances is the interactive website of commonly abused drugs posted by the U.S. National Institute on Drug Abuse (NIDA) at https://www.drugabuse.gov/drugs-abuse/commonly-abused-drugs-charts

Alcohol

The word "alcohol" refers to different types of chemicals: isopropyl (rubbing), methyl, butyl, and ethyl. Each of these can be used for cleaning/sterilizing purposes or burned as fuels. Only ethyl alcohol, also called ethanol, is safe for human consumption in controlled amounts and if it is not "denatured" with toxic additives: ethanol/ethyl alcohol is toxic when consumed in excess. Ethanol is the psychoactive ingredient in alcoholic beverages like wine, beer, and spirits/hard liquor which differ in terms of their alcohol content/concentration and other ingredients or additives.

When consumed, ethanol molecules begin to be broken down (metabolized) by an enzyme called alcohol dehydrogenase (ADH) and others (Zakhari, n.d.). This metabolic process results in the alcohol turning into acetaldehyde and water. Acetaldehyde is the toxic substance responsible for many of the negative health effects associated with drinking: it is carcinogenic (https://pubs.niaaa.nih.gov/publications/aa72.htm), contributes to liver disease (see Chapters 3 and 27) and contributes to "hangover" symptoms (nausea and headache). Acetaldehyde is subsequently metabolized by another enzyme, aldehyde dehydrogenase (ALDH), and eventually excreted from the body. Genetics play a significant role in controlling production of the metabolizing enzymes (ADH and ALDH), reflecting one mechanism in individual differences in alcohol responses (see Chapter 5).

Use

Alcohol is most often consumed in a beverage, although it can be administered intravenously as a medical intervention. Recently, powdered forms have appeared on the market in some global regions (e.g. Japan, Germany, the Netherlands) and are not legally distributed in others (e.g. many states in the United States and Australia). Concerns over the powdered form include greater potential for overdose, risks associated with consuming it in undiluted form, and difficulty in controlling access in restricted venues or by youth because of its portability.

The concentration of alcohol in a liquid beverage is indicated worldwide through its "alcohol by volume" (ABV) measure—milliliters of pure ethanol in 100 milliliters of the beverage (at 68 °F/20 °C)—with this proportion converted to a percentage value. For example, 40% is a typical ABV value for tequila, vodka, and rum. The "proof" value conveys similar information but has greater variability by nation. For example, in the United States, proof is two times the ABV (40% ABV is 80 proof); in the United Kingdom, proof is 1.75 times ABV (40% ABV is 70 proof).

Standard drink measurement

An important piece of information about alcohol consumption in practice and research concerns the amount individuals drink. Asking "how many drinks" someone consumed is unfortunately imprecise for determining their ethanol exposure: "I had one drink"

25

could mean very different circumstances. Servers and even entire countries differ in terms of serving sizes/pour volume, as well as strength of preferred beverages (e.g. beer versus malt liquor, wine versus sake, or different hard liquors) (Bloomfield, Stockwell, Gmel, & Rehn, 2003). For example, one beer might mean a 12 oz can, 16 oz pint, 24 oz Pilsner, or 40 oz bottle; beers vary in their alcohol content, as well (e.g. 4.2% ABV in Light/Lite beer to "strong brews" with 29–67% ABV). To address this confusion, the U.S. National Institute on Alcohol Abuse and Alcoholism (NIAAA, 2016) published a standard drink measure protocol based on 14 grams of pure ethanol per drink equivalent; the WHO applies a criterion of 10 grams adopted in most European nations (see Chapter 3), and other countries vary within the range across these two metrics (Ritchie & Roser, 2018).

Effects

Alcohol is a central nervous system (CNS) depressant (see next section on CNS depressants). For this reason (and others) combining alcohol with other substances can be dangerous (see section on drug interactions) and alcohol can impair mental and physical functions to the point where driving and other activities become dangerous to self and others. Alcohol is also a known teratogen—meaning that it disrupts fetal development (see Chapters 3, 11, 12, and 26).

Alcohol is considered an addictive substance (alcohol use disorder, AUD), and is associated with the development of tolerance and withdrawal symptoms (see later sections on these topics). The NIAAA has produced guidelines related to what constitutes low risk for AUD; these guidelines differ for men and women based on body mass, body composition, and how alcohol becomes metabolized (see Table 2.2). Drinking at higher levels (e.g. more than four standard drink equivalents on any day or 14 per week for men, more than three on any day or seven per week for women) is considered at-risk or heavy drinking—the risk of developing an alcohol use disorder and other problems. For example, 50% of individuals engaged in two or more heavy drinking days per week have an AUD (NIAAA, 2016). Low-risk drinking standards address not only the risk of developing an AUD, but also multiple detrimental health effects (see Chapter 3). There is no level of alcohol consumption that is entirely safe, particularly among pregnant women and adolescents (see Chapter 13).

Table 2.2 Low-risk drinking limits for men and women (adapted from NIAAA, 2016)

	Men	Women	Men or Women over Age 65
On any single day	No more than four standard drink equivalents AND	No more than three standard drink equivalents AND	No more than three standard drink equivalents AND
Per week	No more than 14 standard drink equivalents	No more than seven standard drink equivalents	No more than seven standard drink equivalents

Less or no alcohol may be best depending on health, medications, and how alcohol affects you; none is recommended for adolescents and pregnancy women

Statistics

This chapter began with alcohol because, worldwide, it is the most commonly used psychoactive substance (see Chapter 3). The majority of individuals (at least in the United States) either do not drink at all or do so at low-risk levels (35% and 37% respectively); 28% drink at levels that place them at risk for AUD or other serious health consequences (NIAAA, 2016). For information on the global statistics related to alcohol use, misuse, use disorder, and fetal exposure, see Chapter 3.

Sedative-hypnotics and CNS depressants

Central nervous system (CNS) depressants work by decreasing brain activity, usually through neurotransmitter actions like enhancing effects of GABA (gamma-aminobutyric acid). As a result, these substances have a calming effect on anxiety and acute stress reactions and can induce drowsiness in persons experiencing a sleep disorder. As medications, these types of drugs are used in treating certain mental health conditions (i.e. anxiolytics to treat anxiety, panic, acute stress disorders). Common forms of sedative-hypnotic and CNS depressants other than alcohol include (NIDA, 2018a):

- benzodiazepines (e.g. Valium®/diazepam, Klonopin®/clonazepam, Xanax®/alprazolam, Halcion®/triazolam, Prosom®/estazolam);
- barbiturates (e.g. phenobarbital, pentobarbitol); and
- non-benzodiazepine sedative-hypnotics/sleep aids (Ambien®/zolpidem, Lunesta®/eszopiclone, Sonata®/zaleplon).

Less commonly accessed but potentially misused are drugs used for anesthesia purposes. For example, propofol was sensationalized as contributing to the death of singer Michael Jackson.

Use

Most commonly, substances in this class are consumed orally, although one form of misuse involves crushing pills or emptying capsules and inhaling ("snorting") or injecting them.

Effects

In addition to the previously noted effects on anxiety and sleep, CNS depressants also cause mental confusion, poor concentration, and memory difficulties. These substances work on other parts of the body, too: for example, slowing the breathing rate and lowering blood pressure. This makes them potentially dangerous in overdose or combination with other breathing suppression substances like alcohol. They also affect reaction times and coordination, thus driving or engaging in other precision-demanding physical activities may become significantly impaired. Sedative-hypnotic and CNS depressant drugs are associated with a risk of developing dependence, hence a substance use disorder, as well as tolerance and withdrawal symptoms with cessation (see later section concerning these processes and the withdrawal risks associated with these drugs). Because of their sedative and hypnotic (amnesic) effects, some of these drugs are sometimes used in the perpetration of sexual assault crimes (e.g. GHB (gamma hydroxybutyrate), Rohypnol®, ketamine as "date rape" drugs) and can cause death to the victim through overdose and combination with alcohol (see https://www.womenshealth.gov/a-z-topics/date-rape-drugs).

Statistics

It is difficult to locate global statistics concerning misuse of these substances. According to the United Nations Office on Drugs and Crime (UNODC, 2018), comparing the latest available data for various countries, annual prevalence rates for sedative/tranquilizer misuse were greatest in Czechia (19.50), Croatia (17.30), Italy (13.8), Lithuania (13.4), Northern Ireland (10.30), and the former Yugoslav Republic (10.0). In the United States, an estimated 0.5% of the population aged 12 years and older (1.35 million persons) illicitly used sedatives during the past year (SAMHSA, 2018). The Centers for Disease Control and Prevention (CDC, 2018) reported 11,537 benzodiazepine-related deaths in the United States, the vast majority of which also included an opioid/narcotic.

Cannabis

As discussed in Chapter 31, the name cannabis is preferred over marijuana for substances from *cannabis sativa* or *cannabis indica* plants. Various parts of the plant may be used: leaves, flowers, stems, and seeds (see https://www.drugabuse.gov/publications/drugfacts/marijuana). Second only to alcohol, cannabis is the most widely used psychoactive substance in the world (WHO, 2016). Cannabinoid receptors occur naturally in the human brain, controlling neurotransmitter release when acted on by introducing cannabinoid substances or by endocannabinoids that are naturally produced by the human body. Cannabinoids have recognized medical uses recognized in many, but not all, countries: cannabis remains a Schedule 1 drug in the U.S. DEA classification system because of its high potential for abuse and the absence of recognized medical uses in the United States. This, however, is changing as increasing evidence supporting its efficacy in treating numerous physical and mental health conditions evolves.

The primary cannabinoid having psychoactive effects is THC (delta-9-tetrahydrocannabinol); CBD (cannabidiol) and CBN (cannabinol) are non-psychoactive cannabinoids, although CBD and some of the other 100 or more cannabinoids may modify THC's effects (WHO, 2016). It is difficult to determine dose exposure to THC in cannabis use because (1) different strains and growing conditions produce different concentrations, (2) different preparation methods affect THC concentrations (e.g. marijuana, hashish resin, hash oil, and parts of the plant used), (3) amounts used/inhaled in any administration vary, and (4) other products may be combined (WHO, 2016). Cannabis potency worldwide varies markedly and in Europe and the United States has been increasing since 1980, particularly during the past decade, from approximately 2% THC content to 16% or greater (WHO, 2016).

Use

Cannabis is commonly used by smoking or otherwise inhaling vapors which releases the psychoactive chemicals quickly to the brain. Products from the cannabis plant may be consumed in food, chewed, or drunk, as well. Other psychoactive substances are sometimes consumed with cannabis (e.g. alcohol, stimulants, opioids).

Effects

The primary psychoactive effects of cannabis are intoxication, euphoria, relaxation, and distorted sensory perception (see Chapter 23). These effects potentially contribute to accidental injury (impaired balance/coordination and cognition/judgment). Some individuals and/or circumstances of use are more susceptible to prolonged cannabis-induced psychosis that persists after the active ingredients have been completely metabolized (Grewal & George, 2017). Alternatively, acute cannabis intoxication is a diagnosable condition in the DSM-5 and ICD-11 (see Chapter 1). Both conditions are distinct from cannabis use disorder, which is also a clinically diagnosed condition affecting an estimated 4–8% of adults during their lifetime (WHO, 2016). Evidence concerning the potential for harm with fetal exposure is mixed (Ross, Graham, Money, & Stanwood, 2015). Finally, mode of administration may prove to be an important factor as the hundreds of chemicals in the cannabis plant may have respiratory health implications when smoked/inhaled.

Statistics

Like alcohol, rates of cannabis use vary markedly by global region. The prevalence for cannabis use is greatest in the following countries (UNODC, 2018): Israel (27.0), United States (17.0), Chile (15.1), Canada (14.73), Nigeria (14.3), and New Zealand (13.89). Cannabis dependence appears more frequently in high-income countries (1–2% of population) compared to the global estimate which is less than 0.5%, or about 13.1 million persons (WHO, 2016).

Hallucinogenic and dissociative substances

Hallucinogens are substances that distort a person's perceptions and recognition of reality—particularly visual and auditory perception. For this reason, they are sometimes referred to as psychotomimetic—mimicking psychosis. Examples include LSD (lysergic acid diethylamide), psilocybin ("magic" mushrooms), mescaline (peyote cactus), and DMT (ayahuasca). Naturally occurring and manufactured/synthesized substances may cause hallucinogenic effects produced through their actions on brain neurotransmitters (particularly serotonin) and perception/mental processes.

Dissociative substances also alter a person's experience of reality, inducing a sense of disconnection from reality and/or being out of control of one's body and environment (see https://www.drugabuse.gov/publications/drugfacts/hallucinogens). Dissociatives include both synthesized and naturally occurring substances, such as PCP (phencyclidine; Angel Dust), ketamine, dextromethorphan (DXM), and salvia (*salvia divinorum* plant). Some dissociatives have or have had medical applications, primarily as forms of anesthesia.

Both hallucinogenic and dissociative substances vary greatly in terms of potency, both because of differences in their active ingredients/chemicals and preparation processes. Their addictive potential is largely unknown, although addiction is a recognized possibility for some of these substances.

Use

Most hallucinogens listed here are consumed orally (swallowed, chewed, or dissolved on tongue/cheek tissue). Some are used in native/natural medicine practices, and some are used in spiritual rituals. Any might be misused recreationally. Dissociative substances are also consumed orally, but some may be inhaled/smoked, and PCP may also be injected.

Effects

In addition to the main effect of altered perceptions, many hallucinogenic substances also cause increased heart rate, blood pressure, and body temperature. They may also cause sleep disorder, and possibly paranoia/panic. Hallucinogenic experiences may persist or recur ("flashback") well after the active ingredients have been fully metabolized. Dissociative substances can also cause hallucinations and increased heart rate, blood pressure, and body temperature. They may also cause numbness, amnesia, disorientation, inability to move, and trouble breathing. Anxiety and depression (including suicidal thoughts) may persist long-term after a period of regular use.

Statistics

Global statistics are lacking in terms of hallucinogenic and dissociative substances. In part, this is due to the tremendous cultural variations in their medicinal and spiritual/ritual use and where they naturally occur. In addition, they are not as commonly used/misused as some other classes of substance. The 2017 NSDUH data included lifetime use figures for specific types of hallucinogens (SAMHSA, 2018). Among persons aged 12 and older, 15.5% had used any type of hallucinogen/dissociative in their lifetime, with the most commonly reported being LSD (9.6%), psilocybin mushrooms (8.8%), and ecstasy (MDMA). Between 1.3% and 2.8% had used PCP, peyote, mescaline, ketamine, or salvia.

Stimulants

The stimulant category encompasses a broad range of commonly misused substances, including amphetamines, methamphetamine, cocaine, and nicotine. Globally, many naturally occurring stimulant substances are used for medical, psychiatric, and nonmedical reasons, such as chewing betel nuts in some Asian and Pacific regions and coca leaves in parts of South America. Although these practices may have significant health consequences (e.g. oral cancer), they are not usually included in reports of psychoactive substance misuse. Caffeine is included here because it is considered the most widely used stimulant in the world (NIDA, 2014). While these various substances seem unrelated, they all have certain effects in common and when consumed together the effects (and side effects) are amplified. Stimulant substances are sometimes consumed together with other types of drugs (polydrug use) to alter the experience: for example, a combination of heroin and cocaine or methamphetamine. The addictive potential for stimulant drugs is associated with their effect on neurotransmitter action (especially dopamine and norepinephrine) affecting the brain's reward centers (see Chapter 4).

Amphetamines

Amphetamine and amphetamine-like drugs are used to treat a variety of medical and psychiatric conditions, including attention deficit disorder with or without hyperactivity (ADD/ADHD), such as Adderall® (dextroamphetamine), Ritalin® and Concerta® (methylphenidate), and Dexedrine® (dextroamphetamine). Amphetamines (e.g. benzadrine, Dexamyl/Drinamyl) were used historically to treat depression and narcolepsy, and as weight loss aids, as well as being distributed to members of the military (Rasmussen, 2008). These drugs are generally swallowed in pill or capsule form, but can be "snorted," smoked, or injected, as well. The psychoactive effects of stimulant substances include increased alertness/focus, wakefulness, reaction times, sexual libido, and positive affect (including euphoria); they can also produce restlessness, sleeplessness, irritability, and anxiety (see Chapter 23). High doses can cause irregular heart rate, dangerously high body temperature, or seizure (NIDA, 2018c). Amphetamine-induced psychosis is also a possibility with cumulative dosing over time and tends to disappear with drug cessation. Fetal exposure may negatively impact growth and neurodevelopment well into childhood (Ross et al., 2015).

Many amphetamines have high addictive and abuse potential, thus have been replaced by less addictive drugs in medical treatment protocols. Globally, the highest reported prevalence of amphetamine misuse (UNODC, 2018) was in the United States (2.95%); in other countries for which current data were available, prevalence was below 2%.

Methamphetamine

Very similar to amphetamines, methamphetamine is a synthetically manufactured CNS stimulant (meth, ice, crystal, crystal meth, yaba, yama, shabau, tik; Stoneberg, Shukla, & Magness, 2018), with high addictive potential because of its rapid effect, releasing high levels of dopamine in the brain's reward centers (NIDA, 2019; see Chapter 4). Vast amounts of misused methamphetamine are produced in illegal, foreign, or clandestine "labs." In multiple nations, just as methamphetamine is a controlled substance, so too are some of the chemicals used in its manufacture (precursor production controls). Methamphetamine production is additionally a public health and social work concern because of its contamination and explosion/fire potential. Globally, methamphetamine is the second most commonly used illicit drug and involves international trafficking patterns (Stoneberg et al., 2018).

Methamphetamine is most often smoked, swallowed, "snorted," or injected. While the "high" occurs quickly, it persists for a relatively long time (8–12 hours or more) compared to the brief duration of cocaine's effects. In addition to rapid dopamine release, the effects of methamphetamine exposure include rapid breathing and heart rate, increased body temperature and blood pressure, decreased appetite, and increased activity/wakefulness. Long-term use is associated with addiction, extreme weight loss, severe dental problems ("meth mouth"), sleep disorder, mental changes (confusion, memory loss, anxiety, paranoia, hallucinations), violent behavior, and changes in the immune system (e.g. causing a worsening of HIV consequences) (NIDA, 2019). Methamphetamine taken with opioids contributes to a greater risk of fatal overdose events, as well (NIDA, 2019). Fetal exposure is associated with growth retardation and abnormal brain development (Ross et al., 2015).

Cocaine

Leaves of the coca plant are the source of the powerful stimulant known as cocaine (coke, crack, blow, rock, snow). Cocaine powder is usually "snorted" through the nose, rubbed on the gums for absorption, or dissolved and then injected. Crack (freebase) cocaine is a processed crystal form, which is typically heated and inhaled or smoked. The psychoactive effects of cocaine use are similar to other stimulant substances: euphoria and mental alertness. Cocaine's psychoactive effects are primarily related to its action on dopamine in the brain, and its addictive potential is relatively strong because of its rapid, strong impact on the brain's reward system (NIDA, 2018b). Furthermore, because its psychoactive effects wear off rapidly, individuals may engage in repeat dosing over a lengthy period to sustain the effects, prolonging side effect exposure, as well.

Tolerance, withdrawal, overdose, and addiction occur with cocaine, and cocaine is sometimes used in combination with other drugs (e.g. heroin, fentanyl, marijuana, and other stimulants). In the short term, cocaine use may trigger fast heart rate, increased body temperature and blood pressure (potentially causing a stroke), tremors, nausea, restlessness, irritability, paranoia, hypersensitivity to sensory stimuli, and "bizarre, unpredictable, and violent behavior" (NIDA, 2018b). While injection increases the risk of exposure to infection and infectious diseases, cocaine use without needles can, as well, because impaired judgment may contribute to risky sexual contact with partners who are infected. Furthermore, cocaine may alter the immune system response to HIV allowing the virus to reproduce, thereby accelerating disease progression (NIDA, 2018b). Fetal exposure is known to interfere with growth and neurodevelopment (Ross et al., 2015).

In the United States during 2017, 14.9% of persons aged 12 and older reported having used cocaine at some point during their lifetime, 2.2% within the past year, and 0.8% in the past month; the rate of substance use disorder involving cocaine during the past year (reported in 2017) was 0.4% (SAMHSA, 2018). Globally, cocaine use rates were greater than 2% in the United States, the United Kingdom, Australia, Albania, the Netherlands, and Spain (UNODC, 2018).

Nicotine

Tobacco products, from the leaves of tobacco plants, are a common source of nicotine. The psychoactive effect of nicotine is primarily through triggering a rapid release of the body's naturally present epinephrine, which acts on the brain reward system (through dopamine circuits), and some effect on endorphin release (causing mild, brief euphoria) (NIDA, 2018d). Most commonly smoked (cigarette, cigar, pipe, hookah), tobacco is also chewed (absorbed through oral tissues) or inhaled through the nose ("snuff"). Not only is the nicotine potentially harmful, but also many other harmful chemicals naturally occur in tobacco, and tobacco is sometimes smoked in combination with other psychoactive substances. Producers of tobacco products may also enhance the effects of nicotine with additives. Nicotine is available in gum and skin patches, intended for use as a means of weaning a person off dependency on tobacco products by following a step-down dosing protocol to minimize withdrawal symptoms and manage cravings. However, many individuals using these products continue their use at steady levels as an alternative to smoking, not as a step-down recovery process.

Similarly, e-cigarettes using liquid nicotine (highly concentrated) are marketed as an alternative to tobacco products. However, marketing claims have led to significant misconceptions safety of electronic cigarettes (e-cigarettes, vaping). Whether consumed as tobacco or e-cigarettes, nicotine remains a highly addictive substance. Furthermore, e-cigarettes may be carcinogenic, just like tobacco products, and reports of burns, fires, and explosions from the delivery mechanisms have occurred, as well. Tobacco and liquid nicotine pose a danger to children who access them, with serious consequences (nicotine poisoning) because of the relative dose to their smaller and non-tolerant bodies. Adolescents in one U.S. community who used e-cigarettes were at greater risk of cigarette smoking in the future than those who did not (Bold et al., 2017). The developing adolescent brain is harmed by exposure to nicotine, in any form, as is a developing fetus (https://www.cdc.gov/tobacco/basic_information/e-cigarettes/index.htm).

Cancer and lung diseases are well-recognized health risks associated with smoking tobacco products. Not only is the person who actively smokes at risk (first-hand smoke), so too are individuals sharing the immediate environment when smoking takes place (second-hand or passive smoke exposure). Infants and young children may also be susceptible to smoking residue that forms on hard and soft surfaces with which they come into contact (e.g. carpeting and upholstery in the home and automobile, or a caregiver's hair, skin, and clothing), placing them at risk for respiratory problems even if they are not present when smoking occurs (Jacob et al., 2017). Fetal exposure occurs both through mothers' active and passive smoking, and is associated with growth and neurodevelopment deficits (Ross et al., 2015).

Worldwide, an estimated 8.32 million deaths in 2017 were attributable to active and passive (second-hand) smoking combined (7.10 and 1.22 million respectively; https://our worldindata.org/smoking). In 2017 the lifetime reported use of tobacco products in the United States was 62.7% of persons aged 12 and older (SAMHSA, 2018); the past-year and past-month rates were lower but remained relatively high (27.5% and 22.4% respectively). These numbers are despite 64.4% believing a great risk of harm is associated with smoking one or more packs of cigarettes daily (SAMHSA, 2018). Globally, over 1.1 billion people were estimated to smoke tobacco in 2016 with the highest rates occurring in Europe and portions of Southeast Asia and the Western Pacific (https://www.who.int/gho/tobacco/use/en/).

Caffeine

Caffeine is the most commonly used psychostimulant used around the world (Reyes & Cornelis, 2018), and is generally consumed in safe amounts (Meredith, Juliano, Hughes, & Griffiths, 2013). However, literature is mixed as to what constitutes "safe" limits on caffeine intake, especially habitual consumption. Caffeine produces its psychoactive effects through similar mechanisms to the other stimulants discussed: increased dopamine levels in the brain. Caffeine content in coffee, tea, soft drinks, energy drinks, and chocolate (and mate in South America) differ as a function of the species and growing condition of plants from which it is derived, as well as preparation procedures and other ingredients with which it might be combined. Caffeine in powdered form is available in some countries, which increases the potential for fatal overdosing.

Energy drinks and energy shots are widely consumed by adolescents and emerging adults (https://nccih.nih.gov/health/energy-drinks) with energy shots providing highly concentrated liquid doses of caffeine. The amount of caffeine in different products (and packaging sizes) varies markedly. These products often contain additional energizing substances, including excessive amounts of sugar. A considerable number of U.S. emergency department visits during 2011 involved energy drinks combined with other substances, particularly alcohol, marijuana, prescription medicines, and over-the-counter products (https://nccih.nih.gov/health/energy-drinks). Regular use of energy drinks/shots may result in disrupted sleep patterns which could contribute to other physical and mental health concerns. These products are consumed around the world.

The topic is discussed here because caffeine use disorder and withdrawal are recognized in diagnostic systems (see Chapter 1 and Appendix A); developing caffeine tolerance is possible, as well (Meredith et al., 2013). In moderation, caffeine is generally safe; high doses increase the risk of problems associated with some other stimulant substances: increased heart rate, agitation/anxiety, and withdrawal symptoms. It is of questionable safety to a developing fetus (Ross et al., 2015), and may have a negative impact on the developing adolescent brain, as well. An estimated 68% of adolescents and 18% of children under the age of 10 consume energy drinks (WHO, 2014).

Based on sales data, caffeine consumption appears to be greatest in North America and Europe, followed by Latin America and the Caribbean; rates in Asia and the Pacific and Africa were less than half or one-third (respectively) the rate in North America (Reyes & Cornelis, 2018).

Opioids

Opioids are substances that interact with naturally occurring opioid receptors in the human body and are either derived from opium or synthetically constructed/manufactured; opiates are the subset of opioids derived from opium. For example, morphine is produced from the seed pods of opium poppies and heroin is made from morphine (NIDA, 2018e). The opium poppy is most heavily harvested in Southeast and Southwest Asia, Mexico, and Columbia. The medical use of opioids is to provide pain relief; narcotics are opioid substances used to treat moderate to severe pain. Common types include heroin and prescription drugs like oxycodone, hydrocodone, codeine, morphine, and fentanyl, as well as combination medications (e.g. aspirin or acetaminophen plus opioid, such as Percodan, Percocet, or Tylox). Opioids are powerfully psychoactive and addictive, with chronic use accompanied by tolerance and withdrawal.

Use

Heroin ("horse," "smack") is generally injected, smoked, or sniffed/snorted. Prescription misuse of opioids generally involves pills which are either swallowed or crushed and injected or snorted. Some forms are meant to be absorbed through the skin in a controlled dose, such as the fentanyl patch, or to be administered intravenously (IV) under medical supervision. Heroin and other opioids are frequently combined with other substances to amplify their effects or to counter some of their side effects.

Drugs like fentanyl or carfentanil may be added to heroin or other substances to amplify their effects and increase trafficking profits (Taxel, 2019). Because these two substances are many times more potent than the primary substance, their addition greatly increases the risk of overdose.

Opioid overdose can be reversed by administering naloxone (Narcan® or Evzio®) by injection or nasal spray, when this drug is available in sufficient amounts at the scene. As an opioid antagonist, naloxone binds to opioid receptors in the body and blocks the opioid effects; the amount needed depends on the dose and strength of the opioid involved in the overdose event. Methadone (an opioid) and buprenorphine (an opioid partial agonist) are used to treat opioid use disorder (see Chapter 19) as part of a medication-assisted treatment protocol (MAT).

Effects

Their psychoactive effect comes from the release of dopamine to the pleasure areas of the brain, rewarding the behavior (see Chapters 4 and 6). The greatest acute danger is the effect of slowing (or stopping) a person's breathing. Other opioid effects include sleepiness, confusion, nausea, constipation, pneumonia, and over time, insomnia and increased sensitivity to pain; heroin use may also lead to liver and kidney disease (NIDA, 2018e; see Chapter 23). Depending on the mode of administration, opioid misuse may increase the risk of infection and infectious disease exposure. Physical dependence on opioids can develop even when used as medically prescribed; a person may become dependent on the class of substances, such that heroin and prescription misuse may become intertwined depending on a person's access to the different substances. Evidence in the United States (2011) indicates that an estimated 4–6% of individuals engaged in opioid prescription misuse eventually switched to heroin and about 80% of individuals using heroin first engaged in opioid prescription misuse (NIDA, 2018e).

Statistics

UNODC (2018) data discriminate between opiates and opioids. Opioid misuse prevalence is greatest in the United States, Serbia, Australia, Afghanistan, and Pakistan. Opiate prevalence is greatest in Iran, Afghanistan, Seychelles, Poland, Scotland, and Azerbaijan. In the United States, 2017 data indicated that 4.2% of individuals aged 12 or older (over 11 million) engaged in opioid misuse (heroin or prescription opioids) during the past year; 1.3% (3.5 million) during the past month (SAMHSA, 2018). Heroin use in the past month was reported by 0.2% (almost 500,000); important to note is that past-year substance use disorder involving heroin was also reported by 0.2% (SAMHSA, 2018). Opioid-related deaths in the United States increased by over 290% in the 15 years between 2001 and 2016, from 0.4% of all deaths to 1.5%, and represented 20% of deaths among 24- to 35-year-olds during 2016 (Gomes, Tadrous, Mamdani, Paterson, & Juurlink, 2018). In 2017, the U.S. Department of Health and Human Services declared the opioid crisis a public health emergency, stating that over 130 individuals died every day (47,600 in a year) from opioid-related drug overdose and problems of opioid addiction, as well as newborns experiencing withdrawal syndrome (see Chapter 10), were also of great concern (https://www.hhs.gov/opioids/about-the-epidemic/index.html).

Inhalants

A wide range of chemicals are gases at room temperature, which is the definition of high or extreme volatility. These means that these chemicals are easily inhaled when a person is exposed. Inhalants are substances that are typically misused only by inhaling, which is how they differ from substances that are inhaled as smoke or "snorted" up the nose. Inhalants have a high potential for health damage, including death. Unfortunately, many of these chemicals are easily accessed as they are produced and distributed as legal, inexpensive, common household and workplace products: for instance, cleaning solvents, nail polish remover, lighter fluid, markers, adhesives, spray paints, paint thinner/remover, and aerosol deodorant or hair products. Nitrites are inhalants, too, sold as video head cleaner, room odorizer, leather cleaner, or liquid aroma (NIDA, 2017). A few misused prescription-controlled inhalants are meant to be used in medical, veterinary, or dental practice as part of an anesthesia protocol (e.g. nitrous oxide, ether, chloroform).

Use

Inhalant misuse involves breathing in fumes through the nose or mouth (sniffing or huffing). To concentrate the dose exposure, the fumes may be gathered in a plastic bag or balloon (bagging) to be inhaled more quickly. "Although the high that inhalants produce usually lasts just a few minutes, people often try to make it last by continuing to inhale again and again over several hours" (NIDA, 2017). Thus, the potential for overdose is great; coma or death may occur with only one exposure.

Effects

The psychoactive effects of inhalant misuse include intoxication, euphoria, hallucinations (NIDA, 2017). Additionally, the chemical exposure slows brain activity and can cause dizziness, slurred speech, and loss of coordination. With continued use, but possibly even with one exposure, inhalants can cause irreversible damage to internal organs (liver, kidney, respiratory system), as well as brain damage, seizures, coma, and for the heart to stop beating. Addiction is possible (though not common), accompanied by withdrawal symptoms, sleep disturbance, and mood changes.

Statistics

Current global statistics concerning inhalant misuse are difficult to locate. A 1995 monograph indicated that the problem of inhalant abuse was present and growing in many countries of Asia and the Pacific region, Bolivia, Brazil, Columbia, Hungary, Japan, Mexico, Nigeria, Peru, the United Kingdom, and the United States (Kozol, Sloboda, & de la Rosa, 1995). The 2017 NSDUH data included information concerning reported lifetime use of different forms of inhalants. Overall, 9.3% of individuals aged 12 years and older reported having used inhalants, the most common being nitrous oxide/"whippits" (4.7%). Less common, but not negligible, were the rates reported for use of amyl nitrite/"poppers" (2.5%), felt-tip markers (2.3%), gasoline or lighter fluid (1.1%), glue/shoe polish/toluene (1.1%), computer cleaner/air duster (1.0%), spray paints (0.7%), lacquer thinner/paint solvents (0.6%), cleaning fluid (0.5%), or other aerosol sprays (0.5%). In the United States, inhalant use is most common among young adolescents, dropping in prevalence with older groups: past-year use occurred among 4.60% of 8th graders, 2.40% of 10th graders, and 1.60% of 12th graders participating in the 2018 Monitoring the Future Study (Miech et al., 2019).

Conclusions

This chapter provides social workers and other professionals with an orientation to seven commonly misused types of psychoactive substances and prescription drug misuse: alcohol, sedative-hypnotics and central nervous system depressants, cannabis, hallucinogens, stimulants, opioids, and inhalants. Each type was introduced in terms of what they are, how they are commonly used/misused, their effects, and relevant global statistics. Additional important concepts were introduced, as well: how psychoactive substances are classified in different systems, the impact of a substance's mode of administration, polydrug use, and basic pharmacokinetic and psychopharmacology (tolerance, withdrawal) principles. Understanding the nature of these different types of substances and substance-related principles helps readers understand topics discussed throughout this handbook, and helps inform their work with individuals, families, and communities.

References

Bakhshaee, M., Khadivi, E., Sadr, M. S., & Esmatinia, M. F. (2013). Nasal septum perforation due to methamphetamine abuse. *Iranian Journal of Otorhinolaryngology, 25*(70), 53–56.

Binswanger, I. A., Nowels, C., Corsi, K. F., Glanz, J., Long, J., Booth, R. E., & Steiner, J. F. (2012). Return to drug use and overdose after release from prison: A qualitative study of risk and protective factors. *Addiction Science & Clinical Practice, 7*(1), 1–9. doi:10.1186/1940-0640-7-3

Bloomfield, K., Stockwell, T., Gmel, G., & Rehn, N. (2003). *International comparisons of alcohol consumption*. National Institute on Alcohol Abuse and Alcoholism (NIAAA). Retrieved from https://pubs.niaaa.nih.gov/publications/arh27-1/95-109.htm

Bold, K. W., Kong, G., Camenga, D. R., Simon, P., Cavallo, D. A., Morean, M. E., & Krishnan-Sarin, S. (2017). Trajectories of e-cigarette and conventional cigarette use among youth. *Pediatrics, 141*(1). doi:10.1542/peds.2017-1832

Centers for Disease Control and Prevention (CDC). (2018). Multiple cause of death 1999–2018, Figure 2: National drug overdose deaths. National Center for Health Statistics on CDC WONDER Online Database (December). https://d14rmgtrwzf5a.cloudfront.net/sites/default/files/national_drug_overdose_deaths_through_2017.pdf

Gomes, T., Tadrous, M., Mamdani, M. M., Paterson, J. M., & Juurlink, D. N. (2018). *JAMA Network Open, 1*(2), e180217. doi:10.1001/jamanetworkopen.2018.0217

Greene, D. (2005). Total necrosis of the intranasal structures and soft palate as a result of nasal inhalation of crushed OxyContin. *Ear Nose & Throat Journal, 84*(8), 512–516. doi:10.1177/014556130508400814

Grewal, R. S., & George, T. P. (2017). Cannabis-induced psychosis: A review. *Psychiatric Times, 34*(7) (July 14). Retrieved from https://www.psychiatrictimes.com/substance-use-disorder/cannabis-induced-psychosis-review

Jacob, P., Benowitz, N. L., Destaillats, H., Gundel, L., Hang, B., Martins-Green, M., . . . Whitehead, T. P. (2017). Thirdhand smoke: New evidence, challenges, and future directions. *Chemical Research in Toxicology, 30*(1), 270–294. doi:10.1021/acs.chemrestox.6b00343

Jones, C. M. (2013). Heroin use and heroin risk behavior among nonmedical users of prescription opioid pain relievers—United States, 2002–2004 and 2008–2010. *Drug and Alcohol Dependency, 132*(1–2), 95–100. doi:10.1016/j.drugalcdep.2013.01.007

Kozol, N., Sloboda, Z., & de la Rosa, M. (1995). *Epidemiology of inhalant abuse: An international perspective*. NIDA Research Monograph 148. Rockville, MD: U.S. Department of Health and Human Services, National Institutes of Health. doi:10.1037/e495812006-001

Meredith, S. E., Juliano, L. M., Hughes, J. R., & Griffiths, R. R. (2013). Caffeine use disorder: A comprehensive review and research. *Journal of Caffeine Research, 3*(3), 114–130. doi:/10.1089/jcr.2013.0016

Miech, R. A., Johnston, L. D., O'Malley, P. M., Bachman, J. G., Schulenberg, J. E., & Patrick, M. E. (2019). *Monitoring the future national survey results on drug use, 1975–2018: Volume I, secondary school students*. Ann Arbor, MI: Institute for Social Research, The University of Michigan. Retrieved from http://monitoringthefuture.org//pubs/monographs/mtf-vol1_2018.pdf

National Institute on Alcohol Abuse and Alcoholism (NIAAA). (1995). *Alcohol and tolerance*. Alcohol Alert No. 28 PH 356 (April). Retrieved from https://pubs.niaaa.nih.gov/publications/aa28.htm

National Institute on Alcohol Abuse and Alcoholism (NIAAA). (revised 2016). Rethinking drinking: Alcohol and your health, NIH Publication No. 15-3770. Retrieved from https://pubs.niaaa.nih.gov/publications/RethinkingDrinking/Rethinking_Drinking.pdf or https://www.niaaa.nih.gov/sites/default/files/publications/Rethinking_Drinking.pdf

National Institute on Drug Abuse (NIDA). (2014). *Adolescent caffeine use and cocaine sensitivity*. National Institutes of Health, U.S. Department of Health and Human Services. Retrieved from https://www.drugabuse.gov/news-events/latest-science/adolescent-caffeine-use-and-cocaine-sensitivity

National Institute on Drug Abuse (NIDA). (2017). *Inhalants*. National Institutes of Health, U.S. Department of Health and Human Services. Retrieved from https://www.drugabuse.gov/publications/drugfacts/inhalants

National Institute on Drug Abuse (NIDA). (2018a). *Prescription CNS depressants*. National Institutes of Health, U.S. Department of Health and Human Services. Retrieved from https://www.drugabuse.gov/publications/drugfacts/prescription-cns-depressants

National Institute on Drug Abuse (NIDA). (2018b). *Cocaine*. National Institutes of Health, U.S. Department of Health and Human Services. Retrieved from https://www.drugabuse.gov/publications/drugfacts/cocaine

National Institute on Drug Abuse (NIDA). (2018c). *Prescription stimulants*. National Institutes of Health, U.S. Department of Health and Human Services. Retrieved from https://www.drugabuse.gov/publications/drugfacts/prescription-stimulants

National Institute on Drug Abuse (NIDA). (2018d). *Tobacco, nicotine, and e-cigarettes*. National Institutes of Health, U.S. Department of Health and Human Services. Retrieved from https://www.drugabuse.gov/publications/research-reports/tobacco-nicotine-e-cigarettes/introduction

National Institute on Drug Abuse (NIDA). (2018e). *Opioid facts for teens*. National Institutes of Health, U.S. Department of Health and Human Services. Retrieved from https://www.drugabuse.gov/publications/opioid-facts-teens/faqs-about-opioids

National Institute on Drug Abuse (NIDA). (2019). *Methamphetamine*. National Institutes of Health, U.S. Department of Health and Human Services. Retrieved from https://www.drugabuse.gov/publications/drugfacts/methamphetamine

Pennings, E. J., Leccese, A. P., & Wolff, F. A. (2002). Effects of concurrent use of alcohol and cocaine. *Addiction, 97*(7), 773–783. doi:10.1046/j.1360-0443.2002.00158.x

Rasmussen, N. (2008). America's first amphetamine epidemic 1929–1971: A quantitative and qualitative retrospective with implications for the present. *American Journal of Public Health, 98*(6), 974–985. doi:10.2105/AJPH.2007.110593

Reyes, C. M., & Cornelis, M. C. (2018). Caffeine in the diet: Country-level consumption and guidelines. *Nutrients, 10*(11), 1722. doi:10.3390/nu10111772

Ritchie, H., & Roser, M. (2018). Alcohol consumption. Published online at OurWorldInData.org. Retrieved from https://ourworldindata.org/alcohol-consumption

Ritchie, H., & Roser, M. (2019). Substance use. Published online at OurWorldInData.org. Retrieved from https://ourworldindata.org/substance-use

Ross, E. J., Graham, D. L., Money, K. M., & Stanwood, G. D. (2015). Developmental consequences of fetal exposure to drugs: What we know and what we still musts learn. *Neuropharmacology, 40*(1), 61–87. doi:10.1038/npp.2014.147

Salaspuro, M. P. (2003). Alcohol consumption and cancer of the gastrointestinal tract. *Best Practice & Research Clinical Gastroenterology, 17*(4), 679–694. doi:10.1016/S1521-6918(03)00035-0

Stoneberg, D. M., Shukla, R. K., & Magness, M. B. (2018). Global methamphetamine trends: An evolving problem. *International Criminal Justice Review, 28*(2), 136–161. doi:10.1177/1057567717730104

Substance Abuse and Mental Health Administration (SAMHSA). (2018). *Results from the 2017 National survey on drug use and health: Detailed tables.* U.S. Department of Health and Human Services. Retrieved from https://www.samhsa.gov/data/sites/default/files/cbhsq-reports/NSDUHDetailedTabs2017/NSDUHDetailedTabs2017.htm#lotsect1pe

Taxel, S. (2019, May 7). Fentanyl facts and fictions: A safety guide for first responders. *Journal of Emergency Medical Services.* Retrieved from https://www.jems.com/articles/2019/05/fentanyl-facts-and-fiction-a-safety-guide-for-first-responders.html

United Nations Office on Drugs and Crime (UNODC). (2018). *World drug report 2018. Statistics and data.* Retrieved from https://dataunodc.un.org/

World Health Organization (WHO). (2014). *Energy drinks cause concern for health of young people.* Geneva, Switzerland: World Health Organization. Retrieved from http://www.euro.who.int/en/health-topics/disease-prevention/nutrition/news/news/2014/10/energy-drinks-cause-concern-for-health-of-young-people

World Health Organization (WHO). (2016). *The health and social effects of nonmedical cannabis use.* Geneva, Switzerland: World Health Organization. Retrieved from https://www.who.int/substance_abuse/publications/cannabis/en/

Zakhari, S. (n.d.). *Overview: How is alcohol metabolized by the body?* Retrieved from https://pubs.niaaa.nih.gov/publications/arh294/245-255.htm

3

Global alcohol epidemiology

Focus on women of childbearing age

Svetlana Popova, Jürgen Rehm and Kevin Shield

Background

The harmful use of alcohol is a causal factor in more than 200 disease and injury conditions, as measured by International Statistical Classification of Diseases and Related Health Problems, 11th Revision (ICD-11) codes, and affects the risk of communicable and noncommunicable diseases (Rehm, Gmel et al., 2017). According to the World Health Organization (WHO), alcohol affects the risk of diseases and conditions as a result of (1) the amount of alcohol consumed, (2) the patterns in which alcohol is consumed, (3) the lifetime history of alcohol consumption, and (4) the presence of harmful agents other than ethanol (WHO, 2018b). Alcohol also interacts with societal and political factors (development and macro-economic profiles, cultural and societal values, public health policies, alcohol availability and marketing), as well as with individual vulnerability factors (age and gender, genetic and familial factors, socio-economic status, and smoking, diet and other risk modifying factors) (WHO, 2018b). A significant, pervasive, and persistent alcohol-related public health concern is the potential impact of alcohol use and alcohol use disorders among women of childbearing age and during pregnancy (see also Chapters 11, 12, and 26). Accordingly, this chapter outlines alcohol consumption among women of childbearing age (15–49 years of age) (Manthey et al., 2019; WHO, 2019). Furthermore, this chapter outlines diseases and injuries causally related to alcohol consumption, and consequential deaths and disability-adjusted life years (DALYs) lost, a measure of both premature mortality and disability (WHO, 2018b).

Global alcohol consumption data

Global data on alcohol consumption and alcohol use disorders (AUDs) are based on information obtained from the Global Information System on Alcohol and Health (Poznyak et al., 2014; WHO, 2019). Two different measurement indices are used.

Alcohol per capita consumption (APC)

Globally, the most consistently accurate and widely available measurement of alcohol consumption is adult (≥15 years of age) *per capita* consumption of ethanol (Bloomfield, Stockwell, Gmel, & Rehn, 2003; Gmel & Rehm, 2004; Poznyak et al., 2014). APC is used to monitor alcohol consumption and set health targets by the United Nations (UN) (United Nations, 2015, 2016), the WHO (WHO, 2010), and the Organisation for Economic Co-operation and Development (OECD) (2019). In particular, the UN's Sustainable Development Goals call for a 10% reduction in the harmful use of alcohol by 2025 (United Nations, 2015, 2016). For information on how this target can be achieved, see information on the WHO's Best Buy policies (increases in alcohol taxation, availability restrictions and marketing restrictions; see Begun, Clapp, & The Alcohol Misuse Grand Challenges Collective, 2015; Chisholm et al., 2018).

Due to biases in survey design, study participation, and participant's responses, data on APC consumption from alcohol surveys are thought to underestimate APC consumption by more than 50% (Shield & Rehm, 2012). However, APC consumption statistics are differentiated by age and sex (i.e. stratified) using nationally representative survey data on the prevalence of individuals who currently consume alcohol (i.e. during the past year) and the average amount of alcohol they consumed daily (WHO, 2018b). Unless otherwise noted, the following data are excerpted from the Global Status Report on Alcohol and Health (GSRAH) 2018 (WHO, 2018b) and the Global Information System on Alcohol and Health (WHO, 2018a).

Prevalence

Data on the prevalence of current alcohol consumption (one standard drink during the past year), former alcohol consumption (one standard drink but not within the past year), lifetime abstention, heavy episodic drinking (consumption of 60 grams of alcohol or more during the past 30 days on at least one drinking occasion), and the prevalence AUDs, harmful alcohol use, and alcohol dependence (AD) were obtained from systematic reviews and meta-analyses of population surveys which measured alcohol drinking statuses and AUDs at the population level (for information on how alcohol consumption has been modeled, see Kehoe, Gmel, Shield, Gmel, & Rehm, 2012; Rehm et al., 2010).

APC

In 2016, global APC consumption was estimated to be 6.4 liters, representing a stable APC from 2010 when APC consumption was also 6.4 liters (WHO, 2018a; see Table 3.1). However, between 2016 and 2025, based on previous trends in data, APC is projected to increase by 9.4% to 7.0 liters. This projection is based on forecasted increases in alcohol consumption in the WHO regions of the Americas (8.0–8.4 liters), the Western Pacific (7.3–8.1 liters), and South-East Asia (4.5–6.2 liters) (global regions based on the WHO regional definitions from: https://www.who.int/healthinfo/global_burden_disease/definition_regions/en/).

APC by women

Stratified by gender global APC consumption among women was estimated to be 2.3 liters in 2016; APC consumption among men was estimated to be 10.5 liters. Among women, APC consumption ranged from 0.1 liters in the Eastern Mediterranean region, to 4.2 liters in

Table 3.1 Adult *per capita* consumption and the prevalence of current drinking, former drinking, lifetime abstention, and heavy episodic drinking in 2016

Regions	Adult per capita Consumption (liters)				Per capita Consumption (liters) among Women 15–49 Years of Age	Drinking Prevalence (%: Women 15–49 Years of Age)			
	Men	Women	Total	Ratio		Current Drinking	Former Drinking	Lifetime Abstention	Heavy Episodic Drinking
Global	10.5	2.3	6.4	4.6	2.3	32.1	56.7	11.3	8.7
WHO regions									
African	10.7	2.0	6.3	5.4	2.1	21.7	69.4	9.0	7.6
American	13.3	2.9	8.0	4.5	3.1	42.9	25.0	32.0	10.5
Eastern Mediterranean	1.0	0.1	0.6	10.8	0.1	1.3	97.8	0.9	0.1
European	16.0	4.2	9.8	3.8	4.6	53.9	30.3	15.9	18.7
South-East Asia	7.6	1.3	4.5	5.7	1.4	22.5	70.5	7.0	5.2
Western Pacific	11.9	2.6	7.3	4.7	2.8	42.7	49.6	7.6	10.7
World Bank regions									
Low-income economies	6.6	1.1	3.8	5.8	1.2	17.4	73.8	8.8	5.5
Lower-middle-income economies	7.9	1.4	4.7	5.5	1.5	20.6	71.3	8.1	5.0
Upper-middle-income economies	11.5	2.5	7.0	4.6	2.7	37.6	50.7	11.8	10.4
High-income economies	15.6	4.0	9.8	3.9	4.5	60.7	18.4	20.9	17.3

Source: Data were obtained from the Global Information System on Alcohol and Health (WHO, 2018a).

the European region. Furthermore, APC consumption among women was highest in countries with high-income economies (4.0 liters), followed by upper-middle-income economies (2.5 liters), lower-middle-income economies (1.4 liters), and low-income economies (1.1 liters). The ratio of men's to women's APC in 2016 was estimated to be 4.6 globally; highest in the Eastern Mediterranean region (10.8) and lowest in the European region (3.8). Assuming a prospective trend of convergence of gendered alcohol use (Bloomfield, Gmel, Neve, & Mustonen, 2001), consumption by women is expected to continue to increase in regions where currently there exists a large discrepancy in the amount of alcohol consumed by men and by women.

Among women of childbearing age, 2016 global APC consumption was estimated to be 2.3 liters; this consumption varied widely, ranging from 0.1 liters in the Eastern Mediterranean region to 4.6 liters in the European region. Furthermore, APC consumption among these women was highest in countries with high-income economies (4.5 liters), followed by upper-middle-income economies (2.7 liters), lower-middle-income economies (1.5 liters), and low-income economies (1.2 liters).

Current and heavy episodic drinking

In 2016, 44.0% of adults globally had consumed at least one standard drink of alcohol within the past year; 53.7% of adult men and 32.4% of adult women consumed alcohol in the past year. In 2016, 17.0% of the global adult population engaged in heavy episodic drinking (HED), defined as consuming at least 60 grams or more on at least one occasion in the past 30 days; 27.0% of men and 6.4% of women engaged in HED. A European standard drink contains approximately 10 grams of alcohol, and a U.S. standard drink contains 14 grams.

Heavy drinking by women of childbearing age

Globally, in 2016, 32.1% of women of childbearing age consumed alcohol in the past year, and 8.7% engaged in HED. The prevalence of current drinking among these women was lowest in the Eastern Mediterranean region (1.3%) and highest in the European region (53.9%). Similarly, the prevalence of HED among these women was lowest in the Eastern Mediterranean region (0.1%) and highest in the European region (18.7%). Furthermore, the prevalence rates of women aged 15–49 years who currently consume alcohol and HED were highest in countries with high-income economies (60.7% consume alcohol, 17.3% HED), followed by upper-middle-income economies (37.6% consume alcohol, 10.4% HED), lower-middle-income economies (20.6% consume alcohol, 5.0% HED), and low-income economies (17.4% consume alcohol, 5.5% HED).

Alcohol use disorders

Data concerning HED, AUDs, and AD are utilized by policy makers when determining public health policies and allocating treatment resources (Grant et al., 2015; WHO, 2018b); see Chapter 1 and Appendix A for defining characteristics of AUD. Currently, the majority of individuals experiencing these highly prevalent, highly comorbid, and disabling disorders go untreated.

In 2016, the prevalence of AUDs among adults was 5.1%, while the prevalence of AD was 2.6% (WHO, 2018b). Stratified by sex, the prevalence of AUDs and AD among adult men was 8.6% and 4.5% respectively, and among adult women was 1.7% and 0.8% respectively. Among adult women, the prevalence of AUDs was lowest in the Eastern Mediterranean region (0.2%) and highest in the European region (3.5%). Similarly, among adult women, the prevalence of AD was lowest in the Eastern Mediterranean region (0.1%) and highest in the European region (1.5%). Stratified by income, the prevalence rates of AUDs and AD were highest in countries with very high-income economies (5.0% AUDs and 2.4% AD), while the prevalence of AUDs was lowest in lower-middle-income economies (0.6% AUDs), and the prevalence of AD was lowest in low-income economies (0.3%).

Alcohol use during pregnancy

Alcohol use during pregnancy has been established as a risk factor for many adverse pregnancy outcomes, including stillbirth (Kesmodel, Wisborg, Olsen, Henriksen, & Secher, 2002), spontaneous abortion (Henriksen et al., 2004), premature birth (Albertsen, Andersen, Olsen, & Grønbæk, 2004; Kesmodel, Olsen, & Secher, 2000; Patra et al., 2011), intrauterine growth retardation (Patra et al., 2011; Yang et al., 2001), low birthweight (O'Callaghan, O'Callaghan, Najman, Williams, & Bor, 2003; Patra et al., 2011) and fetal alcohol spectrum disorder (FASD; see Chapters 11, 12, and 26). Many countries raise awareness concerning the detrimental consequences of alcohol consumption during pregnancy in the form of clinical guidelines (examples include Danish National Board of Health, 2010; French Ministry of Youth Affairs and Sports, 2015; National Health and Medical Research Council, 2009; Society of Obstetricians and Gynaecologists of Canada [Carson, Leach, & Murphy, 2018]; U.S. Centers for Disease Control and Prevention, 2005; and WHO's 2014 guidelines for the management of substance use during pregnancy [WHO, 2014]). Despite these public health efforts, about 10% of women worldwide consume alcohol while pregnant (Popova, Lange, Probst, Gmel, & Rehm, 2017a, 2017b).

According to a recent study (Popova et al., 2017a), the highest prevalence of alcohol use during pregnancy occurs in the WHO European Region (25.2%; see Table 3.2). This is

Table 3.2 Global prevalence in 2012 of any amount of alcohol use and of heavy episodic drinking (four or more drinks on a single occasion) during pregnancy, and of FAS and FASD among the general population, by WHO region (Popova et al., 2018)

Region	Alcohol Use (Any Amount) during Pregnancy (%)[a]	Heavy Episodic Drinking during Pregnancy (%)[b]	FAS (per 10,000)	FASD (per 10,000)[c]
Global	9.8	–	14.6	77.3
WHO region				
African	10.0	3.1	14.8	78.3
American	11.2	2.8	16.6	87.9
Eastern Mediterranean	0.2	–	0.2	1.3
European	25.2	2.7	37.4	198.2
South-East Asia	1.8	–	2.7	14.1
Western Pacific	8.6	1.8	12.7	67.4

Source: Popova, Lange, Poznyak et al. (2019).

Notes
a The prevalence of any amount of alcohol use during pregnancy is inclusive of the prevalence of binge drinking during pregnancy.
b It was not possible to estimate the prevalence of binge drinking during pregnancy for the Eastern Mediterranean Region and South-East Asia Region due to a lack of available data for countries in these regions, and, therefore, the global prevalence could not be estimated.
c The prevalence of FASD is inclusive of the prevalence of FAS.

not surprising; according to the latest Global Status Report on Alcohol and Health (WHO, 2018b), almost all major alcohol indicators, including prevalence, level of consumption, rates of alcohol use and HED, and AUDs, are the highest in the European region. Additionally, the five countries with the highest prevalence rates of alcohol use among pregnant women also occur in the European region: Ireland (60.4%), Belarus (46.6%), Denmark (45.8%), United Kingdom (41.3%), and Russia (36.5%). The lowest prevalence of alcohol use during pregnancy was estimated to be among women in the Eastern Mediterranean Region (50 times lower than the global average) and in the South-East Asia Region (five times lower than the global average); in these regions, a large proportion of the population abstains from alcohol use, especially the female population (WHO, 2014).

In addition to alarmingly high rates of alcohol consumption during pregnancy, it has also been established that over 25% of the women who consume any alcohol during pregnancy engage in binge drinking, defined as consuming four or more drinks on a single occasion (Lange, Probst, Rehm, & Popova, 2017; Popova et al., 2017b). The highest prevalence of binge drinking during pregnancy was estimated to be in the African region (3.1%), while the Western Pacific region had the lowest prevalence of binge drinking during pregnancy (1.8%). The proportion of pregnant women who engaged in binge drinking during pregnancy, among women who drank any amount of alcohol, was estimated to range from 10.7% in the European region to 31.0% in the African region. The five countries with the highest estimated prevalence of binge drinking during pregnancy were Paraguay (13.9%), Moldova (10.6%), Ireland (10.5%), Lithuania (10.5%), and the Czech Republic (9.4%).

Estimates presented in this section reflect the general populations of the respective countries. However, prevalence rates of alcohol use during pregnancy have been reported to be much higher among some sub-populations. For example, the prevalence of alcohol use during pregnancy among Inuit women in northern Quebec (Canada) was reported to be 60.5%, which is over ten times higher than the estimate for the general population of Canada (Fraser, Muckle, Abdous, Jacobson, & Jacobson, 2012).

Fetal alcohol syndrome (FAS) and fetal alcohol spectrum disorder (FASD)

Overall, these estimates are very troubling, as binge drinking is the most detrimental pattern of drinking during pregnancy and is a direct cause of FASD. The prevalence of FASD in the Western Cape Province of South Africa, a region known for wine production and a high prevalence of binge drinking among women, has been reported to be 135–208 per 1,000 (13.5–20.8%) among first-grade students—one of the highest FASD prevalence rates in the world (May et al., 2013).

In line with the prevalence of alcohol use during pregnancy, the prevalence rates of FAS (fetal alcohol syndrome) and FASD (fetal alcohol spectrum disorders) were estimated to be highest in the European region at 37.4 per 10,000 and 198.2 per 10,000 respectively, and lowest in the Eastern Mediterranean region at 0.2 per 10,000 and 1.3 per 10,000 respectively. Global prevalence rates of FAS and FASD among the general population were estimated to be 14.6 per 10,000 and 77.3 per 10,000 respectively. The five countries with the highest FAS prevalence per 10,000 were Belarus (69.1), Italy (82.1), Ireland (89.7), Croatia (115.2), and South Africa (585.3). The five countries with the lowest FAS prevalence (less than 0.05 per 10,000) were Oman, United Arab Emirates, Saudi Arabia, Qatar, and Kuwait (all in the Eastern Mediterranean Region). The five countries with the highest FASD prevalence were South Africa (111.1 per 1,000), Croatia (53.3 per 1,000), Ireland (47.5 per 1,000), Italy (45.0 per 1,000), and Belarus (36.6 per 1,000).

FASD prevalence in sub-populations

A recent systematic review and meta-analysis revealed that certain sub-populations, such as children in care, correctional, special education, specialized clinical, and Aboriginal populations, experience a significantly higher prevalence of FASD compared to the general population (see Figure 3.1). This trend poses a great service and cost burden across various systems of care, reflecting a substantial global health problem (Popova, Lange, Shield, Burd, & Rehm, 2019). The pooled prevalence of FASD among children in out-of-home care/foster care in Chile was estimated to be 31.2% and 25.2% in the United States. The pooled prevalence of FAS (the most severe form of FASD) was estimated to be 9.6% among children in care in Russia. The pooled FASD prevalence among Aboriginal populations was estimated to be 4.4% and estimated to be 14.7% among adults in the Canadian correctional system.

FASD prevalence rates among these sub-populations far exceed rates among the general population. Compared to the recently estimated 7.7 per 1,000 global prevalence of FASD in the general population (Lange, Probst, Gmel et al., 2017), prevalence in the selected sub-populations were 10- to 40-times higher. For example, the prevalence among children in care was 32-times higher in the United States and 40-times higher in Chile, the prevalence among adults in the Canadian correctional system was 19-times higher, and the prevalence among special education populations in Chile was over 10-times higher.

Furthermore, prevalence rates reported in individual studies (some not meta-analyzed) are even higher, and more alarming. For instance, the prevalence of FASD among children with intellectual disabilities in care in Chile was 62% (Mena, Navarrete, Avila, Bedregal, & Berríos, 1993), over 52% among adoptees from Eastern Europe (Landgren, Svensson, Strömland, & Grönlund, 2010), and about 40% among children residing in orphanages in Lithuania (Kuzmenkovienė, Prasauskienė, & Endzinienė, 2012). The highest prevalence estimates of FAS, ranging between 46% and 68%, were reported in Russian orphanages for children with developmental abnormalities (Legonkova, 2011). Additionally, the prevalence

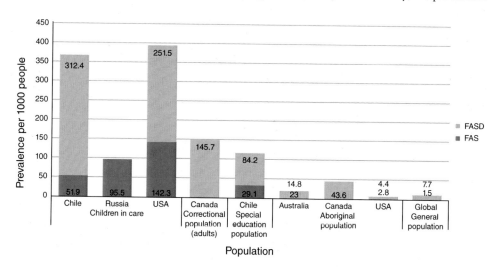

Figure 3.1 Pooled prevalence of FAS and FASD among selected sub-populations, by country and in the general global population

Source: Based on data from Popova, Lange, Poznyak et al. (2019).

of FASD among youth in correctional services was over 23% in Canada (Fast, Conry, & Loock, 1999), and over 14% among United States populations in psychiatric care (Bell & Chimata, 2015). Children are often placed in foster care, orphanages, or for adoption due to unfavorable circumstances, such as parental alcohol and/or drug use, child maltreatment, abandonment, and young maternal age (see Chapter 23). These circumstances suggest a higher likelihood of prenatal alcohol exposure among children in care (Burd, Cohen, Shah, & Norris, 2011).

Appropriate social work interventions, as well as diagnostic and support services, must be applied at an early age for individuals with FASD to decrease their chances of becoming involved with the legal system, either as victims or as offenders. One estimate suggests that, on any given day in a specific year, children and adolescents with FASD are 19 times more likely to be incarcerated compared to children and adolescents without FASD (Popova, Lange, Bekmuradov, Mihic, & Rehm, 2011). Lastly, high prevalence rates of FASD among special education populations and in specialized clinical populations are not surprising, given that individuals with FASD are at greater risk of having learning difficulties and mental health problems, as well as experiencing developmental delays (Popova, Lange, Poznyak et al., 2019).

High prevalence rates of alcohol consumption during pregnancy and FASD within Aboriginal populations must especially be examined within the historical context and socio-demographic reality of this marginalized sub-population—colonization, intergenerational trauma, and residential school experiences. These factors contribute to the high prevalence of alcohol use, both in general and during pregnancy (Sotero, 2006; Szlemko, Wood, & Thurman, 2006). For example, the prevalence rates of alcohol use during pregnancy in the Aboriginal populations of the United States and Canada were approximately three and four times higher, respectively, compared to the general population (Popova, Lange, Probst, Parunashvili, & Rehm, 2017). Even more alarmingly, approximately 20% of women in the Aboriginal populations who consumed alcohol during pregnancy engaged in binge drinking as compared to 3% in the general population in both countries (Popova et al., 2017).

Disease burden attributable to alcohol consumption

Estimates of alcohol-attributable (AA) deaths and disability-adjusted life years (DALYs) lost are used to assess the impact of alcohol on health at the population level and the need for public health policies to reduce the harmful consumption of alcohol and resulting burden of disease.

The diseases, conditions, and injuries causally related to alcohol consumption are outlined in Table 3.3. The number of AA deaths and DALYs lost were estimated based on (1) diseases and injuries where alcohol is a necessary cause, such as AUDs (i.e. diseases and injuries which are 100% attributable to alcohol), and (2) diseases and injuries where alcohol is a component cause, where under a counterfactual scenario of no alcohol consumption a fraction of the disease or injury would not occur. For diseases and injuries where alcohol is a component cause, the fractions of AA deaths and DALYs lost were estimated using a Levin-based methodology by combining data on alcohol consumption with corresponding relative risk (RR) estimates obtained from systematic reviews and meta-analyses (Levin, 1953).

According to the WHO's GSRAH (WHO, 2018b), 3 million deaths every year result from the harmful use of alcohol, representing 5.3% of all deaths globally. Overall, 5.1% of the global burden of disease and injury is attributable to alcohol, as measured in DALYs lost. Among women

Table 3.3 Causes of death and disability causally related to alcohol consumption[a]

Diseases and injuries

Communicable diseases
  Tuberculosis, HIV/AIDS, Lower respiratory infections
Noncommunicable diseases
  Malignant neoplasms
    Lip and oral cavity, pharyngeal cancers (excluding nasopharyngeal), esophagus cancer, colon and rectum cancers, liver cancer, breast cancer, larynx cancer
  Diabetes mellitus
  Alcohol use disorders
  Epilepsy
  Cardiovascular diseases
    Hypertensive heart disease, Ischemic heart disease, Ischemic stroke, Hemorrhagic stroke, Cardiomyopathy, myocarditis, endocarditis
  Digestive diseases
    Cirrhosis of the liver
  Pancreatitis
Injuries
  Unintentional injuries
    Road injury, poisonings, falls, fire, heat and hot substances, drowning, exposure to mechanical forces, other unintentional injuries
  Intentional injuries
    Self-harm, interpersonal violence

Source: Based on the conclusions of the review by Rehm, Gmel et al. (2017).

Note
a   Alcohol is also causally related to atrial fibrillation and flutter, esophageal varice, and psoriasis, and major depressive disorder.

15–49 years of age, alcohol was responsible for 150,466 deaths in 2016, representing 4.6% of all deaths, and 12,711,001 DALYs lost, representing 3.5% of all DALYs lost (see Table 3.4).

Geographically, among women 15–49 years of age, alcohol caused the largest number of age-standardized deaths in the African region (17.2 deaths per 100,000 people) and the European region (14.1 deaths per 100,000), while the Eastern Mediterranean (0.6 deaths per 100,000 people) and Western Pacific (5.0 deaths per 100,000) regions experienced the lowest AA death burdens (see Figure 3.2). Furthermore, the age-standardized AA death burden was highest in countries with low-income economies (10.1 deaths per 100,000), followed by lower-middle-income economies (8.7 deaths per 100,000), upper-middle-income economies (7.4 deaths per 100,000), and high-income economies (5.8 deaths per 100,000; see Figure 3.3). Of note is the age-standardized burden of AA communicable, maternal, perinatal, and nutritional conditions in the African region (5.0 deaths per 100,000), as well as in countries with lower-middle-income economies (1.9 deaths per 100,000), and upper-middle-income economies (1.6 deaths per 100,000 people). The burden of AA deaths in the African region as well as in countries with lower- and lower-middle-income economies is greatly affected by the underlying high risk of tuberculosis, HIV/AIDS, and lower respiratory diseases in this region and these countries (WHO, 2018b).

Table 3.4 Deaths and disability-adjusted life years lost globally in 2016, by cause, among women 15–49 years of age

Cause of Death and/or Disability	Deaths				Disability-Adjusted Life Years Lost			
	Burden	AA Burden	Population-Attributable Fraction (%)	Age-Standardized AA Burden Rate Per 100,000 People	Burden	AA Burden	Population-Attributable Fraction (%)	Age-Standardized AA Burden Rate Per 100,000 People
All causes	3,214,365	150,466	4.7	7.9	365,440,152	12,711,001	3.5	673.2
Communicable, maternal, perinatal, and nutritional conditions	1,084,733	18,915	1.7	1.0	92,615,606	1,144,052	1.2	60.6
Tuberculosis	152,436	12,258	8.0	0.6	9,435,283	750,085	7.9	39.7
HIV AIDS	302,730	3,657	1.2	0.2	18,542,354	222,320	1.2	11.8
Lower respiratory infections	85,382	3,000	3.5	0.2	5,078,643	171,647	3.4	9.1
Noncommunicable diseases	1,559,340	67,905	4.4	3.6	227,975,977	6,594,617	2.9	348.5
Malignant neoplasms	564,475	10,202	1.8	0.5	29,921,215	524,761	1.8	27.4
Diabetes mellitus	53,707	-3,143	-5.9	-0.2	7,307,617	-476,918	-6.5	-24.9
Alcohol use disorders	8,440	8,440	100.0	0.4	3,538,984	3,538,984	100.0	187.5
Epilepsy	24,456	1,381	5.6	0.1	3,265,894	178,901	5.5	9.5
Cardiovascular diseases	441,412	13,097	3.0	0.7	26,589,893	663,026	2.5	34.8
Digestive diseases	167,234	37,929	22.7	2.0	11,491,598	2,165,863	18.8	114.2
Injuries	570,293	63,646	11.2	3.4	44,848,570	4,972,331	11.1	264.2
Unintentional injuries	315,315	45,064	14.3	2.4	27,567,796	3,776,856	13.7	200.7
Intentional injuries	254,978	18,582	7.3	1.0	17,280,774	1,195,476	6.9	63.5

Source: Data were obtained from the Global Information System on Alcohol and Health (WHO, 2018a).
AA: Alcohol-Attributable.

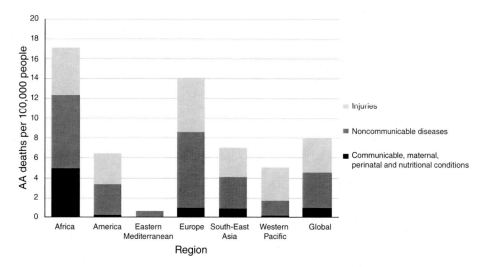

Figure 3.2 Age-standardized alcohol-attributable deaths in 2016 among women 15–49 years of age, by World Health Organization region

Source: Based on data from the Global Information System on Alcohol and Health (WHO, 2018a).

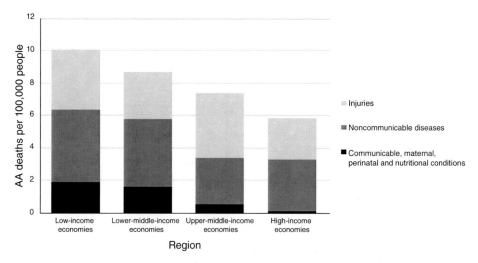

Figure 3.3 Age-standardized alcohol-attributable deaths in 2016 among women 15–49 years of age, by World Bank income regions

Source: Based on data from the Global Information System on Alcohol and Health (WHO, 2018a).

Similar to the AA death burden, the age-standardized AA DALYs lost burden among women 15–49 years of age was highest in the European (1,307 DALYs lost per 100,000 people) and African (1,226 DALYs lost per 100,000 people) regions and lowest in the Eastern Mediterranean region (158 DALYs lost per 100,000 people; see Figure 3.4). Furthermore, the age-standardized burden of AA DALYs lost was highest in countries with low-income economies (799 DALYs lost per 100,000 people), followed by lower-middle-income economies (685 DALYs lost per 100,000 people), upper-middle-income economies

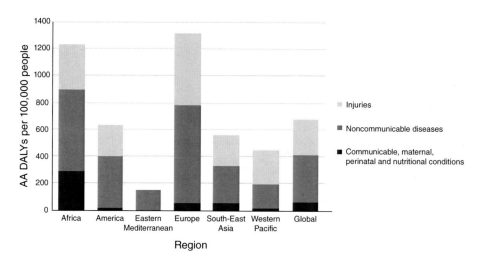

Figure 3.4 Age-standardized alcohol-attributable disability-adjusted life years lost in 2016 among women 15–49 years of age, by World Health Organization region

Source: Based on data from the Global Information System on Alcohol and Health (WHO, 2018a).

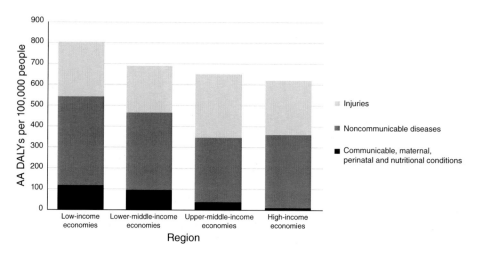

Figure 3.5 Age-standardized alcohol-attributable disability-adjusted life years lost in 2016, by World Bank income regions

Source: Based on data from the Global Information System on Alcohol and Health (WHO, 2018a).

(650 DALYs lost per 100,000 people), and high-income economies (617 DALYs lost per 100,000 people; see Figure 3.5). As with the burden of AA deaths, the age-standardized burden of communicable, maternal, perinatal, and nutritional conditions was particularly high in the African region (288 DALYs lost per 100,000 people) as well as in countries with lower- and lower-middle-income economies (112 and 95 DALYs lost per 100,000 people respectively).

Alcohol and risk of communicable diseases

Alcohol consumption affects the risk of communicable diseases through multiple mechanisms. First, alcohol consumption (in particular HED) negatively impacts the immune system (MacGregor, 1986). Second, alcohol increases the risk of HIV infection through a decrease in the probability of using a condom during sexual intercourse (Rehm, Probst, Shield, & Shuper, 2017; Rehm, Shield, Joharchi, & Shuper, 2012) and of HIV deaths through decreased adherence to antiretroviral therapy (Hendershot, Stoner, Pantalone, & Simoni, 2009). As result, among women of childbearing age, alcohol was responsible in 2016 for 18,915 and 1,144,052 communicable disease deaths and DALYs lost, respectively. Furthermore, alcohol was responsible for 8.0% of all tuberculosis deaths, 1.2% of all HIV/AIDS deaths, and 3.5% of all lower respiratory infection deaths.

Alcohol and risk of noncommunicable diseases

Animal, biological, and epidemiological studies demonstrated sufficient causal evidence that alcohol consumption affects the risk of malignant neoplasms (cancers), diabetes mellitus, AUDs, epilepsy, cardiovascular diseases, and digestive diseases (Rehm, Gmel et al., 2017). For instance, the link between alcohol and esophageal cancer and cardiac carcinoma was first observed in 1910 (Lamy, 1910). Furthermore, the International Agency for Research on Cancer (IARC, 2012) and the World Cancer Research Fund/American Institute for Cancer Research (WCRF/AICR, 2018) have attributed the highest level of causal evidence to the association between alcohol consumption and the risk of developing cancer. In particular, alcohol is causally associated with cancers of the oral cavity, oropharynx, hypopharynx, esophagus, colon, rectum, liver and intrahepatic bile duct, larynx, and breast (IARC, 2012; WCRF/AICR, 2018). In 2016, among women 15–49 years of age, alcohol caused 10,202 cancer deaths and 524,761 cancer DALYs lost, representing 1.8% of all cancer deaths and 1.8% of all cancer DALYs lost. Furthermore, although not modeled, alcohol exposure between menarche and the first pregnancy may increase the risk of breast cancer more than alcohol consumption later in life due to undifferentiated nulliparous breast tissue being more susceptible to carcinogens (Liu et al., 2013).

The antioxidative properties of resveratrol (i.e. the red wine chemical) have received media attention for their anti-carcinogenic properties. However, for every cancer case that the resveratrol in wine prevents, 100,000 cancer cases are caused by ethanol (i.e. the margin of exposure of resveratrol is estimated to be 100,000) (Shield, Soerjomataram, & Rehm, 2016).

At lower doses of alcohol consumption, there is a decrease in the risk of diabetes mellitus through increased insulin sensitivity (Hendriks, 2007), and possibly through other pathways such as increase in the levels of alcohol metabolites (Sarkola, Iles, Kohlenberg-Mueller, & Eriksson, 2002). However, at higher doses of alcohol consumption, there has been an observed increase in the risk of diabetes mellitus. As a result, alcohol consumption has a "J" shaped relationship with the risk of diabetes mellitus (Knott, Bell, & Britton, 2015). At the global level, alcohol had a net protective effect on diabetes mortality and morbidity in 2016, preventing 3,143 diabetes deaths and 476,918 diabetes DALYs lost.

The consumption of alcohol increases the predisposition for epileptic seizures; alcohol withdrawal following heavy alcohol consumption has a kindling effect which lowers the threshold for the inducing of an epileptic episode (Ballenger & Post, 1978). Other causal pathways for epileptic seizures include cerebral atrophy, as well as cerebrovascular infarctions, lesions, and head traumas (Rathlev, Ulrich, Delanty, & D'Onofrio, 2006). As a result, among women 15–49 years of age, alcohol consumption in 2016 caused 1,381 epilepsy deaths and 178,901 epilepsy DALYs lost, representing 5.5% and 5.6% of epilepsy deaths and epilepsy DALYs lost, respectively.

Although not modeled in the GSRAH, heavy alcohol use related causally to major depressive disorders (Rehm, Gmel et al., 2017). Alcohol use is also associated with worsening the depression course, and outcomes such as suicide, as well as impaired social functioning and decreased health-care utilization (Sullivan, Fiellin, & O'Connor, 2005). Additionally, depressive disorders increase alcohol use and can cause AUDs, thus worsening depressive symptoms (Boden & Fergusson, 2011).

Alcohol has both detrimental and protective effects on cardiovascular diseases. In particular, low-dose alcohol consumption decreased the risks of both ischemic heart disease and ischemic stroke (Patra et al., 2010; Roerecke & Rehm, 2012). This protective effect is hypothesized to be mediated through increases in blood concentrations of high-density lipoprotein, as the result of cellular signaling effects, decreases in the ability of platelets to form blood clots, and blood clot dissolution (Zakhari, 1997). However, this protective effect is not observed for HED (Roerecke & Rehm, 2012). Alcohol has a detrimental effect on cardiovascular diseases by causing abnormalities and disruptions in the electro-chemical signals that coordinate the heartbeat and heart rate. As a result, alcohol has been associated with an increased risk of hypertensive heart disease, hemorrhagic stroke, and cardiomyopathy (Rehm, Gmel et al., 2017). At the global level, alcohol had a net negative effect in 2016 on cardiovascular diseases, causing 13,097 cardiovascular disease deaths and 663,026 cardiovascular disease DALYs lost among women 15–49 years of age, representing 0.7% of all cardiovascular disease deaths and 2.5% of all cardiovascular disease DALYs lost.

Alcohol consumption has been observed to increase the risk of both liver cirrhosis and pancreatitis. In particular, the breakdown of ethanol in the liver through oxidative and non-oxidative pathways, and the resulting production of acetaldehyde, increased risk of fatty liver, alcoholic hepatitis, and cirrhosis (Tuma & Casey, 2003). Alcohol consumption increases the risk of pancreatitis through the same pathways as for liver cirrhosis; in particular, alcohol metabolism results in damage to pancreatic acinar cells (Vonlaufen, Wilson, Pirola, & Apte, 2007). Based on these risk relationships, among women of childbearing age, alcohol was estimated to have caused 37,929 digestive disease deaths and 2,165,863 DALYs lost during 2016, representing 22.7% of all digestive disease deaths and 18.8% of DALYs lost.

Alcohol and risk of injury

Alcohol increases the risk of injury as a result of psychomotor (Dawson & Reid, 1997) and executive functioning impairment (Giancola, 2000), with the risk of injury being dependent on the person(s) who contribute to the injury, the vehicle/agent which causes the injury, and the environment where the injury takes place (Haddon Jr., 1980; Rivara, Koepsell, Jurkovich, Gurney, & Soderberg, 1993). In particular, alcohol consumption has been linked to an increase in the risk of road and other unintentional injuries, as well as risk of self-harm and interpersonal violence (Rehm, Gmel et al., 2017). Overall, among women 15–49 years of age, AA injuries caused a total of 63,646 injury deaths and 4,972,331 injury DALYs lost, representing 11.2% and 11.1% of all injury deaths and DALYs lost, respectively.

Alcohol harms by socio-economic status

Although not accounted for in the 2018 GSRAH estimations, when standardized based on the grams consumed, alcohol has been shown to impact individuals of lower socio-economic statuses to a greater extent (Probst, Roerecke, Behrendt, & Rehm, 2014). This is due to multiple factors, including the interaction with other risk factors, such as tobacco, obesity, and hepatitis infection, and by access to and utilization of health-care resources (WHO, 2018c).

Public health guidelines for low-risk alcohol consumption

As alcohol consumption has both protective and detrimental effects on health, the question remains as to what constitutes low-risk drinking; the information on which to make such a determination is inconsistent. Low-risk drinking guidelines are often determined by a group of independent experts, and/or community stakeholders, such as blue-ribbon committees, and are based on average alcohol consumption RR curves for all-cause or selected disease mortality (Shield et al., 2017). This is problematic as it does not consider non-fatal outcomes caused by alcohol, such as AUDs (Rehm, Gmel et al., 2017), and all-cause mortality RRs are estimated based on large, non-representative cohort studies constructed based on the ease of following up participants. As a result, these estimates are based on data which over-represent deaths occurring in the middle-class population compared to other segments of the general population (Shield et al., 2017).

Recent data from the 2016 Global Burden of Disease study suggest that there is no safe level of drinking (i.e. even at low levels of alcohol consumption there is a net detrimental effect on health) (GBD 2016 Alcohol Collaborators, 2018). However, there may be a net protective effect at lower alcohol consumption amounts (not engaging in HED) (Shield & Rehm, 2019) due to the protective effects of alcohol on the risks of diabetes mellitus, ischemic heart disease, and ischemic stroke (Rehm, Gmel et al., 2017).

Conclusions

Alcohol has a net negative impact on health at the population level, impacting the risk of over 230 diseases and injuries. Accordingly, the harmful effects of alcohol should be recognized globally as a large public health problem warranting attention from social workers and health-care professionals. Evidence-supported efforts should be made to educate the general population (women and men, children and teenagers) about the risks of alcohol use, especially binge and frequent drinking, and especially during pregnancy. Moreover, prevention initiatives, aimed at reducing alcohol misuse and alcohol use during and before pregnancy, should be implemented around the world. Social workers and health-care providers are well positioned to fulfill a crucial role in reducing the harms associated with alcohol misuse, and in primary prevention of prenatal alcohol exposure.

References

Albertsen, K., Andersen, A.-M. N., Olsen, J., & Grønbæk, M. (2004). Alcohol consumption during pregnancy and the risk of preterm delivery. *American Journal of Epidemiology, 159*(2), 155–161. doi:10.1093/aje/kwh034

Ballenger, J. C., & Post, R. M. (1978). Kindling as a model for alcohol withdrawal syndromes. *The British Journal of Psychiatry, 133*(1), 1–14. doi:10.1192/bjp.133.1.1

Begun, A. L., Clapp, J. D., & The Alcohol Misuse Grand Challenges Collective. (2015). *Reducing and preventing alcohol misuse and its consequences: A grand challenge for social work.* American Academy of Social Work & Social Welfare Working Paper No. 14. Retrieved from http://grandchallengesf orsocialwork.org/wp-content/uploads/2015/12/WP14-with-cover.pdf

Bell, C. C., & Chimata, R. (2015). Prevalence of neurodevelopmental disorders among low-income African Americans at a clinic on Chicago's South Side. *Psychiatric Services, 66*(5), 539–542. doi:10.1176/appi.ps.201400162

Bloomfield, K., Gmel, G., Neve, R., & Mustonen, H. (2001). Investigating gender convergence in alcohol consumption in Finland, Germany, The Netherlands, and Switzerland: A repeated survey analysis. *Substance Abuse, 22*(1), 39–53. doi:10.1080/08897070109511444

Bloomfield, K., Stockwell, T., Gmel, G., & Rehn, N. (2003). International comparisons of alcohol consumption. *Alcohol Research and Health, 27*(1), 95–109.

Boden, J. M., & Fergusson, D. M. (2011). Alcohol and depression. *Addiction, 106*(5), 906–914. doi:10.1111/j.1360-0443.2010.03351.x

Burd, L., Cohen, C., Shah, R., & Norris, J. (2011). A court team model for young children in foster care: The role of prenatal alcohol exposure and fetal alcohol spectrum disorders. *Journal of Psychiatry and Law, 39*(1), 179–191. doi:10.1177/009318531103900107

Carson, N., Leach, L., & Murphy, K. J. (2018). A re-examination of Montreal cognitive assessment (MoCA) cutoff scores. *International Journal of Geriatric Psychiatry, 33*(2), 379–388. doi:10.1002/gps.4756

Centers for Disease Control and Prevention. (2005). *Advisory on alcohol use during pregnancy. A 2005 message to women from the US surgeon general.* Retrieved from: https://www.cdc.gov/ncbddd/fasd/documents/sg-advisory.pdf

Chisholm, D., Moro, D., Bertram, M., Pretorius, C., Gmel, G., Shield, K., & Rehm, J. (2018). Are the "best buys" for alcohol control still valid? An update on the comparative cost-effectiveness of alcohol control strategies at the global level. *Journal of Studies on Alcohol and Drugs, 79*(4), 514–522. doi:10.15288/jsad.2018.79.514

Danish National Board of Health. (2010). *Healthy habits before, during and after pregnancy. 1st English edition (translated from 2nd Danish edition).* Retrieved from https://www.sst.dk/-/media/Udgivelser/2015/Sunde-vaner-fremmedsprog/Sunde_vaner_2015_Engelsk.ashx

Dawson, D., & Reid, K. (1997). Fatigue, alcohol and performance impairment. *Nature, 388*(6639), 235. doi:10.1038/40775

Fast, D. K., Conry, J., & Loock, C. A. (1999). Identifying fetal alcohol syndrome among youth in the criminal justice system. *Journal of Developmental and Behavioral Pediatrics, 20*(5), 370–372. doi:10.1097/00004703-199910000-00012

Fraser, S. L., Muckle, G., Abdous, B. B., Jacobson, J. L., & Jacobson, S. W. (2012). Effects of binge drinking on infant growth and development in an Inuit sample. *Alcohol, 46*(3), 277–283. doi:10.1016/j.alcohol.2011.09.028

French Ministry of Youth Affairs and Sports. (2015). *Health comes with eating and moving: The food guide for pregnancy.* Retrieved from http://www.mangerbouger.fr/content/download/3817/101729/version/4/file/1059.pdf

GBD 2016 Alcohol Collaborators. (2018). Alcohol use and burden for 195 countries and territories, 1990–2016: A systematic analysis for the global burden of disease study 2016. *Lancet, 392*(10152), 1015–1035. doi:10.1016/S0140-6736(18)31310-2

Giancola, P. R. (2000). Executive functioning: A conceptual framework for alcohol-related aggression. *Experimental and Clinical Psychopharmacology, 8*(4), 576. doi:10.1037/1064-1297.8.4.576

Gmel, G., & Rehm, J. (2004). Measuring alcohol consumption. *Contemporary Drug Problems, 31*, 467. doi:10.1177/009145090403100304

Grant, B. F., Goldstein, R. B., Saha, T. D., Chou, S. P., Jung, J., Zhang, H., . . . Huang, B. (2015). Epidemiology of DSM-5 alcohol use disorder: Results from the national epidemiologic survey on alcohol and related conditions III. *JAMA Psychiatry, 72*(8), 757–766. doi:10.1001/jamapsychiatry.2015.0584

Haddon Jr., W. (1980). Advances in the epidemiology of injuries as a basis for public policy. *Public Health Reports, 95*(5), 411–421.

Hendershot, C. S., Stoner, S. A., Pantalone, D. W., & Simoni, J. M. (2009). Alcohol use and antiretroviral adherence: Review and meta-analysis. *Journal of Acquired Immune Deficiency Syndromes, 52*(2), 180. doi:10.1097/QAI.0b013e3181b18b6e

Hendriks, H. F. (2007). Moderate alcohol consumption and insulin sensitivity: Observations and possible mechanisms. *Annals of Epidemiology, 17*(5), S40–S42. doi:10.1016/j.annepidem.2007.01.009

Henriksen, T. B., Hjollund, N. H., Jensen, T. K., Bonde, J. P., Andersson, A.-M., Kolstad, H., . . . Olsen, J. (2004). Alcohol consumption at the time of conception and spontaneous abortion. *American Journal of Epidemiology, 160*(7), 661–667. doi:10.1093/aje/kwh259

International Agency for Research on Cancer. (2012). *IARC monographs on the evaluation of carcinogenic risks to humans. Volume 96–100E personal habits and indoor combustions.* Lyon, France: International Agency for Research on Cancer.

Kehoe, T., Gmel, G., Shield, K. D., Gmel, G., & Rehm, J. (2012). Determining the best population-level alcohol consumption model and its impact on estimates of alcohol-attributable harms. *Population Health Metrics, 10*(1), 1. doi:10.1186/1478-7954-10-6

Kesmodel, U., Olsen, S. F., & Secher, N. J. (2000). Does alcohol increase the risk of preterm delivery? *Epidemiology, 11*(5), 512–518. doi:10.1097/00001648-200009000-00005

Kesmodel, U., Wisborg, K., Olsen, S. F., Henriksen, T. B., & Secher, N. J. (2002). Moderate alcohol intake during pregnancy and the risk of stillbirth and death in the first year of life. *American Journal of Epidemiology, 155*(4), 305–312. doi:10.1093/aje/155.4.305

Knott, C., Bell, S., & Britton, A. (2015). Alcohol consumption and the risk of type 2 diabetes: A systematic review and dose-response meta-analysis of more than 1.9 million individuals from 38 observational studies. *Diabetes Care, 38*(9), 1804–1812. doi:10.2337/dc15-0710

Kuzmenkovienė, E., Prasauskienė, A., & Endzinienė, M. (2012). The prevalence of fetal alcohol spectrum disorders and concomitant disorders among orphanage children in Lithuania. *Journal of Population Therapeutics and Clinical Pharmacology, 19*(3), e423.

Lamy, L. (1910). Étude clinique et statistique de 134 cas de cancer de l'oesophage et du cardia. *Archives des maladies de L'Appareil Digestif, 4*, 451–475.

Landgren, M., Svensson, L., Strömland, K., & Grönlund, M. A. (2010). Prenatal alcohol exposure and neurodevelopmental disorders in children adopted from eastern Europe. *Pediatrics, 125*(5), e1178–e1185. doi:10.1542/peds.2009-0712

Lange, S., Probst, C., Gmel, G., Rehm, J., Burd, L., & Popova, S. (2017). Global prevalence of fetal alcohol spectrum disorder among children and youth: A systematic review and meta-analysis. *JAMA Pediatrics, 171*(10), 948–956. doi:10.1001/jamapediatrics.2017.1919

Lange, S., Probst, C., Rehm, J., & Popova, S. (2017). Prevalence of binge drinking during pregnancy by country and world health organization region: Systematic review and meta-analysis. *Reproductive Toxicology, 73*, 214–221. doi:10.1016/j.reprotox.2017.08.004

Legonkova, S. V. (2011) *Kliniko-funktcionalnaia kharakteristika fetal-nogo alkogolnogo sindroma u detei rannego vozrasta (Clinicaland functional characteristics of fetal alcohol syndrome in early childhood).* Doctoral dissertation, St. Peterburg's State Paediatric Medical Academy, St. Peterburg, Russia.

Levin, M. L. (1953). The occurrence of lung cancer in man. *Acta Union International Contra, 9*, 531–541.

Liu, Y., Colditz, G. A., Rosner, B., Berkey, C. S., Collins, L. C., Schnitt, S. J., . . . Tamimi, R. M. (2013). Alcohol intake between menarche and first pregnancy: A prospective study of breast cancer risk. *Journal of the National Cancer Institute, 105*(20), 1571–1578. doi:10.1093/jnci/djt213

MacGregor, R. R. (1986). Alcohol and immune defense. *JAMA, 256*(11), 1474–1479. doi:10.1001/jama.1986.03380110080031

Manthey, J., Shield, K. D., Rylett, M., Hasan, O. S., Probst, C., & Rehm, J. (2019). Global alcohol exposure between 1990 and 2017 and forecasts until 2030: A modelling study. *Lancet, 393*(10190), 2493–2502. doi:10.1016/S0140-6736(18)32744-2

May, P. A., Blankenship, J., Marais, A. S., Gossage, J. P., Kalberg, W. O., Barnard, R., . . . Buckley, D. (2013). Approaching the prevalence of the full spectrum of fetal alcohol spectrum disorders in a South African population-based study. *Alcoholism, Clinical and Experimental Research, 37*(5), 818–830. doi:10.1111/acer.12033

Mena, M., Navarrete, P., Avila, P., Bedregal, P., & Berríos, X. (1993). Alcohol drinking in parents and its relation with intellectual score of their children. *Revista Medica de Chile, 121*(1), 98–105.

National Health and Medical Research Council. (2009). *Australian guidelines to reduce health risks from drinking alcohol.* Retrieved from https://www.nhmrc.gov.au/about-us/publications/australian-guidelines-reduce-health-risks-drinking-alcohol

O'Callaghan, F. V., O'Callaghan, M., Najman, J. M., Williams, G. M., & Bor, W. (2003). Maternal alcohol consumption during pregnancy and physical outcomes up to 5 years of age: A longitudinal study. *Early Human Development, 71*(2), 137–148. doi:10.1016/S0378-3782(03)00003-3

Organisation for Economic Co-operation and Development. (2019). *OECD data: Alcohol consumption*. Retrieved from https://data.oecd.org/healthrisk/alcohol-consumption.htm

Patra, J., Bakker, R., Irving, H., Jaddoe, V. W., Malini, S., & Rehm, J. (2011). Dose–response relationship between alcohol consumption before and during pregnancy and the risks of low birthweight, preterm birth and small for gestational age (SGA)—A systematic review and meta-analyses. *BJOG: An International Journal of Obstetrics and Gynaecology, 118*(12), 1411–1421. doi:10.1111/j.1471-0528.2011.03050.x

Patra, J., Taylor, B., Irving, H., Roerecke, M., Baliunas, D., Mohapatra, S., & Rehm, J. (2010). Alcohol consumption and the risk of morbidity and mortality for different stroke types—A systematic review and meta-analysis. *BMC Public Health, 10*(1), 258. doi:10.1186/1471-2458-10-258

Popova, S., Lange, S., Bekmuradov, D., Mihic, A., & Rehm, J. (2011). Fetal alcohol spectrum disorder prevalence estimates in correctional systems: A systematic literature review. *Canadian Journal of Public Health. Revue Canadienne de Santé Publique, 102*(5), 336–340. doi:10.1007/BF03404172

Popova, S., Lange, S., Poznyak, V., Chudley, A. E., Shield, K., Murray, M., . . . Rehm, J. (2019). Population-based prevalence of fetal alcohol spectrum disorder in Canada. *BMC Public Health, 19*, 845.

Popova, S., Lange, S., Probst, C., Gmel, G., & Rehm, J. (2017a). Estimation of national, regional, and global prevalence of alcohol use during pregnancy and fetal alcohol syndrome: A systematic review and meta-analysis. *Lancet Global Health, 5*(3), e290–e299. doi:10.1016/S2214-109X(17)30021-9

Popova, S., Lange, S., Probst, C., Gmel, G., & Rehm, J. (2017b). Global prevalence of alcohol use and binge drinking during pregnancy, and fetal alcohol spectrum disorder. *Biochemistry and Cell Biology, 96*(2), 237–240. doi:10.1139/bcb-2017-0077

Popova, S., Lange, S., Probst, C., Parunashvili, N., & Rehm, J. (2017). Prevalence of alcohol consumption during pregnancy and fetal alcohol spectrum disorders among the general and Aboriginal populations in Canada and the United States. *European Journal of Medical Genetics, 60*(1), 32–48. doi:10.1016/j.ejmg.2016.09.010

Popova, S., Lange, S., Shield, K., Burd, L., & Rehm, J. (2019). Prevalence of fetal alcohol spectrum disorder among special subpopulations: A systematic review and meta-analysis. *Addiction, 114*(7), 1150–1172. doi:10.1111/add.14598

Poznyak, V., Fleischmann, A., Rekve, D., Rylett, M., Rehm, J., & Gmel, G. (2014). The world health organization's global monitoring system on alcohol and health. *Alcohol Research: Current Reviews, 35*(2), 244–249.

Probst, C., Roerecke, M., Behrendt, S., & Rehm, J. (2014). Socioeconomic differences in alcohol-attributable mortality compared with all-cause mortality: A systematic review and meta-analysis. *International Journal of Epidemiology, 43*(4), 1314–1327. doi:10.1093/ije/dyu043

Rathlev, N. K., Ulrich, A. S., Delanty, N., & D'Onofrio, G. (2006). Alcohol-related seizures. *Journal of Emergency Medicine, 31*(2), 157–163. doi:10.1016/j.jemermed.2005.09.012

Rehm, J., Gmel, G., Gmel, G., Hasan, O., Imtiaz, S., Popova, S., . . . Samokhvalov, A. (2017). The relationship between different dimensions of alcohol use and the burden of disease—An update. *Addiction, 112*(6), 968–1001. doi:10.1111/add.13757

Rehm, J., Kehoe, T., Gmel, G., Stinson, F., Grant, B., & Gmel, G. (2010). Statistical modeling of volume of alcohol exposure for epidemiological studies of population health: The US example. *Population Health Metrics, 8*(1), 1. doi:10.1186/1478-7954-8-3

Rehm, J., Probst, C., Shield, K., & Shuper, P. (2017). Does alcohol use have a causal effect on HIV incidence and disease progression? A review of the literature and a modeling strategy for quantifying the effect. *Population Health Metrics, 15*(1), 4. doi:10.1186/s12963-017-0121-9

Rehm, J., Shield, K. D., Joharchi, N., & Shuper, P. A. (2012). Alcohol consumption and the intention to engage in unprotected sex: Systematic review and meta-analysis of experimental studies. *Addiction, 107*(1), 51–59. doi:10.1111/j.1360-0443.2011.03621.x

Rivara, F. P., Koepsell, T. D., Jurkovich, G. J., Gurney, J. G., & Soderberg, R. (1993). The effects of alcohol abuse on readmission for trauma. *Journal of the American Medical Association, 270*(16), 1962–1964. doi:10.1001/jama.1993.03510160080033

Roerecke, M., & Rehm, J. (2012). The cardioprotective association of average alcohol consumption and ischaemic heart disease: A systematic review and meta-analysis. *Addiction, 107*(7), 1246–1260. doi:10.1111/j.1360-0443.2012.03780.x

Sarkola, T., Iles, M. R., Kohlenberg-Mueller, K., & Eriksson, C. P. (2002). Ethanol, acetaldehyde, acetate, and lactate levels after alcohol intake in white men and women: Effect of 4-methylpyrazole. *Alcoholism, Clinical and Experimental Research, 26*(2), 239–245. doi:10.1111/j.1530-0277.2002.tb02530.x

Shield, K. D., Gmel, G., Gmel, G., Mäkelä, P., Probst, C., Room, R., & Rehm, J. (2017). Lifetime risk of mortality due to different levels of alcohol consumption in seven European countries: Implications for low-risk drinking guidelines. *Addiction, 112*(9), 1535–1544. doi:10.1111/add.13827

Shield, K. D., & Rehm, J. (2012). Difficulties with telephone-based surveys on alcohol consumption in high-income countries: The Canadian example. *International Journal of Methods in Psychiatric Research, 21*(1), 17–28. doi:10.1002/mpr.1345

Shield, K. D., & Rehm, J. (2019). Alcohol and the global burden of disease. *Lancet, 393*(10189), 2390. doi:10.1016/S0140-6736(19)30726-3

Shield, K. D., Soerjomataram, I., & Rehm, J. (2016). Alcohol use and breast cancer: A critical review. *Alcoholism, Clinical and Experimental Research, 40*(6), 1166–1181. doi:10.1111/acer.13071

Sotero, M. (2006). A conceptual model of historical trauma: Implications for public health practice and research. *Journal of Health Disparities Research and Practice, 1*(1), 93–108.

Sullivan, L. E., Fiellin, D. A., & O'Connor, P. G. (2005). The prevalence and impact of alcohol problems in major depression: A systematic review. *American Journal of Medicine, 118*(4), 330–341. doi:10.1016/j.amjmed.2005.01.007

Szlemko, W. J., Wood, J. W., & Thurman, P. J. (2006). Native Americans and alcohol: Past, present, and future. *Journal of General Psychology, 133*(4), 435–451. doi:10.3200/GENP.133.4.435-451

Tuma, J., & Casey, C. A. (2003). Dangerous byproducts of alcohol breakdown-focus on adducts. *Alcohol Research and Health, 27*, 285–290.

United Nations. (2015). *Transforming our world: The 2030 agenda for sustainable development.* Retrieved from New York: https://www.unfpa.org/resources/transforming-our-world-2030-agenda-sustainable-development

United Nations. (2016). *Sustainable development goals: 17 goals to transform our world.* Retrieved from https://www.un.org/development/desa/disabilities/envision2030.html

Vonlaufen, A., Wilson, J. S., Pirola, R. C., & Apte, M. V. (2007). Role of alcohol metabolism in chronic pancreatitis. *Alcohol Research and Health, 30*(1), 48–54.

World Cancer Research Fund/American Institute for Cancer Research. (2018). *Diet, nutrition, physical activity and cancer: A global perspective. The third expert report.* Retrieved from https://www.wcrf.org/dietandcancer

World Health Organization. (2010). *Global strategy to reduce harmful use of alcohol consumption.* Retrieved from https://www.who.int/substance_abuse/activities/gsrhua/en/

World Health Organization. (2014). *Guidelines for the identification and management of substance use and substance use disorders in pregnancy.* Retrieved from https://www.who.int/substance_abuse/publications/pregnancy_guidelines/en/

World Health Organization. (2018a). *Global information system on alcohol and health.* Retrieved from https://www.who.int/gho/alcohol/en/

World Health Organization. (2018b). *Global status report on alcohol and health, 2018.* Retrieved from https://www.who.int/substance_abuse/publications/global_alcohol_report/en/

World Health Organization. (2018c). *WHO global status report on road safety 2018.* Retrieved from https://www.who.int/violence_injury_prevention/road_safety_status/2018/en/

World Health Organization. (2019). *Sexual and reproductive health: Infertility definitions and terminology.* Retrieved from https://www.who.int/reproductivehealth/topics/infertility/definitions/en/

Yang, Q., Witkiewicz, B. B., Olney, R. S., Liu, Y., Davis, M., Khoury, M. J., . . . Erickson, J. D. (2001). A case-control study of maternal alcohol consumption and intrauterine growth retardation. *Annals of Epidemiology, 11*(7), 497–503. doi:10.1016/S1047-2797(01)00240-X

Zakhari, S. (1997). Alcohol and the cardiovascular system: Molecular mechanisms for beneficial and harmful action. *Alcohol Health and Research World, 21*(1), 21–29.

4

Overview of addiction and the brain

Aaron M. White and George F. Koob

Background

In the United States, roughly 18.7 million adults (7.6% of the population) struggle with a substance use disorder each year involving alcohol, prescription medications, illicit drugs, or a combination (see Table 4.1). Costs associated with alcohol and other drug misuse exceed $740 billion annually, mainly due to lost productivity, healthcare and crime. In 2017, more than 70,000 individuals died from drug overdoses, and estimates suggest at least 88,000 die from alcohol misuse each year (NIDA, 2017). Globally, alcohol contributes to roughly 3 million deaths (5.3% of all deaths) each year and other substances are involved in 452,000 deaths (0.8% of all deaths) (World Drug Report, 2018).

Individuals experiencing severe substance use disorders, commonly called addictions, were long viewed as morally compromised or weak willed (Botticelli & Koh, 2016). Neurobiological research beginning in the second half of the 20th century helped change our understanding of addiction by shedding light on the mechanisms underlying its development. Studies indicating that addiction is rooted in brain changes continue to reduce the stigma of addiction

Table 4.1 Prevalence of substance use disorders in the United States

	Number	%
Illicit drugs	6,800,000	2.8
Marijuana	3,500,000	1.4
Cocaine	947,000	0.4
Rx opioids	1,580,000	0.6
Heroin	648,000	0.3
Sedatives	188,000	0.1
Alcohol	14,062,000	5.7
Illicit drugs or alcohol	18,708,000	7.6

Substance use disorder is defined as meeting DSM-IV criteria for illicit drug or alcohol abuse or dependence (Source: SAMHSA, 2018, NSDUH 2017 data for ages 18+).

and provide support for incorporating treatment for substance use disorders into mainstream healthcare. Still, fewer than one in ten individuals experiencing an alcohol use disorder and two in ten experiencing any substance use disorder in the United States receive help each year, and stigma remains a common barrier to treatment (Hammarlund, Crapanzano, Luce, Mulligan, & Ward, 2018; SAMHSA, 2018). In this chapter, we explore the concept of addiction, the neurobiology underlying its development, and treatment options addressing the root causes.

What is addiction?

The term addiction evolved from the Latin verb *addicere*, originally meaning "to speak to" and later referring to "indebtedness and enslavement." The noun, *addictus*, referred to the person who was indebted or enslaved. Early Romans recognized that gambling, as well as excessive alcohol use, could enslave an individual. During the 1700s and 1800s, the word addiction had a mainly positive connotation. The 1828 version of Webster dictionary defined addiction as, "The act of devoting or giving up in practice; the state of being devoted" (Rosenthal & Faris, 2019). A century later, the 1933 Oxford English Dictionary defined addiction similarly, as a "formal giving over or delivery by sentence of court. Hence, a surrender or dedication of anyone to a master" (Alexander & Schweighofer, 1998). More recent usage of the term typically conveys a negative connation, indicating that a person continues to engage in a compulsive behavior despite harm to their well-being.

The American Psychiatric Association defined addiction to substances as,

> a complex condition, a brain disease that is manifested by compulsive substance use despite harmful consequence. People with addiction (severe substance use disorder) have an intense focus on using a certain substance(s), such as alcohol or drugs, to the point that it takes over their life. They keep using alcohol or a drug even when they know it will cause problems.
>
> *(American Psychiatric Association, 2017)*

A recent report on addiction in the United States from the Surgeon General defined addiction as, "The most severe form of substance use disorder, associated with compulsive or uncontrolled use of one or more substances. Addiction is a chronic brain disease that has the potential for both recurrence (relapse) and recovery" (SAMHSA, 2016, p. 1–6).

Based on neuroscience research, drug addiction has been described as a

> chronically relapsing disorder characterized by: (1) compulsion to seek and take the drug, (2) loss of control in limiting intake, and (3) emergence of a negative emotional state (e.g., dysphoria, anxiety, irritability) reflecting a motivational withdrawal syndrome when access to the drug is prevented. Drug addiction has been conceptualized as a disorder involving elements of both impulsivity and compulsivity that yield a composite addiction cycle composed of three stages: "binge/intoxication", "withdrawal/ negative affect", and "preoccupation/anticipation" (craving).
>
> *(Koob & Le Moal, 1997, p. 217)*

The question often arises whether addiction is a brain disease or whether it simply reflects maladaptive learning. The answer appears to be both. Addiction involves maladaptive learning leading to the development and repetition of substance-related habits. But addiction is more than just a bad habit. The disease aspect of addiction stems from what happens when systems governing motivation and decision-making are forced to adapt in ways that manifest in an irrational drive to continue substance use in the face of potentially fatal consequences. In other words, addiction turns brain systems central to survival against an individual, often hastening mortality. Except in extreme cases, addiction does not involve a *loss* of free will. Most individuals struggling with even severe substance use disorder are not mindless automatons locked in stimulus-response relationships with drugs. However, the combination of changes that occur as addiction unfolds can make it extremely difficult, if not impossible, to escape the cycle on one's own, and often free will involves asking for and accepting help (Churchland & Witkowski, 2014).

Clinically, alcohol and other substance use disorders occur on a spectrum. The fifth edition of the DSM, the DSM-5 (American Psychiatric Association, 2013), divides substance use disorders into mild, moderate, and severe based upon the severity of symptoms, with moderate and severe considered consistent with the concept of addiction (see Chapter 1 and Appendix A).

Neurobiology of addiction

One hallmark of all organ systems in the body is adaptability. Every organ, and indeed every cell, can alter its functioning in some way to maintain overall balance, or homeostasis. The cardiovascular and pulmonary systems adjust to high altitudes and increased physical exertion with changes that ensure sufficient delivery of oxygen to tissues. In the brain, plasticity in the face of demands allows us to learn new skills, form social bonds, and develop habits that aid in survival. The powerful reinforcement that substance use provides leads to changes in the brain that promote further substance use, despite often serious consequences. Adjustments made by the brain to maintain balance in the face of repeated substance use result in physiological dependence. In the following sections, we explore the basics of brain function, examine the neural substrates of reinforcement and habit development, and discuss how changes in the brain following repeated drug use manifest in the addiction cycle.

Brain function

The brain is a roughly three-pound organ comprised of two primary cell types: neurons and glia. Neurons are the information processing units of the brain (see Figure 4.1). Each neuron has a cell body, or soma, extensions called dendrites, and an axon. Dendrites receive signals in the form of chemical messengers called neurotransmitters from other neurons. The axon is longer, often extending great distances away from the soma, in some cases several feet, and allows neurons in one brain area to communicate with cells in other areas.

To communicate with other cells, a neuron generates an electrochemical impulse, called an action potential, which travels down the axon. When the action potential reaches the end of the axon, neurotransmitters are released into a gap between neurons called a synapse. The neurotransmitters float through the synapse and attach to protein receptors on the next cell, typically on the dendrites. Sometimes a neurotransmitter signals that the post-synaptic cell should send its own signal, not send signals, grow, or even die. There are nearly 100,000,000,000 neurons in the human brain, each forming synapses with potentially thousands of other cells, creating a vast communication network throughout the

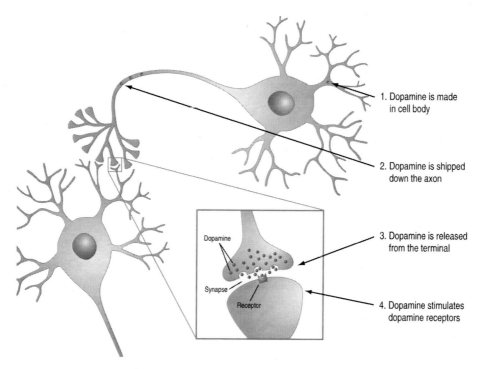

1. Dopamine is made in cell body

2. Dopamine is shipped down the axon

3. Dopamine is released from the terminal

4. Dopamine stimulates dopamine receptors

Figure 4.1   Communication between two neurons across a synapse using the neurotransmitter dopamine. Dopamine plays roles in learning to attach incentive salience (value) to stimuli

Source: SAMHSA (2016).

brain, as well as between the brain, muscles, and organs in the periphery of the body (Herculano-Houzel, 2009).

The second category of cells in the brain are glial cells, which come in several types and serve critical roles in brain function and brain health. Microglia are involved in the immune response to infections and help clean up debris from dead cells. Astrocytes form a key part of the blood–brain barrier that regulates the flow of molecules in and out of the brain. Through a process called myelination, oligodendrocytes (a type of astrocyte) wrap their appendages around the axons of neurons, thereby insulating axonal membranes and facilitating the transmission of action potentials. Without myelin, action potentials would not travel as far or fast, severely limiting both the speed and complexity of communication in the brain.

Most research examining the neurobiology of addiction has focused on the roles of neurons. These roles will be explored throughout this chapter. The role of glial cells in addiction is poorly understood but under intense investigation (Linker, Cross, & Leslie, 2019). Neurons and glial cells in the brain comprise several hundred regions linked to each other in neurocircuits (Glasser et al., 2016). In contrast to the myth that most people only use 10% of their brains, every brain area contributes to behavior and survival in some way (Boyd, 2008). In this chapter, we will focus on a subset of brain neurocircuits involved in reinforcement, incentive salience, the development of habits, negative affect and executive function, all of which contribute to the development of the three-stage cycle of addiction (see Figure 4.2).

Overview of the addiction cycle and its neurobiological substrates

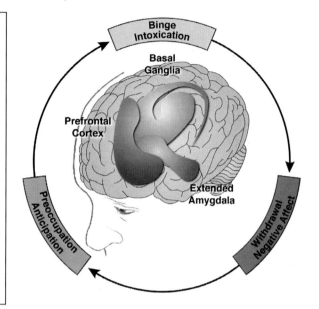

Binge/intoxication
The person engages in substance use to experience its rewarding or pleasurable effects and reduce emotional discomfort.

Withdrawal/negative affect
The person experiences emotional discomfort (e.g., anxiety, dysphoria, irritability) when the alcohol wears off.

Preoccupation/anticipation
The person experiences strong urges (cravings) to drink, especially when exposed to stimuli associated with the substance (e.g., sight of drug paraphernalia) or stressful experiences.

Figure 4.2 Alterations in brain function as a result of repeated substance use manifest in the cycle of addiction

Source: SAMHSA (2016), Zorrilla and Koob (2019); adapted with permission from Koob and Volkow (2010).

Reinforcement and addiction

> What do [humans] demand of life and wish to achieve in it? The answer to this can hardly be in doubt. They strive after happiness; they want to become happy and to remain so. This endeavor has two sides, a positive and a negative aim. It aims, on the one hand, at an absence of pain and unpleasure, and, on the other, at the experiencing of strong feelings of pleasure.
>
> *(Freud, 1930, p. 21)*

Many animal species are born hardwired with behavioral responses allowing them to locate food and mates without experience. In contrast, humans are imbued with the motivation to drink, eat, and find mates, but the specifics of how those objectives are accomplished are highly influenced by experience and the learning that results. Frogs dart their tongues at black specs, presuming the specs are flies. If all black specs disappear, frogs are in trouble. Humans, on the other hand, learn from experience which types of foods to eat and how to procure them. One strength of basing most behaviors on hardwired scripts is that offspring can hit the ground running shortly after birth and begin the business of making a living and surviving. Humans, in contrast, have protracted periods of vulnerability during which adults are needed to protect and teach them. The obvious benefit is malleability: humans can adapt to conditions that require behavioral flexibility, without which the species would not survive. If black specs disappeared, humans would just find something else to eat.

To help determine which behaviors are worth repeating, the brain uses a combination of circuits to monitor behavioral outcomes and provide feedback. In nature, eating a novel food for the first time can be a risky endeavor. If it turns out the food is safe, feedback in the form of a small increase in pleasure and/or a decrease in the discomfort of hunger reinforces the choice and increases the likelihood of eating that food again (see Chapter 6). Initial responses to substances of abuse and the transition to addiction can be explained in part by the principles of reinforcement. Receiving desirable feedback in response to substance use is a powerful motivator for repeating the behavior and, after addiction develops, is a key driver of the addiction cycle. Two primary forms of reinforcement, positive and negative, are involved in the development and maintenance of addiction.

Positive reinforcement

Positive reinforcement refers to an increase in the likelihood of repeating behaviors based on the outcome, such as when a behavior leads to a reward. Substances with abuse potential produce reward in the form of pleasure, which reinforces the choice to use them. Indeed, the ancient Sumerians referred to the opium poppy as *Hul Gil*, or the "joy plant." Until the mid-20th century, it remained entirely unknown how substances such as opium produce pleasure. That changed with a serendipitous discovery in the 1950s, when Dr. James Olds and a graduate student named Peter Milner, both psychologists, performed a set of experiments in which small wires were implanted in various lower brain areas in rats. After implanting one such electrode, a rat was placed in an open area and allowed to explore. Periodically, the researchers passed a small amount of electric current through the electrode and into the brain. They noticed that the rat returned to the location where the electric current was last applied. The team then demonstrated that rats would quickly learn to press levers by themselves in order to receive the stimulation. In their 1954 manuscript, Olds and Milner stated that "the control exercised over the animal's behavior by means of this reward is extreme, possibly exceeding that exercised by any other reward previously used in animal experimentation" (p. 426). They suggested that the experience of reward in response to a wide range of behaviors might originate from a common brain origin.

Subsequent studies revealed that the most pronounced reinforcement came from stimulation near the ventral tegmental area (VTA) located in the midbrain (see Figure 4.2). The VTA sends signals, via the neurotransmitter dopamine, to another deep-seated structure called the nucleus accumbens, located in the basal ganglia. Together, the VTA and its projections to the nucleus accumbens and the frontal cortex comprise the key components of the mesocorticolimbic dopamine system. This system is strongly activated both on the initial delivery of reward and in anticipation of reward (Schultz, 1998). Activation of this circuitry leads to positive reinforcement, meaning animals tend to repeat behaviors that result in activity here. It appears that the rate and magnitude of the dopamine release is positively associated with the intensity of the subjective reward that follows an event (Volkow et al., 2010). Steep increases in dopamine activity at dopamine D1 receptors play key roles in learning to associate the reward with drug-related cues, such as the sight or smell of a drug.

Initially, when a reward is received, dopamine release from the VTA into the nucleus accumbens increases, presumably contributing to the pleasure associated with the reward and increasing the individual's attention to what is happening. If a cue precedes the reward, the dopaminergic neurons in the VTA eventually begin to fire in response to the cue and not the reward itself. If the cue is presented but the reward does not follow, dopaminergic neurons temporarily become less active, signaling a discrepancy between the expected and actual outcome.

The increase in dopamine levels in the nucleus accumbens in response to drugs of abuse can surpass the activation produced by natural reinforcers such as eating, drinking, or copulating (Di Chiara & Imperato, 1988; Volkow et al., 2010). Supraphysiological activation of the reward system leads the brain to attach an abnormally high level of incentive salience, or value, to stimuli associated with substances. In one study, the more alcohol college students reported drinking during a typical week, the greater the increase in activity in the VTA, as well as in the orbitofrontal region of the prefrontal cortex (see Figure 4.3), in response to alcohol-related images (Courtney, Rapuano, Sargent, Heatherton, & Kelley, 2018). The orbitofrontal cortex is involved in learning about stimuli associated with reinforcement and registering the magnitude of importance, or salience, of those stimuli.

Attribution of incentive salience to drug-related cues contributes prominently to driving the binge/intoxication stage of the addiction cycle. Increased dopamine release in response to these drug-related cues, whether real or imagined, can trigger craving, or a strong desire for the drug. Craving is central to preoccupation/anticipation stage of the addiction cycle that precedes an episode of binging and becoming intoxicated.

While dopamine levels increase in the nucleus accumbens in rewarded behaviors, dopamine is not alone in triggering feelings of pleasure (Koob, 2014; Koob & Volkow, 2016). In humans, positron emission tomography (PET) studies demonstrated that intoxicating doses of alcohol and other drugs release endorphins (endogenous opioid peptides) into the nucleus accumbens (Mitchell et al., 2012). Similar findings have been observed in laboratory studies using animal models (Olive, Koenig, Nannini, & Hodge, 2001). Further, blocking opioid receptors in the nucleus accumbens decreases the self-administration of alcohol and other drugs, such as opioids and cannabinoids, suggesting that the amount of reward these substances provide diminishes when opioid receptors are blocked (Nestler, 2005).

The strong effects of drugs on the reward system are met with neuroadaptations aimed at reducing their impact. Over time, the reward activity triggered by substances diminishes due to tolerance, often leading to an increase in use as a means of regaining the original

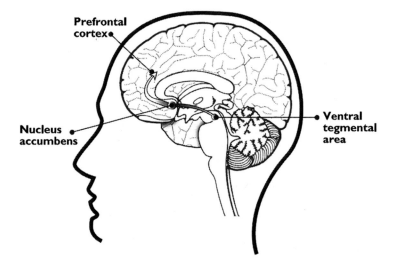

Figure 4.3 Brain areas involved in learning about the rewarding effects of substances, assigning incentive salience (value) to substance-related cues, and regulating the motivation to repeat rewarded behaviors

Source: NIDA (2011).

reinforcement level. The brain is not able to reduce reward-related activity only to the drugs being used: chronic substance use also leads to a blunted response to natural rewards, such as food and sex (Volkow et al., 2010). One mechanism for such blunted responses is engagement of an antireward system in the brain, which helps return activated reward circuits to baseline and becomes more active as addiction develops. In a subsequent section, we explore how neuroadaptations in the mesocorticolimbic reward pathway and other areas contributes to the development of the addiction cycle.

Negative reinforcement

I have absolutely no pleasure in the stimulants in which I sometimes so madly indulge. It has not been in the pursuit of pleasure that I have periled life and reputation and reason. It has been the desperate attempt to escape from torturing memories, from a sense of insupportable loneliness and a dread of some strange impending doom.

(Edgar Allen Poe quoted by Whitman, 1860, p. 76, retrieved from https://www.eapoe.org/works/letters/p4811030.htm)

When considering the role of reinforcement in shaping substance use behaviors, positive reinforcement (e.g. repeating drug use due to the resulting euphoria) is often the main focus. But positive reinforcement is not the only form of reinforcement the brain uses to shape behavior (see Chapter 6). Negative reinforcement, an increase in the likelihood of repeating a behavior if it leads to the reduction of a negative state, plays a prominent role, as well. It is important to note that negative reinforcement differs from punishment, which involves a decrease in the likelihood of engaging in a behavior due to an uncomfortable outcome. As an example of the difference, the application of physical pain in response to a behavior reduces the chances of engaging in a behavior again (punishment), whereas the removal of physical pain increases the chances of repeating the behavior (negative reinforcement).

A common source of negative reinforcement from substance use stems from temporary reductions in stress-related brain activity. Threatening stimuli, such as from predators or traumatic memories, activate the central nucleus of the amygdala. The amygdala then prepares the body for action in several ways. It signals the hypothalamus to increase sympathetic nervous system activity, resulting in release of epinephrine (adrenaline) from the adrenal medulla, or middle of the adrenal glands, located just above the kidneys. Epinephrine triggers an increase in heart rate and blood pleasure, shifts blood flow to the muscles, and leads to an increase in attention to threatening stimuli: the well-known "fight or flight" response. The amygdala also signals the hypothalamus to release corticotropin-releasing factor (CRF) into the pituitary gland, causing the pituitary to release adrenocorticotropin-releasing hormone (ACTH) into peripheral circulation. ACTH stimulates the release of cortisol from the adrenal cortex, or outer part of the adrenal gland. Cortisol increases blood sugar levels by triggering gluconeogenesis in the liver. It also reduces inflammation and increases attention to, and memory for, emotionally arousing (e.g. threat-related) information (Putman & Roelofs, 2011). Normally, when receptors in the hypothalamus detect sufficiently high levels of circulating cortisol, release of CRF and ACTH decreases, and the system returns to balance.

Many abused substances suppress activity in the amygdala and temporarily dampen the stress response and the psychological discomfort that goes with it, providing powerful negative reinforcement and increasing motivation to use the drug again. Unfortunately, neuroadaptations following repeated substance use result in increased stress-related brain activity during withdrawal and a heightened reactivity to stress-related stimuli. With prolonged activation, the response of the amygdala to stress-related neurotransmitters, such as CRF, can become hypersensitized, leading to a greater than normal reaction and more emotional discomfort, even when CRF levels are not elevated. Adaptations in stress circuits are central to driving the withdrawal/negative affect stage of the addiction cycle and increase the likelihood of stress-related relapse during recovery (Koob, 2014).

Several substances with abuse potential also provide negative reinforcement by reducing physical pain. In addition to producing euphoria by activating opioid receptors in the nucleus accumbens and reducing anxiety by dampening activity in the amygdala, opioids reduce physical pain in part by acting in brainstem regions such as the periaqueductal gray (PAG). Injecting opioids directly into the PAG produces pain relief (Loyd & Murphy, 2009). Opioids, alone or in combination with sedatives like alcohol or benzodiazepines, also can suppress vital reflex centers in the brainstem that control respiration, leading to death (van der Schrier et al., 2017). Because of overlap in how alcohol and opioids reduce physical pain, chronic use of either results in tolerance to and a reduction in the negative reinforcing effects of both drugs (He & Whistler, 2011; Shurman, Koob, & Gutstein, 2010). As an example of cross-tolerance between alcohol and opioids, a history of frequent drinking is associated with a need for higher doses of opioids to control post-operative pain following abdominal surgery (Kao et al., 2017).

Habit formation and the shift from impulsive toward compulsive substance use

> The more of the details of our daily life we can hand over to the effortless custody of automatism, the more our higher powers of mind will be set free for their own proper work.
> *(James, 1890, retrieved from https://fs.blog/2013/05/william-james-on-habit/)*

In addition to playing important roles in positive reinforcement in response to substance use, dopamine activity during substance use plays a central role in developing the habits involved in obtaining and consuming drugs. Initially, drug use is goal-directed and voluntary. As with other new behaviors, the prefrontal cortex helps individuals weigh the pros and cons of a decision to engage in the behavior and proceed accordingly. But the brain has a more energy efficient strategy for choosing behavior patterns that frees up cognitive functions for other purposes: habit formation.

Initial, goal-directed substance use involves, among other circuits, neuronal projections from the orbitofrontal cortex to the dorsomedial striatum (DMS). While engaging in goal-direct behaviors, neurons in the DMS become active. As the behavior is repeated, activity in the DMS quiets and neurons in the dorsolateral striatum (DLS) become active at the beginning and end of the familiar action sequence. This pattern in the DLS, known as task-bracketing, becomes strengthened with successive repetitions as the habit becomes more deeply engrained (Lipton, Gonzales, & Citri, 2019). The brain appears to "chunk" the behaviors involved in a habit such that activation of the first behavior in the sequence initiates the others (Smith & Graybiel, 2016). In laboratory studies, if the DLS is damaged, rodents can still engage in goal-directed actions, but the behaviors will not become habitual. In contrast, damaging the DMS leads to faster formation of habits and interferes with goal-directed control over the activity.

The ability to engage in goal-directed activities and habit formation develop in parallel, such that habit circuits do not replace the circuits used to accomplish tasks in a goal-directed manner. As such, habitual behaviors usually can be brought under voluntary control when needed. For example, when encountering a detour during a daily commute, circuits involved in deliberation and goal-directed behavior can override the DLS circuits that govern the sequence of actions that normally get us home. Reasserting cognitive control over behavior becomes much more difficult as habits become increasingly well-established and overlearned, as is the case with habits involved in addictions.

In their review of the neuroscience of habit formation, Smith and Graybiel (2016) discussed how, as habits develop, the tendency to repeat the behaviors becomes increasingly contingent on positive outcomes and less sensitive to undesirable outcomes. They examined a population of neurons in the DLS that monitors the outcomes of a behavioral choice. They suggested that, as habits form, registration of a negative outcome (no reward) is devaluated and registration of a rewarded behavior (e.g. food) becomes overvalued, allowing habits to persist despite sometimes negative outcomes.

> Though the population sizes of both of these subsets [of DLS neurons] are similar during training, we find a striking shift during overtraining and habit formation: the number of neurons responding to errors after incorrect runs falls to near zero, whereas the number of neurons responding to rewards after correct runs increases proportionally. Thus, outcome signaling of errors is almost gone, but outcome signaling after correct responses remains strong.
>
> *(Smith & Graybiel, 2016, p. 38)*

Such a shift could help explain the persistence of behaviors involved in a range of addictions, including gambling and substance use disorders, in the face of inconsistent reinforcement and undesirable outcomes. Even intermittent positive outcomes can reinforce the habit and keep it going.

The powerful positive reinforcement from drugs of abuse and the strength of the learning that results contribute to habit development and, eventually, to compulsive drug use, defined by a maladaptive persistence of drug use despite adverse consequences (Dalley, Everitt, & Robbins, 2011). According to Zorrilla and Koob (2019):

> Behavior that is impulsive... is defined as an action that is instigated suddenly without forethought of potential consequences... Externally, impulsivity may appear as acting hastily, capriciously, or on whims and prioritizing immediate gains vs. later outcomes. Behavior that is compulsive... is defined as an action that results from or is related to an irresistible urge, whereby irresistibility can be operationalized as behavior that persists despite aversive or incorrect outcomes. A compulsive behavior is often experienced as outside of one's control and, even during its performance, can be intrusive, unwanted, and ego-dystonic.
>
> *(p. 2)*

As Lipton et al. (2019) state:

> The central characteristic of compulsions and addictions is the continued pursuit of a previously rewarding stimulus, despite its clear current association with adverse consequences... This hallmark of addiction, action performance in spite of punishment, can be viewed as an extreme of habitual behavior.
>
> *(p. 2)*

In sum, the brain develops habit circuits for engaging in often repeated and reinforced behaviors. Once initiated, the behavioral patterns tend to complete regardless of the outcome. It appears that the brain places more emphasis on positive rather than negative outcomes for sustaining established habits. While habits certainly increase the efficiency of actions and can contribute to health, when the actions are maladaptive, habit formation can help trap people in unhealthy cycles.

Overview of key brain areas involved in addiction

Basal Ganglia—Group of structures that play important roles in coordinating body movements, learning routine behaviors and forming habits. Two sub-regions are particularly important in substance use disorders: The **nucleus accumbens** is involved in motivation and the experience of reward and the **dorsal striatum** is involved in forming habits.

Extended Amygdala—Regulates reactions to stress including the "fight or flight" response and negative emotions like anxiety and irritability. While initially calmed by many substances, activity here can increase during periods of abstinence, motivating further use.

Prefrontal Cortex—Located at the front of the brain and is responsible for "executive functions" such as the ability to organize thoughts and activities, prioritize tasks, manage time, make decisions, and regulate emotions and impulses.

Source: SAMHSA (2016). Facing Addiction in America: The Surgeon General's Report on Alcohol, Drugs, and Health.

Opponent processes, allostasis, and the dark side of addiction

But Socrates sat up on his couch and bent his leg and rubbed it with his hand, and while he was rubbing it, he said, "What a strange thing, my friends, that seems to be which men call pleasure! How wonderfully it is related to that which seems to be its opposite, pain, in that they will not both come to a man at the same time, and yet if he pursues the one and captures it he is generally obliged to take the other also, as if the two were joined together in one head... Just so it seems that in my case, after pain was in my leg on account of the fetter [shackle], pleasure appears to have come following after."

(Plato, 1966; retrieved from https://www.loebclassics.com/view/plato_philosopher-phaedo/1914/pb_LCL036.209.xml?readMode=recto&result=2&rskey=3w67cc)

As mentioned previously, each cell in the human body is capable of altering its activity in an effort to maintain stable functioning in the face of changing circumstances. This process, known as homeostasis, can be viewed as a resistance to deviating from the baseline state of an organism. For example, thermoregulation allows mammals to maintain an ideal internal temperature despite fluctuations in the temperature outside. To aid in maintaining homeostasis, the brain utilizes feedback loops that counter fluctuations in one direction with fluctuations in the opposite direction. When the hypothalamus senses a drop in body temperature, it initiates changes in heart rate, blood flow, muscle movement, and metabolism to bring the body temperature back to the preferred level. An increase in body temperature above the normal level is met with sweating and an increase in blood flow to the skin to aid in cooling.

Similar efforts are made to maintain hedonic homeostasis, or an appropriate level of pleasure. Changes in neuronal activity in reward areas in response to repeated substance use were hypothesized in Solomon's opponent process theory (Koob, Markou, Weiss, & Schulteis, 1993). Solomon and Corbit (1974) postulated that hedonic states, once initiated, are automatically modulated by the central nervous system with mechanisms that reduce the intensity of the hedonic feelings. This theory suggests that drugs initiate two opposing motivational processes. The *a-process*, the initial acute effect of a drug, was hypothesized to be opposed or counteracted by a slower *b-process* that returns brain systems to homeostasis. With repeated exposure to drugs, the a-process becomes smaller and the b-process becomes larger, appears sooner, lasts longer, and masks the a-process. If a drug initially produces pleasure (a-process), repeated use leads to a reduction in pleasure following the drug and an increase in dysphoria when the drug wears off (b-process), motivating further drug use. The underlying changes both within and between brain regions lead to dependence, a reliance on the drug for normal functioning, and withdrawal symptoms upon removal of the drug.

According to Koob (2009):

> The a-process in drug use consists of positive hedonic responses, occurs shortly after presentation of a stimulus, correlates closely with the intensity, quality, and duration of the reinforcer, and shows tolerance. In contrast, the b-process in drug use appears after the a-process has terminated, consists of negative hedonic responses, and is sluggish in onset, slow to build up to an asymptote, slow to decay, and gets larger with repeated exposure.
>
> *(p. 3)*

When systems in the body are pushed beyond the range of homeostasis for extended periods of time, they might be forced to settle into new states of balance outside of the original equilibrium. This new balance is called *allostasis* (Sterling & Eyer, 1988) and can be defined as "the integrative adaptive processes maintaining stability through change, a stability that is not within the normal homeostatic range" (Koob & Le Moal, 2001, p. 101). Allostasis results from, and subsequently contributes to, addiction. The powerful initial effects of substances on reward and stress circuitry are simply not sustainable. Remaining in a state of heightened pleasure and low vigilance and anxiety would threaten the ability of an animal to effectively recognize and respond to threats, locate mates, protect offspring, find food sources, and engage in other critical behaviors. As a result, the brain adjusts in order to minimize the impact of the drug and settles into a new balance that involves less than normal reward function and higher than normal stress-related brain function.

Chronic deviations from normal can produce a burden, or allostatic load, on the body leading to further dysfunction. McEwen and Stellar (1993) defined allostatic load as "the cost of chronic exposure to fluctuating or heightened neural or neuroendocrine response resulting from repeated or chronic environmental challenge that an individual reacts to as being particularly stressful" (p. 2093). For instance, reductions in reward activity and heightened stress reactivity can strain the body and contribute to illness (Koob & Le Moal, 2001). Due to the neuroadaptations underlying allostatic changes following repeated substance use, a drug that once caused deviations from the homeostatic state (the old normal) is now necessary to maintain activity in the allostatic state (the new normal) even if doing so is detrimental to the well-being of the individual (Koob & Le Moal, 1997). In essence, many of the symptoms of addiction can be viewed as a consequence of allostasis.

As an example of shifts in brain function and motivational processes during the development of addiction, let us examine changes in dopamine activity in the mesocorticolimbic reward pathway (a-process) and changes in CRF activity in the hypothalamus and amygdala (b-process). The initial reinforcing effects of alcohol and other drugs involve activation of the mesocorticolimbic dopamine neurons. Chronic alcohol consumption is associated with the decreased activity of dopaminergic neurons in the ventral tegmental area and decreased dopamine release in the nucleus accumbens (Weiss et al., 1996). This represents a weakening of the a-process. Initial reinforcement from alcohol and other drugs also involves dampening of activity in the amygdala, reductions in CRF release in the amygdala and hypothalamus, and calming of the stress response in general. However, repeated use leads to an increase in the magnitude and duration of activity in stress-related circuits and increased sensitivity to stress-related neurotransmitters like CRF. These adaptations, which represent a strengthening of the b-process, help keep reward-related activity in check.

Increased CRF release in the amygdala has been observed in withdrawal from a variety of drugs, including alcohol, opioids, THC (tetrahydrocannabinol), cocaine, and nicotine (George et al., 2007; Merlo Pich et al., 1995). It appears that, as addiction develops, increased CRF activity during abstinence plays a central role in motivating substance use aimed at negative reinforcement. In animal models, symptoms of anxiety following withdrawal from alcohol, cocaine, nicotine, cannabinoids, opiates, and benzodiazepines can be reversed by administering compounds that block CRF activity directly into the brain (Baldwin, Rassnick, Rivier, Koob, & Britton, 1991; Zorrilla, Logrip, & Koob, 2014). The role of CRF in driving alcohol consumption in individuals experiencing alcohol dependence was recently demonstrated by de Guglielmo and colleagues (2019), who showed that temporarily inactivating CRF-containing neurons in the central nucleus of the amygdala of rodents reduced the amount of alcohol rats consumed during alcohol withdrawal.

Another key contributor to the reduction in reward activity and increase in discomfort that develops with repeated drug use is the dynorphin-kappa system, which has the dual action of suppressing the incentive salience system and activating the stress system. As previously noted, activation of dopaminergic neurons in the VTA results in elevated dopamine levels in the nucleus accumbens and incentive salience for the stimuli paired with that activation. Following the increases in dopamine, there is an elevation in the level of a neurotransmitter called dynorphin. Dynorphin acts on a type of opioid receptor called the kappa opioid receptor (KOR). While activation of *mu* opioid receptors, either by endorphins or prescription or illicit opioids, results in euphoria, activation of KOR by dynorphin is generally aversive. Dopamine released by VTA neurons into the nucleus accumbens activates smaller neurons in the area that generate dynorphin. These smaller neurons release dynorphin back onto the cells that released the dopamine, thereby inhibiting further dopamine release (Threlfell & Cragg, 2011). Dynorphin also appears to be integral in the stress response, and release of dynorphin occurs during exposure to a wide range of stressful stimuli (Chavkin, 2013). Repeated activation of the reward system leads to an increase in activity at KORs in an effort to return reward function to homeostatic levels (Karkhanis, Holleran, & Jones, 2017). Heightened levels of stress-related activity, including elevated levels of dynorphin, during periods of abstinence contribute to the emergence of a negative state known as the "dark side" of addiction, in which emotional misery (hyperkatifeia) during the withdrawal/negative affect stage of the addiction cycle motivates further drug use in an effort to find relief (Koob & Le Moal, 2001). In essence, while early drug use is maintained by positive reinforcement, continued drug use during addiction is maintained by negative reinforcement.

To use again or not to use again—that is the question during the preoccupation/anticipation stage of addiction

Between substance use episodes, an individual must decide whether to engage in substance use again. Such decision-making is made difficult by the emotional misery that emerges during periods of abstinence. As discussed previously, initial substance use might be motivated by a desire to feel pleasure and reduce emotional discomfort, but the transition from limited use to addiction involves an increase in stress-related brain activity and a shift in motivation to engage in substance use to relieve suffering. The neuroadaptations that occur, including elevated levels of stress-related transmitters, such as CRF, and increased activity in the dynorphin-κ opioid system, all contribute to feelings of restlessness, agitation, and anxiety (Koob et al., 2014). In addition, reductions in reward circuit activity contribute to feelings of dysphoria and hypohedonia (reduced ability to experience pleasure). Previously rewarding activities, such as eating a delicious meal or spending time with loved ones, can fail to register as rewarding. Collectively, these changes can make it very difficult for the brain's frontal lobes to regulate the motivation to engage in substance use and increase the likelihood that a person will become intoxicated again, repeating the addiction cycle.

Early in the development of drug-related habits, the prefrontal cortex is able to weigh the pros and cons of the choice, wielding its influence over decision-making. Going to happy hour might sound alluring but the prefrontal cortex might ultimately decide against it due to an early workday, family responsibilities, or insufficient funds. Choosing not to engage in substance use becomes much harder as addiction develops due to a combination of strong incentive salience attributed to drug-related cues (real or remembered), deficits in pleasure, and increases in emotional misery. In the case of some drugs (e.g. alcohol), direct damage to the prefrontal circuits that mediate executive functions makes it even harder to remain abstinent. Relapse, or reinstatement of drug use, is a central feature of addiction and can be placed in this stage of the addiction cycle.

When struggling with substance use, cravings can make it challenging to maintain abstinence. Craving, which was added as a criterion for substance use disorders in the DSM-5, can lead to relapse under some circumstances (Hasin et al., 2013). The strong incentive salience given to drug-related cues means that either seeing or recalling drug-related images can activate the urge to approach and consume them. Relative to control groups, individuals experiencing drug use disorders showed increased activity in the medial prefrontal cortex, nucleus accumbens, and VTA in response to drug-related cues (MacNiven et al., 2018). Greater activation of the nucleus accumbens is associated with a shorter time to relapse. It appears that, in response to drug-related cues, the prefrontal cortex sends excitatory signals, via the neurotransmitter glutamate, to the VTA. Glutamate stimulates VTA neurons to release dopamine into the nucleus accumbens and the prefrontal cortex, which increases motivation to use the substance. Via glutamate, the prefrontal cortical areas also activate habit circuits in the dorsal striatum. In this way, drug-related cues tap into circuits mediating the goal-directed consumption of drugs and trigger the habits involved in using them.

Craving levels and the likelihood that craving will lead to substance use fluctuate based on several factors. Individuals experiencing substance use disorders often can modulate the intensity of their cravings and decrease the likelihood of acting on them at that moment. Engaging the prefrontal cortical areas that mediate executive functions in activities inconsistent with the urge to use substances can help a person wait out the craving. In one study (Dulin & Gonzalez, 2017), the use of a smart phone application that helped individuals experiencing alcohol use disorder distract themselves or wait out ("surf") the craving significantly reduced the likelihood that a craving would lead to use. In a clever study using fMRI (Karch et al., 2015), researchers reported that, among participants experiencing alcohol use disorder, alcohol-related cues caused increases in activity in several brain areas, including the anterior cingulate gyrus, dorsolateral prefrontal cortex, and insula. While being scanned, study participants were shown a graphical depiction of the current level of brain activity in response to alcohol-related or neutral cues. Through neurofeedback, they were trained to reduce activity levels in these areas which produced small reductions in craving during cue exposure.

Craving magnitude and its influence on behavior also depends on an individual's current emotional state. As Berridge and O'Doherty (2014) noted, "Incentive salience integrates two separate input factors to generate decision utility in the moment of re-encounter with cues for a reward that could potentially be chosen: (i) current physiological/neurobiological state; (ii) previously learned associations about the reward cue" (p. 342). In this way, the magnitude of the drive to use substances in response to drug-related cues can vary depending on what else is going on in an individual's life. For example, individuals experiencing heroin dependence spent more time looking at heroin-related images, rather than non-drug cues, after being exposed to depressing statements and music (Hogarth et al., 2019). The tendency to attend to heroin-related cues in response to stressors was more common in subjects who reported using heroin to cope with negative affect. When individuals engaged in heavy social drinking were exposed to a stressful laboratory condition (e.g. a mock job interview with a five-minute speech and a math problem), self-reported levels of stress, craving in response to alcohol-related cues, and the amount of money they were willing to pay for alcohol all increased (Amlung & MacKillop, 2014). In another study, individuals self-identifying as tending to drink alcohol to cope with negative affect showed an increase in attention to alcohol-related cues when exposed to mild stress in a laboratory (Field & Quigley, 2009). Miller, Hersen, Eisler, and Hilsman (1974) reported that a stressful laboratory condition caused "alcoholics," but not "non-alcoholics," to respond faster in an operant task in order to receive more alcohol. Higley et al. (2011) reported that a higher level of stress-induced craving in a laboratory task early in recovery was associated with shorter times to relapse among individuals in treatment for alcohol dependence.

An increased tendency to engage in drug-related behaviors in response to the strong incentive value of drug-related cues, and a decrease in the ability to inhibit such responses, particularly when faced with stressors in daily life, helps keep an individual stuck in the cycle of addiction. Given the powerful impact of stress on the motivation to repeat substance use, learning to cope with stress is a key component of recovery from substance use disorders.

Implications for treatment and recovery

Because the positive and negative reinforcement provided by substances maintains the habits underlying the binge/intoxication stage of the addiction cycle, the use of medications (see Chapter 19), like the opioid receptor antagonist naltrexone, that reduce the pleasure produced by drugs of abuse can help weaken reinforcement for engaging in the behavior and slowly reduce the incentive salience of drug-related cues. A meta-analysis of human laboratory studies involving naltrexone administration to individuals engaged in heavy drinking concluded that naltrexone reduced alcohol self-administration and craving compared to placebo (Hendershot, Wardell, Samokhvalov, & Rehm, 2017). Such effects could help, over time, loosen the grip of addiction.

The hyperkatifeia and physical misery that follow cessation of drug use in the withdrawal/negative affects stage make it challenging for individuals struggling with addiction to withstand the urge to use again (Koob & Volkow, 2010). Medications and behavioral therapies that reduce the hyperalgesia and hyperkatifeia associated with withdrawal might be helpful here. For instance, withdrawal from alcohol leads to an increase in the release of the excitatory neurotransmitter, glutamate, and subsequent increased activity at a type of glutamate receptor known as the NMDA receptor. These changes are thought to contribute to symptoms of alcohol withdrawal, including seizures, cravings, mood, and sleep disturbances (Mason & Heyser, 2010). Acamprosate, a medication approved for the treatment of alcohol use disorder, appears to inhibit activity at NMDA receptors and reduces some of the physical and emotional suffering of protracted withdrawal (Maisel, Blodgett, Wilbourne, Humphreys, & Finney, 2013). As such, acamprosate and other medications that act on the withdrawal/negative affect stage of addiction may reduce the drive to use substance for negative reinforcement.

Medications that work directly and safely on hyperactivity in the amygdala and the elevated CRF that follows are lacking but could play critical roles in reducing the drive to use substances and helping addicted individual escape the cycle (Mason, 2017). In animal models, administering a CRF antagonist (compound that blocks the effects of CRF) directly into the central nucleus of the amygdala of alcohol-dependent rats reduces alcohol self-administration (Funk, O'Dell, Crawford, & Koob, 2006). And temporarily inactivating CRF-containing neurons in the central nucleus of the amygdala of alcohol-dependent rats reduced the amount of alcohol consumed during withdrawal (de Guglielmo et al., 2019). Medications that reduce elevated CRF activity during withdrawal could prove very beneficial in addressing the withdrawal/negative affect stage of the addiction cycle.

Over time, with repeated substance use, the frontal lobes become preoccupied with substance use, and become less effective at regulating urges to use, particularly if the individual is under stress (Sinha, Garcia, Paliwal, Kreek, & Rounsaville, 2006). As such, therapeutic approaches that teach mindfulness, meditation, heart rate variability training, urge surfing, and other techniques that help an individual learn to tolerate and calm the stress response are helpful in treating addiction (Garland & Howard, 2018; see Chapter 21). Such strategies could reduce the likelihood of returning to substance use and repeating the cycle of addiction. Learning new habits involving healthy stimulus–response relationships, such as driving to the gym after work instead of the bar or pub, and deriving positive reinforcement from something other than alcohol, can help individuals wrestling with addiction learn healthy, appropriate strategies for obtaining positive reinforcement and coping with stress (Lynch, Peterson, Sanchez, Abel, & Smith, 2013)

Summary

Addiction involves maladaptive learning in which strong positive and negative reinforcement shapes drug seeking and consumption, and cues associated with the drug to take on incentive salience, leading to powerful motivation to approach and consume substances when the cues are present. As the behaviors involved in substance use are repeated, initiation of drug seeking and consumption shifts from conscious, goal-directed, and voluntary to habits initiated by stimulus–response relationships with drug-related cues.

The perturbations in brain activity involved in reinforcement, such as changes in the reward neurotransmitter systems (positive reinforcement) in the nucleus accumbens and the brain stress systems (negative reinforcement) in the central nucleus of the amygdala, caused by drugs are much larger than the changes produced by natural reinforcers such as food and social bonding. As a result, reinforcement circuits in the brain adapt to minimize the impact.

Opponent processes lead to a blunted response of the reward system to both the drug that was used and normal, healthy reinforcers like food. And the negative reinforcement provided by dampening of activity in the amygdala gives rise to an increase in stress-related brain activity during periods of abstinence, which contributes to sleep problems and stress-induced relapse. These antireward processes also involve elevated CRF and an increase in the dynorphin-kappa system as addiction develops. An increase in motivation to consume drugs to contend with physical and emotional (hyperkatifeia) discomfort during abstinence is referred to as the "dark side" of addiction.

In severe cases, the neuroadaptations underlying the development of addiction can lead an individual to repeat continually a three-stage cycle—binging/intoxication, withdrawal/negative affect, and preoccupation/anticipation. Breaking the cycle of addiction involves strategies that address the three stages. Just as maladaptive learning and neuroadaptations lead to addiction, the ability of the brain to reverse these neuroadaptations and to change with experience can be used to establish healthy behavior patterns that facilitate recovery. In essence, neuroadaptations in response to substance use can trap a person in the cycle of addiction, but neuroadaptations involving new, healthy behaviors can help get them out.

References

Alexander, B. K., & Schweighofer, A. R. F. (1998). Defining "addiction." In J. A. Schaler (Ed.), *Drugs: Should we legalize, decriminalize or deregulate?* (pp. 215–234). Amherst, NY: Prometheus Books.

American Psychiatric Association. (2017). What is addiction? Available: https://www.psychiatry.org/patients-families/addiction/what-is-addiction

American Psychiatric Association, DSM-5 Task Force. (2013). *Diagnostic and statistical manual of mental disorders: DSM-5™* (5th ed.). Arlington, VA: American Psychiatric Publishing, Inc.

Amlung, M., & MacKillop, J. (2014). Understanding the effects of stress and alcohol cues on motivation for alcohol via behavioral economics. *Alcoholism: Clinical & Experimental Research, 38*(6), 1780–1789. doi:10.1111/acer.12423

Baldwin, H. A., Rassnick, S., Rivier, J., Koob, G. F., & Britton, K. T. (1991). CRF antagonist reverses the "anxiogenic" response to ethanol withdrawal in the rat. *Psychopharmacology (Berl), 103*(2), 227–32. doi:10.1007/BF02244208

Berridge, K. C., & O'Doherty, J. P. (2014). From experienced utility to decision utility. In P. W. Glimcher & F. Ernst (Eds.), *Neuroeconomics* (2nd ed., pp. 335–351). San Diego, CA: Academic Press. doi:10.1016/B978-0-12-416008-8.00018-8

Botticelli, M. P., & Koh, H. K. (2016). Changing the language of addiction. *JAMA, 316*(13), 1361–1362. doi:10.1001/jama.2016.11874

Boyd, R. (2008). Do people only use 10 percent of their brains? *Scientific American* (February 7). Retrieved from https://www.scientificamerican.com/article/do-people-only-use-10-percent-of-their-brains/

Chavkin, C. (2013). Dynorphin—Still an extraordinarily potent opioid peptide. *Molecular Pharmacology, 83*(4), 729–736. doi:10.1124/mol.112.083337

Churchland, P., & Witkowski, J. (2014). A conversation with Patricia Churchland. *Cold Spring Harbor Symposia on Quantitative Biology, 79*, 263–265. doi:10.1101/sqb.2014.79.06.

Courtney, A. L., Rapuano, K. M., Sargent, J. D., Heatherton, T. F., & Kelley, W. M. (2018). Reward system activation in response to alcohol advertisements predicts college drinking. *Journal of Studies on Alcohol & Drugs, 79*(1), 29–38. doi:10.15288/jsad.2018.79.29

Dalley, J. W., Everitt, B. J., & Robbins, T. W. (2011). Impulsivity, compulsivity, and top-down cognitive control. *Neuron, 69*, 680–694. doi:10.1016/j.neuron.2011.01.020

de Guglielmo, G., Kallupi, M., Pomrenze, M. B., Crawford, E., Simpson, S., Schweitzer, P., . . . George, O. (2019). Inactivation of a CRF-dependent amygdalofugal pathway reverses addiction-like behaviors in alcohol-dependent rats. *Nature Communications, 10*(1238), 1–10. doi:10.1038/s41467-019-09183-0

Di Chiara, G., & Imperato, A. (1988). Drugs abused by humans preferentially increase synaptic dopamine concentrations in the mesocorticolimbic system of freely moving rats. *Proceedings of the National Academy of Sciences, 85*(14) 5274–5278. doi:10.1073/pnas.85.14.5274

Dulin, P. L., & Gonzalez, V. M. (2017). Smartphone-based, momentary intervention for alcohol cravings amongst individuals with an alcohol use disorder. *Psychology of Addictive Behavior, 31*(5), 601–607. doi:10.1037/adb0000292

Field, M., & Quigley, M. (2009). Mild stress increases attentional bias in social drinkers who drink to cope: A replication and extension. *Experimental and Clinical Psychopharmacology, 17*(5), 312–319. doi:10.1037/a0017090

Freud, S. (1930). *Civilization and its discontents.* Translation by James Strachey Retrieved from https://faculty.georgetown.edu/irvinem/theory/Freud-CivDis.html

Funk, C. K., O'Dell, L. E., Crawford, E. F., & Koob, G. F. (2006). Corticotropin-releasing factor within the central nucleus of the amygdala mediates enhanced ethanol self-administration in withdrawn, ethanol-dependent rats. *Journal of Neuroscience, 26,* 11324–11332. doi:10.1523/JNEUROSCI.3096-06.2006

Garland, E. L., & Howard, M. O. (2018). Mindfulness-based treatment of addiction: Current state of the field and envisioning the next wave of research. *Addiction Science & Clinical Practice, 13*(14). doi:10.1186/s13722-018-0115-3

George, O., Ghozland, S., Azar, M. R., Cottone, P., Zorrilla, E. P., Parsons, L. H., . . . Koob, G. F. (2007). CRF–CRF1 system activation mediates withdrawal-induced increases in nicotine self-administration in nicotine-dependent rats. *Proceedings of the National Academy of Science, 104*(43), 17198–17203. doi:10.1073/pnas.0707585104

Glasser, M. F., Coalson, T. S., Robinson, E. C., Hacker, C. D., Harwell, J., Yacoub, E., . . . Van Essen, D. C. (2016). A multi-modal parcellation of human cerebral cortex. *Nature, 536*(7615), 171–178. doi:10.1038/nature18933

Hammarlund, R., Crapanzano, K. A., Luce, L., Mulligan, L., & Ward, K. M. (2018). Review of the effects of self-stigma and perceived social stigma on the treatment-seeking decisions of individuals with drug- and alcohol-use disorders. *Substance Abuse and Rehabilitation, 9,* 115–136. Published 2018 November 23. doi:10.2147/SAR.S183256

Hasin, D. S., O'Brien, C. P., Auriacombe, M., Borges, G., Bucholz, K., Budney, A., . . . Grant, B. F. (2013). DSM-5 criteria for substance use disorders: Recommendations and rationale. *American Journal of Psychiatry, 170*(8), 834–851. doi:10.1176/appi.ajp.2013.12060782

He, L., & Whistler, J. L. (2011). Chronic ethanol consumption in rats produces opioid antinociceptive tolerance through inhibition of mu opioid receptor endocytosis. *PLoS One, 6*(5): e19372. doi:10.1371/journal.pone.0019372

Hendershot, C. S., Wardell, J. D., Samokhvalov, A. V., & Rehm, J. (2017). Effects of naltrexone on alcohol self-administration and craving: Meta-analysis of human laboratory studies. *Addiction Biology, 22*(6), 1515–1527. doi:10.1111/adb.12425

Herculano-Houzel, S. (2009). The human brain in numbers: A linearly scaled-up primate brain. *Frontiers in Human Neuroscience, 3,* 31. doi:10.3389/neuro.09.031.2009

Higley, A. E., Crane, N. A., Spadoni, A. D., Quello, S. B., Goodell, V., & Mason, B. J. (2011). Craving in response to stress induction in a human laboratory paradigm predicts treatment outcome in alcohol-dependent individuals. *Psychopharmacology, 218*(1), 121–129. doi:10.1007/s00213-011-2355-8

Hogarth, L., Hardy, L., Bakou, A., Mahlberg, J., Weidemann, G., Cashel, S., & Moustafa, A. A. (2019). Negative mood induction increases choice of heroin versus food pictures in opiate-dependent individuals: Correlation with self-medication coping motives and subjective reactivity. *Frontiers in Psychiatry, 10,* 274. doi:10.3389/fpsyt.2019.00274

Kao, S. C., Tsai, H. I., Cheng, C. W., Lin, T. W., Chen, C. C., & Lin, C. S. (2017). The association between frequent alcohol drinking and opioid consumption after abdominal surgery: A retrospective analysis. *PloS One, 12*(3), e0171275. doi:10.1371/journal.pone.0171275

Karch, S., Keeser, D., Hümmer, S., Paolini, M., Kirsch, V., & Karali, T. (2015). Modulation of craving related brain responses using real-time fMRI in patients with alcohol use disorder. *PLoS One, 10*(7), e0133034. doi:10.1371/journal.pone.0133034

Karkhanis, A., Holleran, K. M., & Jones, S. R. (2017). Dynorphin/kappa opioid receptor signaling in preclinical models of alcohol, drug, and food addiction. *International Review of Neurobiology, 136,* 53–88. doi:10.1016/bs.irn.2017.08.001

Koob, G. F. (2009). The role of CRF and CRF-related peptides in the dark side of addiction. *Brain Research, 1314,* 3–14. doi:10.1016/j.brainres.2009.11.008

Koob, G. F. (2014). Neurocircuitry of alcohol addiction: Synthesis from animal models. *Handbook of Clinical Neurology, 125,* 33–54. doi:10.1016/B978-0-444-62619-6.00003-3

Koob, G. F., Buck, C. L., Cohen, A., Edwards, S., Park, P. E., Schlosburg, J. E., . . . George, O. (2014). Addiction as a stress surfeit disorder. *Neuropharmacology, 76*(Part B), 370–382. doi:10.1016/j.neuropharm.2013.05.024

Koob, G. F. & Le Moal, M. (1997). Drug abuse: Hedonic homeostatic dysregulation. *Science, 278*(5335), 52–58. doi:10.1126/science.278.5335.52

Koob, G. F. & Le Moal, M. (2001). Drug addiction, dysregulation of reward, and allostasis. *Neuropsychopharmacology, 24*, 97–129. doi:10.1016/S0893-133X(00)00195-0

Koob, G. F., Markou, A., Weiss, F., & Schulteis, G. (1993). Opponent process and drug dependence: Neurobiological mechanisms. *Seminars in Neuroscience, 5*, 351–358. doi:10.1016/S1044-5765(05)80043-0

Koob, G. F., & Volkow, N. D. (2016). Neurobiology of addiction: A neurocircuitry analysis. *Lancet Psychiatry, 3*(8), 760–773. doi:10.1016/S2215–0366(16)00104-8

Koob G. F., & Volkow, N. D. (2010). Neurocircuitry of addiction. *Neuropsychopharmacology Review, 35*, 217–238.

Linker, K. E., Cross, S. J., & Leslie, F. M. (2019). Glial mechanisms underlying substance use disorders. *European Journal of Neuroscience, 50*(3), 2574–2589. doi:10.1111/ejn.14163

Lipton, D. M., Gonzales, B. J., & Citri, A. (2019). Dorsal striatal circuits for habits, compulsions and addictions. *Frontiers in Systems Neuroscience, 13*, 28. doi:10.3389/fnsys.2019.00028

Loyd, D. R., & Murphy, A. Z. (2009). The role of the periaqueductal gray in the modulation of pain in males and females: Are the anatomy and physiology really that different? *Neural Plasticity*, Article ID 462879. doi:10.1155/2009/462879

Lynch, W. J., Peterson, A. B., Sanchez, V., Abel, J., & Smith, M. A. (2013). Exercise as a novel treatment for drug addiction: A neurobiological and stage-dependent hypothesis. *Neuroscience & Biobehavioral Reviews, 37*(8), 1622–1644. doi:10.1016/j.neubiorev.2013.06.011

MacNiven, K. H., Jensen, E., Borg, N., Padula, C. B., Humphreys, K., & Knutson, B. (2018). Association of neural responses to drug cues with subsequent relapse to stimulant use. *JAMA Network Open, 1*(8), e186466. doi:10.1001/jamanetworkopen.2018.6466

Maisel, N. C., Blodgett, J. C., Wilbourne, P. L., Humphreys, K., & Finney, J. W. (2013). Meta-analysis of naltrexone and acamprosate for treating alcohol use disorders: When are these medications most helpful? *Addiction, 108*(2), 275–293. doi:10.1111/j.1360-0443.2012.04054.x

Mason, B. J. (2017). Emerging pharmacotherapies for alcohol use disorder. *Neuropharmacology, 122*, 244–253. doi:10.1016/j.neuropharm.2017.04.032

Mason, B. J., & Heyser, C. J. (2010). Acamprosate: A prototypic neuromodulator in the treatment of alcohol dependence. *CNS & Neurological Disorders Drug Targets, 9*(1), 23–32. doi:10.2174/187152710790966641

McEwen, B. S., & Stellar, E. (1993). Stress and the individual. Mechanisms leading to disease. *Archives of Internal Medicine, 153*(18), 2093–2101. doi:10.1001/archinte.1993.00410180039004

Merlo Pich, E., Lorang, M., Yeganeh, M., Rodriguez de Fonseca, F., Raber, J., Koob, G. F., & Weiss, F. (1995). Increase of extracellular corticotropin-releasing factor-like immunoreactivity levels in the amygdala of awake rats during restraint stress and ethanol withdrawal as measured by microdialysis. *Journal of Neuroscience, 15*(8), 5439–5447. doi:10.1523/JNEUROSCI.15-08-05439.1995

Miller, P. M., Hersen, M., Eisler, R. M., & Hilsman, G. (1974). Effects of social stress on operant drinking of alcoholics and social drinkers. *Behaviour Research and Therapy, 12*(2), 67–72. doi:10.1016/0005-7967(74)90094-1

Mitchell, J. M., O'Neil, J. P., Janabi, M., Marks, S. M., Jagust, W. J., & Fields, H. L. (2012). Alcohol consumption induces endogenous opioid release in the human orbitofrontal cortex and nucleus accumbens. *Science Translational Medicine, 4*, 116ra6. doi:10.1126/scitranslmed.3002902

National Institute of Drug Abuse (NIDA). (2011). Mind over matter: Teacher's guide. Retrieved from https://teens.drugabuse.gov/teachers/mind-matters/teachers-guide

National Institute of Drug Abuse (NIDA). (2017). Trends & statistics. Retrieved from https://www.drugabuse.gov/related-topics/trends-statistics.

Nestler, E. J. (2005). Is there a common molecular pathway for addiction? *Nature Neuroscience, 8*, 1445–1449. doi:10.1038/nn1578

Olds, J., & Milner, P. (1954). Positive reinforcement produced by electrical stimulation of septal area and other regions of the rat brain. *Journal of Comparative and Physiological Psychology, 47*(6), 419–427. doi:10.1037/h0058775

Olive, M. F., Koenig, H. N., Nannini, M. A., & Hodge, C. W. (2001). Stimulation of endorphin neurotransmission in the nucleus accumbens by ethanol, cocaine, and amphetamine. *Journal of Neuroscience, 21*(23):RC184. doi:10.1523/JNEUROSCI.21-23-j0002.2001

Plato (1966). *Plato in twelve volumes.* Vol. 1 translated by Harold North Fowler. Introduction by W. R. M. Lamb. Cambridge, MA: Harvard University Press; London, UK: William Heinemann Ltd.

Putman, P., & Roelofs, K. (2011). Effects of single cortisol administrations on human affect reviewed: Coping with stress through adaptive regulation of automatic cognitive processing. *Psychoneuroendocrinology, 36*(4), 439–448. doi:10.1016/j.psyneuen.2010.12.001

Rosenthal, R.J., & Faris, S.B. (2019). The etymology and early history of 'addiction'. Addiction Research & Theory, 27(5), 437–449. https://doi.org/10.1080/16066359.2018.1543412

Schultz, W. (1998). Predictive reward signal of dopamine neurons. *Journal of Neurophysiology, 80*(1), 1–27. doi:10.1152/jn.1998.80.1.1

Shurman, J., Koob, G. F., & Gutstein, H. B. (2010). Opioids, pain, the brain, and hyperkatifeia: A framework for the rational use of opioids for pain. *Pain Medicine, 11*(7), 1092–1098. doi:10.1111/j.1526-4637.2010.00881.x

Sinha, R., Garcia, M., Paliwal, P., Kreek, M. J., & Rounsaville, B. J. (2006). Stress-induced cocaine craving and hypothalamic-pituitary-adrenal responses are predictive of cocaine relapse outcomes. *Archives of General Psychiatry, 63*(3), 324–331. doi:10.1001/archpsyc.63.3.324

Smith, K. S., & Graybiel, A. M. (2016). Habit formation. *Dialogues in Clinical Neuroscience, 18*(1), 33–43.

Solomon, R. L., & Corbit, J. D. (1974). An opponent-process theory of motivation. I. Temporal dynamics of affect. *Psychological Review, 81*(2), 119–145. doi:10.1037/h0036128

Sterling, P., & Eyer, J. (1988). Allostasis: A new paradigm to explain arousal pathology. In S. Fisher & J. T. Reason (Eds.). *Handbook of life stress, cognition, and health* (pp. 629–649). Chichester, NY: Wiley.

Substance Abuse and Mental Health Services Administration (SAMHSA). (2016). *Facing addiction in America: The surgeon general's report on alcohol, drugs, and health.* Washington, DC: US Department of Health and Human Services.

Substance Abuse and Mental Health Services Administration (SAMHSA). (2018). *Key substance use and mental health indicators in the United States: Results from the 2017 national survey on drug use and health* (HHS Publication No. SMA 18–5068, NSDUH Series H-53). Rockville, MD: Center for Behavioral Health Statistics and Quality. Retrieved from https://www.samhsa.gov/data/report/2017-nsduh-annual-national-report

Threlfell, S., & Cragg, S. J. (2011). Dopamine signaling in dorsal versus ventral striatum: The dynamic role of cholinergic interneurons. *Frontiers in Systems Neuroscience, 5*(11). doi:10.3389/fnsys.2011.00011

van der Schrier, R., Roozekrans, M., Olofsen, E., Aarts, L., van Velzen, M., de Jong, M., . . . Niesters, M. (2017). Influence of ethanol on oxycodone-induced respiratory depression: A dose-escalating study in young and elderly individuals. *Anesthesiology, 126*(3), 534–542. doi:10.1097/ALN.0000000000001505

Volkow, N. D., Wang, G. J., Fowler, J. S., Tomasi, D., Telang, F., & Baler, R. (2010). Addiction: Decreased reward sensitivity and increased expectation sensitivity conspire to overwhelm the brain's control circuit. *BioEssays: News and Reviews in Molecular, Cellular and Developmental Biology, 32*(9), 748–755. doi:10.1002/bies.201000042

Weiss, F., Parsons, L. H., Schulteis, G., Hyytiä, P., Lorang, M. T., Bloom, F. E., & Koob, G. F. (1996). Ethanol self-administration restores withdrawal-associated deficiencies in accumbal dopamine and 5-hydroxytryptamine release in dependent rats. *Journal of Neuroscience, 16*(10), 3474–3485. doi:10.1523/JNEUROSCI.16-10-03474.1996

World Drug Report. (2018). United Nations publication, Sales No. E.18.XI.9.

Zorrilla, E. P., & Koob, G. F. (2019). Impulsivity derived from the dark side: Neurocircuits that contribute to negative urgency. *Frontiers in Behavioral Neuroscience, 13.* doi:10.3389/fnbeh.2019.00188

Zorrilla, E. P., Logrip, M. L., & Koob, G. F. (2014). Corticotropin releasing factor: A key role in the neurobiology of addiction. *Frontiers in Neuroendocrinology, 35*(2), 234–244. doi:10.1016/j.yfrne.2014.01.001

5

The role of genes and environments in shaping substance misuse

Cristina B. Bares and Karen G. Chartier

Background

The development of substance misuse and addictive behaviors during adolescence and early adulthood involves multiple factors. Whether or not individuals encounter problems with using substances, like alcohol and tobacco, is due to genes, environment factors, and gene-environment interactions. Contemporary disease models of addiction highlight biological contributions to addictive behaviors. This chapter summarizes existing studies concerning the effects of genes and gene-environment interactions on substance misuse and substance use disorders. Recognizing and understanding the genetic factors and the role of gene-environment interactions in determining addictive behavior outcomes contributes to the development of robustly informed strategies for diagnosis, intervention, and prevention.

We first define and describe the developmental and conceptual frameworks for gene-environment interplay that guide our examination of genetic and environmental influences on tobacco and alcohol use. We focus on these two substances because most young people who smoke tobacco products become adults who smoke, and alcohol remains the most widely used psychoactive substance among U.S. adolescents and emerging adults (NCCDPH, 2012). Subsequently, we review studies that inform our knowledge regarding how genes and genes together with environments contribute to the initiation and maintained use of these substances: twin and other family studies, as well as studies utilizing measured genetic markers. Concluding implications are then discussed.

Developmental perspective

The developmental perspective helps us understand milestones for substance use/misuse and recognize that relationships between genetic and environmental factors change across life stages. Models to understand human development and behavior have long included the influence of "nature" and "nurture" in interaction (Sameroff, 2009). These models explain the degree to which innate qualities or aspects of environmental exposures are responsible for variations in behavior and development. "Phenotype" is the term used for describing observable outcomes of substance use and misuse (see Table 5.1).

Table 5.1 Glossary of terms

Term	Definition
Additive genetic effects	The proportion of variance attributed to the influence of genes derived from a structural equation model
Allele	One of two possible versions at a DNA base
Chromosomes	DNA molecule is packaged into tightly packed structures
Dizygotic	Twins who develop out of two fertilized eggs
DNA	Deoxyribonucleic acid; the hereditary material in humans and other organisms
Gene	Sections of DNA that code for making proteins or are noncoding and instead control gene activity
GWAS	Genome-wide association study
Minor allele frequency	The second most frequent allele
Monogenic disease	A disease that arises due to variation or mutation in a single gene
Monozygotic	Twins who develop out of one fertilized egg
Mutation	A difference in the genetic sequence found in most people
Non-shared environmental effects	The proportion of variance attributed to the influence of contexts that are unique to each individual twin derived from a structural equation model
Phenotype	An observable, outward behavior or trait
Polygenic disease	A disease that arises due to variation in multiple genes
Shared environmental effects	The proportion of variance attributed to the influence of environments that twins share with one another derived from a structural equation model
Single nucleotide polymorphism	A difference in a single DNA base
Univariate genetic model	A structural equation model that separates the variance of one variable into additive genetic, shared environmental and unique environmental components

Note: Most definitions obtained from the U.S. National Library of Medicine Genetics Home Reference.

Applying a developmental perspective to substance use problems indicates that through a combination of transactional processes between nature and nurture, substance misuse results from individual level factors, environmental exposures, and their combined effect (Schulenberg, Patrick, Maslowsky, & Maggs, 2014). Developmentally, behaviors at one point in time might result from either intrinsically mediated individual characteristics or extrinsic environmental exposures, currently or from a previous point in development.

Two developmentally defined phenotypes for tobacco and alcohol use are (1) onset of substance use and (2) regular use, or the point when substance use begins occurring at regular intervals. Following initiation to tobacco or alcohol use, common by age 16 (NIAAA, 2017), many individuals progress to using these substances on a regular basis while others do not. It is therefore important to evaluate whether the same genetic factors or gene-environment interplay influences someone to both initiate and maintain substance use, thereby differentiating individuals at increasing levels of risk for tobacco- and alcohol-related consequences. Although substance use disorders are rare outcomes during adolescence, early initiation of substance use is a risk factor for substance use disorders during adulthood, and the mechanisms involved span many systems from genetic predispositions to the social context (Dodge et al., 2009).

Variation in genetically influenced individual characteristics is developmentally linked with rates of cigarette and alcohol use during adolescence. At the individual level, increased rates relate to a cluster of behaviors typified by childhood externalizing behaviors (Dubow, Boxer, & Huesmann, 2008; Lynskey & Fergusson, 1995; Zucker, 2008), adolescent externalizing disorders (Merline, Jager, & Schulenberg, 2008) and low levels of behavioral inhibition (Dubow et al., 2008). Childhood externalizing behaviors have emerged as part of an early-developing chain of behaviors that manifests during childhood and transforms into problematic levels of alcohol use during adolescence (Karriker-Jaffe, Lönn, Cook, Kendler, & Sundquist, 2018). More recently, additional nuance has been contributed through recognition that a series of genetic vulnerabilities can emerge within various types of social contexts and play a role in the etiology of substance use disorders.

Models of gene × environment interplay

Studies extend the idea that genetic predisposition and environmental exposures interact with one another and contribute to increases in alcohol use (Sher et al., 2010) and tobacco use (Chen et al., 2009). Several models explain different ways in which genes and environments are expected to influence addictive behaviors and other psychiatric conditions: additive, interactive, and correlational models (Kendler & Eaves, 1986). An additive model predisposes that environmental conditions and genetic risk have mutually exclusive effects; they both independently increase the risk of developing a problematic behavior or illness. The next two models describe how genetic and environmental effects interrelate or jointly influence risk.

Under the interactive model, the effect of genes depends on the level of environmental exposure and vice versa. This is often referred to as a "gene-by-environment" interaction, indicating that genes can control individuals' sensitivity to environmental effects or, alternatively, whether environmental exposure enhances or buffers genetic effects. In other words, individuals experiencing equal genetic risk could develop the problem in risky but not in healthy environments (see Chapters 7 and 39). A correlational model, also called a "gene-environment correlation," suggests a third possible relationship between genetic and environmental effects. Under this model, genetic predisposition influences an individual's exposure to particular environmental conditions. An often-used example is that individuals predisposed toward externalizing behaviors are more likely to seek out peers who engage in deviant behaviors, using tobacco and alcohol as well as other substances. This predisposition influences environmental exposure to additional risk factors.

Behavioral genetic studies

How are genetic effects and their relationships with environments assessed? We begin by describing how study designs involving twins and adopted families are useful for teasing apart genetic and environmental effects. Twin and family studies (Plomin, DeFries, McClearn, & McGuffin, 2000; Turkheimer, 2000) contributed to our understanding that genes and environments together play a role in numerous traits and complex behaviors, to varying degrees. The typical twin study design includes recruiting related individuals who share either their genes or their environments with one another to varying degrees. Twin studies take advantage of the fact that twins can either be monozygotic ("identical") or dizygotic ("fraternal") and share either almost 100% (monozygotic twins) or, on average, 50% (dizygotic twins) of their genetic makeup (see Table 5.2). A trait or a behavior is thought to be under genetic control if monozygotic twins are more than twice as phenotypically

Table 5.2 Source of overlap by rearing environment and sibling type

| | Reared Together | | | | Reared Apart | | | |
| | Sibling Type | | | | Sibling Type | | | |
Overlap	Monozygotic Twins (%)	Dizygotic Twins (%)	Full Siblings (%)	Half Siblings (%)	Monozygotic Twins (%)	Dizygotic Twins (%)	Full Siblings (%)	Half Siblings (%)
Genetic	100	avg 50	avg 50	avg 25	100	avg 50	avg 50	avg 25
Environmental	100	100	100	50	0	0	0	0

similar to one another than are dizygotic twins. When reared in the same family, twins and full siblings are thought to share about 100% of the familial environment. Thus, the effect of the familial (shared) environment is assumed to be the same for monozygotic and dizygotic twins who grow up together.

Evidence concerning the magnitude of genetic and rearing environment influences on substance use outcomes also comes from studies in which individuals are reared away from their biological parents, thereby reducing a twin study confound where parents provide both genetic and rearing environment influences. Two types of study designs fall in this category: studies of twins reared apart and studies of adopted individuals. In studies of twins reared apart, one twin is raised by an adoptive parent and the degree of similarity on any behavior or trait between the offspring and biological parent is computed and compared to the trait similarity between the offspring and adoptive parent. Similarly, in non-twin adoption studies, the behavior or trait of adopted offspring is compared to both that of their biological and adoptive parents (Lynskey, Agrawal, & Heath, 2010). Although fewer in number, studies of twins reared apart (Grove et al., 1990; Kendler, Thornton, & Pedersen, 2000) and studies of adopted individuals (Cadoret, Troughton, O'Gorman, & Heywood, 1986; Cloninger, Bohman, & Sigvardsson, 1981; McGue, Sharma, & Benson, 1996; Osler, Holst, Prescott, & Sørensen, 2001) have provided additional information regarding the effect of the rearing environment on various traits and complex behaviors. A review of the result of these studies is available elsewhere (Hopfer, Crowley, & Hewitt, 2003).

Twin-based studies are more frequently used than adoption studies to describe genetic and environmental effects for substance misuse. Behavioral genetic studies examine the heritability of a behavior or trait: the contribution of genes to that behavior or trait while also providing an estimate of the degree to which the environment influences the behavior or trait under study. Data from twin studies decompose observed behavioral variance into three latent components: additive genetic effects, shared environmental effects, and non-shared environmental effects. These three latent components are included in a structural equation model with certain constraints and heritability is reflected in the resulting proportion of variance due to additive genetic effects (Neale & Cardon, 1992).

Substance use and additive gene × environment effects

Twin studies have examined the magnitude of genetic and shared environmental effects on the initiation and regular use of various substances across developmental periods beginning in adolescence and continuing to adulthood (see Table 5.3 for exemplars). Heritability of the initiation of tobacco and alcohol use during adolescence appears to depend on the specific ages measured in each study. For example, alcohol initiation has a heritability of 0% in studies of 13–16-year-olds (Maes et al., 1999) but 35% in studies involving slightly older (16–18-year-old) participants (Han, McGue, & Iacono, 1999). The regular use of alcohol has a heritability of about 40%, again depending on the study. For tobacco initiation, heritability in general ranges between 36% (Han et al., 1999) and 80% (Maes et al., 1999; Sartor et al., 2015), and for regular tobacco use ranges between 40% and 50%. Additional evidence from these studies suggests that environmental (shared and non-shared) influences play a stronger role than additive genetic effects for a broad category of behaviors during early adolescence, including substance misuse (Burt, 2009; Kendler, Prescott, Myers, & Neale, 2003).

The trend appears to be one of heritability increasing with age, as evidenced by one of few twin studies to assess the effect of genes on tobacco use across different adolescent age ranges (Bares, Kendler, & Maes, 2015). A study of various twin studies across the globe demonstrated that the effect of genes on tobacco initiation during adolescence ranges between 15% and 45% (Maes et al., 2017) and tends to increase across adolescence into adulthood. This finding is consistent with previous studies showing a decrease in the role of the shared environment on substance use across adolescence (Bares et al., 2015; Kendler, Schmitt, Aggen, & Prescott, 2008), suggesting a developmentally or age-specific interplay of genes and environments.

The shared environment, or factors within a family context shared by twins, contributes independently of genes to the risk of initiating and using tobacco or alcohol during early adolescence (Han et al., 1999; Kendler et al., 2008; Maes et al., 2017; Meyers et al., 2014; Rose, Dick, Viken, & Kaprio, 2001). Some alcohol initiation studies show a relatively large effect of the shared environment during adolescence (Maes et al., 1999), while others, using smaller age ranges, show a more moderate influence (Han et al., 1999). Regular alcohol use appears to be under moderate genetic influence during adolescence (Kendler et al., 2008; Rose et al., 2001). The shared environment effect wanes in influence as individuals move into adulthood (Bares et al., 2015; Maes et al., 1999). Taken together, evidence from the reviewed twin studies suggests that genetic effects are smaller for the initiation of use than for the regular use of substances, indicating a larger role when adolescents start to drink or use tobacco for environmental conditions like access to alcohol (e.g. through older siblings, other family members, or peers). There also exists a similar shift, from stronger environmental contributions to stronger genetic contributions across the developmental stages of adolescence to young adulthood.

Interactive gene × environment effects

Two approaches using a twin study design can test whether the contribution of genes and environments on a behavior interact or interrelate in other ways. First, the effect of genes on substance use phenotype can be compared among twin pairs raised in different types of environments. We would assess the behavior of individuals (Twin 1 and Twin 2) within the same family raised in either low- or high-risk environments. Applying univariate genetic models to these data would result in estimates of heritability and shared environmental influences for each environment type (i.e. low- and high-risk) that can then be tested for equivalence across the two groups. These studies provide answers concerning whether heritability of particular behaviors is the same or different in environments varying in degree of risk.

A second approach to assessing the interplay between environmental and genetic effects requires the use of twin data where aspects of participants' social context were measured. In such a twin study, the effect of the measured social context can be statistically regressed onto

Table 5.3 Studies examining heritability and shared environmental influence of alcohol and tobacco

Substance	Behavior Assessed	Heritability[b]	Shared Environment[b]	Developmental Period	Source Study
Alcohol	Initiation[a]	0%	71%	Adolescence (13–16)	Maes et al. (1999)
Alcohol	Initiation[a]	35%	46%	Adolescence (17–18)	Han et al. (1999)
Alcohol	Regular use	74%	0%	Adolescence (13–16)	Vaes et al. (1999)
Alcohol	Regular use	0% (adolescence); 40% (young adulthood-adulthood)[b]	40% (adolescence); (young adulthood); (adulthood)[b]	Adolescence, young adulthood, adulthood	Kendler et al. (2008)
Alcohol	Regular use	33% (age 16) 49% (age 17); 50% (age 18.5)	37% (age 16); 20% (age 17); 14% (age 18.5)	Adolescence (16–18.5)	Rose et al. (2001)
Tobacco	Initiation[a]	84%	0%	Adolescence (13–16)	Maes et al. (1999)
Tobacco	Initiation (African Americans)[a,c]	50%	46%	Adolescence (13–19)	Sartor et al. (2015)
Tobacco	Initiation (European Americans)[a,c]	51%	12%	Adolescence (13–19)	Sartor et al. (2015)
Tobacco	Initiation[a]	36%	44%	Adolescence (17–18)	Han et al. (1999)
Tobacco	Initiation[a]	42% (ages 14–15); 43% (ages 16–17); 84% (ages 18–25); 87% (ages 26–33)	46% (ages 14–15); 10% (ages 16–17); 0% (ages 18–25); 0% (ages 26–33)	Adolescence, young adulthood	Bares et al. (2015)
Tobacco	Regular use	82%	0%	Adolescence (13–16)	Maes et al. (1999)
Tobacco	Regular use	0% (adolescence); 40% (young adulthood); 40% (adulthood)	45% (adolescence); 30% (young adulthood); 20% (adulthood)	Adolescence, young adulthood, adulthood	Kendler et al. (2008)

Notes
a Initiation defined as having ever used this substance.
b Age-specific estimates available from source.
c Only females were included in sample.

the behavior of interest, as well as the additive genetic, shared environmental, and unique environmental effects. Applying univariate genetic models to these data yields estimates of the effect of each component and can be followed up with tests of nested models that indicate whether each component contributes significant variance to the behavior of interest.

Fewer studies have examined changes in heritability across various types of environmental exposure compared to the number of twin studies evaluating the independent contributions of genetic and environmental effects. The social environment exposures studied and described here include both proximal factors, like peer and family influences, as well as community-level variables.

In one study of community variables using the first approach, environmental exposure was operationalized in two separate ways: first computing the expenditures each community spent on alcohol, then the amount of residential stability in each community. Some twins (Kaprio, Pulkkinen, & Rose, 2002) came from families residing in communities with a high level of alcohol expenditures and others from communities spending low amounts on alcohol. The heritability of alcohol use frequency among young adults was higher in communities with greater expenditures on alcohol and greater residential mobility (in and out of the communities) where young adults resided (Dick, Rose, Viken, Kaprio, & Koskenvuo, 2001). An additional study suggested that greater alcohol density surrounding communities where adolescents resided is associated with increased heritability (Slutske, Deutsch, & Piasecki, 2018), that is, genetic effects on alcohol use are stronger for individuals who live near more alcohol retail outlets. Studies employing the second approach, including a measured environmental variable in a twin model to directly test its effect on the trait, showed that parental monitoring can alter, in this case reduce, the heritability of cigarette use (Dick et al., 2007). Similarly, studies suggest greater genetic effects on alcohol use during adolescence among individuals receiving low levels of parental monitoring and affiliating with friends and peers expressing high levels of deviant behavior (Kendler, Gardner, & Dick, 2011).

Molecular genomic studies

Since Mendel's discoveries concerning the transmission of traits between parents and offspring, the world has a broader, deeper understanding of the genetic basis of many human traits and behaviors. Inside each human cell (except eggs and sperm), DNA sequences (genes) are contained within 23 pairs of chromosomes on which various numbers and types of genes are located. The Human Genome Project was undertaken to understand the architecture of genes, their variants (alleles), and their role in many human traits and disorders. The human genome contains genetic instructions for our physical, physiological, and behavioral traits in over 20,000 genes (NHGRI, 2018). Although sequencing the human genome demonstrated that humans share 99.9% of our genomes, individuals differ from each other in multiple ways.

Genomes can vary at a single place, single nucleotide polymorphism (SNP), or at many places in large SNP groups (hundreds or more). There exist an estimated 4–5 million SNPs across the human genome: the most common type of genetic variation. Other types of genetic variation include the insertion, deletion, inversion, or duplication of DNA sequences. SNPs exist mostly in between genes, but SNPs within or near genes tend to serve a more direct role in affecting a gene's function. At most SNP locations, individuals carry an allele pair, and it is this variation (for simplicity, we refer to the symbols AA, Aa, and aa to designate variants at each location) that is examined to estimate relationships with substance use phenotypes.

The basic concept is that researchers seek to determine if an allele pattern (AA, Aa, or aa) is associated with increased risk or protection for substance use behaviors. We encourage readers interested in learning more about this topic to refer to resources provided by the U.S. National Library of Medicine's Genetics Home Reference.

The genetics of substance misuse

Advances since completion of the Human Genome Project in 2003 (NHGRI, 2018) include identification of specific genetic variants involved in monogenic diseases like sickle cell disease (Chial, 2008) and the exploration of multiple genes (polygenic) in complex traits and illnesses including height (NHGRI, 2017) or addiction (Goldman, Oroszi, & Ducci, 2005). Studies examining the relationship of genetic variation to substance misuse and substance use disorders have passed through stages. Early studies, called candidate gene studies, focused on exploring the effect of individual genes suspected of playing a role in substance misuse or use disorders. Candidate genes were selected based on their biological function and presumed relevance to the phenotype of interest.

These studies highlighted associations between: (1) genes involved in modifying neuronal excitability through a neurotransmitter involved in muscle regulation (e.g. *CHRM2*) and alcohol use (Dick et al., 2011); (2) genes involved in the speed through which neurons communicate (e.g. acetylcholine receptor genes *CHRNA5, CHRNA3, CHRNA4, CHRNB3*) and tobacco use (Bierut et al., 2007; Saccone et al., 2007); and (3) associations between genes that control dopamine receptors and the use of alcohol (Agrawal & Lynskey, 2009; Creemers et al., 2011). Candidate gene studies are viewed with caution given that their findings have not always replicated across studies (Chanock et al., 2007; Munafo & Flint, 2004) or they produced null findings. Notable exceptions to the lackluster results for candidate genes in the field of alcohol research are related to the *GABRA* gene that controls the GABA neurotransmitter (Edenberg et al., 2004; Long et al., 1998; Zinn-Justin & Abel, 1999) and the genes involved in the metabolism of alcohol (e.g. *ADH1B, ADH1C,* and *ALDH2*), which have consistently replicated across various samples (Edenberg, Gelernter, & Agrawal, 2019). Regardless, these studies indicate the complexity of genetic influence on substance misuse and substance use disorders.

More recently, genomic work focused on exploring the entire genome in a hypothesis-free approach called genome-wide association studies (GWAS). In GWAS, common variants with a minor allele frequency of 5% or greater are searched across the entire genome without a prior hypothesis, not querying specific gene variants or sequences (Kitsios & Zintzaras, 2009). GWAS conducted in the addiction field have uncovered specific gene variants associated with various substance use phenotypes like the number of cigarettes smoked per day, heavy versus light tobacco use, nicotine dependence, maximum alcoholic drinks in 24 hours, and alcohol use disorder (Hancock, Markunas, Bierut, & Johnson, 2018). Genetic variants involved in substance-specific metabolism pathways such as those involved in the metabolism of nicotine (e.g. *CYP2A6* genetic variants) (Chenoweth et al., 2016; O'Loughlin et al., 2004) and alcohol (e.g. *ADH1B* genetic variants) (Hurley & Edenberg, 2012) have been identified and/or further replicated through genome-wide association studies. Because early GWAS often involved relatively small sample sizes, replicated variants tended to be those with larger effect sizes. A lesson learned from studying psychiatric conditions like schizophrenia (PGC, 2014), major depression (Wray et al., 2018), and bipolar disorder (Stahl et al., 2019) was that identification of genetic markers associated with complex diseases, involving many variants or small effects, requires very large sample sizes—in the magnitude of 100s of thousands of participants. This has been possible through large consortiums of researchers collaborating to pool their samples in GWAS meta-analyses. For a review of the findings of this most recent stage of gene discovery in alcohol use, see the work of Edenberg, Gelernter, and Agrawal (2019).

Molecular gene-by-environment research

Having reviewed some of the basic ideas in genetics and gene discovery efforts, we turn our attention to describing molecular gene-by-environment (G×E) research for tobacco and alcohol use. These studies began with candidate G×E approaches, and more recently have applied a polygenic score approach as a solution to the shortcomings of candidate G×E studies (Dick et al., 2015). Complex genetic traits like tobacco and alcohol misuse are linked to many genetic markers with small effects, and a polygenic score (PGS) is an effective tool for aggregating these effects. PGSs are calculated for each study participant representing a weighted total of the risk and protective alleles that they carry and are then analyzed in gene-by-environment relationships.

Candidate G×E examples

An often-used example of how social norms in the macro-level environment can alter genetic effects on alcohol use is research conducted among Japanese individuals who are more likely to carry an allele (*ALDH2*2*) involved in the metabolism of alcohol (Goedde, Harada, & Agarwal, 1979). This allele is considered protective against alcohol dependence because its actions generate unpleasant physical reactions to alcohol consumption (Harada, Agarwal, Goedde, & Ishikawa, 1983). Among three cohorts of Japanese individuals, alcohol dependence rates differed depending on whether they carried the protective allele (Higuchi et al., 1994). However, over time as social norms around alcohol consumption changed and promoted social/business drinking, rates of alcohol dependence increased even among individuals who carried the protective *ALDH2*2* (Higuchi et al., 1994). Similar to reviewed twin studies, more proximal relationships are important in changing the effect of genes on substance use and related behaviors. For example, researchers showed a reduced effect for the protective *ADH1B* allele and for *ALDH2*2* protection when adolescents had siblings who drank (Irons, Iacono, Oetting, & McGue, 2012) or when most or all of their peers drank alcohol (Olfson et al., 2014).

Based on earlier studies of depression and post-traumatic stress disorder, genes also influence how individuals respond to social stressors, including drinking to cope. Variations in genes associated with greater sensitivity to stressors (e.g. *FKBP5* and *SLC6A4*) strengthen the influence of negative life events and early life trauma on alcohol misuse (Kranzler et al., 2012; Lieberman et al., 2016). It is notable that individuals most vulnerable to social stressors may also benefit the most from environmental enhancements (Belsky & Pluess, 2009; Belsky & van Ijzendoorn, 2017), such as parental monitoring and participation in prevention interventions (Brody, Chen, & Beach, 2013; Trucco, Villafuerte, Heitzeg, Burmeister, & Zucker, 2016).

Polygenic scores and G×E study

Using a PGS approach, Salvatore and colleagues (2014) presented evidence of both gene-environment interaction and correlation in an adolescent sample: low parental monitoring and high peer deviance strengthened genetic effects on alcohol problems, and higher polygenic scores were positively associated with greater levels of peer deviance. Musci, Uhl, Maher, and Ialongo (2015) similarly demonstrated that parent (low parental monitoring) and peer relationships (having more peers engaged in substance use) moderated polygenetic effects on adolescent tobacco use. While these two studies replicated both twin-based and candidate gene studies, the convergence of evidence enabled a higher comfort with their implications for substance misuse prevention and intervention strategies.

Implications

We believe there are many practical implications for social work and other professions of research concerning the genetic and gene-environment interaction basis of substance misuse. Risk perception for health and disease is a complex, cognitive undertaking. For some diseases, better comprehension of risk is associated with greater likelihood of screening and adherence to preventative treatments (McCaul, Schroeder, & Reid, 1996). An accurate understanding of the genetic basis of problems and diseases involves understanding the double meaning implied in the concept of "genetic basis." Hereditary problems said to "run in families" can be observed in multiple generations. The current state of genomics concerning substance misuse and substance use disorders is focused on understanding which inherited genetic variants are involved. However, variants in DNA sequence may not have been passed down from one generation to the next; they may represent new mutations.

Recent attention has been devoted to personalizing medicine, creating individual-specific treatments based on an individual's unique genetic sequence rather than providing a treatment meant to work for the average patient. However, until GWAS on substance use phenotypes gather samples sufficiently large to identify variants of very small effects, we will not know the full effect of the genetic contributions to substance use behaviors and substance use disorders, or their applicability to specific treatment and prevention efforts. GWAS focuses on common variants; other methods need to be utilized to examine the relationship of rare variants to substance use phenotypes.

In addition, greater diversity is necessary in gene discovery studies. Genomic research has been primarily conducted with European ancestry populations (Hancock et al., 2018), and even fewer gene-by-environment studies include individuals of non-European ancestry populations (Chartier, Karriker-Jaffe, Cummings, & Kendler, 2017). This is problematic because GWAS results associated with greater liability to substance misuse and substance use disorders may not generalize to the other major population groups, such as individuals of African, American (being from the Americas), East Asian, and South Asian ancestry as defined by the 1000 Genomes Project (IGSR, 2018). First, the frequency with which alleles are present in these population groups can differ (Gabriel et al., 2002; Manolio, Brooks, & Collins, 2008) and, when a variant or gene is found to increase or decrease liability for substance misuse, it may be population specific. For example, the *ALDH2*2* variant, which is involved in the metabolism of alcohol and is protective against alcohol problems, is mostly found in individuals of East Asian ancestry and rarely in other populations (Hurley & Edenberg, 2012). Second, over-reliance on one ancestry group as the basis for understanding the genomic architecture of problems with substance use means that researchers are creating an imbalance in the knowledge generated. It is therefore critical to include greater proportions of diverse populations in research (Tekola-Ayele & Rotimi, 2015; Tishkoff et al., 2009); social work research can play a significant role in understanding the factors that may encourage other diverse populations to participate in genomic research (Werner-Lin, McCoyd, Doyle, & Gehlert, 2016).

As the technology to conduct genetic tests and genomic sequencing becomes more affordable (NHGRI, 2016) and more widely available to greater proportions of the population, the issues of fully understanding the implications of this information with clients and their clinicians becomes more important. Family disease history has been most informative for uncovering the hereditary basis of monogenic and highly penetrant genetic diseases but can also be informative for more common diseases (Yoon, Scheuner, & Khoury, 2003). Even as methods for creating polygenic risk scores are developed, family history of substance use may be more informative than genetic information (Yan et al., 2014) at identifying individuals at greater risk for substance misuse. Due to their novelty and perceived utility, on receiving genetic testing results, individuals often discuss these with family (Ashida et al., 2009; Kaphingst et al., 2012) as their individual results may have implications for family members. They also discuss results with friends (Ashida et al., 2009), which presents an opportunity to promote healthy lifestyles for themselves, their families, and broader social networks (Koehly & McBride, 2010). Important issues between clinicians and their clients should continue to be discussed such as the idea that our genetic makeup is not deterministic and the important role (agency) that an individual has in changing their own behavior. Studies have revealed that when presented with genetic information, individuals who use tobacco may not be motivated to quit (McClure, 2001; Waters, Ball, Carter, & Gehlert, 2014) if they consider their behavior as being determined by something outside of their control (i.e. their genes). Information about which genes are associated with increased risk for a disease can be augmented by also providing information regarding environmental risk factors for substance use behaviors. A list of which environmental risk factors can be changed and those that are less amenable to change can spark discussion between clinicians and clients and empower clients to gain control of their health behaviors.

Having an understanding of their risk due to family history of alcohol use may result in more positive intervention outcomes for reducing alcohol use among college students (Neale et al., 2018). For tobacco use and cancer risks, modifiable risk factors may include decreasing smoking frequency and the reduction of second-hand exposure, while exposure to contaminants at work may be less amenable to change. For harmful substance use, parental monitoring and reducing exposure to deviant or substance-using peers may be more amenable, while changing neighborhood exposures may be less amenable, unless the entire community and macro-level institutions and organizations are included in the effort (Gravely et al., 2017; Schneider, Buka, Dash, Winickoff, & O'Donnell, 2016).

As diagnostic tools are developed (Valdez, Coates, St Pierre, Grossniklaus, & Khoury, 2011; Weigl et al., 2018) to help individuals understand their relative risk for developing a disorder, it is important to consider how family health history, individual's genetic risk, and both distal and proximal environmental exposures are used in assessing and modifying substance use behaviors. More research in this area will be facilitated as results on the genetics of addiction continue to emerge.

Conclusions

The genomics field is uncovering the genetic sequences relevant for substance misuse and substance use disorders. Both genetic and environmental factors and their interaction are responsible for their onset and persistence, although the level of contribution from each changes across development. This evidence has profound implications for the development of prevention and treatment interventions at the individual, family, community, and larger-system levels. Few studies allow for an exploration of the interaction and correlation between genes and environments using polygenic approaches. The information available about how to lessen substance use risk will not be complete until more studies adequately describe which combinations of genes and environments are the riskiest or most protective against the development of substance misuse and substance use disorders. This knowledge may be useful in helping individuals understand their own personal vulnerability, risks, and protection status, and guide more informed behavioral health decisions.

References

Agrawal, A., & Lynskey, M. T. (2009). Candidate genes for cannabis use disorders: Findings, challenges and directions. *Addiction, 104*(4), 518–532. doi:10.1111/j.1360-0443.2009.02504.x

Ashida, S., Koehly, L. M., Roberts, J. S., Chen, C. A., Hiraki, S., & Green, R. C. (2009). Disclosing the disclosure: Factors associated with communicating the results of genetic susceptibility testing for Alzheimer's disease. *Journal of Health Communication, 14*(8), 768–784. doi:10.1080/10810730903295518

Bares, C. B., Kendler, K. S., & Maes, H. H. (2015). Developmental changes in genetic and shared environmental contributions to smoking initiation and subsequent smoking quantity in adolescence and young adulthood. *Twin Research and Human Genetics, 18*(5), 497–506. doi:10.1017/thg.2015.48

Belsky, J., & Pluess, M. (2009). Beyond diathesis stress: Differential susceptibility to environmental influences. *Psychological Bulletin, 135*(6), 885. doi:10.1037/a0017376

Belsky, J., & van Ijzendoorn, M. H. (2017). Genetic differential susceptibility to the effects of parenting. *Current Opinion in Psychology, 15*, 125–130. doi:10.1016/j.copsyc.2017.02.021

Bierut, L. J., Madden, P. A., Breslau, N., Johnson, E. O., Hatsukami, D., Pomerleau, O. F., . . . Ballinger, D. G. (2007). Novel genes identified in a high-density genome wide association study for nicotine dependence. *Human Molecular Genetics, 16*(1), 24–35. doi:10.1093/hmg/ddl441

Brody, G. H., Chen, Y. F., & Beach, S. R. (2013). Differential susceptibility to prevention: GABAergic, dopaminergic, and multilocus effects. *Journal of Child Psychology and Psychiatry, 54*(8), 863–871. doi:10.1111/jcpp.12042

Burt, S. A. (2009). Rethinking environmental contributions to child and adolescent psychopathology: A meta-analysis of shared environmental influences. *Psychological Bulletin, 135*(4), 608. doi:10.1037/a0015702

Cadoret, R. J., Troughton, E., O'Gorman, T. W., & Heywood, E. (1986). An adoption study of genetic and environmental factors in drug abuse. *Archives of general psychiatry, 43*(12), 1131–1136. doi:10.1001/archpsyc.1986.01800120017004

Chanock, S. J., Manolio, T., Boehnke, M., Boerwinkle, E., Hunter, D. J., Thomas, G., . . . Bailey-Wilson, J. E. (2007). Replicating genotype–phenotype associations. *Nature, 447*(7145), 655. doi:10.1038/447655a

Chartier, K. G., Karriker-Jaffe, K. J., Cummings, C. R., & Kendler, K. S. (2017). Environmental influences on alcohol use: Informing research on the joint effects of genes and the environment in diverse US populations. *The American Journal on Addictions, 26*(5), 446–460. doi:10.1111/ajad.12478

Chen, L. S., Johnson, E. O., Breslau, N., Hatsukami, D., Saccone, N. L., Grucza, R. A., . . . Goate, A. M. (2009). Interplay of genetic risk factors and parent monitoring in risk for nicotine dependence. *Addiction, 104*(10), 1731–1740. doi:10.1111/j.1360-0443.2009.02697.x

Chenoweth, M. J., Sylvestre, M. P., Contreras, G., Novalen, M., O'Loughlin, J., & Tyndale, R. F. (2016). Variation in CYP2A6 and tobacco dependence throughout adolescence and in young adult smokers. *Drug Alcohol Depend, 158*, 139–146. doi:10.1016/j.drugalcdep.2015.11.017

Chial, H. (2008). Mendelian genetics: Patterns of inheritance and single-gene disorders. *Nature Education, 1*(1), 63.

Cloninger, C. R., Bohman, M., & Sigvardsson, S. (1981). Inheritance of alcohol abuse. Cross-fostering analysis of adopted men. *Archive of General Psychiatry, 38*(8), 861–868. doi:10.1001/archpsyc.1981.01780330019001

Creemers, H. E., Harakeh, Z., Dick, D. M., Meyers, J. L., Vollebergh, W. A., Ormel, J., . . . Huizink, A.C. (2011). DRD2 and DRD4 in relation to regular alcohol and cannabis use among adolescents: Does parenting modify the impact of genetic vulnerability? The TRAILS study. *Drug and Alcohol Dependence, 115*(1–2), 35–42. doi:10.1016/j.drugalcdep.2010.10.008

Dick, D. M., Agrawal, A., Keller, M. C., Adkins, A., Aliev, F., Monroe, S., . . . Sher, K. J. (2015). Candidate gene–environment interaction research: Reflections and recommendations. *Perspectives on Psychological Science, 10*(1), 37–59. doi:10.1177/1745691614556682

Dick, D. M., Meyers, J. L., Latendresse, S. J., Creemers, H. E., Lansford, J. E., Pettit, G. S., . . . Goate, A. (2011). CHRM2, parental monitoring, and adolescent externalizing behavior: Evidence for gene–environment interaction. *Psychological Science, 22*(4), 481–489. doi:10.1177/0956797611403318

Dick, D. M., Pagan, J. L., Viken, R., Purcell, S. M., Kaprio, J., Pulkkinen, L., & Rose, R. J. (2007). Changing environmental influences on substance use across development. *Twin Research and Human Genetics, 10*(2), 315–326. doi:10.1375/twin.10.2.315

Dick, D. M., Rose, R. J., Viken, R. J., Kaprio, J., & Koskenvuo, M. (2001). Exploring gene–environment interactions: Socioregional moderation of alcohol use. *Journal of Abnormal Psychology, 110*(4), 625–632. doi:10.1037/0021-843X.110.4.625

Dodge, K. A., Malone, P. S., Lansford, J. E., Miller, S., Pettit, G. S., & Bates, J. E. (2009). A dynamic cascade model of the development of substance-use onset. *Monographs of the Society for Research in Child Development, 74*(3), vii–119. doi:10.1111/j.1540-5834.2009.00528.x

Dubow, E. F., Boxer, P., & Huesmann, L. R. (2008). Childhood and adolescent predictors of early and middle adulthood alcohol use and problem drinking: The Columbia county longitudinal study. *Addiction, 103*, 36–47. doi:10.1111/j.1360-0443.2008.02175.x

Edenberg, H. J., Dick, D. M., Xuei, X., Tian, H., Almasy, L., Bauer, L. O., . . . Jones, K. (2004). Variations in GABRA2, encoding the α2 subunit of the GABAA receptor, are associated with alcohol dependence and with brain oscillations. *The American Journal of Human Genetics, 74*(4), 705–714. doi:10.1086/383283

Edenberg, H. J., Gelernter, J., & Agrawal, A. (2019). Genetics of alcoholism. *Current Psychiatry Reports, 21*(4), 26. doi:10.1007/s11920-019-1008-1

Gabriel, S. B., Schaffner, S. F., Nguyen, H., Moore, J. M., Roy, J., Blumenstiel, B., . . . Altshuler, D. (2002). The structure of haplotype blocks in the human genome. *Science, 296*(5576), 2225–2229. doi:10.1126/science.1069424

Goedde, H. W., Harada, S., & Agarwal, D. (1979). Racial differences in alcohol sensitivity: A new hypothesis. *Human Genetics, 51*(3), 331–334. doi:10.1007/BF00283404

Goldman, D., Oroszi, G., & Ducci, F. (2005). The genetics of addictions: Uncovering the genes. *Nature Reviews Genetics, 6*(7), 521–532. doi:10.1038/nrg1635

Gravely, S., Giovino, G. A., Craig, L., Commar, A., D'Espaignet, E. T., Schotte, K., & Fong, G. T. (2017). Implementation of key demand-reduction measures of the WHO framework convention on tobacco control and change in smoking prevalence in 126 countries: An association study. *The Lancet Public Health, 2*(4), e166–e174. doi:10.1016/S2468-2667(17)30045-2

Grove, W. M., Eckert, E. D., Heston, L., Bouchard Jr, T. J., Segal, N., & Lykken, D. T. (1990). Heritability of substance abuse and antisocial behavior: A study of monozygotic twins reared apart. *Biological Psychiatry, 27*(12), 1293–1304. doi:10.1016/0006-3223(90)90500-2

Han, C., McGue, M. K., & Iacono, W. G. (1999). Lifetime tobacco, alcohol and other substance use in adolescent Minnesota twins: Univariate and multivariate behavioral genetic analyses. *Addiction, 94*(7), 981–993. doi:10.1046/j.1360-0443.1999.9479814.x

Hancock, D. B., Markunas, C. A., Bierut, L. J., & Johnson, E. O. (2018). Human genetics of addiction: New insights and future directions. *Current Psychiatry Reports, 20*(2), 8. doi:10.1007/s11920-018-0873-3

Harada, S., Agarwal, D. P., Goedde, H. W., & Ishikawa, B. (1983). Aldehyde dehydrogenase isozyme variation and alcoholism in Japan. *Pharmacology Biochemistry and Behavior, 18*, 151–153. doi:10.1016/0091-3057(83)90163-6

Higuchi, S., Matsushita, S., Imazeki, H., Kinoshita, T., Takagi, S., & Kono, H. (1994). Aldehyde dehydrogenase genotypes in Japanese alcoholics. *The Lancet, 343*(8899), 741–742. doi:10.1016/S0140-6736(94)91629-2

Hopfer, C. J., Crowley, T. J., & Hewitt, J. K. (2003). Review of twin and adoption studies of adolescent substance use. *Journal of the American Academy of Child & Adolescent Psychiatry, 42*(6), 710–719. doi:10.1097/01.CHI.0000046848.56865.54

Hurley, T. D., & Edenberg, H. J. (2012). Genes encoding enzymes involved in ethanol metabolism. *Alcohol Research, 34*(3), 339–344.

International Genome Sample Resource (IGSR). (2018). Retrieved from http://www.international genome.org/category/population/

Irons, D. E., Iacono, W. G., Oetting, W. S., & McGue, M. (2012). Developmental trajectory and environmental moderation of the effect of ALDH2 polymorphism on alcohol use. *Alcoholism: Clinical and Experimental Research, 36*(11), 1882–1891. doi:10.1111/j.1530-0277.2012.01809.x

Kaphingst, K. A., Goodman, M., Pandya, C., Garg, P., Stafford, J., & Lachance, C. (2012). Factors affecting frequency of communication about family health history with family members and doctors in a medically underserved population. *Patient Education and Counseling, 88*(2), 291–297. doi:10.1016/j.pec.2011.11.013

Kaprio, J., Pulkkinen, L., & Rose, R. J. (2002). Genetic and environmental factors in health-related behaviors: Studies on Finnish twins and twin families. *Twin Research and Human Genetics, 5*(5), 366–371. doi:10.1375/136905202320906101

Karriker-Jaffe, K. J., Lönn, S. L., Cook, W. K., Kendler, K. S., & Sundquist, K. (2018). Chains of risk for alcohol use disorder: Mediators of exposure to neighborhood deprivation in early and middle childhood. *Health & Place, 50*, 16–26. doi:10.1016/j.healthplace.2017.12.008

Kendler, K. S., & Eaves, L. J. (1986). Models for the joint effect of genotype and environment on liability to psychiatric illness. *American Journal of Psychiatry, 143*(3), 279–289. doi:10.1176/ajp.143.3.279

Kendler, K. S., Gardner, C., & Dick, D. M. (2011). Predicting alcohol consumption in adolescence from alcohol-specific and general externalizing genetic risk factors, key environmental exposures and their interaction. *Psychological Medicine, 41*(7), 1507–1516. doi:10.1017/s003329171000190x

Kendler, K. S., Prescott, C. A., Myers, J., & Neale, M. C. (2003). The structure of genetic and environmental risk factors for common psychiatric and substance use disorders in men and women. *Archives of General Psychiatry, 60*(9), 929–937. doi:10.1001/archpsyc.60.9.929

Kendler, K. S., Schmitt, E., Aggen, S. H., & Prescott, C. A. (2008). Genetic and environmental influences on alcohol, caffeine, cannabis, and nicotine use from early adolescence to middle adulthood. *Archives of General Psychiatry, 65*(6), 674–682. doi:10.1001/archpsyc.65.6.674

Kendler, K. S., Thornton, L. M., & Pedersen, N. L. (2000). Tobacco consumption in Swedish twins reared apart and reared together. *Archives of General Psychiatry, 57*(9), 886–892. doi:10.1001/archpsyc.57.9.886

Kitsios, G. D., & Zintzaras, E. (2009). Genome-wide association studies: Hypothesis-"free" or "engaged"? *Translational Research, 154*(4), 161–164. doi:10.1016/j.trsl.2009.07.001

Koehly, L. M., & McBride, C. M. (2010). Genomic risk information for common health conditions: Maximizing kinship-based health promotion. In K. P. Tercyak (Ed.), *Handbook of genomics and the family: Psychosocial context for children and adolescents* (pp. 407–433). New York, NY: Springer Science + Business Media. doi:10.1007/978-1-4419-5800-6_17

Kranzler, H. R., Scott, D., Tennen, H., Feinn, R., Williams, C., Armeli, S., . . . Covault, J. (2012). The 5-HTTLPR polymorphism moderates the effect of stressful life events on drinking behavior in college students of African descent. *American Journal of Medical Genetics Part B: Neuropsychiatric Genetics, 159*(5), 484–490. doi:10.1002/ajmg.b.32051

Lieberman, R., Armeli, S., Scott, D. M., Kranzler, H. R., Tennen, H., & Covault, J. (2016). FKBP5 genotype interacts with early life trauma to predict heavy drinking in college students. *American Journal of Medical Genetics Part B: Neuropsychiatric Genetics, 171*(6), 879–887. doi:10.1002/ajmg.b.32460

Long, J. C., Knowler, W. C., Hanson, R. L., Robin, R. W., Urbanek, M., Moore, E., . . . Goldman, D. (1998). Evidence for genetic linkage to alcohol dependence on chromosomes 4 and 11 from an autosome-wide scan in an American Indian population. *American Journal of Medical Genetics, 81*(3), 216–221. /doi:10.1002/(SICI)1096-8628(19980508)81:3<216::AID-AJMG2>3.0.CO;2-U

Lynskey, M. T., Agrawal, A., & Heath, A. C. (2010). Genetically informative research on adolescent substance use: Methods, findings, and challenges. *Journal of the American Academy of Child & Adolescent Psychiatry, 49*(12), 1202–1214. doi:10.1016/j.jaac.2010.09.004

Lynskey, M. T., & Fergusson, D. M. (1995). Childhood conduct problems, attention deficit behaviors, and adolescent alcohol, tobacco, and illicit drug use. *Journal of Abnormal Child Psychology, 23*(3), 281–302. doi:10.1007/BF01447558

Maes, H. H., Prom-Wormley, E., Eaves, L. J., Rhee, S. H., Hewitt, J. K., Young, S., . . . Neale, M. C. (2017). A genetic epidemiological mega analysis of smoking initiation in adolescents. *Nicotine & Tobacco Research, 19*(4), 401–409. doi:10.1093/ntr/ntw294

Maes, H. H., Woodard, C. E., Murrelle, L., Meyer, J. M., Silberg, J. L., Hewitt, J. K., . . . Carbonneau, R. (1999). Tobacco, alcohol and drug use in eight-to sixteen-year-old twins: The Virginia twin study of adolescent behavioral development. *Journal of Studies on Alcohol and Drugs, 60*(3), 293. doi:10.15288/jsa.1999.60.293

Manolio, T. A., Brooks, L. D., & Collins, F. S. (2008). A HapMap harvest of insights into the genetics of common disease. *Journal of Clinical Investigation, 118*(5), 1590–1605. doi:10.1172/jci34772

McCaul, K. D., Schroeder, D. M., & Reid, P. A. (1996). Breast cancer worry and screening: Some prospective data. *Health Psychology, 15*(6), 430. doi:10.1037/0278-6133.15.6.430

McClure, J. B. (2001). Are biomarkers a useful aid in smoking cessation? A review and analysis of the literature. *Behavioral Medicine, 27*(1), 37–47. doi:10.1080/08964280109595770

McGue, M., Sharma, A., & Benson, P. (1996). Parent and sibling influences on adolescent alcohol use and misuse: Evidence from a US adoption cohort. *Journal of Studies on Alcohol, 57*(1), 8–18. doi:10.15288/jsa.1996.57.8

Merline, A., Jager, J., & Schulenberg, J. E. (2008). Adolescent risk factors for adult alcohol use and abuse: Stability and change of predictive value across early and middle adulthood. *Addiction, 103*, 84–99. doi:10.1111/j.1360-0443.2008.02178.x

Meyers, J. L., Salvatore, J. E., Vuoksimaa, E., Korhonen, T., Pulkkinen, L., Rose, R. J., . . . Dick, D. M. (2014). Genetic influences on alcohol use behaviors have diverging developmental trajectories: A prospective study among male and female twins. *Alcoholism: Clinical & Experimental Research, 38*(11), 2869–2877. doi:10.1111/acer.12560

Munafo, M. R., & Flint, J. (2004). Meta-analysis of genetic association studies. *Trends in Genetics, 20*(9), 439–444. doi:10.1016/j.tig.2004.06.014

Musci, R. J., Uhl, G., Maher, B., & Ialongo, N. S. (2015). Testing gene × environment moderation of tobacco and marijuana use trajectories in adolescence and young adulthood. *Journal of Consulting & Clinical Psychology, 83*(5), 866–874. doi:10.1037/a0039537

NCCDPH. (2012). *Preventing tobacco use among youth and young adults: A report of the surgeon general.* Atlanta, GA: Centers for Disease Control and Prevention (US).

Neale, M. C., & Cardon, L. (1992). *Methodology for genetic studies of twins and families* (Vol. 67). Springer Science & Business Media. doi:10.1007/978-94-015-8018-2

Neale, Z. E., Salvatore, J. E., Cooke, M. E., Savage, J. E., Aliev, F., Donovan, K. K., . . . Dick, D. M. (2018). The utility of a brief web-based prevention intervention as a universal approach for risky alcohol use in college students: Evidence of moderation by family history. *Frontiers in Psychology, 9*, 747. doi:10.3389/fpsyg.2018.00747

National Human Genome Research Institute (NHGRI). (2016). The cost of sequencing a genome. Retrieved from https://www.genome.gov/about-genomics/fact-sheets/Sequencing-Human-Genome-Cost.

National Human Genome Research Institute (NHGRI). (2017). Is height determined by genetics? Retrieved from https://ghr.nlm.nih.gov/primer/traits/height

National Human Genome Research Institute (NHGRI). (2018). What is the human genome project? Retrieved from https://www.genome.gov/human-genome-project/What

National Institute on Alcohol Abuse and Alcoholism (NIAAA). (2017). *Underage drinking.* National Institute on Alcohol Abuse and Alcoholism. Retrieved from https://pubs.niaaa.nih.gov/publications/UnderageDrinking/UnderageFact.htm

Olfson, E., Edenberg, H. J., Nurnberger Jr., J., Agrawal, A., Bucholz, K. K., Almasy, L. A., . . . Kramer, J. R. (2014). An ADH1B variant and peer drinking in progression to adolescent drinking milestones: Evidence of a gene-by-environment interaction. *Alcoholism: Clinical and Experimental Research, 38*(10), 2541–2549. doi:10.1111/acer.12524

O'Loughlin, J., Paradis, G., Kim, W., DiFranza, J., Meshefedjian, G., McMillan-Davey, E., . . . Tyndale, R. F. (2004). Genetically decreased CYP2A6 and the risk of tobacco dependence: A prospective study of novice smokers. *Tobacco Control, 13*(4), 422–428. doi:10.1136/tc.2003.007070

Osler, M., Holst, C., Prescott, E., & Sørensen, T. I. (2001). Influence of genes and family environment on adult smoking behavior assessed in an adoption study. *Genetic Epidemiology, 21*(3), 193–200. doi:10.1002/gepi.1028

Plomin, R., DeFries, J., McClearn, G., & McGuffin, P. (2000). *Behavioral genetics.* New York, NY: Worth Publishers.

Psychiatric Genomics Consortium (PGC) Schizophrenia Working Group. (2014). Biological insights from 108 schizophrenia-associated genetic loci. *Nature, 511*(7510), 421–427. doi:10.1038/nature13595

Rose, R. J., Dick, D. M., Viken, R. J., & Kaprio, J. (2001). Gene–environment interaction in patterns of adolescent drinking: Regional residency moderates longitudinal influences on alcohol use. *Alcoholism: Clinical & Experimental Research, 25*(5), 637–643. doi:10.1111/j.1530-0277.2001.tb02261.x

Saccone, S. F., Hinrichs, A. L., Saccone, N. L., Chase, G. A., Konvicka, K., Madden, P. A. F., . . . Bierut, L. J. (2007). Cholinergic nicotinic receptor genes implicated in a nicotine dependence association study targeting 348 candidate genes with 3713 SNPs. *Human Molecular Genetics, 16*(1), 36–49. doi:10.1093/hmg/ddl438

Salvatore, J. E., Aliev, F., Edwards, A. C., Evans, D. M., Macleod, J., Hickman, M., . . . Dick, D. M. (2014). Polygenic scores predict alcohol problems in an independent sample and show moderation by the environment. *Genes (Basel), 5*(2), 330–346. doi:10.3390/genes5020330

Sameroff, A. (2009). *The transactional model of development: How children and contexts shape each other.* Washington, DC: American Psychological Association. doi:10.1037/11877-000

Sartor, C. E., Grant, J. D., Agrawal, A., Sadler, B., Madden, P. A. F., Heath, A. C., & Bucholz, K. K. (2015). Genetic and environmental contributions to initiation of cigarette smoking in young African-American and European-American women. *Drug and Alcohol Dependence, 157*, 54–59. doi:10.1016/j.drugalcdep.2015.10.002

Schneider, S. K., Buka, S. L., Dash, K., Winickoff, J. P., & O'Donnell, L. (2016). Community reductions in youth smoking after raising the minimum tobacco sales age to 21. *Tobacco Control, 25*(3), 355–359. doi:10.1136/tobaccocontrol-2014-052207

Schulenberg, J., Patrick, M. E., Maslowsky, J., & Maggs, J. L. (2014). The epidemiology and etiology of adolescent substance use in developmental perspective. In M. Lewis & K. D. Rudolph (Eds.), *Handbook of developmental psychopathology* (pp. 601–620). Boston, MA: Springer. doi:10.1007/978-1-4614-9608-3_30

Sher, K. J., Dick, D. M., Crabbe, J. C., Hutchison, K. E., O'Malley, S. S., & Heath, A. C. (2010). Consilient research approaches in studying gene × environment interactions in alcohol research. *Addiction Biology, 15*(2), 200–216. doi:10.1111/j.1369-1600.2009.00189.x

Slutske, W. S., Deutsch, A. R., & Piasecki, T. M. (2018). Neighborhood alcohol outlet density and genetic influences on alcohol use: Evidence for gene–environment interaction. *Psychological Medicine, 49*(3), 474–482. doi:10.1017/S0033291718001095

Stahl, E. A., Breen, G., Forstner, A. J., McQuillin, A., Ripke, S., Trubetskoy, V., . . . Sklar, P. (2019). Genome-wide association study identifies 30 loci associated with bipolar disorder. *Nature Genetics, 51*(5), 793–803. doi:10.1038/s41588-019-0397-8

Tekola-Ayele, F., & Rotimi, C. N. (2015). Translational genomics in low- and middle-income countries: Opportunities and challenges. *Public Health Genomics, 18*(4), 242–247. doi:10.1159/000433518

Tishkoff, S. A., Reed, F. A., Friedlaender, F. R., Ehret, C., Ranciaro, A., Froment, A., . . . Doumbo, O. (2009). The genetic structure and history of Africans and African Americans. *Science, 324*(5930), 1035–1044.

Trucco, E. M., Villafuerte, S., Heitzeg, M. M., Burmeister, M., & Zucker, R. A. (2016). Susceptibility effects of GABA receptor subunit alpha-2 (GABRA2) variants and parental monitoring on externalizing behavior trajectories: Risk and protection conveyed by the minor allele. *Developmental Psychopathology, 28*(1), 15–26. doi:10.1017/s0954579415000255

Turkheimer, E. (2000). Three laws of behavior genetics and what they mean. *Current Directions in Psychological Science, 9*(5), 160–164. doi:10.1111/1467-8721.00084

Valdez, R., Coates, R. J., St Pierre, J., Grossniklaus, D., & Khoury, M. J. (2011). Knowledge gaps remain in the use of family health history in public health. *Public Health Genomics, 14*(2), 94–95. doi:10.1159/000294583

Waters, E. A., Ball, L., Carter, K., & Gehlert, S. (2014). Smokers' beliefs about the tobacco control potential of "a gene for smoking": A focus group study. *BMC Public Health, 14*(1), 1218. doi:10.1186/1471-2458-14-1218

Weigl, K., Chang-Claude, J., Knebel, P., Hsu, L., Hoffmeister, M., & Brenner, H. (2018). Strongly enhanced colorectal cancer risk stratification by combining family history and genetic risk score. *Clinical Epidemiology, 10*, 143–152. doi:10.2147/clep.s145636

Werner-Lin, A., McCoyd, J. L., Doyle, M. H., & Gehlert, S. J. (2016). Leadership, literacy, and translational expertise in genomics: Challenges and opportunities for social work. *Health & Social Work, 41*(3), e52–e59. doi:10.1093/hsw/hlw022

Wray, N. R., Ripke, S., Mattheisen, M., Trzaskowski, M., Byrne, E. M., Abdellaoui, A., . . . Sullivan, P. F. (2018). Genome-wide association analyses identify 44 risk variants and refine the genetic architecture of major depression. *Nature Genetics, 50*(5), 668–681. doi:10.1038/s41588-018-0090-3

Yan, J., Aliev, F., Webb, B. T., Kendler, K. S., Williamson, V. S., Edenberg, H. J., . . . Dick, D. M. (2014). Using genetic information from candidate gene and genome-wide association studies in risk prediction for alcohol dependence. *Addiction Biology, 19*(4), 708–721. doi:10.1111/adb.12035

Yoon, P. W., Scheuner, M. T., & Khoury, M. J. (2003). Research priorities for evaluating family history in the prevention of common chronic diseases. *American Journal of Preventive Medicine, 24*(2), 128–135. doi:10.1016/S0749-3797(02)00585-8

Zinn-Justin, A., & Abel, L. (1999). Genome search for alcohol dependence using the weighted pairwise correlation linkage method: Interesting findings on chromosome 4. *Genetic Epidemiology, 17*(Suppl 1), S421–S426. doi:10.1002/gepi.1370170771

Zucker, R. A. (2008). Anticipating problem alcohol use developmentally from childhood into middle adulthood: What have we learned? *Addiction, 103*, 100–108. doi:10.1111/j.1360-0443.2008.02179.x

6

Psychological models of addictive behavior

Audrey L. Begun

Background

A best-practice for planning comprehensive interventions to address substance misuse and other addictive behaviors involves establishing a logic model showing logical connections between a theory of change, designed intervention elements and processes, and intervention outcomes (Fraser, Richman, Galinsky, & Day, 2009). In formulating intervention logic models, practitioners, program planners, policy makers, and evaluators first need to identify the theoretical models that inform their interventions. Previous chapters have detailed theories, models, and evidence regarding the "bio" aspects of the biopsychosocial perspective on addictive behaviors (Chapters 4 and 5). This chapter places emphasis on major psychological theories, models, and evidence that explain or predict the development and persistence of addictive behaviors, as well as theories of change to guide intervention development and implementation. Social context theories and models are presented in Chapter 7.

Psychological models are broadly defined in this chapter. Theories and models related to internal mental processes are included, dealing with thoughts, beliefs, emotions, motivation, and learning. While emphasis is on internal psychological processes, it is critically important to remain aware of the interactive nature of relationships between mind and brain and the inherent difficulty in separating biological and social context processes from psychological processes in an integrated biopsychosocial framework. For example, learning and memory are mental processes both implemented and affected by neurobiological processes and neuroanatomy of the brain—mind and brain influence behavior together (Moreira-Almeida & Santos, 2012). Additionally, internal psychological processes and external environmental contexts represent mutual and iterative forces of influence. For example, experiences with family and other members of the social context shape individuals' thoughts, attitudes, beliefs, values, learning, and behavior, and vice versa: the individual has influence on the social environment, as well. Nine types of theories/models of psychological processes are presented: cognitive, information processing, developmental, psychodynamic, personality, learning/social learning, expectancies, reasoned behavior, and motivation in the change process.

Cognition (cognitive theory)

Cognition is concerned with the mental processes involved in a person's knowledge, thoughts, and understanding of their experiences—both what and how individuals think. As such, cognitive processes have great potential to mediate human behavior. Treatment strategies based on theories or models of the role that cognition plays in addictive behavior (e.g. cognitive behavior[al] therapy, rational emotive therapy, cognitive skill building) have a common assumption: "Certain cognitive, emotional, and social skills are particularly useful for voluntarily steering one's path out of addiction" (Heather et al., 2018, p. 251). Rotgers (2012) identified a set of common basic assumptions among cognitive behavioral (CB) models and interventions related to substance use disorders, most of which could be applied to other forms of addictive behavior:

- human behavior is largely learned;
- learning processes leading to problematic behaviors also apply to changing these behaviors (classical conditioning, operant conditioning, modeling);
- environmental context factors play a major role in determining behavior;
- learning principles apply to changing covert behaviors (e.g. thoughts and feelings), not just overt behaviors;
- critical to changing behavior is the practice of new behaviors within the contexts where they will be performed;
- each individual person is unique and must be assessed with consideration of their experienced contexts;
- "The cornerstone of adequate treatment is a thorough CB assessment" (p. 114); and
- "A strong working alliance is crucial to effective behavior change, regardless of therapy technique" (p. 115).

Figure 6.1 depicts the role cognition plays as a mediator of behavior.

Information processing

The information processing model comes from cognitive psychology and helps explain (1) what a person "knows" about a substance, and (2) how a person's substance use might affect behavior through its influence on perception, short- and long-term memory, and information retrieval. Not only does this model have implications for information/education intervention and how individuals behave while under the acute influence of certain substances, it also has behavior implications for long-term substance use and the period of recovery from a substance use disorder. How information processing relates to other forms of addictive behavior is not yet well understood.

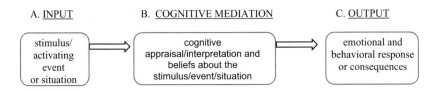

Figure 6.1   Cognitive behavior model (adapted from Ellis, 1991)

Information uptake

For information, stimuli, events, or experiences to have an impact on an individual's behavior, several things need to happen in the processing of the information. First, the person needs to be exposed to the information or other stimulus. Next, the person must attend to and perceive the stimulus through one or more of the five senses. Third, the experience or information needs to be stored in long-term memory, the first step of which involves short-term memory retention, and the second which involves "transfer" to long-term memory. Fourth, to influence behavior, the information must be retrieved at the appropriate time, which involves both the ability to recall the information and the act of retrieval as a response to cues for its application. Under these circumstances and through these mechanisms, available information can positively or negatively influence behavior and performance (Figure 6.2).

Distortion of information processes

In addition to trauma or acute crisis events, psychoactive substances can have profound effects on information processing steps: perception, memory, and retrieval. For example, information processing is slowed among men exhibiting chronic excessive alcohol consumption compared to men who do not drink alcohol excessively, beginning with perception and carrying through the decision-making and response (behavior) phases (Kaur, Walia, Grewal, & Negpal, 2016). Fortunately, affected cognitive functions improve in many individuals during months to years of abstinent recovery (Cabé et al., 2015). In addition, evidence suggests that individuals in early recovery may not effectively process information delivered through treatment/intervention efforts with a heavy cognitive component—these strategies are better processed a few weeks into recovery (NIAAA, 2001). Furthermore, evidence concerning state-dependent learning suggests that retrieval of information learned while under the influence of alcohol or other substances may be more difficult when a person is in a different (normal) state of consciousness than while under the influence of the same or similar substances; vice versa, what is learned under normal conditions may not be recalled when in an altered state (Overton, 1984). Thus, a person in recovery may need to relearn what was originally learned while under the influence of substances.

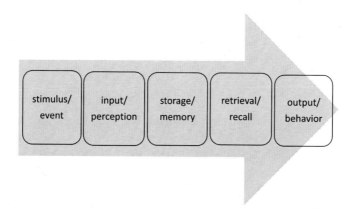

Figure 6.2 Information processing model

Developmental theory

Developmental theory and science related to addictive behavior comes in two major forms: life course development impact and developmental trajectories of addiction. These both are examined next.

Impact of addictive behavior on life course development and addictive behavior

Engaging in addictive behavior at different points in the life course has differential potential impact on subsequent development. While exposure to substances at any developmental period is potentially influential, certain periods are more sensitive than others to persistent developmental impact. For example, as discussed in Chapters 10, 11, and 12, the entire prenatal/fetal development period is characterized by peak sensitivity for persistent cognitive, physical, and neurobehavioral challenges related to exposure to alcohol and other substances. Or, for example, the risk of developing a substance use disorder in the cases of tobacco, alcohol, or cannabis is "robustly associated" with early first use of these substances (Richmond-Rakerd et al., 2016). Evidence also indicates that among U.S. adolescents and emerging adults (aged 13–21 years), for each year that initiation of substance use was delayed, the lifetime likelihood of developing a substance use disorder declined by 4–5% (Grant & Dawson, 1998).

Investigators reported that alcohol use disorder during adolescence predicted substance use disorder (alcohol or other drugs) and symptoms of other psychiatric disorders (depression and antisocial personality disorder) at age 24 years in a U.S. general population sample (Rohde, Lewinsoh, Kahler, Seeley, & Brown, 2001). Similarly, in a German general population sample, repeated (cumulative) cannabis use during adolescence and emerging adulthood (14–24 years old) predicted persistent cannabis use 10 years later (2.8 times higher risk); using other illicit substances as well compounded the risk (4.4 times), and cannabis dependence in the initial period remained relatively stable 10 years later (Perkonigg et al., 2007). Despite these reported odds, it is important to note that the probability was never 100%: many individuals eventually decreased or stopped their use/misuse of these substances over time.

Developmental trajectories of addictive behaviors

During the 1950s and 1960s E. Morton Jellinek concluded that the "disease" of alcoholism follows a four-stage natural course that can be applied as a typology to describe drinking behavior patterns: pre-alcoholic, early alcoholic, middle alcoholic, and late alcoholic. He argued that these stages are qualitatively different from one another and described symptoms associated with each. His work was based on retrospective surveys completed by men recruited through Alcoholics Anonymous (AA) programs. A great deal of criticism followed in the literature (see Chapter 1), noting that the trajectory of progressive worsening is not universal across the population, a great deal of clinical heterogeneity exists (Moss, Chen, & Yi, 2007), and weaknesses in the data and methodology Jellinek used. More recent studies demonstrated the dynamic, constantly changing nature of addictive behaviors: "Addiction can be viewed as a trajectory that emerges, becomes ingrained, and then in most cases evolves further (people quit or learn to control their use) over time" (Heather et al., 2018, p. 251). Yakhnich and Michael (2016) described the trajectory as a process beginning with occasional use of substances and ending with addiction, recognizing that many individuals "mature out" of excessive use at points along the trajectory.

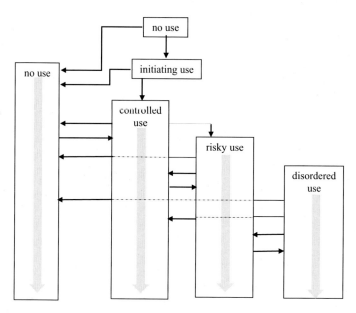

Figure 6.3   Developmental trajectories of substance use

A 60-year longitudinal study of college-aged men whose drinking patterns were identified as "alcoholism" demonstrated widely varied patterns in later adulthood, including stable abstinence, non-problematic/controlled drinking, alcohol abuse, or death (Vaillant, 2003). A typical substance misuse trajectory begins during adolescence or emerging adulthood, declines or escalates during emerging and early adulthood—where it may or may not meet criteria for a substance use disorder—then either declines or extends into adulthood, possibly but not necessarily meeting criteria as a substance use disorder (see Figure 6.3).

The important aspects of this diagram are: (1) the multiple pathways/trajectories that occur, and (2) the iterative nature of the trajectories, such as moving back and forth between controlled, risky, disordered, and no use. It is also important to note that the probability of different trajectories is affected by a host of individual-specific factors, as well as the "addictive potential" of different substances involved (Upah, Jacob, & Price, 2015) and individuals' different histories of change attempts over the life course (Begun, Berger, & Salm-Ward, 2011). Similarly, no single, "natural" trajectory to/through recovery exists, and there are a multitude of addiction "careers" in individuals' relationships or involvement with substances over their lifetimes following the emergence of a substance use disorder (DiClemente, 2006).

Multiple factors play a role in "positive outcome" trajectories, including engaging in treatment. For example, U.S. combat veterans who experienced both posttraumatic stress disorder and hazardous drinking behavior (alcohol) were less likely to continue hazardous drinking despite persistent/unremitting PTSD symptoms 11 months later if they had engaged in treatment addressing their alcohol use, particularly if they also had experienced negative consequences associated with their heavy drinking (Possemato et al., 2017). The field also recognizes "natural" recovery is a studied phenomenon whereby many individuals change their problematic alcohol or other substance use without engagement of formal treatment systems (DiClemente, 2006; Robins, 1993; Sobell, Ellingstad, & Sobell, 2000), or by combining formal, informal, and natural recovery systems in their change efforts (Begun et al., 2011).

Psychodynamic theory

Cavaiola (2009) summarized three facets of psychodynamic and psychoanalytic models of substance misuse and addiction. First, oral addictive behaviors (e.g. drinking, smoking) might be explained in terms of individuals' reactions to fixation caused by either over or under stimulation of the oral zone during the oral stage of psychosexual development. Second, substance misuse may be an attempt to escape the intrapsychic conflict caused by tension between the uncensored id and an overly harsh super ego. Third, substance misuse could be an attempt to cope with the formation of insecure attachments early in childhood or ego deficits/personality defects (see section below on personality theory). This rationale underlies the self-medication hypothesis of substance misuse: individuals turn to substance use (and perhaps other addictive behaviors) to "numb" the psychic pain that results from insecure attachment or ego deficits. This line of thinking has been extended to the experience of trauma more generally—not only are the events contributing to insecure attachment and ego deficits, other psychically traumatizing experiences may also account for a person's attempts to self-medicate or engage in addictive behaviors that may reflect a form of self-destructive behavior in response to psychic trauma and conflict (McNeece & DiNitto, 2012).

One problem with relying on psychodynamic theories of addictive behavior is that the mechanisms and constructs involved are difficult to operationalize and difficult to objectively measure in systematic research efforts; thus, "empirical support of psychodynamic theory is scanty" (McNeece & DiNitto, 2012, p. 28). A second problem with these theories is that the presumed "causes" are experienced by a large number of individuals who do not engage in problematic substance use or other addictive behaviors. Third, the historical events are so distant from expression of the problem with addictive behaviors (even by decades), that retrospective accounts are heavily relied on in research, despite their methodological limitations. Fourth, in terms of implications for treatment: "Many counselors warn that a nondirective approach that focuses solely on the patients' development of insight into their problems neglects the addictive power of alcohol or other drugs" (McNeece & DiNitto, 2012, p. 28). However, intervention based on psychodynamic principles *may* be appropriately combined with other forms of intervention that address additional aspects of the problem (McNeece & DiNitto, 2012).

Personality theory

Some evidence exists to suggest that certain personality traits are more common among individuals who misuse substances compared to others—particularly in terms of low levels of conscientiousness and high levels of phobia, impulsivity/disinhibition, difficulty delaying gratification, disagreeableness, sensation seeking, valuing nonconformity/tolerance of deviance, social alienation, antisocial behavior, and a sense of heightened stress (Kotov, Gamez, Schmidt, & Watson, 2010; Nathan, 1988). These common personality and antisocial behavior traits, however, are not conclusive evidence for the existence of a predisposing "addictive personality" described in some clinical literature, nor are they supportive of antisocial personality as a precursor to a substance use disorder (Nathan, 1988). These traits appear in association with multiple disorders, as well as among persons who never develop any disorders (Kotov et al., 2010). Instead of personality, these represent either vulnerability factors for developing problems with substance use (Franques, Auriacombe, &

Tignol, 2000) or sequelae of substance misuse. The take-home messages about personality and addictive behavior are:

- "Within the field of substance abuse, it is now widely admitted that the addictive personality does not exist" (Franques et al., 2000, p. 68); and
- "The term addictive personality needs to be retired permanently from use by the alcohol and drug (AOD) treatment field. The term engenders confusion and misunderstanding and undermines our ability to help individuals with AOD problems" (Amodeo, 2015, p. 1031).

Learning theory

Learning theory presents both classical and operant conditioning processes as explanation of how addictive behavior patterns might develop, be maintained and become extinguished. It also reflects an intersection between psychological, social, and biological mechanisms, as learning (psychological) evidenced by changes within the brain (biological) results from interactions with the environment (social).

Classical conditioning

Classical conditioning principles help explain how environmental cues might trigger a person's craving to engage in an addictive behavior that has previously been experienced positively. Just as Pavlov's dogs developed an anticipatory salivation response to a previously unpaired stimulus (a ringing bell) when it was repeatedly associated with food, a person might develop a conditioned response to stimuli associated with an addictive substance or activity seeing a cold, foamy glass of beer on television might trigger a person's anticipation of the feelings experienced with drinking (a drinking craving); holding poker chips or dice might trigger a person's learned gambling urge; being around drug paraphernalia or people with whom one used drugs in the past might trigger a person's anticipatory craving to use again.

Environmental cues can become craving triggers through classical conditioning processes, with exposure to those triggering cues increasing the risk of relapse to engage in the addictive behavior again. This is called a cue-induced response (see Figure 6.4). Triggering cues may involve any combination of the five senses (sight, sound, taste, feel, and smell) or internal states (e.g. anxiety, loneliness, boredom, depression, mania). For example, a woman in treatment for substance use disorder described loud rock music as a trigger for her craving to use alcohol and marijuana because she first "learned" to enjoy these substances at rock concerts. Regardless of its nature, craving cues trigger "abnormally strong desires to engage in addictive behaviours," though not necessarily leading to subsequent use (Heather, 2017, p. 32).

One goal in cognitive behavioral therapy (CBT) is to help individuals identify their personal triggers and develop strategies for managing situations where these might be encountered. This is an important consideration, as craving cues are often person-specific: what serves as a craving cue to one person might be neutral to another.

Cue-exposure treatment is also based on the classical conditioning learning model of addictive behavior where the circumstances surrounding substance use become paired with the unconditioned response to the substance use. Exposures to the circumstances "may generate craving and motivate drug-seeking behavior" (Conklin & Tiffany, 2002, p. 156). The logic

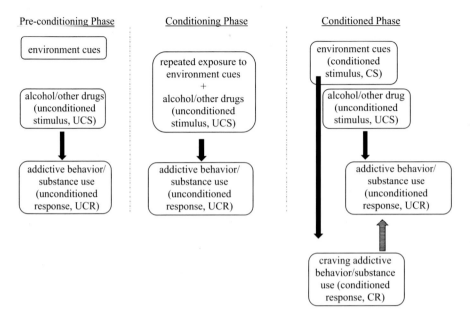

Figure 6.4 Classical conditioning of craving cues and relapse triggers

behind cue-exposure treatment is that carefully guided, repeated exposure of an individual to the triggering stimuli, without that individual experiencing the unconditioned response, will eventually break the conditioned link, thereby reducing the power of the stimuli to trigger craving and relapse to use. However, "unlearning" is less likely than "re-learning" through classical conditioning processes. In other words, the original learned association continues to exist once developed, but new, competing associations may be introduced through cue-replacement methods. A meta-analytic review concluded that little systematic evidence exists for the consistent effectiveness of cue-exposure addiction treatment alone (Conklin & Tiffany, 2002).

Operant conditioning

In this model, initiation of an addictive behavior is presumed to be a voluntary choice (e.g. beginning to drink alcohol or engage in gambling activities). The consequences experienced when engaging in that behavior determine the future probability of repeating or continuing to engage in that behavior. Operant conditioning functions through reinforcement paradigms (see Figure 6.5). Two types of consequences reinforce (reward) behavior—delivering a positive stimulus or removing a negative stimulus—and two types punish the behavior— delivering a negative stimulus or removing a positive stimulus. Reinforcing consequences increase the probability of repeating the behavior and punishing consequences decrease that probability. For example, when an adolescent experiences peer approval for sharing a smoke with them, combined with the positive feelings nicotine induces, smoking is positively reinforced; when a person experiencing high levels of stress or anxiety finds that using marijuana removes those negative emotions, marijuana use is negatively reinforced; when a person becomes sick from drinking excessive amounts of alcohol, binge drinking is punished. Unfortunately, experiencing acute withdrawal symptoms when abstaining from use of an addictive

Label	Consequence	Effect
Positive Reinforcement	provide favorable stimulus (reward)	increased probability of repeating behavior
Negative Reinforcement	remove unfavorable stimulus (reward)	increased probability of repeating behavior
Punishment	provide unfavorable stimulus _or_ remove favorable stimulus	decreased probability of repeating behavior

Figure 6.5   Reinforcement paradigm in operant conditioning

substance punishes abstinence challenges a person's attempts to avoid the addictive behavior that has previously been rewarding.

In theory, a learned behavior can also be extinguished through applying a different reinforcement paradigm. In other words, if a person ceases to experience the "positive" consequences of engaging in an addictive behavior, over time the person learns to no longer engage in that behavior. This is the logic behind some of the medications developed to treat substance use disorders (see Chapter 19). For example, naltrexone acts to block the "high" a person is used to experiencing when drinking alcohol, thus reducing or eliminating the positive reinforcement associated with drinking. Over time, the individual who continues to drink learns that drinking is no longer pleasurable, thus reducing the urge to engage in this particular addictive behavior—a form of behavior extinction.

A medication like disulfiram (e.g. Antabuse) operates on a different set of operant conditioning principles. A person dosed with disulfiram will quickly develop unpleasant physical effects from consuming alcohol—intense flushing, nausea/vomiting, headache, and heart palpitations. The negative, punishing consequence "teaches" the person an aversion to drinking alcohol. This treatment, however, is only effective if the medication is consistently taken, so that the punishment is consistently experienced in association with drinking. Intermittent reinforcement interferes significantly with the learned extinction process.

A tricky aspect of operant conditioning is that rewards and punishments can be somewhat idiosyncratic to the individual: what is rewarding to some is not to others. Second, the sequence of consequences is an important consideration. If a reinforcing consequence (e.g. peer approval) is experienced first, then a punishing consequence (e.g. hangover) comes later, the first consequence may have greater influence over future behavior. Another tricky aspect has to do with the timing of consequences: if too much time passes between the behavior and the consequence, the power of the consequence to shape behavior is weakened. This can, to some extent, be attenuated in humans through use of cognitive mechanisms and symbolic rewards, such as tokens delivered immediately that lead to a tangible reward later. These operant conditioning principles underlie contingency management (CM) therapy where abstinence behaviors are reinforced through material rewards.

Social learning theory

Social learning theory, initially proposed by Albert Bandura, represents an extension of learning theory based on how learning differs among human beings compared to animal models where learning theory was originally refined. The major relevant principles relate to principles surrounding observational learning. First, humans can learn by observing others' behavior and its consequences; they do not need to experience the consequences themselves, first-hand. Second, humans learn complex behaviors by observing and imitating behaviors modeled by others. Observational learning not only teaches specific behaviors but can also transfer to entire class of behaviors. For example, smoking cigarettes might be the specific behavior modeled, but the observer may learn a general class of smoking behaviors (cigarettes, marijuana, hookah, e-cigarettes) as a result. Social learning theory informs interventions designed to shape the learning environment—providing "positive" behavior models, removing "negative" behavior models, and emphasizing positive consequences experienced by positive behavior models and negative consequences experienced by negative behavior models. Many scholars place social learning theory in the social context domain; behavior models are part of the experienced social environment, but internal psychological processes determine their impact on individual behavior which explains why here it is included with psychological models.

An important consideration in social learning theory concerns the salience of behavior models to the individual learning through observation. A person is likely to imitate behaviors exhibited by others who they deem relevant and highly salient to themselves. For some individuals, this might be a parent, sibling, or other close family member. For others, these potential models may be less salient than peer models or models presented in the media (e.g. television, movies, music, social media). Observing consequences experienced by behavior models helps establish expectancies about the likely results of engaging in those behaviors themselves.

Expectancies

Expectancies help explain why individuals opt to engage in certain behaviors. This model relies on cognitive processes where the individual evaluates the likely outcomes and consequences of engaging in a specific behavior. For example, if a person expects to feel exhilaration from using a certain drug, the probability of using it increases. However, if a person expects to feel sick or to be shamed or punished if caught using that drug, the probability of using it decreases. Evidence generally, but not entirely consistently, supports the association between alcohol use expectancies and drinking outcomes (Jones, Corbin, & Fromme, 2001): expecting positive consequences is associated with greater consumption, and expecting negative consequences is associated with lower consumption. Furthermore, several studies demonstrated that holding negative alcohol expectancies is associated with better alcohol treatment outcomes compared to having positive drinking consequence expectancies at treatment initiation (Jones et al., 2001).

An important aspect of expectancies concerns where these expectancy conclusions originate. This is, where the model connects to social learning. Expectancies may develop from observing consequences experienced by others. Expectancies may also develop from direct messages delivered through public awareness/education efforts. An individual's expectancies are learned from an early age—young children have demonstrated both positive and negative drinking expectancies (Donovan, Molina, & Kelly, 2009)—and "positive expectancies of alcohol's effects predict initiation of drinking, intention to drink, and drinking rates among middle-school students" (Hesselbrock & Hesselbrock, 2006, p. 101). Another important aspect of expectancies is that individuals are presented with many conflicting messages, resulting in decisional dilemmas that they need to resolve concerning the relative salience and prioritization of the different messages received. This leads to consideration of the health beliefs and behavioral economics models described next.

Theories of rational, reasoned, or planned behavior

A group of theories and models explain addictive behaviors in terms of individuals making reasoned, rational decisions about using substances—substance use and not using are intentional choices. Different theories in this category focus on different aspects of these choices. Models relying on reasoned action processes assume that behavior is directly determined by a person's intentions—influencing intentions is a means of influencing behavioral choices—and intentions are influenced by attitudes, beliefs, expectancies, and social norms about the behavior choices.

Health beliefs model

The health beliefs model underlies a great deal of public health intervention logic. In essence, the model suggests that choices individuals make regarding health-affecting behaviors (e.g. using substances or quitting their use) depend on the person's beliefs concerning the relative advantages and disadvantages of those behaviors. Six principles related to this model are that individuals evaluate (LaMorte, 2018): (a) their perceived susceptibility to the risks associated with the behavior; (b) their perceptions about the severity of the associated risks; (c) the perceived benefits of the behavior and of alternatives to the behavior; (d) perceived barriers to engaging in a recommended action; (e) the presence of cues to engage in such an analysis (e.g. symptoms) and take positive action; and (f) sense of self-efficacy for successfully engaging in recommended behaviors. Educational and informational interventions are founded on health belief model premises where the expectation is that people will choose healthy behavior alternatives if they are provided information about what is good and bad for them by someone they trust, awareness of their personal risks and cues to action, and how they can be effective in promoting their own health.

While health beliefs model interventions can address knowledge aspects of health-related behaviors, they are not sufficient to address other factors influencing addictive behaviors. Cognitive processes operate within the complex of biological (addictive) processes, learning and social learning processes, potentially impaired information processing, and the other psychological and social factors discussed in this chapter.

Behavioral economics theory

Like the health beliefs model, behavioral economics theory relies on persons making rational decisions, choosing between their available behavioral options. Specifically, a person decides to engage in an addictive behavior if perceiving it as a course of action that will meet a need better than other available options (McNeece & DiNitto, 2012). Research in this arena points to a number of factors that potentially bias decisions when the "default" decision is a clear, rational choice (e.g. not engaging in unhealthy behaviors). Samson (2018) summarizes the literature by including these factors: (a) the prospect of giving something up is harder to accept than the prospect of what will be gained; (b) limited knowledge or understanding of elements involved; (c) affect and feelings about the options; (d) uneven salience of the different pieces of information and options; (e) inertia and pressure to maintain the "status quo;" (f) perceptions about time and timeliness regarding the options and their potential outcomes; (g) optimism/pessimism about the options and their own self-efficacy for each; (h) the experienced social context, social norms, and social pressures; and (i) cognitive dissonance in terms of "goodness-of-fit" each option holds regarding their own self-perceptions.

Behavioral economic decisions are individual- and situation-specific; decisions made in one context are not necessarily generalizable to other situations, even by the same individual. This kind of model informs intervention development either by changing the cost-benefit ratio (e.g. increasing price of substances such as through taxes or reduced availability), or helping individuals re-value the costs and benefits of engaging in addictive behaviors (Murphy, MacKillop, Vuchinic, & Tucker, 2012). In addition, evidence suggests that where individuals place the relative cost and benefit values (their demand curves) may predict problem severity and responsiveness to treatment (Murphy et al., 2012).

Motivation and behavior change process

Since the 1980s, health psychologists and scholars in many disciplines have gathered and analyzed a great deal of data describing the process of change engaged by individuals experiencing problematic addictive or other intentional behaviors (e.g. tobacco or alcohol use; intimate partner violence), as well as persons attempting to initiate health-promoting behaviors (e.g. dieting or exercising). This category is not about the etiology or development of problematic addictive behavior but concerns the mechanisms by which these problematic behaviors might be changed. Because the observations and conclusions regarding the processes by which people change cross theoretical, intervention model, and disciplinary lines, it is titled a transtheoretical model of behavior change (TMBC), first proposed by Carlo DiClemete and James Prochaska (see, e.g. Prochaska, DiClemente, & Norcross, 1992).

Motivation to change one's addictive behavior is an important aspect of intervention logic models based on the presumption that these are intentional behaviors with the potential to be intentionally changed. Three principles come together in the TMBC to inform "best fit" strategies for intentionally changing behavior: decisional balance, self-efficacy for change, and stages of the change process. These concepts underlie motivational interviewing practices and interventions (e.g. motivational enhancement therapy), as well as efforts to match specific treatment strategies to change readiness and motivation.

Decisional balance

Decisional balance is about the four forces operating simultaneously as individuals contemplate making a change in behavior—engaging or not engaging in an addictive behavior, for example (see Figure 6.6). Exploring all four facets of decisional balance plays a significant role in motivational interviewing.

Self-efficacy for change

At the same time individuals are mentally calculating the pros and cons of both changing and not changing their addictive behavior, they develop estimations regarding their ability to make a desired change come into play. These estimations reflect their sense of self-efficacy for changing the behavior: low self-efficacy impedes the change process; high self-efficacy helps.

Forces against Change	Forces for Change
Positive aspects/consequences of not changing; positives of the behavior	Negative aspects/consequences of the behavior
Negative aspects of changing the behavior	Positive aspects/consequences of changing the behavior
Low self-efficacy for making change	High self-efficacy for making change

Figure 6.6 Decisional balance and self-efficacy factors for and against behavior change

Stages of change

The stages of change element of the TMBC summarizes much of the data: each of five stages in the change process is characterized by certain beliefs, attitudes, intentions, and behaviors (Connors, DiClemente, Velasquez, & Donovan, 2013). It is important to note that individuals do not necessarily move in a linear progression through the stages: "In the addictions, cycling or recycling is normative—individuals often 'successfully' attempt to change a problem numerous times before the change is stable" (Connors et al., 2013, p. 13). Precontemplation actually precedes any change orientation—it is characterized by either a lack of recognizing that a problem exists or a lack of self-efficacy for making change. The next stages are contemplation, preparation for action, action, and maintenance. Relapse is recognized as a commonly occurring feature of the overall change process and is best viewed as an opportunity to learn from the event to support the change goals rather than as a failed change attempt. A great deal of literature describes these stages and associated intervention approaches for work with individuals and groups (e.g. Connors et al., 2013; Velasquez, Crouch, Stephens, & DiClemente, 2016).

Conclusions

Various psychological models explaining the development or maintenance of problematic addictive behaviors, and/or mechanisms of change, help inform the logic behind interventions applied by social workers and other health, behavioral health, and mental health professionals. These psychological models include processes related to thoughts, beliefs, motivation, and learned behavior. It is important to keep in mind that they operate in conjunction with biological and social context forces.

References

Amodeo, M. (2015). The addictive personality. *Substance Use & Misuse, 50,* 1031–1036.

Begun, A. L., Berger, L. K., & Salm-Ward, T.C. (2011). Using a lifecourse context for exploring alcohol change attempts and treatment efforts among individuals with alcohol dependency. *Journal of Social Work Practice in the Addictions, 11*(2), 101–123. doi:10.1080/1533256X.2011.567945

Cabé, N., Laniepce, A., Ritz, L., Lannuzel, C., Boudehent, C., Bavret, F., . . . Pitel, A. L. (2015). Cognitive impairments in alcohol dependence: From screening to treatment improvements. *Encepahle, 42*(1), 74–81. (English translation).

Cavaiola, A. A. (2009). Psychological models of addiction. In G. L. Fisher & N. A. Roget (Eds.), *Encyclopedia of substance abuse prevention, treatment, & recovery* (pp. 720–723). Los Angeles, CA: Sage.

Conklin, C. A., & Tiffany, S. T. (2002). Applying extinction research and theory to cue-exposure addiction treatments. *Addiction, 97,* 155–167. doi:10.1046/j.1360-0443.2002.00014.x

Connors, G. J., DiClemente, C. C., Velasquez, M. M., & Donovan, D. M. (2013). *Substance abuse treatment and the stages of change: Selecting and planning interventions* (2nd ed.). New York, NY: Guilford.

DiClemente, C. C. (2006). Natural change and the troublesome use of substances: A life-course perspective. In W. R. Miller & K. M. Carroll (Eds.), *Rethinking substance abuse: What the science shows, and what we should do about it* (pp. 81–96). New York, NY: Guilford.

Donovan, J. E., Molina, B. S. G., & Kelly, T. M. (2009). Alcohol outcome expectancies as socially shared and socialized beliefs. *Psychology of Addictive Behaviors, 32*(2), 248–259. doi:10.1037/a0015061

Ellis, A. (1991). The revised ABC's of rational-emotive therapy (RET). *Journal of Rational-Emotive and Cognitive-Behavior Therapy, 9*(3), 139–172. doi:10.1007/BF01061227

Franques, P., Auriacombe, M., & Tignol, J. (2000). Addiction and personality. *Encephale, 26*(1), 68–78. (Translation from French). Retrieved from https://www.ncbi.nlm.nih.gov/pubmed/10875064

Fraser, J. W., Richman, J. M., Galinsky, M. J., & Day, S. H. (2009). *Intervention research: Developing social programs.* New York, NY: Oxford University Press, Pocket Guides to Social Work Research Methods.

Grant, B. F., & Dawson, D. A. (1998). Age of onset of drug use and its association with DSM-IV drug abuse and dependence: Results from the national longitudinal alcohol epidemiologic survey. *Journal of Substance Abuse, 10*(2), 163–173. doi:10.1016/S0899-3289(99)80131-X

Heather, N. (2017). Is the concept of compulsion useful in the explanation or description of addictive behavior and experience? *Addictive Behavior Reports, 6*, 15–38. doi:10.1016/j.abrep.2017.05.002

Heather, N., Best, D., Kawalek, A., Field, M., Lewis, M., Rotgers, F., . . . Heim, D. (2018). Challenging the brain disease model of addiction: European launch of the addiction theory network. *Addiction Research & Theory, 26*(4), 249–255. doi:10.1080/16066359.2017.1399659

Hesselbrock, V. M., & Hesselbrock, M. N. (2006). Developmental perspectives on the risk for developing substance abuse problems. In W. R. Miller & K. M. Carroll (Eds.), *Rethinking substance abuse: What the science shows, and what we should do about it*. New York, NY: Guilford.

Jones, B. T., Corbin, W., & Fromme, K. (2001). A review of expectancy theory and alcohol consumption. *Addiction, 96*(1), 57–72. doi:10.1046/j.1360-0443.2001.961575.x

Kaur, V., Walia, L., Grewal, S., & Negpal, S. (2016). A comparative study of information processing time in chronic alcoholic and non-alcoholic men. *International Journal of Research in Medical Sciences, 4*(11), 4812–4815. doi:10.18203/2320-6012.ijrms20163771

Kotov, R., Gamez, W., Schmidt, F., & Watson, D. (2010). Linking "big" personality traits to anxiety, depressive, and substance use disorders: A meta-analysis. *Psychological Bulletin, 136*(5), 768–821. doi:10.1037/a0020327

LaMorte, W. W. (2018). Behavioral change models: The health beliefs model. Retrieved from http://sphweb.bumc.bu.edu/otlt/MPH-Modules/SB/BehavioralChangeTheories/BehavioralChange-Theories2.html

McNeece, C. A., & DiNitto, D. M. (2012). *Chemical dependency: A systems approach* (4th ed.). New York, NY: Pearson.

Moreira-Almeida, A., & Santos, F. S. (Eds.). (2012). *Exploring frontiers of the mind-brain relationship*. New York, NY: Springer. doi:10.1007/978-1-4614-0647-1

Moss, H. B., Chen, C. M., & Yi, H. Y. (2007). Subtypes of alcohol dependence in a nationally representative sample. *Drug and Alcohol Dependence, 91*, 149–158. doi:10.1016/j.drugalcdep.2007.05.016

Murphy, J. G., MacKillop, J., Vuchinic, R. E., & Tucker, J. A. (2012). The behavioral economics of substance abuse. In S. T. Walters & F. Rotgers (Eds.), *Treating substance abuse: Theory and technique* (pp. 48–80). New York, NY: Guilford.

Nathan, P. E. (1988). The addictive personality is the behavior of the addict. *Journal of Consulting and Clinical Psychology, 56*(2), 183–188. doi:10.1037/0022-006X.56.2.183

National Institute on Alcohol Abuse and Alcoholism (NIAAA). (2001). *Cognitive impairment and recovery from alcoholism*. Alcohol Alert, No. 53. Rockville, MD: U.S. Department of Health and Human Services.

Overton, D. A. (1984). State dependent learning and drug discriminations. In L. L. Iverson, S. D. Iverson, & S. Snyder (Eds.), *Drugs, neurotransmitters, and behavior* (pp. 59–127). New York, NY: Springer. doi:10.1007/978-1-4615-7178-0_2

Perkonigg, A., Goodwin, R. D., Fiedler, A., Behrendt, S., Beesdo, K., Lieb, R., & Wittchen, H. U. (2007). The natural course of cannabis use, abuse and dependence during the first decades of life. *Addiction, 103*, 439–449. doi:10.1111/j.1360-0443.2007.02064.x

Possemato, K., Maisto, S. A., Wade, M., Barrie, K., Johnson, E. M., & Ouimette, P. C. (2017). Natural course of co-occurring PTSD and alcohol use disorder among recent combat veterans. *Journal of Traumatic Stress, 30*, 279–287. doi:10.1002/jts.22192

Prochaska, J. O., DiClemente, C. C., & Norcross, J. C. (1992). In search of how people change: Applications to addictive behaviors. *American Psychologist, 47*, 1102–1114. doi:10.1037/0003-066X.47.9.1102

Richmond-Rakerd, L.S., Slutske, W.S., Lynskey, M.T., Agrawal, A., Maddern, P.A.F., Bucholz, K.K., . . . Martin, N. G. (2016). Age at first use and later substance use disorder: Shared genetic and environmental pathways for nicotine, alcohol, and cannabis. *Journal of Abnormal Psychology, 125*(7), 946–959. doi:10.1037/abn0000191

Robins, L. N. (1993). Vietnam veterans' rapid recovery from heroin addiction: A fluke or normal expectation? *Addiction, 88*(8), 1041–1054. doi:10.1111/j.1360-0443.1993.tb02123.x

Rohde, P., Lewinsoh, P. M., Kahler, C. W., Seeley, J. R., & Brown, R. A. (2001). Natural course of alcohol use disorder from adolescence to young adulthood. *Journal of the American Academy of Child & Adolescent Psychiatry, 40*(1), 83–90. doi:10.1097/00004583-200101000-00020

Rotgers, F. (2012). Cognitive-behavioral theories of substance abuse. In S. T. Walters & F. Rotgers (Eds.), *Treating substance abuse: Theory and technique* (3rd ed., pp. 113–137). New York, NY: Guilford.

Samson, A. (2018). An introduction to behavioral economics. Retrieved from https://www.behavioral economics.com/resources/introduction-behavioral-economics/

Sobell, L. C., Ellingstad, T. P., & Sobell, M. B. (2000). Natural recovery from alcohol and drug problems: Methodological review of the research with suggestions for future directions. *Addiction, 95*(5), 749–764. doi:10.1046/j.1360-0443.2000.95574911.x

Upah, R., Jacob, T., & Price, R. K. (2015). Trajectories of lifetime comorbid alcohol and other drug use disorders through midlife. *Journal of Studies on Alcohol and Drugs, 76*, 721–732. doi:10.15288/jsad.2015.76.721

Vaillant, G. (2003). A 60-year follow-up of alcoholic men. *Addiction, 98*, 1043–1051. doi:10.1046/j.1360-0443.2003.00422.x

Velasquez, M. M., Crouch, C., Stephens, N. S., & DiClemente, C. C. (2016). *Group treatment for substance abuse: A stages-of-change therapy manual* (2nd ed.). New York, NY: Guilford Press.

Yakhnich, L., & Michael, K. (2016). Trajectories of drug abuse and addiction development among FSU immigrant drug users in Israel. *Journal of Cross-Cultural Psychology, 47*(8), 1130–1153. doi:10.1177/0022022116660764

Social environmental contexts
of addictive behavior

Audrey L. Begun, Cristina B. Bares and Karen G. Chartier

Background

The social context of human development and behavior represents one of three pillars in the biopsychosocial framework so critical to social work and other disciplines/professions. In social work, this is partially reflected in the person-in-environment perspective. Scholars sometimes refer to sociocultural theories of human development, addressing the impact on individual behavior of interactions with social systems: family, peers, communities, institutions, and other actors in the social environment. However necessary to understanding and intervening around addictive behaviors, "sociocultural" and person-in-environment theories alone are not sufficient to carry the full weight of the biopsychosocial framework's "social" domain. Broader environmental or ecological thinking incorporates multiple levels of social and physical context factors—for instance, social determinants of health is a contemporary term encompassing "conditions in the places where people live, learn, work, and play [that] affect a wide range of health risks and outcomes" (CDC, 2018). Contributing to the complex biopsychosocial understanding of how addictive behaviors develop, are maintained, and ultimately change is consideration of the myriad social and physical environments everyone is exposed to, and that can be either protective against or "predisposing" toward substance use and related problems (Kendler & Eaves, 1986).

This kind of environmental or ecological perspective provides a useful lens through which to view the interactions between various micro-, meso-, and macro-level factors in their influences on addictive behavior. The social and physical contexts represent mechanisms through which the environment may modify individuals' genetic and other biological vulnerability or resilience around engaging in addictive behaviors such as substance misuse and developing a substance use disorder (see Chapters 4, 5, and 39). For instance, social and environmental factors may compound biological and psychological vulnerabilities or impart resilience by invoking constraints or triggers, thereby operating to enable, trigger, disrupt, or strengthen biological or psychological effects.

In this chapter, we examine several theories and models of sociocultural, social context, and physical environment for their relevance to understanding addictive behavior, particularly substance misuse and substance use disorders. The chapter first introduces key concepts: social determinants, circularity of influence, environmental impact mechanisms (social control, social triggers), and proximal versus distal factors. Next explored are principles and examples concerning the role of social systems, social norms, and stigma, followed by an analysis of how environments and genetics interact to influence substance use outcomes. Several specific social domains are identified (family systems, supervision, relationships; peers and relationships with delinquent peers; school and workplace; neighborhood and community; culture; and policy) and conclusions with relevance to social work and other professions are presented.

Key concepts

Social determinants

Social determinants of health (SDOH) include a wide range of social, economic, and environmental forces that influence population health outcomes (Browne et al., 2017). A phenomenon such as poverty has a pervasive influence on health outcomes (CDC, 2018), largely through its impact on behavior, exposure, and opportunity. For example, poverty, with its accompanying adversities and deprivations may create an experience of chronic stress, which is a known contributor to substance misuse and relapse (Shaw, Egan, & Gillespie, 2007; Sinha, 2008). In addition, drug trafficking in neighborhoods experiencing high poverty levels enhances individuals' access to substances and exposure to models of substance misuse behavior. Furthermore, low-income communities are disproportionately targeted with alcohol and tobacco marketing (Scott, Cohen, Schonlau, Farley, & Bluthenthal, 2008) and poverty may affect access to treatment for substance-related problems. These examples demonstrate that social determinants of health can be important intervention targets: health behaviors and health outcomes (such as substance misuse and its consequences) can be altered by directly or indirectly influencing relevant social determinants (Browne et al., 2017). For instance, among American Indian adults in one community whose families received income supplement payments when they were adolescents (as a result of casino operations in their community), initially observed improvements in mental health and substance use resistance, better than among comparison groups, persisted over time (Costello, Erkanli, Copeland, & Angold, 2010).

Circularity of influence

Individuals' development and behavior are influenced, to a great degree, by their interactions with elements in their social and physical environments.

However, individuals are not necessarily passively influenced by their environments. Individuals also may actively influence environments and make choices between environmental options. The circularity of influence concept gets at the multi-directional and iterative nature of transactions (as opposed to interactions) between individuals and their social/physical contexts (Shelton, 2019). This is important, for example, in intervention strategies designed around prevention, principles of empowerment, and coping skills training.

Environmental impact mechanisms

Environments exert influence on substance use behaviors through two mechanisms: social control and social triggers.

Social control

Social control mechanisms involve increased or reduced opportunities to engage in the substance use/misuse—increasing or reducing access to alcohol, tobacco, or cannabis is a social control example. Evidence that social control mechanisms impact substance use behavior includes studies demonstrating the effect of restrained substance use by parents and other parenting behaviors, such as monitoring and norm setting, on delaying or preventing adolescent substance use and substance-related risk behavior (Carpenter, Dobkin, & Warman, 2016; Cook & Tauchen, 1984; Hawkins, Catalano, & Miller, 1992). Opportunities to engage in substance use are also influenced by access to substances. Considering U.S. 12th-grade students' perceptions about access to different types of substances (in 2018), adolescents perceived having easy or very easy access to marijuana (79.7%), alcohol (85.5%), cigarettes (75.1%), and vaping devices (80.5%), despite policies designed to restrict under-aged access (Monitoring the Future Study, Miech et al., 2019).

Social triggers

Social trigger mechanisms are aspects of the environment that amplify or dampen the behavior (exposure to violence and its associated stressors, for example), thereby acting as a "trigger" promoting substance use and other related behaviors (Shih et al., 2015).

Evidence surrounding factors that act as social trigger mechanisms includes consistently identified relationships between adverse childhood events (ACEs) and substance misuse (Sartor et al., 2018).

Proximal and distal factors

Social control and social trigger mechanisms most often studied are proximal in nature: they were present in the immediate physical and temporal context. But distal (macro-level) social control mechanisms also occur. For example, policy increases in legal drinking age (Wagenaar & Toomey, 2002) and the age individuals can legally obtain tobacco (Schneider, Buka, Dash, Winickoff, & O'Donnell, 2016) are social control actions shown to decrease substance use. Retail advertisements for alcohol and tobacco products provide additional examples: greater numbers of these advertisements in environments surrounding individuals too young to legally purchase them is, nevertheless, associated with their increased use (Kirchner et al., 2015). In the case of tobacco use in the United States, individual states can set policies regarding the taxation, advertisement, and use in public places of tobacco products.

Studies show significant associations in tobacco use with variations in state taxation of, and in restrictions on, the use of tobacco products (Luke, Stamatakis, & Brownson, 2000) and in the density of retail outlets that sell tobacco (Cantrell et al., 2015; Novak, Reardon, Raudenbush, & Buka, 2006). For example, a greater proportion of high school students who are daily cigarette smokers is observed in those U.S. states that have minimal regulations on the sale of tobacco to minors (Botello-Harbaum et al., 2009).

Social systems

Anthropologists argue that substance use can only be properly understood when placed within a social context including family, peer, school, work, economic, political, cultural, and religious/spiritual systems (Hunt & Barker, 2001). The terms environment and environmental exposures broadly refer to aspects of the immediate social context, like parent-child and peer relationships, as well as community-level or more distal factors, like societal substance use/ misuse norms, tobacco and alcohol outlet density, and laws/regulatory frameworks. Consistent with a multi-level, ecological perspective of where health risk factors reside (Boardman, Daw, & Freese, 2013; Bronfenbrenner, 1996), the contexts within which individuals are raised, live, and work, as well as the policies and physical spaces that constrain or permit their behavioral choices, are all important to substance use initiation and progression to problematic substance use. Recovery is heavily influenced by social processes and occurs within social contexts, as well (Heather et al., 2018).

The social system within which an individual exists, develops, and functions is comprised of multiple, nested, inter-connected, interacting fields defined in the social ecological "develecology" model (Shelton, 2019; see Figure 7.1). The most immediate and regular (proximal) social context interactions occur between the individual and the microsystem, often comprised of close family members, friends, school or work mates, and others in regular, significant contact.

The mesosystem involves interactions between microsystem elements and settings where the individual functions: family interactions with neighbors or teachers in school/employers in the workplace, for example. The exosystem has more indirect influence on the individual: these are interactions with settings rather than individuals, such as a healthcare setting (rather than an individual provider). Macrosystem elements are the most distal to an individual yet they exert influence on these nested systems which, in turn, affect individuals: for instance, policies or cultural mores that dictate opportunities for what happens at the exosystem or macrosystem level of interaction. These nested systems also operate within a temporal context (chronosystem), meaning that each subsystem and the whole social system are dynamic and potentially changing over time, and the system's past, present, and future are all relevant. The chronosystem also helps explain why cohort matters: for example, why the experience of adolescent substance use might be very different when comparing adolescent cohorts from 1969, 1979, 1989, 1999, 2009, and 2019.

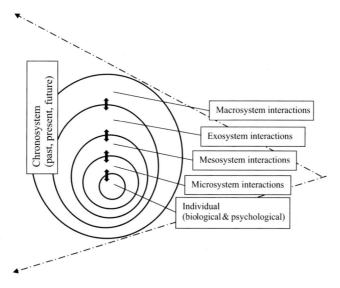

Figure 7.1 Social ecological model (adapted from Bronfenbrenner's work; see Shelton, 2019)

In terms of substance use, substance misuse, substance use disorders, and recovery, social systems are critically important considerations. When considering the initial phases of substance use, adolescents report active involvement with friends who use alcohol (Chassin, Pillow, Curran, Molina, & Barrera Jr, 1993) in a pattern that holds from adolescence until young adulthood (Piehler, Véronneau, & Dishion, 2012). Friends and peers are also important in efforts at quitting substance use at various points including adolescence and in adulthood (Mohr, , Averna, Kenny, Del Boca, 2001; Valente et al., 2007). The recovery process is similarly influenced by individuals in social contexts. For example, a person in recovery from an alcohol use disorder engages in daily microsystem (proximal) interactions with family, friends, and co-workers. These significant others (SOs) may either support the individual's recovery effort or engage in substance misuse themselves, serving as an influence against recovery. A major advantage offered by mutual help programs (e.g. Alcoholics Anonymous) involves inserting significant others who support recovery into an individual's immediate social network (microsystem interactions) and creating recovery support context options (meso- and exosystem interactions). Formal treatment may occur as mesosystem interactions with a provider, shaped in part by interactions with the exosystem (e.g. program/agency features). This all occurs within the macrosystem of culture, economics, history, policy, and other distal forces that influence interactions among the micro-, meso-, and exosystems (e.g. treatment coverage, policies, and social stigma).

Social contexts and environments have a significant impact on substance use and related behavior, as well. For example, drinking setting (public bars versus private parties) is related to drinking behavior, at least among college students (Clapp, Reed, Holmes, Lange, & Voas, 2006): having many intoxicated other people in public or private settings, and having drinking games or illicit substances also available in private party settings, was associated with individuals' higher alcohol consumption.

Social norms

Social norms are a social group's set of behavioral expectations, defining what is acceptable or unacceptable behavior. Norms can fluctuate under different circumstances and are culturally determined. For example, drinking to excess may be "accepted" behavior at certain parties but not approved at a religious ceremony involving wine. Social norms vary over time and by geographical region. For instance, a review of literature concluded that in North America younger birth cohorts were more likely to engage in heavy episodic drinking (and develop alcohol use disorders) than earlier cohorts, but this trend was not reflective of women's drinking patterns in Australia or Western Europe (Keyes, Li, & Hasin, 2011). Social norms may differ by gender and age, as well—intoxication may be accepted in young adults but not middle-aged adults, or by men but not women. Social norms define boundaries about initiating use and socially acceptable patterns of use—when, where, by whom, how much— including attitudes about intoxication, substance use disorders, and the recovery process. For example, women's reported reasons for limiting their drinking declined in importance between 2000 and 2010 (Karriker-Jaffe, Greenfield, Mulia, & Zemore, 2018): women were less likely to identify health concerns, upsetting family/friends, and religion as reasons to limit their alcohol use.

The U.S. Monitoring the Future study (Miech et al., 2019) has provided informative data about social norms in students' disapproval for specific substance use behaviors (see Table 7.1). The percentage of students disapproving of substance use depends on the substance involved (heroin use was disapproved of at much higher rates than alcohol, marijuana, or

Table 7.1 Disapproval by 12th graders of people aged 18 or older doing the following (adapted from Monitoring the Future [Miech et al., 2019], Table 14)

Substance use behavior	Percent disapprove or strongly disapprove
Marijuana	
Trying once or twice	41.1
Smoking occasionally	49.2
Smoking regularly	66.7
Alcohol	
Trying one or two drinks	31.3
Taking one or two drinks nearly every day	74.7
Taking four or five drinks nearly every day	91.7
Having five or more drinks once or twice each weekend	75.8
Nicotine	
Smoking one or more packs of cigarettes per day	89.0
Vaping with nicotine occasionally	59.2
Vaping with nicotine regularly	70.9
Heroin	
Trying heroin once or twice	95.0
Taking heroin occasionally	96.4
Taking heroin regularly	96.8

nicotine products) and the frequency of use (regular use was disapproved of at higher rates than "trying" or occasional use). Students also reported stark differences between what they perceived as their friends' and parents' attitudes toward the possibility they would engage in each of these behaviors: they generally believed their parents would be more disapproving than their friends (Miech et al., 2019).

Understanding social norms is important because there exists a significant association between norms about substance use/misuse and actual substance use behavior, at least among adolescents (Eisenberg, Toumbourou, Catalano, & Hemphill, 2014). While family and peer group social norms may help inform assessment and intervention at the individual level, this is also a potentially rewarding target for prevention and behavior change interventions at the community and societal level. For example, mass media campaigns may have positive impact on health risk behaviors such as driving while intoxicated, tobacco use, or parents talking to their children about substance misuse (Wakefield, Loken, & Hornik, 2010).

Stigma

Stigma reflects a type of negative social attitude or stereotype about a type of person or behavior. Stigma about persons engaged in substance misuse or experiencing substance use disorder potentially affects their opportunities and willingness to engage in formal or informal treatment to address substance-related problems, thereby increasing their marginalization and exacerbating "both structural and individual-level barriers to treatment and help-seeking" (Kulesza et al., 2016). Explicit bias refers to the beliefs, attitudes, and social norms of which someone is conscious and aware, whereas implicit bias reflects those lying outside of conscious awareness and intentional control; explicit and implicit bias may not fully align even within the same person's belief systems. For example, explicit belief that persons engaged in substance misuse (particularly injecting drugs) deserve help rather than punishment may not persist at the implicit level (Kulescza et al., 2016).

Encountering stigma is commonly reported among persons experiencing substance use disorders, having a profound and pervasive impact on their everyday lives, social relationships, and healthcare experiences (Fraser et al., 2017). Stigma is also an internalized experience: stigmatized individuals often regard themselves in stigmatized and shaming ways (Fraser et al., 2017). Stigma potentially has a considerable impact on public perceptions that inform policy, as well. A randomized experiment involving presentation of vignettes depicting either untreated or successfully treated addiction demonstrated the potential power of framing addiction as a treatable health condition: compared to untreated addiction vignettes, portrayals of successful treatment were followed by greater belief in the effectiveness of treatment and less willingness to discriminate against persons with a drug addiction, leading to the conclusion that stigma against these individuals can be reduced and public perceptions of treatment effectiveness can be enhanced (McGinty, Goldman, Pescosolido, & Barry, 2015).

Specific contexts

Family systems, functions, and roles

One of the most important social contexts for human development and behavior is the family system (Bronfenbrenner, 1986). A considerable body of literature demonstrates the role of various family characteristics and behaviors in the emergence and sustainment of individuals' alcohol or other substance use/misuse. For example, poor parenting (Moffitt, Caspi, Dickson, Silva, & Stanton, 1996) and specific family stressors such as experiencing parental unemployment and marital difficulties increased conduct problems and other behaviors linked to adolescent substance use (Bøe, Serlachius, Sivertsen, Petrie, & Hysing, 2018) and alcohol use (King & Chassin, 2008). Adolescents lacking parental support (Stice, Barrera, & Chassin, 1993) and experiencing low levels of parental monitoring (Hill, Hawkins, Catalano, Abbott, & Guo, 2005) were more likely to use substances, possibly due to greater opportunities to select similarly involved friends and peers or being open to their influences. As individuals age, attaining important family social role transitions, like marriage or other cohabiting relationships (Bachman et al., 2014; Kandel, 1980; O'Malley, 2004), is often associated with individuals' reduction in substance use, perhaps due to the greater responsibility these relationships place on individuals or social pressure from partners concerning what constitutes appropriate levels of substance use. This pattern of "maturing" out of substance misuse is less likely if an adolescent's misuse has progressed to the point of a substance use disorder, however: "For the majority of adolescents, [alcohol use disorders] are not benign conditions that resolve over time" (Rohde, Lewinsohn, Kahler, Seeley, & Brown, 2001).

Parental substance misuse not only affects the quality of parenting behavior (see Chapter 23) and parental monitoring of their sons' and daughters' behavior, it also creates a drinking environment modeling substance misuse (see Chapter 6 on social learning), communicates ambiguous social norms concerning substance misuse, increases children's and adolescents' access to substances, and potentially exposes children/adolescents to ACEs, including crime, violence, neglect/maltreatment, and poverty conditions (Fang & McNeil, 2017). Similarly, parental behaviors around establishing clear, unambiguous prohibitive norms concerning substance use/misuse, parental monitoring, and warm, positive relationships with their sons and daughters are protective factors. For example, positive father-child relationships decreased the likelihood that adolescents used alcohol and was more important than family structure (living together or not, and father figure available) in African American families (Jordan & Lewis, 2005). It is important to note that the opposite does not seem to be consistently true across studies: negative parent-child relationships did not necessarily predict adolescent alcohol use in high-quality studies (Visser, de Winter, & Reijneveld, 2012). This suggests that other impactful social environment and gene × environment influences may be at play.

Family influences on alcohol misuse include both family environment and genetic influences (see Chapter 5). The family drinking environment (modeling, norms, and access) and genetic vulnerability are independently associated with alcohol problems in both adolescents and adults (Chartier, Hesselbrock, & Hesselbrock, 2010; Light, Irvine, & Kjerulf, 1996; Zucker, Ellis, & Fitzgerald, 1994). Kendler et al. (2015), for example, demonstrated that the parent-child transmission of alcohol problems was associated with both stepparents (i.e. non-biological relatives) who resided in the home and biological parents who never resided in the home. The risk for developing alcohol problems is highest among individuals with densely affected families. This can be measured by a higher proportion of affected biological family members, particularly among first-degree relatives, relative to total family members or by other genetic "red flags" that indicate affected biological relatives over multiple generations and on both maternal and paternal sides of the family (Dawson, Hartford, & Grant, 1992; Hill, Blow, Young, & Singer, 1994; Kendler, Ohlsson, Sundquist, & Sundquist, 2018; Lieb et al., 2002; Milne, et al., 2008; Stoltenberg, Mudd, Blow, & Hill, 1998; Turner et al., 1993). Among college students, having a greater family density of alcohol problems related to experiencing more negative consequences from drinking (Powers, Berger, Fuhrmann, & Fendrich, 2017). Adults with a family history of alcohol problems reported being more likely to transition from at-risk drinking to alcohol use disorder, experience a recurrent course of alcohol problems, and drink despite health problems like liver disease (Beseler, Aharonovich, Keyes, & Hasin, 2008; Elliott, Stohl, & Hasin, 2017; Milne et al., 2009).

Family systems are important not only in the initiation and course of addictive behaviors like substance use/misuse, but also in recovery (see Chapters 22 and 24). According to family systems theory, families are characterized by the following (Begun, Hodge, & Early, 2017):

- families are greater than the sum of the parts—meaning that the "family" has identity, character, and meaning beyond the individuals of which it is comprised;
- change in any part of the system affects the entire system—a family member's fluctuating behavior (as a function of substance use/withdrawal) will have an impact on everyone else in the system and create stress for the system struggling to achieve a certain degree of stability, predictability, and homeostasis: similarly, a person's changes with the recovery process also reverberate throughout the system, and may create new sources of stress despite being a positive sort of change;
- subsystems are incorporated in the larger family system—couples, parent/child, and sibling relationships are important examples, but complex systems may also include ex-, step-, and pseudo- family relationships, as well: some families view their family member as being engaged in a unique subsystem relationship with the source of the addictive behavior (e.g. substances, gambling, gaming) and supportive SOs are critical in the recovery process (see Chapters 18 and 29);

- family systems are embedded in larger social systems, including extended family and the other micro-, meso-, and macro-systems previously discussed—the family system engages with other social systems, whether healthy or not, and excessive isolation produced as a result of stigma or other isolating processes is unhealthy for families; and
- family systems are dynamic over time—their past, present, and future realities and aspirations are all relevant.

Role theory is also relevant in understanding how family systems function and how a family member's substance misuse might be experienced. The family functions as a unit serving both the demands of the social environment ("external agencies") and the needs of its internal members (Begun et al., 2017). While their specific tasks and how they accomplish them vary by culture, context, time, and circumstances, key functions concern procuring, producing, and distributing resources to meet members' basic needs (food, shelter, protection) and socialization of members into their family and societal roles (including social norms and establishing an identity as a family). Family dysfunction is determined by the extent to which these functions fail to be met. A partner's or parent's addictive behavior can threaten any or all these functions, jeopardizing the health and well-being of the family as a whole and/or individual members. The concept of compensatory parenting warrants social workers' attention, as significant others may step in to help fulfill roles and functions absented by a family member engaged in substance misuse or other addictive behavior. These positive, stable compensatory relationships represent important aspects in a child's or adolescent's resilience (e.g. see Chapter 25 concerning "Grandfamilies"). Social workers can help foster the support provided by SOs and in compensatory parenting situations by helping participants understand their roles and develop the requisite knowledge, skills, and attitudes to fulfill these functions. They can also help family systems adapt and adjust to the changes in family process and subsystems that occur during the recovery process.

Peers

Environments that shape substance initiation, progression of substance use disorder (SUD), and recovery include the behaviors of friend networks and peers. Studies among adolescents report that substance use initiation and escalation to problematic levels of substance use are strongly associated with friends' and peers' use of drugs (Vink, 2016). Adolescents are more likely to regularly use cigarettes if more than half of their peer network do so, if one or two of their best friends smoke, or if a large proportion of their school smoke cigarettes (Alexander, Piazza, Mekos, & Valente, 2001; Mrug, Gaines, Su, & Windle, 2010; Mrug & McCay, 2013).

Similar findings have been reported when other drugs like alcohol and marijuana are examined (Henry, Slater, & Oetting, 2005; Pinchevsky et al., 2012; Poelen, Scholte, Willemsen, Boomsma, & Engels, 2007). Relative to the influence of other individuals in their social networks, the most robust predictor of initiating substances came from adolescents' friends and peer network (Bahr, Hoffmann, & Yang, 2005; Fergusson, Boden, & Horwood, 2008).

Peers not only are a key force in the initiation of substances, acting as mechanisms to reduce social control, but are also instrumental in assisting in recovery. Peer support for recovery from substance use disorders has been reported to instill a sense of hope and well-being (Ratzlaff, McDiarmid, Marty, & Rapp, 2006), increased engagement (Davidson, Bellamy, Guy, & Miller, 2012), and decreased substance use (Davidson et al., 2012) among individuals in treatment. In the college setting where students with substance use disorders are often considered a hidden group (Woodford, 2001), peers support is a key component of campus recovery programs (Laudet, Harris, Kimball, Winters, & Moberg, 2014). Similar efforts have been developed for adolescents at risk for substance use disorder and are delivered by young adult peers (Paquette, Pannella Winn, Wilkey, Ferreira, & Donegan, 2019).

Neighborhood & community

Decades of social science research point to neighborhood environment conditions shaping daily experiences, health-related behavior, and health outcomes, neighborhood conditions like frequent movement of residents into and out of neighborhoods, the collective efficacy that neighbors feel toward where they live, poverty, crime, and violence (Dishion, Capaldi, & Yoerger, 1999). The cumulative effect of these daily experiences erodes social ties among community members, increasing social isolation (Wang, Phillips, Small, & Sampson, 2018) and resulting in greater stress (McEwen, 1998; McEwen & Stellar, 1993; Theall, Drury, & Shirtcliff, 2012).

Research concerning social environments and substance use has tended to emphasize more proximal factors (e.g. family and peers), although more distal neighborhood/community structural and social processes are quite relevant (Warner, 2016). Structural aspects include ease of access to substances, modeling of substance use by others, and targeted advertising. Certain social determinants also operate at the neighborhood/community level, such as neighborhood socioeconomic status: residing in disadvantaged neighborhoods was associated with higher odds of adults using tobacco and women's use of other drugs (Karriker-Jaffe, 2013). Initiation of marijuana use and the trajectory of ongoing use by emerging adults are related to neighborhood type, "above and beyond traditional demographic correlates of substance use and key individual, family, and peer risk and protective factors" (Warner, 2016, p. 48). Community norms regarding substance use appear to have little effect on marijuana or alcohol use by adolescents, but exposure to violence, and particularly the experience of violence victimization, was associated with a significant increase in the likelihood of marijuana use (Fagan, Wright, & Pinchevsky, 2015). Neighborhood context may have a nuanced, indirect effect on substance use behavior, as well, by amplifying or attenuating the effects of more proximal influences such as parent and peer substance use and perceptions of harm related to substance use (Zimmerman & Farrell, 2017).

Culture

Cultural environments associated with race/ethnicity, national origin, religion/spirituality, and other identities influence a person's behavior and attitudes about substance use and misuse. These influences occur through multiple mechanisms (see Chapter 15). For example, a strong cultural identity or closeness to one's culture of origin can be protective against susceptibility to alcohol and substance use behaviors (Banks, Winningham, Wu, & Zapolski, 2019; Perreira et al., 2019), while among immigrant populations, acculturation or adapting to the practices and values of the new dominant culture can be a risk factor for alcohol use and related problems—depending on norms held in the original and new cultures. Mediational mechanisms for acculturation are reductions of family closeness and an increased association with substance-using peers (Bacio, Lau, & Mays, 2013; Iwamoto, Kaya, Grivel, & Clinton, 2016; Gil, Wagner, & Vega, 2000). Some individuals engage in substance use in response to acculturative stress or to instances of discrimination and isolation (Alamilla et al., 2019; Gilbert & Zemore, 2016), particularly those born in the United States to immigrant parents. However, closeness with one's cultural identity may not be protective if it is associated with a wetter drinking culture or more permissive drinking norms and behaviors in the country of origin (Cook, Mulia, & Karriker-Jaffe, 2012).

Religiosity also plays a vital role in establishing norms related to substance use. Some religious denominations have norms that discourage drinking, including Islam and evangelical protestant religions. As a result, Muslim countries globally have the lowest prevalence rates of alcohol use (Michalak & Trocki, 2006), and in the United States, residents in Southern states consistently have the lowest rates of alcohol use compared to residents of states in the Midwest, West, and Northeast. Conversely, having no religious affiliation and a Catholic affiliation are associated with an increased risk for alcoholism and heavier drinking compared to other denominations (Heath et al., 1997; Michalak, Trocki, & Bond, 2007). The combination of having both strong spiritual beliefs and greater religious involvement provides a particularly strong protection against heavy drinking (Brechting et al., 2010; Hodge, Andereck, & Montoya, 2007; Holt, Roth, Huang, & Clark, 2015). By enabling individuals to manage stressful experiences, using prayer to cope is inversely associated with alcoholism (Borders, Curran, Mattox, & Booth, 2010). The protective relationship between religiosity and alcohol use may also arise because individuals with greater religiosity belong to low- or non-drinking social networks (Ford & Kadushin, 2002) or have greater self-control over personal thoughts, emotions, and behaviors (DeWall et al., 2014).

Interactions

Various environmental and social context factors, including at different system levels, interrelate and interact in different ways. For example, not only do parental monitoring and peer relationships influence adolescents' use of various substances (Dick & Kendler, 2012; Sher et al., 2010), high levels of parental monitoring weakens the strong influence of associating with peers engaged in substance misuse (Marschall-Levesque, Castellanos-Ryan, Vitaro, & Seguin, 2014). Not only are such interactions observed at the proximal (micro/mesosystem) level, factors at the macro-level work together, as well. For instance, when electronic cigarettes were first introduced in the United States, the Federal Drug and Alcohol Administration did not yet regulate them as tobacco products (macrosystem), leading to dramatic use rates among youth who could not legally purchase combustible cigarettes (Cobb, Byron, Abrams, & Shields, 2010), including even greater increases among low-income individuals in rural settings (Pesko & Robarts, 2017).

Gene-environment interplay

Not only are social workers concerned with interactions between different levels of social and physical environments, they are also concerned with interaction between social and other domains: the biological and psychological rounding out a biopsychosocial perspective (see Chapter 1). For example, genetic variation may affect the risk of substance use by moderating an individual's susceptibility to social stressors (Chartier et al., 2014). Evidence supporting social trigger mechanisms depends on the specific genetic markers examined. For example, there is evidence for an interaction between childhood abuse and genetic risk related to some (Ducci et al., 2008; Goyal et al., 2016; Kaufman et al., 2007) but not in all genetic markers (Enoch et al., 2010). Joint effects between genes and adverse life events have also been demonstrated for only some sex and racial/ethnic subgroups: African American females (Kranzler et al., 2012) and White males (Sartor, Wang, Xu, Kranzler, & Gelernter, 2014). Gene × environment interaction effects for heavy drinking may depend on when in development an environmental factor was encountered, for instance, early life trauma but not past-year trauma or stress when examined among college students (Lieberman et al., 2016). Notably, individuals most biologically vulnerable to social stressors may also be those who benefit the most from environmental enhancements (Belsky & Pluess, 2009; Belsky & van Ijzendoorn, 2017). Two teams tested this hypothesis (Brody, Chen, & Beach, 2013; Trucco, Villafuerte, Heitzeg, Burmeister, & Zucker, 2016), demonstrating that genes influencing the effects of the neurotransmitter GABA moderated the benefit of parental monitoring and prevention efforts on substance use and related behaviors.

Conclusions

Understanding the social context and physical environment influences on substance misuse rounds out the biopsychosocial perspective prevalent in this book. Gene × environment interactions explain a great deal of the individual variation in substance use behavior, including the development of and recovery from substance use disorder. Environmental conditions have a great deal of power to modify genetic and psychological influences and physical/mental health outcomes, with social determinants operating at all social ecological levels, from micro- to macro-levels and from the most proximal to distal factors, as well. The social context operates through various mechanisms including social control and social trigger forces that can either serve protective or exacerbating functions. However, it is important to recognize that individuals are not simply responding to their social and physical environments, but they also play active roles in shaping those environments, particularly the most proximal contexts (circularity of influence).

Addictive behaviors, as any type of complex behavior, cannot be fully understood outside of the social systems within which individuals develop and function. These social systems influence the initiation of addictive behaviors, their maintenance, and recovery processes. Important proximal social systems include family and peers. Much of their influence operates through learning and social learning mechanisms (see Chapter 6). Parental addictive behavior not only influences children, adolescents, and emerging adults through imitation/modeling, but also communicates acceptance norms and provides easier access to engage in these behaviors. Parental substance misuse can also impair effective parenting behavior, including parental supervision which is important in deterring or delaying adolescent substance use initiation.

Social and cultural norms represent another mechanism through which addictive behaviors are influenced. These norms can impose restraint on an individual's behavior, acting as a protective force. Unfortunately, deviance norms can encourage addictive behavior, as well. Social norms are communicated through a vast array of media, including messages communicated by family, peers, co-workers, social institutions, advertising, and entertainment sources (television, movies, social media, and others), and such messaging can be ambiguous. Religiosity and spirituality represent social context forces with potential (but no guarantee) for resisting pressure to engage in addictive behaviors.

Family members, friends, and peer support persons within the proximal social system can play a crucial role in supporting individuals' attempts to change their addictive behavior (supportive significant others, SOs) and as part of the process of recovery from an addictive disorder. Social stigma related to addictive behavior can inhibit an individual's efforts to self-identify as having a problem with and seek help to change the behavior. Furthermore, stigma concerning (in)effectiveness of treatment approaches can further encourage or discourage individuals' recovery efforts.

Together, the wide array of social context and physical environment factors related to addictive behavior play significant roles in the emergence, expression, and recovery from addictive behavior problems. While much is known about various aspects of the social context, a paucity of evidence exists to thoroughly assess the full range of risk and protective environments from micro- to macro-level and proximal to distal in nature.

References

Alamilla, S. G., Barney, B. J., Small, R., Wang, S. C., Schwartz, S. J., Donovana, R. A., & Lewis, C. (2019). Explaining the immigrant paradox: The influence of acculturation, enculturation, and acculturative stress on problematic alcohol consumption. *Behavioral Medicine, (January 5)*, 1–13. doi:10.1080/08964289.2018.1539945

Alexander, C., Piazza, M., Mekos, D., & Valente, T. (2001). Peers, schools, and adolescent cigarette smoking. *The Journal of Adolescent Health: Official Publication of the Society for Adolescent Medicine, 29*(1), 22–30. doi:10.1016/S1054-139X(01)00210-5

Bachman, J. G., O'Malley, P. M., Schulenberg, J. E., Johnston, L. D., Bryant, A. L., & Merline, A. C. (2002). *The decline of substance use in young adulthood: Changes in social activities, roles, and beliefs.* Mahwah, NJ: Lawrence Erlbaum Associates.

Bacio, G. A., Lau, A. S., & Mays, V. M. (2013). Drinking initiation and problematic drinking among Latino adolescents: Explanations of the immigrant paradox. *Psychology of Addictive Behaviors, 27*(1), 14–22. doi:10.1037/a0029996

Bahr, S. J., Hoffmann, J. P., & Yang, X. (2005). Parental and peer influences on the risk of adolescent drug use. *Journal of Primary Prevention, 26*(6), 529–551. doi:10.1007/s10935-005-0014-8

Banks, D. E., Winningham, R. D., Wu, W., & Zapolski, T. C. B. (2019). Examination of the indirect effect of alcohol expectancies on ethnic identity and adolescent drinking outcomes. *American Journal of Orthopsychiatry, 89*(5), 600–608. doi:10.1037/ort0000390

Begun, A. L., Hodge, A. I., & Early, T. J. (2017). A family systems perspective in prisoner reentry. In S. Stojkovic (Ed.), *Prisoner reentry* (pp. 85–144). New York, NY: Palgrave Macmillan. doi:10.1057/978-1-137-57929-4_3

Belsky, J., & Pluess, M. (2009). Beyond diathesis stress: Differential susceptibility to environmental influences. *Psychological bulletin, 135*(6), 885. doi:10.1037/a0017376

Belsky, J., & van Ijzendoorn, M. H. (2017). Genetic differential susceptibility to the effects of parenting. *Current Opinion in Psychology, 15*, 125–130. doi:10.1016/j.copsyc.2017.02.021

Beseler, C.L., Aharonovich, E., Keyes, K.M., & Hasin, D.S. Adult transition from at-risk drinking to alcohol dependence: The relationship of family history and drinking motives. *Alcoholism: Clinical & Experimental Research, 32*(4), 607–616. doi:10.1111/j.1530-0277.2008.00619.x

Boardman, J. D., Daw, J., & Freese, J. (2013). Defining the environment in gene-environment research: Lessons from social epidemiology. *American Journal of Public Health, 103* (Suppl. 1), S64–S72. doi:10.2105/ajph.2013.301355

Bøe, T., Serlachius, A. S., Sivertsen, B., Petrie, K. J., & Hysing, M. (2018). Cumulative effects of negative life events and family stress on children's mental health: The Bergen child study. *Social Psychiatry and Psychiatric Epidemiology, 53*(1), 1–9. doi:10.1007/s00127-017-1451-4

Borawski, E. A., Ievers-Landis, C. E., Lovegreen, L. D., & Trapl, E. S. (2003). Parental monitoring, negotiated unsupervised time, and parental trust: The role of perceived parenting practices in adolescent health risk behavior. *Journal of Adolescent Health, 33*(2), 60–70. doi:10.1016/S1054-139X(03)00100-9

Borders, T. F., Curran, G. M., Mattox, R., & Booth, B. M. (2010). Religiousness among at-risk drinkers: Is it prospectively associated with the development or maintenance of an alcohol-use disorder? *Journal of Studies on Alcohol and Drugs, 71*, 136–142. doi:10.15288/jsad.2010.71.136

Botello-Harbaum, M. T., Haynie, D. L., Iannotti, R. J., Wang, J., Gase, L., & Simons-Morton, B. (2009). Tobacco control policy and adolescent cigarette smoking status in the United States. *Nicotine & Tobacco Research, 11*(7), 875–885. doi:10.1093/ntr/ntp081

Brechting, E. H., Brown, T. L., Salsman, J. M., Sauer, Se. E., Holeman, V. T., & Carlson, C. R. (2010). The role of religious beliefs and behaviors in predicting underage alcohol use. *Journal of Child & Adolescent Substance Abuse, 19*, 324–334. doi:10.1080/1067828X.2010.502494

Brody, G. H., Chen, Y. F., & Beach, S. R. (2013). Differential susceptibility to prevention: GABAergic, dopaminergic, and multilocus effects. *Journal of Child Psychology and Psychiatry, 54*(8), 863–871. doi:10.1111/jcpp.12042

Bronfenbrenner, U. (1986). Ecology of the family as a context for human development: Research perspectives. *Developmental Psychology, 22*(6), 723–742. doi:10.1037/0012-1649.22.6.723

Bronfenbrenner, U. (1996). *The ecology of human development: Experiments by nature and design.* Cambridge, MA: Harvard University Press.

Browne, T., Gehlert, S., Andrews, C. M., Zebrack, B. J., Walther, V. N., . . . Merighi, J. R. (2017). *Strengthening health care systems: Better health across America.* American Academy of Social Work & Social Welfare, Grand Challenges for Social Work Initiative Working Paper No. 22. Retrieved from http://grandchallengesforsocialwork.org/wp-content/uploads/2017/11/WP22.pdf

Cantrell, J., Pearson, J. L., Anesetti-Rothermel, A., Xiao, H., Kirchner, T. R., & Vallone, D. (2015). Tobacco retail outlet density and young adult tobacco initiation. *Nicotine & Tobacco Research, 18*(2), 130–137. doi:10.1093/ntr/ntv036

Carpenter, C. S., Dobkin, C., & Warman, C. (2016). The mechanisms of alcohol control. *Journal of Human Resources, 51*(2), 328–356. doi:10.3368/jhr.51.2.0314-6240R

Centers for Disease Control and Prevention (CDC). (2018). *Social determinants of health: Know what affects health.* Retrieved from www.cdc.gov/socialdeterminants/index.htm

Chartier, K. G., Hesselbrock, M. N., & Hesselbrock, V. M. (2010). Development and vulnerability factors in adolescent alcohol use. *Child and Adolescent Psychiatric Clinics of North America, 19*(3), 493–504. doi:10.1016/j.chc.2010.03.004

Chartier, K. G., Scott, D. M., Wall, T. L., Covault, J., Karriker-Jaffe, K. J., Mills, B. A., . . . Arroyo, J. A. (2014). Framing ethnic variations in alcohol outcomes from biological pathways to neighborhood context. *Alcohol: Clinical & Experimantl Research, 38*(3), 611–618. doi:10.1111/acer.12304

Chassin, L., Pillow, D. R., Curran, P. J., Molina, B. S., & Barrera, M. (1993). Relation of parental alcoholism to early adolescent substance use: A test of three mediating mechanisms. *Journal of Abnormal Psychology, 102*(1): 3. doi:10.1037/e500402006-010

Clapp, J. D., Reed, M. B., Holmes, M. R., Lange, J. E., & Voas, R. B. (2006). Drunk in public, drink in private: The relationship between college students, drinking environments and alcohol consumption. *The American Journal of Drug and Alcohol Abuse, 32*, 275–285. doi:10.1080/00952990500481205

Cobb, N. K., Byron, M. J., Abrams, D. B., & Shields, P. G. (2010). Novel nicotine delivery systems and public health: The rise of the "e-cigarette." *American Journal of Public Health, 100*(12), 2340–2342. doi:10.2105/AJPH.2010.199281

Cook, P. J., & Tauchen, G. (1984). The effect of minimum drinking age legislation on youthful auto fatalities, 1970–1977. *Journal of Legal Studies, 13*(1), 169–190. doi:10.1086/467738

Cook, W. K., Mulia, N., & Karriker-Jaffe, K. (2012). Ethnic drinking cultures and alcohol use among Asian American adults: Findings from a national survey. *Alcohol, 47*(3), 340–348. doi:10.1093/alcalc/ags017

Costello, E. J., Erkanli, A., Copeland, W., & Angold, A. (2010). Association of family income supplements in adolescence with development of psychiatric and substance use disorders in adulthood among an American Indian population. *JAMA, 303*(19), 1954–1960. doi:10.1001/jama.2010.621

Davidson, L., Bellamy, C., Guy, K., & Miller, R. (2012). Peer support among persons with severe mental illnesses: A review of evidence and experience. *World Psychiatry, 11*(2), 123–128. doi:10.1016/j.wpsyc.2012.05.009

Dawson, D. A., Harford, T. C., & Grant, B. F. (1992). Family history as a predictor of alcohol dependence. *Alcoholism: Clinical & Experimental Research, 16*(3), 572–575.

DeWall, C. N., Pond, R. S., Carter, E. C., McCullough, M. E., Lambert, N. M., Fincham, F. D., & Nezlek, J. B. (2014). Explaining the relationship between religiousness and substance use: Self-control matters. *Journal of Personality and Social Psychology, 107*, 339–351. doi:10.1037/a0036853

Dick, D. M., & Kendler, K. S. (2012). The impact of gene–environment interaction on alcohol use disorders. *Alcohol Research: Current Reviews, 34*(3), 318.

Dishion, T. J., Capaldi, D. M., & Yoerger, K. (1999). Middle childhood antecedents to progressions in male adolescent substance use: An ecological analysis of risk and protection. *Journal of Adolescent Research, 14*(2), 175–205. doi:10.1177/0743558499142003

Dixon, M.A., & Chartier, K.G. (2016). Alcohol use patterns among urban and rural residents. *Alcohol Research: Current Reviews, 38*(1), 69–77.

Ducci, F., Enoch, M. A., Hodgkinson, C., Xu, K., Catena, M., Robin, R. W., & Goldman, D. (2008). Interaction between a functional MAOA locus and childhood sexual abuse predicts alcoholism and antisocial personality disorder in adult women. *Mol Psychiatry, 13*(3), 334–347. doi:10.1038/sj.mp.4002034

Eisenberg, M. E., Toumbourou, J. W., Catalano, R. F., & Hemphill, S. A. (2014). Social norms in the development of adolescent substance use: A longitudinal analysis of the international youth development study. *Journal of Youth and Adolescence, 43*(9), 1486–1497. doi:10.1007/s10964-014-0111-1

Elliott, J. C., Stohl, M., & Hasin, D. S. (2017). Drinking despite health problems among individuals with liver disease across the United States. *Drug & Alcohol Dependence, 176*, 28–32. doi:10.1016/j.drugalcdep.2017.03.008

Enoch, M. A., Hodgkinson, C. A., Yuan, Q., Shen, P. H., Goldman, D., & Roy, A. (2010). The influence of GABRA2, childhood trauma, and their interaction on alcohol, heroin, and cocaine dependence. *Biological Psychiatry, 67*(1), 20–27. doi:10.1016/j.biopsych.2009.08.019

Fagan, A. A., Wright, E. M., & Pinchevsky, G. M. (2015). Exposure to violence, substance use, and neighborhood context. *Social Science Research, 49*, 314–326. doi:10.1016/j.ssresearch.2014.08.015

Fang, L., & McNeil, S. (2017). Is there a relationship between adverse childhood experiences and problem drinking behaviors? Findings from a population-based sample. *Public Health, 150*, 34–42. doi:10.1016/j.puhe.2017.05.005

Fergusson, D. M., Boden, J. M., & Horwood, L. J. (2008). The developmental antecedents of illicit drug use: Evidence from a 25-year longitudinal study. *Drug and alcohol dependence, 96*(1–2), 165–177. doi:10.1016/j.drugalcdep.2008.03.003

Ford, J., & Kadushin, C. (2002). Between sacral belief and moral community: A multidimensional approach to the relationship between religion and alcohol among whites and blacks. *Sociological Forum, 17*, 255–279. doi:10.1023/A:1016089229972

Fraser, S., Pienaar, K., Dilkes-Frayne, E., Moore, D., Kokanovic, R., Treloar, C., & Dunlop, A. (2017). Addiction stigma and biopolitics of liberal modernity: A qualitative analysis. *The International Journal on Drug Policy, 44*, 192–201. doi:10.1016/j.drugpo.2017.02.005

Gil, A. G., Wagner, E. F., & Vega, W. A. (2000). Acculturation familism, and alcohol use among Latino adolescent males: Longitudinal relations. *Journal of Community Psychology 28*, 443–458. doi:10.1002/1520-6629(200007)28:4<443::AID-JCOP6>3.0.CO;2-A

Gilbert, P. A., & Zemore, S. E. (2016). Discrimination and drinking: A systematic review of the evidence. *Social Science and Medicine, 161*, 178–194. doi:10.1016/j.socscimed.2016.06.009

Goyal, N., Aliev, F., Latendresse, S. J., Kertes, D. A., Bolland, J. M., Byck, G. R., . . . Dick, D. M. (2016). Genes involved in stress response and alcohol use among high-risk African American youth. *Substance Abuse, 37*(3), 450–458. doi:10.1080/08897077.2015.1134756

Hawkins, J. D., Catalano, R. F., & Miller, J. Y. (1992). Risk and protective factors for alcohol and other drug problems in adolescence and early adulthood: Implications for substance abuse prevention. *Psychological Bulletin, 112*(1), 64–105. doi:10.1037/0033-2909.112.1.64

Heath, A. C., Bucholz, K. K., Madden, P. A. F., Dinwiddie, S. H., Slutske, W. S., Bierut, L. J., . . . Martin, N. G. (1997). Genetic and environmental contributions to alcohol dependence risk in a national twin sample: Consistency of findings in women and men. *Psychological Medicine, 27*, 1381–1396. doi:10.1017/S0033291797005643

Heather, N., Best, D., Kawalek, A., Field, M., Lewis, M., Rotgers, F., . . . Heim, D. (2018). Challenging the brain disease model of addiction: European launch of the addiction theory network. *Addiction Research & Theory, 26*(4), 249–255. doi:10.1080/16066359.2017.1399659

Henry, K. L., Slater, M. D., & Oetting, E. R. (2005). Alcohol use in early adolescence: The effect of changes in risk taking, perceived harm and friends' alcohol use. *Journal of Studies on Alcohol, 66*(2), 275–283. doi:10.15288/jsa.2005.66.275

Hill, E. M., Blow, F. C., Young, J. P., & Singer, K. M. (1994). Family history of alcoholism and childhood adversity: Joint effects on alcohol consumption and dependence. *Alcoholism: Clinical & Experimental Research, 18*(5), 1083–1090. doi:10.1111/j.1530-0277.1994.tb00085.x

Hill, K. G., Hawkins, J. D., Catalano, R. F., Abbott, R. D., & Guo, J. (2005). Family influences on the risk of daily smoking initiation. *Journal of Adolescent Health, 37*(3), 202–210.

Hunt, G., & Barker, J. C. (2001). Socio-cultural anthropology and alcohol and drug research: Towards a unified theory. *Social Science & Medicine, 53*(2), 165–188. doi:10.1016/j.jadohealth.2004.08.014

Hodge, D. R., Andereck, K., & Montoya, H. (2007). The protective influence of spiritual-religious lifestyle profiles on tobacco use, alcohol use, and gambling. *Social Work Research, 31*, 211–219. doi:10.1093/swr/31.4.211

Holt, C. L., Roth, D. L., Huang, J., & Clark, E. M. (2015). Gender differences in the roles of religion and locus of control on alcohol use and smoking among African Americans. *Journal of Studies on Alcohol and Drugs, 76*, 482–492. doi:10.15288/jsad.2015.76.482

Iwamoto, D. K., Kaya, A., Grivel, M., & Clinton, L. (2016). Under-researched demographics: Heavy episodic drinking and alcohol-related problems among Asian Americans. *Alcohol Research, 38*(1), 17–25.

Jordan, L. C., & Lewis, M. (2005). Paternal relationship quality as a protective factor: Preventing alcohol use among African American adolescents. *Journal of Black Psychology, 31*(2), 152–171 doi:10.1177/0095798405274881

Kandel DB. (1980). Drug and drinking behavior among youth. *Annual Review of Sociology, 6*(1), 235–285. doi:10.1146/annurev.so.06.080180.001315

Karriker-Jaffe, K. J. (2011). Areas of disadvantage: A systematic review of effects of area-level socioeconomic status on substance use outcomes. *Drug and Alcohol Review, 30*(1), 84–95. doi:10.1111/j.1465-3362.2010.00191.x

Karriker-Jaffe, K. J. (2013). Neighborhood socioeconomic status and substance use by U.S. adults. *Drug and Alcohol Dependence, 133*(1), 212–221. doi:10.1016/j.drugalcdep.2013.04.033

Karriker-Jaffe, K. J., Greenfield, T. K., Mulia, N., & Zemore, S. E. (2018). Ten-year trend in women's reasons for abstaining or limiting drinking: The 2000 and 2010 United States National Alcohol Surveys. *Journal of Women's Health, 27*(5), 665–675. doi:10.1089/jwh.2017.6613

Kaufman, J., Yang, B. Z., Douglas-Palumberi, H., Crouse-Artus, M., Lipschitz, D., Krystal, J. H., & Gelernter, J. (2007). Genetic and environmental predictors of early alcohol use. *Biological Psychiatry, 61*(11), 1228–1234. doi:10.1016/j.biopsych.2006.06.039

Kendler, K. S., & Eaves, L. J. (1986). Models for the joint effect of genotype and environment on liability to psychiatric illness. *The American Journal of Psychiatry, 143*(3), 279–289. doi:10.1176/ajp.143.3.279

Kendler, K. S., Gardner, C., & Dick, D. M. (2011). Predicting alcohol consumption in adolescence from alcohol-specific and general externalizing genetic risk factors, key environmental exposures and their interaction. *Psychological Medicine, 41*(7), 1507–1516. doi:10.1017/s003329171000190x

Kendler, K. S., Ji, J., Edwards, A. C., Ohlsson, H., Sundquist, J., & Sundquist, K. (2015). An extended Swedish national adoption study of alcohol use disorder. *JAMA Psychiatry, 72*(3), 211–218. doi:10.1001/jamapsychiatry.2014.2138

Kendler, K. S., Ohlsson, H., Sundquist, J., & Sundquist, K. (2018). Transmission of alcohol use disorder across three generations: A Swedish national study. *Psychological Medicine, 48*(1), 33–42. doi:10.1017/S0033291717000794

Keyes, K. M., Li, G., & Hasin, D. S. (2011). Birth cohort effects and gender differences in alcohol epidemiology: A review and synthesis. *Alcohol: Clinical & Experimental Research, 35*(12), 2101–2112. doi:10.1111/j.1530-0277.2011.01562.x

King, K. E., Morenoff, J. D., & House, J. S. (2011). Neighborhood context and social disparities in cumulative biological risk factors. *Psychosomatic Medicine, 73*(7), 572. doi:10.1097/PSY.0b013e318227b062

King, K. M., & Chassin, L. (2008). Adolescent stressors, psychopathology, and young adult substance dependence: A prospective study. *Journal of Studies on Alcohol and Drugs, 69*(5), 629–638. doi:10.15288/jsad.2008.69.629

Kirchner, T. R., Villanti, A. C., Cantrell, J., Anesetti-Rothermel, A., Ganz, O., Conway, K. P., . . . Abrams, D. B. (2015). Tobacco retail outlet advertising practices and proximity to schools, parks and public housing affect Synar underage sales violations in Washington, DC. *Tobacco Control, 24*(e1), e52–e58. doi:10.1136/tobaccocontrol-2013-051239

Kranzler, H. R., Scott, D., Tennen, H., Feinn, R., Williams, C., Armeli, S., . . . Covault, J. (2012). The 5-HTTLPR polymorphism moderates the effect of stressful life events on drinking behavior in college students of African descent. *American Journal of Medical Genetics Part B: Neuropsychiatric Genetics, 159*(5), 484–490. doi:10.1002/ajmg.b.32051

Kulesza, M., Matsuda, M., Ramirez, J. J., Werntz, A. J., Teachman, B. A., & Lindgren, K. P. (2016). Towards greater understanding of addiction stigma: Intersectionality with race/ethnicity and gender. *Drug and Alcohol Dependence, 169*, 85–91. doi:10.1016/j.drugalcdep.2016.10.020

Laudet, A., Harris, K., Kimball, T., Winters, K. C., & Moberg, D. P. (2014). Collegiate recovery communities program: What do we know and what do we need to know? *Journal of Social Work Practice in the Addictions, 14*(1), 84–100. doi:10.1080/1533256X.2014.872015

Lieb, R., Merikangas, K. R., Hofler, M., Pfister, H., Isensee, B., & Wittchen, H. U. (2002). Parental alcohol use disorders and alcohol use and disorders in offspring: A community study. *Psychological Medicine, 32*(1), 63–78. doi:10.1017/S0033291701004883

Lieberman, R., Armeli, S., Scott, D. M., Kranzler, H. R., Tennen, H., & Covault, J. (2016). FKBP5 genotype interacts with early life trauma to predict heavy drinking in college students. *American Journal of Medical Genetics Part B: Neuropsychiatric Genetics, 171*(6), 879–887. doi:10.1002/ajmg.b.32460

Light, J. M., Irvine, K. M., & Kjerulf, L. (1996). Estimating genetic and environmental effects of alcohol use and dependence from a national survey: A "quasi-adoption" study. *Journal of Studies on Alcohol, 57*(5), 507–520. doi:10.15288/jsa.1996.57.507

Lui, P. P., & Zamboanga, B. L. (2018a). Acculturation and alcohol use among Asian Americans: A meta-analytic review. *Psychology of Addictive Behaviors, 32*(2), 173–186. doi:10.1037/adb0000340

Lui, P. P., & Zamboanga, B. L. (2018b). A critical review and meta-analysis of the associations between acculturation and alcohol use outcomes among Hispanic Americans. *Alcoholism: Clinical & Experimental Research, 42*(10), 1841–1862. doi:10.1111/acer.13845

Luke, D. A., Stamatakis, K. A., & Brownson, R. C. (2000). State youth-access tobacco control policies and youth smoking behavior in the United States. *American Journal of Preventive Medicine, 19*(3), 180–187. doi:10.1111/acer.13845

Marschall-Levesque, S., Castellanos-Ryan, N., Vitaro, F., & Seguin, J. R. (2014). Moderators of the association between peer and target adolescent substance use. *Addictive Behavior, 39*(1), 48–70. doi:10.1016/j.addbeh.2013.09.025

McEwen, B. S. (1998). Protective and damaging effects of stress mediators. *New England Journal of Medicine, 338*(3), 171–179. doi:10.1056/NEJM199801153380307

McEwen, B. S., & Stellar, E. (1993). Stress and the individual: Mechanisms leading to disease. *Archives of Internal Medicine, 153*(18), 2093–2101. doi:10.1001/archinte.1993.00410180039004

McGinty, E. E., Goldman, H. H., Pescosolido, B., & Barry, C. L. (2015). Portraying mental illness and drug addiction as treatable health conditions: Effects of a randomized experiment on stigma and discrimination. *Social Science & Medicine, 126*(2015), 73–85. doi:10.1016/j.socscimed.2014.12.010

Michalak, L. & Trocki, K. (2006). Alcohol and Islam: An overview. *Contemporary Drug Problems, 33*(4), 523–562. doi:10.1177/009145090603300401

Michalak, L., Trocki, K., & Bond, J. (2007). Religion and alcohol in the U.S. national alcohol survey: How important is religion for abstention and drinking? *Drug and Alcohol Dependence, 87*, 268–280. doi:10.1016/j.drugalcdep.2006.07.013

Miech, R. A., Johnston, L. D., O'Malley, P. M., Bachman, J. G., Schulenberg, J. E., & Patrick, M. E. (2019). *Monitoring the Future national survey results on drug use. Data tables and figures.* Retrieved from http://www.monitoringthefuture.org/data/data.html

Milne, B. J, Caspi, A., Harrington, H., Poulton, R., Rutter, M., & Moffitt, T. E. (2009). Predictive value of family history on severity of illness: The case for depression, anxiety, alcohol dependence, and drug dependence. *Archives of General Psychiatry, 66*(7), 738–747. doi:10.1001/archgenpsychiatry.2009.55

Milne, B. J., Moffitt, T. E., Crump, R., Poulton, R., Rutter, M., Sears, M. R., . . . Caspi, A. (2008). How should we construct psychiatric family history scores? A comparison of alternative approaches from the Dunedin Family Health History Study. *Psychological Medicine, 38*(12), 1793–1802. doi:10.1017/S0033291708003115

Moffitt, T. E., Caspi, A., Dickson, N., Silva, P., & Stanton, W. (1996). Childhood-onset versus adolescent-onset antisocial conduct problems in males: Natural history from ages 3 to 18 years. *Development and Psychopathology, 8*(2), 399–424. doi:10.1017/S0954579400007161

Mohr, C. D., Averna, S., Kenny, D. A., Del Boca, F. K. (2001). "Getting by (or getting high) with a little help from my friends": An examination of adult alcoholics' friendships. *Journal of Studies on Alcohol, 62*(5), 637–645. doi:10.15288/jsa.2001.62.637

Mrug, S., Gaines, J., Su, W., & Windle, M. (2010). School-level substance use: Effects on early adolescents' alcohol, tobacco, and marijuana use. *Journal of Studies on Alcohol and Drugs, 71*(4), 488–495. doi:10.15288/jsad.2010.71.488

Mrug, S., & McCay, R. (2013). Parental and peer disapproval of alcohol use and its relationship to adolescent drinking: Age, gender, and racial differences. *Psychology of Addictive Behaviors, 27*(3), 604–614. doi:10.1037/a0031064

Novak, S. P., Reardon, S. F., Raudenbush, S. W., & Buka, S. L. (2006). Retail tobacco outlet density and youth cigarette smoking: A propensity-modeling approach. *American Journal of Public Health, 96*(4), 670–676. doi:10.2105/AJPH.2004.061622

O'Malley, P. M. (2004). Maturing out of problematic alcohol use. *Alcohol Research & Health, 28*(4), 202–205.

Paquette, K. L., Pannella Winn, L. A., Wilkey, C. M., Ferreira, K. N., & Donegan, L. R. W. (2019). A framework for integrating young peers in recovery into adolescent substance use prevention and early intervention. *Addictive Behavior, 99*, 106080. doi:10.1016/j.addbeh.2019.106080

Perreira, K. M., Marchante, A. N., Schwartz, S. J., Isasi, C. R., Carnethon, M. R., Corliss, H. L., . . . Delamater, A. M. (2019). Stress and resilience: Key correlates of mental health and substance use in the Hispanic community health study of Latino youth. *Journal of Immigrant and Minority Health, 21*(1), 4–13. doi:10.1007/s10903-018-0724-7

Pesko, M. F., & Robarts, A. M. (2017). Adolescent tobacco use in urban versus rural areas of the United States: The influence of tobacco control policy environments. *Journal of Adolescent Health, 61*(1), 70–76. doi:10.1016/j.jadohealth.2017.01.019

Piehler, T. F., Véronneau, M. H., & Dishion, T. J. (2012). Substance use progression from adolescence to early adulthood: Effortful control in the context of friendship influence and early-onset use. *Journal of Abnormal Child Psycholog, 40*(7), 1045–1058. doi:10.1007/s10802-012-9626-7

Pinchevsky, G. M., Arria, A. M., Caldeira, K. M., Garnier-Dykstra, L. M., Vincent, K. B., & O'Grady, K. E. (2012). Marijuana exposure opportunity and initiation during college: Parent and peer influences. *Prevention Science, 13*(1), 43–54. doi:10.1007/s11121-011-0243-4

Poelen, E. A., Scholte, R. H., Willemsen, G., Boomsma, D. I., & Engels, R. C. (2007). Drinking by parents, siblings, and friends as predictors of regular alcohol use in adolescents and young adults: A longitudinal twin-family study. *Alcohol & Alcoholism, 42*(4), 362–369. doi:10.1093/alcalc/agm042

Powers, G., Berger, L., Fuhrmann, D., & Fendrich, M. (2017). Family history density of substance use problems among undergraduate college students: Associations with heavy alcohol use and alcohol use disorder. *Addictive Behavior, 71*, 1–5. doi:10.1016/j.addbeh.2017.02.015

Ratzlaff, S., McDiarmid, D., Marty, D., & Rapp, C. (2006). The Kansas consumer as provider program: Measuring the effects of a supported education initiative. *Psychiatric Rehabilitation Journal, 29*(3), 174–182. doi:10.2975/29.2006.174.182

Rohde, P., Lewinsohn, P. M., Kahler, C. W., Seeley, J. R., & Brown, R. A. (2001). Natural course of alcohol use disorders from adolescence to young adulthood. *Journal of the American Academy of Child & Adolescent Psychiatry, 40*(1), 83–90. doi:10.1097/00004583-200101000-00020

Sampson, R. J., Raudenbush, S. W., & Earls, F. (1997). Neighborhoods and violent crime: A multilevel study of collective efficacy. *Science, 277*(5328), 918–924. doi:10.1126/science.277.5328.918

Sartor, C. E., Grant, J. D., Few, L. R., Werner, K. B., McCutcheon, V. V., Duncan, A. E., . . . Heath, A. C. (2018). Childhood trauma and two stages of alcohol use in African American and European American women: Findings from a female twin sample. *Prevention Science, 19*(6), 795–804. doi:10.1007/s11121-017-0838-5

Sartor, C. E., Wang, Z., Xu, K., Kranzler, H. R., & Gelernter, J. (2014). The joint effects of ADH1B variants and childhood adversity on alcohol related phenotypes in African-American and European-American women and men. *Alcoholism: Clinical and Experimental Research, 38*(12), 2907–2914. doi:10.1097/00004583-200101000-00020

Schneider, S. K., Buka, S. L., Dash, K., Winickoff, J. P., & O'Donnell, L. (2016). Community reductions in youth smoking after raising the minimum tobacco sales age to 21. *Tobacco Control, 25*(3), 355–359. doi:10.1136/tobaccocontrol-2014-052207

Scott, M. M., Cohen, D. A., Schonlau, M., Farley, T. A., & Bluthenthal, R. N. (2008). Alcohol and tobacco marketing: Evaluating compliance with outdoor advertising guidelines. *American Journal of Preventive Medicine, 35*(3), 203–209. doi:10.1016/j.amepre.2008.05.026

Shaw, A., Egan, J., & Gillespie, M. (2007). *Drugs and poverty: A literature review.* Glasgow: Scottish Drugs Forum (SDF) and the Scottish Association of Alcohol and Drug Action Teams (SAADAT). Retrieved from http://www.sdf.org.uk/wp-content/uploads/2017/03/Drugs_Poverty_Literature_Review_2007.pdf

Shelton, L. G. (2019). *The Bronfenbrenner Primer: A Guide to Develecology.* New York, NY: Routledge.

Sher, K. J., Dick, D. M., Crabbe, J. C., Hutchison, K. E., O'Malley, S. S., & Heath, A. C. (2010). Consilient research approaches in studying gene × environment interactions in alcohol research. *Addiction Biology, 15*(2), 200–216. doi:10.1111/j.1369-1600.2009.00189.x

Shih, R. A., Mullins, L., Ewing, B. A., Miyashiro, L., Tucker, J. S., Pedersen, E. R., . . . D'Amico, E. J. (2015). Associations between neighborhood alcohol availability and young adolescent alcohol use. *Psychology of Addictive Behaviors, 29*(4), 950. doi:10.1037/adb0000081

Sinha, R. (2008). Chronic stress, drug use, and vulnerability to addiction. *Annals of the New York Academy of Sciences, 1141*, 105–130. doi:10.1196/annals.1441.030

Stice, E., Barrera, M., & Chassin, L. (1993). Relation of parental support and control to adolescents' externalizing symptomatology and substance use: A longitudinal examination of curvilinear effects. *Journal of Abnormal Child Psychology, 21*(6), 609–629. doi:10.1007/BF00916446

Stoltenberg, S. F., Mudd, S. A., Blow, F. C., & Hill, E. M. (1998). Evaluating measures of family history of alcoholism: Density versus dichotomy. *Addiction, 93*(10), 1511–1520. doi:10.1046/j.1360-0443.1998.931015117.x

Theall, K. P., Drury, S. S., & Shirtcliff, E. A. (2012). Cumulative neighborhood risk of psychosocial stress and allostatic load in adolescents. *American Journal of Epidemiology, 176* (Suppl_7), S164–S174. doi:10.1093/aje/kws185

Trucco, E. M., Villafuerte, S., Heitzeg, M. M., Burmeister, M., & Zucker, R. A. (2016). Susceptibility effects of GABA receptor subunit alpha-2 (GABRA2) variants and parental monitoring on externalizing behavior trajectories: Risk and protection conveyed by the minor allele. *Developmental Psychopathology, 28*(1), 15–26. doi:10.1017/s0954579415000255

Turner, W. M., Cutter, H. S., Worobec, T. G., O'Farrell, T. J., Bayog, R. D., & Tsuang, M. T. (1993). Family history models of alcoholism: Age of onset, consequences and dependence. *Journal of Studies on Alcohol, 54*(2), 164–171. doi:10.15288/jsa.1993.54.164

Valente, T. W., Ritt-Olson, A., Stacy, A., Unger, J. B., Okamoto, J., & Sussman S. (2007). Peer acceleration: Effects of a social network tailored substance abuse prevention program among high-risk adolescents. *Addiction, 102*(11), 1804–1815. doi:10.1111/j.1360-0443.2007.01992.x

Vink, J. M. (2016). Genetics of addiction: Future focus on gene x environment interaction? *Journal of Studies on Alcohol and Drugs, 77*(5), 684–687. doi:10.15288/jsad.2016.77.684

Visser, L., de Winter, A. F., & Reijneveld, S. A. (2012). The parent-child relationship and adolescent alcohol use: A systematic review of longitudinal studies. *BMC Public Health, 12,* 886. doi:10.1186/1471-2458-12-886

Wagenaar, A. C., & Toomey, T. L. (2002). Effects of minimum drinking age laws: Review and analyses of the literature from 1960 to 2000. *Journal of Studies on Alcohol, Supplement* (14), 206–225. doi:10.15288/jsas.2002.s14.206

Wakefield, M. A., Loken, B., & Hornik, R. C. (2010). Use of mass media campaigns to change health behaviour. *Lancet, 376*(9748), 1261–1271. doi:10.1016/S0140-6736(10)60809-4

Wang, Q., Phillips, N. E., Small, M. L., & Sampson, R. J. (2018). Urban mobility and neighborhood isolation in America's 50 largest cities. *Proceedings of the National Academy of Sciences, 115*(30), 7735–7740. doi:10.1073/pnas.1802537115

Warner, T. D. (2016). Up in smoke: Neighborhood contexts of marijuana use from adolescence through young adulthood. *Journal of Youth and Adolescence, 45*(1), 35–53. doi:10.1007/s10964-015-0370-5

Woodford, M.S. (2001). *Recovering college students' perspectives: Investigating the phenomenon of recovery from substance abuse among undergraduate students.* Doctoral dissertation, University of Virginia.

Zemore, S. E., Karriker-Jaffe, K. J., Mulia, N., Kerr, W. C., Ehlers, C. L., Cook, W. K., . . . Greenfield, T. K. (2018). The future of research on alcohol-related disparities across U.S. racial/ethnic groups: A plan of attack. *Journal of Studies on Alcohol and Drugs, 79*(1), 7–21. doi:10.15288/jsad.2018.79.7

Zimmerman, G. M., & Farrell, C. (2017). Parents, peers, perceived risk of harm, and the neighborhood: Contextualizing key influences on adolescent substance use. *Journal of Youth and Adolescence, 46*(1), 228–247. doi:10.1007/s10964-016-0475-5

Zucker, R. A., Ellis, D. A., & Fitzgerald, H. E. (1994). Developmental evidence for at least two alcoholisms. I. Biopsychosocial variation among pathways into symptomatic difficulty. *Annals of the New York Academy of Science, 708,* 134–146. doi:10.1111/j.1749-6632.1994.tb24706.x

Gambling disorder
The first behavioral addiction

Lia Nower, Devin Mills and Wen Li (Vivien) Anthony

Background

In the United States, the expansion of legalized gambling beyond Las Vegas and Atlantic City began in the 1990s with pooled lotteries and floating casinos but escalated significantly with the growing popularity of the Internet and smart phones. Most individuals who gamble do so for recreation only. However, a meaningful proportion of individuals who gamble experience a wide range of adverse consequences, including stress-induced health problems (Morasco & Petry, 2006); criminality and bankruptcy (see Nower & Blaszczynski, 2013, for a review); and elevated rates of family violence (Afifi, Brownridge, MacMillian, & Sareen, 2010; Suomi et al., 2013), sometimes resulting in suicide or familicide (Anderson, Sisask, & Varnik, 2011). Children of individuals experiencing gambling problems are likely to develop addictions, mental health problems such as anxiety and depression (See Kourgiantakis, Saint-Jacques, & Tremblay, 2013, for a review), and to act out at school. All of these consequences occur in systems where social workers practice.

Unfortunately, social work is largely absent from advocacy and prevention efforts around gambling. Practitioners in social work and other fields view gambling as harmless recreation (Sansanwal, Derevensky, & Gavriel-Fried, 2016), and schools of social work continue to train students in identifying and treating only substance use disorders, despite changes in diagnostic classifications to acknowledge gambling disorder as an addiction. This chapter provides an overview of problem gambling and gambling disorder for social workers, including: (a) terminology and history of the disorder; (b) prevalence of problem gambling and gambling disorder; (c) etiological influences; (d) comorbidity; (e) diagnosis and treatment; and (f) implications and emerging issues.

Terminology and history of the disorder

Gambling disorder is a "spectrum" disorder, with individuals shifting from lower (recreational) to higher (disorder) levels of pathology across their lifetimes, and, sometimes, back again (Custer & Milt, 1985). The progression across the spectrum typically occurs in three phases: the winning phase, the losing phase, and the desperation phase (Custer & Milt, 1985).

Typically, an early win, series of wins, or positive emotional state resulting from gambling fuel continued play in the "winning phase," which invariably leads to mounting losses in the "losing phase," and negative consequences, including criminality, in the "desperation phase."

There exists a lack of clarity in gambling research around terms used to refer to non-recreational gambling. In social work, we conscientiously attempt to avoid labels, opting instead for person-first language. However, gambling studies has largely been a domain inhabited by scholars in psychiatry, psychology, and public health with a disease-focus, and, therefore, individuals who gamble are referred to as "gamblers" and those who endorse problem symptomatology as "problem gamblers." The absence of clinical criteria for individuals who report symptoms of problem gambling but fail to meet clinical criteria provides an added confound. As a result, "problem gambler" is typically used in the literature as a catch-all phrase, applied to sub-threshold problem gamblers and, sometimes, to those who meet criteria as well. Where possible, we will opt to substitute person-first language in this chapter, however, for brevity and accuracy, we will also use the existing terminology in the field.

Gambling disorder is a secret addiction. Most problem gamblers can hide the scope of their financial devastation from friends and families until it is too late to remediate the damage. Thus, problem gambling has remained largely under-recognized since it was first identified in the writings of Freud (1928). Gambling to excess has long been viewed as a vice, with those who develop problems as "degenerates," lacking in self-control; for example, Moran (1970) argued that gambling only becomes a problem when the money runs out. Those who experience gambling problems, however, dispute that characterization, referring to their behavior as "compulsive" and beyond their volitional control (Custer & Milt, 1985).

Tension in the field is reflected in the evolution of the diagnostic criteria for gambling disorder. Sigmund Freud (1928) was the first to identify excessive gambling as a treatable illness. However, the medical community largely ignored the disorder until 1979 when the World Health Organization (WHO) identified "pathological gambling" as a psychiatric illness in the International Classification of Diseases (ICD-9; WHO, 1979). The next year, the American Psychiatric Association (APA) added pathological gambling to the third edition of the *Diagnostic and Statistical Manual of Mental Disorders* (DSM-III; APA, 1980).

Initially, the APA classified pathological gambling as an impulse control disorder, along with kleptomania, trichotillomania, explosive temper disorder, and pyromania. Counselors working in the field disputed this classification, arguing that gambling was an addictive behavior analogous to substance use disorders. While the classification remained unchanged, criteria evolved in the DSM-III-R (APA, 1987) to include parallels with substance addictions (i.e. preoccupation, tolerance, withdrawal, loss of control). All versions of the diagnostic criteria have retained two hallmark characteristics of gambling disorder: (a) "chasing," that is, repeated attempts to relive a win or recoup a loss, and (b) "bailouts," borrowing from family, friends and others to address growing debt. Subsequent publications of the DSM, editions IV (APA, 1994) and IV-R (APA, 2000), retained a hybrid-criteria of addiction and behavioral criteria.

In subsequent years, psychiatric researchers began documenting the neurobiological similarities between individuals experiencing gambling and those experiencing substance use disorders, which share similar clinical expression, brain origin, comorbidity, and physiology (Goudriaan, Oosterlaan, de Beurs, & Van den Brink, 2004, 2006; Grant, Potenza, Weinstein, & Gorelick, 2010; Potenza, 2006, 2008). These findings informed a conceptual shift in DSM-5 (APA, 2013), which reclassified "Gambling Disorder" as an addictive disorder in the "Substance-Related and Addictive Disorders" chapter and removed the commission of criminal acts from the criteria. This change in classification failed to provide guidance on how to classify sub-threshold problem gamblers, individuals who fail to meet full clinical criteria for gambling disorder but manifest significant problems with the behavior.

Prevalence across populations

In the United States, epidemiological studies have consistently reported that 80–90% of adults gamble at some point in their lives and 60–80% report gambling within the past year, with rates of gambling disorder of about 2% (past year to 3% lifetime) (Kessler et al., 2008; National Opinion Research Center, 1999; Welte, Barnes, Wieczorek, Tidwell, & Parker, 2002). However, in states like New Jersey, which has a long history of gambling and a wide range of gambling opportunities, rates are significantly higher. For example, a recent New Jersey prevalence study found that about 6% of residents who gamble would likely meet criteria for gambling disorder with an additional 15% reporting symptoms of problem gambling (Nower, Volberg, & Caler, 2017).

Attempts to reconcile disparities in prevalence rates are confounded by the lack of classification for sub-threshold problem gamblers as well as the wide variation in clinical versus epidemiological assessment instruments. However, the breadth of studies in both the United States and other countries suggest that U.S. rates are around the median for worldwide rates, which range from 0.12% to 7.6%, depending on methodologies, screening instruments, and time frames (Calado & Griffiths, 2016; Williams, Volberg, & Stevens, 2012). In addition, a number of studies have consistently reported higher rates of gambling problems and disorder among racial and ethnic minorities: Native Americans (Alegría et al., 2009; Martins, Lee, Kim, Letourneau, & Storr, 2014); Asians (Kong et al., 2013; Toyama et al., 2014); Hispanics/Latinos (Barry, Stefanovics, Desai, & Potenza, 2011a; Caler, Garcia, & Nower, 2017), and African American/Blacks (Alegría et al., 2009; Barry, Stefanovics, Desai, & Potenza, 2011b; Welte et al., 2002). In addition, homeless individuals (Matheson, Devotta, Wendaferew, & Pedersen, 2014; Nower, Eyrich-Garg, Pollio & North, 2015) and war veterans (See Levy & Tracy, 2018, for a review) who gamble at problem levels have exhibited significantly higher rates of gambling disorder, as well as mental health, substance use, and personality disorders.

Decades of research demonstrate that gambling typically begins at home and early gambling correlates with later onset of gambling (Kundu et al., 2013; Nower, Derevensky, & Gupta, 2004), as well as other problems: sexual behavior before age 18 (Martins et al., 2014), substance misuse (Nower, Derevensky et al., 2004), decreased academic performance (Vitaro, Brendgen, Girard, Dionne, & Boivin, 2018), and delinquent behaviors (Vitaro, Brendgen, Ladouceur, & Tremblay, 2001). In the United States and Canada, between 70% and 85% of underage youth report past-year gambling and 4–6% endorse serious symptoms of disorder (Blinn-Pike, Worthy, & Jonkman, 2010; Chalmers & Willoughby, 2006). Worldwide, rates of both gambling participation and gambling problems vary widely, due primarily to methodological inconsistencies including the lack of sub–clinical cut-scores. One recent review estimated that 0.2–12.3% of youth meet diagnostic criteria for problem gambling across five continents (Calado, Alexandre, & Griffiths, 2017). Recent legalization of online sports wagering, as well as the pervasive availability of gambling through smart phones, could increase the risk of youth gambling, as youth can wager with parents and friends or utilize the online accounts of those who are of legal gambling age if an adult grants them access. This is particularly troubling because rates of problem gambling typically peak in young adulthood with youth of college age. A meta-analysis of college-age gambling studies reported that more than 6% of college students met clinical criteria for gambling disorder, and an additional 10% reported serious gambling problems—rates nearly three times that of adults (Nowak, 2018). These and other studies portend serious implications from the increasing availability of online gambling opportunities, as tech-savvy youth are able to evade geo-fencing and other platform safeguards designed to protect them.

Etiological influences

Researchers have proposed a number of etiological models to explain the development of gambling problems, among them: social reward (Ocean & Smith, 1993), behavioral (Weatherly & Dixon, 2007), cognitive behavioral (Sharpe, 2002), and neurobiological and genetic factors (Ibáñez, Blanco, & Sáiz-Ruiz, 2002; Ibáñez, Blanco, de Castro, Fernandez-Piqueras, & Sáiz-Ruiz, 2003; Potenza, 2013). The most widely cited etiological model is the pathways model (Blaszczynski & Nower, 2002), a common conceptual framework for research studies (Allami et al., 2017; Balodis, Thomas, & Moore, 2014; Nower, Martins, Lin, & Blanco, 2013; Valleur et al., 2016). The pathways model asserts that the accessibility, availability, and acceptability of gambling opportunities contribute to the initiation of gambling. In addition, positive experiences in the gambling environment as well as erroneous cognitions about the nature of randomness, odds, and probabilities fuel persistence in play.

Apart from these common factors, the pathways model asserts that the development of gambling problems is distinguished by distinct sub-groups of risk factors that lead to problem gambling: problem gamblers in Pathway 1 typically begin gambling for social or other reasons and develop problems due primarily to the conditioning effects of continued gambling over time. In contrast, Pathway 2 problem gamblers report pre-morbid mental health comorbidity and gamble primarily to cope with stress or to escape aversive mood states. Gamblers in Pathway 3 typically present with high levels of impulsivity, risk-taking, and antisocial traits; therefore, gambling is but one of many pleasure-seeking activities. These factors were comprehensively explored by the authors of the Gambling Pathways Questionnaire (GPQ; Nower & Blaszczynski, 2017), cited in a later section, which provided empirical support for the model but suggest that motivational factors (e.g. coping with stress, searching for meaning) and child maltreatment and trauma are key factors in the development and maintenance of gambling problems.

As suggested by the pathways model, a proportion of individuals experiencing gambling problems have genetic and/or biological vulnerabilities that predispose them to sensation seeking and risk-taking, fueled by the release of dopamine which mediates pleasure responses of the brain (Clark & Dagher, 2014; Comings et al., 2001). Studies cite evidence for the familial transmission of problem gambling, alcohol use disorder (Slutske, Ellingson, Richmond-Rakerd, Zhu, & Martin, 2013), and negative emotionality in family members (Slutske, Cho, Piasecki, & Martin, 2013; Slutske et al, 2014), suggesting that environmental factors and inherited genetic traits such as impulsivity (Clark et al., 2012) likely play a role in the development of gambling disorder in a proportion of gamblers (Slutske, Moffitt, Poulton, & Caspi, 2012).

Specifically, several studies reported that parental gambling is a key predictor of problem gambling behavior among youth (Kundu et al., 2013; Nower, Derevensky et al., 2004). Parents who gamble at problem levels are significantly more likely to have children who demonstrate impulsive, hyperactive, and/or inattentive behaviors (Carbonneau, Vitaro, Brendgen, & Tremblay, 2018). Youth who gamble with their parents or believe their parents have a problem, even if untrue, have the highest rates of gambling problems (King, Abrams, & Wilkinson, 2010; Leeman et al., 2014; Vitaro & Wanner, 2011). These findings are particularly troublesome in light of the fact that gambling is generally viewed by parents and educators as harmless activity (Campbell, Derevensky, Meerkamper, & Cutajar, 2011; Derevensky, St-Pierre, Temcheff, & Gupta, 2014). For example, one study of parents with children ages 13–18 found that most parents had little knowledge of gambling-related harms and viewed gambling as a relatively unimportant issue compared to other potentially risky behaviors (Campbell et al., 2011). Similarly, teachers of middle and high school students in another study viewed gambling as the least serious of a list of activities affecting youth, and half of the participants indicated that gambling in school can constitute a good learning activity (Derevensky et al., 2014).

Of particular interest to social workers, childhood maltreatment and trauma appear to serve as an underlying motivation for gambling in some groups, fueling a desire for escape and mental disengagement. Studies report that problem gamblers, compared to recreational gamblers, are more likely to report childhood sexual, physical, and emotional abuse (Black, Shaw, McCormick, & Allen, 2012; Hodgins et al., 2010; Petry & Steinberg, 2005). Those gamblers, in turn, report higher rates of comorbid disorders (Leppink & Grant, 2015) and use gambling as a stress-coping strategy which, in turn, compounds stress due to mounting debts.

Finally, a common element across all individuals experiencing gambling problems is the presence of cognitive distortions during play. Gamblers typically misperceive their chances of winning based primarily on three erroneous beliefs: the "illusion of control," the belief that they can control a random outcome (Langer, 1975); "gambler's fallacy," the belief that, as losses increase, wins also will increase (Tversky & Kahneman, 1971); and "biased evaluation," the tendency to accept wins at face value but explain away losses (Gilovich, 1983). Those beliefs support the notion that a number is "due" or "hot," that machines on casino aisles pay more than others, or that small credit increases on a machine are wins, even though, overall, the player is losing money. Combined with other etiological risk factors, these cognitions encourage continued play and lead to the development of disorder.

Comorbidity

It is well established in the gambling literature that a majority of problem gamblers report comorbid mental health and substance use disorders, particularly alcohol and/or drug use disorders, nicotine dependence, anxiety and/or depression, post-traumatic stress disorder, and/or personality disorders, even after controlling for gender, race, and other sociodemographic factors (Håkansson, Karlsson, & Widinghoff, 2018; Nower et al., 2013; Schluter et al., 2019; for a review, see Dowling et al., 2015). Of particular concern, a number of studies have reported that problem gamblers experience higher rates of suicidality than any other addiction—as high as 81% in one study—and are three times more likely to report suicidality than the general population (Newman & Thompson, 2007; Wong, Kwok, Tang, Blaszczynski, & Tse, 2014). These findings are consistent across studies with youth (Nower, Gupta, et al., 2004), college students (Stuhldreher, Stuhldreher, & Forrest, 2007), and adults (Nower & Blaszczynski, 2008). By the time families learn of a member's gambling losses, it is often too late to save their cars, homes, or jobs. Faced with the prospect of facing the loved ones they have betrayed problem gamblers often contemplate or resort to self-harm.

Diagnosis and treatment

Given that Gambling Disorder is a relatively novel addiction to most social workers, many educators and students are unfamiliar with current screening tools used in gambling research and practice. As outlined above, the diagnosis has undergone significant changes since its introduction in 1980, and commonly used tools such as the South Oaks Gambling Screen (SOGS; Lesieur & Blume, 1987) are long outdated. Increasing identification of gamblers in social work settings will require a two-step approach: introducing a very brief screen to "flag" those with potential gambling problems, and following positive screening with a problem severity measure for classification and an etiology measure to assist in individualizing treatment. The following instruments are currently used by gambling researchers and treatment providers internationally.

Screening instruments

For decades, there was only one measure of problem gambling and gambling disorder: the SOGS (Lesieur& Blume, 1987), a 20-item screen based on the DSM-III. The SOGS had satisfactory reliability but yielded high rates of false positives in some populations (Stinchfield, 2013). As a result, other measures were developed with greater reliability, particularly in differentiating among levels of problem gambling (for a detailed review of all measures, see Caler, Garcia, & Nower, 2016). Currently utilized measures include:

- The Problem Gambling Severity Index (Ferris & Wynne, 2001): a nine-item screen for problem severity, demonstrating high internal consistency and validity, used internationally for both epidemiological and clinical populations.
- The NODS—CLiP (National Opinion Research Center DSM-IV Screen for Gambling Problems Control, Lying, and Preoccupation brief screen) (Toce-Gerstein, Gerstein, & Volberg, 2009) and NODS PERC (NODS Preoccupation, Escape, Risked Relationships, and Chasing brief screen) (Volberg, Munck, & Petry, 2011): validated three- and four-item screening instruments, based on a longer instrument used in the 1998 U.S. general population survey and based on the DSM. The CLiP is intended for use in mental health settings and PERC is more discriminating for those experiencing comorbid substance use disorders (See Himelhoch et al., 2015).
- The Gambling Pathways Questionnaire (GPQ; Nower & Blaszczynski, 2017): a 48-item valid and reliable etiological screening instrument, used to group gamblers into subgroups by risk factors. It is intended for use with a problem severity measure.

Treatment outcomes

Published systematic reviews and meta-analyses have evaluated gambling treatment outcomes (Petry, Ginley, & Rash, 2017; Pickering, Keen, Entwistle, & Blaszczynski, 2018; Yakovenko & Hodgins, 2016). Cognitive behavioral therapy (CBT) remains the most empirically supported approach (see reviews by Blaszczynski & Nower, 2013; Fortune & Goodie, 2012). Seminal studies on the effectiveness of CBT and gambling are by Ladouceur, Sylvain, Letarte, Giroux, and Jacques (1998), who established that individuals restructure gambling-related cognitions, primarily through education about concepts of randomness and the independence of events, the odds of winning, and the futility of common cognitive fallacies that initiate or maintain problem gambling behavior. They concluded that interventions that also incorporate problem solving and relapse-prevention along with CBT are the most successful at decreasing gambling severity (Ladouceur et al., 1998; Sylvain, Ladouceur & Boisvert, 1997).

Other treatment approaches have demonstrated mixed results, including motivational enhancement (Hodgins, Currie, & el-Guebaly, 2001; Ledgerwood et al., 2013) and brief motivational treatments (Hodgins, Currie, el-Guebaly, & Peden, 2004); motivational interviewing, which is more effective when combined with CBT (Petry et al., 2017); personalized feedback (Marchica & Derevensky, 2016; Yakovenko & Hodgins, 2016); mindfulness-enhanced cognitive therapy (Toneatto, Pillai, & Courtice, 2014); meditation awareness training (Shonin, Van Gordon, & Griffiths, 2014); and imaginal desensitization (Blaszczynski & Nower, 2013). Studies fail to provide strong support for the use of specific medications for the treatment of gambling disorder (Bartley & Bloch, 2013; Yakovenko & Hodgins, 2016).

Implications and emerging issues for social work

A significant emerging issue for social work is the advent of interactive technologies that allow 24/7 access to gambling opportunities, irrespective of age. This is particularly critical in light of the recent legalization of sports wagering in the United States, which appeals to youth, and a growing overlap between gambling and video gaming (see Chapter 9). Historically, the gambling industry uses the term "gaming" for "gambling," which traditionally involves wagering on chance outcomes for money. In contrast, researchers typically reserve the term "gaming" for video game play without money bets. However, video game developers increasingly blur the lines between gaming and gambling by embedding gambling elements in video games to generate more income. Such monetization tactics include:

- Social casino games: gambling-themed video games, which are free to play and hosted by social media sites (e.g. Facebook), casual games with gambling elements, and practice modules of online casino games, which "prime" players to transition to a gambling environment (Gainsbury, Hing, Delfabbro & King, 2014).
- Loot boxes (also called "loot crates" or "loot chests"): virtual items that can be purchased with real money for a chance to win valuable in-game items to enhance play. As with gambling, loot box contents are determined by chance. Preliminary data suggest loot box purchases are related to higher frequency of video gaming and online gambling engagement, which, in turn, increase the risk of developing problem video gaming and gambling (Li, Mills, & Nower, 2019).
- "Skin" betting: virtual, decorative items in video games, which can be purchased and traded with money through an online market place or a third-party service, as a stake in a bet on the outcome of gambling activities or professional video game matches (i.e. eSports) based on chance. Skin betting has been associated with higher problem gambling severity (Macey & Hamari, 2019).

These new technologies introduce children and youth to gambling elements at a very young age and prime them for the crossover to gambling with money. The conditioning effects of such reinforcement schedules can fuel persistence and the initiation of problem Internet/video gaming behavior (see Chapter 9). King, Delfabbro, Kaptsis, and Zwaans (2014) examined the relationship of adolescent gambling to free gambling sites and social media and reported that adolescents aged 12–17 with a history of gambling in simulated activities were at highest risk of developing gambling disorder. Social workers should be well educated on emerging technologies and their potential impact on the early onset of addictive behaviors among children, adolescents, and young adults.

Future directions for advocacy and practice

Gambling is a popular and poorly understood behavior with the potential to cause irreparable harm to individuals and their families, particularly those who lack the financial ability to recover from significant losses. Social workers are a critical but largely absent voice in advocacy and policymaking efforts around this issue, even though gambling disorder adversely affects populations of central interest to social work. Few social work programs offer gambling-specific training, incorporate gambling into courses focused on addiction, or prepare practitioners to deliver evidence-based screening or treatment. Social workers in child welfare, health/mental health, and school settings generally lack the skills to identify and address problem gambling, and, as a result, are largely unable to help children of problem gamblers who may develop addictions themselves. In the United States, for example, organizations focused on social work practice and research have yet to make gambling disorder a priority or to broaden their focus from substance misuse to include all addictive behaviors. In contrast, the Australia Association of Social Work has published a position paper and regularly conducts advocacy and training on problem gambling; notably, gambling tops the list of social problem targets on their website (www.aasw.asn.au). Given that social workers are at the forefront of many care systems, it is critical to broaden our focus and train new social workers to anticipate and address problems that accompany rapidly evolving technology.

Social work is well positioned to partner with those most affected by the unintended adverse consequences of gambling in settings where they will likely encounter them: child welfare agencies, mental health settings, emergency rooms, schools, family violence shelters, human service organizations, community agencies, homeless shelters, and the criminal justice system. As interactive forms of gambling and gaming continue to expand, and players become engaged at younger ages, it is critical for social workers to become stakeholders in this growing area of public health concern.

References

Afifi, T. O., Brownridge, D. A., MacMillian, H., & Sareen, J. (2010). The relationship of gambling to intimate partner violence and child maltreatment in a nationally representative sample. *Journal of Psychiatric Research, 44*(5), 331–337. doi:10.1016/j.jpsychires.2009.07.010

Alegría, A. A., Petry, N. M., Hasin, D. S., Liu, S. M., Grant, B. F., & Blanco, C. (2009). Disordered gambling among racial and ethnic groups in the US: Results from the national epidemiologic survey on alcohol and related conditions. *CNS Spectrums, 14*(03), 132–143. doi:10.1017/S1092852900020113

Allami, Y., Vitaro, F., Brendgen, M., Carbonneau, R., Lacourse, É., & Tremblay, R. E. (2017). A longitudinal empirical investigation of the pathways model of problem gambling. *Journal of Gambling Studies, 33*(4), 1153–1167. doi:10.1007/s10899-017-9682-6

American Psychiatric Association. (1980). *Diagnostic and statistical manual of mental disorders* (3rd ed.). Washington, DC.: American Psychiatric Association.

American Psychiatric Association. (1987). *Diagnostic and statistical manual of mental disorders* (3rd ed., text rev.). Washington, DC: Authors.

American Psychiatric Association. (1994). *Diagnostic and statistical manual of mental disorders* (4th ed.). Washington, DC: Authors.

American Psychiatric Association. (2000). *Diagnostic and statistical manual of mental disorders* (4th ed., text rev.). Washington, DC: Authors.

American Psychiatric Association. (2013). *Diagnostic and statistical manual of mental disorders* (5th ed.). Arlington, VA: Authors. doi:10.1176/appi.books.9780890425596

Anderson, A., Sisask, M., & Värnik, A. (2011). Familicide and suicide in a case of gambling dependence. *The Journal of Forensic Psychiatry & Psychology, 22*(1), 156–168. doi:10.1080/14789949.2010.518244

Balodis, S. R. S., Thomas, A. C., & Moore, S. M. (2014). Sensitivity to reward and punishment: Horse race and EGM gamblers compared. *Personality and Individual Differences, 56*, 29–33. doi:10.1016/j.paid.2013.08.015

Barry, D. T., Stefanovics, E. A., Desai, R. A., & Potenza, M. N. (2011a). Gambling problem severity and psychiatric disorders among Hispanic and white adults: Findings from a nationally representative sample. *Journal of Psychiatric Research, 45*(3), 404–411. doi:10.1016/j.jpsychires.2010.07.010

Barry, D. T., Stefanovics, E. A., Desai, R. A., & Potenza, M. N. (2011b). Differences in the associations between gambling problem severity and psychiatric disorders among black and white adults: Findings from the national epidemiologic survey on alcohol and related conditions. *The American Journal on Addictions, 20*(1), 69–77. doi:10.1111/j.1521-0391.2010.00098.x

Bartley, C. A., & Bloch, M. H. (2013). Meta-analysis: Pharmacological treatment of pathological gambling. *Expert Review of Neurotherapeutics, 13*(8), 887–894. doi:10.1586/14737175.2013.814938

Black, D. W., Shaw, M. C., McCormick, B. A., & Allen, J. (2012). Marital status, childhood maltreatment, and family dysfunction: A controlled study of pathological gambling. *Journal of Clinical Psychiatry, 73*(10), 1293–1297. doi:10.4088/JCP.12m07800

Blaszczynski, A., & Nower, L. (2002). A pathways model of problem and pathological gambling. *Addiction, 97*(5), 487–499. doi:10.1046/j.1360-0443.2002.00015.x

Blaszczynski, A. & Nower, L. (2013). Cognitive-behavioral therapy: Translating research into clinical practice. In D. C. S. Richard, A. Blaszczynski, & L. Nower (Eds.), *The Wiley-Blackwell handbook of disordered gambling* (pp. 204–220). New York, NY: Wiley-Blackwell. doi:10.1002/9781118316078.ch9

Blinn-Pike, L., Worthy, S. L., & Jonkman, J. N. (2010). Adolescent gambling: A review of an emerging field of research. *Journal of Adolescent Health, 47*(3), 223–236. doi:10.1016/j.jadohealth.2010.05.003

Calado, F., Alexandre, J., & Griffiths, M. D. (2017). Prevalence of adolescent problem gambling: A systematic review of recent research. *Journal of Gambling Studies, 33*(2), 397–424. doi:10.1007/s10899-016-9627-5

Calado, F., & Griffiths, M. D. (2016). Problem gambling worldwide: An update and systematic review of empirical research (2000–2015). *Journal of Behavioral Addictions, 5*(4), 592–613. doi:10.1556/2006.5.2016.073

Caler, K., Garcia, J. R. V., & Nower, L. (2016). Assessing problem gambling: A review of classic and specialized measures. *Current Addiction Reports, 3*(4), 437–444. doi:10.1007/s40429-016-0118-7

Caler, K. R., Garcia, J. R. V., & Nower, L. (2017). Problem gambling among ethnic minorities: Results from an epidemiological study. *Asian Journal of Gambling Issues and Public Health, 7*(1), 7. doi:10.1186/s40405-017-0027-2

Campbell, C., Derevensky, J., Meerkamper, E., & Cutajar, J. (2011). Parents' perceptions of adolescent gambling: A Canadian national study. *Journal of Gambling Issues, 25*, 36–53. http://jgi.camh.net/doi/pdf/10.4309/jgi.2011.25.4

Carbonneau, R., Vitaro, F., Brendgen, M., & Tremblay, R. E. (2018). The intergenerational association between parents' problem gambling and impulsivity-hyperactivity/inattention behaviors in children. *Journal of Abnormal Child Psychology, 46*(6), 1203–1215. doi:10.1007/s10802-017-0362-x

Chalmers, H., & Willoughby, T. (2006). Do predictors of gambling involvement differ across male and female adolescents? *Journal of Gambling Studies, 22*(4), 373–392. doi:10.1007/s10899-006-9024-6

Clark, C. A., & Dagher, A. (2014). The role of dopamine in risk taking: A specific look at Parkinson's disease and gambling. *Frontiers in Behavioral Neuroscience, 8*, 196. doi:10.3389/fnbeh.2014.00196

Clark, L., Stokes, P. R., Wu, K., Michalczuk, R., Benecke, A., Watson, B. J., . . . & Lingford-Hughes, A. R. (2012). Striatal dopamine D2/D3 receptor binding in pathological gambling is correlated with mood-related impulsivity. *Neuroimage, 63*(1), 40–46. doi:10.1016/j.neuroimage.2012.06.067

Comings, D. E., Gade-Andavolu, R., Gonzalez, N., Wu, S., Muhleman, D., Chen, C., Koh, P., & Rosenthal, R. J. (2001). The additive effect of neurotransmitter genes in pathological gambling. *Clinical Genetics, 60*(2), 107–116. doi:10.1034/j.1399-0004.2001.600204.x

Custer, R., & Milt, H. (1985). *When luck runs out: Help for compulsive gamblers and their families.* New York, NY: Facts on File.

Derevensky, J. L., St-Pierre, R. A., Temcheff, C. E., & Gupta, R. (2014). Teacher awareness and attitudes regarding adolescent risky behaviours: Is adolescent gambling perceived to be a problem? *Journal of Gambling Studies, 30*(2), 435–451. doi:10.1007/s10899-013-9363-z

Dowling, N. A., Cowlishaw, S., Jackson, A. C., Merkouris, S. S., Francis, K. L., & Christensen, D. R. (2015). Prevalence of psychiatric co-morbidity in treatment-seeking problem gamblers: A systematic review and meta-analysis. *Australian and New Zealand Journal of Psychiatry, 49*(6), 519–539. doi:10.1177/0004867415575774

Ferris, J. A., & Wynne, H. J. (2001). *The Canadian problem gambling index* (pp. 1–59). Ottawa, Canada: Canadian Centre on Substance Abuse.

Fortune, E. E., & Goodie, A. S. (2012). Cognitive distortions as a component and treatment focus of pathological gambling: A review. *Psychology of Addictive Behaviors, 26*(2), 298–310. doi:10.1037/a0026422

Freud, S. (1928). Dostoevsky and parricide. In J. Strachey (Ed.), *Complete psychological works of Sigmund Freud*. London, UK: Hogarth Press.

Gainsbury, S., Hing, N., Delfabbro, P. H., & King, D. L. (2014). A taxonomy of gambling and casino games via social media and online technologies. *International Gambling Studies, 14*(2), 196–213. doi:10.1556/2006.5.2016.073

Gilovich, T. (1983). Biased evaluation and persistence in gambling. *Journal of Personality and Social Psychology, 44*(6), 1110–1126. doi:10.1037/0022-3514.44.6.1110

Goudriaan, A. E., Oosterlaan, J., de Beurs, E., & Van den Brink, W. (2004). Pathological gambling: A comprehensive review of biobehavioral findings. *Neuroscience & Biobehavioral Reviews, 28*(2), 123–141. doi:10.1016/j.neubiorev.2004.03.001

Goudriaan, A. E., Oosterlaan, J., de Beurs, E., & Van Den Brink, W. (2006). Neurocognitive functions in pathological gambling: A comparison with alcohol dependence, Tourette syndrome and normal controls. *Addiction, 101*(4), 534–547. doi:10.1111/j.1360-0443.2006.01380.x

Grant, J. E., Potenza, M. N., Weinstein, A., & Gorelick, D. A. (2010). Introduction to behavioral addictions. *The American Journal of Drug and Alcohol Abuse, 36*(5), 233–241. doi:10.3109/00952990.2010.491884

Håkansson, A., Karlsson, A., & Widinghoff, C. (2018, September). Primary and secondary diagnoses of gambling disorder and psychiatric comorbidity in the Swedish health care system—A nationwide register study. *Frontiers in Psychiatry, 9*, 1–9. doi:10.3389/fpsyt.2018.00426.

Himelhoch, S. S., Miles-McLean, H., Medoff, D. R., Kreyenbuhl, J., Rugle, L., Bailey-Kloch, M., . . . Brownley, J. (2015). Evaluation of brief screens for gambling disorder in the substance use treatment setting. *The American Journal on Addictions, 24*(5), 460–466. doi:10.1111/ajad.12241

Hodgins, D. C., Currie, S.R., & el-Guebaly, N. (2001). Motivational enhancement and self-help treatments for problem gambling. *Journal of Consulting and Clinical Psychology, 69*(1), 50-57. doi:10.1037/0022-006X.69.1.50

Hodgins, D. C., Currie, S., el-Guebaly, N., & Peden, N. (2004). Brief motivational treatment for problem gambling: A 24-month follow-up. *Psychology of Addictive Behaviors, 18*(3), 293–296. doi:10.1037/0893-164X.18.3.293

Hodgins, D. C., Schopflocher, D. P., el-Gueblay, N., Casey, D. M., Smith, G. J., Williams, R. J., & Wood, R. T. (2010). The association between childhood maltreatment and gambling problems in a community sample of adult men and women. *Psychology of Addictive Behaviors, 24*(3), 548–554. doi:10.1037/a0019946

Ibáñez, A., Blanco, C., de Castro, I. P., Fernandez-Piqueras, J., & Sáiz-Ruiz, J. (2003). Genetics of pathological gambling. *Journal of Gambling Studies, 19*(1), 11–22. doi:10.1023/A%3A1021271029163

Ibáñez, A., Blanco, C., & Sáiz-Ruiz, J. (2002). Neurobiology and genetics of pathological gambling. *Psychiatric Annals, 32*(3), 181–185. doi:10.3928/0048-5713-20020301-07

Kessler, R. C., Hwang, I., LaBrie, R., Petukhova, M., Sampson, N. A., Winters, K. C., & Shaffer, H. J. (2008). DSM-IV pathological gambling in the national comorbidity survey replication. *Psychological Medicine, 38*(9), 1351–1360. doi:10.1017/S0033291708002900

King, D. L., Delfabbro, P. H., Kaptsis, D., & Zwaans, T. (2014). Adolescent simulated gambling via digital and social media: An emerging problem. *Computers in Human Behavior, 31*, 305–313. doi:10.1016/j.chb.2013.10.048

King, S. M., Abrams, K., & Wilkinson, T. (2010). Personality, gender, and family history in the prediction of college gambling. *Journal of Gambling Studies, 26*(3), 347–359. doi:10.1007/s10899-009-9163-7

Kong, G., Tsai, J., Pilver, C. E., Tan, H. S., Hoff, R. A., Cavallo, D. A., . . . Potenza, M. N. (2013). Differences in gambling problem severity and gambling and health/functioning characteristics among Asian-American and Caucasian high-school students. *Psychiatry Research, 210*(3), 1071–1078. doi:10.1016/j.psychres.2013.10.005

Kourgiantakis, T., Saint-Jacques, M. C., & Tremblay, J. (2013). Problem gambling and families: A systematic review. *Journal of Social Work Practice in the Addictions, 13*(4), 353–372. doi:10.1080/1533256X.2013.838130

Kundu, P. V., Pilver, C. E., Desai, R. A., Steinberg, M. A., Rugle, L., Krishnan-Sarin, S., & Potenza, M. N. (2013). Gambling-related attitudes and behaviors in adolescents having received instant (scratch) lottery tickets as gifts. *Journal of Adolescent Health, 52*(4), 456–464. doi:10.1016/j.jadohealth.2012.07.013

Ladouceur, R., Sylvain, C., Letarte, H., Giroux, I., & Jacques, C. (1998). Cognitive treatment of pathological gamblers. *Behaviour Research and Therapy, 36,* 1111–1119. doi:10.1016/S0005-7967(98)00086-2

Langer, E. J. (1975). The illusion of control. *Journal of Personality and Social Psychology, 32*(2), 311 328. doi:10.103//0022-3514.32.2.311

Ledgerwood, D. M., Arfken, C. L., Wiedemann, A., Bates, K. E., Holmes, D., & Jones, L. (2013). Who goes to treatment? Predictors of treatment initiation among gambling help-line callers. *The American Journal on Addictions, 22*(1), 33–38. doi:10.1111/j.1521-0391.2013.00323.x

Leeman, R. F., Patock-Peckham, J. A., Hoff, R. A., Krishnan-Sarin, S., Steinberg, M. A., Rugle, L. J., & Potenza, M. N. (2014). Perceived parental permissiveness toward gambling and risky behaviors in adolescents. *Journal of Behavioral Addictions, 3*(2), 115–123. doi:10.1556/JBA.3.2014.012

Leppink, E. W. & Grant, J. E. (2015). Traumatic event exposure and gambling: Associations clinical, neurocognitive, and personality variables. *Annals of Clinical Psychiatry, 27*(1), 16–24.

Lesieur, H., & Blume, S. (1987). The South Oaks gambling screen (SOGS): A new instrument for the identification of pathological gamblers. *American Journal of Psychiatry, 144*(9), 1184–1188. doi:10.1176/ajp.144.9.1184

Levy, L., & Tracy, J. K. (2018). Gambling disorder in veterans: A review of the literature and implications for future research. *Journal of Gambling Studies, 34*(4), 1205–1239. doi:10.1007/s10899-018-9749-z

Li, W., Mills, D., & Nower, L. (2019). The relationship of loot box purchases to problem video gaming and problem gambling. Manuscript submitted for publication. doi:10.1016/j.addbeh.2019.05.016

Macey, J., & Hamari, J. (2019). eSports, skins and loot boxes: Participants, practices and problematic behaviour associated with emergent forms of gambling. *New Media & Society, 21*(1), 20–41. doi:10.1177/1461444818786216

Marchica, L., & Derevensky, J. L. (2016). Examining personalized feedback interventions for gambling disorders: A systematic review. *Journal of Behavioral Addictions, 5*(1), 1–10. doi:10.1556/2006.5.2016.006

Martins, S. S., Lee, G. P., Kim, J. H., Letourneau, E. J., & Storr, C. L. (2014). Gambling and sexual behaviors in African-American adolescents. *Addictive Behaviors, 39*(5), 854–860. doi:10.1016/j.addbeh.2014.02.002

Matheson, F. I., Devotta, K., Wendaferew, A., & Pedersen, C. (2014). Prevalence of gambling problems among the clients of a Toronto homeless shelter. *Journal of Gambling Studies, 30*(2), 537–546. doi:10.1007/s10899-014-9452-7

Moran, E. (1970). Pathological gambling. *British Journal of Hospital Medicine, 4,* 59–70. doi:10.1192/bjp.116.535.593

Morasco, B. J., & Petry, N. M. (2006). Gambling problems and health functioning in individuals receiving disability. *Disability and Rehabilitation, 28*(10), 619–623. doi:10.1080/09638280500242507

National Opinion Research Center. (1999). *Gambling impact and behavior study. Report to the national gambling impact study commission.* Chicago, IL: Authors.

Newman, S. C., & Thompson, A. (2007). The association between pathological gambling and attempted suicide: Findings from a national survey in Canada. *Canadian Journal of Psychiatry, 52*(9), 605–612. doi:10.1177/070674370705200909

Nowak, D. E. (2018). A meta-analytical synthesis and examination of pathological and problem gambling rates and associated moderators among college students, 1987–2016. *Journal of Gambling Studies, 34*(2), 465–498. doi:10.1007/s10899-017-9726-y

Nower, L., & Blaszczynski, A. (2008). Characteristics of problem gamblers 56 years of age or older: A statewide study of casino self-excluders. *Psychology and Aging, 23*(3), 577–584. doi:10.1037/a0013233

Nower, L., & Blaszczynski, A. (2013). Legal and financial issues and disordered gambling. In D. C. S. Richard, A. Blaszczynski, & L. Nower (Eds.), *The Wiley-Blackwell handbook of disordered gambling* (pp. 386–399). New York, NY: Wiley-Blackwell. doi:10.1002/9781118316078.ch18

Nower, L., & Blaszczynski, A. (2017). Development and validation of the gambling pathways questionnaire (GPQ). *Psychology of Addictive Behaviors, 31*(1), 95–109. doi:10.1037/adb0000234

Nower, L., Derevensky, J. L., & Gupta, R. (2004). The relationship of impulsivity, sensation seeking, coping, and substance use in youth gamblers. *Psychology of Addictive Behaviors, 18*(1), 49–55. doi:10.1037/0893-164X.18.1.49

Nower, L., Eyrich-Garg, K. M., Pollio, D. E., & North, C. S. (2015). Problem gambling and homelessness: Results from an epidemiologic study. *Journal of Gambling Studies, 31*(2), 533–545. doi:10.1007/s10899-013-9435-0

Nower, L., Gupta, R., Blaszczynski, A., & Derevensky, J. (2004). Suicidality ideation and depression among youth gamblers: A preliminary examination of three studies. *International Gambling Studies, 4*(1), 69–80. doi:10.1080/1445979042000224412

Nower, L., Martins, S. S., Lin, K. H., & Blanco, C. (2013). Subtypes of disordered gamblers: Results from the national epidemiologic survey on alcohol and related conditions. *Addiction, 108*(4), 789–798. doi:10.1111/add.12012

Nower, L., Volberg, R. A., & Caler, K. R. (2017). *The prevalence of online and land-based gambling in New Jersey. Report to the New Jersey division of gaming enforcement.* New Brunswick, NJ: Authors.

Ocean, G., & Smith, G. J. (1993). Social reward, conflict, and commitment: A theoretical model of gambling behavior. *Journal of Gambling Studies, 9*(4), 321–339. doi:10.1007/BF01014625

Petry, N. M., Ginley, M. K., & Rash, C. J. (2017). A systematic review of treatments for problem gambling. *Psychology of Addictive Behaviors, 31*(8), 951–961. doi:10.1037/adb0000290

Petry, N. M., & Steinberg, K. L. (2005). Childhood maltreatment in male and female treatment-seeking pathological gamblers. *Psychology of Addictive Behaviors, 19*(2), 226–229. doi:10.1037/adb0000290

Pickering, D., Keen, B., Entwistle, G., & Blaszczynski, A. (2018). Measuring treatment outcomes in gambling disorders: A systematic review. *Addiction, 113*(3), 411–426. doi:10.1111/add.13968

Potenza, M. N. (2006). Should addictive disorders include non-substance-related conditions? *Addiction, 101*(s1), 142–151. doi:10.1111/j.1360-0443.2006.01591.x

Potenza, M. N. (2008). The neurobiology of pathological gambling and drug addiction: An overview and new findings. *Philosophical Transactions of the Royal Society B: Biological Sciences, 363*(1507), 3181–3189. doi:10.1098/rstb.2008.0100

Potenza, M. N. (2013). Neurobiology of gambling behaviors. *Current Opinion in Neurobiology, 23*(4), 660–667. doi:10.1016/j.conb.2013.03.004

Sansanwal, R. M., Derevensky, J. L., & Gavriel-Fried, B. (2016). What mental health professionals in Israel know and think about adolescent problem gambling. *International Gambling Studies, 16*(1), 67–84. doi:10.1080/14459795.2016.1139159

Schluter, M. G., Kim, H. S., Poole, J. C., Hodgins, D. C., McGrath, D. S., Dobson, K. S., & Taveres, H. (2019). Gambling-related cognitive distortions mediate the relationship between depression and disordered gambling severity. *Addictive Behaviors, 90*(October 2018), 318–323. doi:10.1016/j.addbeh.2018.11.038

Sharpe, L. (2002). A reformulated cognitive–behavioral model of problem gambling: A biopsychosocial perspective. *Clinical Psychology Review, 22*(1), 1–25. doi:10.1016/S0272-7358(00)00087-8

Shonin, E., Van Gordon, W., & Griffiths, M. D. (2014). Cognitive behavioral therapy (CBT) and meditation awareness training (MAT) for the treatment of co-occurring schizophrenia and pathological gambling: A case study. *International Journal of Mental Health and Addiction, 12*(2), 181–196. doi:10.1007/s11469-013-9460-3

Slutske, W. S., Cho, S. B., Piasecki, T. M., & Martin, N. G. (2013). Genetic overlap between personality and risk for disordered gambling: Evidence from a national community-based Australian twin study. *Journal of Abnormal Psychology, 122*(1), 250–255. doi:10.1037/a0029999

Slutske, W. S., Deutsch, A. R., Richmond-Rakerd, L. S., Chernyavskiy, P., Statham, D. J., & Martin, N. G. (2014). Test of a potential causal influence of earlier age of gambling initiation on gambling involvement and disorder: A multilevel discordant twin design. *Psychology of Addictive Behaviors, 28*(4), 1177–1189. doi:10.1037/a0035356

Slutske, W. S., Ellingson, J. M., Richmond-Rakerd, L. S., Zhu, G., & Martin, N. G. (2013). Shared genetic vulnerability for disordered gambling and alcohol use disorder in men and women: Evidence from a national community-based Australian twin study. *Twin Research and Human Genetics, 16*(02), 525–534. doi:10.1017/thg.2013.11

Slutske, W. S., Moffitt, T. E., Poulton, R., & Caspi, A. (2012). Undercontrolled temperament at age 3 predicts disordered gambling at age 32: A longitudinal study of a complete birth cohort. *Psychological Science, 23*(5), 510–516. doi:10.1177/0956797611429708

Stinchfield, R. (2013). A review of problem gambling assessment instruments and brief screens. In D. C. S. Richard, A. Blaszczynski, & L. Nower (Eds.), *The Wiley-Blackwell handbook of disordered gambling* (pp. 165–203). New York, NY: Wiley-Blackwell. doi:10.1002/9781118316078.ch8

Stuhldreher, W. L., Stuhldreher, T. J., & Forrest, K. Y. (2007). Gambling as an emerging health problem on campus. *Journal of American College Health, 56*(1), 75–88. doi:10.3200/JACH.56.1.75-88

Suomi, A., Jackson, A. C., Dowling, N. A., Lavis, T., Patford, J., Thomas, S. A., . . . Cockman, S. (2013). Problem gambling and family violence: Family member reports of prevalence, family impacts and family coping. *Asian Journal of Gambling Issues and Public Health, 3*(1), 1–15. doi:10.1186/2195-3007-3-13

Sylvain, C., Ladouceur, R., & Boisvert, J. (1997). Cognitive and behavioral treatment of pathological gambling: A controlled study. *Journal of Consulting and Clinical Psychology, 65*, 727–732. doi:10.1037/0022-006X.65.5.727

Toce-Gerstein, M., Gerstein, D. R., & Volberg, R. A. (2009). The NODS–CLiP: A rapid screen for adult pathological and problem gambling. *Journal of Gambling Studies, 25*(4), 541–555. doi:10.1007/s10899-009-9135-y

Toneatto, T., Pillai, S., & Courtice, E. L. (2014). Mindfulness-enhanced cognitive behavior therapy for problem gambling: A controlled pilot study. *International Journal of Mental Health and Addiction, 12*(2), 197–205. doi:10.1007/s11469-014-9481-6

Toyama, T., Nakayama, H., Takimura, T., Yoshimura, A., Maesato, H., Matsushita, S., . . . Higuchi, S. (2014). Prevalence of pathological gambling in Japan: Results of national surveys of the general adult general population in 2008 and 2013. *Alcohol and Alcoholism, 49*(suppl 1), i17–i17. doi:10.1093/alcalc/agu052.75

Tversky, A., & Kahneman, D. (1971). Belief in the law of small numbers. *Psychological Bulletin, 76*, 105–110. doi:10.1037/h0031322

Valleur, M., Codina, I., Vénisse, J. L., Romo, L., Magalon, D., Fatséas, M., . . . Groupe, J. E. U. (2016). Towards a validation of the three pathways model of pathological gambling. *Journal of Gambling Studies, 32*(2), 757–771. doi:10.1007/s10899-015-9545-y

Vitaro, F., Brendgen, M., Girard, A., Dionne, G., & Boivin, M. (2018). Longitudinal links between gambling participation and academic performance in youth: A test of four models. *Journal of Gambling Studies, 34*(3), 881–892. doi:10.1007/s10899-017-9736-9

Vitaro, F., Brendgen, M., Ladouceur, R., & Tremblay, R. E. (2001). Gambling, delinquency, and drug use during adolescence: Mutual influences and common risk factors. *Journal of Gambling Studies, 17*(3), 171–190. doi:10.1023/A:1012201221601

Vitaro, F., & Wanner, B. (2011). Predicting early gambling in Children. *Psychology of Addictive Behaviors, 25*(1), 118–126. doi:10.1037/a0021109

Volberg, R. A., Munck, I. M., & Petry, N. M. (2011). A quick and simple screening method for pathological and problem gamblers in addiction programs and practices. *The American Journal on Addictions, 20*(3), 220–227. doi:10.1111/j.1521-0391.2011.00118.x

Weatherly, J. N., & Dixon, M. R. (2007). Toward an integrative behavioral model of gambling. *Analysis of Gambling Behavior, 1*(1), 4–18.

Welte, J. W., Barnes, G. M., Wieczorek, W. F., Tidwell, M. C., & Parker, J. (2002). Gambling participation in the U.S.—Results from a national survey. *Journal of Gambling Studies, 18*(4), 313–337. doi:10.1023/A:1021019915591

Williams, R. J., Volberg, R. A., & Stevens, R. M. (2012). *The population prevalence of problem gambling: Methodological influences, standardized rates, jurisdictional differences, and worldwide trends.* Guelph, Canada: Ontario Problem Gambling Research Centre.

Wong, P. W., Kwok, N. C., Tang, J. Y., Blaszczynski, A., & Tse, S. (2014). Suicidal ideation and familicidal-suicidal ideation among individuals presenting to problem gambling services: A retrospective data analysis. *Crisis: The Journal of Crisis Intervention and Suicide Prevention, 35*(4), 219–232. doi:10.1027/0227-5910/a000256

World Health Organization. (1979). *International classification of diseases-9th revision (ICD-9).* Geneva: World Health Organization.

Yakovenko, I., & Hodgins, D. C. (2016). Latest developments in treatment for disordered gambling: Review and critical evaluation of outcome studies. *Current Addiction Reports, 3*(3), 299–306. doi:10.1007/s40429-016-0110-2

Internet Gaming Disorder and problematic technology use

Wen Li (Vivien) Anthony, Devin Mills and Lia Nower

Background

Social work has not, to date, adequately addressed behavioral, process addictions. Research has established that gambling disorder can activate the brain's mesolimbic dopaminergic system, leading to persistent and compulsive behavior, in much the same way as psychoactive substances (Grant, Potenza, Weinstein, & Gorelick, 2010). These and other scientific results led the American Psychiatric Association (APA) in 2013 to reclassify gambling disorder from an impulse control disorder to an addictive disorder, analogous to substance use disorder in the fifth edition of the *Diagnostic and Statistical Manual of Mental Disorders* (DSM-5; APA, 2013). Acknowledgment by the medical profession that behavioral addictions exist and can cause the same degree of harm as substance use disorders has fueled research concerning other potentially addictive behaviors. In particular, there exists concern over the potential psychosocial harms of excessive and problematic technology use (e.g. Internet, video gaming, social media), particularly among youth. The importance of this emerging area of research is further evidenced by an observed overlap between gambling and video gaming: aspects of video gaming may "prime" youth to spend increasing amounts of money in gambling activities that are dependent on random chance (see Chapter 8 for more information).

Technology is a ubiquitous part of today's society, and underlying almost all interactive technologies is the Internet. More than 3.7 billion people worldwide accessed the Internet in 2017, which is a 933.8% increase over the number of Internet users in 2000 (World Internet Usage and Population Statistics, 2017). Whether for school, work, entertainment, socializing, bill payment, or general information, access to the Internet is critical to everyday life in many parts of the world. Increasing reliance on the Internet has spawned concerns about problematic Internet usage and Internet addiction (Young, 1998, 2004), exacerbated by the widespread use of mobile devices and smartphones that provide 24/7 Internet access (Taylor & Silver, 2019). Although research in this area is in its infancy, it is important to familiarize social workers and other professionals with the diagnostic features, risk factors, and emerging intervention programs related to problematic technology use.

Table 9.1 Popular video game genres and video game titles

Video Game Genres/Subgenres	Video Game Titles
Role play games (RPG)	
Japanese (JRPG)	Final Fantasy
Computer (CRPG)	Skyrim
Action (ARPG)	Dark Souls
Massive multiplayer online games (MMO)	
MMORPG	World of Warcraft
MMO action	Grand Theft Auto (GTA) Online
Multiplayer online battle arena games (MOBA)	League of Legends (LOL), DOTA
Shooter games (first- and third person)	Gears of War, Call of Duty, Halo, Counter Strike: Global Offensive (CS:GO)
Battle royale games	PlayerUnknown's Battlegrounds (PUBG), Fortnite
Action/Adventure games	
Horror/Survival	Resident Evil
Stealth	Metal Gear Solid
Platformer	Super Mario Odyssey, Uncharted, Sonic
Open world	Grand Theft Auto (GTA)
Strategy games	
Real-time strategy games	StarCraft
Turn-base strategy games	Civilization
Simulation games	SIMs, Football Manager, Truck Simulator
Puzzle/casual games	Candy Crush Saga, Angry Birds
Card trading games	Hearthstone
Gambling-themed games/social casino games	Texas Hold'em
Sports/racing games	Madden NFL, FIFA, Forza
Fighting games	Street Fighter, Super Smash Bros
Sandbox games	Minecraft, Terraria

Defining (Internet) gaming

The general terms *video* or *digital gaming* refer to a form of interactive, digital entertainment, played on a variety of devices, including computers, game consoles (e.g. SONY® PlayStation systems, Microsoft® Xbox systems, and Nintendo® Switch), and mobile devices. Video gaming is a major entertainment activity; more than 2 billion people worldwide play video games (Newzoo, 2018). Individuals can play video games offline or on the Internet across multiple devices either alone or with other people. The APA adopts the terminology "Internet gaming" to distinguish this condition from gambling and because online gaming is associated with more problems (Petry, Rehbein, Ko, & O'Brien, 2015). However, online gambling is often dubbed as "Internet gaming" by the gambling industry. This chapter applies the terminology "video/Internet gaming" to refer to the overall classification of video or digital game playing (see Table 9.1 for popular video games).

Defining and assessing Internet Gaming Disorder
(IGD) and problematic technology use

The growth of interactive media has fostered a reliance on the technology, for some, to an excessive degree that causes harm. Problematic video gaming and other technology use is broadly defined as a persistent and pathological pattern of video game playing or technology use that contributes to impaired functioning (Petry, Zajac, & Ginley, 2018; Spada, 2014). Despite evidence that problematic video gaming and technology use share similar symptoms to substance use disorders (e.g. diminished control, tolerance, psychological withdrawal), some researchers and professionals conceptualize these problems as types of behavioral addiction (e.g. Griffiths, 2005; Young, 1998), but others theorize these problems as symptoms of underlying psychological distress (Caplan, 2002; Davis, 2001).

Complicating the discussion is difficulty in distinguishing an addiction to specific uses of the Internet from a generalized Internet addiction (Davis, 2001). Some scholars argue that the Internet is merely a medium or "channel" through which individuals express addictive behaviors: for example, users are not addicted to the Internet but to viewing of pornography (Wéry & Billieux, 2017), engaging with social media (Andreassen, Torsheim, Brunborg, & Pallesen, 2012), shopping (Duroy, Gorse, & Lejoyeux, 2014), gambling (see Chapter 6), or video gaming (Petry et al., 2014). As a result, the term "Internet addiction" has little utility as a diagnosis and may prove to be a confound which overlaps with other categories (Starcevic, 2013; Van Rooij, Ferguson, Van De Mheen, & Schoenmakers, 2017).

These debates notwithstanding, the DSM-5 proposed "Internet Gaming Disorder (IGD)" as a condition for further study (APA, 2013), while the *International Classification of Diseases* (ICD-11) (WHO, 2018) officially recognized "Gaming Disorder" as a diagnosable condition. The APA limited its potential classification to Internet gaming, in contrast to including other types of problematic technology use, and proposed nine diagnostic criteria to assess IGD that loosely parallel those for gambling disorder (APA, 2013). Research applying the proposed DSM-5 criteria has reported IGD prevalence rates ranging from less than 1 to 6% of adolescents and adults (Fam, 2018; Lemmens, Valkenburg, & Gentile, 2015; Przybylski, Weinstein, & Murayama, 2016). The criteria for Gaming Disorder outlined in the ICD-11 references a loss of control over digital or video gaming, a preference for video gaming over other obligations, and a continuation of video gaming despite negative consequences (WHO, 2018). Both definitions emphasize repetitive use of video games, often with other players, which leads to significant functional impairment. However, nothing in either of the DSM-5 or ICD-11 criteria or definitions precludes classifying online gambling (also dubbed "Internet gaming" by the gambling industry) from inclusion under either category. Research in this area is still emerging amid continued debate in the literature over the proper focus of study (Aarseth et al., 2017; Griffiths et al., 2016; Van Rooij et al., 2018).

Several measures have been developed to assess IGD and validated in both research and clinical settings. The nine-item short-form of the Internet Gaming Disorder Scale (IGDS-SF9; Pontes & Griffiths, 2015) is the most widely used. It demonstrates sound reliability and validity, as well as measurement invariance (e.g. Pontes, Stavropoulos, & Griffiths, 2017). The scale, compared in Table 9.2 to the proposed DSM-5 criteria, measures frequency of Internet gaming-related symptoms over the past 12 months on a 5-point scale ranging from *Never* to *Very Often*. A cutoff score of 21 is presently recommended for IGD diagnosis based on recent results from an Italian sample (Monacis, Palo, Griffiths, & Sinatra, 2016). The scale could also be scored using a dichotomous Yes/No format in which

Table 9.2 An example of assessment for Internet Gaming Disorder

DSM-5 Criteria	IGDS9-SF Item
Preoccupation	1. Do you feel preoccupied with your gaming behavior? (Some examples: Do you think about previous gaming activity or anticipate the next gaming session? Do you think gaming has become the dominant activity in your daily life?)
Withdrawal	2. Do you feel more irritability, anxiety or even sadness when you try to either reduce or stop your gaming activity?
Tolerance	3. Do you feel the need to spend increasing amount of time engaged gaming in order to achieve satisfaction or pleasure?
Loss of control	4. Do you systematically fail when trying to control or cease your gaming activity?
Loss of interest	5. Have you lost interests in previous hobbies and other entertainment activities as a result of your engagement with the game?
Continue playing despite harms	6. Have you continued your gaming activity despite knowing it was causing problems between you and other people?
Lying	7. Have you deceived any of your family members, therapists or others because the amount of your gaming activity?
Escape	8. Do you play in order to temporarily escape or relieve a negative mood (e.g., helplessness, guilt, anxiety?)
Risk of relationships or opportunities	9. Have you jeopardized or lost an important relationship, job or an educational or career opportunity because of your gaming activity?

endorsing five or more criteria would be indicative of IGD. No instrument has been validated to screen for IGD in clinical setting.

In addition to assessing IGD, a variety of research measures have also been developed that purport to measure Internet addiction (e.g. Young's Internet Addiction Test, see Young, 1998), smartphone addiction (e.g. the Smartphone Addiction Scale, see Kwon et al., 2013), and social media addiction (e.g. the Bergen Facebook Addiction Scale, see Andreassen et al, 2012; Table 9.3). Criteria in these measures largely overlap with substance use disorders and IGD assessment, such as preoccupation, tolerance, withdrawal, using technology for mood regulation, and negative outcomes associated with addictive behaviors.

Table 9.3 An example of assessment for social media addiction

Criteria	Bergen Facebook Addiction Scale
Salience	1. Spent a lot of time thinking about Facebook or planned use of social media
Tolerance	2. Felt an urge to use social media more and more
Mood modification	3. Used social media in order to forget about personal problems
Relapse	4. Tried to cut down on the use of social media without success
Withdrawal	5. Become restless or troubled if you have been prohibited from using social media
Conflict	6. Used social media so much that it has had a negative impact on your job or studies

Risk factors and comorbidities of IGD and problematic technology use

The etiology and negative consequences of IGD and other problematic technology use can be understood from a holistic and multifactorial perspective: neurobiological changes, personality traits, psychological and cognitive factors, and social and cultural influences. Brand, Young, Laier, Wölfling, and Potenza (2016) proposed an interaction of person-affect-cognition-execution (I-PACE) model that explains IGD and Internet addiction as a consequence of interactions between neurobiological and psychological contributions, coping styles and cognitive biases, and affective and cognitive responses to triggers in combination with reduced executive functioning. Results from the current literature are largely limited to cross-sectional investigations of risk factors and comorbidities implicated in the development and maintenance of IGD and other problematic technology use.

Neurological risks and processes

Medical research has observed neuroadaptation and brain structure changes associated with altered reward processing and impaired impulse control among individuals who develop IGD and problematic technology use, similar to changes observed among individuals with psychoactive drug addiction. For example, Internet gaming activated similar brain regions associated with cues and reward systems as those for nicotine and cocaine dependence, including the orbitofrontal cortex, anterior cingulate and medial frontal cortex, and nucleus accumbens (e.g. Han et al., 2011; Ko et al., 2009; Ko, Liu, Yen, Chen, & Lin, 2013). Activation of the brain's dopaminergic system is hypothesized to increase an individual's sensitivity to reward from Internet gaming and technology use and to cue-induced urges. Symptoms such as tolerance and withdrawal result from reward deficiency due to decreased dopaminergic activity associated with a persistent and pathological pattern of technology use or gaming (Hou et al., 2012). Excessive Internet gaming and other technology use are also associated with impaired neurocognitive functioning across various domains, including increases in impulsivity and cognitive-bias and decreases in behavioral response inhibition related to enhanced brain activity in prefrontal areas (e.g. Decker & Gay, 2011, Littel et al., 2012; Lorenz et al., 2013). Similar neurocognitive impairments are experienced with substance use disorders.

Personality traits

Personality traits associated with IGD and other problematic technology use are similar to those of individuals identified with substance use disorders (Kotov, Gamez, Schmidt, & Watson, 2010). Specifically, higher neuroticism is associated with greater IGD, and problematic Internet and social media use, whereas higher conscientiousness is associated with less severity of IGD and other problematic technology use (Braun, Stopfer, Müller, Beutel, & Egloff, 2016; Gervasi et al., 2017; Mehroof & Griffiths, 2010; Müller, Beutel, Egloff, & Wölfling, 2014). High neuroticism indicates a tendency to experience greater anxiety and negative affect, and increased reactivity to emotions (Costa & McCrae, 1992; DeYoung, Quilty, & Peterson, 2007). As such, individuals evidencing high neuroticism may use Internet or video games as part of a maladaptive coping process (Mehroof & Griffiths, 2010). Low conscientiousness reflects deficits in self-control and greater impulsivity, specifically a lack of planning and organization (DeYoung et al., 2007). Individuals with low locus of control and high impulsivity are particularly vulnerable to IGD and other problematic technology use (Chak & Leung, 2004; Lee et al., 2012; Mehroof & Griffiths, 2010). In addition, high sensation-seeking, an underlying characteristic of substance use disorders, is found to be associated with IGD and Internet addiction (Mehroof & Griffiths, 2010).

Comorbid psychopathology

IGD and problematic technology use are associated with depression, anxiety, and suicidal ideation (Andreassen et al., 2016; Männikkö, Ruotsalainen, Miettunen, Pontes, & Kääriäinen, 2017). These psychological harms are generally consistent across different cultures (Cheng, Cheung, & Wang, 2018). In addition, IGD and problematic technology use increase the risk of obesity due to insufficient physical activity and unhealthy snacking while playing, and result in sleep disturbances and fatigue (Lam, 2014; Männikkö et al., 2017). Incidents have also been reported of individuals dying from exhaustion and cardiopulmonary-related deaths after gaming-marathons or binge-gaming sessions (e.g. Rudd, 2012). In addition, individuals evidencing problematic technology use often experience impaired social functioning and interpersonal relationships (Kerkhof, Finkenauer, & Muusses 2011; Li, O'Brien, Snyder, & Howard, 2015). Like substance and gambling disorders, psychological and physical harms that stem from IGD and problematic technology use often exacerbate an individual's maladaptive patterns of gaming and/or technology use.

Internalized maladaptive cognitions and expectancies

Internalized, maladaptive cognitions are a significant risk factor for IGD and other problematic technology use (Davis, 2001; Forrest, King, & Delfabbro, 2017; King & Delfabbro, 2016; LaRose & Eastin, 2004). Video gaming-related maladaptive cognitions include overvaluing video game involvement relative to other life domains (e.g. video gaming rewards or experiences matter more than rewards or experiences outside of video gaming), possessing a "sunk cost bias" regarding gaming involvement (e.g. continuing to play due to perceiving a large investment of resources toward gaming), gaming-contingent sense of self-worth (e.g. I feel worthless when offline), and gaming to increase social acceptance (e.g. I am respected because of my video gaming skills) (Delfabbro & King, 2015). Additionally, individuals may expect Internet and social media use to offer a relief from a problem, a path to intimate online relationships that cannot be achieved in the real world, or a feeling of value that can only be attained within a virtual online community (LaRose & Eastin, 2004). These outcome expectancies are formed prior to individuals' endorsement of motivations for problematic video gaming and technology use.

Motivations

Various motivations underlie both IGD and problematic technology use. In general, playing video games for any reason not directly associated with the pleasure of gaming itself places individuals at risk for IGD (Mills, Milyavskaya, Heath, & Derevensky, 2018). For instance, stronger motivations to compete through video gaming or use video games as a means of coping with daily stressors are strong predictors of IGD (Ballabio et al., 2017; Király et al., 2015; Yee, 2006). Likewise, motivations for problematic social media use similarly focus on coping or escaping aversive mood states, socialization, and mood enhancement (Marino, Gini, Vieno, & Spada, 2018; Ryan, Chester, Reece, & Xenos, 2014). These motivations are related to expectancies or beliefs that individuals have regarding the outcomes of their video gaming and technology use. Individuals problematically playing video games may be doing so to satisfy basic needs that may be met only through playing video game (Mills, Milyavskaya, Mettler, & Heath, 2018). Thus, enthusiastic gamers may struggle to manage their gaming involvement when their environment prevents them from meeting these basic needs, alluding to video gaming being a primary path for basic need satisfaction.

Family environment

The family environment is another etiological precursor to IGD and problematic technology use. Adolescents from single-parent families are at greater risk for IGD and Internet addiction (Rehbein & Baier, 2013). High family functioning and positive parent-child relationships are protective factors against the development of IGD and problematic technology use among youth and young adults across different cultural contexts (Li, Garland, & Howard, 2014; Schneider, King, & Delfabbro, 2017).

Higher levels of family satisfaction and family warmth, and lower levels of family conflict, also ameliorate the probability of developing IGD and Internet addiction (Schneider et al., 2017). Children from well-functioning families, experiencing positive parent-child relationships, are more likely also to have parental mediation of their video gaming and technology use. Parental mediation occurs when parents engage in conversations with their children about gaming and technology use, set rules regulating gaming and technology use, and monitor the content of video games and online activities. Higher levels of parental supervision during childhood predict lower rates of IGD and problematic technology use among adolescents (Rehbein & Baier, 2013). Moreover, new studies investigating the intergenerational influence of IGD report that the frequency of parental gaming, combined with play accompanied by their children, predicts adolescent problematic Internet gaming (Wu et al., 2016).

Evidence-informed interventions for IGD and problematic technology use

Interventions developed for substance and gambling disorders informed more targeted approaches for addressing IGD and problematic technology use. One highly salient difference between substance use disorders and problematic technology use concerns the extent to which technology has become an integrated aspect of modern life. For that reason, a harm reduction versus abstinence-based approach to treatment is recommended, shifting the treatment goal toward facilitating a responsible and healthy pattern of video gaming and technology use. Harm reduction is at the core of various psychotherapeutic interventions for IGD and problematic technology use, including cognitive-behavioral therapy (CBT), motivational interviewing (MI), mindfulness-based interventions, family-based therapy, and multilevel interventions. Preliminary evidence suggests that harm reduction approaches may be efficacious psychotherapeutic interventions for IGD and problematic technology use (King et al., 2017). However, multi-site randomized control trials (RCT) with large samples that replicate the efficacy of these interventions are needed to confirm best practice approaches.

Cognitive-behavioral therapy (CBT)

CBT is widely applied in treating problems with addictive behaviors. Key processes underlying the effectiveness of CBT are a focus on interrupting and redirecting addictive behaviors by identifying situational triggers and associated feelings, changing addiction-related maladaptive thoughts and beliefs, and reducing positive expectancies for addictive behaviors (McHugh, Hearon, & Otto, 2010). CBT holds promise as an effective means of reducing IGD and problematic technology use by modifying individuals' maladaptive cognitions (e.g. "I am only able to make meaningful personal connections through video games/Internet"), as well as modifying escape-oriented coping styles, thereby enhancing self-efficacy and life/social skills to better regulate video gaming and technology use.

CBT has been adapted for Internet addiction and successfully pilot tested among adolescents and adults from different countries (King et al., 2017). Young (2007) first proposed applying CBT in treating Internet addiction via three therapeutic components: behavior modification, cognitive restructuring, and harm reduction. This CBT model, administered in 12 weekly individual sessions, successfully reduced adults' problematic Internet use and improved interpersonal relationships at six months following completion of the intervention (Young, 2013). Moreover, Du, Jiang, and Vance (2010) applied a RCT design to examine an eight-session group-administered CBT intervention among Chinese adolescents experiencing Internet addiction. The CBT intervention showed sustained reductions in problematic Internet use at six months post-intervention follow-up. Overall, meta-analysis revealed that CBT demonstrates better outcomes in reducing the amount of time spent on the Internet and the level of co-occurring depressive symptoms compared to other types of psychosocial treatments (Winkler, Dörsing, Rief, Shen, & Glombiewski, 2013).

Motivational interviewing (MI)

MI is a person-centered approach that can activate clients' motivation and commitment to change by exploring and reinforcing reasons for change, resolving ambivalence about change, and strengthening individuals' commitment to change their addictive behaviors (Miller & Rollnick, 2012). MI could reinforce individuals' motivation to reduce their problematic video gaming and technology use and promote individuals' self-efficacy for change vis-à-vis regulating their video gaming behavior and technology use (O'Brien, Li, Snyder, & Howard, 2016). MI often combines with CBT and other treatment models, enhancing individuals' self-efficacy for change and coping skills by capitalizing on their commitment to change and reinforcing pro-social values (Van Rooij, Zinn, Schoenmakers, & Van de Mheen, 2012). For example, one study in China found that a brief Internet-based intervention, combining CBT and MI components, had a greater effect on reducing Internet addiction than did psychoeducation (Su, Fang, Miller, & Wang, 2011).

Mindfulness-based intervention

Mindfulness-based interventions have become popular in treating both substance (Li, Howard, Garland, McGovern, & Lazar, 2017; see Chapter 21) and gambling disorders (see Chapter 8). Mindfulness-based interventions target cognitive mechanisms implicated in IGD and problematic technology use: (a) mindfulness could facilitate individual's cognitive flexibility in Internet gaming and technology use, which could reduce excessive and problematic patterns of engagement; (b) mindfulness training could enhance individual's awareness of triggers and urges for gaming and technology use and increase coping strategies for craving (e.g. urge surfing technique, see Marlatt & Gordon, 1985); (c) mindful reappraisal could produce a non-judgmental attitude toward negative moods and emotions and enhance the ability to accept a distressing experience, which, in turn, could reduce the use of Internet gaming/technology for escapism-oriented coping, and (d) meditation could increase the sense of reward from other pleasant events in place of Internet gaming and technology use (Li et al., 2018). One RCT adapted Mindfulness-Oriented Recovery Enhancement/MORE (Garland, 2013) to address IGD, and found that this eight-week group-administered treatment demonstrates effects in reducing IGD symptoms, craving for Internet gaming, and maladaptive gaming-related cognitions (Li et al., 2017, 2018). In addition to formal mindfulness treatment, meditation training is combined with reality therapy to reduce IGD and intertemporal decision impulsivity (Yao et al., 2017).

Family-based therapy

Family-based therapy takes into account environmental context factors (e.g. family functioning and parent–child relationships) which play an important role in addictive behaviors, particularly among adolescents and young adults (see Chapters 13 and 14). Family-based therapy includes parents and their children, addressing problems by: (a) increasing parental awareness and mediation of their children's problematic gaming/technology use; (b) teaching problem-solving and communication skills to improve family functioning and parent–child relationships; and (c) enhancing social and emotional support from parents for their children's behavior change. Empirical studies with Korean and Chinese youth concluded that family-based therapy reduced adolescents' problematic gaming and technology use, maladaptive cognitions associated with Internet gaming/technology use, and amount of time spent gaming (Han, Kim, Lee, & Renshaw, 2012; Liu et al., 2015). Notably, one study reported reduced brain activity in response to gaming-related cues and increased brain activity in response to family affection among adolescents who received family-based therapy (Han et al., 2012).

Multi-level and multi-modality intervention

It is possible that a multi-level intervention approach may prove the most efficacious in the long term for addressing IGD and problematic technology use. A multi-level framework integrates individual and family counseling, peer support, and community and school support networks to simultaneously address multiple factors underlying the development and maintenance of IGD and problematic technology use (Pallesen, Lorvik, Bu, & Molde, 2015; Shek, Tang, & Lo, 2009). Moreover, therapeutic residential treatment programs that apply multi-modality therapies are used to address IGD and problematic technology use in the United States and Korea (e.g. Sakuma et al., 2017).

Such programs provide a technology-free environment for individuals who evidence severe symptoms and psychosocial impairments. For example, reStart® Life (Washington State) is one such therapeutic community, providing varied treatment options for adolescents and adults experiencing different types of problematic technology use: individual- and group-based psychotherapies, family-based therapy, mindfulness meditation and yoga practice, and vocational rehabilitation focusing on computer skills.

Conclusions

The field of behavioral addictions, including those that occur in cyberspace gaming, is relatively new and emerging. The medical field finally recognizes gambling disorder as the first behavioral addiction, and the WHO recently classified (video) gaming disorder as diagnosable addictive behavior. Despite these strides, social work pays insufficient attention to technology-related addictive behaviors capable of inducing the same biopsychosocial consequences and harms as substance misuse. Social workers have a unique opportunity to position ourselves as leaders in this field through research, policy, practice, and educational initiatives because we serve populations most at risk of developing IGD and problematic technology use.

To that end, social work programs need to integrate behavioral addiction content into courses focused on psychopathology and substance use disorders, as well as human development curriculum related to adolescence and emerging adulthood. That, in turn, will inform and encourage future social work professionals to identify and address IGD and related behavioral addictions, including routinely screening for misuse of interactive media among clients and families. In addition, social workers' greater awareness of IGD and problematic technology use could inspire research to focus on this developing area in the future, an area currently dominated by psychologists. Social work research into the developmental risks and protective factors for IGD and problematic technology use, longitudinal consequences of the disorder on individuals, families, and communities, and best practices for intervention is urgently needed. Social workers are uniquely positioned to develop and implement evidence-based screening tools and treatment strategies, based on experience with family systems, which could bring new and effective approaches for addressing these problems. Social workers can then utilize the research evidence to advocate at institutional and policy levels for age-appropriate safeguards in video games and interactive media correlated with higher levels of disorder, as well as better treatment access and options for health/mental health promotion to alleviate factors pressing for development of these disorders.

References

Aarseth, E., Bean, A. M., Boonen, H., Colder Carras, M., Coulson, M., Das, D., . . . Haagsma, M. C. (2017). Scholars' open debate paper on the World Health Organization ICD-11 gaming disorder proposal. *Journal of Behavioral Addictions, 6*(3), 267–270. doi:10.1556/2006.5.2016.088

American Psychiatric Association. (2013). *Diagnostic and statistical manual of mental disorders* (5th ed.). Arlington, VA: American Psychiatric Association. doi:10.1176/appi.books.9780890425596

Andreassen, C. S., Billieux, J., Griffiths, M. D., Kuss, D. J., Demetrovics, Z., Mazzoni, E., & Pallesen, S. (2016). The relationship between addictive use of social media and video games and symptoms of psychiatric disorders: A large-scale cross-sectional study. *Psychology of Addictive Behaviors, 30*(2), 252–262. doi:10.1037/adb0000160

Andreassen, C. S., Torsheim, T., Brunborg, G. S., & Pallesen, S. (2012). Development of a Facebook addiction scale. *Psychological Reports, 110*(2), 501–517. doi:10.2466/02.09.18.PR0.110.2.501-517

Ballabio, M., Griffiths, M. D., Urbán, R., Quartiroli, A., Demetrovics, Z., & Király, O. (2017). Do gaming motives mediate between psychiatric symptoms and problematic gaming? An empirical survey study. *Addiction Research & Theory, 25*(5), 397–408. doi:10.1080/16066359.2017.1305360

Brand, M., Young, K. S., Laier, C., Wölfling, K., & Potenza, M. N. (2016). Integrating psychological and neurobiological considerations regarding the development and maintenance of specific Internet-use disorders: An interaction of person-affect-cognition-execution (I-PACE) model. *Neuroscience & Biobehavioral Reviews, 71*, 252–266. doi:10.1016/j.neubiorev.2016.08.033

Braun, B., Stopfer, J. M., Müller, K. W., Beutel, M. E., & Egloff, B. (2016). Personality and video gaming: Comparing regular gamers, non-gamers, and gaming addicts and differentiating between game genres. *Computers in Human Behavior, 55*, 406–412. doi:10.1016/j.chb.2015.09.041

Caplan, S. E. (2002). Problematic Internet use and psychosocial well-being: Development of a theory-based cognitive-behavioral measurement instrument. *Computer and Human Behavior, 18*, 553–575. doi:10.1016/S0747-5632(02)00004-3

Chak, K., & Leung, L. (2004). Shyness and locus of control as predictors of Internet addiction and Internet use. *CyberPsychology & Behavior, 7*(5), 559–570. doi:10.1089/cpb.2004.7.559

Cheng, C., Cheung, M. W., L., & Wang, H. (2018). Multinational comparison of Internet gaming disorder and psychosocial problems versus well-being: Meta-analysis of 20 countries. *Computers in Human Behavior, 88*, 153–167. doi:10.1016/j.chb.2018.06.033

Costa, P. T., & McCrae, R. R. (1992). Normal personality assessment in clinical practice: The NEO personality inventory. *Psychological Assessment, 4*(1), 5–13. doi:10.1037/1040-3590.4.1.5

Davis, R. A. (2001). A cognitive-behavioral model of pathological Internet use. *Computers in Human Behavior, 17*, 187–195. doi:10.1016/S0747-5632(00)00041-8

Decker, S. A., & Gay, J. N. (2011). Cognitive-bias toward gaming-related words and disinhibition in world of Warcraft gamers. *Computers in Human Behavior, 27*(2), 798–810. doi:10.1016/j.chb.2010.11.005

Delfabbro, P., & King, D. (2015). On finding the C in CBT: The challenges of applying gambling-related cognitive approaches to video-gaming. *Journal of Gambling Studies, 31*(1), 315–329. doi:10.1007/s10899-013-9416-3

DeYoung, C. G., Quilty, L. C., & Peterson, J. B. (2007). Between facets and domains: 10 aspects of the Big Five. *Journal of Personality and Social Psychology, 93*(5), 880–896. doi:10.1037/0022-3514.93.5.880

Du, Y., Jiang, W., & Vance, A. (2010). Longer-term effect of randomized, controlled group cognitive behavioural therapy for Internet addiction in adolescent students in Shanghai. *Australian and New Zealand Journal of Psychiatry, 44*, 2, 129–134. doi:10.3109/00048670903282725

Duroy, D., Gorse, P., & Lejoyeux, M. (2014). Characteristics of online compulsive buying in Parisian students. *Addictive Behaviors, 39*(12), 1827–1830. doi:10.1016/j.addbeh.2014.07.028

Fam, J. Y. (2018). Prevalence of Internet gaming disorder in adolescents: A meta-analysis across three decades. *Scandinavian Journal of Psychology, 59*(5), 524–531. doi:10.1111/sjop.12459

Forrest, C. J., King, D. L., & Delfabbro, P. H. (2017). Maladaptive cognitions predict changes in problematic gaming in highly-engaged adults: A 12-month longitudinal study. *Addictive Behaviors, 65*, 125–130. doi:10.1016/j.addbeh.2016.10.013

Garland, E. L. (2013). *Mindfulness-oriented recovery enhancement for addiction, stress, and pain.* Washington, DC: NASW Press.

Gervasi, A. M., La Marca, L., Lombardo, E., Mannino, G., Iacolino, C., & Schimmenti, A. (2017). Maladaptive personality traits and Internet addiction symptoms among young adults: A study based on the alternative DSM-5 model for personality disorders. *Clinical Neuropsychiatry, 14*(1), 20–28.

Grant, J. E., Potenza, M. N., Weinstein, A., & Gorelick, D. A. (2010). Introduction to behavioral addictions. *The American Journal of Drug and Alcohol Abuse, 36*(5), 233–241. doi:10.3109/00952990.2010.491884

Griffiths, M. (2005). A 'components' model of addiction within a biopsychosocial framework. *Journal of Substance Use, 10*(4), 191–197. doi:10.1080/14659890500114359

Griffiths, M. D., Van Rooij, A. J., Kardefelt-Winther, D., Starcevic, V., Király, O., Pallesen, S., . . . King, D. L. (2016). Working towards an international consensus on criteria for assessing Internet gaming disorder: A critical commentary on Petry et al. (2014). *Addiction, 111*(1), 167–175. doi:10.1111/add.13057

Han, D. H., Bolo, N., Daniels, M. A., Arenella, L., Lyoo, I. K., & Renshaw, P. F. (2011). Brain activity and desire for Internet video game play. *Comprehensive Psychiatry, 52*, 88–95. doi:10.1016/j.comppsych.2010.04.004

Han, D. H., Kim, S. M., Lee, Y. S., & Renshaw, P. F. (2012). The effect of family therapy on the changes in the severity of on-line game play and brain activity in adolescents with on-line game addiction. *Psychiatry Research: Neuroimaging, 202*(2), 126–131. doi:10.1016/j.pscychresns.2012.02.011

Hou, H., Jia, S., Hu, S., Fan, R., Sun, W., Sun, T., & Zhang, H. (2012). Reduced striatal dopamine transporters in people with Internet addiction disorder. *BioMed Research International, 2012*, 1–5. doi:10.1155/2012/854524

Kerkhof, P., Finkenauer, C., & Muusses, L. D. (2011). Relational consequences of compulsive Internet use: A longitudinal study among newlyweds. *Human Communication Research, 37*, 147–173. doi:10.1111/j.1468-2958.2010.01397.x

King, D. L., & Delfabbro, P. H. (2016). The cognitive psychopathology of Internet gaming disorder in adolescence. *Journal of Abnormal Child Psychology, 44*(8), 1635–1645. doi:10.1007/s10802-016-0135-y

King, D. L., Delfabbro, P. H., Wu, A. M., Doh, Y. Y., Kuss, D. J., Pallesen, S., . . . Sakuma, H. (2017). Treatment of Internet gaming disorder: An international systematic review and CONSORT evaluation. *Clinical Psychology Review, 54*, 123–133. doi:10.1016/j.cpr.2017.04.002

Király, O., Urbán, R., Griffiths, M. D., Ágoston, C., Nagygyörgy, K., Kökönyei, G., & Demetrovics, Z. (2015). The mediating effect of gaming motivation between psychiatric symptoms and problematic online gaming: An online survey. *Journal of Medical Internet Research, 17*(4), e88. doi:10.2196/jmir.3515

Ko, C. H., Liu, G. C., Hsiao, S., Yen, J. Y., Yang, M. J., Lin, W. C., . . . Chen, C. S. (2009). Brain activities associated with gaming urge of online gaming addiction. *Journal of Psychiatric Research, 43*, 739–747. doi:10.1016/j.jpsychires.2008.09.012

Ko, C. H., Liu, G. C., Yen, C. F., Chen, C. S., & Lin, W. C. (2013). The brain activations for both cue-induced gaming urge and smoking craving among subjects comorbid with Internet gaming addiction and nicotine dependence. *Journal of Psychiatric Research, 47*, 486–493. doi:10.1016/j.jpsychires.2012.11.008

Kotov, R., Gamez, W., Schmidt, F., & Watson, D. (2010). Linking "big" personality traits to anxiety, depressive, and substance use disorders: A meta-analysis. *Psychological Bulletin, 136*(5), 768–821. doi:10.1037/a0020327

Kwon, M., Lee, J. Y., Won, W. Y., Park, J. W., Min, J. A., Hahn, C., . . . Kim, D. J. (2013). Development and validation of a smartphone addiction scale (SAS). *PloS One, 8*(2), e56936. doi:10.1371/journal.pone.0056936

Lam, L.T. (2014). Internet gaming addiction, problematic use of the internet, and sleep problems: A systematic review. *Current Psychiatry Reports, 16*(4), 444.

LaRose, R., & Eastin, M. S. (2004). A social cognitive theory of Internet uses and gratifications: Toward a new model of media attendance. *Journal of Broadcasting & Electronic Media, 48*, 358–377. doi:10.1207/s15506878jobem4803_2

Lee, H. W., Choi, J. S., Shin, Y. C., Lee, J. Y., Jung, H. Y., & Kwon, J. S. (2012). Impulsivity in Internet addiction: A comparison with pathological gambling. *Cyberpsychology, Behavior, and Social Networking, 15*(7), 373–377. doi:10.1089/cyber.2012.0063

Lemmens, J. S., Valkenburg, P. M., & Gentile, D. A. (2015). The Internet gaming disorder scale. *Psychological Assessment, 27*(2), 567–582. doi:10.1037/pas0000062

Li, W., Garland, E. L., & Howard, M. O. (2014). Family factors in Internet addiction among Chinese youth: A systematic review of English- and Chinese-language studies. *Computers in Human Behavior, 31*, 393–411. doi:10.1016/j.chb.2013.11.004

Li, W., Garland, E. L., McGovern, P., O'Brien, J. E., Tronnier, C., & Howard, M. O. (2017). Mindfulness-oriented recovery enhancement for Internet gaming disorder in US adults: A stage I randomized controlled trial. *Psychology of Addictive Behaviors, 31*(4), 393–402. doi:10.1037/adb0000269

Li, W., Garland, E. L., O'Brien, J. E., Tronnier, C., McGovern, P., Anthony, B., & Howard, M. O. (2018). Mindfulness-oriented recovery enhancement for video game addiction in emerging adults: Preliminary findings from case reports. *International Journal of Mental Health and Addiction, 16*, 928–945. doi:10.1007/s11469-017-9765-8

Li, W., Howard, M. O., Garland, E. L., McGovern, P., & Lazar, M. (2017). Mindfulness treatment for substance misuse: A systematic review and meta-analysis. *Journal of Substance Abuse Treatment, 75*, 62–96. doi:10.1016/j.jsat.2017.01.008

Li, W., O'Brien, J. E., Snyder, S. M., & Howard, M. O. (2015). Characteristics of Internet addiction/pathological Internet use in US university students: A qualitative-method investigation. *PloS One, 10*(2), e0117372. doi:10.1371/journal.pone.0117372

Littel, M., Van den Berg, I., Luijten, M., Van Rooij, A. J., Keemink, L., & Franken, I. H. (2012). Error processing and response inhibition in excessive computer game players: An event-related potential study. *Addiction Biology, 17*(5), 934–947. doi:10.1111/j.1369-1600.2012.00467.x

Liu, Q. X., Fang, X. Y., Yan, N., Zhou, Z. K., Yuan, X. J., Lan, J., & Liu, C. Y. (2015). Multi-family group therapy for adolescent Internet addiction: Exploring the underlying mechanisms. *Addictive Behaviors, 42*, 1–8. doi:10.1016/j.addbeh.2014.10.021

Lorenz, R. C., Krüger, J. K., Neumann, B., Schott, B. H., Kaufmann, C., Heinz, A., & Wüstenberg, T. (2013). Cue reactivity and its inhibition in pathological computer game players. *Addiction Biology, 18*(1), 134–146. doi:10.1111/j.1369-1600.2012.00491.x

Männikkö, N., Ruotsalainen, H., Miettunen, J., Pontes, H. M., & Kääriäinen, M. (2017). Problematic gaming behaviour and health-related outcomes: A systematic review and meta-analysis. *Journal of Health Psychology*, 1–15. doi:10.1177/1359105317740414

Marino, C., Gini, G., Vieno, A., & Spada, M. M. (2018). A comprehensive meta-analysis on problematic Facebook use. *Computers in Human Behavior, 83*, 262–277. doi:10.1016/j.chb.2018.02.009

Marlatt, G. A., & Gordon, J. R. (1985). *Relapse prevention: Maintenance strategies in the treatment of addictive behaviors.* New York, NY: Guilford.

McHugh, R. K., Hearon, B. A., & Otto, M. W. (2010). Cognitive behavioral therapy for substance use disorders. *Psychiatric Clinics, 33*(3), 511–525. doi:10.1016/j.psc.2010.04.012

Mehroof, M., & Griffiths, M. D. (2010). Online gaming addiction: The role of sensation seeking, self-control, neuroticism, aggression, state anxiety, and trait anxiety. *Cyberpsychology, Behavior, and Social Networking, 13*(3), 313–316. doi:10.1089/cyber.2009.0229

Miller, W. R., & Rollnick, S. (2012). *Motivational interviewing: Helping people change.* New York, NY: Guilford Press.

Mills, D. J., Milyavskaya, M., Heath, N. L., & Derevensky, J. L. (2018). Gaming motivation and problematic video gaming: The role of needs frustration. *European Journal of Social Psychology, 48*(4), 551–559. doi:10.1002/ejsp.2343

Mills, D. J., Milyavskaya, M., Mettler, J., Heath, N. L., & Derevensky, J. L. (2018). How do passion for video games and needs frustration explain time spent gaming?. *British Journal of Social Psychology, 57*(2), 461–481. doi:10.1111/bjso.12239

Monacis, L., Palo, V. D., Griffiths, M. D., & Sinatra, M. (2016). Validation of the Internet gaming disorder scale-short-form (IGDS9-SF) in an Italian-speaking sample. *Journal of Behavioral Addictions, 5*(4), 683–690. doi:10.1556/2006.5.2016.083

Müller, K. W., Beutel, M. E., Egloff, B., & Wölfling, K. (2014). Investigating risk factors for Internet gaming disorder: A comparison of patients with addictive gaming, pathological gamblers and healthy controls regarding the big five personality traits. *European Addiction Research, 20*(3), 129–136. doi:10.1159/000355832

Newzoo. (2018). *2018 global games market report.* San Francisco, CA: Newzoo America.

O'Brien, J. E., Li, W., Snyder, S. M., & Howard, M. O. (2016). Problem Internet overuse behaviors in college students: Readiness-to-change and receptivity to treatment. *Journal of Evidence-Informed Social Work, 13*(4), 373–385. doi:10.1080/23761407.2015.1086713

Pallesen, S., Lorvik, I. M., Bu, E. H., & Molde, H. (2015). An exploratory study investigating the effects of a treatment manual for video game addiction. *Psychological Reports, 117*(2), 490–495. doi:10.2466/02.PR0.117c14z9

Petry, N. M., Rehbein, F., Gentile, D. A., Lemmens, J. S., Rumpf, H. J., Mößle, T., . . . O'Brien, C. P. (2014). An international consensus for assessing Internet gaming disorder using the new DSM-5 approach. *Addiction, 109*(9), 1399–1406. https://doi.org/10.1111/add.12457

Petry, N. M., Rehbein, F., Ko, C. H., & O'Brien, C. P. (2015). Internet gaming disorder in the DSM-5. *Current Psychiatry Reports, 17*(9), 72. doi:10.1007/s11920-015-0610-0

Petry, N. M., Zajac, K., & Ginley, M. K. (2018). Behavioral addictions as mental disorders: To be or not to be? *Annual Review of Clinical Psychology, 14*, 399–423. doi:10.1146/annurev-clinpsy-032816-045120

Pontes, H. M., & Griffiths, M. D. (2015). Measuring DSM-5 Internet gaming disorder: Development and validation of a short psychometric scale. *Computers in Human Behavior, 45*, 137–143. doi:10.1016/j.chb.2014.12.006

Pontes, H. M., Stavropoulos, V., & Griffiths, M. D. (2017). Measurement invariance of the Internet gaming disorder scale-short-form (IGDS9-SF) between the United States of America, India and the United Kingdom. *Psychiatry Research, 257*, 472–478. doi:10.1016/j.psychres.2017.08.013

Przybylski, A. K., Weinstein, N., & Murayama, K. (2016). Internet gaming disorder: Investigating the clinical relevance of a new phenomenon. *American Journal of Psychiatry, 174*(3), 230–236. doi:10.1176/appi.ajp.2016.16020224

Rehbein, F., & Baier, D. (2013). Family-, media-, and school-related risk factors of video game addiction. *Journal of Media Psychology, 25*(3), 118–128. doi:10.1027/1864-1105/a000093

Rudd, A. (2012, July 18). Diablo death: Teenager dies after playing video game for 40 hours without eating or sleeping. *Mirror.* Retrieved from http://www.mirror.co.uk/news/world-news/diablo-iii-death-teenager-dies-1147472

Ryan, T., Chester, A., Reece, J., & Xenos, S. (2014). The uses and abuses of Facebook: A review of Facebook addiction. *Journal of Behavioral Addictions, 3*(3), 133–148. doi:10.1556/JBA.3.2014.016

Schneider, L. A., King, D. L., & Delfabbro, P. H. (2017). Family factors in adolescent problematic Internet gaming: A systematic review. *Journal of Behavioral Addictions, 6*(3), 321–333. doi:10.1556/2006.6.2017.035

Shek, D. T., Tang, V. M., & Lo, C. Y. (2009). Evaluation of an Internet addiction treatment program for Chinese adolescents in Hong Kong. *Adolescence, 44*, 359–374.

Spada, M. M. (2014). An overview of problematic Internet use. *Addictive Behaviors, 39*(1), 3–6. doi:10.1016/j.addbeh.2013.09.007

Starcevic, V. (2013). Is Internet addiction a useful concept? *Australian & New Zealand Journal of Psychiatry, 47*(1), 16–19doi:10.1177/0004867412461693

Su, W., Fang, X., Miller, J. K., & Wang, Y. (2011). Internet-based intervention for the treatment of online addiction for college students in China: A pilot study of the healthy online self-helping center. *Cyberpsychology, Behavior, and Social Networking, 14*(9), 497–503. doi:10.1089/cyber.2010.0167

Sakuma, H., Mihara, S., Nakayama, H., Miura, K., Kitayuguchi, T., Maezono, M., . . . Higuchi, S. (2017). Treatment with the self-discovery camp (SDiC) improves Internet gaming disorder. *Addictive Behaviors, 64*, 357–362. doi:10.1016/j.addbeh.2016.06.013

Taylor, K., & Silver, L. (2019, February 5). *Smartphone ownership is growing rapidly around the world, but not always equally.* Pew Research Center. Retrieved from http://www.pewglobal.org/2019/02/05/smartphone-ownership-is-growing-rapidly- around-the-world-but-not-always-equally/

Van Rooij, A. J., Ferguson, C. J., Colder Carras, M., Kardefelt-Winther, D., Shi, J., Aarseth, E., . . . Deleuze, J. (2018). A weak scientific basis for gaming disorder: Let us err on the side of caution. *Journal of Behavioral Addictions, 7*(1), 1–9. doi:10.1556/2006.7.2018.19

Van Rooij, A. J., Ferguson, C. J., Van de Mheen, D., & Schoenmakers, T. M. (2017). Time to abandon Internet addiction? Predicting problematic Internet, game, and social media use from psychosocial well-being and application use. *Clinical Neuropsychiatry, 14*(1), 113–121. doi:10.1007/s11469-010-9295-0

Van Rooij, A. J., Zinn, M. F., Schoenmakers, T. M., & Van de Mheen, D. (2012). Treating Internet addiction with cognitive-behavioral therapy: A thematic analysis of the experiences of therapists. *International Journal of Mental Health and Addiction, 10*(1), 69–82. doi:10.1007/s11469-010-9295-0

Wéry, A., & Billieux, J. (2017). Problematic cybersex: Conceptualization, assessment, and treatment. *Addictive Behaviors, 64*, 238–246. doi:10.1016/j.addbeh.2015.11.007

Winkler, A., Dörsing, B., Rief, W., Shen, Y., & Glombiewski, J. A. (2013). Treatment of Internet addiction: A meta-analysis. *Clinical Psychology Review, 33*(2), 317–329. doi:10.1016/j.cpr.2012.12.005

World Health Organization. (2018). *International classification of diseases (ICD) 11th revision.* Geneva: Authors.

World Internet Usage and Population Statistics. (2017). Retrieved from http://www.internetworldstats.com/stats.htm

Wu, C. S. T., Wong, H. T., Yu, K. F., Fok, K. W., Yeung, S. M., Lam, C. H., & Liu, K. M. (2016). Parenting approaches, family functionality, and Internet addiction among Hong Kong adolescents. *BMC Pediatrics, 16*, 130. doi:10.1186/s12887-016-0666-y

Yao, Y. W., Chen, P. R., Chiang-shan, R. L., Hare, T. A., Li, S., Zhang, J. T., . . . Fang, X. Y. (2017). Combined reality therapy and mindfulness meditation decrease intertemporal decisional impulsivity in young adults with Internet gaming disorder. *Computers in Human Behavior, 68*, 210–216. doi:10.1016/j.chb.2016.11.038

Yee, N. (2006). Motivations for play in online games. *CyberPsychology & Behavior, 9*(6), 772–775. doi:10.1089/cpb.2006.9.772

Young, K. S. (1998). Internet addiction: The emergence of a new clinical disorder. *Cyberpsychology & Behavior, 1*(3), 237–244. doi:10.1089/cpb.1998.1.237

Young, K. S. (2004). Internet addiction: A new clinical phenomenon and its consequences. *American Behavioral Scientist, 48*(4), 402–415. doi:10.1177/0002764204270278

Young, K. S. (2007). Cognitive behavior therapy with Internet addicts: Treatment outcomes and implications. *CyberPsychology & Behavior, 10*(5), 671–679. doi:10.1089/cpb.2007.9971

Young, K. S. (2013). Treatment outcomes using CBT-IA with Internet-addicted patients. *Journal of Behavioral Addictions, 2*(4), 209–215. doi:10.1556/JBA.2.2013.4.3

Introduction to Section II
Addictive behavior across the lifespan and specific populations

A social worker's understanding of addictive behaviors depends on recognizing individual differences in what each person brings to any situation. Individual differences reflect cultural diversity broadly defined (ethnicity, age, gender/gender identity, religion/spirituality, ability/disability, national origin, and more). Diversity in individual characteristics, experiences, developmental trajectories, and exposure to various environmental and social determinants all contribute to the tremendous heterogeneity in addictive behavior and outcomes observed in practice and research.

The chapters included in Section II explore aspects of human diversity with implications for understanding addictive behaviors. Several chapters focus on different periods of the life span. The first three address the effects of prenatal exposure to alcohol or opioids beginning from when the children are very young infants (Chapter 10 on neonatal abstinence syndrome and Chapter 11 on fetal alcohol exposure). Chapter 12 is unique in that it expresses the views and experiences of several young adults who began life prenatally exposed to alcohol. The next three chapters address addictive behavior during adolescence (Chapter 13 on the adolescent brain), emerging adulthood (Chapter 14), and older adulthood (Chapter 15).

The final two chapters move away from the lifespan perspective and focus on other aspects of human diversity. Chapter 16 applies a health disparities framework in exploring addictive behavior in relation to race/ethnicity, gender, and disability status. Chapter 17 applies minority stress theory in examining addictive behavior experiences among LGBTQ+ populations at four different developmental periods: adolescence, emerging adulthood, middle adulthood, and older adulthood. The purpose of the Section II chapters is to help inform social work interventions with the expectation that these can be age and culturally relevant and responsive. These specific population groups were selected because of their global presence and significance, the strength of evidence concerning these groups, and the relative neglect of these groups in social work education concerning addictive behaviors.

10

Neonatal abstinence syndrome

Recognition, management, and prevention

Kristina M. Reber, Amy B. Schlegel,
Erica F. Braswell and Edward G. Shepherd

Background

Neonatal abstinence syndrome (NAS) is a condition of opiate withdrawal in newborn babies first described in literature of the mid-1970s (Finnegan, Kron, Connaughton, & Emich, 1975). Although it was relatively rare for several decades, its incidence has increased markedly in conjunction with the use of both legal and illicit opiates in the United States and internationally (Ko et al., 2016; Kuehn, 2018; Patrick, Davis, Lehmann, & Cooper, 2015). NAS affects all demographic and racial groups.

Epidemiology of NAS

The rate of maternal opiate usage during pregnancy increased by almost a factor of five in the United States between 2000 and 2009, while rates of NAS increased from 1.5 cases per 1,000 live births to 6 per 1,000 live births between 1999 and 2013 (Sanjanwala & Harper, 2019; Wachman, Schiff, & Silverstein, 2018). The U.S. incidence of both maternal opiate usage and NAS is highly variable across geographic areas: from 0.7 per 1,000 live births in Hawaii to over 30 per 1,000 live births in West Virginia (Committee on Obstetric Practice, 2017; Ko et al., 2016; McQueen & Murphy-Oikonen, 2016). Increases in NAS have been most pronounced in rural and suburban areas versus urban areas, with increases of 1.2–7.5 per 1,000 live births in rural areas of the United States compared to 1.4–4.8 per 1,000 live births in urban areas between 2004 and 2013 (Patrick et al., 2019). As expected, areas with high rates of opiate prescribing have high rates of opioid use disorder (OUD) and NAS. Similarly, OUD during pregnancy is widely variable based on geography, with rates ranging from 0.7 per 1,000 deliveries in the District of Columbia to almost 50 per 1,000 deliveries in Vermont (Ko et al., 2016).

Although international data are relatively limited compared to the United States, there is evidence that OUD and NAS occur with a similar frequency in the United States, Canada, England, and Australia (Davies et al., 2016). There is essentially no reported data in the medical literature regarding NAS in developing nations. Estimates suggest that all regions of the world have at least some OUD, but prevalence figures are difficult to obtain due to punitive drug policies and political instability (Peacock et al., 2018). Nevertheless, it is safe to assume that NAS exists in most countries and regions, and as misuse of opiates increases so will the incidence of NAS.

NAS rates are influenced by the same social determinant factors that influence OUD: for example, regions with higher unemployment and shortages of mental health care have higher NAS rates (Liu, Kong, Leslie, & Corr, 2019). Fortunately, while the risk of opiate misuse during pregnancy is driven by the same risk factors as for non-pregnant women, rates of use are lower among pregnant women than non-pregnant women. Women younger than 26 years of age are more likely to use opiates during pregnancy than are women 26 years and older, but both groups are less likely to misuse opiates than non-pregnant women of similar age groups (Rosenthal & Baxter, 2019; Sanjanwala & Harper, 2019). Other social determinate risk factors for opiate use during pregnancy include poverty, absence of other children under age five in the household, and lack of commercial or any health insurance; however, it is critical to understand that opiate misuse during pregnancy and subsequent NAS is increasing among women and babies across every race, ethnicity, and socioeconomic group (Krans & Patrick, 2016).

Costs of NAS

Medical and societal costs of NAS are substantial. Such costs include direct expenditures for health care, typically in the hospital setting, and indirect costs like lost wages due to missed work. Direct medical costs related to NAS in the United States are estimated between $500 million and $1.5 billion annually, largely driven by the cost of initial newborn hospitalizations which are typically as long as 20 days for affected babies (Corr & Hollenbeak, 2017; Patrick et al., 2012).

NAS effects

Although NAS is nearly uniformly treatable and survivable, with most babies remaining clinically stable throughout treatment, in utero exposure to opiates occurs at critical periods of fetal neurodevelopment and is associated with alterations in neurodevelopmental and health outcomes. NAS causes a number of physiologic derangements concentrated in the central nervous system, the autonomic nervous system (which controls "fight or flight" responses), and the gastrointestinal system. Symptoms include jitteriness, irritability, fussiness, diarrhea, sweating, poor sleep, skin irritation from constant movements, and in rare cases, seizures and death (McQueen & Murphy-Oikonen, 2016). Babies experiencing NAS can be very difficult to care for due to their symptoms and are at risk for many complications and maltreatment after discharge (Liu et al., 2019; Uebel et al., 2015). Additionally, societal costs include infants experiencing NAS being more likely than others to be placed in foster care or with relatives (Prindle, Hammond, & Putnam-Hornstein, 2018).

Long-term outcomes for infants with NAS are unclear, although there is concern that chronic fetal exposure to opiates may lead to developmental delays and/or behavioral problems. Given the marked increase in incidence of NAS, however, it is quite clear that longitudinal neurodevelopmental follow-up is imperative to identify and provide therapy for any emerging delays or behavioral difficulties (Patrick et al., 2016).

Opioids are known to impair fetal neurodevelopment and function. They accelerate brain cell death (neuronal apoptosis) (Hu, Sheng, Lokensgard, & Peterson, 2002), alter myelination which is critical to nerve cell functioning (Sanchez, Bigbee, Fobbs, Robinson, & Sato-Bigbee, 2008; Vestal-Laborde, Eschenroeder, Bigbee, Robinson, & Sato-Bigbee, 2014), and affect neurotransmitter "brain chemistry" systems (Robinson, Maher, Wallace, & Kunko, 1997). Chronic in utero opiate exposure is associated with a significantly smaller mean head circumference at birth, as well (Towers et al., 2019).

Because of the research design and statistical challenges of isolating independent effects of exposure to the developing fetus from additional environmental and medical risk factors, later neurodevelopmental effects of chronic in utero opiate exposure and NAS remain largely unknown. Lower socioeconomic status, poor prenatal care, and comorbid substance exposure—all associated with maternal OUD rates—are also associated with negative impacts on neurodevelopmental outcomes independent of NAS. Emerging bodies of work, however, suggest that independent of socioeconomic factors, in utero opiate exposure is associated with risk for future cognitive, language, attention, and visual deficiencies, and poorer academic outcomes. Toddlers treated for NAS at birth demonstrated lower neurodevelopmental scores than age matched peers (Merhar et al., 2018); however, post-birth environmental influences cannot be ruled out as contributing factors. Infants exposed to opiates in utero demonstrated abnormalities in motor rigidity and dysregulated motor patterns that persisted into toddlerhood and demonstrated decreased social responsivity, attention span, and social engagement (Bernstein, Jeremy, Hans, & Marcus, 1984). In utero exposure to opiates, along with other misused substances, is associated with poor neurobiological organization during infancy, placing infants at risk for physiological and behavior regulation problems, which can impact early learning (Conradt et al., 2013). Again, these studies are unable to fully separate biological and post-birth environmental influences on infant development and behavior.

It is unclear if maternal opioid use is associated with congenital anomalies or birth defects, as existing studies demonstrated conflicting findings (Bada et al., 2005; McQueen & Murphy-Oikonen, 2016). The overall rate of such anomalies or birth defects is very low across studies, however; thus, it is generally believed to be safe to prescribe opiates during pregnancy under carefully controlled circumstances (Committee on Obstetric Practice, 2017). The most common complication of opioid administration under these circumstances is NAS in the newborn, which can be successfully treated with proven regimens. The incidence of NAS requiring pharmacological treatment in babies is variable, with rates from about 30% to 94% reported in the literature (Committee on Obstetric Practice, 2017; McQueen & Murphy-Oikonen, 2016). Historically, such treatment often resulted in extended hospital stays for affected babies, but recent advances in care have reduced length of stay to under 14 days in many centers (Sanlorenzo, Stark, & Patrick, 2018; Wachman, Grossman, et al., 2018).

Social determinants and confounding factors

There exists an increased probability of poverty, food insecurity, malnutrition, lower levels of education among U.S. families of children experiencing NAS. Concern for the additional impacts of these factors on neurodevelopment in infants with a history of NAS is supported by higher cognitive scores in children affected by NAS subsequently raised by foster or adoptive families (Merhar et al., 2018). This highlights the importance of early neurodevelopmental screening and intervention programs, family education, and access to resources and support for children affected by maternal OUD.

Physical health and well-being in children with a history of NAS is an additional concern: as many as 25% may not receive necessary healthcare during the first two years (Callaghan, Crimmins, & Schweitzer, 2011). Conversely, they are at increased risk of re-hospitalization during childhood for maltreatment, trauma, and mental and behavioral disorders (Uebel et al., 2015). Infant and childhood mortality in children with a history of in utero opioid exposure is increased as well. Epidemiological studies suggest that this risk persists until adolescence and is due to neglect, maltreatment, and trauma with causes of death including SIDS, accidents, and assault (Uebel et al., 2015). This combined evidence reinforces the potential importance of social worker roles as part of the team assisting these babies and their families.

Identifying NAS

NAS is an unusual syndrome as it involves both mother and fetus, but typically does not manifest in the infant until after delivery. This occurs because fetal opiate levels are maintained by maternal usage in utero, as opiates move freely from the mother's to the fetus' circulation via the placenta. As a result of maternal opiate levels over time, the fetus becomes habituated to high opiate levels (Committee on Obstetric Practice, 2017; McQueen & Murphy-Oikonen, 2016); the infant's immature organ systems are inefficient at processing the drugs, resulting in a relatively higher circulating exposure. Once the infant is born, the supply of opiates is immediately halted as the umbilical cord is cut, and the infant's opiate levels drop steadily over several days. The time required for opiate levels to drop is variable and depends on a number of factors, including the baby's intrinsic drug metabolism rate, genetics, and type of opiate exposure. Infants exposed to short-acting opiates (e.g. heroin) typically suffer withdrawal symptoms more rapidly than infants exposed to longer-acting opiates like methadone. Unfortunately, even within acceptable maternal dosing guidelines, the timing, incidence, and severity of NAS are unpredictable: some babies exposed to relatively low doses may experience severe NAS, while other babies exposed even to higher doses may not (Hudak, Tan, Committee on Drugs, Committee on Fetus and Newborn, & American Academy of Pediatrics, 2012).

Screening

NAS may present as late as five days after birth, and it is therefore important that all babies at risk for NAS are monitored carefully in the hospital during that time (Smirk, Bowman, Doyle, & Kamlin, 2014). The American College of Obstetrics and Gynecology (ACOG) and other women's health organizations have recently emphasized universal screening across all populations based on validated screening tools for alcohol, opiate use, and alcohol or opioid use disorders (AUD or OUD), to minimize stigma and stereotyping, as well as promote early identification, and referral to treatment when indicated. Validated screening instruments are available for use with obstetric populations. Confidentiality and benefit to the mother-infant dyad should be emphasized in the screening and feedback process (Reddy, Davis, Ren, & Greene, 2017). Social workers trained in administering alcohol and other drug use screening protocols may play an important role in maternal-child health teams.

Diagnosing NAS

Testing newborns for drug biomarkers and metabolites can offer objective evidence of in utero exposure when suggested by maternal screening results or infant behavior. Results of toxicology or drug tests can assist clinicians in medical decision-making surrounding monitoring for and treatment of NAS. They can also have social and legal implications given the risks to the fetus of uncontrolled maternal opiate use (Martins, Oppolzer, Santos, Barroso, & Gallardo, 2019). No test captures exposure across the entire gestational period and most are unable to assess magnitude of exposure (Polak, Kelpin, & Terplan, 2019). Neonatal urine and meconium testing are generally efficient with standardized laboratory protocols. An optimal neonatal urine drug screen is obtained from the first urine after delivery; however, urine screening in the neonate may reflect only recent exposure. Many substances are quickly metabolized and subsequently undetectable (Hudak et al., 2012). Substances metabolized by the liver and kidney can concentrate in the meconium, which can detect exposure that occurred during the months before birth (Hudak et al., 2012). Neonatal meconium testing is the gold standard for detecting in utero drug exposure, however tissue testing of the umbilical cord is an emerging alternative, offering an extended window of exposure (Martins et al., 2019), as well as possible opportunities for universal exposure testing. Currently, availability of laboratory tests remains institution-dependent.

Clinicians caring for infants born to mothers experiencing OUD should be trained in recognizing and assessing signs and symptoms of NAS. While nearly all infants exposed to opiates in utero demonstrate some signs and symptoms of NAS, there exists variability in the proportion that will develop symptoms severe enough to require pharmacological intervention. The expression and course of NAS is variable and may be dependent on a host of factors, including: type, amount, and purity of opioid used; duration of exposure; maternal drug metabolism; dyad-specific placental transfer; gestational age at birth; concomitant exposure to other substances; breast/breastmilk feeding; genetic variation; and comorbid medical conditions (Brandt & Finnegan, 2017; Sutter, Leeman, & Hsi, 2014). For example, NAS following exposure to heroin is typically more rapid (4–24 hours) compared to methadone (24–48 hours), which is earlier than buprenorphine exposure (48–72 hours) (Zelson, Rubio, & Wasserman, 1971). Infants of mothers actively using non-prescribed opiates may present differently than those whose mothers are enrolled in opioid maintenance therapy (OMT) involving pharmacotherapy. Preterm babies with immature neurologic systems may demonstrate a different clinical withdrawal picture than those born at term. Concomitant in utero exposure to nicotine, benzodiazepines, SSRI antidepressant medications, and other psychotropic or neuroactive medications can impact the timing, degree, and trajectory of an individual baby's NAS course, sometimes significantly exacerbating withdrawal.

Any baby with known (or highly suspected) in utero opiate exposure should be monitored in a newborn or special-care nursery setting where clinicians are trained in standardized symptom-assessment methods. The American Academy of Pediatrics recommends observation, including standardized assessment or scoring of withdrawal symptoms, for 3 days for short-acting opioids and up to 5–7 days for long-acting opioids (Hudak et al., 2012). NAS scoring tools are used to objectively assess signs and symptoms of withdrawal and to determine when an infant meets the threshold for initiation, escalation, and weaning of pharmacological therapies (Sutter et al., 2014). Tools are typically based on presence/absence and severity of specific symptoms in three general categories: central nervous system, autonomic nervous system, and gastrointestinal system. These tools include the commonly used Modified Finnegan Neonatal Abstinence Scoring system, as well as others such as the Lipsitz Neonatal Drug-Withdrawal Scoring System, the Neonatal Withdrawal Inventory, and the Neonatal Narcotic Withdrawal Index (Finnegan, Connaughton, Kron, & Emich, 1975; Grossman, Lipshaw, Osborn, & Berkwitt, 2018; Hudak et al., 2012; Sutter et al., 2014). Institution-specific protocols utilizing standardized assessment tools and quality-assurance practices may enhance internal validity across clinicians and high-quality care of the neonate with NAS; however, concerns exist regarding the complexity of available scoring tools and the subjectivity of their use. Literature indicates the value of simplified, less subjective tools such as the "Eat, Sleep, Console" assessment tool (Grossman et al., 2018). Regardless of which tool a hospital chooses to use, thoughtful protocol development and regular assessor-training targeting high inter-observer reliability are critical.

Treating NAS

Effective treatments for NAS exist; however, all such treatments require accurate diagnosis and careful, repeated assessments. The basis of treatment for active NAS is careful administration of opiates to eliminate or minimize symptoms (Hudak et al., 2012). Once symptoms are controlled, these medications are steadily weaned until the baby no longer requires treatment and is discharged (Wachman, Schiff, et al., 2018). This treatment approach is most successful when there exists a strong partnership between the mother and the healthcare team, including social workers since social evaluation and support are critical components of ongoing care.

Infants experiencing NAS require treatment

Once an infant is diagnosed with NAS based on maternal history, toxicology screening, and symptom severity scoring tools, the next step is treatment which requires a multidisciplinary, multifaceted approach (McQueen & Murphy-Oikonen, 2016). Babies experiencing NAS treated in healthcare systems that developed and used standard treatment protocols were shown to have shorter lengths of stay (Asti, Magers, Keels, Wispe, & McClead, 2015; Loudin et al., 2017; Patrick et al., 2016; Walsh et al., 2018). Management of these infants should be undertaken in a stepwise approach depending on severity of symptoms. The first step in the treatment pathway should be non-pharmacological with escalation to pharmacological intervention only if/when the former does not provide adequate support for the infant (Hudak et al., 2012; Siu & Robinson, 2014; Velez & Jansson, 2008; Wiles, Isemann, Ward, Vinks, & Akinbi, 2014).

Non-pharmacological treatment

Non-pharmacological interventions to treat NAS should start immediately after birth. First, these infants benefit from skin-to-skin time with mother, father, or other caregivers. Skin-to-skin contact helps regulate the infant's external stimulation and autonomic nervous system. Skin-to-skin time has the added benefits of increased maternal/paternal/caregiver-infant dyad bonding and helps aid mothers' breastmilk production (Moore, Bergman, Anderson, & Medley, 2016; Pritham, 2013). Other aspects of the non-pharmacological intervention pathway focus on keeping the infant in a low-stimulation environment with dim lighting and decreased noise stimulation. Initial interventions that decrease the environmental stimulation for the infant improve neurodevelopmental outcomes and minimize the need and duration of pharmacological treatment: measures that reduce environmental and auto-stimulation (e.g. tight swaddling, responding in a timely manner to infant cues regarding hunger and discomfort, and providing positions that comfort the infant, such as swaying or rocking). The best uses of non-pharmacological interventions are dependent on the individual infant's symptoms (Grossman, Seashore, & Holmes, 2017; Hudak et al., 2012; McQueen & Murphy-Oikonen, 2016; Siu & Robinson, 2014; Wiles et al., 2014).

It is also important to encourage parents/family members of infants with NAS to play an active role in their care during the hospitalization period (Howard et al., 2017; McQueen & Murphy-Oikonen, 2016). A non-pharmacological intervention that enables better family involvement is providing parental rooming-in care, where parents are able to hold and re-spond to their infant's cues. It also allows for family education opportunities on how to suc-cessfully and safely provide care and engage in interventions once discharged (Holmes et al., 2016; McQueen, 2018; Wiles et al., 2014). However, due to the increased time required for this initial hospitalization, the decreased ability for some institutions to provide a place for the post-partum discharged mother to stay, and the economic/social burden this can place on families, there are times when parents/family members are not present to hold the infant. Research has shown the benefit of using volunteers to hold NAS patients (Grossman et al., 2017; McQueen & Murphy-Oikonen, 2016).

Engagement with ancillary services is beneficial for maximizing non-pharmacological support. Occupational Therapists (OT), Physical Therapists (PT), and Speech Language Pathologists (SLP) can aid in the feeding of infants with NAS who may have frantic and/or dysregulated suck-swallow-breath patterns (Gewolb, Fishman, Qureshi, & Vice, 2004; LaGasse et al., 2003). These therapists can provide positional support that decreases the infant's auto-stimulation, along with providing developmental support to improve neuro-developmental outcomes (Maguire, Shaffer-Hudkins, Armstrong, & Clark, 2018). Music therapists and massage therapists can provide noise and physical stimulation in a soothing, low-stimulating way (Grossman & Berkwitt, 2019; Maguire, 2014). All of these therapists, along with social workers, can provide education to families in preparation for the transi-tion home.

Nutrition as non-pharmacological therapy

Infants experiencing NAS are at risk for poor growth and failure to thrive due to two differ-ent symptoms. First, some NAS infants have dysregulated feedings and may be very frantic, poor nipple feeders (Gewolb et al., 2004; LaGasse et al., 2003). Second, these infants experi-ence increased energy expenditure, thus increased caloric needs (Hudak et al., 2012; Maguire et al., 2018). Many of these infants need more frequent feeding schedules and often consume larger volumes in a 24-hour period based on weight than infants not exposed to opioids.

It is important to promote breast or breastmilk feeding prior to and following the baby's birth when NAS is anticipated. Contraindications to the use of maternal breastmilk in-clude continued illicit drug use and HIV positivity; however, for mothers in an OMT pro-gram, breastmilk is best. When infants prenatally exposed to opioids receive breastmilk from mothers in OMT programs, their withdrawal symptoms can be lessened by the opioid in the maternal breastmilk. In addition, breastfeeding and/or breastmilk production improves the mother-infant dyad bond. When a mother provides breastmilk for her hospitalized newborn, it allows her to maintain a sense of control in a situation where otherwise she may feel a lack of control and belonging (Dryden, Young, Campbell, & Mactier, 2012; Jansson et al., 2008; McQueen & Murphy-Oikonen, 2016; McQueen, Murphy-Oikonen, Gerlach, & Montelpare, 2011; Pritham, 2013; Wiles et al., 2014).

It is also important for the care team to recognize an infant's feeding symptoms related to withdrawal and provide appropriate feeding modifications on an individualized basis. Some infants with NAS cannot regulate their suck-swallow-breathe pattern to consume adequate nutrition from nipple feeds. In these cases, a feeding tube may be warranted until the withdrawal symptoms decrease to allow effective oral feeding (Grossman & Berkwitt, 2019). On the other end of the spectrum are infants with hyperphagia (increased appetite). It is important to follow the infant's cues, allowing on-demand feeding, to decrease irritability and auto-stimulation due to hunger.

In addition to on-demand feeding, increased calorie feedings are helpful in managing over-stimulation from hunger cues. The increased calories improve the growth trajectory of infants experiencing NAS. Enriched feedings of 22–27 calories/ounce are used by various institutions, with breastmilk and standard infant formulas generally running around 20 calories/ounce (Bogen, Hanusa, Baker, Medoff-Cooper, & Cohlan, 2018). Due to gastrointestinal symptoms of opioid withdrawal, such as vomiting and diarrhea, some institutions provide a low lactose or "sensitive" formula instead of a standard newborn formula; low-lactose formula should be in increased-calorie form to promote healthy growth and minimize failure to thrive risk (McQueen & Murphy-Oikonen, 2016; Walsh et al., 2018).

Pharmacological intervention

After maximizing non-pharmacological interventions, if an infant continues to exhibit signs of significant withdrawal, the next step is pharmacological management while continuing to maximize non-pharmacological interventions (Grossman & Berkwitt, 2019; Walsh et al., 2018). Multiple studies showed that use of an opioid agonist to treat opioid withdrawal is the ideal first-line therapy to treat NAS. Three main opioid agonists are used to treat NAS withdrawal symptoms: morphine, methadone, and buprenorphine (Grossman & Berkwitt, 2019; Hudak et al., 2012; Kocherlakota, 2014; Kraft & van den Anker, 2012; Osborn, Jeffery, & Cole, 2010; Patrick, Kaplan, Passarella, Davis, & Lorch, 2014).

- Morphine currently remains the most commonly used opioid receptor agonist to treat NAS. It is a full *mu*-opioid receptor agonist. Based on the half-life of morphine, dosing interval is every three to four hours. There is the added benefit of ease in titration due to its need for frequent dosing related to the shorter half-life relative to other medications; however, it must be gradually weaned to minimize the recurrence of withdrawal symptoms (Hudak et al., 2012; Kocherlakota, 2014; Raffaeli et al., 2017; Wiles et al., 2014).
- Methadone is the second most common medication used to treat infants with NAS. Like morphine, it is a full *mu*-opioid receptor agonist, but it has a much longer half-life of 25–30 hours. Because of its long half-life, methadone is typically dosed once a day. The longer half-life provides the advantage of more stable levels but has the disadvantage of being harder to titrate (Kocherlakota, 2014; Raffaeli et al., 2017; Wiles et al., 2014). Some institutions use methadone to transition from the inpatient setting to outpatient treatment to complete the weaning process (Wiles et al., 2014).
- Buprenorphine is the newest of the three opioid receptor agonists used in the treatment of NAS. Unlike morphine and methadone, it is a partial *mu*-opioid receptor agonist. This medication is given sublingually (under the tongue). The half-life of buprenorphine is between that of morphine and methadone (Hall et al., 2016; Kraft et al., 2011; Raffaeli et al., 2017). Research in the use of buprenorphine has shown less abuse potential in adults and a decrease in respiratory depression (Kraft et al., 2011; Raffaeli et al., 2017).

Pharmacological management can be divided into three phases: initiation/escalation, weaning, and backslide. The time-frame for moving from one phase to another is dependent on two things: the institution's protocol and the medication used to treat withdrawal symptoms (i.e. morphine, methadone, or buprenorphine). The initiation/escalation phase begins as soon as non-pharmacological measures have failed to adequately control an infant's withdrawal symptoms and continues until symptoms are controlled on a consistent dose. The weaning phase commences once a baby has succeeded on a stable dose of opioid withdrawal treatment for a set amount of time. Discontinuation of medication occurs for some; however, some infants experience worsening of symptoms and require transition in a backslide phase. Backsliding involves escalation of medication doses after a weaning dose failure (Asti et al., 2015; Hall et al., 2015; Kocherlakota, 2014; Kraft & van den Anker, 2012). Progressing to treatment with an opioid agonist and a second medication, usually deemed adjunct therapy, is sometimes required. Clonidine and phenobarbital are both commonly used as adjunct therapies to treat babies with NAS.

Is one opioid agonist superior to the others?

This is an area where most practitioners treating NAS agree that more research is needed, including as related to the length of stay and long-term developmental outcomes. At this time, there is insufficient evidence to conclusively promote the use of one opiate versus another (Hall et al., 2016; Hudak et al., 2012; Kraft et al., 2011; Kraft & van den Anker, 2012; McQueen & Murphy-Oikonen, 2016; Patrick et al., 2014; Raffaeli et al., 2017; Wachman, Schiff, et al., 2018; Wiles et al., 2014). Currently, there are several clinical trials evaluating approaches to treat NAS (for more information, see ClinicalTrials.gov).

Adjunct therapy

At times the use of one medication does not control withdrawal symptoms of NAS or escalation of the opioid receptor agonist used at the institution reaches maximum allowed dose. At these times, use of a second medication is needed to control symptoms. The most commonly used secondary, or adjunct, medications used are clonidine and phenobarbital. Use of an adjunct therapy typically is associated with prolonged hospitalizations.

The overall approach

Another important aspect of the care of infants experiencing NAS and their families is to ensure a non-judgmental atmosphere as the infant's care cannot effectively occur without family involvement (McQueen & Murphy-Oikonen, 2016; Patrick et al., 2016; Smith, Wilson, & Committee on Substance Use and Prevention, 2016; Walsh et al., 2018). Most women using illicit drugs or in an OMT program have experienced substantial trauma in their lives; showing empathy in a non-judgmental way empowers them to actively engage with the team caring for their infants (Liebschutz et al., 2002; McHugo et al., 2005; Najavits, Weiss, & Shaw, 1997; Saia et al., 2016).

Preventing NAS

Pregnancy provides a unique and important opportunity for interaction between healthcare providers to identify, partner with, and treat women with substance use disorders: practices recommended by ACOG. In addition, ACOG practice guidelines emphasize prevention by avoiding opiate administration during pregnancy when possible.

Treating a mother's OUD during pregnancy

Identifying and treating mothers experiencing OUD during the prenatal period is key in optimizing both medical and social health outcomes for the mother-infant dyad. Pregnancy may be one of the few periods that a woman presents for routine healthcare, highlighting the important opportunity for intervention (Reddy et al., 2017). Recognized factors associated with maternal substance misuse during pregnancy include poor prenatal care, previous unexplained fetal demise, placental abruption, unexplained intrauterine growth failure, maternal hypertension, and precipitous labor (Hudak et al., 2012; Sutter et al., 2014). While universal maternal drug testing continues to raise questions of clinical feasibility and ethical acceptability, some institutions have successfully utilized these practices to improve identification of infants at risk for developing NAS (Wexelblatt et al., 2015) and maternal access to prenatal substance abuse treatment.

The standard of medical care for OUD during pregnancy is medication-assisted therapy (MAT) or opioid maintenance treatment (OMT). The most common pharmacotherapies for OUD during pregnancy are methadone and buprenorphine: both are effective at preventing maternal withdrawal symptoms and complications, and both seem to improve the mother's adherence to prenatal care and addiction treatment programs (Jancaitis et al., 2019). ACOG recommends that adequate prenatal and postpartum psychosocial supports are key components of healthcare for these mothers to optimize substance use disorder treatment and prevention of relapse (Committee on Obstetric Practice, 2017).

While medically assisted withdrawal may be considered in specific cases, there is a high rate of relapse, physical stress to the pregnant patient, and concern for fetal stress and unknown harm (Zuspan, 1978). Many neonatal outcomes are positively impacted by initiation of OMT and utilization of prenatal substance abuse programs; both OUD and OMT result in fetal opioid exposure and associated risk of neonatal abstinence syndrome. The difference is that circumstances may be more controlled with OMT exposure. Long-term maternal health remains a central goal of OUD identification and treatment during pregnancy. The long-term implications of OMT and maternal well-being can include improvement in current and future pregnancy outcomes, enhanced management of comorbid maternal physical and psychiatric conditions, decreased infectious disease risk, minimization of complications of OUD, and improved access to social support networks for individual and family health. While it would be intuitively beneficial to wean a pregnant mother from substance use during pregnancy, such attempts increase risks to the mother and the pregnancy. Thus, care teams should engage with pregnant women through opiate maintenance programs during the pregnancy. Once the baby is delivered, attempts can be made to reduce or eliminate substance misuse in partnership with each woman (Committee on Obstetric Practice, 2017).

Roles for social work practice and advocacy

Safe and stable housing is integral to addiction recovery (Mericle, Mahoney, Korcha, Delucchi, & Polcin, 2019). Communities have recognized that for a mother to be effective in the care of her neonate, she must be successful in her own addiction recovery. Safe housing and food stability are associated with improved success in overcoming addiction (Rose-Jacobs et al., 2019).

Pregnant women experiencing OUD should have access to interdisciplinary prenatal substance abuse programs. Ideally, these programs include maternal psychiatric and abstinence support care during and after pregnancy, OMT using methadone or buprenorphine, consistent medical prenatal care, promotion of breastfeeding, and anticipatory support and social planning for care of the mother-infant dyad during the post-partum period (Johnson & Jones, 2018; Reddy et al., 2017). OMT has been associated with improved compliance with prenatal care, higher neonatal birth weights, lower rates of intrauterine growth restriction, and decreased preterm birth, fetal mortality, and neonatal death (Reddy et al., 2017);

additionally, there exists a positive association with likelihood of neonatal discharge home with parents (Reddy et al., 2017).

Treatment for the postpartum mother and infant with NAS should focus on treatment for the mother-infant dyad. Postpartum mothers are often discharged from the hospital prior to the release of their baby who is being monitored for NAS. Infants requiring pharmacological therapy often require an intensive or special-care admission for closer monitoring, leading to prolonged separation of the mother and infant. Several studies have demonstrated that babies have less-severe NAS symptoms and are less likely to require pharmacotherapy when allowed to room-in with mother, and rooming-in allows for more successful bonding and results in greater likelihood that the babies will remain in their mother's custody at the time of discharge (Newman et al., 2015). Howard et al. (2017) observed 86 mother-infant dyads and reported that maximum parental presence (100%) was associated with a nine-day shorter length of stay, and a nine-day reduction in length of treatment. Rooming-in has been associated with higher rates of breastfeeding, reduced pharmacological treatment, and fewer admission to the NICU for infants exposed to opiates in utero (Abrahams et al., 2007). Innovative hospital systems are creating new approaches to allow mothers to remain with their babies to continue providing the optimal non-pharmacological interventions, including breastfeeding, skin-to-skin contact, maternal-infant bonding, and consistent care from the same caregiver.

Programs in some communities offer an opportunity for babies to be discharged on medication in a setting outside of the hospital. These settings are often more "home-like" and welcoming to mothers who are in therapy for their opiate addiction. These centers provide comprehensive support for mothers including therapy, parenting education, life skills education, and social work services to help navigate transition back into the community.

Future directions

While improvements have been made in the care provided to pregnant women using opiates and their neonates experiencing NAS, there are emerging opportunities to optimize care. These opportunities include personalized, tailored treatments based on genetic variations. Personalized, targeted therapies based on specific fetal drug exposure and an understanding of how genetic variations impact opiate pharmacokinetics will likely improve efficiency and potentially shorten pharmacological treatment. There exists increasing evidence that genetics play an important role in the severity and optimal treatment of neonatal abstinence syndrome. Single-nucleotide polymorphisms (SNPs) of the *mu*-opioid receptor (OPRM1) and catechol-o-methyltransferase (COMT genes) in adults are associated with an increased risk for opioid addiction (Sanlorenzo et al., 2018). Newborns with these SNPs likely have a prolonged length of stay for NAS treatment (Wachman et al., 2013). Genetic variations can also impact how the placenta regulates fetal exposure and lead to variable responses of the fetus and neonate to opiate exposure and treatment. Elucidating the influence of genetics on the pharmacodynamics related to fetal exposure and newborn treatment will help us to predict the risk for NAS and individualize treatment for affected newborns (Lewis, Dinh, & Leeder, 2015).

Conclusions

Practitioners should maintain a high index of suspicion to ensure that the diagnosis of prenatal opiate exposure is not missed (Committee on Obstetric Practice, 2017; Kuehn, 2018). Once such a diagnosis is established, it is critical that the health care team work with the mother and ensure that she is provided non-judgmental, empathetic care. A multidisciplinary approach including parental participation is important to prevent short- and long-term problems associated with a maternal history of opiate addiction and an infant with neonatal abstinence syndrome. Social work services should guide caregivers and parents through the optimal discharge scenario in consultation with local children's protective services. It is important not only that the mother is engaged in a maintenance addiction therapy program but also that she has the support systems in place to assure her continued success. These support systems include medical and addiction support prenatally and post-partum, psychological interventions, education in parenting skills, safe and secure housing, and other human services/community resources as needed to support the mother, baby, and family system in the short and long term. Successful treatment of addiction will require a multidisciplinary community commitment. These resources include readily available prenatal care and opiate addiction treatment for women. Pregnant woman experiencing OUD must be supported in their addiction recovery and reassured that they will have the support they need to overcome their addiction and ultimately care for their newborn. Postpartum women should be encouraged to remain in their maintenance addiction programs and engaged with the care of their infant. Ideally, community resources will be available to support engagement of the mother-infant dyad throughout the post-partum period and beyond for safe transition back into the community.

References

Abrahams, R. R., Kelly, S. A., Payne, S., Thiessen, P. N., Mackintosh, J., & Janssen, P. A. (2007). Rooming-in compared with standard care for newborns of mothers using methadone or heroin. *Canadian Family Physician, 53*(10), 1722–1730.

Asti, L., Magers, J. S., Keels, E., Wispe, J., & McClead, R. E., Jr. (2015). A quality improvement project to reduce length of stay for neonatal abstinence syndrome. *Pediatrics, 135*(6), e1494–e1500. doi:10.1542/peds.2014-1269

Bada, H. S., Das, A., Bauer, C. R., Shankaran, S., Lester, B. M., Gard, C. C., . . . Higgins, R. (2005). Low birth weight and preterm births: Etiologic fraction attributable to prenatal drug exposure. *Journal of Perinatology, 25*(10), 631–637. doi:10.1038/sj.jp.7211378

Bernstein, V., Jeremy, R. J., Hans, S. L., & Marcus, J. (1984). A longitudinal study of offspring born to methadone-maintained women. II. Dyadic interaction and infant behavior at 4 months. *American Journal of Drug and Alcohol Abuse, 10*(2), 161–193. doi:10.3109/00952998409002779

Bogen, D. L., Hanusa, B. H., Baker, R., Medoff-Cooper, B., & Cohlan, B. (2018). Randomized clinical trial of standard-versus high-calorie formula for methadone-exposed infants: A feasibility study. *Hospital Pediatrics, 8*(1), 7–14. doi:10.1542/hpeds.2017-0114

Brandt, L., & Finnegan, L. P. (2017). Neonatal abstinence syndrome: Where are we, and where do we go from here? *Current Opinions in Psychiatry, 30*(4), 268–274. doi:10.1097/YCO.0000000000000334

Callaghan, T., Crimmins, J., & Schweitzer, R. D. (2011). Children of substance-using mothers: Child health engagement and child protection outcomes. *Journal of Paediatrics and Child Health, 47*(4), 223–227. doi:10.1111/j.1440-1754.2010.01930.x

Committee on Obstetric Practice. (2017). Committee opinion No. 711: Opioid use and opioid use disorder in pregnancy. *Obstetrics and Gynecology, 130*(2), e81–e94. doi:10.1097/AOG.0000000000002235

Conradt, E., Sheinkopf, S. J., Lester, B. M., Tronick, E., LaGasse, L. L., Shankaran, S., . . . Maternal Lifestyle Study. (2013). Prenatal substance exposure: Neurobiologic organization at 1 month. *Journal of Pediatrics, 163*(4), 989–994. doi:10.1016/j.jpeds.2013.04.033

Corr, T. E., & Hollenbeak, C. S. (2017). The economic burden of neonatal abstinence syndrome in the United States. *Addiction, 112*(9), 1590–1599. doi:10.1111/add.13842

Davies, H., Gilbert, R., Johnson, K., Petersen, I., Nazareth, I., O'Donnell, M., . . . Gonzalez-Izquierdo, A. (2016). Neonatal drug withdrawal syndrome: Cross-country comparison using hospital administrative data in England, the USA, Western Australia and Ontario, Canada. *Archives of Disease in Childhood: Fetal and Neonatal Edition, 101*(1), F26–F30. doi:10.1136/archdischild-2015-308948

Dryden, C., Young, D., Campbell, N., & Mactier, H. (2012). Postnatal weight loss in substitute methadone-exposed infants: Implications for the management of breast feeding. *Archives of Disease in Childhood: Fetal and Neonatal Edition, 97*(3), F214–F216. doi:10.1136/adc.2009.178723

Finnegan, L. P., Connaughton, J. F., Jr., Kron, R. E., & Emich, J. P. (1975). Neonatal abstinence syndrome: Assessment and management. *Addictive Diseases, 2*(1–2), 141–158.

Finnegan, L. P., Kron, R. E., Connaughton, J. F., & Emich, J. P. (1975). Assessment and treatment of abstinence in the infant of the drug-dependent mother. *International Journal of Clinical Pharmacology and Biopharmacy, 12*(1–2), 19–32.

Gewolb, I. H., Fishman, D., Qureshi, M. A., & Vice, F. L. (2004). Coordination of suck-swallow-respiration in infants born to mothers with drug-abuse problems. *Developmental Medicine and Child Neurology, 46*(10), 700–705. doi:10.1111/j.1469-8749.2004.tb00984.x

Grossman, M. & Berkwitt, A. (2019). Neonatal abstinence syndrome. *Seminars in Perinatology.* doi:10.1053/j.semperi.2019.01.007

Grossman, M., Lipshaw, M. J., Osborn, R. R., & Berkwitt, A. K. (2018). A novel approach to assessing infants with neonatal abstinence syndrome. *Hospital Pediatrics, 8*(1), 1–6. doi:10.1542/hpeds.2017-0128

Grossman, M., Seashore, C., & Holmes, A. V. (2017). Neonatal abstinence syndrome management: A review of recent evidence. *Reviews on Recent Clinical Trials, 12*(4), 226–232. doi:10.2174/15748871 12666170816144818

Hall, E. S., Isemann, B. T., Wexelblatt, S. L., Meinzen-Derr, J., Wiles, J. R., Harvey, S., & Akinbi, H. T. (2016). A cohort comparison of buprenorphine versus methadone treatment for neonatal abstinence syndrome. *Journal of Pediatrics, 170*, 39–44. doi:10.1016/j.jpeds.2015.11.039

Hall, E. S., Wexelblatt, S. L., Crowley, M., Grow, J. L., Jasin, L. R., Klebanoff, M. A., . . . Walsh, M. C. (2015). Implementation of a neonatal abstinence syndrome weaning protocol: A multicenter cohort study. *Pediatrics, 136*(4), e803–e810. doi:10.1542/peds.2015-1141

Holmes, A. V., Atwood, E. C., Whalen, B., Beliveau, J., Jarvis, J. D., Matulis, J. C., & Ralston, S. L. (2016). Rooming-in to treat neonatal abstinence syndrome: Improved family-centered care at lower cost. *Pediatrics, 137*(6). doi:10.1542/peds.2015-2929

Howard, M. B., Schiff, D. M., Penwill, N., Si, W., Rai, A., Wolfgang, T., . . . Wachman, E. M. (2017). Impact of Parental Presence at Infants' Bedside on Neonatal Abstinence Syndrome. *Hospital Pediatrics, 7*(2), 63–69. doi:10.1542/hpeds.2016-0147

Hu, S., Sheng, W. S., Lokensgard, J. R., & Peterson, P. K. (2002). Morphine induces apoptosis of human microglia and neurons. *Neuropharmacology, 42*(6), 829–836. doi:10.1016/S0028-3908(02)00030-8

Hudak, M. L., Tan, R. C., Committee on Drugs, Committee on Fetus and Newborn, & American Academy of Pediatrics. (2012). Neonatal drug withdrawal. *Pediatrics, 129*(2), e540–e560. doi:10.1542/peds.2011-3212

Jancaitis, B., Kelpin, S., Masho, S., May, J., Haug, N. A., & Svikis, D. (2019). Factors associated with treatment retention in pregnant women with opioid use disorders prescribed methadone or electing non-pharmacological treatment. *Women and Health*, 1–11. doi:10.1080/03630242.2019.1610829

Jansson, L. M., Choo, R., Velez, M. L., Harrow, C., Schroeder, J. R., Shakleya, D. M., & Huestis, M. A. (2008). Methadone maintenance and breastfeeding in the neonatal period. *Pediatrics, 121*(1), 106–114. doi:10.1542/peds.2007-1182

Johnson, A. J., & Jones, C. W. (2018). Opioid use disorders and pregnancy. *Obstetrics and Gynecology Clinics of North America, 45*(2), 201–216. doi:10.1016/j.ogc.2018.01.008

Ko, J. Y., Patrick, S. W., Tong, V. T., Patel, R., Lind, J. N., & Barfield, W. D. (2016). Incidence of neonatal abstinence syndrome—28 states, 1999–2013. *MMWR: Morbidity and Mortality Weekly Report, 65*(31), 799–802. doi:10.15585/mmwr.mm6531a2

Kocherlakota, P. (2014). Neonatal abstinence syndrome. *Pediatrics, 134*(2), e547–e561. doi:10.1542/peds.2013-3524

Kraft, W. K., Dysart, K., Greenspan, J. S., Gibson, E., Kaltenbach, K., & Ehrlich, M. E. (2011). Revised dose schema of sublingual buprenorphine in the treatment of the neonatal opioid abstinence syndrome. *Addiction, 106*(3), 574–580. doi:10.1111/j.1360-0443.2010.03170.x

Kraft, W. K., & van den Anker, J. N. (2012). Pharmacologic management of the opioid neonatal abstinence syndrome. *Pediatric Clinics of North America, 59*(5), 1147–1165. doi:10.1016/j.pcl.2012.07.006

Krans, E. E., & Patrick, S. W. (2016). Opioid use disorder in pregnancy: Health policy and practice in the midst of an epidemic. *Obstetrics and Gynecology, 128*(1), 4–10. doi:10.1097/AOG.0000000000001446

Kuehn, B. (2018). Opioid use disorder during pregnancy. *JAMA, 320*(12), 1232. doi:10.1001/jama.2018.13546

LaGasse, L. L., Messinger, D., Lester, B. M., Seifer, R., Tronick, E. Z., Bauer, C. R., . . . Liu, J. (2003). Prenatal drug exposure and maternal and infant feeding behaviour. *Archives of Disease in Childhood: Fetal and Neonatal Edition, 88*(5), F391–F399. doi:10.1136/fn.88.5.F391

Lewis, T., Dinh, J., & Leeder, J. S. (2015). Genetic determinants of fetal opiate exposure and risk of neonatal abstinence syndrome: Knowledge deficits and prospects for future research. *Clinical Pharmacology and Therapeutics, 98*(3), 309–320. doi:10.1002/cpt.159

Liebschutz, J., Savetsky, J. B., Saitz, R., Horton, N. J., Lloyd-Travaglini, C., & Samet, J. H. (2002). The relationship between sexual and physical abuse and substance abuse consequences. *Journal of Substance Abuse Treatment, 22*(3), 121–128. doi:10.1016/S0740-5472(02)00220-9

Liu, G., Kong, L., Leslie, D. L., & Corr, T. E. (2019). A longitudinal healthcare use profile of children with a history of neonatal abstinence syndrome. *Journal of Pediatrics, 204*, 111–117. doi:10.1016/j.jpeds.2018.08.032

Loudin, S., Werthammer, J., Prunty, L., Murray, S., Shapiro, J. I., & Davies, T. H. (2017). A management strategy that reduces NICU admissions and decreases charges from the front line of the neonatal abstinence syndrome epidemic. *Journal of Perinatology, 37*(10), 1108–1111. doi:10.1038/jp.2017.101

Maguire, D. (2014). Care of the infant with neonatal abstinence syndrome: Strength of the evidence. *Journal of Perinatal and Neonatal Nursing, 28*(3), 204–211; quiz E203-204. doi:10.1097/JPN.0000000000000042

Maguire, D., Shaffer-Hudkins, E., Armstrong, K., & Clark, L. (2018). Feeding infants with neonatal abstinence syndrome: Finding the sweet spot. *Neonatal Network, 37*(1), 11–18. doi:10.1891/0730-0832.37.1.11

Martins, F., Oppolzer, D., Santos, C., Barroso, M., & Gallardo, E. (2019). Opioid use in pregnant women and neonatal abstinence syndrome—A review of the literature. *Toxics, 7*(1). doi:10.3390/toxics7010009

McHugo, G. J., Caspi, Y., Kammerer, N., Mazelis, R., Jackson, E. W., Russell, L., . . . Kimerling, R. (2005). The assessment of trauma history in women with co-occurring substance abuse and mental disorders and a history of interpersonal violence. *Journal of Behavioral Health Services and Research, 32*(2), 113–127. doi:10.1007/BF02287261

McQueen, K. A. (2018). 'Rooming-in' could be an effective non-pharmacological treatment for infants with neonatal abstinence syndrome. *Evidence-Based Nursing, 21*(4), 110. doi:10.1136/eb-2018-102948

McQueen, K. A., & Murphy-Oikonen, J. (2016). Neonatal abstinence syndrome. *New England Journal of Medicine, 375*(25), 2468–2479. doi:10.1056/NEJMra1600879

McQueen, K., Murphy-Oikonen, J., Gerlach, K., & Montelpare, W. (2011). The impact of infant feeding method on neonatal abstinence scores of methadone-exposed infants. *Advances in Neonatal Care, 11*(4), 282–290. doi:10.1097/ANC.0b013e318225a30c

Merhar, S. L., McAllister, J. M., Wedig-Stevie, K. E., Klein, A. C., Meinzen-Derr, J., & Poindexter, B. B. (2018). Retrospective review of neurodevelopmental outcomes in infants treated for neonatal abstinence syndrome. *Journal of Perinatology, 38*(5), 587–592. doi:10.1038/s41372-018-0088-9

Mericle, A. A., Mahoney, E., Korcha, R., Delucchi, K., & Polcin, D. L. (2019). Sober living house characteristics: A multilevel analyses of factors associated with improved outcomes. *Journal of Substance Abuse Treatment, 98*, 28–38. doi:10.1016/j.jsat.2018.12.004

Moore, E. R., Bergman, N., Anderson, G. C., & Medley, N. (2016). Early skin-to-skin contact for mothers and their healthy newborn infants. *Cochrane Database of Systematic Reviews, 11*, CD003519. doi:10.1002/14651858.CD003519.pub4

Najavits, L. M., Weiss, R. D., & Shaw, S. R. (1997). The link between substance abuse and posttraumatic stress disorder in women—A research review. *American Journal on Addictions, 6*(4), 273–283. doi:10.3109/10550499709005058

Newman, A., Davies, G. A., Dow, K., Holmes, B., Macdonald, J., McKnight, S., & Newton, L. (2015). Rooming-in care for infants of opioid-dependent mothers: Implementation and evaluation at a tertiary care hospital. *Canadian Family Physician, 61*(12), e555–e561.

Osborn, D. A., Jeffery, H. E., & Cole, M. J. (2010). Opiate treatment for opiate withdrawal in newborn infants. *Cochrane Database of Systematic Reviews, 10*, CD002059. doi:10.1002/14651858.CD002059.pub3

Patrick, S. W., Davis, M. M., Lehmann, C. U., & Cooper, W. O. (2015). Increasing incidence and geographic distribution of neonatal abstinence syndrome: United States 2009 to 2012. *Journal of Perinatology, 35*(8), 650–655. doi:10.1038/jp.2015.36

Patrick, S. W., Faherty, L. J., Dick, A. W., Scott, T. A., Dudley, J., & Stein, B. D. (2019). Association among county-level economic factors, clinician supply, metropolitan or rural location, and neonatal abstinence syndrome. *JAMA, 321*(4), 385–393. doi:10.1001/jama.2018.20851

Patrick, S. W., Kaplan, H. C., Passarella, M., Davis, M. M., & Lorch, S. A. (2014). Variation in treatment of neonatal abstinence syndrome in US children's hospitals, 2004–2011. *Journal of Perinatology, 34*(11), 867–872. doi:10.1038/jp.2014.114

Patrick, S. W., Schumacher, R. E., Benneyworth, B. D., Krans, E. E., McAllister, J. M., & Davis, M. M. (2012). Neonatal abstinence syndrome and associated health care expenditures: United States, 2000–2009. *JAMA, 307*(18), 1934–1940. doi:10.1001/jama.2012.3951

Patrick, S. W., Schumacher, R. E., Horbar, J. D., Buus-Frank, M. E., Edwards, E. M., Morrow, K. A., . . . Soll, R. F. (2016). Improving care for neonatal abstinence syndrome. *Pediatrics, 137*(5). doi:10.1542/peds.2015-3835

Peacock, A., Leung, J., Larney, S., Colledge, S., Hickman, M., Rehm, J., . . . Degenhardt, L. (2018). Global statistics on alcohol, tobacco and illicit drug use: 2017 status report. *Addiction, 113*(10), 1905–1926. doi:10.1111/add.14234

Polak, K., Kelpin, S., & Terplan, M. (2019). Screening for substance use in pregnancy and the newborn. *Seminars in Fetal & Neonatal Medicine.* doi:10.1016/j.siny.2019.01.007

Prindle, J. J., Hammond, I., & Putnam-Hornstein, E. (2018). Prenatal substance exposure diagnosed at birth and infant involvement with child protective services. *Child Abuse and Neglect, 76*, 75–83. doi:10.1016/j.chiabu.2017.10.002

Pritham, U. A. (2013). Breastfeeding promotion for management of neonatal abstinence syndrome. *Journal of Obstetric, Gynecologic, and Neonatal Nursing, 42*(5), 517–526. doi:10.1111/1552-6909.12242

Raffaeli, G., Cavallaro, G., Allegaert, K., Wildschut, E. D., Fumagalli, M., Agosti, M., . . . Mosca, F. (2017). Neonatal abstinence syndrome: Update on diagnostic and therapeutic strategies. *Pharmacotherapy, 37*(7), 814–823. doi:10.1002/phar.1954

Reddy, U. M., Davis, J. M., Ren, Z., Greene, M. F., Opioid Use in Pregnancy, N. A. S., & for the Opioid Use in Pregnancy, Neonatal Abstinence Syndrome, and Childhood Outcomes Workshop Invited Speakers. (2017). Opioid use in pregnancy, neonatal abstinence syndrome, and childhood outcomes: Executive summary of a joint workshop by the Eunice Kennedy Shriver national institute of child health and human development, American congress of obstetricians and gynecologists, American academy of pediatrics, society for maternal-fetal medicine, Centers for disease control and prevention, and the March of Dimes Foundation. *Obstetrics and Gynecology, 130*(1), 10–28. doi:10.1097/AOG.0000000000002054

Robinson, S. E., Maher, J. R., Wallace, M. J., & Kunko, P. M. (1997). Perinatal methadone exposure affects dopamine, norepinephrine, and serotonin in the weanling rat. *Neurotoxicology and Teratology, 19*(4), 295–303. doi:10.1016/S0892-0362(97)00018-4

Rose-Jacobs, R., Trevino-Talbot, M., Lloyd-Travaglini, C., Cabral, H. J., Vibbert, M., Saia, K., & Wachman, E. M. (2019). Could prenatal food insecurity influence neonatal abstinence syndrome severity? *Addiction, 114*(2), 337–343. doi:10.1111/add.14458

Rosenthal, E. W., & Baxter, J. K. (2019). Obstetric management of women with opioid use disorder. *Seminars in Perinatology.* doi:10.1053/j.semperi.2019.01.006

Saia, K. A., Schiff, D., Wachman, E. M., Mehta, P., Vilkins, A., Sia, M., . . . Bagley, S. (2016). Caring for pregnant women with opioid use disorder in the USA: Expanding and improving treatment. *Current Obstetrics and Gynecology Reports, 5*, 257–263. doi:10.1007/s13669-016-0168-9

Sanchez, E. S., Bigbee, J. W., Fobbs, W., Robinson, S. E., & Sato-Bigbee, C. (2008). Opioid addiction and pregnancy: Perinatal exposure to buprenorphine affects myelination in the developing brain. *Glia, 56*(9), 1017–1027. doi:10.1002/glia.20675

Sanjanwala, A. R., & Harper, L. M. (2019). Opioid use disorder in pregnancy. *Clinical Obstetrics and Gynecology, 62*(1), 191–207. doi:10.1097/GRF.0000000000000419

Sanlorenzo, L. A., Stark, A. R., & Patrick, S. W. (2018). Neonatal abstinence syndrome: An update. *Current Opinion in Pediatrics, 30*(2), 182–186. doi:10.1097/MOP.0000000000000589

Siu, A., & Robinson, C. A. (2014). Neonatal abstinence syndrome: Essentials for the practitioner. *Journal of Pediatric Pharmacology and Therapeutics, 19*(3), 147–155. doi:10.5863/1551-6776-19.3.147

Smirk, C. L., Bowman, E., Doyle, L. W., & Kamlin, C. O. (2014). How long should infants at risk of drug withdrawal be monitored after birth? *Journal of Paediatrics and Child Health, 50*(5), 352–355. doi:10.1111/jpc.12513

Smith, V. C., Wilson, C. R., & Committee on Substance Use and Prevention. (2016). Families affected by parental substance use. *Pediatrics, 138*(2). doi:10.1542/peds.2016-1575

Sutter, M. B., Leeman, L., & Hsi, A. (2014). Neonatal opioid withdrawal syndrome. *Obstetrics and Gynecology Clinics of North America, 41*(2), 317–334. doi:10.1016/j.ogc.2014.02.010

Towers, C. V., Hyatt, B. W., Visconti, K. C., Chernicky, L., Chattin, K., & Fortner, K. B. (2019). Neonatal head circumference in newborns with neonatal abstinence syndrome. *Pediatrics, 143*(1). doi:10.1542/peds.2018-0541

Uebel, H., Wright, I. M., Burns, L., Hilder, L., Bajuk, B., Breen, C., . . . Oei, J. L. (2015). Reasons for rehospitalization in children who had neonatal abstinence syndrome. *Pediatrics, 136*(4), e811–e820. doi:10.1542/peds.2014-2767

Velez, M., & Jansson, L. M. (2008). The opioid dependent mother and newborn dyad: Non-pharmacologic care. *Journal of Addiction Medicine, 2*(3), 113–120. doi:10.1097/ADM.0b013e31817e6105

Vestal-Laborde, A. A., Eschenroeder, A. C., Bigbee, J. W., Robinson, S. E., & Sato-Bigbee, C. (2014). The opioid system and brain development: Effects of methadone on the oligodendrocyte lineage and the early stages of myelination. *Developmental Neuroscience, 36*(5), 409–421. doi:10.1159/000365074

Wachman, E. M., Grossman, M., Schiff, D. M., Philipp, B. L., Minear, S., Hutton, E., . . . Whalen, B. L. (2018). Quality improvement initiative to improve inpatient outcomes for neonatal abstinence syndrome. *Journal of Perinatology, 38*(8), 1114–1122. doi:10.1038/s41372-018-0109-8

Wachman, E. M., Hayes, M. J., Brown, M. S., Paul, J., Harvey-Wilkes, K., Terrin, N., . . . Davis, J. M. (2013). Association of OPRM1 and COMT single-nucleotide polymorphisms with hospital length of stay and treatment of neonatal abstinence syndrome. *JAMA, 309*(17), 1821–1827. doi:10.1001/jama.2013.3411

Wachman, E. M., Schiff, D. M., & Silverstein, M. (2018). Neonatal abstinence syndrome: Advances in diagnosis and treatment. *JAMA, 319*(13), 1362–1374. doi:10.1001/jama.2018.2640

Walsh, M. C., Crowley, M., Wexelblatt, S., Ford, S., Kuhnell, P., Kaplan, H. C., . . . Ohio Perinatal Quality Collaborative. (2018). Ohio perinatal quality collaborative improves care of neonatal narcotic abstinence syndrome. *Pediatrics, 141*(4), e20170900. doi:10.1542/peds.2017-0900

Wexelblatt, S. L., Ward, L. P., Torok, K., Tisdale, E., Meinzen-Derr, J. K., & Greenberg, J. M. (2015). Universal maternal drug testing in a high-prevalence region of prescription opiate abuse. *Journal of Pediatrics, 166*(3), 582–586. doi:10.1016/j.jpeds.2014.10.004

Wiles, J. R., Isemann, B., Ward, L. P., Vinks, A. A., & Akinbi, H. (2014). Current management of neonatal abstinence syndrome secondary to intrauterine opioid exposure. *Journal of Pediatrics, 165*(3), 440–446. doi:10.1016/j.jpeds.2014.05.010

Zelson, C., Rubio, E., & Wasserman, E. (1971). Neonatal narcotic addiction: 10 year observation. *Pediatrics, 48*(2), 178–189.

Zuspan, F. P. (1978). Drug addiction in pregnancy: An invitational symposium. *Journal of Reproductive Medicine, 20*(6), 301–302.

11

Fetal alcohol spectrum disorder
Evidence, theory, and current insights

Christine Loock, Elizabeth Elliott and Lori Vitale Cox

Background

Fetal Alcohol Spectrum Disorder (FASD) is a pervasive, complex condition, often camouflaged and missed by social service and health professionals. FASD represents a continuum of effects encompassing physical, developmental, emotional, and behavioral consequences resulting from prenatal alcohol exposure (PAE). FASD occurs all over the world, across all ethnic groups, and in every stratum of society, although higher risk groups are identifiable. The functional consequences of FASD are heterogeneous but, regardless of the individual's needs, FASD has impacts across the lifespan.

PAE is common (see Chapter 3), but factors leading to alcohol use during pregnancy are complex and variable. PAE may disrupt the development of vital organs, including the developing brain, and may result in FASD. The risk of developing FASD depends on unpredictable interactions between PAE and other factors, including genetics, epigenetics, and environment (see Chapter 5), but FASD is preventable if the root causes of alcohol use during pregnancy can be mitigated and prenatal alcohol exposure avoided. Through earlier diagnosis and intervention, adopting a strengths-based approach, and being cognizant of the social determinants of health (SDoH), collaborative approaches can mitigate primary effects of FASD and secondary adverse outcomes. Lifelong support is required to assist with navigating physical health, mental health, disability, employment, legal, and family services and accommodating for challenges in adaptive skills, including activities of daily living (ADL), self-care, employment, and housing. In this chapter we define FASD and highlight the role of social workers in prevention, earlier identification, and support of individuals and families to navigate complex systems. This enables individuals with FASD to maximize their potential, lessens secondary adverse outcomes, and supports families and communities in the process. We briefly review the history and prevalence of PAE and FASD, provide recommendations for reframing our professional jargon through use of respectful language, and consider trauma, disability, and culturally informed practices. We describe common (universal) elements of the medical diagnosis of FASD, functional impacts, and secondary adverse outcomes in FASD, and provide recommendations for a collaborative approach to shared care and decision making to improve outcomes.

Key points

Twelve key points related to prenatal alcohol exposure and fetal alcohol spectrum disorder include the following (also see Chapter 3).

- PAE is common and can be harmful to mother and child: "No amount of alcohol consumption can be considered safe during pregnancy" (U.S. Surgeon General 2005 Advisory on Alcohol Use in Pregnancy, https://www.cdc.gov/ncbddd/fasd/documents/surgeon-genbookmark.pdf).
- FASD is a complex, pervasive condition frequently missed by health and social service providers, affecting 5–25% of individuals receiving social work services.
- There exists a higher prevalence of FASD among potentially more vulnerable "subpopulations," including individuals with a history of foster care, adoption, specialized chronic health needs, special education, or involvement with corrections (Popova, Lange, Shield, Burd, & Rehm, 2019).
- Risk for FASD is increased when PAE occurs in high quantity and/or frequency (binge patterns), when alcohol absorption is increased (e.g. through fasting, poor nutrition, low body weight), and when there is concurrent exposure to smoking or other substances (May & Gossage, 2011).
- Not all PAE results in measurable effects or a diagnosis of FASD. Outcomes are unpredictable due to complex interactions between dose and timing of alcohol exposure, other exposures, maternal/fetal genetics, epigenetics, metabolism, placental function, and pre- and post-natal environment (Kobor & Weinberg, 2011; Thomas, Warren, & Hewitt, 2010).
- Individuals with FASD have a pattern of brain function which may affect all aspects of development—physical, intellectual, emotional, and social—and result in early developmental delays, challenging behaviors, and difficulties in learning and adaptive skills (Mattson, Schoenfeld, & Riley, 2001; O'Connor, 2014).
- FASD is primarily a Neurodevelopmental Disorder (ND) and diagnosis requires assessment by a multidisciplinary team (Chudley et al., 2005; IOM, 1996).
- FASD is frequently described as a "prenatally acquired brain injury" and an "invisible disability," as many individuals may not show other physical signs. Persons with FASD are often perceived as *being the problem*, as opposed to being recognized as *having a disability.*
- While recognized as one of the most common causes of developmental disability worldwide, the majority of individuals diagnosed with FASD do not have intellectual impairment (IQ score below 70) and may be excluded from education and disability support services if defined solely by IQ score (Streissguth, Barr, Kogan, & Bookstein, 1996).
- It is never too late to make a FASD diagnosis. The brain is "plastic" and new skills can be learned; however, early intervention may mitigate secondary adverse outcomes and increase developmental potential (Heckman & Masterov, 2007; Thomas, Warren, & Hewitt, 2010).
- Everyone working with individuals in child welfare and juvenile/adult justice systems should collaborate with medical, mental health, and disability services, and adopt policies that acknowledge the effects of PAE and better assist individuals with FASD (ABA, 2012).
- Social workers can play a key role across the lifespan in helping individuals with FASD and their families navigate health and social support services (Badry & Choate, 2015).

What is FASD?

During the three decades after the term Fetal Alcohol Syndrome (FAS) was coined, it became evident that a spectrum of problems may result from PAE. By 2000, the term FASD emerged as an umbrella term to encompass a range of diagnoses and disabilities associated with PAE and in 2005 FASD was incorporated into formal clinical guidelines (Chudley et al., 2005; Streissguth & O'Malley, 2000). The key feature of FASD is brain injury resulting in neurodevelopmental impairment, manifesting as behavioral, learning, developmental, and emotional problems. Facial or other physical anomalies and growth deficiencies are variable. A diagnosis of FASD requires documentation of multiple, pervasive, and significant functional impairments involving several domains of brain function, and measurement and validation through a multidisciplinary assessment.

FASD is clinically heterogenous

FASD does not invariably follow PAE because the FASD phenotype depends on a complex interplay between factors—exposure, timing, dose, and frequency of PAE, maternal and fetal genetics, epigenetics, and maternal stress (Kobor & Weinberg, 2011). Clinical outcomes are modified by post-natal exposures including early childhood trauma and adverse childhood events (ACEs) (Felitti et al., 1998). Even with similar levels of PAE, clinical outcomes among offspring may differ, including greater concordance between identical and non-identical twins (Astley Hemingway et al., 2019; Streissguth & Dehaene, 1993). The timing of PAE in the first trimester is an important determinant for a range of alcohol-related birth defects. The characteristic (sentinel) facial features associated with FASD begin to develop within three weeks after conception, before many women know they are pregnant (Astley & Clarren, 2000; Sulik, Johnston, & Webb, 1981).

Certain groups are at higher risk of FASD including individuals: whose siblings have FASD; with mothers experiencing alcohol misuse disorders; in foster, adoptive, or out-of-home care, including orphanages; living in disadvantaged communities; in contact with the justice system or in juvenile detention; or, with developmental problems of unexplained etiology (Fast, Conry, Loock, 1999; Popova, Lange, Shield et al., 2019). Although universal screening is not indicated, targeted screening for PAE, developmental delay, and sentinel facial features may be indicated for high risk groups (Astley, Stachowiak, Clarren, & Clausen, 2002; Fast et al., 1999).

Defining the spectrum: diagnostic terminology

Several international guidelines have been published to assist in the diagnosis of FASD. All recommend diagnosis by a multidisciplinary team and development of interconnected processes for screening and referral across systems including: primary health, psychology, psychiatry, counseling, social work, allied health, education, and vocational training. From a social work and frontline perspective, the various diagnostic systems are more alike than different. Because there are multiple guidelines, various terms have been used to describe PAE effects (see Table 11.1).

Currently, in the United States, South Africa, and parts of Europe, the term FASD is used as an umbrella term which includes the diagnostic groups of FAS, Partial FAS (pFAS), alcohol-related neurodevelopmental disorder (ARND), and alcohol-related birth defects (ARBD) (Hoyme et al., 2016). ARBD are birth defects that have been associated with PAE

Table 11.1 Terms used internationally to describe FASD and its diagnostic categories

FAS	Fetal Alcohol Syndrome (Jones & Smith, 1973)
FAE	Possible Fetal Alcohol Effects (1980s)—lacked operational criteria (Sokol & Clarren, 1989)
FASD	Fetal Alcohol Spectrum Disorder(s) note: pluralized in US to Disorders (2005–present)
pFAS	Partial Fetal Alcohol Syndrome (partial or atypical, requires some but not all predictive physical findings including facial features) (IOM, 1996)
ARBD	Alcohol-Related Birth Defects (major congenital anomalies vary, and not always present) (Sokol & Clarren, 1989)
ARND	Alcohol-Related Neurodevelopmental Disorder (no physical biomarkers) (Chudley et al., 2005; Hoyme et al., 2016; IOM, 1996)
ND-PAE	Neurodevelopmental Disorder associated with PAE (APA, 2013; Astley, 2004)

in human and animal models and include congenital heart, cranial-facial, renal, neural tube/ spinal, and skeletal defects. In contrast, the Canadian, Australian, New Zealand, and Scottish guidelines use FASD as a diagnostic term, with two diagnostic sub-groups:

- FASD with the three sentinel facial features that are highly predictive of the diagnosis (this equates to FAS) and
- FASD with fewer than three of these facial features (this includes pFAS and ARND).

These guidelines recommend recording alcohol-related birth defects and growth impairment, but do not require them for a diagnosis. The updated Canadian FASD Guidelines address diagnosis across the lifespan. This has led the way for individuals with FASD to become more active in leadership and advocacy for FASD-informed adolescent and adult diagnosis and services (Cook et al., 2015; see Chapter 12).

Global efforts are underway, led by researchers, clinicians, and other stakeholders to adopt a global approach and develop universal FASD diagnostic guidelines that are valid, reliable, flexible, and relevant for all jurisdictions (see Elliott & Loock at https://dentistry-ipce.sites. olt.ubc.ca/files/2019/04/Precon_Loock.pdf). It is beyond the scope of this chapter to review and compare the current international FASD diagnostic systems. For a detailed comparison of current diagnostic systems, refer to the 2015 Canadian Guidelines Supplement Appendix A: examples of the interface with other diagnostic systems (Cook et al., 2015). In the absence of current consensus, we recommend that readers access and use guidelines relevant to their own country.

Epidemiology and costs of FASD and PAE

Rates of FASD vary depending on location, population, and method of ascertainment, but are in line with the prevalence of PAE (see Chapter 3). Recent research indicates that FASD rates within the general population may be much higher than originally estimated. May et al. (2013) identified the five countries with the highest FASD prevalence as South Africa (11.1%), Croatia (5.3%), Ireland (4.8%), Italy (4.5%), and Belarus (3.6%). In a 2018 study of a representative Toronto area school population, rates of FASD were 2–3% (Popova, Lange, Shield et al., 2019). A large study of school-age children in the United States indicated that the conservative prevalence estimate in the United States was 1.1–5.0%, with a weighted prevalence estimate of 3.1–9.9% (or as high as approximately one in ten children) (May et al., 2018).

FASD results in enormous financial costs for the individual, family, and society. The economic impact of FASD has been studied in Canada and the United States. Loss of productivity from illness, disability, and premature mortality was the highest overall contributor to FASD-attributable costs (41%), followed by corrections (29%) and health (10%) system involvement (Popova, Lange, Burd, & Rehm, 2016; Popova, Stade, Bekmuradov, Lange, & Rehm, 2011; Stade et al., 2009). Estimates do not include chronic health and other costs to individuals, their families, and communities, especially when diagnosis and interventions are not available. Because of the higher prevalence of FASD among sub-populations (e.g. 10–40% higher in specialized health and education, foster care, corrections), there may be greater burden of costs across various systems of care, representing a "substantial global health problem" (Popova, Lange, Shield, Burd, & Rehm, 2019).

Prenatal alcohol exposure (PAE)

Most international guidelines recommend abstinence from alcohol for women who are planning pregnancy, pregnant, or breastfeeding (Carson et al., 2010; Chudley et al., 2005; Cook et al., 2015; NHMRC, 2009; Warren, 2015). Despite this advice and the known harms of PAE, alcohol use during pregnancy remains common. Detailed prevalence data from the World Health Organization (WHO) show approximately 10% of pregnancies worldwide are associated with PAE and 25% of pregnant women who drink any alcohol consume four or more drinks on an occasion (see Chapter 3). However, rates vary significantly by geographic region and socio-economic status, with highest rates among women from high-income countries (see Chapter 3). Alcohol use during pregnancy is most prevalent in the WHO European region and lowest in the South-East Asia and Eastern-Mediterranean regions. Significant increases in alcohol use during pregnancy have been observed in South America, Africa, and Asia.

Individual country data indicate that rates of any alcohol use during pregnancy are much higher than 10% in certain sub-populations. Reported prevalence rates of PAE are higher in more isolated or disadvantaged communities, including Indigenous communities in Australia and South Africa (Fitzpatrick et al., 2015; May et al., 2013). PAE is reported in up to 60% of Inuit women in northern Quebec, Canada (Popova, Lange, Poznyak et al., 2019). Similar rates have been reported in urban areas, including Melbourne and Sydney, Australia (McCormack et al., 2017; Muggli et al., 2017).

What contributes to PAE?

Pregnancy is a powerful motivator for women to stop using alcohol; many women abstain or cut down on alcohol use once they know they are pregnant. However, approximately half of all pregnancies in middle- to high-income countries are unplanned, frequently resulting in unintended PAE during the first trimester after conception, before pregnancy recognition. Some clinicians perceive FASD to be primarily a problem for children of women with alcohol use disorders or belonging to sub-populations of marginalized or oppressed groups. However, higher socio-economic status is a strong predictor of PAE, and it is likely that FASD is underdiagnosed in educated, financially secure groups (McCormack et al., 2017; see Chapter 3). Reasons for continued alcohol use during pregnancy are many, including intrinsic and extrinsic factors. Intrinsic factors, such as family history and possible genetic predispositions to alcohol use disorder, are detailed elsewhere (Astley & Clarren, 2000; see Chapters 4, 5, and 6). Extrinsic factors include social determinants of health/

SDoH (e.g. overcrowded housing, unemployment, poor access to education and health care), a history of ACEs, smoking and other substance use, mental health concerns, alcohol use by partners and family members, and exposure to intimate partner or sexual violence (see Chapters 7, 34, and 35). The impact of early-life trauma including child abuse, neglect, and historic trauma (e.g. forced removal from family, displacement from traditional lands, war, and famine) may also be transmitted over generations via "epigenetic" mechanisms (Kobor & Weinberg, 2011).

Reframing the language and jargon of PAE and FASD

Many professionals are reluctant to ask about PAE for fear of stigmatizing women or damaging their relationship with their client; others do not know how to ask, what to advise, or where to refer, indicating the need for building skills and knowledge. The consensus of health professionals is that when possible, the use of the term "prenatal alcohol exposure" is preferable to "maternal alcohol use during pregnancy" because it acknowledges alcohol as the cause of harm to the unborn child. It highlights that women drink alcohol for many reasons and that there is no place for stigma, shame, or blame. In an effort to decrease stigma regarding PAE and promote dignity among individuals with FASD and their families, international meetings held in Vancouver, Canada have challenged assumptions and changed the conversations about FASD by including the voices of parents and lived experiences of adults with FASD (Choate, & Hiemstra, 2017). Recommendations from the "Mapping the Gaps" Report from Manitoba, Canada, include reframing and refocusing our dialog on FASD to avoid ascribing blame, shame, hopelessness, and fatalism (see the FrameWorks Institute's "Seeing the Spectrum: Mapping the Gaps between Expert and Public Understandings of Fetal Alcohol Spectrum Disorder in Manitoba" at http://www.fasdcoalition.ca/wp-content/uploads/2017/09/Seeing-the-Spectrum-May-2017-pdf). This includes shifting from a focus on the individual to a focus on the context, including community factors and values that led to PAE. Core values promoted as solutions include: community interdependence, resourcefulness to create change, pragmatic harm reduction approaches, and healthy public policy to address root causes associated with multiple social determinants. Guidelines to help change public and professional language are under development in several jurisdictions (see the "Language Guide for Promoting Dignity for those impacted by FASD" developed with the Canada Northwest FASD Partnership at http://www.fasdcoalition.ca/wp-content/uploads/2016/10/LAEO-Language-Guide.pdf).

Social determinants, adversity, and FASD

Relevant to social workers, many individuals with FASD have experienced ACEs including early-life trauma, separation, family dysfunction, and substance use at home. Additional adverse SDoH include overcrowding, financial and social poverty, and lack of access to quality health care and education. There is emerging evidence suggesting that FASD results from the interactive effects of PAE and stress hormones (Hellemans, et al., 2010; Kobor & Weinberg, 2011). Some clinicians discuss FASD in the context of "Family Adversity and Stress/System Disorders" because PAE may also be a marker of environmental adversities and physiological stress. A survey of over 200 participants from the 2019 International FASD Conference in Vancouver revealed universal agreement that FASD is associated with historical or continued adverse SDoH (see Elliott & Loock at https://dentistry-ipce.sites.olt.ubc.ca/files/2019/04/Precon_Loock.pdf).

An historical perspective on Fetal Alcohol Syndrome (FAS)

For centuries and in many cultures, at various times, PAE has been described as either harmful or safe (Sullivan, 1899; Warren, 2015). For example, the response to a reader's question about the effects of a father's alcoholism at the time of conception was: "… drunkards come frequently from families with hereditary moronism, and this heredity accounts for the moronism of the drunkard's offspring rather than germ damage from alcohol" (JAMA, 1946, p. 419); presumably this theory extended to the mother, as well. Similarly, belief that the placenta could filter out alcohol and protect the fetus from harm was once promoted, as well (Ritchie, 1975). The harms of PAE were "rediscovered" during the 1960s in France among 127 infants born to "*des parents alcoholiques*" (Lemoine, Harousseau, Borteyru, & Menuet, 1968).

Jones and Smith in Seattle were the first to apply the name FAS to the constellation of characteristic facial features, developmental problems, and growth failure observed among children with high levels of PAE (Jones & Smith, 1973). Alcohol is now well recognized as a teratogen (a substance that may disrupt normal development of the embryo and fetus resulting in physical or birth defects) and neurotoxin (a substance that may interfere with or injure the developing brain and nervous system and cause intellectual and other functional impairment).

How much is too much?

Since the precise lower threshold for PAE effects including FASD is unknown, pregnant women are advised to abstain from all alcohol use if possible (Loock, Conry, Cook, Chudley, & Rosales, 2005). The alcohol guideline used in Canada (Box 1) provides advice to women who are pregnant or planning pregnancy (Guideline 4) similar to that provided elsewhere, including the United Kingdom, United States, and Australia.

Box 1: Canada's low risk drinking guidelines (Butt et al., 2011, pp. 8, 20)

Guideline 1: Recommends <u>no</u> exposure in certain situations including … "working; making important decisions; if pregnant or planning to be; before breastfeeding; while responsible for the care or supervision of others …"

Guideline 4: The safest option during pregnancy or when planning to become pregnant is to not drink alcohol at all. Alcohol in the mother's blood stream can harm the developing fetus. While the risk from light consumption during pregnancy appears very low, there is no threshold of alcohol use in pregnancy that has been definitively proven to be safe.

Screening and referral for PAE and FASD

All women should be asked screening questions regarding their current and past alcohol consumption in a sensitive and culturally appropriate manner. "The public should be informed that alcohol screening and support for women at risk is part of routine women's health care" (Carson et al., 2010). Several screening tools for alcohol use and PAE are sensitive and specific: CRAFFT (Knight, Sherritt, Harris, Gates, & Chang, 2006; Loock et al., 2005) for adolescent women; the modified CAGE (Cut-Down, Annoyed, Guilty, Eye-Opener) questions; T-ACE which adds an alcohol tolerance question (Sokol, Martier, & Ager, 1989); TWEAK which adds a "worried" question for pregnant and nonpregnant women (Chan, Pristach, Welte, & Russell, 1993); and the three-item Alcohol Use Disorders Identification Test—Consumption Questions (AUDIT-C) (Bush, Kivlahan, McDonnell, Fihn, & Bradley, 1998).

Social work roles in screening, early identification and referral

Social workers may be uniquely qualified to screen, intervene, and provide support when working with women of childbearing age or with sub-populations identified as having a higher prevalence of FASD (Kotrla & Martin, 2009; Popova, Lange, Shield et al., 2019). Although social workers are not expected to diagnose FASD, it is important they recognize and understand the predisposing ACEs, SDoH history, and functional neurodevelopmental features requiring further assessment or support, as well as where/how to refer families for these services.

For many individuals with FASD and their families, the social worker plays a key role in translating the components of a FASD diagnosis into a support strategy that avoids stigma and enables the person with FASD to navigate services throughout life. In their various roles (e.g. support for disability and chronic health needs, child welfare, youth outreach, mental health and addiction, adult and family services for housing and food insecurity), social workers may also be the first to identify signs associated with unrecognized PAE or missed FASD, and to make a referral for diagnosis.

Social work screening and referral for FASD

Social work clients should be referred for screening or multidisciplinary assessment for FASD in the following situations:

- Known PAE in the presence of a history of developmental, cognitive, neurobehavioral, or other functional differences. History of growth delay, failure to thrive, or other physical characteristic should be included in the referral if available.
- Siblings or other first-degree relatives with PAE or FASD.
- In the absence of known PAE (e.g. in individuals who have experienced family separation or been placed in foster or adoptive care), facial features would justify referral for assessment. The presence of three sentinel facial features is both sensitive and specific for FASD (Astley et al., 2002).

A non-judgmental approach avoiding stigma and shame is required for discussing a referral for FASD assessment, at all ages and in all settings, for birth, foster, and adopted clients. In addition to PAE, information regarding social adversity, family health, and other risk factors for PAE are essential. It is also important that a referral includes as much information as possible regarding other potential exposures and possible genetic factors to assist with diagnostic accuracy and to consider and exclude other confounding or concurrent conditions.

FASD diagnostic systems: global perspectives

In the 1990s, two major diagnostic systems emerged: the Institute of Medicine (IOM) guidelines (1996) and the University of Washington 4-digit Diagnostic System (Astley & Clarren, 2000). In 2005, the two were harmonized in the Canadian Guidelines, which provided

Table 11.2 Common elements of diagnostic criteria for FASD specified in various guidelines[a]

Element of Diagnostic Criteria	Notes
Prenatal alcohol exposure (PAE)	Some guidelines specify a minimum PAE
Neurodevelopmental impairment	Significant, permanent, pervasive, with multiple domains of dysfunction. Most guidelines define the level and number of domains of impairment required
Sentinel facial features (may or may not be present)	Sentinel features: narrow palpebral fissure, flat/smooth philtrum, thin upper lip
Growth deficiency (may or not be present)	Required in some, not all guidelines for a diagnosis of FAS
Other birth defects (may or not be present)	Should be documented and for some guidelines contribute to a diagnosis of ARBD
Exclusion of other causes of neurodevelopmental impairment	Genetic disorders, exposure to other teratogens
Document co-morbidities	Includes organic diseases, SDoH, ACEs, PTSD, and other pre-existing diagnoses

a Most guidelines recommend use of the University of Washington lip-philtrum guides and facial Dx software (Astley, 2004). Some guidelines recommend use of the four-digit diagnostic code (Astley, 2004). PTSD refers to post-traumatic stress disorder.

the first consensus criteria for diagnosing the full spectrum of neurodevelopmental effects (Chudley et al., 2005). The 2005 Canadian Guidelines were updated to include all ages and have been adapted for use elsewhere including the Commonwealth countries of New Zealand, Australia, and Scotland (Bower & Elliott, 2016; Cook et al., 2015; Rogan, 2010; SIGN, 2019). The common features of the diagnosis of FASD, relevant for all diagnostic systems, are presented in Table 11.2. Other criteria required for the diagnosis in some systems include growth impairment.

Functional neurodevelopmental domains

The criteria for marked or significant neurodevelopmental impairment differ across international FASD guidelines. Several Commonwealth nations have adapted the Canadian Guidelines approach in which significant impairment in at least three of ten specified functional domains is required for a FASD diagnosis. Impairment is defined as a score on a validated assessment tool of two or more standard deviations from the mean (see Table 11.3). In the

Table 11.3 Ten common domains for assessment and possible functional outcomes (Adapted from Cook et al., 2015)

1. Brain structure/neurology	Small head size, low tone, seizures, etc.
2. Motor skills	Clumsy, poor coordination, weak pencil grip
3. Language	Weak receptive and/or expressive language
4. Cognition	Weak cause/effect and quantitative reasoning
5. Academic achievement	Mathematics, reading, & writing disorders
6. Memory	Impaired memory
7. Attention	ADHD, distractible
8. Executive functioning	Poor planning, organization, & making choices
9. Affect (mood) regulation	Anxious, depressed, withdrawn, labile
10. Adaptive function	Poor grooming, self-care, & safety skills

Hoyme guidelines, used by several U.S. teams and internationally, the number of domains of impairment required is not specified and the cut-point for abnormality is 1.5 standard deviations (Hoyme et al., 2016).

The DSM-V and social work roles

The American Psychiatric Association's Diagnostic and Statistical Manual (DSM) approach to the diagnosis and classification of FASD interfaces closely with current social work practice (APA, 2013; Hagan, et al., 2016). Similar to the available diagnostic guidelines, this diagnostic approach requires information on PAE, sentinel physical features, plus a neuro-behavioral constellation of abnormalities in three "Super-Domains" which must manifest during childhood and cause significant impairment or distress:

- *Neurocognitive*—difficulty with thinking and memory (e.g. trouble planning or forgetting material previously learned);
- *Self-regulation*—behavior problems (e.g. severe tantrums, mood issues, and difficulty shifting attention from one task to another); and
- *Adaptive*—Difficulty with day-to-day living (e.g. dressing for the weather, playing with others as a child, or social interactions and understanding social cues as an adult) (Hagan et al., 2016).

This DSM approach may also be useful for pre-screening and earlier referral to multidisciplinary diagnostic teams by social workers and other allied health professionals (see Table 11.4).

The DSM-5 diagnostic category 315.8 also has special significance for mental health and social service professionals supporting youth in juvenile justice systems who have been in care, where access to prenatal/early life history and multidisciplinary diagnosis is often limited. Prior to DSM-5, FASD was often "invisible" to forensic psychologists as it was not recognized nor coded for in their diagnostic manuals and assessments. Inclusion of FASD as ND-PAE in the DSM-5 opens the door for consideration of FASD in the courts.

Table 11.4 DSM-5 criteria for neurodevelopment disorder associated with PAE (APA, 2013; Hagan et al., 2016)

---

1. *Prenatal alcohol exposure (PAE): 'more than minimal'* [where *'more than minimal'* is defined as greater than 13 drinks per month or more than 2 alcoholic drinks in one sitting]
2. Neurodevelopmental Disorder
   - Neurocognitive domain (n = 1): IQ, executive functioning, memory, visual-spatial reasoning skills and their ability to learn
   - Self-regulation domain (n = 1): attention, mood, behavior, impulses
   - Adaptive domain (n=2): communication, daily living skills, motor skills, and social skills
3. Onset in childhood
4. Causes extensive and significant impairment or distress in multiple areas of functioning

If unknown PAE add physical characteristics (biomarkers) e.g.
- Characteristic [Sentinel] Facial features
- Growth Parameters (height, weight, head size)
- Brain imaging (when available in future)

Preventing secondary adverse outcomes through earlier diagnosis

The Streissguth "Secondary Disability" study described multiple adverse challenges and outcomes among adolescents and adults with FASD, including problems with mental health, independent living, and the justice system (Streissguth et al., 1996; see Table 11.5). Many "secondary" effects might be modified by earlier intervention and hence were not considered "primary" impacts or disabilities related to PAE (Streissguth et al., 2004). Newer research suggests that some secondary effects, such as mental health and social communication, may actually be "primary" effects (O'Connor, 2014; O'Connor & Paley, 2009).

Functional needs and supports for FASD

In supporting individuals with FASD, social workers should occupy a key navigating role. Just as diagnosis is multidisciplinary, support for FASD requires both multidisciplinary and intersectoral approaches, often involving health, education, vocational, legal, child welfare, and other community services. Social workers should consider the following important principles:

- early diagnosis is crucial and early intervention results in optimal outcomes (Heckman & Masterov, 2007);
- misdiagnosis can exacerbate problems (Chasnoff, Wells, & King, 2015);
- neurodevelopmental impairments are the key features of FASD—many individuals will not exhibit characteristic facial or other physical signs, and if they do, these may be "unremarkable," making FASD an "invisible disability;"
- significant mental health and behavioral phenomena (e.g. mood and anxiety, impulse control, ADHD, other externalizing behaviors, and suicidality) may also be related to the brain injury in FASD (O'Connor, 2014; O'Connor & Paley, 2009);

Table 11.5 Secondary conditions or outcomes: Prevalence from the longitudinal "secondary disabilities" study of FAS and FAE [FASD] (Streissguth et al., 1996)

Secondary outcomes
Mental health problems: over 90%; may be primary or secondary (O'Connor, 2014)

Onset Age 12 and older
- Disrupted schooling: 60%
- Trouble with the law: 60%
- Confinement: 50% (e.g. inpatient psychiatric/chemical dependency/or incarceration)
- Inappropriate sexual behavior: 50%
- Alcohol and drug problems: 35%

Age 21 and older
- Dependent living: 80%
- Problems with employment: 80%

Protective factors and strengths
- Stable and nurturing home for over 73% of life
- Remaining in each living situation for at least 2.8 years
- Never having experienced violence
- Having basic needs met for at least 13% of life
- Diagnosis of FAS/FAE [FASD] before age 6 years
- Having a diagnosis of full FAS, rather than "FAE" [less visible forms of FASD]
- Being eligible for developmental disability (DD) services (relates to above)

- FASD is over-represented child welfare and legal/justice settings (ABA, 2012; Fast et al., 1999; Lange, Shield, Rehm, & Popova, 2013; TRC, 2015);
- FASD affects individuals in all aspects of life and across the lifespan; many struggle to live and work independently (Streissguth et al., 1996; see Chapter 12);
- FASD is not "genetic," though the root causes of PAE may be intergenerational (Astley & Clarren, 2000; Kobor & Weinberg, 2011);
- approaches to diagnosis and support in racialized and oppressed communities must be culturally appropriate and acceptable to families and communities; and
- persons with FASD require respect, understanding, empathy, advocacy, and sustained support. "FASD means you may have trouble making choices. It doesn't mean you can't succeed" (Barr & Streissguth, personal communication to Loock, 1989).

The indigenous Canadian FASD "two-eyed seeing" medicine wheel

Dr. Lori (Vitale) Cox and the Traditional Healer Noel Milliea, members of the Indigenous community team called the Eastern Door, have developed a diagnostic wheel for FASD and related conditions called the "Two-Eyed Seeing" (TES) Wheel. This tool uses a traditional Medicine Wheel framework for assessment that includes mental, physical, emotional, and social-spiritual domains (see https://canfasd.ca/topics/indigenous/). "Two-Eyed Seeing" is a concept developed by Mi'gmag elders Murdena and Albert Marshall. The elders suggested that when one eye looks with a scientific lens and the other with a traditional lens, there will be more depth in the perspective.

Half of the TES wheel is a template to record the measurements needed for FASD diagnosis using the medically accepted diagnostic criteria of the IOM, Canadian Guidelines, and DSM-5. The other half looks at FASD as a life-time disorder, reflecting other factors that might contribute to how PAE might be expressed in an individual, a family, and a community system. For instance, there is consideration of paternal alcohol use, secondary conditions, residential schooling, and a generational family trauma component extending back three generations. The TES approach to diagnosis within communities encourages clinicians and social workers to consider both nature and nurture, and epigenetic and trans-generational effects when approaching and supporting individuals and families with FASD. This respects the spiritual, physical, emotional, and mental domains while providing a visual representation of key components of global, current FASD diagnostic systems.

Reframing our shared approach for FASD

To optimize care for individuals and families with FASD, we must re-frame our approaches. Social pediatrics is an equity-oriented philosophy and practice that seeks to address social determinants such as income, housing, education, social capital, and environment that are critical mediators of child and youth health (Tyler et al., 2018). Working in the FASD field requires a "RICH" approach—Responsive, Inter-disciplinary/Intersectoral, [individual and family] Centered, Collaborative/Community and Holistic—that extends well beyond pediatrics into adult health and support systems (Loock, Suleman, Lynam, Scott, & Tyler, 2016).

In FASD the primary disability cannot be "cured" but early intervention, diagnosis, and support can change outcomes and mitigate "secondary" conditions. We must adapt our practices and the environment, rather than expect to "change" the individual.

We need to support all parents. Many parents (birth, foster and adoptive) feel ostracized or blamed for "poor parenting" and even blame themselves for adverse secondary outcomes.

Biological parents may need higher levels of support (Mitchell, 2017), with ongoing mental health and substance use problems, higher rates of ACEs, and untreated mental health needs including Post-traumatic Stress Disorder and agoraphobia. Problems are exacerbated by social isolation and living with co-dependent partners who do not support their decreased alcohol use (Astley & Clarren, 2000).

We have a responsibility to change our approach in all social systems to meet the challenges of FASD. This may require professional training, adapting professional practice, reframing our language and jargon, and developing community interventions for prevention and support. It is possible to unknowingly perpetuate structural violence on individuals who do not have access to diagnosis, and whose problem behaviors are viewed as defiant or deviant, as opposed to part of their disability. We must overcome the lack of diagnostic capacity and current misdiagnosis, close the gaps in our systems, and prevent silos (e.g. lack of resources to adapt educational environments, including resorting to suspension and exclusion; and lack of outreach and prevention services).

Social workers may require additional training and specific information on screening for PAE and FASD, referral processes, and local services (Badry & Choate, 2015). Social systems must be responsive and focus on promoting resilience. Resilience should be viewed as both internal and external; however, in FASD it is more about external supports and services than trying to change the underlying neurodevelopmental disorder.

> The science of resilience is clear: The social, political and natural environments in which we live are far more important to our health, fitness, finances and time management than our individual thoughts, feelings or behaviours.
>
> *(Ungar, 2019)*

Healthy public policy applies to FASD

Sir Michael Marmot (2010) recommended the following six policy objectives for reducing health inequalities—they can directly apply to FASD prevention, treatment, and support services, as well:

- give every child the best start in life;
- enable all children young people and adults to maximize their capabilities and have control over their lives;
- create fair employment and good work for all;
- ensure a healthy standard of living for all;
- create and develop healthy and sustainable places and communities; and
- strengthen the role and impact of ill health prevention (e.g. focusing public health interventions such as smoking cessation programs and alcohol reduction on reducing the social gradient).

Conclusions

In this chapter we have highlighted salient messages regarding PAE and FASD for social workers, summarized diagnostic guidelines and identified examples of useful approaches for professionals working with individuals and families with FASD. The term FASD encompasses a wide range of primary and secondary physical, mental, and behavioral effects that may result from PAE. Ideally, the diagnosis and management of FASD requires a multidisciplinary approach. Although most frequently diagnosed in early childhood, FASD is not a "pediatric" disability, but a lifelong condition. As outlined in Chapter 12, it may result in chronic health, mental health, and legal-justice problems which require a cross-sectorial response.

The community social worker, in partnership with primary health care teams and specialists, is well positioned to be a catalyst for referrals for diagnostic assessment and prevention of PAE. The social worker may also play a key role in coordinating clinic services, making connections with education, justice, and other services, and providing resources and referrals for peer-support to improve outcomes and mitigate secondary conditions. "It takes a village" to address FASD. Solutions to inequities in outcomes should include a "social pediatric" perspective, with diagnostic and treatment services linked across sectors for more responsive services and supports (Loock, Suleman, Lynam, Scott, & Tyler, 2016; Tyler et al., 2018). In revisioning our health and social service delivery systems, accessible services must be embedded in "resource-rich, supportive social environments that foster resiliency" (Ungar, 2019). Services must enable access to earlier identification and support services that reduce inequities and maximize human potential (Marmot, 2010).

Every individual with FASD is unique and a multidisciplinary approach can activate relevant systems to develop individualized support plans. Outcomes are influenced, and can be significantly improved, by social and environmental factors. As one young adult with FASD pointed out, we must not assume that the destiny is set for a person with FASD at birth:

> FASD is an origin story; it is not a destination.
>
> *C. J. Lutke (personal communication to Loock, 2019)*

Acknowledgments

The authors wish to acknowledge our clinical, social work, and research colleagues who have contributed to this review, as well as the trust, reciprocity, and knowledge shared by patients and families living with FASD, with special recognition to Ms. Jan Lutke, Ms. Kristina Hiemstra, and the Adult Leadership Committee of FASD Change Makers, for their wisdom, patience, and experience.

References

American Bar Association (ABA). (2012). *FASD resolution and report*. Retrieved from https://www.americanbar.org/groups/public_interest/child_law/resources/attorneys/fasd-resolution/

American Psychiatric Association (APA). (2013). *Diagnostic and statistical manual of mental disorders, version 5 (DSM-5)*. Washington, DC: American Psychiatric Association. doi:10.1176/appi.books.9780890425596

Astley, S. J. (2004). *Diagnostic guide for fetal alcohol spectrum disorders: The 4-digit diagnostic code* (3rd ed.). Seattle: University of Washington Publication Services. Retrieved from http://depts.washington.edu/fasdpnhtmls/4-digit-code.htm

Astley, S. J., & Clarren, S. K. (2000). Diagnosing the full spectrum of fetal alcohol-exposed individuals: Introducing the 4-digit diagnostic code. *Alcohol and Alcoholism, 35*(4), 400–410. doi:10.1093/alcalc/35.4.400

Astley, S. J., Stachowiak, J., Clarren, S. K., & Clausen, C. (2002). Application of the fetal alcohol syndrome facial photographic screening tool in a foster care population. *Journal of Pediatrics, 141*, 712–717. doi:10.1093/alcalc/35.4.400

Astley Hemingway, S. J., Bledsoe, J. M., Davies, J. K., Brooks, A., Jirikowic, T., Olson, E. M., & Thorne, J. C. (2019). Twin study confirms virtually identical prenatal alcohol exposures can lead to markedly different fetal alcohol spectrum disorder outcomes-fetal genetics influences fetal vulnerability. *Advances in Pediatric Research, 5*(23). doi:10.24105/apr.2019.5.23

Badry, D., & Choate, P., (2015). Fetal alcohol spectrum disorder: A disability in need of social work education, knowledge and practice. *Social Work & Social Sciences Review, 17*(3), 20–32.

Bower, C., & Elliott, E. J., on behalf of the Steering Group. (2016). *Australian guide to the diagnosis of Fetal Alcohol Spectrum Disorder (FASD).* Report to the Australian Government Department of Health. Retrieved from https://www.fasdhub.org.au/fasd-information/assessment-and-diagnosis/guide-to-diagnosis/

Bush, K., Kivlahan, D.R., McDonnell, M.B., Fihn, S.D., & Bradley, K.A. (1998). The AUDIT alcohol consumption questions (AUDIT-C): An effective brief screening test for problem drinking. *Archives of Internal Medicine, 158*(16), 1789–1795.

Butt, P., Beirness, D., Gliksman, L., Paradis, C., & Stockwell, T. (2011). *Alcohol and health in Canada: A summary of evidence and guidelines for low-risk drinking.* Ottawa, Canada: Canadian Centre on Substance Abuse.

Carson, G., Cox, L. V., Crane, J., Croteau, P., Graves, L., Kluka, S., . . . Society of Obstetricians and Gynaecologists of Canada. (2010). Alcohol use and pregnancy consensus clinical guidelines. *Journal of Obstetrics and Gynaecology Canada, 32,* S1–S31. doi:10.1016/S1701-2163(16)34633-3

Chan, A.K., Pristach, E.A., Welte, J.W., & Russell, M. (1993). Use of the TWEAK test in screening for alcoholism/heavy drinking in three populations. *Alcoholism: Clinical and Experimental Research, 6,* 1188–1192. doi: 10.1111/j.1530-0277.1993.tb05226.x

Chasnoff, I. J., Wells, A. M., & King, L. (2015). Misdiagnosis and missed diagnoses in foster and adopted children with prenatal alcohol exposure. *Pediatrics, 135*(2), 264–270. doi:10.1542/peds.2014-2171. Epub 2015, January 12.

Choate, P., & Hiemstra, K. (Eds.). (2017). *Let's talk stigma and stereotypes—Where do we begin?* Preconference summary. Paper presented at the 7th International Conference on Fetal Alcohol Spectrum Disorder Research, Results and Relevance. Retrieved from https://www.interprofessional.ubc.ca/files/2018/06/FASD2017_Stigma_and_Stereotypes_Summary.pdf

Chudley, A. E., Conry, J., Cook, J. L., Loock, C., Rosales, T., & LeBlanc, N. (2005). Fetal alcohol spectrum disorder: Canadian guidelines for diagnosis. *Canadian Medical Association Journal, 172*(5 Suppl), S1–S21. doi:10.1503/cmaj.1040302

Cook, J. L., Green, C. R., Lilley, C. M., Anderson, S. M., Baldwin, M. E., Chudley, A. E., . . . Rosales, T. (2015). Fetal alcohol spectrum disorder: A guideline for diagnosis across the lifespan. *Canadian Medical Association Journal, 188*(3), 191–197. doi:10.1503/cmaj.141593

Fast, D. K., Conry, J., & Loock, C. A. (1999). Identifying fetal alcohol syndrome among youth in the criminal justice system. *Journal of Developmental & Behavioral Pediatrics, 20*(5), 370–32.

Felitti, V. J., Anda, R. F., Nordenberg, D., Williamson, D. F., Spitz, A. M., Edwards, V., . . . Marks, J. S. (1998). Relationship of childhood abuse and household dysfunction to many of the leading causes of death in adults. The adverse childhood experiences (ACE) study. *American Journal of Preventive Medicine, 14*(4), 245–258.

Fitzpatrick, J., Latimer, J., Ferreira, M. L., Carter, M., Oscar, J., Martiniuk, A. L., . . . Elliott, E. J. (2015). Prevalence and patterns of alcohol use in pregnancy in remote Western Australian communities: The Lililwan project. *Drug and Alcohol Review, 34*(3), 329–339. doi:10.1111/dar.12232

Hagan, J., Balachova, T., Bertrand, J., Chasnoff, I., Dang, E., Fernandez-Baca, D., . . . on behalf of Neurobehavioral Disorder Associated with Prenatal Alcohol Exposure Workgroup, American Academy of Pediatrics. (2016). Neurobehavioral disorder associated with prenatal alcohol exposure. *Pediatrics, 138*(4), e20151553. doi:10.1542/peds.2015-1553

Heckman, J. J., & Masterov, D. V. (2007). The productivity argument for investing in young children. *Review of Agricultural Economics, 29*(3), 446–493. doi:10.1111/j.1467-9353.2007.00359.x

Hellemans, K. G. C., Silwowkka, J. A., Verma, P., Yoon, V. E., Yu, W., & Weinberg, J. (2010). Prenatal alcohol exposure: Fetal programming and later life vulnerability to stress, depression and anxiety disorders. *Neuroscience & Biobehavioral Reviews, 34,* 791–807. doi:10.1016/j.neubiorev.2009.06.004

Hoyme, H. E., Kalberg, W. O., Elliott, A. J., Blankenship, J., Buckley, D., Marais, A. S., . . . May, P.A. (2016). Updated clinical guidelines for diagnosing fetal alcohol spectrum disorders. *Pediatrics, 138*(2), e20154256. doi: 10.1542/peds.2015-4256.

Institute of Medicine (IOM). (1996). *Fetal alcohol syndrome: Diagnosis, epidemiology, prevention, and treatment.* Washington, DC: National Academy Press.

Jones, K. L., & Smith, D. W. (1973). Recognition of the fetal alcohol syndrome in early infancy. *Lancet, 302*(7836), 999–1001. doi:10.1016/S0140-6736(73)91092-1

Journal of the American Medical Association (JAMA). (1946). Queries and minor notes: Effect of alcoholism at the time of conception. *JAMA, 132*(7), 419. doi:10.1001/jama.1946.02870420059030

Knight, J. R, Sherritt, L., Harris, S. K., Gates, E. C., & Chang, G. (2006). Validity of brief alcohol screening tests among adolescents: A comparison of the AUDIT, POSIT, CAGE, and CRAFFT. *Alcoholism: Clinical and Experimental Research, 27*(1), 67–73. doi:10.1111/j.1530-0277.2003.tb02723.x

Kobor, M. S., & Weinberg, J. (2011). Focus on epigenetics and fetal alcohol spectrum disorders. *Alcohol Research & Health, 34,* 29–37.

Kotrla, K., & Martin, S. (2009). Fetal alcohol spectrum disorders: A social worker's guide for prevention and intervention. *Social Work in Mental Health, 7*(5), 494–507. doi:10.1080/15332980802466565

Lange, S., Shield, K., Rehm, J., & Popova, S. (2013). Prevalence of fetal alcohol spectrum disorders in child care settings: A meta-analysis. *Pediatrics, 132*(4), e980–e995. doi:10.1542/peds.2013-0066

Lemoine, P., Harousseau, H., Borteyru, J. P., & Menuet, J. C. (1968). Les enfants de parents alcooliques: Anomolies observees. A propos de 127 cas. *Ouest Medical, 21,* 476–482.

Loock, C., Conry, J., Cook, J. L., Chudley, A. E., & Rosales, T. (2005). Identifying fetal alcohol spectrum disorder in primary care. *Canadian Medical Association Journal, 172*(5), 628–630. doi:10.1503/cmaj.050135

Loock, C., Suleman, S., Lynam, J., Scott, L., & Tyler, I. (2016). Linking in and linking across using a RICHER model: Social pediatrics and inter professional practices at UBC. *University of British Columbia Medical Journal, 7*(2), 7–9.

Marmot, M. (Chair). (2010). The Marmot review: Fair society, healthy lives. Strategic review of health inequalities in England post-2010. Retrieved from http://www.instituteofhealthequity.org/resources-reports/fair-society-healthy-lives-the-marmot-review/fair-society-healthy-lives-full-report-pdf.pdf

Mattson, S. N., Schoenfeld, A. M., & Riley, E. P. (2001). Teratogenic effects of alcohol on brain and behavior. *Alcohol Research & Health, 25*(3), 185–191.

May, P. A., Blankenship, J., Marais, A. S., Gossage, J. P., Kalberg, W. O., Barnard, R., . . . Buckley, D. (2013). Approaching the prevalence of the full spectrum of fetal alcohol spectrum disorders in a South African population-based study. *Alcoholism, Clinical and Experimental Research, 37*(5), 818–830. doi:10.1111/acer.12033

May, P. A., Chambers, C. D., Kalberg, W. O., Zellner, J., Feldman, H., Buckley, D., . . . Hoyme, H. E. (2018). Prevalence of fetal alcohol spectrum disorders in 4 US communities. *JAMA, 319*(5), 474–482. doi:10.1001/jama.2017.21896

May, P. A., & Gossage, J.P. (2011). Maternal risk factors for fetal alcohol spectrum disorders. *Alcohol Research & Health, 34*(1), 16–23.

McCormack, C., Hutchinson, D., Burns, L., Wilson, J., Elliott, E., Allsop, S., . . . Mattick, R. (2017). Prenatal alcohol consumption between conception and recognition of pregnancy. *Alcohol: Clinical & Experimental Research, 41*(2), 369–378. doi:10.1111/acer.13305.

Mitchell, K. (2017). *Living stigma—How social media anonymity and the words we use sustain stigma.* Presented at The 7th International Conference on Fetal Alcohol Spectrum Disorder Research, Results and Relevance. Retrieved from https://www.interprofessional.ubc.ca/files/2018/06/FASD2017_Stigma_and_Stereotypes_Summary.pdf

Muggli, E., Matthews, H., Penington, A., Claes, P., O'Leary, C., Forster, D., . . . Halliday, J. (2017). Association between prenatal alcohol exposure and craniofacial shape of children at 12 months of age. *JAMA Pediatrics, 171*(8), 771–780. doi:10.1001/jamapediatrics.2017.0778

National Health and Medical Research Council of Australia (NHMRC). (2009). *Australian guidelines to reduce health risks from drinking alcohol.* Commonwealth of Australia: National Health and Medical Research Council. Retrieved from https://alcoholthinkagain.com.au/Portals/0/documents/publications/Resources%20for%20Health%20Professionals/Nhmrc-Guidelines.pdf

O'Connor, M. J. (2014). Mental health outcomes associated with prenatal alcohol exposure: Genetic and environmental factors. *Current Developmental Disorders Reports, 1*(3), 181–188. doi:10.1007/s40474-014-0021-7

O'Connor, M. J., & Paley, B. (2009). Psychiatric conditions associated with prenatal alcohol exposure. *Developmental Disabilities Research Review, 15,* 225–234. doi:10.1002/ddrr.74

Popova, S., Lange, S., Burd, L., & Rehm, J. (2016). The economic burden of fetal alcohol spectrum disorder in Canada in 2013. *Alcohol and Alcoholism, 51*(3), 367–375. doi:10.1093/alcalc/agv117

Popova, S., Lange, S., Poznyak, V., Chudley, A. E., Shield, K., Murray, M., . . . Rehm, J. (2019). Population-based prevalence of fetal alcohol spectrum disorder in Canada. *BMC Public Health, 19,* 845. doi:10.1186/s12889-019-7213-3

Popova, S., Lange, S., Shield, K., Burd, L., & Rehm, J. (2019). Prevalence of fetal alcohol spectrum disorder among special subpopulations: A systematic review and meta-analysis. *Addiction, 114,* 1150–1172. doi:10.1111/add.1459

Popova, S., Stade, B., Bekmuradov, D., Lange, S., & Rehm, J. (2011). What do we know about the economic impact of fetal alcohol spectrum disorder? A systematic literature review. *Alcohol & Alcoholism, 46*(4), 490–497. doi:10.1093/alcalc/agr029

Ritchie, J. M. (1975). The aliphatic alcohols. In L. S. Goodman & A. Gillman (Eds.), *The pharmacological basis of theraputics* (5th ed., p. 142). New York, NY: Macmillan.

Rogan, C. (2010). *Towards multidisciplinary diagnostic service for fetal alcohol spectrum disorder.* Auckland, New Zealand: Alcohol Healthwatch.

Scottish Intercollegiate Guidelines Network (SIGN). (2019). *Children and young people exposed prenatally to alcohol.* Edinburgh, Scotland: SIGN (SIGN Publication No. 156). Retrieved from http://www.sign.ac.uk

Sokol, R. J., & Clarren, S. K. (1989). Guidelines for use of terminology describing the impact of prenatal alcohol on the offspring. *Alcoholism: Clinical and Experimental Research, 13*(4), 597–598. doi:10.1111/j.1530-0277.1989.tb00384.x

Sokol, R. J., Martier, S. S., & Ager, J. W. (1989). The T-ACE questions: Practical prenatal detection of risk-drinking. *American Journal of Obstetrics and Gynecology, 160*, 863–871. doi:10.1016/0002-9378(89)90302-5

Stade, B., Ali, A., Bennett, D., Campbell, D., Johnston, M., Lens, C., . . . Koren, G. (2009). The burden of prenatal exposure to alcohol: Revised measurement of cost. *Canadian Journal of Clinical Pharmacology, 16*(1), e91–e102.

Streissguth, A. P., Barr, H. M., Kogan, J., & Bookstein, F. L. (1996). *Understanding the occurrence of secondary disabilities in clients with fetal alcohol syndrome (FAS) and fetal alcohol effects (FAE).* Final report to the Centers for Disease Control and Prevention. Seattle: University of Washington, Fetal Alcohol and Drug Unit.

Streissguth, A. P., Bookstein, F. L., Barr, H. M., Sampson, P. D, O'Malley, K., & Young, J. K. (2004). Risk factors for adverse life outcomes in fetal alcohol syndrome and fetal alcohol effects. *Journal of Developmental & Behavioral Pediatrics, 25*(4), 228–238. doi:10.1097/00004703-200408000-00002

Streissguth, A. P., & Dehaene, P. (1993). Fetal alcohol syndrome in twins of alcoholic mothers: Concordance of diagnosis and IQ. *American Journal of Medical Genetics, 47*, 857–861. doi:10.1002/ajmg.1320470612

Streissguth, A. P., & O'Malley, K. (2000). Neuropsychiatric implications and long-term consequences of fetal alcohol spectrum disorders. *Seminars in Clinical Neuropsychiatry, 5*(3), 177–90. doi:10.1053/scnp.2000.6729

Sulik, K. K., Johnston, M. C., & Webb, M. A. (1981). Fetal alcohol syndrome: Embryogenesis in a mouse model. *Science, 214*, 936–938. doi:10.1126/science.6795717

Sullivan, W. C. (1899). A note on the influence of maternal inebriety on the offspring. *Journal of Mental Science, 45*(190), 489–503. doi:10.1192/bjp.45.190.489

Thomas, J. D., Warren, K., & Hewitt, B. (2010). Fetal alcohol spectrum disorders from research to policy. *Alcohol Research & Health, 33*(1–2), 118–126.

Truth and Reconciliation Commission of Canada (TRC). (2015). Call to action, No. 33 (FASD). Retrieved from https://www.rcaanc-cirnac.gc.ca/eng/1524502695174/1557513515931

Tyler, I., Lynam, J., O'Campo, P., Manson, H., Lynch, M., Dashti, B., . . . Loock, C. (2018). It takes a village: A realist synthesis of social pediatrics program. *International Journal of Public Health, 64*(5), 691–701. doi:10.1007/s00038-018-1190-7

Ungar, M. (2019, May 25). Put down the self-help book. Resilience is not a DIY endeavour. *The Globe and Mail.* Retrieved from https://www.theglobeandmail.com/opinion/article-put-down-the-self-help-books-resilience-is-not-a-diy-endeavour

Warren, K. (2015). A review of the history of attitudes toward drinking in pregnancy. *Alcoholism: Clinical and Experimental Research, 39*(7), 1110–1117. doi:10.1111/acer.12757

12

The lay of the land

Fetal alcohol spectrum disorder (FASD) as a whole-body diagnosis

Myles Himmelreich, C. J. Lutke and Emily Travis Hargrove

Background

Myles Himmelreich, CJ Lutke, Emily Travis Hargrove, and a group of other adults with Fetal Alcohol Spectrum Disorder (FASD) were dining together at an FASD Conference and started talking about health issues they experienced. As more and more health problems were mentioned, and more and more individuals said, "Oh, I have that!" they began to realize that all of them experienced numerous similar health problems. Myles wrote down the words: "FASD, health issues, body," and they all wondered: "Is there a connection? Is it a coincidence that we all have these problems or is there more to it?" Thus was born the idea of a survey that sought to answer these questions.

Fetal Alcohol Spectrum Disorder (FASD) is an umbrella term describing the broad range of physical, neurobiological, physiological, cognitive, behavioral, adaptive, and functional effects that can occur in an individual prenatally exposed to alcohol. While extensive research since 1973, when FASD was first described, has documented adverse consequences of prenatal alcohol exposure across multiple domains, the majority of studies have involved children (Moore & Riley, 2015). Other than a large body of research utilizing animal models, less is known about long-term consequences of prenatal alcohol exposure as individuals transition into adolescence and adulthood, and even less is known about the immune and health effects. This is a large gap in the FASD field, and the lack of information in these areas has resulted in negative effects on the health and well-being of individuals with FASD. Research is urgently needed to understand the long-term developmental trajectory of individuals with FASD, including associated health risks (Moore & Riley, 2015).

This chapter reports results from an anonymous, community-based health survey developed by Myles, CJ, and Emily, three adults with FASD, to find answers to questions raised during their dinner meeting. This is the first extensive exploration of the broad health issues in adults with FASD, and it is their story to tell in relation to the important findings of the survey, the questions and issues raised, and what they believe is needed to ensure the health and well-being of individuals, particularly adults, with FASD.

In consultation with individuals Myles, CJ, and Emily know, including other adults with FASD and professionals working in the FASD field, they identified 25 areas for investigation and developed more than 260 questions to interrogate these areas. The questions were reviewed for content and presentation bias, and with assistance from professionals in software and programming, the survey was assembled and prepared for online distribution. Myles, CJ, and Emily then reached out again to individuals they know, community-based groups, support groups, social media groups, FASD diagnostic clinics, social service agencies, and others to help distribute the survey broadly within Canada and the U.S. Distribution was facilitated because Myles, CJ, and Emily are known, respected, and trusted within the FASD community. Within six months, they had more than 500 responses; ultimately, 612 individuals completed the survey. Of these, when incomplete surveys and surveys with other issues were removed, responses from 541 people were analyzed. The frequency of the health issues reported among adults with FASD were compared to prevalence rates in the general population reported in reliable sources (including the U.S. Centers for Disease Control and Prevention (CDC), Statistics Canada, National Institutes of Health (NIH), the World Health Organization (WHO), Mayo Clinic, Thyroid Foundation of Canada, Sjögren's Syndrome Foundation, and scientific journals listed in PubMed). Survey results were presented at the Seventh International Conference on Fetal Alcohol Spectrum Disorder Research; this presentation is available at the UBC Interprofessional Continuing Education (IPCE) website: http://interprofessional.ubc.ca/webcasts/fasd2017/

Several caveats are noted by the authors: (1) As their survey questions did not ask about a timeframe for each specific health issue, the responses received likely reflect lifetime frequencies; (2) From the 541 surveys, prevalence cannot be generalized across *all* individuals with FASD since the survey methodology did not involve a random population sample; (3) Where it existed and where it could be important (e.g. high blood pressure), general population data for the 18–44 age group were utilized, as most respondents were in that age range; (4) In a few cases, incidence data are reported for the general population if prevalence data were not available; this must be considered in making comparison for those cases between individuals with FASD (frequency data) and those in the general population; (5) Myles, CJ, and Emily recognize the possibility of some errors in how they calculated or interpreted data from the literature if specific prevalence numbers were not presented in the sources used; (6) For each survey question respondents could reply "Yes," "No," or "Unsure." In calculating frequencies for individuals with FASD, the authors excluded "Unsure" responses (i.e. they did not subtract the number "Unsure" from the total of "Yes plus No);" thus, specific calculations may underestimate actual frequencies.

Overall, the survey results indicate higher frequencies among individuals with FASD of almost every health issue listed, and in many cases, many times higher, than prevalence rates in the general population. This speaks to the need for a broader understanding that FASD involves not only brain, behavior, and mental health issues, but is, as adults with FASD will tell you, a "whole body diagnosis." We hope that the information in this chapter will help to get this message out.

The health survey

Respondent demographics

Respondents ranged in age from ≤16 to greater than 60 years, with the greatest number of individuals in the 16–40-year range, and an average age of 27.5 years (Table 12.1). The sample was reasonably balanced by gender, with 52.8% females and 45.5% males, and including 0.8% "other" and 1.0% "rather not say."

Table 12.1 Respondent demographics

Diagnosis	%
FAS	47.8
pFAS	8.0
ARND	17.4
FAE	9.9
Static encephalopathy PAE	7.9
Other	9.8
Age	
<16	7.6
16–19	20.3
20–30	43.4
31–40	16.3
41–50	5.7
51–59	4.4
>60	2.2

A range of FASD diagnoses was reported by these individuals: 47.8% had been diagnosed with fetal alcohol syndrome (FAS) and 17% with alcohol-related neurodevelopmental disorder (ARND); the remaining ~35% were diagnosed with pFAS (partial FAS, 8.0%), FAE (fetal alcohol effects, 9.9%), static encephalopathy PAE (prenatal alcohol exposure, 7.9%), and Other (9.8%, including FASD, FAS Atypical, and Neurobehavioral Disorder PAE) (Table 12.1). Each respondent provided the name of their diagnosing physician and/or clinic. Individuals were asked about access to health care: 85.8% in Canada (similar to general population statistics of 84.2% [Statistics Canada, 2019]) and 78% in the United States (somewhat lower than general population statistics of 87.6% [National Center for Health Statistics, 2019]) had a family doctor, 18.5% a nurse practitioner, and 82.5% a dentist. Other reported health professionals included: psychiatrist (37.9%), mental health therapist (33.3%), psychologist (24.5%), endocrinologist (6.5%), allergist (6.7%), cardiologist (8.8%), occupational therapist (8.4%), speech therapist (6.3%), and physical therapist (7.7%). These numbers suggest that, despite having access to health care and support services, many adults with FASD still have numerous health problems. However, although acknowledging access to a health professional, it is unclear how often they engaged with each health provider or whether they were correctly assessed/diagnosed.

Specific health issues identified in the survey

Congenital disorders and growth/developmental alterations

Congenital disorders are also known as congenital anomalies, congenital malformations, or birth defects (World Health Organization, 2017) and include structural or functional abnormalities that occur prenatally; these may be identified prior to or at birth or later in life. Congenital disorders can be caused by single gene defects, chromosomal disorders, nutrient deficiencies, or exposure to environmental teratogens, including drugs and alcohol.

In 1996, the Institute of Medicine (IOM) of the National Academy of Sciences published a report detailing results of a study mandated by the U.S. Congress, entitled *Fetal Alcohol Syndrome: Diagnosis, Epidemiology, Prevention, and Treatment* (Stratton, Howe, & Battaglia,1996).

In reviewing and evaluating the diagnostic criteria for FAS and related conditions, the IOM developed five diagnostic categories. Categories 4 and 5, alcohol-related birth defects (ARBD), and alcohol-related neurodevelopmental disorder (ARND) identified physical and behavioral/cognitive (respectively) deficits, resulting from prenatal exposure to alcohol. Of particular relevance, ARBDs included cardiac, skeletal, renal, ocular, and auditory anomalies, malformations, and dysplasias. This category also included "Other," noting that "virtually every malformation has been described in some patient with FAS" (Stratton et al., 1996, p. 77). More recently, O'Leary and colleagues (2011) reported a fourfold increased risk of birth defects classified as ARBDs after heavy prenatal alcohol exposure during the first trimester but no association between low or moderate prenatal alcohol exposure and birth defects.

Survey results related to congenital diseases/disorders involving the heart, musculoskeletal system, dental/oral health, vision, and hearing are discussed below. Here, we present data on congenital, growth and developmental disorders including cleft lip and/or palate, spina bifida, cerebral palsy, autism spectrum disorder (ASD), and alterations in body weight and growth (Tables 12.2 and 12.3). The increased frequency of these problems in adults with FASD compared to the general population prevalence is noteworthy (Cragan et al., 1995; Fryar, Carroll, & Ogden, 2018).

Particular highlights include: a markedly increased frequency of cleft lip or palate, spina bifida, and cerebral palsy; a frequency of ASD 6.6 times higher than in the general population (with this frequency of ASD in individuals with FASD, one might question the frequency of FASD in those diagnosed with ASD); 38.2% of respondents showed growth delay during childhood; and a high occurrence of being underweight as adults.

Table 12.2 Congenital disorders

Disease/Disorder/ Condition	General Prevalence (%)	FASD Frequency (%)	Times Higher
Cleft lip or palate	0.1	2.6	26.0
Cleft palate	0.05–0.06		
Spinal (sacral) dimple	4.8	5.3	1.1
Spina bifida/spina bifida occulta	0.1	1.9	19.0
Cerebral palsy	0.15–0.4	3.4	12.4

Table 12.3 Growth and development alterations

Disease/Disorder/ Condition	General Prevalence (%)	FASD Frequency (%)	Times Higher
Growth delay as child		38.2	
Treated for GH deficiency		1.6	
Low weight (i.e. lose weight easily or can't gain weight)	1.5	14.7–21.5	12.1
Overweight/obese		27.4	
Overweight	31.8		
Obese	40.0		
Severe obesity	8.0		
Autism/Asperger's (ASD)	2.24	14.7	6.6

Immune system and autoimmune disorders

The immune system comprises special organs, tissues, and cells that work together to protect the body from diseases and infections through a variety of mechanisms. Organs and tissues of the immune system include the bone marrow, spleen, thymus, tonsils, mucus membranes, and skin. White blood cells (leukocytes) are immune system cells produced in the bone marrow, maturing there or in the thymus and other lymphoid organs, and normally migrating into various organs to fight infectious agents.

However, sometimes the immune system attacks the body's own organs, tissues, and cells, resulting in an autoimmune disease or disorder. While the causes of many autoimmune diseases remain unknown, a person's genetics in combination with a variety of adverse environmental exposures, including infections, drugs, and toxic agents, likely play a role (Lerner, Jeremias, & Matthias, 2016). Treatments may attenuate symptoms in many of these diseases, but cures do not yet exist.

Immune disorders, diseases, and infections

Immune disorders result when a person's immune system function is disrupted. One might be born with a weakened immune system/reduced immune function due to genetic alterations or to exposure to adverse environmental conditions/agents. Sometimes disease can permanently alter immune function even after recovery from the disease itself. The immune system might also be overactive in response to stimulation, such as occurs in allergic reactions. In this survey, acute and chronic immune system diseases/disorders were reported by as few as 2.0% and as many as 77% of respondents, depending on the condition (Table 12.4).

For almost every disease, disorder, or infection, with the exception of sexually transmitted infections (STIs), frequencies in adults with FASD were higher than prevalence rates in the general population. Notably, the frequent reporting of chronic ear infections in adults with FASD is shockingly high. Acute and chronic ear infections are well-studied in children, with the majority occurring in children under 5–7 year of age (Qureishi, Lee, Belfield, Birchall, & Daniel, 2014). Chronic ear infections have a much lower prevalence among adults and are frequently associated with other underlying diagnoses, such as paranasal sinus disease. Thus, it is possible that adults with FASD who present to their health care providers with chronic ear infections are not evaluated and/or treated appropriately (Qureishi et al., 2014). Other infections reported in the survey include *C. difficile*, scarlet fever, cryptosporidium, constant yeast infections, brain infection, H1N1, rectal abscess, UTI (may overlap with reports of bladder infections), tonsillitis, salmonella, shingles, mononucleosis, parotitis, and cellulitis. Together, these results starkly highlight the understudied effects of prenatal alcohol exposure on immune function and health outcomes.

Autoimmune disorders

The more than 80 known autoimmune diseases have an overall prevalence of approximately 5–8% in the general population (Rose, 2017), while approximately 35% of adults with FASD reported having an autoimmune disorder. Eleven of the most common autoimmune diseases were covered in the survey (Table 12.5). Additional autoimmune disorders reported by respondents are also included in the table. Additionally, one case of Sjögren's syndrome was reported. While Sjögren's syndrome has a prevalence of 1.2% in the general population, most individuals are 40 or older when diagnosed; the respondent who reported Sjögren's

Table 12.4 Immune disorders

Disease/Disorder/Condition	General Prevalence (%)	FASD Frequency (%)	[i]Times Higher
Sinusitis	12.5–14.0		
Chronic	14.0	35.4	2.5
Acute	1.3	60.4	46.5
Ear infections (chronic)	0.25[a]	36.7	*146.8*
Chest infections		41.9	
Chronic bronchitis	3.3–3.6		
Colds/year (all ages)	23.65		
Flu/year (all ages)	36.0		
Allergies	27.3[b]	59.1	2.2
Hay fever	7.7–8.1		
Asthma	7.7–8.3[c]	35.9	*4.7*
Carry EpiPen	0.08–2.4	9.6	7.7
Eczema	10.1–10.7[d]	27.7	*2.7*
Fungal infections		25.2	
Pneumonia	1.62	34.8	21.5
Kidney infections	0.01–0.03[e]	16.6	830.0
Bladder infections	20.0–50.0	41.1	2.1
Influenza B	11.37–13.05[f]	11.1	*1.0*
Strep	3.4[g]	40.2	*11.8*
Staph	0.24–0.41[a]	19.2	*80.0*
Eye infections		54.4	
Bone infections	0.01–0.1[a]	2.0	*200.0*
Skin infections	13.5	29.3	
STDs/STIs	34.48	19.5	
Hepatitis (all)		4.7	
A	0.00044–0.00062[f]		
B	0.0065[f]		
C	0.745[f]		
Difficulty with wound healing		24.6	

Notes
a Incidence (adult).
b 12+ years.
c 13.6% ever had.
d 7.2% (adult).
e Of women.
f Incidence.
g Incidence (non-invasive).
h Incidence (community acquired).
i Italics indicate times higher calculated using FASD frequency and incidence in general population.

syndrome was 23. Furthermore, three relatively rare disorders, scleroderma, Goodpasture's syndrome, and Kawasaki disease, a rare inflammatory disease of blood vessels most commonly occurring in infants and young children of Asian or Pacific Island descent, were also more frequent in adults with FASD than in the general population. Type 1 diabetes and thyroid diseases have an autoimmune component but are discussed under endocrine and metabolic disorders.

Table 12.5 Autoimmune disorders

Disease/Disorder/Condition	General Prevalence (%)	FASD Frequency (%)	[c]Times Higher
Overall autoimmune	5.0–8.0	35	4.1
Rheumatoid arthritis	0.6–1.3	6.6	5.4
Lupus	0.05	0.8	6.9
Sarcoidosis	0.05[a]	0.6	*16.0*
Angioedema	0.5	1.4	12.0
Celiac	0.75–1.0	2.2	2.8
Psoriasis	2.4–3.0	7.4	2.5
Ulcerative colitis	0.3–0.95	2.2	2.7
Crohn's disease	0.14–0.83	2.4	3.5
Fibromyalgia	2.0–3.3	5.9	4.9
Gout	3.76–3.9	3.4	2.2
Kawasaki disease	0.001–0.01	1	0.9
Sjögren's syndrome	1.2	0.3	181.8
Scleroderma	0.024	0.32	0.3
Anti-GBM antibody disease (Goodpasture's syndrome)	0.0001–0.00016[b]	0.16	*13.3*

Notes

General prevalence is based on 80 autoimmune disorders; FASD frequency is based on the 11 autoimmune disorders in the survey.

a   Among Caucasians.

b   Incidence—Prevalence unknown.

c   Italics indicate times higher calculated using FASD frequency and incidence in general population.

Organ systems

Cardiovascular system

The U.S. Centers for Disease Control and Prevention (CDC, 2012) estimated the prevalence for all types of heart disease at ~10.6% for adults 18–75+ (4.0% for ages 18–44 and 11.9% for ages 45–64; prevalence rate increases significantly for adults 65+) (CDC, 2017b). Congenital heart defects (CHD) are common birth defects with highly variable severity (Hoffman & Kaplan, 2002). In the United States, over 35,000 children with CHDs are born each year (a prevalence rate of about 1% of infants with a CHD), and thus, the total is approximately 1 million individuals living with CHD (Habbick, Nanson, Snyder, & Casey, 1997; Hoffman & Kaplan, 2002). A literature review (Burd et al., 2007) investigating the comorbid occurrence of CHD and FASD identified 29 studies that together suggested a co-occurrence rate of 28.6%: several hundred to several thousand cases of CHD each year may be due to prenatal alcohol exposure. In the present survey, 7.6% of adults reported a CHD (Table 12.6). Interestingly, a recent study concluded that significant changes in fetal heart function, particularly alterations in heart blood flow, occurred long before structural changes were observed and suggested that mechanical forces created by the altered blood flow may affect developmental processes and lead to structural abnormalities (Karunamuni et al., 2013).

In addition to congenital heart defects, other heart problems identified in the survey included coronary heart disease, hypertension, valvular heart disease, supraventricular tachycardia, cardiomyopathy, heart murmur, myocarditis, heart failure, and heart attacks; other heart problems occurred less frequently (Table 12.6). In addition, 2.7% of individuals reported having had heart surgery as a child and 0.8% reported having had heart surgery as an adult.

Table 12.6 Cardiovascular system

Disease/Disorder/Condition	General Prevalence (%)	FASD Frequency (%)	Times Higher
Heart disease (all types)	10.6–11.5[a]		
Congenital heart defects (CHD)	0.3–1	7.6	11.7
Coronary heart disease	1.2[b]	1.9	1.6
Hypertension	8.4[b]	16.1	1.9
Valvular heart disease	0.7[b]	2.7	3.9
SVT (supraventricular tachycardia)	2	5.7	2.9
Cardiomyopathy	0.036–0.04	0.8	21.1
Heart murmur	10[a]	21	2.1
Heart failure	20[c]	0.4	0.0
Heart attack	1.0–1.8[d]	2.1	1.5
Heart surgery			
As child	0.25	2.7	10.8
As adult		0.8	

Others
Bundle branch block (×5)
Stents
Mitral valve prolapse
Bradycardia
Pulmonary stenosis
Enlarged heart
Enlarged aorta
Lown–Ganong–Levine syndrome
Wolff-Parkinson-White syndrome

Notes
a   Adult.
b   Ages 18–44.
c   Lifetime risk.
d   Ages 20–59.

Musculoskeletal system

The musculoskeletal system provides form, stability, and movement to the human body. It consists of the bones (skeleton), muscles, and joints, as well as tendons, ligaments, and other connective tissues that support and connect tissues and organs. While musculoskeletal disorders can occur through injury or strain, the focus of this survey was on naturally occurring and congenital diseases or disorders. The number of individuals reporting overall chronic joint problems/symptoms was twice that in the general population, and if stratified by age, is seven times that for 18–44-year-olds, and four times that for 45–64-year-olds. Stiff joints, lack of flexibility, and/or limited mobility of some joints was reported by 49.3% of respondents; conversely, 26.3% of respondents reported hypermobile joints and some had experienced one or more episodes of joint dislocation (Table 12.7). Osteoarthritis, osteoporosis, and osteopenia typically increase with age; most available statistics for osteoporosis and osteopenia are for individuals aged 50+. Nevertheless, these disorders were reported in 13.2%, 3.4%, and 5.7%, respectively, of respondents. The number of more minor bone and joint issues as well

Table 12.7 Bones, muscles, joints

Disease/Disorder/Condition	General Prevalence	FASD Frequency (%)	[i]Times Higher
Osteoarthritis		13.2	3.7[h]
	0.2–2.2%[a]		
	3.6–6.9%[b]		
	9.2%[c]		
Osteoporosis	10%	3.4	0.3
	4%[d]		
	16%[e]		
Osteopenia	48%[f]	5.7	*0.1*
Sciatica	13–5.3%	17.2	1.9
Shin splints		23	
Flat feet	~20.0%[g]	34.9	*1.7*
Plantar fasciitis	8.3–10.0%	14.3	1.6
Congenital hip		5.9	
Adult hip dysplasia	5.0–44%	4.9	0.2
Bone spurs		6.3	
Femoral rotation	0.05%	2.2	44.0
Abnormalities of digits			
Clinodactyly	1.0–19%	25	2.5
Camptodactyly	<1.0%	19.9	19.9
Syndactyly	0.05–0.33%	3.9	20.5
Radioulnar synostosis	350 cases in literature	1	
Scoliosis	2.5%[g]	19.5	*7.8*
Missing vertebrae in neck	Rare	1.2	
Fused vertebrae in neck	0.0025%	2.2	880.0
Odontoid anomaly	Rare	2.2	
Pectus excavatum	0.25–0.1%	6.3	36.0
Pectus carinatum	0.067%	3.1	46.3

Other chronic complaints

Joints always hurt

Joints make noise

Joints lock

Joints swell

Cartilage problems (grinding, "crunching" with movement)

Notes

a   Ages 20–39 (PHAC).

b   Ages 40–49 (PHAC).

c   Adult (CDC).

d   Male.

e   Female.

f   Ages 50+.

g   Adult.

h   Compared to adults 20–49.

i   Italics indicate times higher calculated using FASD frequency and incidence in general population.

Myles Himmelreich et al.

as congenital disorders of the skeleton reported is also significantly higher among adults with
FASD than in the general population. Finally, while the annual incidence for broken bones in
the general population, across all ages, is approximately 2.4%, many respondents to the survey
reported having broken one or more bones and many had experienced multiple breaks.

Dental and oral health

In assessing health status, the mouth is often considered separately from the body (Sheiham,
2005). This compartmentalization can have serious consequences, as oral health is integral
and essential to general health (Petersen, 2003; Sheiham, 2005). Oral health problems affect
other disease processes and general health by causing pain and disfigurement, altering diet
and speech, and generally affecting quality of life. Congenital problems involving the mouth
and teeth similarly adversely affect health, quality of life, and general well-being.

Numerous oral and dental problems were reported by adults with FASD in the present survey (Table 12.8). Although more than a third of respondents reported few or no cavities, half
reported having many cavities. This compares to a 31% prevalence of cavities across the U.S.
population (National Center for Health Statistics, 2017a) and a 35% prevalence across Canada
(Canadian Dental Association, 2017). Congenital/developmental and non-congenital/devel-
opmental bone and joint jaw problems were noted by numerous respondents. A final point of
relevance often overlooked is that many individuals with FASD have increased sensitivity to
stimuli, including oral stimuli, which can adversely impact oral hygiene, including brushing
one's teeth, as well as routine dental care, which often must be done in the hospital, and thus
is often put off or neglected.

Table 12.8 Dental and oral health

Disease/Disorder/Condition	General Prevalence (%)	FASD Frequency (%)	[f]Times Higher
Absence of all natural teeth	6.4	7.6[a]	1.2
		10.7[b]	
Extra adult teeth		13.6	
Fused teeth		3.3	
Hypoplastic enamel	9.8–93[c]	19.3	0.4
	2.2–21.6[d]		
Cavities			
Many	35.0[e]	50.6	*1.4*
Few/none		37.1	
High arched palate		22.0	
Tori (overgrowth of bone in the mouth)	7.0–10.0	4.0	0.5
Had braces	33.0	41.7	1.3
Never had but needed braces	20.0	26.7	1.3

Notes
a Never had baby teeth.
b Never had adult teeth.
c Simple (1 tooth).
d Severe (multiple teeth).
e Ages 25–44.
f Italics indicate times higher calculated using FASD frequency and incidence in general population.

Vision and hearing

Vision and hearing problems can markedly impact quality of life, including ability to hear and understand nuances of conversations, interact socially, navigate new situations, read and write, and carry out normal activities of daily living (Crews & Campbell, 2004). Additionally, sensory problems can exacerbate deficits or problems that occur in FASD, including attention, learning, visual-spatial perception, communication, and social behavior, leading individuals to feel confused and frustrated, and to withdraw and become more isolated. This is of particular relevance to social workers and other professionals engaging with adults who have FASD.

Approximately 10.5–14.3% of adults in North America have vision problems (National Center for Health Statistics, 2017b; Statistics Canada, 2018). Stratified further by age, the prevalence for adults 18–44 is 7.2%, with an increase to 13.1% for adults 45–64. Prevalence of hearing problems for adults in North America is approximately 12–15.5% (National Center for Health Statistics, 2017b; Statistics Canada, 2016); stratified by age, the prevalence is 6.0% for adults 18–44, increasing to 17.2% for adults 45–64. In the present survey, adults with FASD reported a large number of eye and vision problems, generally at a frequency significantly higher than that seen in the general population (Table 12.9). Almost 65% of respondents wear glasses or contact lenses, and 12.4% have had eye surgery. In relation to strabismus (misalignment of the eyes), the frequency of exotropia (eyes rotated outward) is twice that of esotropia (eyes "crossed" inward) in the general population, but that frequency is reversed among individuals with FASD. Fewer hearing/auditory problems than vision problems were reported (Table 12.10). Notably, 14.6% of individuals reported hearing loss that began in childhood and 8.1% reported hearing problems that emerged after age 20. The high frequency of chronic ear infections reported in these adults may have contributed to this level of hearing loss.

Table 12.9 Vision

Disease/Disorder/Condition	General Prevalence (%)	FASD Frequency (%)	[c]Times Higher
Myopia	30	48.2	1.6
Astigmatism	4.7	35.6	7.6
Amblyopia	2.0–3.0	21.6	8.6
Ptosis	0.97	8.8	9.1
Strabismus			
Esotropia	1.2	11.4	9.5
Exotropia	2.1	5.1	2.4
"Jittery" vision when reading (Nystagmus?)		20.8	
Problems with depth perception		30.9	
Wear glasses/contacts	40.0–42.0[a] 60[b]	64.9	*1.6*
Eye surgery		12.4	

Notes
a Ages 20–40.
b Ages 40–50.
c Italics indicate times higher calculated using FASD frequency and incidence in general population.

Table 12.10 Hearing

Disease/Disorder/Condition	General Prevalence (%)	FASD Frequency (%)	Times Higher
Hearing loss (as a child)	0.2–0.3	14.6	58.4
Tubes in ears (as a child)	7.0	22.2	3.2
Hearing problems beginning after age 20		8.1	

Reproductive health

Reproductive health refers to the diseases, disorders, and conditions that affect the functioning of the male and female reproductive systems during all stages of life (National Institute of Environmental Health Sciences, 2019). Disorders of the reproductive system can include altered fertility, impotence, menstrual disorders, prostate disorders, and cancers of the female (ovary, uterus, cervix) and male (prostate, testes) reproductive systems. Also included under reproductive health are issues related to birth and health of a baby, including birth defects/congenital anomalies, developmental disorders, low birth weight, and preterm birth. Exposure to toxic or adverse environmental conditions, such as pollutants, toxic agents, drugs and alcohol, may pose a threat to reproductive health (Sadeu, Hughes, Agarwal, & Foster, 2010).

Survey respondents reported numerous reproductive health issues, including infertility, dysmenorrhea, ovarian cysts/polycystic ovaries, and undescended testicles (Table 12.11). Notably, more than 6% of women reported premature menopause, and while not everyone listed the age at which menopause occurred, for those who did report age, 29 individuals reported that menopause occurred in their teens (n = 10), 20s (n = 8) or 30s (n = 11).

Table 12.11 Reproductive health

Disease/Disorder/Condition	General Prevalence (%)	FASD Frequency (%)	[f]Times Higher
Dysmenorrhea	5.0–59.0+[a]	34.8	*1.1*
Ovarian cysts	20	12.9	*0.6*
Premature menopause	1.0[b]	6.6	*6.6*
	5.0[c]		
Undescended testicles	1.0–2.0	5.2	*3.5*
Infertility	6.0–6.7	4.7	*0.7*
For those who had children			
Recurrent miscarriage	2.0[d]	11.1	*5.6*
	1.0%[e]		
Premature Baby	10.0	9.5	
Breast feeding problems		21.3	
Child with special needs	13.0–15.0	16.4	*1.2*

Notes
a   Wide variance.
b   Ages <40.
c   Ages 41–45.
d   2 miscarriages.
e   3 miscarriages.
f   Italics indicate times higher calculated using FASD frequency and incidence in general population.

These numbers contrast with national statistics that list premature menopause (occurring before age 40 or at 41–45 years) affecting approximately 1% of women (Gold et al., 2013; Okeke, Anyaehie, & Ezenyeaku, 2013). Consequences of premature menopause not only relate to reproduction but put women at risk for premature death, neurological diseases, psychosexual dysfunction, mood disorders, osteoporosis, and ischemic heart disease. Finally, for women with FASD who have had children, problems reported in the survey included recurrent miscarriages, breast feeding problems, premature birth of the baby, and having a child with special needs.

Gastrointestinal/digestive system

The digestive system is made up of the gastrointestinal (GI or digestive) tract, liver, pancreas, and gallbladder; these organs help the body digest or break down food into nutrients, which the body uses for energy, growth, and cell repair. Digestive diseases or conditions can be acute, lasting only a short time, or chronic/long-lasting (Lancaster, 1990; National Institute of Diabetes and Digestive and Kidney Diseases, 2012). GI diseases or disorders can cause symptoms ranging from mild discomfort to severe pain that is constant or intermittent, which can be debilitating and seriously interfering with normal daily life and work. Respondents reported numerous GI problems including stomach ulcers, esophageal reflux (GERD—Gastro Esophageal Reflux Disease), irritable bowel syndrome (IBS), chronic diarrhea or constipation, hernias, and appendicitis (Table 12.12). These were generally more common (in some cases double the prevalence) of that observed in the general population (Choung & Saito, 2014).

Endocrine and metabolic diseases/disorders

Endocrine diseases/disorders involve dysregulation of hormone production (e.g. either over- or under-production), and include changes in thyroid, parathyroid, adrenal, pancreatic, ovarian, and testicular hormone regulation. Metabolic diseases/disorders affect the body's normal metabolism, or the process of converting food to energy at the cellular level or the inability to process certain nutrients. These can include inherited diseases/disorders (also known as inborn errors of metabolism) involving defective genes that result in enzyme deficiencies. Such deficiencies can have serious adverse effects and include diseases/disorders such as phenylketonuria (PKU), homocystinuria, cystic fibrosis, and Tay-Sachs disease. Other metabolic diseases/disorders may have less severe consequences involving organs such as the liver or pancreas, or changes in metabolism of key nutrients (e.g. cholesterol/lipoprotein disorders [changes in levels of low- or high-density lipoproteins]), or changes in carbohydrate

Table 12.12 Gastrointestinal/digestive system

Disease/Disorder/Condition	General Prevalence (%)	FASD Frequency (%)	Times Higher
Stomach ulcers (all types)	1.0–6.2	8.4	2.3
Esophageal reflux (GERD)	20.0	42.1	2.1
Irritable bowel syndrome (IBS)	11.2	20	1.8
Chronic diarrhea	5.0	12.7	2.5
Chronic constipation	2.0–27	26.3	1.8

Table 12.13 Endocrine and metabolic diseases/disorders

Disease/Disorder/Condition	General Prevalence (%)	FASD Frequency (%)	[c]Times Higher
Diabetes Type 1	0.34–0.42[a]	1.9	*5.0*
	0.31–0.49[b]		
Diabetes Type 2	8.5	6.0	0.7
Thyroid disease			
Hypothyroidism (clinically evident)	0.03	5.6	186.7
Hyperthyroidism	0.5	1.3	2.6
Parathyroid disease	0.03–0.7	2.1	5.8
High cholesterol			
Total	12.9	16.5	1.3
LDL	31.7		
Hypoglycemia (not related to diabetes)	0.36	31.4	87.2

Notes
a Ages 20–39.
b Ages 40–59.
c Italics indicate times higher calculated using FASD frequency and incidence in general population.

metabolism (e.g. hyper- or hypoglycemia), among others (Golden, Robinson, Saldanha, Anton, & Ladenson, 2009; Service, Cryer, & Vella, 2019).

Survey respondents reported endocrine and metabolic disorders including both Type 1 and Type 2 diabetes, thyroid and parathyroid disorders, as well as hypoglycemia (non-diabetes related) and changes in cholesterol levels (Table 12.13). Notably, hypothyroidism is 186 times higher in adult respondents with FASD than in the general population. As only clinically evident hypothyroidism was tracked, it is possible that hypothyroidism in this population is even more common. Moreover, the statistic for Type 2 diabetes is a general population statistic across the lifespan. Because the average age of respondents was 27.5 years, a frequency of 6.0% for Type 2 diabetes is a stark indicator of the adverse consequences of FASD on endocrine health.

Sleep disorders

Sleep is a critical part of daily life (National Institute of Neurological Disorders and Stroke, 2019), and quality sleep is essential to health. Sleep affects almost every tissue, system, and process in the body, including the brain, heart, and lungs, as well as metabolism, immune function, mood, and disease resistance. Chronic lack of sleep or poor quality sleep increases the risk of high blood pressure, cardiovascular disease, diabetes, depression, and obesity. Up to 80% of children with FASD exhibit alterations in daytime and nighttime functioning, including sleep problems (Jan et al., 2010)that can include short sleep duration, low sleep efficiency, decreased active sleep, increased sleep fragmentation, night awakenings, sleep disordered breathing, and parasomnias (Troese et al., 2008).

There are complex interactions between sleep and daytime behaviors, and it is possible that at least some disruptive daytime behaviors seen in FASD are related to sleep problems (Ipsiroglu et al., 2019). However, in assessing children with FASD for disruptive daytime behaviors, clinicians often fail to ask about, and caregivers fail to report, sleep problems.

Table 12.14 Sleep disorders

Disease/Disorder/Condition	General Prevalence (%)	FASD Frequency (%)	[c]Times Higher
Narcolepsy	0.025–0.05	0.45	12.0
Problems falling asleep	11.9–22.8	70.0	4.0
Problems staying asleep	17.0–26.9	57.6	2.6
Problems sleeping too much		41.7	
Problems sleeping at night		65.7	
Need to sleep during the day		47.4	
Problems waking up in the morning		57.6	
Tired all the time		34.8	
Sleep apnea	9.0–38.0[a]	15.2	0.6
	6.0–17.0[b]		
Restless leg syndrome	7.0–10.0	18.5	2.2
Night sweats		24.7	
Parasomnias			
Night terrors		2.7	
Sleep walking		1.7	
Sleep talking		17.7	
Nightmares		19.4	
Other			
Incontinence due to sleep			
Heart stops while asleep			

Notes
a ≥5 events/hour.
b ≥15 events/hour.
c Italics indicate times higher calculated using FASD frequency and incidence in general population.

This is an even greater issue among adults with FASD where practitioners may lack a broad understanding of FASD and the complex nature of their behavioral and health problems, which often include sleep problems.

There are virtually no data available concerning sleep and sleep disorders among adults with FASD; results of this survey thus provide important new data for the field. Numerous sleep issues and sleep disorders were reported by respondents, often at rates significantly higher than those in the general population (Table 12.14). Treatments or interventions that address these issues could significantly improve day-to-day functioning among adults with FASD.

Mental health and substance use disorders

Mental health provides the basis for emotions, thinking, communication, learning, resilience, and self-esteem (American Psychiatric Association, 2019). Mental health is also key to relationships, personal and emotional well-being, and the ability to contribute to community or society. Positive mental health allows individuals to function effectively in daily life activities, adapt to changes in the environment and life circumstances, and cope with adversity. Mental illnesses are health conditions involving changes in emotion, thinking,

Table 12.15 Mental health disorders

Disease/Disorder/Condition	General Prevalence (%)	FASD Frequency (%)	*d*Times Higher
Dementia (early onset)	0.00–0.0086[a]	0.9	209.3
Mood disorder (any)	8.6–9.7	52.6	5.7
Depression (including MDD)	7.6	67.4	8.9
Anxiety or agitation	19.1[b]	88.4	4.6
Panic disorder	2.7	46.2	17.1
ADHD/ADD	4.4	79.7	18.1
Schizophrenia	0.25–1.1	3.1	4.6
Bipolar disorder	2.8	17	6.1
Agoraphobia	0.9	16.6	18.4
Personality disorder	9.1	16.5	1.8
Oppositional defiant disorder	9.7	27.3	2.8
OCD	1.2	4.4	3.7
Psychosis	0.749[c]	7.9	10.5
Suicide			
Attempted	0.6	29.7	49.5
Suicidal thoughts	4.3		

Notes
a Ages 25–64.
b Any anxiety disorder among U.S. adults.
c Median lifetime risk.
d Italics indicate times higher calculated using FASD frequency and incidence in general population.

behavior, or a combination of these (American Psychiatric Association, 2019), and are often associated with distress and/or impaired ability to function and participate in typical daily life activities. Mental illnesses are not uncommon: as many as 19% of adults in any given year may experience some form of mental illness, and 8.5% may develop a substance use disorder (American Psychiatric Association, 2019). While mental illnesses often can be treated effectively, stigma or discrimination is sometimes attached to mental illness, compounding the stigma individuals with FASD already often face (Bell et al., 2016). Stigma can present a significant barrier to diagnosis and treatment and can adversely impact acceptance by the community as well as health policy and practices (Bell et al., 2016; Canadian Mental Health Association, 2019).

Mental health issues are commonly reported in individuals with FASD (Pei, Denys, Hughes, & Rasmussen, 2011). The results of the present survey support and extend these findings, demonstrating a wide range of mental health disorders (Table 12.15). Particularly noteworthy are the high frequencies of anxiety or agitation (88.4%), panic attacks (46.2%), ADHD/ADD (79.7%), and oppositional defiant disorder (27.3%). A heartbreaking statistic is that 29.7% of respondents had attempted suicide. Other reported mental health issues included: reactive attachment disorder, PTSD, delusional disorder, social anxiety disorder, disruptive mood dysregulation, self-harming, and eating disorders. Of note, four individuals (0.9%) in their 50s or younger reported early-onset dementia, which is medically defined as <64 years (Vieira 2013).

Substance use was also reported at a high level, with a third or more of respondents using alcohol, drugs, or both, as well as cigarettes or marijuana (Table 12.16).

Table 12.16 Substance use disorders

Disease/Disorder/Condition	General Prevalence (%)	FASD Frequency (%)	Times Higher
Alcohol or drugs		37.1	
Alcohol	8.5–25.1		
Drugs	2.0		
Both	1.1		
Cigarettes	14.0–19.4	37.8	2.3
Marijuana	9.5[a]	31.5	3.3
	2.9[b]		

Notes

a Use.

b Substance use disorder (SUD).

Other diseases, disorders, conditions Cancer

In this survey, 18 individuals or 3.75% of respondents reported having had some form of cancer: five during childhood (<18 years), nine at 18–44 years, and four at 45–55 years. According to the CDC (2017a), the overall cancer prevalence rate for adults is 9.4%; stratified by age, it is 2.0% among 18–44-year-olds and 9.9% for those aged 45–64. As the majority of respondents who reported cancer were under 44 years of age, the frequency among these individuals was almost twice the prevalence in the general population. Types of cancer included: cervical, Hodgkin's lymphoma, liver, malignant melanoma, prostate, skin, thyroid, and embryonal rhabdomyosarcoma (see Table 12.17).

Migraine headaches

In this survey, 32.8% of individuals reported having migraines, compared to 11.7–16.2% of adults in the general population (Smitherman, Burch, Sheikh, & Loder, 2013); see Table 12.17.

Seizures

Epilepsy affects approximately 3.4 million Americans (~1.0% of the population); in Canada, the figure is 0.36–0.44% (Gilmour, Ramage-Morin, & Wong, 2016). In addition, the lifetime risk of experiencing a seizure is about 4.0%, although not all will develop epilepsy. Among survey respondents, 20.1% reported having experienced seizures. In addition, 18.9% reported having auditory or visual hallucinations (not due to mental illness).

These are of unknown origin, but could possibly be auras related to seizures or neurological disturbances. Seizures due to alcohol poisoning and alcohol withdrawal also were reported (Table 12.17).

Hernias

Abdominal wall hernias are fairly common (Jenkins & O'Dwyer, 2008; Velasco, García-Urena, Hidalgo, Vega, & Carnero, 1999). Prevalence of umbilical hernias in the adult population is approximately 2%. Hiatal hernias most frequently develop among persons over 50 years of age and have an overall prevalence of 15%; by age 60, up to 60% of people have them to some degree (Cleveland Clinic, n.d.; Yale Medicine, n.d.). Approximately 3.0–5.0%

Table 12.17 Other diseases/disorders/conditions

Disease/Disorder/Condition	General Prevalence (%)	FASD Prevalence (%)	Times Higher
Cancer	9.4[a]	3.75	0.4
Ages 18–44	2.0		1.9
Ages 45–64	9.9		
Migraine headaches	11.7–16.2	32.8	2.4
Seizures (lifetime risk)	4.0	20.1	5.0
Hernias		3.0–5.0	
Umbilical	2.0	5.0	2.5
Hiatal	15.0	3.0	0.2
Inguinal		4.5	
Appendicitis	13.0[b]	45.5	4.3
	10.8[c]		
	7.8[d]		
Tourette syndrome	0.3–0.6	4.4	
Kidney disease	2.1	10.1	4.8

Others
Ehlers Danloss syndrome
Fetal Dilantin syndrome
Reiter's syndrome
Neurofibromatosis (×2)
Thalassemia
Prader Willi syndrome
Thalidomide syndrome
Central core myopathy
Balance translocation chromosomes 2 & 3
Caroli syndrome
Noonan's syndrome
Hemophilia
Klinefelter syndrome
Williams syndrome
Turner's syndrome
Cyclic neutropenia
Duane syndrome
Short Gut syndrome
Proteus syndrome
Several chromosomal anomalies, unspecified

Notes
a   Overall.
b   Ages 20–29.
c   Ages 30–39.
d   Ages 40–49.

of respondents to this survey reported having hernias: 5.0% had umbilical hernias, 4.5% had inguinal hernias, and 3% had hiatal hernias. The occurrence of hiatal hernias in adults with FASD is likely an underestimate as these are often associated with GERD which was reported by more than 42% of respondents (Table 12.17).

Appendicitis

Lifetime risk for appendicitis/appendectomy is 6.7% among women and 8.6% among men (Addiss, Shaffer, Fowler, & Tauxe, 1990). National U.S. estimates of acute appendicitis from 2005 to 2008 was 13% among 20–29-year-olds, 10.8% among 30–39-year-olds, and 7.8% among 40–49-year-olds (Buckius et al., 2012). By contrast, 45.5% of survey respondents (mean age of 27.5) reported appendicitis (Table 12.17).

Tourette syndrome

Tourette syndrome is a neurological disorder characterized by repetitive, stereotyped, involuntary movements, and/or vocalizations called tics (CDC, 2018; National Institute of Neurological Disorders and Stroke, 2012). The exact prevalence of Tourette Syndrome is unknown but estimates suggest a prevalence rate of 0.3–0.6% (CDC, 2018). In this survey, 4.4% of respondents reported having Tourette Syndrome. In addition, some individuals reported transient tics (Table 12.17).

Kidney disease

The CDC estimates a prevalence of 2.1% of adults with diagnosed kidney disease. By contrast, 10.1% of respondents to this survey reported kidney problems/defects, including cysts and stones (Table 12.17).

Pain, touch, taste, and other sensory issues

While not directly health issues, individuals with FASD typically have numerous sensory issues that affect them in their daily lives, and importantly, can interfere with their receiving appropriate health care. For example, pain perception often is altered; in this survey, 53.1% of respondents reported having high pain tolerance and 33.6% reported having low pain tolerance. Such alterations significantly impact both diagnosis and treatment; individuals may not report or even be fully aware of illnesses or injuries, resulting in missed or delayed diagnoses. Where children are concerned, lack of reporting might incur suspicion of abuse or neglect and referral to family services, an issue of particular concern for social workers. Furthermore, tools typically used by physicians and other health professionals to assess pain, such as pain scales, may be ineffective in assessing individuals with FASD. In addition to alterations in pain perception, numerous other sensory issues were reported (Table 12.18). Changes in the sense of taste and smell and abnormal hunger sensations could have detrimental effects on nutrition and subsequently on health. Sensitivity to touch or texture could lead to avoidance of medical care by individuals uncomfortable with being touched, especially by relative strangers.

Table 12.18 Other sensory issues

Disease/Disorder/Condition	General Prevalence	FASD Frequency (%)
Do not feel pain the way others do—High pain tolerance for major things		53.1
Feel more pain than others do even for minor things		33.6
Don't like tags, wrinkles, socks, etc.		74.8
Clothes need to be very tight		16.1

(Continued)

Disease/Disorder/Condition	General Prevalence	FASD Frequency (%)
Clothes need to very loose		46.0
Don't like loud noise (hyperacusis)		63.4
Cannot tolerate bright light		57.5
Difficulty feeling temperature (hot or cold) like others do		54.1
Difficulty regulating temperature (go from too hot to too cold quickly and often)		49.9
No sense of smell		10.1
Disordered sense of smell (things smell different than to others (dysosmia)		28.3
Poor or no sense of taste for many foods (hypoaguesa or aguesa)		10.9
Do not like texture of some/many foods		58.2
Really like spicy hot foods (can taste)		39.1
Like to eat lemons		33.1
Do not feel hunger much		36.6
Skin is very sensitive to stimuli		52.2
Skin itself (not muscles) hurts with use		16.3
Easily overwhelmed (panicky) by crowds, large groups (noise, light, movement, touch)		75.7
Over-reactive to some body sensations and under-reactive to others		68.6

Table 12.19 Executive function issues

Disease/Disorder/Condition	General Prevalence	FASD Frequency (%)
Problems with short-term memory		81.5
Problems with long-term memory		67.5
Difficulty with math or numbers		82.8
Difficulty with calculation		80.0
Difficulty with estimation		82.8
Problems paying attention		90.2
Problems managing money		87.4
Problems making decisions		85.8
Difficulty with judgment		82.8
Difficulty following directions (esp. verbal)		85.2
Problems with time management		81.5
Difficulty understanding what is said to you		71.5
Difficulty reading		48.1
Difficulty understanding what you read		69.0
Dyslexia		13.9

Executive function issues

Issues with executive function can have serious adverse effects on normal activities of daily living and adversely impact health. More than 70% (and as high as 90%) of respondents reported deficits in one or more domains of executive function (Table 12.19). The authors and their colleagues reported serious difficulty concentrating, remembering, and making decisions, as well as independently completing errands (e.g. shopping or visiting a doctor's office) because of physical, mental, or emotional conditions. Executive function is typically evaluated in individuals with FASD. What is often not on the radar, however, are possible adverse spillover effects of deficits in executive function that may interfere with seeking and/ or receiving appropriate health care, which, in turn, may have serious impacts on health outcomes in individuals with FASD.

Conclusions

The findings of the health survey dramatically highlight the significant adverse effects of pre-natal alcohol exposure on long-term vulnerability to diseases or disorders over the life course, above and beyond what has traditionally been described in the literature. Indeed, there could be no more powerful illustration than the present findings of the fact that FASD is not a disorder involving only the brain and behavior but rather is a "whole body" disorder. The survey re-vealed that over a wide range of health conditions, diseases, and disorders, the frequency among respondents with FASD was significantly higher than prevalence rates in the general population, and health issues arose at a much younger age than is typical for adults in the general population. For the authors and other adults with FASD, as well as for professionals in the field who work closely with these individuals, the survey results were not surprising. Yet professionals in a vari-ety of areas who treat or provide services for adults appear to be largely unaware of the physical and mental health problems encountered by adults with FASD. Thus, these problems are often ignored, overlooked, or denied, and individuals may be written off as difficult, noncompliant, whiners, and complainers. Moreover, our health care and human service delivery systems may be ill-equipped to detect and address these prematurely emerging problems.

The survey findings speak to the fact that health (including mental health) issues experi-enced by adults with FASD are real and common, and they provide a heads-up for profes-sionals to listen to both children and adults with FASD and take their complaints seriously. Health care providers need to critically examine diagnostic and laboratory test results, even if numbers are in the normal range, asking whether they are really normal for someone with FASD. Health care providers should also investigate gut symptoms, endocrine function, metabolic disturbances, bone and joint symptoms, complaints of hot flashes, cognitive distur-bances, pain, and more as real events, so that individuals can be treated early on and disease progression can be preempted. Parents and caregivers need to be alert and observant of even small changes in well-being and function of adults with FASD and ensure that they seek care as soon as possible. Social workers engaged in providing family support need to help educate and advocate for these processes.

These survey results are particularly salient to social workers who provide services and support to adults who have FASD. Many adults with FASD, despite leading active and pro-ductive lives, may not be able to assume fully independent lives, including health care respon-sibility. They may not recognize the onset of a health issue, may not feel pain or discomfort in the same way as typically developing adults, and may not have the wherewithal to schedule and organize a provider visit. Similarly, individuals with FASD may need assistance in read-ing prescription labels and understanding how and when to take their medications as well as any indicated restrictions to their activities. Finally, the survey results highlight the fact that health issues appear to occur regardless of early-life environmental conditions: the number and extent of health problems did not differ in those who experienced early-life adversity compared to those who had consistent and supportive early-life environments.

Another issue for social workers and other professionals to consider involves secondary disabilities, defined as "deficits that are not evident at birth but may result from the interaction between primary disabilities (i.e. neuropsychological damage) and the environment" (Pei et al., 2011, p. 439). These can include "mental health disorders, addictions, trouble with the law, difficulty in finding and maintaining stable housing, and problems with employment" (Streissguth, Barr, Kogan, & Bookstein, 1996, p. 30). Current evidence suggests that such mental health, adaptive, and behavioral problems may have, at least in part, a primary origin. As discussed by Pei and colleagues (2011), conceptualization of mental health disorders in FASD (and, in our view, in cognitive, adaptive, and behavioral function as well) is changing to encompass an "integrated, multifactorial model, incorporating several overlapping and related factors including environment, brain impact due to prenatal alcohol exposure, and genetics" (p. 445). It is more and more accepted that "nature" and "nurture" are inextricably intertwined and interact to influence outcomes. That FASD is a whole-body diagnosis is the manifestation of the integrated, multifactorial factors that shape the development of individuals prenatally exposed to alcohol.

We end this chapter with words and thoughts expressed by adults with FASD who developed and participated in the Health Survey. The profound nature of the questions and issues the authors and hundreds of respondents raised is testament to their comprehension, self-awareness, knowledge, and resilience.

1   What do we want to know?
   • Do our bodies age and break down faster?
   • How many disorders are diagnosed as mental health issues when they actually have a physical cause and may be something else?
   • What else is going on and what can be treated?
   • How are our chronically high stress levels related to our health?
   • How can we prevent or minimize health effects?
   • What is the role of chronic inflammation or inflammatory responses in our overall health problems, and how can these be treated?

2   What do we think we need?
   • Access to funded adult diagnosis as a medical "right"
   • Development of health care guidelines for those with FASD across the lifespan
   • Health care services specific to those with FASD—need to develop expertise in health care (would help to lower costs with early and assertive treatment)
   • Development of supported health care and health decision making
   • Recognition of whole-body diagnosis with less emphasis on behavior and mental health as all that is important

Research into health outcomes and issues of individuals with FASD is urgently needed to broaden the conversation and provide a fuller picture of FASD: it is not just a brain, behavior, or mental health issue, but it is a "whole body diagnosis." Research is also needed to provide insights into possible mechanisms underlying these adverse health outcomes and provide a basis for developing targeted interventions and treatments for individuals with FASD. Furthermore, we need to work hard to get these messages out to everyone who provides services or health care for individuals with FASD and advocate for systems change.

Acknowledgments

The authors would like to acknowledge the outstanding assistance, guidance and support of Jan Lutke throughout the process of developing, administering, and analyzing the survey; without her participation, this survey would not have happened. They also acknowledge Michelle Sherbuck for her help in the IT aspects of the project, formatting the survey for the online platform and analyzing the survey results. Thanks also to Parker Holman for expert editing of the chapter and preparing the tables and figure. Finally, they wish to thank Dr. Christine Loock, Dr. Edward Riley, and Dr. Joanne Weinberg for their advice and support on this survey.

References

Addiss, D. G., Shaffer, N., Fowler, B. S., & Tauxe, R. V. (1990). The epidemiology of appendicitis and appendectomy in the United States. *American Journal of Epidemiology, 132*(5), 910–925. doi:10.1093/oxfordjournals.aje.a115734

American Psychiatric Association. (2019). What is mental illness? Retrieved from https://www.psychiatry.org/patients-families/what-is-mental-illness

Bell, E., Andrew, G., Di Pietro, N., Chudley, A. E., N. Reynolds, J., & Racine, E. (2016). It's a Shame! Stigma against fetal alcohol spectrum disorder: Examining the ethical implications for public health practices and policies. *Public Health Ethics, 9*(1), 65–77. doi:10.1093/phe/phv012

Buckius, M. T., McGrath, B., Monk, J., Grim, R., Bell, T., & Ahuja, V. (2012). Changing epidemiology of acute appendicitis in the United States: Study period 1993–2008. *Journal of Surgical Research, 175*(2), 185–190. doi:10.1016/j.jss.2011.07.017

Burd, L., Deal, E., Rios, R., Adickes, E., Wynne, J., & Klug, M. G. (2007). Congenital heart defects and fetal alcohol spectrum disorders. *Congenital Heart Disease, 2*(4), 250–255. doi:10.1111/j.1747-0803.2007.00105.x

Canadian Dental Association. (2017). Oral health: A global perspective. Retrieved June 19, 2019, from The State of Oral Health in Canada website: https://www.cda-adc.ca/stateoforalhealth/global/

Canadian Mental Health Association. (2019). Addressing stigma. Retrieved from https://www.camh.ca/en/driving-change/addressing-stigma

Centers for Disease Control and Prevention. (2012). National health interview survey 2009–2012. Retrieved from Public-use data file and documentation website: https://www.cdc.gov/nationalcenterforhealthstatistics/nationalhealthinterviewsurvey2009-2012/

Centers for Disease Control and Prevention. (2017a). Cancer. Retrieved from National Center for Health Statistics website: https://www.cdc.gov/nchs/fastats/cancer.htm

Centers for Disease Control and Prevention. (2017b). QuickStats: Percentage of adults aged ≥18 years with any hearing loss, ★ by state—National health interview survey, 2014–2016. *MMWR. Morbidity and Mortality Weekly Report, 66*(50), 1389. doi:10.15585/mmwr.mm6650a7

Centers for Disease Control and Prevention. (2018). Tourette syndrome. Retrieved from https://www.cdc.gov/ncbddd/tourette/facts.html

Choung, R. S., & Saito, Y. A. (2014). Epidemiology of irritable bowel syndrome. *GI Epidemiology: Diseases and Clinical Methodology: Second Edition, 6*, 222–234. doi:10.1002/9781118727072.ch20

Cleveland Clinic. (n.d.). Hernia. Retrieved from https://my.clevelandclinic.org/health/diseases/15757-hernia

Cragan, J. D., Roberts, H. E., Edmonds, L. D., Khoury, M. J., Kirby, R. S., Shaw, G. M., . . . Dean, J. H. (1995). Surveillance for anencephaly and spina bifida and the impact of prenatal diagnosis—United States, 1985–1994. *MMWR. CDC Surveillance Summaries : Morbidity and Mortality Weekly Report. CDC Surveillance Summaries, 44*(4), 1–13. Retrieved from http://www.ncbi.nlm.nih.gov/pubmed/7637675

Crews, J. E., & Campbell, V. A. (2004). Vision impairment and hearing loss among community-dwelling older Americans: Implications for health and functioning. *American Journal of Public Health, 94*(5), 823–829. doi:10.2105/ajph.94.5.823

Fryar, C. D., Carroll, M. D., & Ogden, C. L. (2018). *Prevalence of overweight, obesity, and severe obesity among adults aged 20 and over: United States, 1960–1962 through 2015–2016.* Retrieved from https://stacks.cdc.gov/view/cdc/58670

Gilmour, H., Ramage-Morin, P., & Wong, S. L. (2016). Epilepsy in Canada: Prevalence and impact. *Health Reports, 27*(9), 24–30. Retrieved from https://www.statcan.gc.ca

Gold, E. B., Crawford, S. L., Avis, N. E., Crandall, C. J., Matthews, K. A., Waetjen, L. E., . . . Harlow, S. D. (2013). Factors related to age at natural menopause: Longitudinal analyses from SWAN. *American Journal of Epidemiology, 178*(1), 70–83. doi:10.1093/aje/kws421

Golden, S. H., Robinson, K. A., Saldanha, I., Anton, B., & Ladenson, P. W. (2009). Prevalence and incidence of endocrine and metabolic disorders in the United States: A comprehensive review. *Journal of Clinical Endocrinology and Metabolism, 94*(6), 1853–1878. doi:10.1210/jc.2008-2291

Habbick, B. F., Nanson, J. L., Snyder, R. E., & Casey, R. E. (1997). Mortality in foetal alcohol syndrome. *Canadian Journal of Public Health, 88*(3), 181–183. doi:10.1007/bf03403884

Hoffman, J. I. E., & Kaplan, S. (2002). The incidence of congenital heart disease. *Journal of the American College of Cardiology, 39*(12), 1890–1900. Retrieved from http://www.ncbi.nlm.nih.gov/pubmed/12084585; https://doi.org/10.1016/S0735-1097(02)01886-7

Ipsiroglu, O. S., Wind, K., Hung, Y. H. (Amy), Berger, M., Chan, F., Yu, W., . . . Weinberg, J. (2019). Prenatal alcohol exposure and sleep-wake behaviors: Exploratory and naturalistic observations in the clinical setting and in an animal model. *Sleep Medicine, 54*, 101–112. doi:10.1016/j.sleep.2018.10.006

Jan, J. E., Asante, K. O., Conry, J. L., Fast, D. K., Bax, M. C. O., Ipsiroglu, O. S., . . . Wasdell, M. B. (2010). Sleep health issues for children with FASD: Clinical considerations. *International Journal of Pediatrics, 2010*, 1–7. doi:10.1155/2010/639048

Jenkins, J. T., & O'Dwyer, P. J. (2008). Inguinal hernias. *BMJ (Clinical Research Edition), 336*(7638), 269–272. doi:10.1136/bmj.39450.428275.AD

Karunamuni, G., Gu, S., Doughman, Y. Q., Peterson, L. M., Mai, K., McHale, Q., . . .Watanabe, M. (2013). Ethanol exposure alters early cardiac function in the looping heart: A mechanism for congenital heart defects? *American Journal of Physiology-Heart and Circulatory Physiology, 306*(3), H414–H421. doi:10.1152/ajpheart.00600.2013

Lancaster, H. O. (1990). Digestive diseases. In H. O. Lancaster (Ed.), *Expectations of life.* , New York, NY: Springer. doi:10.1007/978-1-4612-1003-0_27

Lerner, A., Jeremias, P., & Matthias, T. (2016). The world incidence and prevalence of autoimmune diseases is increasing. *International Journal of Celiac Disease, 3*(4), 151–155. doi:10.12691/ijcd-3-4-8

Moore, E. M., & Riley, E. P. (2015). What happens when children with fetal alcohol spectrum disorders become adults? *Current Developmental Disorders Reports, 2*(3), 219–227. doi:10.1007/s40474-015-0053-7

National Center for Health Statistics. (2017a). FastStats—Oral and dental health. Retrieved from Table 60 website: https://www.cdc.gov/nchs/fastats/dental.htm

National Center for Health Statistics. (2017b). *Table A-6. Hearing trouble, vision trouble, and absence of teeth among adults aged 18 and over, by selected characteristics: United States, 2017.* Retrieved from https://www.cdc.gov/nchs/data/series/sr

National Center for Health Statistics. (2019). FastStats—Access to health care. Retrieved June 7, 2019, from Centers for Disease Control and Prevention website: https://www.cdc.gov/nchs/fastats/access-to-health-care.htm

National Institute of Diabetes and Digestive and Kidney Diseases. (2012). Primary hyperparathyroidism. NIH Publication No. 12-3425. Retrieved from https://www.niddk.nih.gov/health-information/endocrine-diseases/primary-hyperparathyroidism

National Institute of Environmental Health Sciences. (2019). Environment and health A to Z. NIH Publication # 19-ES-4145. Retrieved from https://www.niehs.nih.gov/health/materials/environment_and_health_a_to_z_508.pdf

National Institute of Neurological Disorders and Stroke. (2012). Tourette syndrome fact sheet. NIH Publication No. 12-2163. Retrieved from https://www.ninds.nih.gov/Disorders/Patient-Caregiver-Education/Fact-Sheets/Tourette-Syndrome-Fact-Sheet

National Institute of Neurological Disorders and Stroke. (2019). Brain basics: Understanding sleep. Retrieved from https://www.ninds.nih.gov/Disorders/Patient-Caregiver-Education/Understanding-Sleep

Okeke, T., Anyaehie, U., & Ezenyeaku, C. (2013). Premature menopause. *Annals of Medical and Health Sciences Research, 3*(1), 90–95. doi:10.4103/2141-9248.109458

O'Leary, C. M., Nassar, N., Kurinczuk, J. J., De Klerk, N., Geelhoed, E., Elliott, E. J., & Bower, C. (2011). Prenatal alcohol exposure and risk of birth defects. *Obstetrical and Gynecological Survey, 66*(2), 88–90. doi:10.1097/OGX.0b013e31821684bc

Pei, J., Denys, K., Hughes, J., & Rasmussen, C. (2011). Mental health issues in fetal alcohol spectrum disorder. *Journal of Mental Health, 20*(5), 473–483. doi:10.3109/09638237.2011.577113

Petersen, P. E. (2003). The world oral health report 2003: Continuous improvement of oral health in the 21st century—The approach of the WHO global oral health programme. *Community Dentistry and Oral Epidemiology, 31*(Suppl 1), 3–23. Retrieved from http://www.ncbi.nlm.nih.gov/pubmed/15015736, doi:10.1046/j.2003.com122.x

Qureishi, A., Lee, Y., Belfield, K., Birchall, J.P., & Daniel, M. (2014). Update on otitis media—Prevention and treatment. *Infection and Drug Resistance, 7*, 15–24. doi: 10.2147/IDR.S39637

Rose, N. R. (2017). Autoimmune diseases. In N. R. Rose (Ed.), *International encyclopedia of public health* (pp. 192–195). Baltimore, MD: The Johns Hopkins Schools of Medicine and Public Health. doi:10.1016/B978-0-12-803678-5.00029-1

Sadeu, J. C., Hughes, C. L., Agarwal, S., & Foster, W. G. (2010). Alcohol, drugs, caffeine, tobacco, and environmental contaminant exposure: Reproductive health consequences and clinical implications. *Critical Reviews in Toxicology, 40*(7), 633–652. doi:10.3109/10408444.2010.493552

Service, F. J., Cryer, P. E., & Vella, A. (2019). Hypoglycemia in adults without diabetes mellitus: Clinical manifestations, diagnosis, and causes. *UpToDate*. Retrieved from https://www.uptodate.com/contents/hypoglycemia-in-adults-without-diabetes-mellitus-clinical-manifestations-diagnosis-and-causes

Sheiham, A. (2005). Oral health, general health and quality of life. *Bulletin of the World Health Organization, 83*(9), 644. Retrieved from https://www.ncbi.nlm.nih.gov/pmc/articles/PMC2626333/pdf/16211151.pdf

Smitherman, T. A., Burch, R., Sheikh, H., & Loder, E. (2013). The prevalence, impact, and treatment of migraine and severe headaches in the United States: A review of statistics from national surveillance studies. Headache: *The Journal of Head and Face Pain, 53*(3), 427–436. doi: 10.1111/head.12074

Statistics Canada. (2016). Health fact sheets hearing loss of Canadians, 2012 to 2015. In *Catalogue no. 82-625-X*. Retrieved from https://www150.statcan.gc.ca/n1/pub/82-625-x/2016001/article/14658-eng.htm

Statistics Canada. (2018). Functional difficulties: Washington group 2017. In *Catalogue no. 82-625-X*. Retrieved from https://www150.statcan.gc.ca/n1/pub/82-625-x/2018001/article/54978-eng.htm

Statistics Canada. (2019). Health fact sheets primary health care providers, 2017. In *Catalogue no. 82-625-X*. Retrieved from https://www150.statcan.gc.ca/n1/pub/82-625-x/2019001/article/00001-eng.htm

Stratton, K., Howe, C., & Battaglia, F. (1996). *Fetal alcohol syndrome: Diagnosis, epidemiology, prevention and treatment*. Washington, DC: National Academy Press.

Streissguth, A. P., Barr, H. M., Kogan, J., & Bookstein, F. L. (1996). *Understanding the occurrence of secondary disabilities in clients with fetal alcohol syndrome (FAS) and fetal alcohol effects (FAE)*. Final Report to the Centers for Disease Control and Prevention (CDC), 96-06. Seattle: University of Washington.

Troese, M., Fukumizu, M., Sallinen, B. J., Gilles, A. A., Wellman, J. D., Paul, J. A., . . . Hayes, M. J. (2008). Sleep fragmentation and evidence for sleep debt in alcohol-exposed infants. *Early Human Development, 84*(9), 577–585. doi:10.1016/j.earlhumdev.2008.02.001

Velasco, M., García-Urena, M. A., Hidalgo, M., Vega, V., & Carnero, F. J. (1999). Current concepts on adult umbilical hernia. *Hernia, 3*(4), 233–239. doi:10.1007/BF01194437

Vieira, R. T. (2013). Epidemiology of early-onset dementia: A review of the literature. *Clinical Practice & Epidemiology in Mental Health, 9*(1), 88–95. doi:10.2174/1745017901309010088

World Health Organization. (2017). Congenital anomalies. *WHO Fact Sheets*. Retrieved from http://www.who.int/mediacentre/factsheets/fs370/en/

Yale Medicine. (n.d.). Hernia repair surgery. Retrieved from https://www.yalemedicine.org/conditions/hernia-repair-surgery/

13

The adolescent brain

Predictors and consequences of substance use

Lindsay R. Meredith and Lindsay M. Squeglia

Background

Adolescence comprises a period of various developmental changes, including social, emotional, physical, and neural, as individuals transition from childhood to adulthood. Adolescence roughly includes the span from 10 to 19 years of age (Inchley et al., 2018); however, this period may need to be expanded due to the fact that, in recent years, young people throughout the world are experiencing earlier onset of puberty and longer time to transition into adult roles, including completing education and entering into marriage (Sawyer, Azzopardi, Wickremarathne, & Patton, 2018; see Chapter 14 on emerging adulthood). Aligned with this, the human brain continues to develop into young adulthood, until around 25 years of age (Pfefferbaum et al., 1994). Large longitudinal studies reported that the brain goes through distinct structural and functional time-specific changes during adolescence with slight differences across gender and brain regions (Giedd, 2008; Giedd et al., 1999; Jernigan, Trauner, Hesselink, & Tallal, 1991; Lenroot et al., 2007; Raznahan et al., 2014; Shaw et al., 2008; Squeglia & Gray, 2016). During this sensitive period of rapid neural changes, healthy brain development is imperative.

Structurally, total brain volume remains steady while gray matter (i.e. neuronal cell bodies) development follows an inverted U-shaped curve, whereby volume increases until early adolescence (12–14 years of age) when gray matter volume then decreases as underutilized neural connections are removed and the brain's efficiency is improved (Bava & Tapert, 2010; Giedd et al., 1999). In contrast, white matter (i.e. neuronal axon tracts) growth continues throughout adolescence, as important neural network connections are developed and optimized (Giedd, 2008; Giorgio et al., 2008). Together, these gray and white matter structural changes lead to enhanced information processing required for higher order cognitive functions.

Functionally, adolescent brains continue to develop as well, with certain functions developing more quickly than others (Squeglia & Gray, 2016). Most prominently, adolescent brains exhibit emotional functionality similar to adult brains; however, cognitive functionality (e.g. decision-making, inhibitory control, planning and working memory) is slower to fully develop (Giedd, 2008). White matter maturation in the frontal regions of the brain is linked with this continued cognitive development, as demonstrated through various neuro-imaging techniques (Bava & Tapert, 2010; Luna, Padmanabhan, & O'Hearn, 2010).

Overview of adolescent substance use

The developing adolescent brain contains more mature reward circuitry than cognitive control circuitry, leaving adolescents vulnerable to engage in risky behaviors, such as substance use (Casey, Glatt, & Lee, 2015; Luna et al., 2010; Raznahan et al., 2014; Squeglia & Cservenka, 2017; Squeglia & Gray, 2016). As such, adolescents exhibit heightened sensitivity to incentives and rewards, while lacking the ability to consistently and effectively regulate their emotions and actions (Somerville, Jones, & Casey, 2010). Thus, initiation rates of alcohol and other substance use escalates dramatically during adolescence, as youth seek out new experiences and become more independent, spending more time with friends outside of the home (Inchley et al., 2018).

Substance use among adolescents is heterogenous, ranging from low, normative use to heavy, pathological use. The average age of initiation for alcohol use among U.S. and Australian teens is 15 years (Aiken et al., 2018; Richmond-Rakerd, Slutske, & Wood, 2017). Alcohol is the most frequently used substance, as it is generally easiest for adolescents to access. Worldwide estimate of adolescents (age 15–19) who drank alcohol in the past month is 27%; higher rates of drinking occur among males and in higher income countries (World Health Organization [WHO], 2018). The highest rates of current alcohol consumption among adolescents occur in the European region (44% reporting past-month drinking), while the lowest rates are observed in the Eastern Mediterranean region (1.2%; WHO, 2018; Inchley et al., 2018). Past-month alcohol use rates among students in the following countries ranged between 8% and 38% of the population: Americas and Western Pacific region, 38%; China, 37% (male) and 21% (female) among high school students (Feng & Newman, 2016); Africa and Southeast Asia, 21%; Japan, 14% among middle and high school students (Morioka et al., 2013); and the United States, 8% among 8th graders and 33% among 12th graders (Johnston et al., 2019). In South Korea, lifetime rates of adolescent alcohol consumption are estimated at 47% (So & Park, 2016). While rates of heavy drinking are highest among 20–24-year-olds, heavy drinking among adolescents remains a concern (WHO, 2018). Thankfully, rates of U.S. adolescent binge drinking (defined as five or more drinks in a setting over the past two weeks) has decreased over the past several decades with current rates at 4% among 8th graders and 14% among 12th graders (Johnston et al., 2019).

Frequency of cannabis use among adolescents is second only to alcohol; almost a quarter of U.S. 12th graders reported use in the past month (Johnston et al., 2019). Across European countries, rates of past-month cannabis use among 15–16-year-olds ranged from 1% to 17% with an average of 7% (EPSAD Group, 2016). Rates of past-year cannabis use among 15–16-year-olds averaged 3% in Asian countries and 7% in African countries according to the 2018 World Drug Report (United Nations Office on Drugs and Crime, 2018). Cannabis is most often smoked through joints, blunts, and bongs, but other methods are becoming increasingly popular, such as vaping or the use of hash oil, which often contains very high concentrations of tetrahydrocannabinol (THC), the main psychoactive component of the cannabis plant (Wilson, Freeman, & Mackie, 2019).

While use of traditional, combustible cigarettes has decreased markedly over the past ten years, use of electronic cigarettes (i.e. e-cigarettes, vapes) has risen exponentially among high schoolers and even more concerningly, among middle school students (Cullen et al., 2018; Johnston et al., 2019). The change in e-cigarette use among U.S. high school seniors from 2017 to 2018 was the greatest one-year increase in use among any substance in the 40+ year history of Monitoring the Future, with 21% of high school seniors reporting vaping (Johnston et al., 2019). In the Russian Federation, lifetime prevalence of e-cigarette use was 27% (Kong, Idrisov, Galimov, Masagutov, & Sussman, 2017). E-cigarettes have significantly lower levels of toxic substances than combustible cigarettes, but research suggests that e-cigarettes may deliver nicotine at higher concentrations (Fadus, Smith, & Squeglia, 2019).

Other types of illicit substance use (i.e. hallucinogens, cocaine, opioids) are relatively uncommon in this age group (Johnston et al., 2019). For example, lifetime use of cocaine is around 3% in European countries (ages 15–24) and 2% in the United States (ages 12–17; United Nations Office on Drugs and Crime, 2018). Lifetime prevalence of any illicit drug use among high school and college students in China is estimated at 2% (Jia, Jin, Zhang, Wang, & Lu, 2018).

Not surprisingly, alcohol and other substance use problems have major global health impacts. Alcohol was the leading cause of premature death and disability among persons aged 15–49 in 2018 (GBD 2016 Alcohol Collaborators, 2018). In the United States alone, the annual economic impact of excessive alcohol consumption is estimated at over $250 billion (Sacks, Gonzales, Bouchery, Tomedi, & Brewer, 2015). These statistics stress the importance of identifying early risk factors for problematic substance use by adolescents, in addition to understanding the causal impacts of substance use on brain and behavior.

A developmental perspective on substance use problems

Emerging research supports the notion that substance use disorders can be developmental problems that begin during adolescence and impact the individual throughout the lifespan (Brown et al., 2008; Squeglia, Boissoneault, Van Skike, Nixon, & Matthews, 2014). Earlier exposure to the neurotoxic effects of alcohol (initiation of use) is associated with higher rates of alcohol use disorders later in life (Dawson, Goldstein, Chou, Ruan, & Grant, 2008; Grant & Dawson, 1997). Several large-scale, multi-site longitudinal studies are currently underway, seeking to illuminate the consequences of substance use on neural and cognitive functioning. The Adolescent Brain Cognitive Development (ABCD) Study is following almost 12,000 U.S. children for a decade to answer longstanding questions about healthy brain development (Volkow et al., 2018), and the National Consortium on Alcohol and NeuroDevelopment in Adolescence (NCANDA) is following over 800 U.S. children to better understand the effects of alcohol use patterns on neuromaturation (Brown et al., 2015). The longest-running of these large-scale studies, run by the IMAGEN Consortium, is following European youth to investigate the neurobiological and genetic basis for reward sensitivity and impulsivity in predicting psychopathology (Schumann et al., 2010). Data from these longitudinal studies will help clarify factors that affect normal brain development.

Predictors and consequences of substance use

This rest of this chapter focuses primarily on predictors and consequences of substance use by adolescents, primarily neural predictors. In order to best understand features that predict substance use and consequences of substance use during adolescence, longitudinal data are necessary. Thus, the majority of covered studies follow youth before and after initiation of substance use. Secondarily, the chapter covers psychosocial and genetic contributors to substance use and the subsequent emergence of disordered use and other related psychopathologies. Given that alcohol and cannabis are the most commonly used substances among youth, much of the relevant research covered here focuses on the effects of these two substances. Future directions for studying the effects of substance use on adolescent brain development are also discussed.

Neural predictors of adolescent substance use

The covered literature emphasizes neurocognition, and structural and functional brain measures.

Neuropsychological predictors

Neurocognitive functioning is measured through neuropsychological assessment in research and clinical settings. These assessments measure general Intellectual Quotient (IQ) or specific neurocognitive domains like attention, working memory, processing speed, or language. Neuropsychological batteries may be performed to identify a learning disability or cognitive impairment from brain injury, medical illness, mental illness, etc., or to measure recovery or response to treatment (Harvey, 2012). Performance on certain neurocognitive measures may predict adolescent engagement in alcohol and cannabis use. Inhibition, which is the ability to suppress an automatic response in order to perform a more appropriate and goal-directed response, has been regularly studied in both adult and adolescent substance use research, given its relation to top-down behavioral control (Lopez-Caneda, Rodriguez Holguin, Cadaveira, Corral, & Doallo, 2014; Squeglia, Jacobus, Nguyen-Louie, & Tapert, 2014; Stavro, Pelletier, & Potvin, 2013). A prospective study, following youth before initiation of substance use until adulthood, collected neuropsychological data and reported that deficits in inhibitory functioning at baseline predicted cannabis and alcohol use by age 18 above and beyond other predictors, such as externalizing behaviors, gender, academic achievement, and family history of substance abuse (Squeglia et al., 2014). Together, these factors accounted for over 20% of the observed variability in adolescent substance use. Another study supported and extended this finding, showing that youth naïve to substances who had high reward sensitivity but low inhibitory control engaged in substance use at an earlier age (Kim-Spoon et al., 2016). These findings suggest that, before ever using alcohol or drugs, youth who have poorer inhibition and higher reward sensitivity are more likely to initiate substance use during adolescence.

Impulsivity is highly linked with poor inhibitory control and can be described as the tendency to act with little forethought and minimal consideration or concern for potential consequences (Moeller, Barratt, Dougherty, Schmitz, & Swann, 2001). Impulsivity was studied in a prospective study well-representative of minorities and families from the lower-middle class. The results showed that lower working memory at baseline significantly predicted increases in alcohol use over the course of the study; however, the effect of working memory on alcohol use was completely mediated by high trait impulsivity (Khurana et al., 2013). This suggests that the relationship between working memory deficits and alcohol use may be better explained by individuals' level of impulsivity (Khurana et al., 2013). Further, the literature shows that poorer executive functioning is predictive of alcohol use initiation in adolescents (Peeters et al., 2015; Squeglia et al., 2017). Thus, reward sensitivity, impulsivity, inhibition, working memory, and more broadly, executive function deficits may serve as risk factors and potential points of intervention for adolescents. For example, the *Preventure programme* is an evidence-based substance use prevention program targeting adolescents at "high risk," those identified as having high levels of impulsivity, sensation seeking, anxiety sensitivity, and hopelessness (Edalati & Conrod, 2019). Of note, none of these studies used cognitive functioning to predict problematic substance use, only amount or presence of substance use. Future research is necessary to determine if specific cognitive abilities predict disordered substance use.

Functional brain precursors

Structural and functional imaging techniques can identify the neural markers that coincide with neurocognitive abilities discussed in the previous section. For instance, researchers use tasks measuring response inhibition or reward sensitivity during functional magnetic resonance imaging (fMRI) to examine the neural activation patterns associated with these domains. This imaging technique, fMRI, is safe, non-invasive, and has high spatial and temporal specificity; brain activation is often measured through blood-oxygen-level-dependent (BOLD) signal, which indirectly measures blood flow in the brain during various tasks (Glover, 2011). In longitudinal studies, researchers can determine if certain patterns of activation found in adolescents prior to substance-use initiation can predict later engagement in substance use. In fact, several prospective studies reported that abnormal neural activation during tasks of inhibition (go/no-go task) predicted future alcohol use, substance use, symptoms of substance dependency, and externalizing symptoms of aggression and hyperactivity (Heitzeg et al., 2014; Mahmood et al., 2013; Norman et al., 2011; Whelan et al., 2014).

Differential brain activation during reward processing may predict future substance use. A Dutch study enrolled both young adults who engaged in heavy cannabis use and those who did not, comparing their neural activation during a monetarily driven reward task during an fMRI scan (Cousijn et al., 2013). Young adults who used cannabis displayed greater activation patterns during "win" trials in executive function and decision-making brain regions; these neural reward patterns predicted rates of cannabis use at six-month follow-up. Larger longitudinal studies are needed to better understand how certain brain patterns incur risk for heavy substance use and how this might interact with co-use of different substances.

Comparable results have been reported for reward processing tasks predicting future alcohol use (Morales, Jones, Ehlers, Lavine, & Nagel, 2018; Nguyen-Louie et al., 2018; Ramage, Lin, Olvera, Fox, & Williamson, 2015; Whelan et al., 2014). Adolescents who were naïve to substances ($N = 51$) but had a positive family history for alcoholism demonstrated greater neural activation while viewing alcohol-related images (Nguyen-Louie et al., 2018), suggesting that adolescents with a genetic predisposition and/or environmental exposure to heavy alcohol use may have different motivational responses to alcohol than those who do not, even prior to engaging in drinking behavior. Further, similar findings have been observed during a risky decision-making task, where heightened activation predicted earlier onset of binge drinking by adolescents (Morales et al., 2018).

Finally, two other precursors of substance-use initiation have been reported, yet research is still limited: (1) variability in brain activation during a visual working memory task (Squeglia et al., 2012, 2017) and (2) variations in default mode network activation during rest (Ramage et al., 2015). Overall, it appears that alterations in neural functioning predate substance use, potentially making some youth more vulnerable to initiating alcohol and other drug use during adolescence.

Structural brain precursors

Structural brain markers, such as gray matter, cortical thickness, and volume, as well as white matter microstructure, may help researchers identify vulnerabilities for developing substance use problems during adolescence and adulthood. A longitudinal study following 40 adolescents, half of whom went on to engage in heavy alcohol drinking at three-year follow-up, revealed structural brain differences (gray matter volume) at baseline (Squeglia, Rinker et al., 2014). Specifically, differences arose in frontal brain region volumes, which are associated with cognitive control. Several other prospective studies supported this finding, where smaller frontal gray matter volume is predictive of drinking later in adolescence (Squeglia et al., 2017; Squeglia, Rinker et al., 2014; Weiland et al., 2014; Whelan et al., 2014); these effects are observed even after controlling for family history of alcohol problems.

Smaller frontal cortical brain volume may also predict youth cannabis use (Cheetham et al., 2012), increased rates of binge drinking, and externalizing symptoms (Brumback et al., 2016). Subcortical reward region volume, including volume of the nucleus accumbens, may predict substance-use initiation, as well (Cheetham et al., 2014; Urosevic et al., 2015). Overall, these results are particularly informative given the well-documented findings displaying altered reward activation among adults who regularly use substances.

Lastly, white matter differences may be implicated in adolescent substance use (Squeglia et al., 2015). White matter integrity, measured through diffusion tensor imaging, indicates the efficiency of connections between regions of the brain. Lower white matter integrity in frontolimbic regions predicted future cannabis use, alcohol use, and other risky behaviors among youth at 18-month follow-up (Jacobus, Thayer et al., 2013). Additionally, altered frontostriatal white matter integrity in early adolescence predicted later binge-drinking behavior and family history of alcoholism (Jones & Nagel, 2019). Overall, structural brain abnormalities in both gray and white matter predate substance use in youth and potentially increase the likelihood of youth engaging in alcohol and drug use during adolescence.

Other risk factors

It is important to emphasize other risk factors, aside from neural and cognitive features, that may contribute to the initiation and abuse of substances. A family history of alcohol or drug problems may moderate the effect of individual differences that are predictive of substance-use initiation (Cservenka, Herting, & Nagel, 2012; Jones, Steele, & Nagel, 2017; Nguyen-Louie et al., 2018). A meta-analysis on the genetic contribution of alcohol use disorder suggests that it is approximately 50% heritable (Verhulst, Neale, & Kendler, 2015). However, it has been very challenging to identify specific genes that substantially contribute to the emergence of disease, as many gene segments each have a very small effect that can interact with the environment (Kiser, Rivero, & Lesch, 2015; Prom-Wormley, Ebejer, Dick, & Bowers, 2017; Rhee et al., 2003). Additionally, personality disorder traits (Rosenstrom et al., 2018), prenatal alcohol exposure (Enoch, 2012), early life stress, socioeconomic status (in a U-shaped curve), and early dating may also confer risk for substance use (Squeglia et al., 2017). Not surprisingly, the presence of psychopathology during adolescence, such as attention deficit hyperactivity disorder (ADHD), conduct disorder symptoms, childhood depression, and externalizing behaviors, can also increase the likelihood that youth will engage in substance use or develop a substance use disorder during adulthood (Lee, Humphreys, Flory, Liu, & Glass, 2011; Meier et al., 2016).

Summary

Overall, the reviewed literature suggests that prior to substance-use initiation, neurocognitive and neural functioning alterations during tasks of reward processing, inhibition/impulsivity, and executive functioning, as well as structural regions associated with these processes, may serve as informative predictors of future substance-use initiation. A greater understanding of precursors for heavy and problematic substance use could provide clinicians with earlier identification of risk factors and targets for intervention. Larger longitudinal studies focusing on predictors of problematic use and substances beyond alcohol and cannabis could facilitate this understanding. Researchers need to distinguish neural and cognitive features from other risk factors, such as family history or externalizing behaviors, to better understand their direct influences and mechanisms of action.

Neural consequences of adolescent substance use

The literature on longitudinal and neuroimaging studies indicates that substance use during adolescence negatively affects brain structure and function, as well as cognition and behavior. Since researchers involved in human studies are unable to experimentally control for amount and type of substance use, the causal effects research is mostly longitudinal and naturalistic observational studies. Among adolescents, while it is common to find those who engage only in alcohol use, it is much less common to find those who engage only in non-alcohol substance use (e.g. adolescents who use *only* cannabis). Thus, it is difficult to untangle the unique effects of cannabis or other non-alcoholic drugs on the brain. Currently, very large and exciting longitudinal studies are underway, which will have sufficient power to detect these nuanced and potentially distinctive drug effects (Brown et al., 2015; Schumann et al., 2010; Volkow et al., 2018).

Neuropsychological alterations

Neuropsychological assessment is one of the most common ways for psychologists to assess academic achievement and cognitive abilities. The results of these assessments can influence the diagnosis of developmental disorders and, therefore, facilitate important educational accommodations and other interventions. Neuropsychological batteries are used in research settings to detect potential effects of substance use on neurocognition and academic abilities. Substance-induced deficits are even more impactful for adolescents than adults, given adolescents' ongoing education, learning, and neural development. Alcohol and smoking behaviors during mid-adolescence may predict lower educational achievement in later years, even after considering other factors such as externalizing behavior and gender (Latvala et al., 2014). One ten-year study found that by early adulthood, individuals who had engaged in heavy substance use displayed poorer visuospatial functioning, working memory, and verbal learning than those who did not (Hanson, Cummins, Tapert, & Brown, 2011; Hanson, Medina, Padula, Tapert, & Brown, 2011). Worsened cognitive functioning was also associated with problematic drug use, including hangovers and withdrawal symptoms (Hanson, Medina et al., 2011). Another longitudinal study found that substance use during adolescence may impair verbal memory and visuospatial ability, but not processing speed or working memory (Nguyen-Louie et al., 2015). This and several other studies have observed a dose-dependent relationship between substance use and cognitive impairment, where larger amounts of substance use were predictive of increasingly greater cognitive impairment (Nguyen-Louie et al., 2015; Hanson, Cummins et al., 2011; Winward, Hanson, Tapert, & Brown, 2014; Nguyen-Louie et al., 2016). However, because alcohol and cannabis use by teens and young adults is heterogeneous, ranging from low to heavy use, more research about dose-dependent effects is warranted, especially when considering clinical implications.

The ongoing legalization of cannabis throughout the United States and other countries has come with increased public interest in understanding the effects of cannabis use on the developing brain and body. Coinciding with cannabis legalization were increased rates of use and younger age of initiation, as well as decreased perceptions of harm (Johnston et al., 2019). Thus, elucidating the effects of cannabis use on adolescent development is of significant interest to researchers, clinicians, and the public. Several longitudinal studies from the United States and New Zealand reported that heavy cannabis use negatively affected neurocognitive functioning, including declines in general intelligence (Jacobus et al., 2015; Meier et al., 2012). However, large datasets from twin siblings indicated no greater long-term cognitive declines for siblings engaged in cannabis use versus their abstinent twins (Jackson et al., 2016). This suggests that more work is needed to disentangle genetic and environmental influences on neurocognition which currently make it difficult to identify the direct neurotoxic effects of cannabis use, even in longitudinal studies.

Functional brain alterations

In addition to identifying predictors of future substance use, functional neuroimaging studies also identified potential effects of substance use on the brains of adolescents during tasks of working memory, inhibitory control, and reward sensitivity. For example, at baseline, youth naïve to substances (ages 12–14) who later went on to engage in heavy alcohol use by late adolescence exhibited less brain activation in parietal and frontal regions than demographically matched youth during a visual working memory and inhibition task (Squeglia et al., 2012; Wetherill, Squeglia, Yang, & Tapert, 2013); by late adolescence, the youth engaged in substance use had greater increases in task-related activation over time. This suggests that adolescents engaged in alcohol use may need to recruit more cognitive control in order to perform similarly on tasks as adolescents who remain abstinent. However, when considering cannabis, another study did not detect activational differences during a working memory task when comparing youth heavily using cannabis to those who do not (Cousijn et al., 2014). Thus, more work is necessary to tease apart the individual neural effects of alcohol, cannabis, and other substances. Continued, heavy alcohol use may also affect youths' reactivity or sensitivity to reward (Brumback et al., 2015; Cservenka, Jones, & Nagel, 2015; Tapert et al., 2003). Number of drinks per drinking day was negatively related to left cerebellar activation during a monetary reward task (Cservenka et al., 2015), and binge drinking was associated with reductions in the dorsal striatum during a decision-making task; these abnormalities may perpetuate future binge drinking (Jones, Cservenka, & Nagel, 2016). One study reported that, after one month of abstinence, adolescents who previously drank heavily no longer exhibited alterations in reward activation to alcohol cues, highlighting the potential for adolescents to benefit from early intervention and recover from the short-term effects of alcohol (Brumback et al., 2015). Overall, alcohol use during adolescence appears to affect neural functioning in the developing brain. More research is needed to understand how cannabis and other substance use might affect youths' brain functioning.

Structural brain alterations

Structural brain markers, such as gray matter cortical thickness and volume and white matter microstructure, may help researchers better understand behavioral and cognitive distinctions between youth who are engaged in heavy substance use and those who are not (Squeglia & Gray, 2016). Researchers reported both gray and white matter alterations in adolescents who drank heavily (Squeglia et al., 2015). Even after controlling for other substance use, youth who drank heavily exhibited abnormal neurodevelopmental trajectories, with tempered increases in white matter volume and accelerated decreases in gray matter volume in their frontal and temporal regions. These results extended previous findings with smaller sample sizes that demonstrated accelerated decreases in gray matter over time among adolescents engaged in heavy drinking (Luciana, Collins, Muetzel, & Lim, 2013; Squeglia, Rinker et al., 2014). Thus, while gray matter decline and white matter growth are normal in typical adolescent brain development, patterns observed among youth who use substances may represent non-beneficial pruning, premature cortical decline, and/or attenuated connective efficiency. An even larger study extended these findings, showing that heavy (but not moderate) alcohol use impacted normal brain growth trajectories; cannabis co-use did not contribute to these effects (Pfefferbaum et al., 2018). Adults who engage in sustained problematic drinking exhibit similar structural alterations and have speeded gray and white matter decline, suggesting accelerated brain aging (Guggenmos et al., 2017; Pfefferbaum et al., 1992; Pfefferbaum et al., 2013).

In contrast, adolescents who predominately used cannabis had greater cortical thickness in frontal and parietal regions, differing in directionality from findings involving adolescents who predominately used alcohol (Squeglia et al., 2015). This suggests that cannabis use may interfere with normal cortical thinning trajectories that are seen throughout the course of a typically developing brain (Jacobus et al., 2016). However, more research is needed to determine whether these results illustrate substance-specific directionality effects, or if other factors may be involved, such as genetics, age of onset, or interactive effects of multiple substances (Squeglia & Gray, 2016). Several other studies also detected substance-induced white matter alterations in adolescents (Gruber, Dahlgren, Sagar, Gonenc, & Lukas, 2014; Shollenbarger, Price, Wieser, & Lisdahl, 2015). For example, youth engaged in regular alcohol and cannabis co-use had less white matter integrity than youth not using substances (Bava, Jacobus, Thayer, & Tapert, 2013; Jacobus, Squeglia, Infante, Bava, & Tapert, 2013). These white matter alterations were associated with poor performance on neurocognitive tests.

Future directions

Prospective, longitudinal designs have greatly increased our knowledge of the complex relationship between adolescent brain development and substance use by parsing pre-existing vulnerabilities and consequential effects of substance use (Squeglia & Gray, 2016). However, larger multi-site studies currently underway could help disentangle the complicated picture of substance co-use, the interactive nature of psychopathology, demographics, health habits, and genetic vulnerabilities, among other important factors related to substance use. The goal of this research is to inform early intervention around problematic substance use by adolescents and young adults. Hopefully, current literature together with future research will help identify specific neurodevelopmental processes and cognitive areas that are most receptive to prevention and treatment efforts.

Certainly, future studies need to make concerted efforts to enroll more adolescents with diverse backgrounds, as substance use predictors and effects may not generalize across ethnicities, cultures, various family structures, or psychopathology profiles. Further, it is necessary to understand substance-specific effects, especially given the dramatic rise in adolescent e-cigarette use and global concerns regarding opioid dependency and associated deaths. Larger studies are positioned to differentiate the specific neural developmental effects of e-cigarettes, opioids, cocaine, hallucinogens, and amphetamines. Understanding the dose-dependent effects of substances will enable better public health information to inform policies regarding limiting amounts of adolescent use and controlling potency of substance-containing products. Specifically, it will be useful to know how adolescent binge drinking compared to lower levels of drinking affects development, as well as how the content of cannabis (i.e. THC/CBD ratio) or amount and administration mechanisms of cannabis use (i.e. method, number of hits) differentially affect cognition and behavior. Better standardization in quantification of substance use is also important, especially for less regulated drugs, such as cannabis and the variety of available cannabis-containing products. Additionally, a better understanding of short- vs. long-term effects of specific substances on neural and cognitive measures is needed. This is especially important from a treatment perspective (improvement from abstinence or decreased use) and when thinking about resilience and neuroplasticity. Researchers can track these changes using neural markers of substance use and understand how an individual is responding to treatment (Cservenka & Nagel, 2016).

Substance use researchers are utilizing advances in technology to push the field forward. Researchers are starting to move away from relying solely on self-report measures of substance use or simple positive/negative urine drug tests, toward quantifying use through more sophisticated biological markers (i.e. blood, urine, saliva, and hair samples), as well as daily reporting or real-time tracking of drug use through youths' smart phones and wearable devices. These nuanced tools will help improve the accuracy and reliability of reports. Another recent area of research has focused on quantification of various chemicals in the brain measured through Magnetic Resonance Spectroscopy (MRS; Cohen-Gilbert, Jensen, & Silveri, 2014). Understanding neurochemical changes could help us better understand the neurobiological effects of substance use, the mechanisms of change, and alterations incurred through psychotherapy or pharmacological treatment. Better neuroimaging standards have also been suggested as an area of future research, such as the importance of scanning under neutral conditions to control for factors like time since last drug use (Feldstein Ewing, Witkiewitz, & Filbey, 2015).

Conclusions

Overall, functional and structural brain measures and neuropsychological assessment help inform prevention and treatment efforts by elucidating the predictors and consequences of substance use on adolescent brain development. For example, poor working memory and inhibitory functioning, as well as altered neural reward processing and decreased white matter integrity in youth, may signal risk for future problematic substance use. Heavy alcohol and cannabis use during adolescence may lead to poorer working memory functioning and cognitive control, as well as altered gray and white matter neurodevelopmental trajectories. Knowing the risk factors for future problematic use will inform prevention efforts, while understanding the mechanisms of substance use potentially will produce more effective treatments for youth.

References

Aiken, A., Clare, P. J., Wadolowski, M., Hutchinson, D., Najman, J. M., Slade, T., . . . Mattick, R. P. (2018). Age of alcohol initiation and progression to binge drinking in adolescence: A prospective cohort study. *Alcoholism: Clinical & Experimental Research, 42*(1), 100–110. doi:10.1111/acer.13525

Bava, S., Jacobus, J., Thayer, R. E., & Tapert, S. F. (2013). Longitudinal changes in white matter integrity among adolescent substance users. *Alcoholism: Clinical & Experimental Research, 37*(Suppl 1), E181–E189. doi:10.1111/j.1530-0277.2012.01920.x

Bava, S., & Tapert, S. F. (2010). Adolescent brain development and the risk for alcohol and other drug problems. *Neuropsychology Review, 20*(4), 398–413. doi:10.1007/s11065-010-9146-6

Brown, S. A., Brumback, T., Tomlinson, K., Cummins, K., Thompson, W. K., Nagel, B. J., . . . Tapert, S. F. (2015). The national consortium on alcohol and neurodevelopment in adolescence (NCANDA): A multisite study of adolescent development and substance use. *Journal of Studies on Alcohol & Drugs, 76*(6), 895–908. doi:10.15288/jsad.2015.76.895

Brown, S. A., McGue, M., Maggs, J., Schulenberg, J., Hingson, R., Swartzwelder, S., . . . Murphy, S. (2008). A developmental perspective on alcohol and youths 16 to 20 years of age. *Pediatrics, 121*(Suppl 4), S290–S310. doi:10.1542/peds.2007-2243D

Brumback, T., Squeglia, L. M., Jacobus, J., Pulido, C., Tapert, S. F., & Brown, S. A. (2015). Adolescent heavy drinkers' amplified brain responses to alcohol cues decrease over one month of abstinence. *Addictive Behavior, 46*, 45–52. doi:10.1016/j.addbeh.2015.03.001

Brumback, T. Y., Worley, M., Nguyen-Louie, T. T., Squeglia, L. M., Jacobus, J., & Tapert, S. F. (2016). Neural predictors of alcohol use and psychopathology symptoms in adolescents. *Developmental Psychopathology, 28*(4pt1), 1209–1216. doi:10.1017/S0954579416000766

Casey, B. J., Glatt, C. E., & Lee, F. S. (2015). Treating the developing versus developed brain: Translating preclinical mouse and human studies. *Neuron, 86*(6), 1358–1368. doi:10.1016/j.neuron.2015.05.020

Cheetham, A., Allen, N. B., Whittle, S., Simmons, J., Yucel, M., & Lubman, D. I. (2014). Volumetric differences in the anterior cingulate cortex prospectively predict alcohol-related problems in adolescence. *Psychopharmacology, 231*(8), 1731–1742. doi:10.1007/s00213-014-3483-8

Cheetham, A., Allen, N. B., Whittle, S., Simmons, J. G., Yucel, M., & Lubman, D. I. (2012). Orbitofrontal volumes in early adolescence predict initiation of cannabis use: A 4-year longitudinal and prospective study. *Biological Psychiatry, 71*(8), 684–692. doi:10.1016/j.biopsych.2011.10.029

Cohen-Gilbert, J. E., Jensen, J. E., & Silveri, M. M. (2014). Contributions of magnetic resonance spectroscopy to understanding development: Potential applications in the study of adolescent alcohol use and abuse. *Developmental Psychopathology, 26*(2), 405–423. doi:10.1017/S0954579414000030

Cousijn, J., Vingerhoets, W. A., Koenders, L., de Haan, L., van den Brink, W., Wiers, R. W., & Goudriaan, A. E. (2014). Relationship between working-memory network function and substance use: A 3-year longitudinal fMRI study in heavy cannabis users and controls. *Addiction Biology, 19*(2), 282–293. doi:10.1111/adb.12111

Cousijn, J., Wiers, R. W., Ridderinkhof, K. R., van den Brink, W., Veltman, D. J., Porrino, L. J., & Goudriaan, A. E. (2013). Individual differences in decision making and reward processing predict changes in cannabis use: A prospective functional magnetic resonance imaging study. *Addiction Biology, 18*(6), 1013–1023. doi:10.1111/j.1369-1600.2012.00498.x

Cservenka, A., Herting, M. M., & Nagel, B. J. (2012). Atypical frontal lobe activity during verbal working memory in youth with a family history of alcoholism. *Drug & Alcohol Dependence, 123*-(1–3), 98–104. doi:10.1016/j.drugalcdep.2011.10.021

Cservenka, A., Jones, S. A., & Nagel, B. J. (2015). Reduced cerebellar brain activity during reward processing in adolescent binge drinkers. *Developmental Cognitive Neuroscience, 16*, 110–120. doi:10.1016/j.dcn.2015.06.004

Cservenka, A., & Nagel, B. J. (2016). Neuroscience of alcohol for addiction medicine: Neurobiological targets for prevention and intervention in adolescents. *Progress in Brain Research, 223*, 215–235. doi:10.1016/bs.pbr.2015.07.027

Cullen, K. A., Ambrose, B. K., Gentzke, A. S., Apelberg, B. J., Jamal, A., & King, B. A. (2018). Notes from the field: Use of electronic cigarettes and any tobacco product among middle and high school students—United States, 2011–2018. *Morbidity and Mortality Weekly Report, 67*(45), 1276–1277. doi:10.15585/mmwr.mm6745a5

Dawson, D. A., Goldstein, R. B., Chou, S. P., Ruan, W. J., & Grant, B. F. (2008). Age at first drink and the first incidence of adult-onset DSM-IV alcohol use disorders. *Alcoholism: Clinical & Experimental Research, 32*(12), 2149–2160. doi:10.1111/j.1530-0277.2008.00806.x

Edalati, H. & Conrod, P. J. (2019). A review of personality-targeted interventions for prevention of substance misuse and related harm in community samples of adolescents. *Front Psychiatry 22*(9), 770. doi:10.3389/fpsyt.2018.00770.

Enoch, M. A. (2012). The influence of gene-environment interactions on the development of alcoholism and drug dependence. *Current Psychiatry Reports, 14*(2), 150–158. doi:10.1007/s11920-011-0252-9

EPSAD Group. (2016). *ESPAD report 2015: Results from the European School Survey Project on Alcohol and Other Drugs.* Publications Office of the European Union, Luxembourg. Retrieved from http://www.espad.org/sites/espad.org/files/ESPAD_report_2015.pdf

Fadus, M. C., Smith, T. T., & Squeglia, L. M. (2019). The rise of e-cigarettes, pod mod devices, and JUUL among youth: Factors influencing use, health implications, and downstream effects. *Drug & Alcohol Dependence, 201,* 85–93. doi:10.1016/j.drugalcdep.2019.04.011

Feldstein Ewing, S. W., Witkiewitz, K., & Filbey, F. M. (2015). *Neuroimaging and psychosocial addiction treatment.* New York, NY: Palgrave Macmillan. doi:10.1057/9781137362650

Feng, Y., & Newman, I. M. (2016). Estimate of adolescent alcohol use in China: A meta-analysis. *Archives of Public Health, 74,* 45. doi:10.1186/s13690-016-0157-5

GBD 2016 Alcohol Collaborators. (2018). Alcohol use and burden for 195 countries and territories, 1990–2016: A systematic analysis for the Global Burden of Disease Study 2016. *Lancet (London, England), 392*(10152), 1015–1035. doi:10.1016/S0140-6736(18)31310-2

Giedd, J. N. (2008). The teen brain: Insights from neuroimaging. *Journal of Adolescent Health, 42*(4), 335–343. doi:10.1016/j.jadohealth.2008.01.007

Giedd, J. N., Blumenthal, J., Jeffries, N. O., Castellanos, F. X., Liu, H., Zijdenbos, A., . . . Rapoport, J. L. (1999). Brain development during childhood and adolescence: A longitudinal MRI study. *Nature Neuroscience, 2*(10), 861–863. doi:10.1038/13158

Giorgio, A., Watkins, K. E., Douaud, G., James, A. C., James, S., De Stefano, N., . . . Johansen-Berg, H. (2008). Changes in white matter microstructure during adolescence. *Neuroimage, 39*(1), 52–61. doi:10.1016/j.neuroimage.2007.07.043

Glover, G. H. (2011). Overview of functional magnetic resonance imaging. *Neurosurgery Clinics of North America, 22*(2), 133–139, vii. doi:10.1016/j.nec.2010.11.001

Grant, B. F., & Dawson, D. A. (1997). Age at onset of alcohol use and its association with DSM-IV alcohol abuse and dependence: Results from the national longitudinal alcohol epidemiologic survey. *Journal of Substance Abuse, 9,* 103–110. doi:10.1016/S0899-3289(97)90009-2

Gruber, S. A., Dahlgren, M. K., Sagar, K. A., Gonenc, A., & Lukas, S. E. (2014). Worth the wait: Effects of age of onset of marijuana use on white matter and impulsivity. *Psychopharmacology, 231*(8), 1455–1465. doi:10.1007/s00213-013-3326-z

Guggenmos, M., Schmack, K., Sekutowicz, M., Garbusow, M., Sebold, M., Sommer, C., . . . Sterzer, P. (2017). Quantitative neurobiological evidence for accelerated brain aging in alcohol dependence. *Translatoional Psychiatry, 7*(12), 1279. doi:10.1038/s41398-017-0037-y

Hanson, K. L., Cummins, K., Tapert, S. F., & Brown, S. A. (2011). Changes in neuropsychological functioning over 10 years following adolescent substance abuse treatment. *Psychology of Addictive Behavior, 25*(1), 127–142. doi:10.1037/a0022350

Hanson, K. L., Medina, K. L., Padula, C. B., Tapert, S. F., & Brown, S. A. (2011). Impact of adolescent alcohol and drug use on neuropsychological functioning in young adulthood: 10-year outcomes. *Journal of Child and Adolescent Substance Abuse, 20*(2), 135–154. doi:10.1080/1067828X.2011.555272

Harvey, P. D. (2012). Clinical applications of neuropsychological assessment. *Dialogues in Clinical Neuroscience, 14*(1), 91–99.

Heitzeg, M. M., Nigg, J. T., Hardee, J. E., Soules, M., Steinberg, D., Zubieta, J. K., & Zucker, R. A. (2014). Left middle frontal gyrus response to inhibitory errors in children prospectively predicts early problem substance use. *Drug & Alcohol Dependence, 141,* 51–57. doi:10.1016/j.drugalcdep.2014.05.002

Inchley, J., Currie, D., Vieno, A., Torsheim, T., Ferreira-Borges, C., Weber, M. M., . . . Breda, J. (2018). *Adolescent alcohol-related behaviours: Trends and inequalities in the WHO European Region, 2002–2014.* Copenhagen, Denmark: WHO Regional Office for Europe.

Jackson, N. J., Isen, J. D., Khoddam, R., Irons, D., Tuvblad, C., Iacono, W. G., . . . Baker, L. A. (2016). Impact of adolescent marijuana use on intelligence: Results from two longitudinal twin studies. *Proceedings of the National Academy of Sciences, 113*(5), E500–E508. doi:10.1073/pnas.1516648113

Jacobus, J., Castro, N., Squeglia, L. M., Meloy, M. J., Brumback, T., Huestis, M. A., & Tapert, S. F. (2016). Adolescent cortical thickness pre- and post marijuana and alcohol initiation. *Neurotoxicology and Teratology, 57,* 20–29. doi:10.1016/j.ntt.2016.09.005

Jacobus, J., Squeglia, L. M., Infante, M. A., Bava, S., & Tapert, S. F. (2013). White matter integrity pre- and post marijuana and alcohol initiation in adolescence. *Brain Science, 3*(1), 396–414. doi:10.3390/brainsci3010396

Jacobus, J., Squeglia, L. M., Infante, M. A., Castro, N., Brumback, T., Meruelo, A. D., & Tapert, S. F. (2015). Neuropsychological performance in adolescent marijuana users with co-occurring alcohol use: A three-year longitudinal study. *Neuropsychology, 29*(6), 829–843. doi:10.1037/neu0000203

Jacobus, J., Thayer, R. E., Trim, R. S., Bava, S., Frank, L. R., & Tapert, S. F. (2013). White matter integrity, substance use, and risk taking in adolescence. *Psychology of Addictive Behavior, 27*(2), 431–442. doi:10.1037/a0028235

Jernigan, T. L., Trauner, D. A., Hesselink, J. R., & Tallal, P. A. (1991). Maturation of human cerebrum observed in vivo during adolescence. *Brain, 114*(Pt 5), 2037–2049. doi:10.1093/brain/114.5.2037

Jia, Z., Jin, Y., Zhang, L., Wang, Z., & Lu, Z. (2018). Prevalence of drug use among students in mainland China: A systematic review and meta-analysis for 2003–2013. *Drug & Alcohol Dependence, 186*, 201–206. doi:10.1016/j.drugalcdep.2017.12.047

Johnston, L. D., Miech, R. A., O'Malley, P. M., Bachman, J. G., Schulenberg, J. E., & Patrick, M. E. (2019). *Monitoring the future national survey results on drug use, 1975–2018: Overview, key findings on adolescent drug use.* Retrieved from http://www.monitoringthefuture.org/pubs.html

Jones, S. A., Cservenka, A., & Nagel, B. J. (2016). Binge drinking impacts dorsal striatal response during decision making in adolescents. *Neuroimage, 129*(Epub), 378–388. doi:10.1016/j.neuroimage.2016.01.044

Jones, S. A., & Nagel, B. J. (2019). Altered frontostriatal white matter microstructure is associated with familial alcoholism and future binge drinking in adolescence. *Neuropsychopharmacology*(Epub). doi:10.1038/s41386-019-0315-x

Jones, S. A., Steele, J. S., & Nagel, B. J. (2017). Binge drinking and family history of alcoholism are associated with an altered developmental trajectory of impulsive choice across adolescence. *Addiction, 112*(7), 1184–1192. doi:10.1111/add.13823

Khurana, A., Romer, D., Betancourt, L. M., Brodsky, N. L., Giannetta, J. M., & Hurt, H. (2013). Working memory ability predicts trajectories of early alcohol use in adolescents: The mediational role of impulsivity. *Addiction, 108*(3), 506–515. doi:10.1111/add.12001

Kim-Spoon, J., Deater-Deckard, K., Holmes, C., Lee, J., Chiu, P., & King-Casas, B. (2016). Behavioral and neural inhibitory control moderates the effects of reward sensitivity on adolescent substance use. *Neuropsychologia, 91*, 318–326. doi:10.1016/j.neuropsychologia.2016.08.028

Kiser, D. P., Rivero, O., & Lesch, K. P. (2015). Annual research review: The (epi)genetics of neurodevelopmental disorders in the era of whole-genome sequencing—Unveiling the dark matter. *Journal of Child Psychology & Psychiatry, 56*(3), 278–295. doi:10.1111/jcpp.12392

Kong, G., Idrisov, B., Galimov, A., Masagutov, R., & Sussman, S. (2017). Electronic cigarette use among adolescents in the Russian Federation. *Substance Use & Misuse, 52*(3), 332–339. doi:10.1080/10826084.2016.1225766

Latvala, A., Rose, R. J., Pulkkinen, L., Dick, D. M., Korhonen, T., & Kaprio, J. (2014). Drinking, smoking, and educational achievement: Cross-lagged associations from adolescence to adulthood. *Drug & Alcohol Dependence, 137*, 106–113. doi:10.1016/j.drugalcdep.2014.01.016

Lee, S. S., Humphreys, K. L., Flory, K., Liu, R., & Glass, K. (2011). Prospective association of childhood attention-deficit/hyperactivity disorder (ADHD) and substance use and abuse/dependence: A meta-analytic review. *Clinical Psychology Review, 31*(3), 328–341. doi:10.1016/j.cpr.2011.01.006

Lenroot, R. K., Gogtay, N., Greenstein, D. K., Wells, E. M., Wallace, G. L., Clasen, L. S., . . . Giedd, J. N. (2007). Sexual dimorphism of brain developmental trajectories during childhood and adolescence. *Neuroimage, 36*(4), 1065–1073. doi:10.1016/j.neuroimage.2007.03.053

Lopez-Caneda, E., Rodriguez Holguin, S., Cadaveira, F., Corral, M., & Doallo, S. (2014). Impact of alcohol use on inhibitory control (and vice versa) during adolescence and young adulthood: A review. *Alcohol & Alcoholism, 49*(2), 173–181. doi:10.1093/alcalc/agt168

Luciana, M., Collins, P. F., Muetzel, R. L., & Lim, K. O. (2013). Effects of alcohol use initiation on brain structure in typically developing adolescents. *American Journal of Drug & Alcohol Abuse, 39*(6), 345–355. doi:10.3109/00952990.2013.837057

Luna, B., Padmanabhan, A., & O'Hearn, K. (2010). What has fMRI told us about the development of cognitive control through adolescence? *Brain and Cognition, 72*(1), 101–113. doi:10.1016/j.bandc.2009.08.005

Mahmood, O. M., Goldenberg, D., Thayer, R., Migliorini, R., Simmons, A. N., & Tapert, S. F. (2013). Adolescents' fMRI activation to a response inhibition task predicts future substance use. *Addictive Behavior, 38*(1), 1435–1441. doi:10.1016/j.addbeh.2012.07.012

Meier, M. H., Caspi, A., Ambler, A., Harrington, H., Houts, R., Keefe, R. S., . . . Moffitt, T. E. (2012). Persistent cannabis users show neuropsychological decline from childhood to midlife. *Proceedings of the National Academy of Sciences, 109*(40), E2657–E2664. doi:10.1073/pnas.1206820109

Meier, M. H., Hall, W., Caspi, A., Belsky, D. W., Cerda, M., Harrington, H. L., . . . Moffitt, T. E. (2016). Which adolescents develop persistent substance dependence in adulthood? Using population-representative longitudinal data to inform universal risk assessment. *Psychological Medicne, 46*(4), 877–889. doi:10.1017/S0033291715002482

Moeller, F. G., Barratt, E. S., Dougherty, D. M., Schmitz, J. M., & Swann, A. C. (2001). Psychiatric aspects of impulsivity. *American Journal of Psychiatry, 158*(11), 1783–1793. doi:10.1176/appi.ajp.158.11.1783

Morales, A. M., Jones, S. A., Ehlers, A., Lavine, J. B., & Nagel, B. J. (2018). Ventral striatal response during decision making involving risk and reward is associated with future binge drinking in adolescents. *Neuropsychopharmacology, 43*(9), 1884–1890. doi:10.1038/s41386-018-0087-8

Morioka, H., Itani, O., Kaneita, Y., Ikeda, M., Kondo, S., Yamamoto, R., . . . Ohida, T. (2013). Associations between sleep disturbance and alcohol drinking: A large-scale epidemiological study of adolescents in Japan. *Alcohol, 47*(8), 619–628. doi:10.1016/j.alcohol.2013.09.041

Nguyen-Louie, T. T., Castro, N., Matt, G. E., Squeglia, L. M., Brumback, T., & Tapert, S. F. (2015). Effects of emerging alcohol and marijuana use behaviors on adolescents' neuropsychological functioning over four years. *Journal of Studies on Alcohol & Drugs, 76*(5), 738–748. doi:10.15288/jsad.2015.76.738

Nguyen-Louie, T. T., Courtney, K. E., Squeglia, L. M., Bagot, K., Eberson, S., Migliorini, R., . . . Pulido, C. (2018). Prospective changes in neural alcohol cue reactivity in at-risk adolescents. *Brain Imaging Behavior, 12*(4), 931–941. doi:10.1007/s11682-017-9757-0

Nguyen-Louie, T. T., Tracas, A., Squeglia, L. M., Matt, G. E., Eberson-Shumate, S., & Tapert, S. F. (2016). Learning and memory in adolescent moderate, binge, and extreme-binge drinkers. *Alcoholism: Clinical and Experimental Research, 40*(9), 1895–1904. doi:10.1111/acer.13160

Norman, A. L., Pulido, C., Squeglia, L. M., Spadoni, A. D., Paulus, M. P., & Tapert, S. F. (2011). Neural activation during inhibition predicts initiation of substance use in adolescence. *Drug & Alcohol Dependence, 119*(3), 216–223. doi:10.1016/j.drugalcdep.2011.06.019

Peeters, M., Janssen, T., Monshouwer, K., Boendermaker, W., Pronk, T., Wiers, R., & Vollebergh, W. (2015). Weaknesses in executive functioning predict the initiating of adolescents' alcohol use. *Developmental Cognitive Neuroscience, 16*, 139–146. doi:10.1016/j.dcn.2015.04.003

Pfefferbaum, A., Kwon, D., Brumback, T., Thompson, W. K., Cummins, K., Tapert, S., . . . Clark, D. B. (2018). Altered brain development trajectories in adolescents after initating drinking. *American Journal of Psychiatry, 175*(4), 370–380. doi:10.1176/appi.ajp.2017.17040469

Pfefferbaum, A., Lim, K. O., Zipursky, R. B., Mathalon, D. H., Rosenbloom, M. J., Lane, B., . . . Sullivan, E. V. (1992). Brain gray and white matter volume loss accelerates with aging in chronic alcoholics: A quantitative MRI study. *Alcoholism: Clinical & Experimental Research, 16*(6), 1078–1089. doi:10.1111/j.1530-0277.1992.tb00702.x

Pfefferbaum, A., Mathalon, D. H., Sullivan, E. V., Rawles, J. M., Zipursky, R. B., & Lim, K. O. (1994). A quantitative magnetic resonance imaging study of changes in brain morphology from infancy to late adulthood. *Archive of Neurology, 51*(9), 874–887. doi:10.1001/archneur.1994.005402 10046012

Pfefferbaum, A., Rohlfing, T., Rosenbloom, M. J., Chu, W., Colrain, I. M., & Sullivan, E. V. (2013). Variation in longitudinal trajectories of regional brain volumes of healthy men and women (ages 10 to 85 years) measured with atlas-based parcellation of MRI. *Neuroimage, 65*, 176–193. doi:10.1016/j.neuroimage.2012.10.008

Prom-Wormley, E. C., Ebejer, J., Dick, D. M., & Bowers, M. S. (2017). The genetic epidemiology of substance use disorder: A review. *Drug & Alcohol Dependence, 180*, 241–259. doi:10.1016/j.drugalcdep.2017.06.040

Ramage, A. E., Lin, A. L., Olvera, R. L., Fox, P. T., & Williamson, D. E. (2015). Resting-state regional cerebral blood flow during adolescence: Associations with initiation of substance use and prediction of future use disorders. *Drug & Alcohol Dependence, 149*, 40–48. doi:10.1016/j.drugalcdep.2015.01.012

Raznahan, A., Shaw, P. W., Lerch, J. P., Clasen, L. S., Greenstein, D., Berman, R., . . . Giedd, J. N. (2014). Longitudinal four-dimensional mapping of subcortical anatomy in human development. *Proceedings of the National Academy of Sciences, 111*(4), 1592–1597. doi:10.1073/pnas.1316911111

Rhee, S. H., Hewitt, J. K., Young, S. E., Corley, R. P., Crowley, T. J., & Stallings, M. C. (2003). Genetic and environmental influences on substance initiation, use, and problem use in adolescents. *Archives of General Psychiatry, 60*(12), 1256–1264. doi:10.1001/archpsyc.60.12.1256

Richmond-Rakerd, L. S., Slutske, W. S., & Wood, P. K. (2017). Age of initiation and substance use progression: A multivariate latent growth analysis. *Psychology of Addictive Behavior, 31*(6), 664–675. doi:10.1037/adb0000304

Rosenstrom, T., Torvik, F. A., Ystrom, E., Czajkowski, N. O., Gillespie, N. A., Aggen, S. H., . . . Reichborn-Kjennerud, T. (2018). Prediction of alcohol use disorder using personality disorder traits: A twin study. *Addiction, 113*(1), 15–24. doi:10.1111/add.13951

Sacks, J. J., Gonzales, K. R., Bouchery, E. E., Tomedi, L. E., & Brewer, R. D. (2015). 2010 national and state costs of excessive alcohol consumption. *American Journal of Preventive Medicne, 49*(5), e73–e79. doi:10.1016/j.amepre.2015.05.031

Sawyer, S. M., Azzopardi, P. S., Wickremarathne, D., & Patton, G. C. (2018). The age of adolescence. *Lancet Child Adolesc Health, 2*(3), 223–228. doi:10.1016/S2352-4642(18)30022-1

Schumann, G., Loth, E., Banaschewski, T., Barbot, A., Barker, G., Buchel, C., . . . IMAGEN Consortium. (2010). The IMAGEN study: Reinforcement-related behaviour in normal brain function and psychopathology. *Molecular Psychiatry, 15*(12), 1128–1139. doi:10.1038/mp.2010.4

Shaw, P., Kabani, N. J., Lerch, J. P., Eckstrand, K., Lenroot, R., Gogtay, N., . . . Wise, S. P. (2008). Neurodevelopmental trajectories of the human cerebral cortex. *Journal of Neuroscience, 28*(14), 3586–3594. doi:10.1523/JNEUROSCI.5309-07.2008

Shollenbarger, S. G., Price, J., Wieser, J., & Lisdahl, K. (2015). Poorer frontolimbic white matter integrity is associated with chronic cannabis use, FAAH genotype, and increased depressive and apathy symptoms in adolescents and young adults. *NeuroImage: Clinical, 8*, 117–125. doi:10.1016/j.nicl.2015.03.024

So, E. S., & Park, B. M. (2016). Health behaviors and academic performance among Korean adolescents. *Asian Nursing Research (Korean Society of Nursing Science), 10*(2), 123–127. doi:10.1016/j.anr.2016.01.004

Somerville, L. H., Jones, R. M., & Casey, B. J. (2010). A time of change: Behavioral and neural correlates of adolescent sensitivity to appetitive and aversive environmental cues. *Brain and Cognition, 72*(1), 124–133. doi:10.1016/j.bandc.2009.07.003

Squeglia, L. M., Ball, T. M., Jacobus, J., Brumback, T., McKenna, B. S., Nguyen-Louie, T. T., . . . Tapert, S. F. (2017). Neural predictors of initiating alcohol use during adolescence. *American Journal of Psychiatry, 174*(2), 172–185. doi:10.1176/appi.ajp.2016.15121587

Squeglia, L. M., Boissoneault, J., Van Skike, C. E., Nixon, S. J., & Matthews, D. B. (2014). Age-related effects of alcohol from adolescent, adult, and aged populations using human and animal models. *Alcoholism: Clinical & Experimental Research, 38*(10), 2509–2516. doi:10.1111/acer.12531

Squeglia, L. M., & Cservenka, A. (2017). Adolescence and drug use vulnerability: Findings from neuroimaging. *Current Opinions in Behavioral Science, 13*, 164–170. doi:10.1016/j.cobeha.2016.12.005

Squeglia, L. M., & Gray, K. M. (2016). Alcohol and drug use and the developing brain. *Current Psychiatry Reports, 18*(5), 46. doi:10.1007/s11920-016-0689-y

Squeglia, L. M., Jacobus, J., Nguyen-Louie, T. T., & Tapert, S. F. (2014). Inhibition during early adolescence predicts alcohol and marijuana use by late adolescence. *Neuropsychology, 28*(5), 782–790. doi:10.1037/neu0000083

Squeglia, L. M., Pulido, C., Wetherill, R. R., Jacobus, J., Brown, G. G., & Tapert, S. F. (2012). Brain response to working memory over three years of adolescence: Influence of initiating heavy drinking. *Journal of Studies on Alcohol & Drugs, 73*(5), 749–760. doi:10.15288/jsad.2012.73.749

Squeglia, L. M., Rinker, D. A., Bartsch, H., Castro, N., Chung, Y., Dale, A. M., . . . Tapert, S. F. (2014). Brain volume reductions in adolescent heavy drinkers. *Developmental Cognitive Neuroscience, 9*, 117–125. doi:10.1016/j.dcn.2014.02.005

Squeglia, L. M., Tapert, S. F., Sullivan, E. V., Jacobus, J., Meloy, M. J., Rohlfing, T., & Pfefferbaum, A. (2015). Brain development in heavy-drinking adolescents. *American Journal of Psychiatry, 172*(6), 531–542. doi:10.1176/appi.ajp.2015.14101249

Stavro, K., Pelletier, J., & Potvin, S. (2013). Widespread and sustained cognitive deficits in alcoholism: A meta-analysis. *Addiction Biology, 18*(2), 203–213. doi:10.1111/j.1369-1600.2011.00418.x

Tapert, S. F., Cheung, E. H., Brown, G. G., Frank, L. R., Paulus, M. P., Schweinsburg, A. D., . . . Brown, S. A. (2003). Neural response to alcohol stimuli in adolescents with alcohol use disorder. *Archives of General Psychiatry, 60*(7), 727–735. doi:10.1001/archpsyc.60.7.727

United Nations, Office on Drugs and Crime (UNODC). (2018). Drugs and age: Associated issues among young people and older people. *World drug report, 2018*. Retrieved from https://www.unodc.org/wdr2018/

Urosevic, S., Collins, P., Muetzel, R., Schissel, A., Lim, K. O., & Luciana, M. (2015). Effects of reward sensitivity and regional brain volumes on substance use initiation in adolescence. *Social Cognitive and Affective Neuroscience, 10*(1), 106–113. doi:10.1093/scan/nsu022

Verhulst, B., Neale, M. C., & Kendler, K. S. (2015). The heritability of alcohol use disorders: A meta-analysis of twin and adoption studies. *Psychological Medicine, 45*(5), 1061–1072. doi:10.1017/S0033291714002165

Volkow, N. D., Koob, G. F., Croyle, R. T., Bianchi, D. W., Gordon, J. A., Koroshetz, W. J., . . . Weiss, S. R. B. (2018). The conception of the ABCD study: From substance use to a broad NIH collaboration. *Developmental Cognitive Neuroscience, 32*, 4–7. doi:10.1016/j.dcn.2017.10.002

Weiland, B. J., Korycinski, S. T., Soules, M., Zubieta, J. K., Zucker, R. A., & Heitzeg, M. M. (2014). Substance abuse risk in emerging adults associated with smaller frontal gray matter volumes and higher externalizing behaviors. *Drug & Alcohol Dependence, 137*, 68–75. doi:10.1016/j.drugalcdep.2014.01.005

Wetherill, R. R., Squeglia, L. M., Yang, T. T., & Tapert, S. F. (2013). A longitudinal examination of adolescent response inhibition: Neural differences before and after the initiation of heavy drinking. *Psychopharmacology, 230*(4), 663–671. doi:10.1007/s00213-013-3198-2

Whelan, R., Watts, R., Orr, C. A., Althoff, R. R., Artiges, E., Banaschewski, T., . . . IMAGEN Consortium. (2014). Neuropsychosocial profiles of current and future adolescent alcohol misusers. *Nature, 512*(7513), 185–189. doi:10.1038/nature13402

Wilson, J., Freeman, T. P., & Mackie, C. J. (2019). Effects of increasing cannabis potency on adolescent health. *Lancet: Child & Adolescent Health, 3*(2), 121–128. doi:10.1016/S2352-4642(18)30342-0

Winward, J. L., Hanson, K. L., Tapert, S. F., & Brown, S. A. (2014). Heavy alcohol use, marijuana use, and concomitant use by adolescents are associated with unique and shared cognitive decrements. *Journal of the International Neuropsychological Society, 20*(8), 784–795. doi:10.1017/S1355617714000666

World Health Organization. (2018). *Global status report on alcohol and health, 2018*. Retrieved from https://www.who.int/substance_abuse/publications/global_alcohol_report/en/

14

Addictive behaviors during emerging adulthood

Eric Wagner, Christine Spadola and Jordan P. Davis

Background

Emerging adulthood is the developmental transition period between adolescence and adulthood, during which expansive and rapid changes in biopsychosocial domains occur. Unfortunately, these changes are accompanied by dramatic elevations in risk for substance use disorder (SUD). Emerging adulthood has the highest SUD risk during the lifespan (Schulenberg & Maggs, 2002; Schulenberg & Zarrett, 2006). This chapter begins by providing a developmental framework for understanding emerging adulthood, with an emphasis on the unique characteristics and challenges of this developmental period which contribute to the elevated risk for substance use problems. Next, we examine prevalence and trends in substance use and SUD among emerging adults, with attention to subgroup variation in risk for substance use problems. We follow this with a review of developmentally appropriate treatment approaches for SUD, considering factors that may directly impact treatment seeking and engagement. We also describe novel areas of research and note marginalized and intersectional subgroups particularly likely to experience SUD. We conclude the chapter with a summary of key points relevant to social work.

Developmental framework

Early developmental theory posited that individuals moved directly from adolescence, the period lasting from puberty through the mid-teens, into early adulthood, spanning from late teens to about age 40 (Erikson, 1950). Through the latter part of the 20th century, developmental theory matured and came to regard the late teens and early 20s as a unique developmental epoch. In 2000, Jeffrey Arnett proposed the *Theory of Emerging Adulthood* to describe the developmental transition between the ages of 18 and 25+ years. Emerging adulthood is an extended period of identity exploration (Arnett, 2000, 2003, 2006) in anticipation of the assumption of traditional adult roles (e.g. career, marriage, buying a home, "settling down," choosing to have children). The transitional and self-exploratory nature of emerging adulthood is accompanied by substantial personality change which can escalate risk for substance use problems (Roberts & Davis, 2016). The notion of emerging adulthood has been embraced in social work, though its popularity appears to have outpaced its thorough empirical examination base (see Coté, 2014; Smith, Dumas, & Davis, 2017).

Dimensions of emerging adulthood

Arnett (2000) discussed five dimensions distinguishing emerging adulthood from earlier and later developmental periods. Below, we discuss each of these dimensions vis-à-vis substance use problems.

Identity exploration

Arnett (2000, 2005) proposed that emerging adulthood is a developmental period of continued identity exploration during which individuals experiment with various life paths related to who they want to be and what they want to do.

Experimentation and possibilities

Emerging adults experiment with possibilities such as career paths, relationships, and higher education, and feel generally positive about their own life goals and opportunities. In terms of substance use, Arnett posits that emerging adults experiment with substances to explore their identity and gain new experiences. In addition, emerging adults' general optimism may translate into believing "nothing bad will happen" as a consequence of using alcohol or other drugs.

Feeling "in between"

Acute awareness of living in between adolescence and adulthood is another defining characteristic of emerging adulthood (Arnett, 2000, 2003, 2006). In the United States, nearly 70% of emerging adults report feeling ambivalent about being a "full adult" (Badger, Nelson, & Barry, 2006). Similar ambivalence among emerging adults has been reported in other developed countries: for example, 55% in Austria (Sirsch, Dreher, Mayr, & Willinger, 2009); 52% in Belgium (Luyckx, Schwartz, Goossens, & Pollock, 2008); 35% in China (Badger et al., 2006); and 26% in India (Seiter & Nelson, 2011). Higher feeling-in-between scores associate with more substance use problems (Smith, Bahar, Cleeland, & Davis, 2014).

Self-focused

Emerging adulthood is a time of increased self-focus, which many scholars believe is a crucial step before assuming adult roles and commitments, such as marriage or buying a house (Shulman & Connolly, 2013). Arnett (2000, 2003, 2006) argued that emerging adulthood involves more freedom, less responsibility, less parental oversight, and more peer approval of risky behavior than any other developmental period. Arnett (2000, 2003, 2006) posited that endorsement of increased self-focus (and, thus, lower other-focus) behaviors allows emerging adults to rationalize heightened substance use during this period. Emerging adults who reported being more other-focused had increased motivation to change problematic drug and alcohol use behavior (Goodman, Henderson, Peterson-Badali, & Goldstein, 2015).

Negativity and instability

Finally, many emerging adults experience new life transitions (e.g. relationships, school, employment, housing) which can interrupt and destabilize identify formation and confidence, leading to negativity/instability. Arnett (2000, 2003, 2006) proposed that emerging adults may use substances to lessen stress and negative feelings associated with this instability.

The general dimensions of emerging adulthood have been linked, conceptually and empirically, to substance use (Arnett, 2005). For example, Baggio, Iglesias, Studer, and Gmel (2015) observed that emerging adults who scored higher on a composite measure of emerging adulthood dimensions experienced more alcohol dependency than emerging adults who scored lower on this measure. Findings, however, are equivocal. Allem, Lisha, Soto, Baezconde-Garbanati, and Unger (2013) found no relation between dimensions of emerging adulthood and substance use. Moreover, scholars have questioned the emerging adulthood construct's generalizability across cultures, socioeconomic status, precocious adult roles (e.g. having children), industrialization, and college attendance.

Recently, Davis, Dumas, Briley, and Sussman (2018) completed a systematic review and meta-analysis of studies assessing associations between substance use and dimensions of emerging adulthood, as measured by the Inventory of the Dimensions of Emerging Adulthood. Across 12 articles included in the meta-analysis, identity exploration , experimentation/possibilities , negativity/instability , and feeling in-between were associated with substance use. While these effects were statistically significant, the effect sizes were relatively small. Among studies that included more college students and assessed alcohol use (versus drug use), associations between dimensions of emerging adulthood and substance use were stronger, suggesting particular utility of the emerging adulthood construct.

Personality change during emerging adulthood

While some dimensions of emerging adulthood appear to be associated with substance use, a large amount of variance remains unexplained. Thus, it is important to consider other psychological theories and constructs that may bear on this period of the lifespan. Modern personality theory has emphasized the five-factor model (BIG Five; for review see McCrae & Costa Jr, 2008), recently expanded to six factors (HEXACO; Ashton et al., 2004; Lee & Ashton, 2004):

- Honesty (H) represents a tendency toward being sincere and fair;
- Emotionality (E) refers to a tendency toward experiencing anxiety, and empathy;
- Extraversion (X) refers to being energetic, talkative, assertive, and enjoying the company of others;
- Agreeableness (A) refers to being good-natured, trustworthy, compassionate, and good-natured;
- Conscientiousness (C) refers to having order and structure, being reliable and dependable, and striving for achievement; and
- Openness to Experience (O) refers to being intelligent, imaginative, and independent-minded (Goldberg, 1992; John & Srivastava, 1999; Pervin & John, 1999; Raynor & Levine, 2009).

Among the HEXACO factors, low conscientiousness is associated with a host of risky behaviors such as substance use (Terracciano, Lockenhoff, Crum, Bienvenu, & Costa, 2008).

Low agreeableness is associated with illicit drug use (e.g. Kilbey, Breslau, & Andreski, 1992; Sáiz, González, Paredes, Martínez, & Delgado, 2001). Studies reported positive associations between openness to experience and current cannabis use (Flory, Lynam, Milich, Leukefeld, & Clayton, 2002; Sher, Bartholow, & Wood, 2000; Terracciano et al., 2008; Trull & Sher, 1994). Higher scores on certain facets of extraversion (e.g. excitement seeking) were also associated with increased substance use (Brooner, Schmidt Jr, & Herbst, 1994; Kornør & Nordvik, 2007; Terracciano et al., 2008; Trémeau et al., 2003). Finally, researchers reported strong associations between low honesty and substance use (Lee, Ashton, & de Vries, 2005). Taken together, substance use appears to be positively associated with personality factors including extraversion and dishonesty, and negatively associated with personality factors including agreeableness, conscientiousness, and openness.

While personality changes are stark during adolescence, changes in traits such as neuroticism, conscientiousness, and agreeableness nearly double during emerging adulthood (see Roberts & Wood, 2006). In a recent theoretical paper, Roberts and Davis (2016) presented a neo-socioanalytic perspective, which conceptualized personality as a developmental construct with both continuity and change across the life span (Roberts, Wood, & Caspi, 2008; Roberts & Mroczek, 2008). In line with this theory, emerging adulthood is a key period for personality growth (Roberts, Walton, & Viechtbauer, 2006; Roberts & Davis, 2016). This growth paves the way for changes that can influence short- and long-term substance use trajectories among emerging adults. Important and somewhat independent influences on substance use include several dimensions of emerging adulthood and several HEXACO factors.

Prevalence and trends

Alcohol and substance use

Emerging adults demonstrated the highest prevalence of substance use, drinking, and binge drinking, among all age cohorts according to U.S. epidemiological data (Grucza et al., 2018; Schulenberg, Johnston, Mieh, O'Malley, Bachman, & Patrick, 2018;). Based on results from the 2017 Monitoring the Future Survey (Johnston et al., 2018), alcohol constituted the most commonly used substance among emerging adults in the United States; 82% of 19–30-year-olds reported past-year drinking, 68% in the past month, and 5.2% daily drinking. Binge drinking was also common in this age group; nearly one-third (31.4%) reported consuming five or more drinks in a row at some point during the last two weeks, 10.9% consumed ten or more drinks in a row, and 3.3% consumed 15 or more drinks in a row. Close to half (41.2%) used illegal drugs at least once during the past year: a 9% jump since 2006. In 2017, marijuana was the illegal drug most commonly used by emerging adults, with 37.5% reporting use in the past year, 23% reporting use in the past month, and 7.8% reporting daily or near daily use. Twenty percent of emerging adults reported using illicit drugs other than marijuana during the past year: 7.8% amphetamines, 5.9% non-crack cocaine, 4.7% tranquilizers, 4.6% hallucinogens, 4.0% nonmedical use of narcotics other than heroin, 3.6% MDMA (molly, ecstasy), 3.4% LSD, and 2.2% sedatives/barbiturates.

Alcohol and substance use disorders

The prevalence of alcohol and substance use disorders is also high among emerging adults. An international study conducted with first-year college students (n = 13,894) from eight industrialized countries reported that 6.3% met criteria for an alcohol use disorder and 3% for a substance use disorder during the past 12 months (Auerbach et al., 2018). It is important to note that, due to varying methodology and time frames of the extant research, international comparisons among prevalence estimates has not been possible.

Subgroup variation

The prevalence of alcohol and drug use among emerging adults varies by gender, current educational status, race/ethnicity, and internalized stigma.

- Gender. Males demonstrated a higher prevalence of alcohol and illicit drug use, as well as alcohol and substance use disorders, compared to females (Johnston et al., 2018). Of note, gender differences in alcohol consumption, especially among adults, has been decreasing over the past several decades.
- College student status. College students in the U.S. demonstrate higher rates of binge drinking than non-college attending emerging adults (33% vs. 28% respectively). However, non-college attending emerging adults tend to demonstrate higher rates of illicit drug use than their college attending peers (Johnston et al., 2018).
- Race/ethnicity. In the United States, Native American emerging adults report high rates of alcohol and drug use (Johnston et al., 2018). Elevated risk for alcohol and substance use problems among indigenous people have been documented in Australia and Canada, as well (Jainullabudeen et al., 2015; Marsh, Coholic, Cote-Meek, & Najavits, 2015). Non-Hispanic white emerging adults also have elevated rates of alcohol and substance use problems, with higher a prevalence of alcohol use and substance use disorders compared to African American, Hispanic/Latinx, and Asian American emerging adults (Adams, Knopf, & Park; 2014; Park, McCoy, Erausquin, & Bartlett, 2018).
- Internalized Stigma. Finally, Native American college students demonstrated higher rates of alcohol use disorders than non-Hispanic white college students (Blanco et al., 2008). This appears to be conditioned by internalized stigma, including Native American college students' self-perceived biological, psychological, or social vulnerabilities related to the "firewater myth" (Gonzalez & Skewes, 2018).

Mental health comorbidities

Emerging adulthood also represents the developmental phase during which mental health disorders most typically first manifest. In the United States, most individuals (75%) who experience a mental health disorder have their first episode during emerging adulthood, by age 24 years (Copeland, Shanahan, Costello, & Angold, 2011; Kessler et al., 2005). International research conducted with 13,894 first-year college students reported that 35.3% had a lifetime anxiety, mood, or substance disorder, and 31.4% a past-year anxiety, mood, or substance disorder (Auerbach et al., 2018).

Substance use disorders commonly co-occur with anxiety disorders, depressive disorders, bipolar disorders, ADHD, borderline personality disorder, antisocial personality disorder, and schizophrenia (see Chapter 33). Research indicates genetic vulnerabilities, epigenetics, neurobiology, environment, exposure to stress, and trauma conspire to produce high comorbidity (National Institute of Drug Abuse, 2018). It is important to note that suicide is a leading cause of death among individuals of any age experiencing substance use disorders, and especially those experiencing co-occurring psychiatric disorders (Becker, Dvorsky, Holdaway, & Luebbe, 2018; Center for Substance Abuse Treatment, 2008; Han et al., 2018). Also, there exists notable subgroup variation in co-occurring disorders. Women, in both emerging adult and adult populations, have a higher prevalence of most mental health disorders, particularly depression and anxiety. Longitudinal research conducted in Brazil also demonstrated higher rates of alcohol and substance use disorders among males, and higher rates of mental health disorders among females (Andreoli et al., 2014; Macinko, Mullachery, Silver, Jimenez, & Libanio Morais Neto, 2015).

SUD treatment for emerging adults

Compared to adults, emerging adults experiencing substance use problems are less likely to: (a) perceive a need for treatment, (b) seek treatment, (c) respond to treatment, or (d) complete treatment (Adams et al., 2014; Bergman, Kelly, Nargiso, & McKowen, 2016). Emerging adults who do receive treatment typically have a history of early-onset and chronic substance use problems; earlier intervention would have reduced the severity of SUDs and risk of relapse (De Girolamo, Dagani, Purcell, Cocchi, & McGorry, 2012). However, when engaged in SUD treatment, emerging adults reap benefits on par with older adults who complete treatment (Bergman et al., 2016).

Among emerging adults experiencing SUD of mild to moderate severity, motivational interviewing, motivational engagement, and cognitive behavioral treatment (CBT) are evidence-based practices with demonstrated effectiveness (see https://www.samhsa.gov/ebp-resource-center/about). Motivational approaches to SUD concentrate on client's ambivalence and avoid confrontation and related tactics that may provoke defensiveness and resistance among individuals experiencing substance use problems (Miller & Rollnick, 1991, 2002, 2013; Wagner, 2013). As noted by the Substance Abuse and Mental Health Service Administration (SAMHSA; see TIP Series, No. 35, 2013), motivational engagement is especially useful for: (a) rapid engagement in medical settings to facilitate referral to treatment; (b) a first session to increase the likelihood that a client will return; (c) planting a seed even if the client does not return; (d) preparation for treatment to increase engagement and participation; (e) a cost-effective primary approach; (f) a complement to other therapies; (g) aiding clients to move beyond initial feelings of anger and resentment; (h) overcoming client defensiveness and resistance; and (i) differing stages of readiness to change. Motivational engagement is well-suited to handle, and leverage for change, emerging adolescents' identity exploration, experimentation with possibilities, self-focus, and negativity and instability.

CBT represents the integration of behavioral theory, cognitive social learning theory, and cognitive therapy (see Chapter 18). The approach is here-and-now focused, action-oriented, problem-focused, and time-limited—all qualities that emerging adults may find especially appropriate. CBT is devoted to identifying distorted ways of thinking impairing day-to-day functioning, modifying thinking toward more adaptive and realistic beliefs, enhancing social skills, and promoting positive healthful behaviors. CBT for substance use problems typically employs functional analysis of substance use behavior, the development of alternative activities to substance use, engagement non-substance-involved stress-coping strategies, setting and achieving goals, and relapse prevention. An overarching goal of CBT is to make clients more aware of their thoughts, feelings, and behaviors and develop skills to end or reduce their substance use, reach their goals, and improve health and well-being. A final attractive feature of CBT is the availability of integrated approaches that treat SUD and co-occurring psychopathology together—such as co-occurring SUD and major depressive disorder (Lydecker et al., 2010) or posttraumatic stress disorder (McGovern, Lambert-Harris, Xie, Meier, McLeman, & Saunders, 2015).

Among emerging adults experiencing SUD of greater severity, residential inpatient or intensive outpatient treatment, supplemented by mutual help groups, has been found to be effective (Bergman, Greene, Slaymaker, Hoeppner, & Kelly, 2014; Kelly, Stout, Greene, & Slaymaker, 2014; Ray, Weisner, & Mertens, 2005; Schuman-Olivier, Greene, Bergman, & Kelly, 2014). Especially in cases of severe SUD and co-occurring psychiatric disorder, residential treatment with integrated detoxification, pharmacological, and psychotherapeutic services is indicated. A growing number of emerging adults are seeking treatment for opioid use disorders, but they are less likely to remain in treatment, cease illicit drug use, or benefit from treatment compared to older clients experiencing opioid use problems (Kelly, Stout, & Slaymaker, 2013).

Bergman and colleagues described reasons why treatment of substance use problems among emerging adults is particularly challenging, including (a) the biopsychosocial idiosyncrasies of this life stage; (b) low initial motivation for treatment engagement and abstinence; (c) the life stage wherein the highest rates of alcohol and other drug use occur; (d) the high likelihood of co-occurring psychiatric problems; (e) a disconnect between service accessibility and lifestyle hours and habits; (f) a life stage (and time in history) when polydrug use is common; and (g) a life stage (and time in history) when peer social influences are profound. Elswick, Fallin-Bennett, Ashford, and Werner-Wilson (2018) also pointed out that financial challenges, financial transitions, and issues of financial (in)dependence associated with emerging adulthood may directly compromise treatment access, utilization, and retention.

Services for addressing substance use problems among emerging adults need to be compassionate, effective, efficient, and culturally, linguistically, and developmentally appropriate. We believe strongly that a novel service model is needed, including an overarching environmental focus on reducing SUD stigma, and increasing awareness, help-seeking, and treatment acceptability among emerging adults. The model would be overlapping with but discrete in culture and expertise from systems for younger or older people. Attention to subthreshold cases (i.e. substance misuse) is essential to reduce the incidence and severity of SUDs through screening, early identification, and accessible in-person, on-line (e.g. Therapy Assistance Online [TAO]), or mobile brief intervention (see Berman, Gajecki, Sinadinovic, & Andersson, 2016). Smartphone and social media platforms are well integrated in the emerging adult lifestyle; assertive mobile detection strategies may be especially helpful for hard-to-reach cases. In addition, activity bracelets, smart watches, and wearable sensors are emergent technologies particularly well-suited for therapeutic applications with emerging adults experiencing substance use problems.

An improved model would also emphasize SUD literacy, which can be surprisingly low even among emerging adults enrolled in college (Rafal, Gatto, & DeBate, 2018). Literacy in the present case refers to the ability to recognize and understand characteristics of SUDs, including risks, causes, and when and how to obtain resources and engage services. Enhancing SUD literacy among key gatekeepers (e.g. managers and supervisors for emerging adults in the workforce, faculty, and residence life staff for emerging adult in college) is also important (see GKT program, Mental Health First Aid [Lipson, Speer, Brunwasser, Hahn, & Eisenberg, 2014]). Gatekeepers need to know about the continuum of substance use behaviors, symptoms of substance misuse and SUD, the prevention and treatment of SUDs, and local and national resources and referral options.

Special consideration: sleep and SUD

Inadequate sleep (e.g. short sleep duration, sleep fragmentation) is receiving increasing attention as a modifiable risk factor for substance use initiation, SUD, and SUD relapse

(Brower, 2001; Chakravorty, Chaudhary, & Brower, 2016; Conroy & Arnedt, 2014; Wong, Brower, & Craun, 2016). Approximately 70% of emerging adults report poor sleep quality or lack of sufficient sleep (Lund, Reider, Whiting, & Prichard, 2010). Prospective preliminary studies identified associations between inadequate sleep and subsequent alcohol and marijuana use, along with substance-related problems, among substance-naïve adolescents and emerging adults (Miller et al., 2018; Wong, Robertson, & Dyson, 2015). Among emerging adults, poor sleep quality, and inadequate sleep are associated with a greater risk for negative consequences related to drinking (Kenney, LaBrie, Hummer, & Pham, 2012). Moreover, binge drinking during adolescence is associated with lower self-reported sleep quality during emerging adulthood (Ehlers, Wills, & Gilder, 2018). Mental health disorders, suicidal ideation, suicide attempts, and completed suicide all are associated with inadequate sleep among emerging adults and adults (Becker et al., 2018; Han et al., 2013; Pigeon, Pinquart, & Conner, 2012; Russell et al., 2019).

Sleep also appears to be an important predictor of long-term response to SUD treatment. Nearly 20 research studies, constituting both subjective and objective (i.e. polysomnography) assessments, documented associations between sleep issues and alcohol use relapse (Brower, 2015; Conroy & Arnedt, 2014). Sleep onset latency, or difficulty falling asleep, is the most common issue associated with alcohol relapse; postulated reasons for the association include impaired decision making and increased sensitivity to stress associated with inadequate sleep (Brower, 2001). Substance use (and withdrawal) is associated with poor sleep (Roehrs, Papineau, Rosenthal, & Roth, 1999; Schierenbeck, Riemann, Berger, & Hornyak, 2008), and SUDs are often comorbid with insomnia (Brower, 2001; Chakravorty et al., 2016; Schierenbeck et al., 2008; Wong et al., 2016).

Special considerations: homeless emerging adults and foster care alumni

Emerging adults who are homeless are at especially heighted risk for substance use problems; SAMHSA estimated that 26% of homeless individuals abuse drugs, and 38% are dependent on alcohol (SAMHSA, 2015). More recently, Foster, Gable, and Buckley (2012) estimated between 38–68% of homeless individuals experience alcohol problems, and 24–37% experience drug problems. Moreover, two-thirds of homeless persons reported alcohol and/or drug use as a major reason for their becoming homeless (Didenko & Pankratz, 2007).

Intersectionality characterizes homeless emerging adults, who disproportionately are racial/ethnic or sexual minorities. LGBTQ+ individuals are up to four times more likely to experience alcohol and substance use problems, and are at much greater risk for homelessness, than heterosexual individuals (Burwick, Gates, Baumgartner, & Friend, 2014; Hatzenbuehler, 2011; Silvestre, Beatty, & Friedman, 2013). Homeless emerging adults may also be foster care alumni, having aged out of the system. Emerging adult foster care alumni demonstrated significantly higher rates of lifetime and past-year alcohol and substance use disorders than individuals never involved in foster care (Braciszewski & Stout, 2012).

Despite their high prevalence of substance use problems, only 9% of homeless individuals perceived SUD treatment as something they needed "right now" (Healing Hands, 2003). Similarly, emerging adults were less motivated to seek SUD treatment and harder to retain in SUD treatment than older adults (Al-Tayyib, Rice, Rhoades, & Riggs, 2014; Bergman et al., 2014). LGBTQ+ individuals experienced substantial barriers to seeking and receiving SUD treatment, which led to low rates of treatment utilization (Allen & Mowbray, 2016). A similar gap between SUD treatment need and availability/utilization existed among foster care alumni (Braciszewski & Stout, 2012). For individuals who simultaneously are emerging adults, homeless, and LGBTQ+, and/or foster care alumni, barriers to seeking, accessing, and completing SUD treatment are compounded.

Conclusions

Emerging adults (ages 18 to 24+ years) experience more substance use problems than any other age group, regardless of gender, race/ethnicity, and international boundaries. Despite this, emerging adults are less likely to seek or receive treatment for their substance-related problems. However, emerging adults can benefit from completing evidence-based treatment for substance use problems, especially when social support for recovery is emphasized.

Emerging adulthood is characterized by identity exploration, experimentation, feeling in between, self-focus, and negativity and instability. These dimensions have been linked, conceptually and empirically, to substance use, and need to be considered when tailoring developmentally appropriate approaches to SUD among emerging adults. Moreover, emerging adulthood is a key time for personality growth that can influence short- and long-term substance use trajectories. Emerging adults also experience more mental health disorders than any other age group and are especially likely to experience co-occurring SUD and psychiatric problems, which complicates SUD treatment. While SUDs among emerging adolescents are multiply determined, sleep dysregulation is receiving growing recognition as a potentially modifiable contributor to substance use problems. Finally, while all emerging adults are at heightened risk for SUD, it is important to note that marginalized and intersectional populations like homeless emerging adolescents are at especially high risk for substance use problems.

Social work course offerings on emerging adults are quite limited. Among the schools of social work with which we are affiliated, there is no course, required or elective, devoted to emerging adults. This needs to change. Emerging adulthood is a remarkably unique developmental period and carries with it a remarkably elevated risk for alcohol and drug use problems, as well as other mental health problems. Strategic course development on emerging adulthood for undergraduate, masters, doctoral, and post-doctoral social work students is urgently needed. Moreover, it is important to recognize that most university students are emerging adults, speaking to the personal relevance of course content addressing emerging adulthood.

References

Adams, S. H., Knopf, D. K., & Park, M. J. (2014). Prevalence and treatment of mental health and substance use problems in the early emerging adult years in the United States: Findings from the 2010 national survey on drug use and health. *Emerging Adulthood, 2*(3), 163–172. doi:10.1177/2167696813513563

Allem, J., Lisha, N. E., Soto, D. W., Baezconde-Garbanati, L., & Unger, J. B. (2013). Emerging adulthood themes, role transitions and substance use among Hispanics in southern California. *Addictive Behaviors, 38*(12), 2797–2800. doi:10.1016/j.addbeh.2013.08.001

Allen, J. L., & Mowbray, O. (2016). Sexual orientation, treatment utilization, and barriers for alcohol related problems: Findings from a nationally representative sample. *Drug and Alcohol Dependence, 161*, 323–330. doi:10.1016/j.drugalcdep.2016.02.025

Al-Tayyib, A. A., Rice, E, Rhoades, H, & Riggs, P. (2014) Association between prescription drug misuse and injection among runaway and homeless youth. *Drug Alcohol Dependence*, 134, 406–409. doi:10.1016/j.drugalcdep.2013.10.027

Andreoli, S. B., Dos Santos, M. M., Quintana, M. I., Ribeiro, W. S., Blay, S. L., Taborda, J. G., & de Jesus Mari, J. (2014). Prevalence of mental disorders among prisoners in the state of Sao Paulo, Brazil. *PloS One, 9*(2), e88836. doi:10.1371/journal.pone.0088836

Arnett, J. J. (2000). Emerging adulthood: A theory of development from the late teens through the twenties. *American Psychologist, 55*(5), 469–480. doi:10.1037/0003-066X.55.5.469

Arnett, J. J. (2003). Conceptions of the transition to adulthood among emerging adults in American ethnic groups. *New Directions for Child and Adolescent Development, 2003*(100), 63–75. doi:10.1002/cd.75

Arnett, J. J. (2005). Developmental context of substance use in emerging adulthood. *Journal of Drug Issues, 35*(2), 235–254. doi:10.1177/002204260503500202

Arnett, J. J. (2006). Emerging adulthood: Understanding the new way of coming of age. In J. J. Arnett, & J. L. Tanner (Eds.), *Emerging adults in America: Coming of age in the 21st century* (pp. 3–19, Chapter xxii, 340 pp.). Washington, DC: American Psychological Association. doi:10.1093/acprof:oso/9780195309379.001.0001

Ashton, M. C., Lee, K., Perugini, M., Szarota, P., de Vries, R. E., Di Blas, L., . . . De Raad, B. (2004). A six-factor structure of personality-descriptive adjectives: Solutions from psycholexical studies in seven languages. *Journal of Personality and Social Psychology, 86*(2), 356–366. doi:10.1037/0022-3514.86.2.356

Auerbach, R. P., Mortier, P., Bruffaerts, R., Alonso, J., Benjet, C., Cuijpers, P., . . . WHO WMH-ICS Collaborators. (2018). WHO world mental health surveys international college student project: Prevalence and distribution of mental disorders. *Journal of Abnormal Psychology, 127*(7), 623–638. doi:10.1037/abn0000362

Badger, S., Nelson, L. J., & Barry, C. M. (2006). Perceptions of the transition to adulthood among Chinese and American emerging adults. *International Journal of Behavioral Development, 30*(1), 84–93. doi:10.1177/0165025406062128

Baggio, S., Iglesias, K., Studer, J., & Gmel, G. (2015). An 8-item short form of the Inventory of dimensions of emerging adulthood (IDEA) among young Swiss men. *Evaluation & the Health Professions, 38*(2), 246–254. doi:10.1177/0163278714540681

Becker, S. P., Dvorsky, M. R., Holdaway, A. S., & Luebbe, A. M. (2018). Sleep problems and suicidal behaviors in college students. *Journal of Psychiatric Research, 99*, 122–128. doi:10.1016/j.jpsychires.2018.01.009

Bergman, B. G., Greene, M. C., Slaymaker, V., Hoeppner, B. B., & Kelly, J. F. (2014). Young adults with co-occurring disorders: Substance use disorder treatment response and outcomes. *Journal of Substance Abuse Treatment, 46*(4), 420–428. doi:10.1016/j.jsat.2013.11.005

Bergman, B. G., Hoeppner, B. B., Nelson, L. M., Slaymaker, V., & Kelly, J. F. (2015). The effects of continuing care on emerging adult outcomes following residential addiction treatment. *Drug and Alcohol Dependence, 153*, 207–214. doi:10.1016/j.drugalcdep.2015.05.017

Bergman, B. G., Kelly, J. F., Nargiso, J. E., & McKowen, J. W. (2016). "The age of feeling in-between": Addressing challenges in the treatment of emerging adults with substance use disorders. *Cognitive and Behavioral Practice, 23*(3), 270–288. doi:10.1016/j.cbpra.2015.09.008

Berman, A. H., Gajecki, M., Sinadinovic, K., & Andersson, C. (2016). Mobile interventions targeting risky drinking among university students: A review. *Current Addiction Reports, 3*, 166–174. doi:10.1007/s40429-016-0099-6

Blanco, C., Okuda, M., Wright, C., Hasin, D. S., Grant, B. F., Liu, S. M., & Olfson, M. (2008). Mental health of college students and their non-college-attending peers: Results from the national epidemiologic study on alcohol and related conditions. *Archives of General Psychiatry, 65*(12), 1429–1437. doi:10.1001/archpsyc.65.12.1429

Braciszewski, J. M., & Stout, R. L. (2012). Substance use among current and former foster youth: A systematic review. *Children and Youth Services Review, 34*(12), 2337–2344. doi:10.1016/j.childyouth.2012.08.011

Brooner, R. K., Schmidt, C. W., Jr., & Herbst, J. H. (1994). In P. T., Jr. Costa & T. A. Widiger (Eds.), *Personality trait characteristics of opioid abusers with and without comorbid personality disorders* (pp. 131–148). Washington, DC: American Psychological Association.

Brower, K. J. (2001). Alcohol's effects on sleep in alcoholics. *Alcohol Research & Health: The Journal of the National Institute on Alcohol Abuse and Alcoholism, 25*(2), 110–125.

Brower, K. J. (2015). Assessment and treatment of insomnia in adult patients with alcohol use disorders. *Alcohol, 49*(4), 417–427. doi: 10.1016/j/alcohol.2014.12.003

Burwick, A., Gates, G., Baumgartner, S., & Friend, D. (2014). *Human services for low-income and at-risk LGBT populations: The knowledge base and research needs (brief)*. Washington, DC: Office of Planning, Research and Evaluation Administration for Children and Families U.S. Department of Health and Human Services.

Center for Substance Abuse Treatment. (2008). *Substance abuse and suicide prevention: Evidence and implications—A white paper* (DHHS Publication No. SMA-08-4352). Rockville, MD: Substance Abuse and Mental Health Services Administration.

Chakravorty. S., Chaudhary, N.S., & Brower, K. J. (2016). Alcohol dependence and its relationship with insomnia and other sleep disorders. *Alcoholism: Clinical Experimental Research, 40*, 2271–2282. doi:10.1111/acer.13217

Conroy, D. A., & Arnedt, J. T. (2014). Sleep and substance use disorders: An update. *Current Psychiatry Reports, 16*(10), 487. doi:10.1007/s11920-014-0487-3

Copeland, W., Shanahan, L., Costello, E. J., & Angold, A. (2011). Cumulative prevalence of psychiatric disorders by young adulthood: A prospective cohort analysis from the Great Smoky Mountains study. *Journal of the American Academy of Child & Adolescent Psychiatry, 50*(3), 252–261. doi:10.1016/j.jaac.2010.12.014

Coté, J. E. (2014). The dangerous myth of emerging adulthood: An evidence-based critique of a flawed developmental theory. *Applied Developmental Science, 18*, 177–188. doi:10.1080/10888691.2014.954451

Davis, J. P., Dumas, T. M., Briley, D. A., & Sussman, S. (2018). A meta-analysis of the association between substance use and emerging adult development using the IDEA scale. *The American Journal on Addictions, 27*(3), 166–176. doi:10.1111/ajad.12707

De Girolamo, G., Dagani, J., Purcell, R., Cocchi, A., & McGorry, P. D. (2012). Age of onset of mental disorders and use of mental health services: Needs, opportunities and obstacles. *Epidemiology and Psychiatric Sciences, 21*(1), 47–57. doi:10.1017/S2045796011000746

Didenko, E., & Pankratz, N. (2007). Substance use: Pathways to homelessness? Or a way of adapting to street life. *Visions: BC's Mental Health and Addictions Journal, 4*(1), 9–10.

Ehlers, C. L., Wills, D., & Gilder, D. A. (2018). A history of binge drinking during adolescence is associated with poorer sleep quality in young adult Mexican Americans and American Indians. *Psychopharmacology, 235*(6), 1775–1782. doi:10.1007/s00213-018-4889-5

Elswick, A., Fallin-Bennett, A., Ashford, K., & Werner-Wilson, R. (2018). Emerging adults and recovery capital: Barriers and facilitators to recovery. *Journal of Addictions Nursing, 29*(2), 78–83. doi:10.1097/JAN.0000000000000218

Erikson, E. H. (1950). *Childhood and society.* New York, NY: W. W. Norton & Co.

Flory, K., Lynam, D., Milich, R., Leukefeld, C., & Clayton, R. (2002). The relations among personality, symptoms of alcohol and marijuana abuse, and symptoms of comorbid psychopathology: Results from a community sample. *Experimental and Clinical Psychopharmacology, 10*(4), 425–434. doi:10.1037/1064-1297.10.4.425

Foster, A., Gable, J., & Buckley, J. (2012). Homelessness in schizophrenia. *Psychiatric Clinics, 35*(3), 717–734. doi:10.1016/j.psc.2012.06.010

Goldberg, L. R. (1992). The development of markers for the big-five factor structure. *Psychological Assessment, 4*(1), 26. doi:10.1037/1040-3590.4.1.26

Gonzalez, V. M., & Skewes, M. C. (2018). Association of belief in the "firewater myth" with strategies to avoid alcohol consequences among American Indian and Alaska Native college students who drink. *Psychology of Addictive Behaviors, 32*(4), 401–409. doi:10.1037/adb0000367

Goodman, I., Henderson, J., Peterson-Badali, M., & Goldstein, A. L. (2015). The relationship between psychosocial features of emerging adulthood and substance use change motivation in youth. *Journal of Substance Abuse Treatment, 52*, 58–66. doi:10.1016/j.jsat.2014.12.004

Grucza, R. A., Sher, K. J., Kerr, W. C., Krauss, M. J., Lui, C. K., McDowell, Y. E., Hartz, S., Virdi, G., & Bierut, L. J. (2018). Trends in adult alcohol use and binge drinking in the early 21st-century United States: A meta-analysis of 6 national survey series. *Alcohol: Clinical & Experimental Research, 42*(10), 1939–1950. doi: 10.111/acer.13859

Han, B., Compton, W. M., Blanco, C., Colpe, L., Huang, L., & McKeon, R. (2018). National trends in the prevalence of suicidal ideation and behavior among young adults and receipt of mental health care among suicidal young adults. *Journal of the American Academy of Child & Adolescent Psychiatry, 57*(1), 20–27. doi:10.1016/j.jaac.2017.10.013

Hatzenbuehler, M. L. (2011). The social environment and suicide attempts in lesbian, gay, and bisexual youth. *Pediatrics, 127*(5), 896. doi:10.1542/peds.2010-3020

Healing Hands. (2003). A comprehensive approach to substance abuse and homelessness. *Healing Hands: A Publication of the HCN Clinicians' Network, 7*, 1–3.

Jainullabudeen, T. A., Lively, A., Singleton, M., Shakeshaft, A., Tsey, K., McCalman, J., . . . Jacups, S. (2015). The impact of a community-based risky drinking intervention (beat da binge) on indigenous young people. *BMC Public Health, 15*, 1319. doi:10.1186/s12889-015-2675-4

John, O. P., & Srivastava, S. (1999). The big five trait taxonomy: History, measurement, and theoretical perspectives. In L. A. Pervin & O. P. John (Eds.), *Handbook of personality: Theory and research* (2nd ed., pp. 102–138, Chapter xiii, 738 pp.). New York, NY: Guilford Press. doi:10.3998/2027.42/148123

Johnston, L. D., Miech, R. A., O'Malley, P. M., Bachman, J. G., Schulenberg, J. E., & Patrick, M. E. (2018). Monitoring the future national survey results on drug use: 1975–2017: Overview, key findings on adolescent drug use. Ann Arbor: Institute for Social Research, The University of Michigan. doi:10.3998/2027.42/148123

Kelly, J. F., Stout, R. L., Greene, M. C., & Slaymaker, V. (2014). Young adults, social networks, and addiction recovery: Post treatment changes in social ties and their role as a mediator of 12-step participation. *PLoS One, 9*(6) doi:10.1371/journal.pone.0100121

Kelly, J. F., Stout, R. L., & Slaymaker, V. (2013). Emerging adults' treatment outcomes in relation to 12-step mutual-help attendance and active involvement. *Drug and Alcohol Dependence, 129*(1–2), 151–157. doi:10.1016/j.drugalcdep.2012.10.005

Kenney, S. R., LaBrie, J. W., Hummer, J. F., & Pham, A. T. (2012). Global sleep quality as a moderator of alcohol consumption and consequences in college students. *Addictive Behaviors, 37*(4), 507–512. doi:10.1016/j.addbeh.2012.01.006

Kessler, R. C., Berglund, P., Demler, O., Jin, R., Merikangas, K. R., & Walters, E. E. (2005). Lifetime prevalence and age-of-onset distributions of DSM-IV disorders in the national comorbidity survey replication. *Archives of General Psychiatry, 62*(6), 593–602. doi:10.1001/archpsyc.62.6.593

Kilbey, M. M., Breslau, N., & Andreski, P. (1992). Cocaine use and dependence in young adults: Associated psychiatric disorders and personality traits. *Drug and Alcohol Dependence, 29*(3), 283–290. doi:10.1016/0376-8716(92)90103-J

Kornør, H., & Nordvik, H. (2007). Five-factor model personality traits in opioid dependence. *BMC Psychiatry, 7*, 6. doi:10.1186/1471-244X-7-37

Lee, K., & Ashton, M. C. (2004). Psychometric properties of the HEXACO personality inventory. *Multivariate Behavioral Research, 39*(2), 329–358. doi:10.1207/s15327906mbr3902_8

Lee, K., Ashton, M.C., & de Vries, R. E. (2005). Predicting workplace deliquency with the HEXACO and five-factor models of personality structure. *Human Performance, 18*(2), 179–197. doi:10.1207/s15327043hup1802_4

Lipson, S.K., Speer, N., Brunwasser, S., Hahn, E., & Eisenberg, D. (2014). Gatekeeper training and access to mental health care at universities and colleges, *Journal of Adolescent Health, 55*, 612–619. doi:10.1016/j.jadohealth.2014.05.009

Lund, H. G., Reider, B. D., Whiting, A. B., & Prichard, J. R. (2010). Sleep patterns and predictors of disturbed sleep in a large population of college students. *Journal of Adolescent Health*, 46(2), 124–132. doi:10.1016/j.jadohealth.2009.06.016

Luyckx, K., Schwartz, S. J., Goossens, L., & Pollock, S. (2008). Employment, sense of coherence, and identity formation: Contextual and psychological processes on the pathway to sense of adulthood. *Journal of Adolescent Research, 23*(5), 566–591. doi:10.1177/0743558408322146

Lydecker, K. P., Tate, S. R., Cummins, K. M., McQuaid, J., Granholm, E., & Brown, S. A. (2010). Clinical outcomes of an integrated treatment for depression and substance use disorders. *Psychology of Addictive Behaviors, 24*(3), 453. doi:10.1037/a0019943

Macinko, J., Mullachery, P., Silver, D., Jimenez, G., & Libanio Morais Neto, O. (2015) Patterns of alcohol consumption and related behaviors in Brazil: Evidence from the 2013 national health survey (PNS 2013). *PLOS One, 10*(7), e0134153. doi:10.1371/journal.pone.0134153

Marsh, T. N., Coholic, D., Cote-Meek, S., & Najavits, L. M. (2015). Blending aboriginal and western healing methods to treat intergenerational trauma with substance use disorder in aboriginal peoples who live in northeastern Ontario, Canada. *Harm Reduction Journal, 12*, 14. doi:10.1186/s12954-015-0046-1

McCrae, R. R., & Costa, P. T., Jr. (2008). The five-factor theory of personality. In O. P. John, R. W. Robins, & L. A. Pervin (Eds.), *Handbook of personality: Theory and research* (3rd ed., pp. 159–181, Chapter xv, 862 pp.). New York, NY: The Guilford Press.

McGovern, M. P., Lambert-Harris, C., Xie, H., Meier, A., McLeman, B., & Saunders, E. (2015). A randomized controlled trial of treatments for co-occurring substance use disorders and post-traumatic stress disorder. *Addiction, 110*, 1194–1204. doi:10.1111/add.12943

Miller, M. B., Chan, W. S., Boissoneault, J., Robinson, M., Staud, R., Berry, R. B., & McCrae, C. S. (2018). Dynamic daily associations between insomnia symptoms and alcohol use in adults with chronic pain. *Journal of Sleep Research, 27*, e12604. doi:10.1111/jsr.12604

Miller, W. R., & Rollnick, S. (1991). *Motivational interviewing: Preparing people to change addictive behavior.* New York, NY: The Guilford Press.

Miller, W. R., & Rollnick, S. (2002). *Motivational interviewing: Preparing people for change* (2nd ed.). New York, NY: The Guilford Press. doi:10.1097/01445442-200305000-00013

Miller, W. R., & Rollnick, S. (2013). *Motivational interviewing third edition helping people change.* New York, NY: The Guilford Press.

National Institute of Drug Abuse (NIDA). (2018, February 27). Common comorbidities with substance use disorders. Retrieved May 23, 2019, from https://www.drugabuse.gov/publications/research-reports/common-comorbidities-substance-use-disorders on 2019, May 23.

Park, E., McCoy, T. P., Erausquin, J. T., & Bartlett, R. (2018). Trajectories of risk behaviors across adolescence and young adulthood: The role of race and ethnicity. *Addictive Behaviors, 76*, 1–7. doi:10.1016/j.addbeh.2017.07.014

Pervin, L. A., & John, O. P. (Eds.). (1999). *Handbook of personality: Theory and research* (2nd ed.). New York, NY: The Guilford Press.

Pigeon, W. R., Pinquart, M., & Conner, K. (2012). Meta-analysis of sleep disturbance and suicidal thoughts and behaviors. *The Journal of Clinical Psychiatry, 73*, e1160–e1167. doi:10.4088/JCP.11r07586

Rafal, G., Gatto, A., & DeBate, R. (2018). Mental health literacy, stigma, and help-seeking behaviors among male college students. *Journal of American College Health, 66*(4), 284–291. doi:10.1080/07448481.2018.1434780

Ray, G. T., Weisner, C. M., & Mertens, J. R. (2005). Relationship between use of psychiatric services and five-year alcohol and drug treatment outcomes. *Psychiatric Services, 56*(2), 164–171. doi:10.1176/appi.ps.56.2.164

Raynor, D. A., & Levine, H. (2009). Associations between the five-factor model of personality and health behaviors among college students. *Journal of American College Health, 58*(1), 73–82. doi:10.3200/JACH.58.1.73-82

Roberts, B. W., & Davis, J. P. (2016). Young adulthood is the crucible of personality development. *Emerging Adulthood*, 1–9. doi:10.1177/2167696816653052

Roberts, B. W., & Mroczek, D. (2008). Personality trait change in adulthood. *Current Directions in Psychological Science, 17*(1), 31–35. doi:10.1111/j.1467-8721.2008.00543.x

Roberts, B. W., Walton, K. E., & Viechtbauer, W. (2006). Patterns of mean-level change in personality traits across the life course: A meta-analysis of longitudinal studies. *Psychological Bulletin, 132*(1), 1–25. doi:10.1037/0033-2909.132.1.1

Roberts, B. W., & Wood, D. (2006). *Personality development in the context of the neo-socioanalytic model of personality* (Chapter 2, pp. 11–39). In D. Mroczek & T. Little (Eds.), *Handbook of personality development.* Mahwah, NJ: Lawrence Erlbaum Associates.

Roberts, B. W., Wood, D., & Caspi, A. (2008). The development of personality traits in adulthood. In O. P. John, R. W. Robins, & L. A. Pervin (Eds.), *Handbook of personality: Theory and research* (3rd ed., pp. 375–398, Chapter xv, 862 pp.). New York, NY: The Guilford Press.

Roehrs, T., Papineau, K., Rosenthal, L., & Roth, T. (1999). Ethanol as a hypnotic in insomniacs: Self administration and effects on sleep and mood. *Neuropsychopharmacology, 20*(3), 279–286. doi:10.1016/S0893-133X(98)00068-2

Russell, K., Allan, S., Beattie, L., Bohan, J., MacMahon, K., & Rasmussen, S. (2019). Sleep problem, suicide and self-harm in university students: A systematic review. *Sleep Medicine Reviews, 44*, 58–69. doi:10.1016/j.smrv.2018.12.008

Sáiz, P. A., González, M. P., Paredes, B., Martínez, S., & Delgado, J. M. (2001). Personalidad y uso–abuso de cocaína [Personality and use–abuse of cocaine]. *Adicciones [Addictions], 13*, 47–59.

Schierenbeck, T., Riemann, D., Berger, M., & Hornyak, M. (2008). Effect of illicit recreational drugs upon sleep: Cocaine, ecstasy and marijuana. *Sleep Medicine Reviews, 12*(5), 381–389. doi:10.1016/j.smrv.2007.12.004

Schulenberg, J. E., & Maggs, J. L. (2002). A developmental perspective on alcohol use and heavy drinking during adolescence and the transition to young adulthood. *Journal of Studies on Alcohol Supplement, S14*, 54–70.

Schulenberg, J. E., Johnston, L. D., O'Malley, P. M., Bachman, J. G., Miech, R. A., & Patrick, M. E. (2018). *Monitoring the future national survey results on drug use, 1975–2017: Volume II, college students and adults ages 19–55*. Ann Arbor: Institute for Social Research, The University of Michigan. Retrieved from http://monitoringthefuture.org/pubs.html#monographs, doi:10.3998/2027.42/146531

Schulenberg, J. E., & Zarrett, N. R. (2006). Mental health during emerging adulthood: Continuity and discontinuity in courses, causes, and functions. In J. J. Arnett & J. L. Tanner (Eds.), *Emerging adults in America: Coming of age in the 21st century*, (p. 135–172). Washington, DC: American Psychological Association. doi: 10.1037/11381-006.

Schuman-Olivier, Z., Greene, M. C., Bergman, B. G., & Kelly, J. F. (2014). Is residential treatment effective for opioid use disorders? A longitudinal comparison of treatment outcomes among opioid dependent, opioid misusing, and non-opioid using emerging adults with substance use disorder. *Drug and Alcohol Dependence, 144*, 178–185. doi:10.1016/j.drugalcdep.2014.09.009

Seiter, L. N., & Nelson, L. J. (2011). An examination of emerging adulthood in college students and nonstudents in India. *Journal of Adolescent Research, 26*(4), 506–536. doi:10.1177/0743558410391262

Sher, K. J., Bartholow, B. D., & Wood, M. D. (2000). Personality and substance use disorders: A prospective study. *Journal of Consulting and Clinical Psychology, 68*(5), 818–829. doi:10.1037/0022-006X.68.5.818

Shulman, S., & Connolly, J. (2013). The challenge of romantic relationships in emerging adulthood: Reconceptualization of the field. *Emerging Adulthood, 1*(1), 27–39. doi:10.1177/2167696812467330

Silvestre, A., Beatty, R. L., & Friedman, M. R. (2013). Substance use disorder in the context of LGBT health: A social work perspective. *Social Work in Public Health, 28*(3–4), 366–376. doi:10.1080/19371918.2013.774667

Sirsch, U., Dreher, E., Mayr, E., & Willinger, U. (2009). What does it take to be an adult in Austria? Views of adulthood in Austrian adolescents, emerging adults, and adults. *Journal of Adolescent Research, 24*(3), 275–292. doi:10.1177/0743558408331184

Smith, D. C., Bahar, O. S., Cleeland, L. R., & Davis, J. P. (2014). Self-perceived emerging adult status and substance use. *Psychology of Addictive Behaviors: Journal of the Society of Psychologists in Addictive Behaviors, 28*(3), 935–941. doi:10.1037/a0035900

Smith, D. C., Dumas, T., & Davis, J. (2017). Emerging adult development and substance use disorders. In D. C. Smith (Ed.), *Emerging adults and substance use disorder treatment: Developmental considerations and innovative approaches*. New York, NY: Oxford University Press. doi:10.1093/med-psych/9780190490782.001.0001

Substance Abuse and Mental Health Services Administration (SAMHSA). (2013). *TIP 35: Enhancing motivation for change in substance abuse treatment*. Publication ID: SMA13-4212. Retrieved from https://store.samhsa.gov/product/TIP-35-Enhancing-Motivation-for-Change-in-Substance-Use-Disorder-Treatment/PEP19-02-01-003

Substance Abuse and Mental Health Services Administration (SAMHSA). (2015). *TIP 55: Behavioral health services for people who are homeless*. Publication ID: SMA15-4734. Retrieved from https://store.samhsa.gov/product/TIP-55-Behavioral-Health-Services-for-People-Who-Are-Homeless/SMA15-4734

Terracciano, A., Löckenhoff, C. E., Crum, R. M., Bienvenu, O. J., & Costa, P. T., Jr. (2008). Five-factor model personality profiles of drug users. *BMC Psychiatry, 8*, 22.

Trémeau, F., Darreye, A., Leroy, B., Renckly, V., Ertlé, S., Weibel, H., . . . Macher, J. (2003). Changements psychologiques au cours d'un traitement de substitution de méthadone, mesurés par l'inventaire de personnalité d'eysenck [Personality changes in opioid-dependent subjects in a methadone maintenance treatment program]. *L'Encéphale: Revue De Psychiatrie Clinique Biologique Et Thérapeutique [The Brain: Review of Clinical and Biological Clinical Psychiatry], 29*(4), 285–292.

Trull, T. J., & Sher, K. J. (1994). Relationship between the five-factor model of personality and axis I disorders in a nonclinical sample. *Journal of Abnormal Psychology, 103*(2), 350–360. doi:10.1037/0021-843X.103.2.350

Wagner, E. (2013). Motivational interviewing. In C. Franklin (Editor in Chief), *Encyclopedia of social work*. Online collaboration between the National Association of Social Workers (NASW Press) and Oxford University Press (OUP). https://oxfordre.com/socialwork/, doi:10.1093/acrefore/9780199975839.013.252

Wong, M. M., Brower, K. J., & Craun, E. A. (2016). Insomnia symptoms and suicidality in the national comorbidity survey—Adolescent supplement. *Journal of Psychiatric Research, 81*, 1–8. doi:10.1016/j.jpsychires.2016.06.004

Wong, M. M., Robertson, G. C., & Dyson, R. B. (2015). Prospective relationship between poor sleep and substance-related problems in a national sample of adolescents. *Alcoholism: Clinical and Experimental Research, 39*(2), 355–362. doi:10.1111/acer.12618

15

Older adults and substance misuse

Paul Sacco, Alexis Kuerbis and Robin Harris

Background

Older adults have typically displayed lower risk of alcohol misuse (Grant et al., 2004), use of other drugs such as cannabis, misuse of medication (Huang et al., 2006), and illicit drug use (Grant et al., 2016) compared with younger age groups. However, over the last two decades, clinicians, researchers, and policy makers have grown concerned about an increase in older adults' unhealthy substance use (West, Severtson, Green, & Dart, 2015), and substance use problems (Jeste et al., 1999, 2018; Patterson & Jeste, 1999). It is likely that the need for treatment in this population will increase as the raw number of older adults grows in proportion to the total population (Vincent & Velkoff, 2010) and generational shifts in attitudes about substance misuse among older adults take hold (Glynn, Bouchard, LoCastro, & Laird, 1985; Lay, King, & Rangel, 2008).

Projections suggest that major increases in illicit drug use (Han, Gfroerer, & Colliver, 2009), substance use disorder (Han, Gfroerer, Colliver, & Penne, 2009), and treatment need (Gfroerer, Penne, Pemberton, & Folsom, 2003) among older adults are coming. Trend analysis of data from U.S. population-based epidemiologic studies is consistent with these projections. In the National Epidemiologic Survey on Alcohol and Related Conditions (NESARC), high risk drinking (exceeding NIAAA guidelines) increased by 65%, and alcohol use disorder increased by 106.7% among adults aged 65 and older between 2001–2002 and 2012–2013: alcohol use disorders were experienced by an estimated 1.5% of older adults in 2001–2002 and 3.1% in 2012–2013 (Grant et al., 2017). Data from the National Survey on Drug Use and Health (NSDUH) identified increasing rates of binge drinking (19.2%) and alcohol use disorder (23.3%) from 2005 to 2014 among adults aged 50 and older (Han, Moore, Sherman, Keyes, & Palamar, 2017). Nonmedical use of cannabis and prescription drugs have also increased among middle aged (aged 50–64) and older adults (65+) (Han, Sherman, et al., 2017; Schepis & McCabe, 2016). Han and colleagues (2017), analyzing data from NSDUH, identified increases in cannabis use from 2.8% in 2006–2007 to 4.8% in 2012–2013. Schepis and McCabe (2016) analyzing data from the NESARC surveys identified similar trends for nonmedical prescription drug use, reporting increases in opioid, tranquilizer, and stimulant misuse among adults aged 50 and older. Rates of treatment for illicit drug use have increased, as well (Arndt, Clayton, & Schultz, 2011). In 1998, older adults made up 2.86% of admissions, which rose to 4.42% in 2008, based on data from the Treatment Episode Dataset.

These changes will no doubt extend over the next three decades with implications for social workers and other behavioral health professionals. These changes are a function of two main forces: cohort differences in alcohol and other drug use among cohorts that will reach older adulthood in coming years, and the broader trend of population aging. Clinicians in aging services will need to be responsive to behavioral health concerns of clients they serve, including alcohol and drug misuse, and behavioral health providers will need to equip themselves with an understanding of life course development and aging phenomena. With this in mind, it is helpful to review key concepts regarding aging and unhealthy substance use.

Alcohol use by older adults

Alcohol is the most commonly used substance among older adults, but rates of use vary by locality, age grouping (e.g. 65+ versus 50+), and definition of current use (e.g. past-month versus past-year use). Among older adults in the United States, 55% of persons over 65 reported past-year drinking (Grant et al., 2017). In a European sample of older adults, 64.7% of men and 51.7% of women aged 65 and older reported current alcohol use (Bosque-Prous et al., 2017). Data from New Zealand indicated that 83% of individuals aged 50+ currently consumed alcohol (Towers et al., 2018). In Wave 1 of the World Health Organization (WHO) Study on Global AGEing and Adult Health (SAGE), rates of current alcohol use among adults 50+ varied substantially from India with 16–74% in Russia (Ahangari, Stewart Williams, & Myléus, 2016).

The relationship of alcohol, aging, and health is complex in that low-level alcohol consumption may not be harmful to older adults and can be considered a socially normative behavior without negative health effects (Byles, Young, Furuya, & Parkinson, 2006). The so-called "J-curve" hypothesis (Shaper, Wannamethee, & Walker, 1988; Skog, 1996) suggests that alcohol use at low levels confers cardiovascular and other health benefits such as lower risk of type II diabetes (Rasouli et al., 2013), lower likelihood of cognitive impairment (Richard et al., 2017), and decreased overall mortality. Nonetheless, as average consumption amounts increase, so do health and mortality risks.

Effects of alcohol on older adults

The aging process itself may put older adults at risk from drinking in amounts considered low risk for younger adults. As one ages, the acute biological effects of alcohol and other drugs becomes more pronounced. With age, one's percentage of body fat increases and volume of water in the body decreases. The capacity of the liver to metabolize alcohol also decreases. These changes render older adults more vulnerable to alcohol's acute effects (Novier, Diaz-Granados, & Matthews, 2015). Older adults may also be at higher risk due to medication and alcohol interactions. A wide variety of medications, such as antidepressants, analgesics, and blood thinners taken with alcohol may lead to harmful interactions (Moore, Whiteman, & Ward, 2007). Because of these risks, the National Institute Alcohol Abuse and Alcoholism (NIAAA) guidelines are lower for individuals aged 65 and older than for those younger men and women. They state that older adults should limit consumption to three or fewer drinks per day and no more than seven drinks in a given week (National Institute on Alcohol Abuse and Alcoholism, 2007).

Continuum of risk

Along the continuum of use, alcohol use disorder (American Psychiatric Association, 2013) is the most severe manifestation of alcohol-related problems. Individuals diagnosed as experiencing an alcohol use disorder endorse two or more DSM-5 alcohol use disorder criteria. There are analogous measures in the International Classification of Diseases (ICD-11: Saunders, Peacock, & Degenhardt, 2018; World Health Organization, 2018) that quantify moderate and severe alcohol-related pathology, but concordance or diagnostic agreement among these two classification systems is not well studied as the DSM-5 and the ICD-11 have recently been updated (see Appendix A). As previously noted, rates of alcohol use disorder among older adults are lower than those among younger age groups but are increasing. The rate of past-year alcohol use disorder among those 65+ was estimated to be 2.3% in a national survey conducted in the United States (Grant et al., 2015). Although DSM diagnosis is a standard construct, research suggests that DSM diagnostic approaches may under-identify older adults who experience less severe alcohol problems (Kuerbis, Hagman, & Sacco, 2013).

Tobacco use by older adults

Although rates of tobacco use in the United States are lower among older adults than younger groups, approximately 11% of older adults (65+) reported using tobacco products some days or every day (Wang et al., 2018) and 4% of older adults met criteria for a past-year tobacco use disorder (Lin et al., 2013). It is common that use of tobacco is associated with other substance use, including at-risk alcohol use (Sacco, Bucholz, & Spitznagel, 2009) and cannabis use (Han, Sherman, et al., 2017). Cigarettes are the most commonly used form of tobacco; 8% of older adults reported using this form of tobacco. Although trend data suggest that tobacco use is declining among older adults and is consistently lower than in younger age groups, it remains a cause of preventable death among older persons (U.S. Department of Health and Human Services, 2014).

Cannabis use by older adults

After alcohol and tobacco, cannabis is the most commonly used substance among older adults in the United States. Using NSDUH data, Han and colleagues (2017) reported that the prevalence of past-year cannabis use increased by 250% between 2006 and 2013 with 1.4% of adults 65+ reporting past-year use. When those in late middle age (50–64) are included, cannabis use rates are higher, ranging from 2.6% (Blazer & Wu, 2009a) to 2.8% (DiNitto & Choi, 2011). Rates of DSM-defined cannabis use disorder are relatively low (0.12%) among older adults.

The advent of cannabis legalization for medical and recreational use in many regions of the United States has affected the older adult population, especially those experiencing pain conditions and previous substance use (Nugent et al., 2017). As more states and countries legalize cannabis, older adults are redefining their relationship to a previously illicit substance (Pacek, Mauro, & Martins, 2015). Social workers need to be aware of the changing regulatory environment of cannabis and its effects on this population.

Medical cannabis and older adults

The use of cannabis for medical purposes may be one driver of use among older adults that is distinct from younger groups. In a study of medical cannabis dispensary patients, older consumers (aged 51–71) reported cannabis use to alleviate chronic conditions while younger consumers (aged 18–30) reported using it to alleviate boredom (Haug et al., 2017). With therapeutic cannabis prescriptions rising, practitioners are concerned about health safety for older adults. Effects from cannabis use include psychosis, harmful neurocognitive effects, coordination problems, and negative heart rhythms (Beauchet, 2018). Limited evidence suggests that cannabis may show promise for conditions that largely affect older adults, such as neuropathic pain, nausea-related side effects of cancer treatments, and motor symptoms of Parkinson's disease (Beauchet, 2018; Minerbi, Häuser, & Fitzcharles, 2019; Nugent et al., 2017).

Nonmedical prescription and illicit drug use by older adults

Compared to alcohol and cannabis use, the misuse of other drugs is relatively low, but polysubstance use (among those in treatment) is increasing among older adults (Chhatre, Cook, Mallik, & Jayadevappa, 2017). In a U.S. national prevalence study, among adults aged 65 and older, less than 1% reported engaging in past-year nonmedical use of prescription drugs (Moore et al., 2009); another study identified a rate of 1.4% for past-year prescription drug misuse among individuals aged 50+ (Blazer & Wu, 2009b). Similar to other drugs, rates of prescription drug misuse are higher among persons in late middle age (50–64) than later adulthood (aged 65+), but less than 1% for cocaine, hallucinogens, inhalants, methamphetamine, and heroin (Blazer & Wu, 2009a). Nonetheless, there exists concern that younger cohorts may stimulate increases in these prevalence rates as they reach older ages (Han, Gfroerer, & Colliver, 2009; Han, Gfroerer, Colliver, et al., 2009).

Older adults and the opioid epidemic

Social workers in the United States and other parts of the world recently witnessed a tremendous rise in opioid-related harm, and older adults are a growing part of this epidemic. Older adult (55+) first-time treatment program admissions for opioid use disorder rose 41.2% from 2004 to 2015 and even more rapidly (53.5%) from 2013 to 2015 (Huhn, Strain, Tompkins, & Dunn, 2018). Older adults in rural areas may be particularly vulnerable to opioid abuse due to work-related injuries and prescription medication sharing; an estimated 10 million adults 65 years and older suffered chronic pain in 2017 from work-related injuries sustained during jobs like farming and coal mining (Martin, 2018).

Interventions with older Adults

To match the wide range of severity in older adult substance misuse, a continuum of interventions are available for this population. Although research is limited, a few strong intervention studies show older adult intervention outcomes equivalent to, and in some cases better than, younger adults' outcomes (Brennan, Nichol, & Moos, 2003; Kuerbis & Sacco, 2013; Satre, Mertens, Areán, & Weisner, 2003, 2004). Assuming that substance use disorders have been properly identified and assessed, selection of an intervention depends on both the setting in which an older adult is served and the severity of presenting symptoms/substance misuse (Sacco & Kuerbis, 2013). Interventions implemented outside specialty substance abuse treatment facilities, such as emergency rooms, senior centers, and primary care offices (Sacco & Kuerbis, 2013; Schonfeld et al., 2010), have been successful in reaching a wide range of vulnerable older adults. The review of interventions below includes treatments for which there exists initial evidence of efficacy and/or effectiveness among this population.

General approach

Older clients respond best to a non-confrontational approach regardless of intervention type (Dupree, Broskowski, & Schonfeld, 1984; Schonfeld & Dupree, 1995, 2002). Open-ended questions and reflections will likely yield in-depth information and effective client engagement. Assessing quantity and frequency of substances used, including pills from friends or consuming alcohol at risky levels, will be vital to understanding which type of intervention is needed. Engaging older adults in discussions about substance use is usually most successful when adopting a harm reduction approach.

Brief intervention (BI)

Effective brief interventions tend to occur in primary care settings, though not exclusively (Fink, Elliot, Tsai, & Beck, 2005; Fleming, Manwell, Barry, Adams, & Stauffacher, 1999; Moore et al., 2011). BIs focus on alcohol, smoking, and prescription medication misuse or abuse, and vary in length from 15 minutes to five one-hour sessions (Barry, Oslin, & Blow, 2001; Kuerbis & Sacco, 2013). Their overall structure includes providing education about the substance and its potential for harm, enhancing motivation for reducing harm, and, when necessary, referring individuals experiencing greatest need to more intensive treatments (Blow & Barry, 2000).

BIs often include normative feedback, in which a person's drinking, smoking, or medication misuse is compared to peers, or personalized feedback, in which a person is informed of their risk level based on a series of short assessments. These types of feedback combined with brief advice to cut back are the most common brief interventions utilized with older adults and appear to be moderately effective to address older adults' drinking (Conigliaro, Kraemer, & McNeil, 2000; Fink et al., 2005; Kuerbis, Hail, Moore, & Muench, 2017; Kuerbis & Sacco, 2013). In the case of smoking cessation, brief interventions with older adults, such as those performed by physicians, showed only modest effects (Zbikowski, Magnusson, Pockey, Tindle, & Weaver, 2012). Outcomes related to prescription medication misuse are not often reported. One exception is the Florida BRITE Project (Brief Intervention and Treatment for Elders; Schonfeld et al., 2010, 2015), which evaluated and treated older adults in the community. For this rather intensive BI, prescription medication misuse decreased among only 32% of participants.

Motivational interventions

BIs are often described as using "motivational components," referring to aspects of Motivational Interviewing (MI; Miller & Rollnick, 2013) or Motivational Enhancement Therapy (MET; Miller, Zweben, DiClemente, & Rychtarik, 1992). MI and MET apply a Rogerian approach in discussing substance use—one that is client-centered and non-judgmental. Additionally, clients are encouraged to make positive, healthy behavior changes. The purpose of MI and MET are to reduce ambivalence about changing an addictive behavior and enhance harm reduction by assisting the client to identify, in his or her own words, the perceived benefits of making a healthy change versus maintaining the unhealthy status quo (Miller & Rollnick,

2013; Sacco & Kuerbis, 2013). The reasons for changing substance use are often unique among older adults and may include maintaining independence, optimal health, and mental capacity (Barry et al., 2001).

While MI and MET are consistent with a non-confrontational, supportive approach and are recommended for use with older adults who use substances (Barry et al., 2001; Center for Substance Abuse Treatment, 1998), there remains a void in empirical evidence supporting use of formal MI or MET in addressing older adults' substance misuse. Meta-analyses demonstrate that MI works differentially across health behaviors and subgroups (Hettema, Steele, & Miller, 2005), and no studies among those that contributed to establishing MI as an evidence-based practice for substance misuse included individuals over age 62 (Hettema et al., 2005). Several studies demonstrated efficacy of MI with older adults targeting other health behaviors (Cummings, Cooper, & Cassie, 2009; Schneider, Wong-Anuchit, Stallings, & Krieger, 2017; Stallings & Schneider, 2018), including smoking cessation (Borrelli et al., 2005; Hokanson, Anderson, Hennrikus, Landon, & Kendall, 2006), and some evidence suggests that it works in the context of case management to engage older adults in more formal treatment (Conigliaro et al., 2000). Rigorous controlled trials involving older adults and MI or MET have yet to be conducted.

Pharmacotherapy

Pharmacological treatments are an increasingly accessible way to facilitate reduced substance use among older adults. Most approved medications are for treatment of alcohol use disorders and smoking cessation, although key medications for opioid use disorder are also available (see Chapter 19). In the United States, disulfram, acamprosate, and naltrexone are currently Food and Drug Administration-approved medications for treating alcohol use disorders; medications such as varenicline (Burstein, Fullerton, Clark, & Faessel, 2006; O'Malley et al., 2018), baclofen (Beraha et al., 2016; Farokhnia et al., 2017), and others are being tested for efficacy across populations. Like other treatments for substance use disorder, medications have not been tested thoroughly for efficacy and safety with older adult patients.

Disulfram

Brand named Antabuse®, disulfram is an aversive agent that increases immediacy and severity of ill effects from ingesting alcohol by increasing acetaldehyde levels (Barrick & Connors, 2002). While used with adults over age 50 with some benefit (Garbutt, West, Carey, Lohr, & Crews, 1999), it has important limitations. Disulfram is only useful with strict adherence to the medication regimen. There is also evidence that it places extra strain on the cardiovascular system within older adults, and thus may be contraindicated (Barrick & Connors, 2002).

Acamprosate

Brand named Campral®, acamprosate is used to reduce craving for and pleasurable effects of alcohol (Tempesta, Janiri, Bignamini, Chabac, & Potgieter, 2000). While acamprosate efficacy has not been tested specifically with individuals 65 and older, one study reported that individuals 45 and older who were not abstinent prior to medication initiation fared better than younger participants (Gueorguieva et al., 2015). There are few reports of adverse effects across populations, thus it is presumed relatively safe among older adults (U.S. National Library of Congress, 2013). However, given higher rates of kidney disease among older adults, dosage adjustments may need to be made.

Naltrexone

Brand named Revia®, naltrexone is the most studied medication used for SUD treatment among older adults (Kuerbis & Sacco, 2013; Oslin, Liberto, O'Brien, Krois, & Norbeck, 1997), and has demonstrated some effectiveness within this population. Naltrexone is an opioid receptor antagonist thought to reduce craving and the pleasurable effects of alcohol (or other substances) by blocking substance-induced dopamine release in the brain (Barrick & Connors, 2002). Naltrexone can be taken in daily tablet (Revia®) or monthly injection (Vivitrol®) form, although only daily naltrexone by tablet has been tested in use with older adults. For older adults, naltrexone is most helpful in preventing relapse to heavy drinking when a person is exposed to alcohol, such as having one drink, compared to when a person remains completely abstinent from alcohol (Oslin et al., 1997; Oslin, Pettinati, & Volpicelli, 2002). Because a large proportion of older adults experience chronic pain for which they are prescribed opioid-based medications, naltrexone may be inappropriate as it blocks the pain management effect of opioids. It can also potentiate pre-existing major depressive disorder symptoms; persons with histories of depression should be identified and closely monitored.

Varenicline and baclofen

Two newer medications (brand named Chantix® and Lioresal®) are emerging as options in the treatment of substance use disorders. While existing studies among general adult populations demonstrated a reduction in drinking (Litten et al., 2013; Plebani et al., 2013) and smoking (Garrison & Dugan, 2009), as well as reduction in smoking and heavy drinking simultaneously (O'Malley et al., 2018), varenicline has yet to be tested with older adults. Baclofen demonstrated some initial efficacy across substances, including alcohol (Reynaud et al., 2017) but results are variable across dosage levels; one potential disadvantage of or contraindication for using baclofen with older adults is the potential side effect of extreme drowsiness (Beraha et al., 2016; Farokhnia et al., 2017).

Medication-assisted treatment (MAT) for opioid use disorder

Methadone and buprenorphine are medications commonly used for treating pain and/or opioid use disorder. Both are considered relatively safe for older adults (Vadivelu & Hines, 2008; Wu, 2018); however, dosage should be adjusted to accommodate issues with polypharmacy or overall substance sensitivity. Methadone is an opioid medication originally engineered to treat pain and now widely used to treat opioid-use disorder. Buprenorphine is an opioid analgesic used to treat pain and is well tolerated among the elderly (Vadivelu & Hines, 2008). Used in combination with naloxone, buprenorphine can be an alternative to methadone.

Nicotine replacement therapy (NRT)

NRT is a common and effective way of treating older adults who use nicotine, particularly when combined with cognitive behavioral therapy (Hall et al., 2009; Zbikowski et al., 2012). NRT involves administration of a small amount of nicotine through either a transdermal patch or gum to stave off withdrawal symptoms as a person attempts to quit smoking or using other nicotine-based products. Evidence from a meta-analysis suggests that NRT is effective for older adults in the short term, yet it may lack efficacy longer term without long-term behavioral counseling (Zbikowski et al., 2012).

Case management

Case and care management models take advantage of nontraditional settings to engage older adults in reducing substance use and/or connecting them to treatment (Sacco & Kuerbis, 2013). Advantages of these models include:

- providing a comprehensive format for addressing medical and psychiatric co-morbidities and other medical complexities (Barry et al., 2001; Center for Substance Abuse Treatment, 1998);
- connecting isolated older adults to needed community resources;
- lessening stigma; and
- broadening the intervention approach to address all aspects of health (Center for Substance Abuse Treatment, 1998).

Case management is shown through program evaluations to be an important tool in working with older adults (D'Agostino, Barry, Blow, & Podgorski, 2006; Lee, Mericle, Ayalon, & Areán, 2009; Levkoff et al., 2004; Oslin et al., 2006; Zanjani et al., 2008), and may be particularly effective at engaging and maintaining older adults in substance abuse treatment (Oslin et al., 2006).

Care modalities

Formal substance abuse treatment is provided on a continuum of intensity across the lifespan and depending on problem severity, from detoxification to outpatient treatment or aftercare (Sacco & Kuerbis, 2013). Ideally, treatment plans are tailored to specific client needs.

Individual and group approaches

For older adults, both individual and group treatments are recommended options. While group treatment can reduce isolation and shame related to substance abuse, group treatment may also inadvertently enhance feelings of isolation and shame due to a lack of elder specific treatment available in the community (Schultz, Arndt, & Liesveld, 2003). Older adults may not identify with younger group members, or they may feel their issues in later life will not be understood by others in the group. Therefore, individual therapy provides an ancillary, private forum for older adults to discuss their unique issues.

Psychotherapeutic approaches

Two specific psychotherapeutic approaches have been explored as possible effective treatments for substance use disorders experienced by older adults: supportive therapy models (STM: Kofoed, Tolson, Atkinson, Toth, & Turner, 1987) and cognitive behavioral treatments (CBT: Dupree et al., 1984; Rice, Longabaugh, Beattie, & Noel, 1993; Schonfeld & Dupree, 1995, 2002; Schonfeld et al., 2000).

Supportive therapy models (STMs)

STMs represent traditional treatment with age-specific modifications that enhance older adults' treatment engagement (Kofoed et al., 1987). STMs were designed to develop a culture of support and successful coping among older adults engaged in substance misuse. Supportive therapies concentrate on building social support, improving self-esteem, and a global approach to treatment planning, addressing multiple biopsychosocial arenas in the client's life (Sacco & Kuerbis, 2013). While there exists relatively little research on age-specific treatments incorporating these techniques, some evidence suggests that older adults demonstrate better outcomes in these settings than in non-adapted settings (Kashner, Rodell, Ogden, Guggenheim, & Karson, 1992; Kofoed et al., 1987; Kuerbis & Sacco, 2013; Rimer et al., 1994).

Cognitive behavioral therapy (CBT)

CBT focuses on identifying and altering problematic patterns of thinking, feeling, and behaving that contribute to problematic substance use (Rotgers, 2003). CBT is delivered via individual or group modalities and shows strong evidence of positive outcomes across populations and age groups (Morgenstern & McKay, 2007). Empirical research also demonstrated that CBT is effective with older adults (Dupree et al., 1984; Hall et al., 2009; Rice et al., 1993; Schonfeld & Dupree, 1995, 2002; Schonfeld et al., 2000), and the Substance Abuse and Mental Health Services Association (SAMHSA) published a CBT substance abuse treatment manual specifically for use with older adults (Center for Substance Abuse Treatment, 1998).

Mutual aid groups

Mutual aid groups, such as Alcoholics Anonymous or Seniors for Sobriety, can be helpful in combating social isolation, shame, and stigma, as well as substance misuse (Sacco & Kuerbis, 2013). Unfortunately, no empirical studies demonstrate the effectiveness of Alcoholics, Narcotics Anonymous, or related groups with older adults (Atkinson & Misra, 2002). In addition, the same barriers to formal treatment may plague participation in mutual aid groups—primarily stigma and shame of needing to attend to these issues in later life in the presence of a younger generation; fear of being misunderstood; and a preference for dealing with problems privately. Knowledge of local elder-friendly meetings may be useful in intervening with older adults. When referring older adults to mutual aid groups, it is important to encourage them to try more than one meeting, prior to deciding whether it is a good fit, since each has a unique tone and feel.

Conclusions

Social workers practicing in either substance use treatment or aging need to embrace behavioral health integration. Older individuals seeking substance abuse treatment also face specific challenges with respect to aging, and older adults served by aging services organizations may present with behavioral health concerns. Practitioners can respond effectively by consistently screening for alcohol and drug misuse in non-specialty care settings, and by recognizing the needs of older clients in formal treatment settings. The key to effectively responding to older adult addictive behavior is a non-stigmatizing approach that embraces that idea that it is never too late to change. Rather than being hopeless, older individuals may do as well as or better than younger people when they seek treatment, if the treatment offered is age appropriate. As clinicians, our job is to be ready and open to helping them, and to advocate for service delivery systems and policies that support effective responses to substance misuse by older adults.

References

Ahangari, A., Stewart Williams, J., & Myléus, A. (2016). Pain and alcohol consumption among older adults: Findings from the World Health Organization study on global AGEing and adult health, Wave 1. *Tropical Medicine & International Health, 21*(10), 1282–1292. doi:10.1111/tmi.12757

American Psychiatric Association. (2013). *Diagnostic and statistical manual of mental disorders, Fifth Edition.* Arlington, VA: American Psychiatric Publishing. doi:10.1176/appi.books.9780890425596

Arndt, S., Clayton, R., & Schultz, S. K. (2011). Trends in substance abuse treatment 1998–2008: Increasing older adult first-time admissions for illicit drugs. *American Journal of Geriatric Psychiatry, 19*(8), 704–711. doi:10.1097/JGP.0b013e31820d942b

Atkinson, R. M., & Misra, S. (2002). Further strategies in the treatment of aging alcoholics. In A. M. Gurnack, R. M. Atkinson, & N. J. Osgood (Eds.), *Treating alcohol and drug abuse in the elderly* (pp. 131–151). New York, NY: Springer.

Barrick, C., & Connors, G. D. (2002). Relapse prevention and maintaining abstinence in older adults with alcohol-use disorders. *Drugs & Aging, 19*(8), 583–594. doi:10.2165/00002512-200219080-00004

Barry, K. L., Oslin, D. W., & Blow, F. C. (2001). *Alcohol problems in older adults.* New York, NY: Springer Publishing Company.

Beauchet, O. (2018). Medical cannabis use in older patients: Update on medical knowledge. *Maturitas, 118*, 56–59. doi:10.1016/j.maturitas.2018.10.010

Beraha, E. M., Salemink, E., Goudriaan, A. E., Bakker, A., de Jong, D., Smits, N., . . . Wiers, R. W. (2016). Efficacy and safety of high-dose baclofen for the treatment of alcohol dependence: A multicentre, randomised, double-blind controlled trial. *European Neuropsychopharmacology, 26*(12), 1950–1959. doi:10.1016/j.euroneuro.2016.10.006

Blazer, D. G., & Wu, L. T. (2009a). The epidemiology of substance use and disorders among middle aged and elderly community adults: National survey on drug use and health (NSDUH). *American Journal of Geriatric Psychiatry, 17*(3), 237–245. doi:10.1097/JGP.0b013e318190b8ef

Blazer, D. G., & Wu, L. T. (2009b). Nonprescription use of pain relievers by middle-aged and elderly community-living adults: National survey on drug use and health. *Journal of the American Geriatrics Society, 57*(7), 1252–1257. doi:10.1111/j.1532-5415.2009.02306.x

Blow, F. C., & Barry, K. (2000). Older patients with at-risk and problem drinking patterns: New developments in brief interventions. *Journal of Geriatric Psychiatry and Neurology, 13*, 115–123. doi:10.1177/089198870001300304

Borrelli, B., Novak, S., Hecht, J., Emmons, K., Papandonatos, G., & Abrams, D. (2005). Home health care nurses as a new channel for smoking cessation treatment: Outcomes from project CARES (community-nurse assisted research and education on smoking). *Preventive Medicine, 41*, 815–821. doi:10.1016/j.ypmed.2005.08.004

Bosque-Prous, M., Brugal, M. T., Lima, K. C., Villalbí, J. R., Bartroli, M., & Espelt, A. (2017). Hazardous drinking in people aged 50 years or older: A cross-sectional picture of Europe, 2011–2013. *International Journal of Geriatric Psychiatry, 32*(8), 817–828. doi:10.1002/gps.4528

Brennan, P. L., Nichol, A. C., & Moos, R. H. (2003). Older and younger patients with substance use disorders: Outpatient mental health service use and functioning over a 12-month interval. *Psychology of Addictive Behaviors, 17*(1), 42–48. doi:10.1037/0893-164X.17.1.42

Burstein, A. H., Fullerton, T., Clark, D. J., & Faessel, H. M. (2006). Pharmacokinetics, safety, and tolerability after single and multiple oral doses of varenicline in elderly smokers. *Journal of Clinical Pharmacology, 46*(11), 1234–1240. doi:10.1177/0091270006291837

Byles, J., Young, A., Furuya, H., & Parkinson, L. (2006). A drink to healthy aging: The association between older women's use of alcohol and their health-related quality of life. *Journal of the American Geriatrics Society, 54*(9), 1341–1347. doi:10.1111/j.1532-5415.2006.00837.x

Center for Substance Abuse Treatment. (1998). *Substance abuse among older adults: Treatment improvement protocol (TIP) Series 26.* Rockville, MD: Substance Abuse and Mental Health Services Administration.

Chhatre, S., Cook, R., Mallik, E., & Jayadevappa, R. (2017). Trends in substance use admissions among older adults. *BMC Health Services Research, 17*(1), 584. doi:10.1186/s12913-017-2538-z

Conigliaro, J., Kraemer, K. L., & McNeil, M. (2000). Screening and identification of older adults with alcohol problems in primary care. *Journal of Geriatric Psychiatry and Neurology, 13*, 106–114. doi:10.1177/089198870001300303

Cummings, S. M., Cooper, R. L., & Cassie, K. M. (2009). Motivational interviewing to affect behavioral change in older adults. *Research on Social Work Practice, 19*(2), 195–204. doi:10.1177/1049731508320216

D'Agostino, C. S., Barry, K. L., Blow, F. C., & Podgorski, C. (2006). Community interventions for older adults with comorbid substance use: The geriatrics addiction program (GAP). *Journal of Dual Diagnosis, 2*(3), 31–43. doi:10.1300/J374v02n03_04

DiNitto, D. M., & Choi, N. G. (2011). Marijuana use among older adults in the USA: User characteristics, patterns of use, and implications for intervention. *International Psychogeriatrics, 23*(05), 732–741. doi:10.1017/S1041610210002176

Dupree, L. W., Broskowski, H., & Schonfeld, L. (1984). The gerontology alcohol project: A behavioral treatment program for elderly alcohol abusers. *The Gerontologist, 24*, 510–516. doi:10.1093/geront/24.5.510

Farokhnia, M., Schwandt, M. L., Lee, M. R., Bollinger, J. W., Farinelli, L. A., Amodio, J. P., . . . Leggio, L. (2017). Biobehavioral effects of baclofen in anxious alcohol-dependent individuals: A randomized, double-blind, placebo-controlled, laboratory study. *Translational Psychiatry, 7*(4), e1108. doi:10.1038/tp.2017.71

Fink, A., Elliot, M. N., Tsai, M., & Beck, J. C. (2005). An evaluation of an intervention to assist primary care physicians in screening and educating older patients who use alcohol. *Journal of American Geriatrics Society, 53*, 1937–1943. doi:10.1111/j.1532-5415.2005.00476.x

Fleming, M. F., Manwell, L. B., Barry, K. L., Adams, W., & Stauffacher, E. A. (1999). Brief physician advice for alcohol problems in older adults: A randomized community-based trial. *The Journal of Family Practice, 48*(5), 378–384.

Garbutt, J. C., West, S. L., Carey, T. S., Lohr, K. N., & Crews, F. T. (1999). Pharmacological treatment of alcohol dependence: A review of the evidence. *JAMA: Journal of the American Medical Association, 281*(14), 1318–1325. doi:10.1001/jama.281.14.1318

Garrison, G. D., & Dugan, S. E. (2009). Varenicline: A first-line treatment option for smoking cessation. *Clinical Therapeutics, 31*(3), 463–491. doi:10.1016/j.clinthera.2009.03.021

Gfroerer, J., Penne, M., Pemberton, M., & Folsom, R. (2003). Substance abuse treatment need among older adults in 2020: The impact of the baby-boom cohort. *Drug and Alcohol Dependence, 69*, 127–135. doi:10.1016/S0376-8716(02)00307-1

Glynn, R. J., Bouchard, G. R., LoCastro, J. S., & Laird, N. M. (1985). Aging and generational effects on drinking behaviors in men: Results from the normative aging study. *American Journal of Public Health, 75*(12), 1413–1419. doi:10.2105/AJPH.75.12.1413

Grant, B. F., Chou, S., Saha, T. D., Pickering, R.P., Kerridge, B.T., Ruan, W.J. . . . Hasin, D. S. (2017). Prevalence of 12-month alcohol use, high-risk drinking, and DSM-IV alcohol use disorder in the United States, 2001–2002 to 2012–2013: Results from the national epidemiologic survey on alcohol and related conditions. *JAMA Psychiatry.* doi:10.1001/jamapsychiatry.2017.2161

Grant, B. F., Dawson, D. A., Stinson, F. S., Chou, S. P., Dufour, M. C., & Pickering, R. P. (2004). The 12-month prevalence and trends in DSM-IV alcohol abuse and dependence: United States, 1991–1992 and 2001–2002. *Drug and Alcohol Dependence, 74*(3), 223–234. doi:10.1016/j.drugalcdep.2004.02.004

Grant, B. F., Goldstein, R. B., Saha, T. D., Chou, S. P., Jung, J., Zhang, H., . . . Hasin, D. S. (2015). Epidemiology of DSM-5 alcohol use disorder: Results from the national epidemiologic survey on alcohol and related conditions III. *JAMA Psychiatry, 72*(8), 757–766. doi:10.1001/jamapsychiatry.2015.0584

Grant, B. F., Saha, T. D., Ruan, W., Risë, B. G., Patricia Chou, S., Jung, J., . . . Deborah, S. H. (2016). Epidemiology of DSM-5 drug use disorder: Results from the national epidemiologic survey on alcohol and related conditions–III. *JAMA Psychiatry, 73*(1), 39–47. doi:10.1001/jamapsychiatry.2015.2132

Gueorguieva, R., Wu, R., Tsai, W. M., O'Connor, P. G., Fucito, L., Zhang, H., & O'Malley, S. S. (2015). An analysis of moderators in the COMBINE study: Identifying subgroups of patients who benefit from acamprosate. *European Neuropsychopharmacology, 25*(10), 1586–1599. doi:10.1016/j.euroneuro.2015.06.006

Hall, S. M., Humfleet, G. L., Munoz, R. F., Reus, V. I., Robbins, J. A., & Prochaska, J. J. (2009). Extended treatment of older cigarette smokers. *Addiction, 104*, 1043–1052. doi:10.1111/j.1360-0443.2009.02548.x

Han, B., Gfroerer, J., & Colliver, J. D. (2009). *An examination of trends in illicit drug use among adults aged 50 to 59 in the United States*. Bethesda, MD: Substance Abuse and Mental Health Services Administration. Retrieved from https://www.datafiles.samhsa.gov/study-publication/examination-trends-illicit-drug-use-among-adults-aged-50-59-united-states-nid14194. https://doi.org/10.1037/e592612009-001

Han, B., Gfroerer, J., Colliver, J. D., & Penne, M. A. (2009). Substance use disorder among older adults in the United States in 2020. *Addiction, 104*(1), 88–96. doi:10.1111/j.1360-0443.2008.02411.x

Han, B. H., Moore, A. A., Sherman, S., Keyes, K. M., & Palamar, J. J. (2017). Demographic trends of binge alcohol use and alcohol use disorders among older adults in the United States, 2005–2014. *Drug and Alcohol Dependence, 170*, 198–207. doi:10.1016/j.drugalcdep.2016.11.003

Han, B. H., Sherman, S., Mauro, P. M., Martins, S. S., Rotenberg, J., & Palamar, J. J. (2017). Demographic trends among older cannabis users in the United States, 2006–13. *Addiction, 112*(3), 516–525. doi:10.1111/add.13670

Haug, N. A., Padula, C. B., Sottile, J. E., Vandrey, R., Heinz, A. J., & Bonn-Miller, M. O. (2017). Cannabis use patterns and motives: A comparison of younger, middle-aged, and older medical cannabis dispensary patients. *Addictive Behaviors, 72*, 14–20. doi:10.1016/j.addbeh.2017.03.006

Hettema, J., Steele, J., & Miller, W. R. (2005). Motivational interviewing. *Annual Review Clinical Psychology, 1*, 91–111. doi:10.1146/annurev.clinpsy.1.102803.143833

Hokanson, J. M., Anderson, R. L., Hennrikus, D. J., Landon, H. A., & Kendall, D. M. (2006). Integrated tobacco cessation counseling in a diabetes self-management training program: A randomized trial of diabetes and reduction of tobacco. *The Diabetes Educator, 32*, 562–570. doi:10.1177/0145721706289914

Huang, B., Dawson, D. A., Stinson, F. S., Hasin, D. S., Ruan, W. J., Saha, T. D., . . . Grant, B. F. (2006). Prevalence, correlates, and comorbidity of nonmedical prescription drug use and drug use disorders in the United States: Results of the national epidemiologic survey on alcohol and related conditions. *Journal of Clinical Psychiatry, 67*(7), 1062–1073. doi:10.4088/JCP.v67n0708

Huhn, A. S., Strain, E. C., Tompkins, D. A., & Dunn, K. E. (2018). A hidden aspect of the U.S. opioid crisis: Rise in first-time treatment admissions for older adults with opioid use disorder. *Drug and Alcohol Dependence, 193*, 142–147. doi:10.1016/j.drugalcdep.2018.10.002

Jeste, D. V., Alexopoulos, G. S., Bartels, S. J., Cummings, J. L., Gallo, J. J., Gottlieb, G. L., . . . Lebowitz, B. D. (1999). Consensus statement on the upcoming crisis in geriatric mental health. *Archives of General Psychiatry, 56*, 848–853. doi:10.1001/archpsyc.56.9.848

Jeste, D. V., Peschin, S., Buckwalter, K., Blazer, D. G., McGuire, M. H., Miller, J., . . . Reynolds, C. F. (2018). Promoting wellness in older adults with mental illnesses and substance use disorders: Call to action to all stakeholders. *The American Journal of Geriatric Psychiatry.* doi:10.1016/j.jagp.2018.03.011

Kashner, M., Rodell, D. E., Ogden, S. R., Guggenheim, F. G., & Karson, C. N. (1992). Outcomes and costs of two VA inpatient treatment programs for older adult alcoholic patients. *Hospital and Community Psychiatry, 43*, 985–989. doi:10.1176/ps.43.10.985

Keating, G. M., & Lyseng-Williamson, K. A. (2010). Varenicline: A pharmacoeconomic review of its use as an aid to smoking cessation. *Pharmacoeconomics, 28*(3), 231–254. doi:10.2165/11204380-000000000-00000

Kofoed, L. L., Tolson, R. L., Atkinson, R. M., Toth, R. L., & Turner, J. A. (1987). Treatment compliance of older alcoholics: An elder-specific approach is superior to "mainstreaming". *Journal of Studies on Alcohol, 48*, 47–51. doi:10.15288/jsa.1987.48.47

Kuerbis, A. N., Hagman, B. T., & Sacco, P. (2013). Functioning of alcohol use disorders criteria among middle-aged and older adults: Implications for DSM-5. *Substance Use & Misuse, 48*(4), 309–322. doi:10.3109/10826084.2012.762527

Kuerbis, A. N., Hail, L., Moore, A. A., & Muench, F. (2017). A pilot study of online feedback for adult drinkers 50 and older: Feasibility, efficacy, and preferences for intervention. *Journal of Substance Abuse Treatment, 77*, 126–132. doi:10.1016/j.jsat.2017.04.004

Kuerbis, A. N., & Sacco, P. (2013). A review of existing treatments for substance abuse among the elderly and recommendations for future directions. *Substance Abuse: Research and Treatment, 7*, 13–37. doi:10.4137/SART.S7865

Lay, K., King, L. J., & Rangel, J. (2008). Changing characteristics of drug use between two older adult cohorts: Small sample speculations on baby boomer trends to come. *Journal of Social Work Practice in the Addictions, 8*(1), 116–126. doi:10.1080/15332560802112078

Lee, H. S., Mericle, A. A., Ayalon, L., & Areán, P. A. (2009). Harm reduction among at-risk elderly drinkers: A site-specific analysis from the multi-site primary care research in substance abuse and mental health for elderly (PRISM-E) study. *International Journal of Geriatric Psychiatry, 24*(1), 54–60. doi:10.1002/gps.2073

Levkoff, S. E., Chen, H., Coakley, E., McDonel Herr, E. C., Oslin, D. W., Katz, I., . . . Ware, J. (2004). Design and sample characteristics of the PRISM-E multisite randomized trial to improve behavioral health care for the elderly. *Journal of Aging and Health, 16*, 3–27. doi:10.1177/0898264303260390

Lin, J. C., Karno, M. P., Grella, C. E., Ray, L. A., Liao, D. H., & Moore, A. A. (2013). Psychiatric correlates of alcohol and tobacco use disorders in US adults aged 65 years and older: Results From the 2001–2002 national epidemiologic survey of alcohol and related conditions. *The American Journal of Geriatric Psychiatry.* doi:10.1016/j.jagp.2013.07.005

Litten, R. Z., Ryan, M. L., Fertig, J. B., Falk, D. E., Johnson, B., Dunn, K. E., . . . NCIG (National Institute on Alcohol Abuse and Alcoholism Clinical Investigations Group) Study Group. (2013). A double-blind, placebo-controlled trial assessing the efficacy of varenicline tartrate for alcohol dependence. *Journal of Addiction Medicine, 7*(4), 277–286. doi:10.1097/ADM.0b013e31829623f4

Martin, C. M. (2018). The other side of the opioid debate: Treating older adults with chronic pain. *The Consultant Pharmacist, 33*(9), 478–483. doi:10.4140/TCP.n.2018.478

Miller, W. R., & Rollnick, S. (2013). *Motivational interviewing: Preparing people for change* (3rd ed.). New York, NY: The Guilford Press.

Miller, W. R., Zweben, A., DiClemente, C. C., & Rychtarik, R. G. (1992). *Motivational enhancement therapy manual: A clinical research guide for therapists treating individuals with alcohol abuse and dependence.* Rockville, MD: National Institute on Alcohol Abuse and Alcoholism.

Minerbi, A., Häuser, W., & Fitzcharles, M.-A. (2019). Medical cannabis for older patients. *Drugs & Aging, 36*(1), 39–51. doi:10.1007/s40266-018-0616-5

Moore, A. A., Blow, F. C., Hoffing, M., Welgreen, S., Davis, J. W., Lin, J. C., . . . Barry, K. L. (2011). Primary care-based intervention to reduce at-risk drinking in older adults: A randomized controlled trial. *Addiction, 106*(1), 111–120. doi:10.1111/j.1360-0443.2010.03229.x

Moore, A. A., Karno, M. P., Grella, C. E., Lin, J. C., Warda, U., Liao, D. H., & Hu, P. (2009). Alcohol, tobacco, and nonmedical drug use in older U.S. adults: Data from the 2001/02 national epidemiologic survey of alcohol and related conditions. *Journal of the American Geriatrics Society, 57*(12), 2275–2281. doi:10.1111/j.1532-5415.2009.02554.x

Moore, A. A., Whiteman, E. J., & Ward, K. T. (2007). Risks of combined alcohol/medication use in older adults. *American Journal of Geriatric Pharmacotherapy, 5*(1), 64–74. doi:10.1016/j.amjopharm.2007.03.006

Morgenstern, J., & McKay, J. (2007). Rethinking the paradigms that inform behavioral treatment research for substance use disorders. *Addiction, 102*, 1377–1389. doi:10.1111/j.1360-0443.2007.01882.x

National Institute on Alcohol Abuse and Alcoholism. (2007). *Helping patients who drink too much: A clinician's guide* (NIH Publication No. 07-3769). Bethesda, MD: National Institutes of Health.

Novier, A., Diaz-Granados, J. L., & Matthews, D. B. (2015). Alcohol use across the lifespan: An analysis of adolescent and aged rodents and humans. *Pharmacology Biochemistry and Behavior, 133*, 65–82. doi:10.1016/j.pbb.2015.03.015

Nugent, S. M., Morasco, B. J., O'Neil, M. E., Freeman, M., Low, A., Kondo, K., . . . Kansagara, D. (2017). The effects of cannabis among adults with chronic pain and an overview of general harms: A systematic review effects of cannabis among adults with chronic pain. *Annals of Internal Medicine, 167*(5), 319–331. doi:10.7326/m17-0155

O'Malley, S. S., Zweben, A., Fucito, L. M., Wu, R., Piepmeier, M. E., Ockert, D. M., . . . Gueorguieva, R. (2018). Effect of varenicline combined with medical management on alcohol use disorder with comorbid cigarette smoking: A randomized clinical trial. *JAMA Psychiatry, 75*(2), 129–138. doi:10.1001/jamapsychiatry.2017.3544

Oslin, D. W., Grantham, S., Coakley, E., Maxwell, J., Miles, K., Ware, J., . . . Zubritsky, C. (2006). PRISM-E: Comparison of integrated care and enhanced specialty referral in managing at-risk alcohol use. *Psychiatric Services, 57*(7), 954–958. doi:10.1176/ps.2006.57.7.954

Oslin, D. W., Liberto, J. G., O'Brien, J., Krois, S., & Norbeck, J. (1997). Naltrexone as an adjunctive treatment for older patients with alcohol dependence. *The American Journal of Geriatric Psychiatry, 5*(4), 324–332. doi:10.1097/00019442-199700540-00007

Oslin, D. W., Pettinati, H., & Volpicelli, J. R. (2002). Alcoholism treatment adherence: Older age predicts better adherence and drinking outcomes. *The American Journal of Geriatric Psychiatry, 10*(6), 740–747. doi:10.1176/appi.ajgp.10.6.740

Pacek, L. R., Mauro, P. M., & Martins, S. S. (2015). Perceived risk of regular cannabis use in the United States from 2002 to 2012: Differences by sex, age, and race/ethnicity. *Drug and Alcohol Dependence, 149*, 232–244. doi:10.1016/j.drugalcdep.2015.02.009

Patterson, T. L., & Jeste, D. V. (1999). The potential impact of the baby boom generation on substance abuse among elderly persons. *Psychiatric Services, 50*(9), 1184–1188. doi:10.1176/ps.50.9.1184

Plebani, J. G., Lynch, K. G., Rennert, L., Pettinati, H., O'Brien, C. P., & Kampman, K. M. (2013). Results from a pilot clinical trial of varenicline for the treatment of alcohol dependence. *Drug and Alcohol Dependence, 133*(2), 754–758. doi:10.1016/j.drugalcdep.2013.06.019

Rasouli, B., Ahlbom, A., Andersson, T., Grill, V., Midthjell, K., Olsson, L., & Carlsson, S. (2013). Alcohol consumption is associated with reduced risk of Type 2 diabetes and autoimmune diabetes in adults: Results from the Nord-Trondelag health study. *Diabetic Medicine, 30*(1), 56–64. doi:10.1111/j.1464-5491.2012.03713.x

Reynaud, M., Aubin, H. J., Trinquet, F., Zakine, B., Dano, C., Dematteis, M., . . . Detilleux, M. (2017). A Randomized, Placebo-Controlled Study of High-Dose Baclofen in Alcohol-Dependent Patients—The ALPADIR study. *Alcohol and Alcoholism, 52*(4), 439–446. doi:10.1093/alcalc/agx030

Rice, C., Longabaugh, R., Beattie, M., & Noel, N. (1993). Age group differences in response to treatment for problematic alcohol use. *Addiction, 88*, 1369–1375. doi:10.1111/j.1360-0443.1993.tb02023.x

Richard, E. L., Kritz-Silverstein, D., Laughlin, G. A., Fung, T. T., Barrett-Connor, E., & McEvoy, L. K. (2017). Alcohol intake and cognitively healthy longevity in community-dwelling adults: The Rancho Bernardo study. *Journal of Alzheimer's Disease* (Preprint), 1–12. doi:10.3233/JAD-161153

Rimer, B., Orleans, C. T., Fleisher, L., Cristinzio, S., Resch, N., Telepchak, J., & Keintz, M. (1994). Does tailoring matter? The impact of a tailored guide on ratings and short-term smoking-related outcomes for older adult smokers. *Health Education Research, 9*, 69–84. doi:10.1093/her/9.1.69

Rotgers, F. (2003). Cognitive-behavioral theories of substance abuse. In F. Rotgers, J. Morgenstern, & S. T. Walters (Eds.), *Treating substance abuse: Theory and technique* (2nd ed., pp. 166–189). New York, NY: The Guilford Press.

Sacco, P., Bucholz, K. K., & Spitznagel, E. L. (2009). Alcohol use among older adults in the national epidemiologic survey on alcohol and related conditions: A latent class analysis. *Journal of Studies on Alcohol and Drugs, 70*(6), 829–838. doi:10.15288/jsad.2009.70.829

Sacco, P., & Kuerbis, A. (2013). Older adults. In M. G. Vaughn & B. E. Perron (Eds.), *Social work practice in the addictions* (pp. 213–229). New York, NY: Springer. doi:10.1007/978-1-4614-5357-4_13

Satre, D. D., Mertens, J. R., Areán, P. A., & Weisner, C. (2003). Contrasting outcomes of older versus middle-aged and younger adult chemical dependency patients in a manged care program. *Journal of Studies on Alcohol, 64*, 520–530. doi:10.15288/jsa.2003.64.520

Satre, D. D., Mertens, J. R., Areán, P. A., & Weisner, C. (2004). Five-year alcohol and drug treatment outcomes of older adults versus middle-aged and younger adults in a managed care program. *Addiction, 99*(10), 1286–1297. doi:10.1111/j.1360-0443.2004.00831.x

Saunders, J. B., Peacock, A., & Degenhardt, L. (2018). Alcohol use disorders in the draft ICD-11, and how they compare with DSM-5. *Current Addiction Reports, 5*(2), 257–264. doi:10.1007/s40429-018-0197-8

Schepis, T. S., & McCabe, S. E. (2016). Trends in older adult nonmedical prescription drug use prevalence: Results from the 2002–2003 and 2012–2013 national survey on drug use and health. *Addictive Behaviors, 60*, 219–222. doi:10.1016/j.addbeh.2016.04.020

Schneider, J. K., Wong-Anuchit, C., Stallings, D., & Krieger, M. M. (2017). Motivational Interviewing and fruit/vegetable consumption in older adults. *Clinical Nursing Research, 26*(6), 731–746. doi:10.1177/1054773816673634

Schonfeld, L., & Dupree, L. W. (1995). Treatment approaches for older problem drinkers. *The International Journal of the Addictions, 30*(13–14), 1819–1842. doi:10.3109/10826089509071057

Schonfeld, L., & Dupree, L. W. (2002). Age-specific cognitive behavioral and self management treatment approaches. In A. M. Gurnack, R. M. Atkinson, & N. J. Osgood (Eds.), *Treating alcohol and drug abuse in the elderly* (pp. 109–130). New York, NY: Springer Publishing Company.

Schonfeld, L., Dupree, L. W., Dickson-Fuhrman, E., Royer, C. M., McDermott, C. H., Rosansky, J. S., . . . Jarvik, L. F. (2000). Cognitive-behavioral treatment of older veterans with substance abuse problems. *Journal of Geriatric Psychiatry and Neurology, 13*, 124–128. doi:10.1177/089198870001300305

Schonfeld, L., Hazlett, R. W., Hedgecock, D. K., Duchene, D. M., Burns, L. V., & Gum, A. M. (2015). Screening, brief intervention, and referral to treatment for older adults with substance misuse. *American Journal of Public Health, 105*(1), 205–211. doi:10.2105/ajph.2013.301859

Schonfeld, L., King-Kallimanis, B. L., Duchene, D. M., Etheridge, R. L., Herrera, J. R., Barry, K. L., & Lynn, N. (2010). Screening and brief intervention for substance misuse among older adults: The Florida BRITE project. *American Journal of Public Health, 100*(1), 108. doi:10.2105/ AJPH.2013.301859

Schultz, S. K., Arndt, S., & Liesveld, J. (2003). Locations of facilities with special programs for older substance abuse clients in the US. *International Journal of Geriatric Psychiatry, 18*(9), 839–843. doi:10.1002/gps.994

Shaper, A. G., Wannamethee, G., & Walker, M. (1988). Alcohol and mortality in British men: Explaining the U-shaped curve. *Lancet, 2*(8623), 1267–1273. doi:10.1016/S0140-6736(88)92890-5

Skog, O. J. (1996). Public health consequences of the J-curve hypothesis of alcohol problems. *Addiction, 91*(3), 325–337. doi:10.1111/j.1360-0443.1996.tb02283.x

Stallings, D. T., & Schneider, J. K. (2018). Motivational interviewing and fat consumption in older adults a meta-analysis. *Journal of Gerontological Nursing, 44*(11), 33–43. doi:10.3928/00989134-20180817-01

Tempesta, E., Janiri, L., Bignamini, A., Chabac, S., & Potgieter, A. (2000). Acamprosate and relapse prevention in the treatment of alcohol dependence: A placebo controlled trial. *Pharmacopsychiatry, 29*, 27–29.

Towers, A., Szabó, Á., Newcombe, D. A. L., Sheridan, J., Moore, A. A., Hyde, M., . . . Savage, C. L. (2018). Hazardous drinking prevalence and correlates in older New Zealanders: A comparison of the AUDIT-C and the CARET. *Journal of Aging and Health, 31*(10), 0898264318794108. doi:10.1177/0898264318794108

U.S. Department of Health and Human Services. (2014). *The health consequences of smoking—50 years of progress: A report of the surgeon general.* Atlanta, GA: Centers for Disease Control and Prevention (US).

U.S. National Library of Congress. (2013). *DailyMed.* Retrieved May 4, 2013, from http://dailymed. nlm.nih.gov/dailymed/about.cfm

Vadivelu, N., & Hines, R. L. (2008). Management of chronic pain in the elderly: Focus on transdermal buprenorphine. *Clinical Interventions in Aging, 3*(3), 421–430. doi:10.2147/CIA.S1880

Vincent, G. K., & Velkoff, V. A. (2010). *The next four decades: The older population in the United States: 2010 to 2050.* Washington, DC: US Department of Commerce, Economics and Statistics Administration, US Census Bureau.

Wang, T. W., Asman, K., Gentzke, A. S., Cullen, K. A., Holder-Hayes, E., Reyes-Guzman, C., . . . King, B. A. (2018). Tobacco product use among adults—United States, 2017. *MMWR. Morbidity and Mortality Weekly Report, 67*(44), 1225–1232. doi:10.15585/mmwr.mm6744a2

West, N. A., Severtson, S. G., Green, J. L., & Dart, R. C. (2015). Trends in abuse and misuse of prescription opioids among older adults. *Drug and Alcohol Dependence, 149*, 117–121. doi:doi:10.1016/j. drugalcdep.2015.01.027

World Health Organization. (2018). International statistical classification of diseases and related health problems. ICD-11. from https://icd.who.int/browse11/l-m/en

Wu, A. (2018). Special considerations for opioid use in elderly patients with chronic pain. *U.S. Pharmacist, 43*(3), 26–30.

Zanjani, F., Mavandadi, S., TenHave, T., Katz, I., Durai, N. B., Krahn, D., . . . Oslin, D. W. (2008). Longitudinal course of substance treatment benefits in older male veteran at-risk drinkers. *The Journal of Gerontology: Series A: Biological Sciences and Medical Sciences, 63A*(1), 98–106. doi:10.1093/ gerona/63.1.98

Zbikowski, S. M., Magnusson, B., Pockey, J. R., Tindle, H. A., & Weaver, K. E. (2012). A review of smoking cessation interventions for smokers aged 50 and over. *Maturitas, 71*, 131–141. doi:10.1016/j. maturitas.2011.11.019

16

Understanding addictive behavior from a human diversity perspective

*Christina C. Tam, Katherine J. Karriker-Jaffe
and Karen G. Chartier*

Background

Wide variations exist in use patterns of alcohol and other psychoactive substances across diverse social groups defined by race/ethnicity, gender, gender/sexual identity, religion, geographical location, and disability status. The most salient social characteristics vary by country. For example, race and ethnicity historically have been critically important in the United States (U.S.), while gender or religion may be more relevant in other countries including those in Asia. This chapter presents outcomes related to substance use—including patterns of use, development of substance use disorders (SUD),[1] and access to treatment—in diverse populations across the globe, and explicates reasons that contribute to highlighted group differences.

Variations in substance use outcomes among groups often are products of social, economic, and environmental circumstances. Inequitable differences are known as *disparities*. The U.S. National Institute on Minority Health and Health Disparities (NIMHD) research framework guides this diversity discussion. A central tenet of this framework is that the environments in which individuals live, play, and work influence their health and well-being. These influences are associated with differential exposure to certain types of environmental contexts and experiences over the lifecourse, based in part on an individual's social markers and social status (Alvidrez, Castille, Laude-Sharp, Rosario, & Tabor, 2019). In addition to having direct effects on substance use and related outcomes, these environments interact with individual biological dispositions, rendering some individuals more vulnerable than others to engaging in addictive behaviors (see Chapter 7).

This chapter begins with an overview of three social categories important for discussing diversity and substance use: race/ethnicity, gender, and disability status. The goal is to highlight the most relevant information for each of these categories as they pertain to alcohol and other substance use prevalence, related problems, and treatment access. The focus of the sections on race/ethnicity and gender are primarily on alcohol, as it is the most widely used substance globally (see Chapter 2). A broader definition of substance use is relevant when considering disability status. The information presented is primarily from studies of adults, but similar factors influence young people. A broad overview of diverse social groups in relation to addictive behaviors is provided, but this is by no means an exhaustive discussion. Therefore, it is likely that intersections of social categories and social status influence addictive behaviors in other ways not described here.

Keeping in mind the intersections across diversity factors that may either protect or place individuals at risk for heavy substance use and related problems, the chapter discusses the NIMHD guiding framework in more detail. After presenting the framework, important determinants from individual to societal levels and examples of how these factors might influence substance use outcomes from a global perspective are highlighted. This chapter concludes with suggestions for social workers that may help promote health equity and reduce disparities. In doing so, this discussion addresses a challenge for social work—to close the health gap and "eradicate health inequalities for future generations" (Walters et al., 2016)— by presenting strategies by which disparities can be ameliorated and sharing lessons learned from one nation to another.

Diverse populations

Before turning attention to how different populations (the groups to which people identify and belong) experience substance use, *intersectionality* is an important concept to highlight: individuals do not belong to one single social group; in fact, a person may identify with multiple social categories (e.g. a racial/ethnic minority woman), which together may influence greater or fewer disparities in addictive behaviors and contribute to differences in problem recognition, experienced consequences, and treatment access. Social workers should keep in mind the contexts in which individuals are embedded based on social indicators such as ethnic heritage, gender, and disability status, each of which may singly or jointly affect risk for substance use and related problems. In addition to describing major trends within each social category (race/ethnicity, gender, disability status), information is presented describing how intersectionality of these categories is related to substance use, heavy use, and related problems.

Racial/ethnic background

Overall, there are significant racial/ethnic differences in substance use patterns (including whether someone uses a substance at all, as well as how often and how much they use it), consequences of use, developing SUDs, and treatment access. While *race* refers to a person's physical characteristics, *ethnicity* refers to cultural factors such as nationality, ancestry, and language. With respect to alcohol in the U.S., non-Hispanic Whites report the highest rates of consumption overall, but alcohol use disorder (AUD)[2] is most prevalent among Native Americans (Delker, Brown, & Hasin, 2016). Illicit drug use is highest among Native Hawaiians/Pacific Islanders and American Indians/Alaskan Natives (Substance Abuse and Mental Health Services Administration, 2014), and the latter group has the highest lifetime rates of dependence, followed by Whites and Blacks/African Americans (Delker, Brown, & Hasin, 2015).

Racial/ethnic disparities in heavy alcohol use and AUD contribute to disproportionate rates of health and social harms (including liver disease and car crashes) among some groups such as Native Americans and Blacks (Chartier, Vaeth, & Caetano, 2013; Delker et al., 2016). However, differences in use patterns do not completely account for all of the differentially negative effects of alcohol associated with health disparities. One U.S. study reported

Blacks and Hispanic Americans experienced higher levels of social consequences from alcohol use compared to Whites at similar levels of consumption (Mulia, Ye, Greenfield, & Zemore, 2009). Therefore, some groups bear disparate rates of addictive behavior consequences not solely reflective of their use patterns. Additionally, a consistent research finding is that Hispanics are less likely to access specialty alcohol/drug treatment (Guerrero, Marsh, Khachikian, Amaro, & Vega, 2013), and this is especially the case among women (Zemore et al., 2014).

The relevance of social constructs such as race/ethnicity depends on the country, and so an international lens is applied to highlight how patterns of substance use vary by race/ethnicity outside the U.S. There are ethnic differences in substance use patterns in Scandinavia, for example, with ethnic Finns in Sweden showing higher rates of alcohol and drug problems than ethnic Swedes (Leão, Johansson, & Sundquist, 2006). In the United Kingdom (U.K.), Afro-Caribbean men and women show lower rates of heavy drinking and alcohol-related problems than their native British counterparts, while some South Asian immigrant groups show higher alcohol-related death rates (Mckeigue & Karmi, 1993); alcohol-related hospital admission rates by ethnicity also differ by geography (Barry, Laverty, Majeed, & Millett, 2015). In some countries, racial/ethnic disparities often are attributed to low socioeconomic status (SES) (Fiscella, Franks, Gold, & Clancy, 2000) and they concentrate in certain geographic areas: low SES is linked to barriers in accessing care for alcohol-related conditions and unhealthy behaviors (e.g. poor diet, smoking) that exacerbate risk for alcohol-related death (Probst, Roerecke, Behrendt, & Rehm, 2014).

Gender

Gender is a social construct based on societal roles. Gender roles are prescribed as ideal behaviors for a person of that specific biological sex. In many societies and cultures, social roles for women often conflict with alcohol consumption or getting drunk, and women may experience stronger social sanctions against drinking than men (Nolen-Hoeksema, 2004). In many Western countries such as the U.S., gender differences in alcohol consumption and heavy drinking largely depend on developmental stage (Keyes et al., 2019). When factoring gender into the discussion on disparities, racial/ethnic differences become more complex. For example, in the U.S., consuming alcohol (versus abstinence) is more common among Whites relative to other racial/ethnic subgroups, and this is especially true for White women relative to Black or Hispanic women, with the latter two having higher rates of lifetime abstinence or very low rates of drinking (Kerr et al., 2017).

Problems with addictive substances manifest differently for women compared to men. Although men have high rates of heavy substance use and SUD across racial/ethnic categories compared to women (Wilsnack, Wilsnack, Gmel, & Kantor, 2018), women experience higher rates of problems attributed to alcohol use (Nolen-Hoeksema, 2004), including physical health problems such as alcohol-related liver disease, certain types of cancers, and other chronic health and cognitive problems. These differences are due to many factors that are not yet entirely understood, including social conditions, body composition, and alcohol metabolism (i.e. women have greater blood alcohol content compared to men after similar levels of consumption). Due to some biological (sex) differences such as varying rates of alcohol metabolism, women often drink for less time before developing AUD and related consequences (called *telescoping*) (Erol & Karpyak, 2015; US Department of Health and Human Services, 2016). In addition to physical health problems related to a woman's own use, in many countries women are also more likely than men to be victims of alcohol-related harm perpetrated by someone else. This includes marital or family problems caused by another drinker (Room et al., 2019). Heavier alcohol use is consistently associated with increased likelihood and severity of intimate partner violence by both genders in many nations (Wilsnack et al., 2018). Alcohol consumption by women of child-bearing age also contributes to the risk for Fetal Alcohol Syndrome and Fetal Alcohol Spectrum Disorders (FASD) (see Chapters 11, 12 and 26).

It is important to consider the unique circumstances regarding treatment for women. Relative to men, women often arrive at addictive behaviors through different pathways, and they have different propensities for relapse, or reappearance of problems after some time without problems. For instance, heavy alcohol use is more likely to be influenced by psychological distress for women than for men (Nolen-Hoeksema, 2004), and returning to alcohol use is more often related to negative emotions for women but to social pressures for men (Erol & Karpyak, 2015). In the U.S. in particular, substance use is a primary reason for women's incarceration and related problems, such as loss of custody of children (Wright, Van Voorhis, Salisbury, & Bauman, 2012) that can affect treatment. Women overall are less likely than men to use treatment services, and women face unique challenges and barriers to care including availability of affordable childcare, lack of services for pregnant women, and difficulties managing a relationship with a partner using substances (Tuchman, 2010). Treatment services provided to incarcerated women generally are not gender-responsive and subsequently fail to meet their needs (Wright et al., 2012).

Disability status

Physical impairments generally limit a person's physical functioning (e.g. sensory impairments, amputation, paralysis), while intellectual impairments are characterized by limitations in cognitive functioning (e.g. Down syndrome, FASD). Unlike physical disabilities, which may emerge at any point in the lifecourse, intellectual disabilities generally originate before the age of 18—not including circumstances such as traumatic brain injuries occurring later in life. The Americans with Disabilities Act (ADA) was enacted in the U.S. as a law protecting individuals experiencing disabilities from discrimination in all areas open to the general public, including health care services. Globally, about 161 countries around the world have signed on to the United Nations Convention on the Rights of People with Disabilities, which affords similar protections as the ADA.

Substance use as a consequence of disability

In terms of addictive behaviors, individuals experiencing disabilities may use substances to cope with pain, isolation, and stigma; others may develop a disability as a result of heavy substance use (Glazier & Kling, 2013; Oslin, 2000). The prevalence of substance use other than alcohol is greater among persons experiencing disabilities compared to those not experiencing disabilities: U.S. estimates from 2010 showed two times the prevalence rate of heavy illicit substance use and a greater likelihood of reporting heavy cannabis use (Glazier & Kling, 2013). Heavy substance use often co-occurs with mental illnesses such as depression or anxiety that could develop as a result of isolation, aging, and declining ability (see Chapters 14 and 32). Age-related chronic pain and physical illnesses are also associated with heavy substance use (Oslin, 2000; Simoni-Wastila & Yang, 2006).

Disability as a consequence of heavy substance use

Substance use and SUD can lead to disability in any phase of life. In contrast to research on persons experiencing disabilities who engage in heavy use of substances other than alcohol, the proportion of persons in the U.S. *without* disabilities who reported past-month binge drinking (defined by the U.S. Centers for Disease Control and Prevention as four and five or more drinks for women and men on an occasion, respectively) typically surpassed the proportion for individuals experiencing disabilities (Kraus, Lauer, Coleman, & Houtenville, 2018). However, heavy drinking is a well-established cause of disabilities, especially among older adults. As the body ages, it becomes more vulnerable to the effects of alcohol, and with age there is a greater risk of stroke and impaired motor functioning that could result in falls, fractures, and head injuries (Mukamal et al., 2004; Oslin, 2000). While heavy drinking leads to alcohol-induced disorders including Korsakoff's syndrome, which causes memory impairment and cognitive defects later in life, drinking at moderate levels may exacerbate preexisting medical and mental health problems (Mahli & Hellerbrand, 2016; Oslin, 2000).

Summary

There are many important differences in patterns of substance use, consequences, and development of SUD across social categories defined by race/ethnicity, gender, and disability status. These differences are due to myriad factors that contribute to disparities in addictive behaviors and associated problems, including key elements found within a guiding framework described below. Accounting for social categories across nations, regions, and cultures generates a rich discussion with many implications for social work practice.

U.S. National Institute of Minority Health and Health Disparities framework

The NIMHD research framework includes both biological and social determinants that contribute to health disparities (Alvidrez et al., 2019). Similar to the biopsychosocial perspective interwoven throughout this handbook, the framework is a multi-level, multi-domain model that includes determinants relevant to addictive behaviors. Rather than exclusively focusing on one particular set of determinants, this framework describes cumulative (those that accumulate across someone's life) and interactive effects (those that have different effects depending on other factors that are present).

Determinants are biological and social. *Biological* determinants include genetic and other intrinsic biological factors that exacerbate propensities for engaging in addictive behaviors and developing SUD. These factors interact with *social* determinants, which are characteristics of different social environments in which people are situated and function. Elements of these contexts may affect individuals' exposure to certain risks and protective factors, as well as their access to resources, such as health care, that may help mitigate risks.

Four levels of influence (see Table 16.1), from individual to societal, interact with domains of influence to affect outcomes for specific individuals, as well as for whole populations. The five domains of influence, spanning the lifecourse from birth to older adulthood, include biological and behavioral factors and the cumulative influences of social and environmental exposures (Alvidrez et al., 2019) that intersect the four levels (individual, interpersonal, community, societal) as *determinants of health*. This framework provides a comprehensive model for social workers to target interventions in order to ameliorate health inequities.

Table 16.1 National Institute of Minority Health and Health Disparities framework (National Institute on Minority Health and Health Disparities (2017). NIMHD Research Framework. Retrieved from https://www.nimhd.nih.gov/about/overview/research-framework.html. Accessed on February 19, 2018.)

		Levels of Influence			
		Individual	*Interpersonal*	*Community*	*Societal*
Domains of Influence (Over the lifecourse)	**Biological**	Biological vulnerability and mechanisms	Caregiver-child interaction Family microbiome	Community illness exposure Herd immunity	Sanitation Immunization Pathogen exposure
	Behavioral	ealth behaviors Coping strategies	Family functioning School/work functioning	Community Functioning	Policies and laws
	Physical/built environment	Personal environment	Household environment School/work environment	Community environment Community resources	Societal structure
	Sociocultural environment	Sociodemographics Limited English Cultural identity Response to discrimination	Social networks Family/peer norms Interpersonal discrimination	Community norms Local structural discrimination	Social norms Societal structural discrimination
	Health care system	Insurance coverage Health literacy Treatment preferences	Patient-clinician relationship Medical decision-making	Availability of services Safety Net services	Quality of care Health care policies
Health outcomes		**Individual health**	**Family/organizational health**	**Community health**	**Population health**

Table 16.2 Example applied to Asian-American populations within the framework

Individual		
Biological		**Biological vulnerabilities and mechanisms.** The ability to metabolize alcohol can affect consumption. East Asians such as Chinese and Koreans are deficient in a particular genetic component that causes facial flushing and other symptoms of discomfort (nausea, headaches, heart palpitations) in response to alcohol. This genetic deficiency can be a protective mechanism that results in lower alcohol consumption. However, this does not eliminate risk of heavy drinking entirely, and drinking by those who experience alcohol-related flushing is associated with greater risk for health consequences like esophageal cancer (Brooks, Enoch, Goldman, Li, & Yokoyama, 2009)
Sociocultural environment		**Cultural identity.** For some Asians, adherence to cultural values, such as Confucian principles that include hard work and face, or the way one's actions reflect on the entire family, may influence decisions about engaging in substance use (Iwamoto, Kaya, Grivel, & Clinton, 2016). This may be especially true for newer immigrants to a receiving nation of a different culture, particularly when there is a priority focus on socioeconomic achievement
Interpersonal		
Behavioral		**Family functioning.** Tensions related to clashing value systems may arise between Asian immigrant parents and their children, and these can manifest in substance use among the younger generation (Kane et al., 2018)
Health care system		**Patient-clinician relationship.** An Asian patient may not be assessed for substance use behaviors because of a general perception that they are in a low-risk group that does not use (Iwamoto et al., 2016). Consequently, Asians with SUD may be overlooked, restricting access to necessary care
Community		
Health care system		**Availability of services.** Service availability may be lacking due to limited language capabilities and cultural congruence among providers and Asian clients (Zemore et al., 2018)
Sociocultural environment		**Community norms.** A neighborhood where there is greater presence of residents who identify with their specific Asian heritage group can protect against substance use due to pervasive norms that uphold more traditional cultural values (Molina et al., 2012)
Societal		
Behavioral		**Policies and laws.** There are policies and laws that may inadvertently facilitate substance use among certain groups. For instance, prior to resettlement in the U.S., some refugees (those who are forcibly displaced) such as those from Bhutan may have spent some time in camps where substance use is rampant as a form of coping with the trauma of resettlement (Luitel, Jordans, Murphy, Roberts, & McCambridge, 2013). This is often because the policies in their home country do not allow reentry or because there are long, uncertain waiting periods prior to resettlement in a new receiving country
Sociocultural environment		**Social norms.** Drinking and drug-using cultures in Asian countries also differ drastically, with certain countries such as South Korea having high levels of per capita alcohol consumption (Iwamoto et al., 2016). These social behavioral norms may persist in their ex-patriate communities in other countries

Example: populations from Asian countries

Groups from countries in Asia who immigrated to the U.S., as a whole, have low alcohol and substance use prevalence and dependence rates compared to U.S. national averages. However, this racial category is comprised of many different heritages, and heterogeneity between ethnic groups in substance use rates are masked within this aggregate grouping. For example, in one study, past-month reports of binge drinking ranged from 8.4% among Chinese Americans to 25.9% among Korean Americans (Wu & Blazer, 2015). Thus, rather than viewing "Asian Americans" as a monolithic entity with low risk for substance use and dependence, practitioners are encouraged to think critically about how each level and domain intersect to influence outcomes for different population subgroups. An example of the framework applied to substance use within U.S. Asian populations is presented in Table 16.2. The goals are first to identify some intersections between levels and domains that are relevant for this group, and then to provide specific examples of health determinants at each intersection.

Determinants of substance use and SUD from a diversity perspective

The following sections emphasize some (but certainly not all) salient determinants of disparities that social workers should consider when working with diverse groups. These determinants are based on the previously presented NIMHD framework. Current findings on addictive behaviors are highlighted within individual, interpersonal, community, and societal determinants that contribute to disparities. While substance use in general and SUD are covered more broadly within the discussion of each determinant, the current state of knowledge on alcohol is detailed with more specific examples.

Individual determinants of substance use and SUD

At the individual level, determinants for each domain include: genetic vulnerability (biological), coping strategies (behavioral), cultural identity (sociocultural environment), and insurance coverage (health care system).

Biological domain: genetic vulnerability

At the most fundamental individual level, genetic mechanisms affect the propensity for substance use and developing SUD. For example, some racial/ethnic differences observed in drinking patterns are explained by different allele frequencies observed across geographic ancestry groups for genes associated with alcohol metabolism. As an aside, the race and ethnicity social constructs often overlap with the major African, European, Asian, and Native American continental ancestries. In the prior example, individuals of East Asian ancestry are more likely to carry the *ALDH2*2* and *ADH1B*2* variants, which protect against alcohol use by causing an unpleasant "flushing" response, nausea, headaches, and elevated heart rate when alcohol is consumed (Zaso, Goodhines, Wall, & Park, 2019). Individuals of other ancestry groups likely carry other genetic variants associated with alcohol metabolism. For instance, different variants of the *ADH1B* gene are associated with AUD among individuals of African descent and European descent, with a low risk allele being more frequent among individuals of African ancestry (see Wall, Luczak, & Hiller-Sturmhöfel, 2016 for a comprehensive review).

Behavioral domain: coping strategies

Individuals may use substances to cope with negative life experiences based on their identification with one or more stigmatized or disadvantaged social groups. One such example pertains to disability status. Compared to others, individuals experiencing disabilities may encounter greater disadvantages including lower income and greater unemployment (Iezzoni, 2011). Further, persons experiencing intellectual disabilities have high rates of co-occurring mental health issues (Chapman & Wu, 2012). These disadvantages may be due to social isolation resulting from having a disability, as well as encountering prejudices and stereotypes about disability. While individuals around the world experiencing disabilities have different experiences with public perception and recognition of their circumstances, heavy substance use can exacerbate risks in adjustment related to employment and educational attainment (Hollar & Moore, 2004; Moore, 2001).

Sociocultural environment domain: cultural identity

Some groups immigrate in pursuit of the "American" (or host country) dream, while others emigrate to escape poverty, disease, environmental destruction, or crime in their country of origin (Renzaho, 2016). Among immigrants, closeness to the culture of origin is perceived as a source of resilience, whereas *acculturation* (adopting the practices and values of a new host culture) is a risk factor for alcohol use, heavy use, and related problems (Lui & Zamboanga, 2018a, 2018b). This is particularly evident among individuals who move from other countries to the U.S. Despite barriers to integration that first-generation immigrants (those born outside the host country) may face, these individuals often fare better on substance use outcomes than members of later generations (Lui & Zamboanga, 2018a, 2018b). For immigrants and their children who experience SUD and its related problems, treatment utilization and retention can be difficult due to linguistic and cultural barriers when acculturation is low (Guerrero et al., 2013).

Health care system domain: income and insurance coverage

In the U.S., although low SES is typically associated with abstinence from alcohol use, individuals in this group who do drink often engage in heavy use (Collins, 2016) and may disproportionately experience more problems related to alcohol use. A multi-country meta-analysis detected stark SES differences in alcohol-related mortality (Probst et al., 2014). In countries with limited health care, SES relates to the availability of care and to disparities in access to SUD treatment services, particularly in nations, states or jurisdictions with limited funding for treatment. In the U.S., for example, a person with higher SES may be able to bypass treatment barriers related to insurance coverage and enroll in a private program; persons with lower SES typically have fewer options for treatment, and there often are long waitlists for public programs (Verissimo & Grella, 2017).

Interpersonal determinants of substance use and SUD

Interpersonal determinants include factors that involve relationships or interactions between people, and they include family functioning (behavioral), interpersonal discrimination (socio-cultural environment), and aspects of the patient-clinician relationship (health care system).

Behavioral domain: family functioning

It is well-established that parenting practices and parent-child relationships bear influence on adolescent substance use (Yap, Cheong, Zaravinos-Tsakos, Lubman, & Jorm, 2017). In some immigrant families, parents and children acculturate at different rates, giving rise to family conflict (Lui, 2015). This conflict can lead to breakdown in family communication and closeness, prompting a young person to turn to substances as a way to cope with family stressors or by enabling access to substances through peers because of lower parental involvement and monitoring (Kane et al., 2018). Childhood trauma is also a risk factor for heavy substance use and SUD. While the strength of the relationship of such stressors with adverse substance use outcomes are similar across groups, some groups encounter higher rates of child abuse and neglect than others, including individuals experiencing disabilities (Jones et al., 2012) and in some American Indian/Alaskan Native communities (Enoch & Albaugh, 2017).

Sociocultural environment: interpersonal discrimination

Instances of interpersonal discrimination occur over multiple contexts and include verbal insults, poor service delivery in settings like shops or restaurants, physical and verbal violence, and social exclusion. Individuals who identify with a minority group (based on gender, race/ethnicity, disability, religion, and/or sexual orientation) may experience isolation or a lack of positive group identity due to discrimination (Gilbert & Zemore, 2016). In response, some individuals engage in health compromising behaviors that include substance use: as instances of discrimination increase, high-risk drinking and AUD also increase (Gilbert & Zemore, 2016). Among racial/ethnic minorities in particular, explanations linking experiences of interpersonal discrimination to heavy alcohol use include feelings of anger, posttraumatic stress disorder (PTSD), and depression (Brondolo, Ver Halen, Pencille, Beatty, & Contrada, 2009; Gilbert & Zemore, 2016). It is noteworthy that Blacks in the U.S. exhibit low rates of substance use early in life, but later in life dependency rates in this group are among the highest compared to other racial/ethnic groups, especially among Black men (Delker et al., 2015). Black Americans also are more likely to encounter legal problems compared to Whites consuming similar levels of alcohol; this may be an effect of the higher levels of discrimination (e.g. police contact, racism) that the former group experiences (Zapolski, Pedersen, McCarthy, & Smith, 2014).

Health care system: patient-clinician relationship

Health provider practices may inadvertently prevent certain individuals from accessing quality treatment, including screening protocols and service provision models ill-suited for an individual's background (c.f. Reinert & Allen, 2007). This includes ignoring special needs of pregnant women or overlooking challenges caused by provider-patient cultural incongruence. *Cultural competence* (compatible behaviors and value systems that allow effective service delivery in cross-cultural settings) is linked to better communication, greater client satisfaction, and better treatment retention among Hispanics (Guerrero et al., 2013). In addition to linguistic and cultural barriers that preclude a client from accessing effective treatment options, discriminatory behavior toward certain groups of people through *implicit bias* (acting on automatic and subconscious assumptions) may result in missed opportunities to address factors that are vital to clients' recovery (Stone & Moskowitz, 2011).

Community determinants of substance use and SUD

Community-level determinants include community functioning (behavioral), community resources (physical/built environment), community norms (sociocultural environment), and availability of services (health care system).

Behavioral domain: community functioning

Community social infrastructure (such as quality schools and recreational facilities) sets the foundation for residents' overall physical and social functioning. Without such structure, a community may lack social order, creating greater opportunities for problems such as substance use and crime/violence associated with distribution. Some communities situated along the U.S.-Mexico border have strained infrastructures of this nature. Border residents are more impoverished, less educated, and underemployed compared to those living in other areas of the U.S. This area is home to two nations with different alcohol and drug policies (Mexico has a lower legal drinking age and easy access to very cheap alcohol) that enable U.S. border residents' greater access (Mills & Caetano, 2016). From a global perspective, some regions experiencing economic, political, and environmental crises contribute to a widening income gap, a lack of community infrastructure, and disparities in substance use: for example, sub-Saharan Africa and the Pacific Islands have recently experienced increases in injection drug use (Degenhardt et al., 2017).

Physical/built environment: community resources

Closely related to community functioning is the availability of community resources preventing substance use disparities. Communities lacking essential physical resources inhibit residents from accessing health and mental health services for addictive behaviors and their consequences. In the U.S., 22% of the American Indian/Alaskan Native population reside on reservations which tend to be located in rural and remote areas (US Department of Health and Human Services, 2018). Compounding this geographic isolation is community disadvantage, as reservations often are characterized by poverty and poor access to adequate health care, educational opportunities, and social services, particularly in the Southwestern and Northern Plains states (Spillane & Smith, 2007; Whitesell, Beals, Crow, Mitchell, & Novins, 2012). Partly due to a lack of essential community resources, American Indians/Alaskan Natives living on reservations in the U.S. have higher rates of SUD compared to those who do not (Whitesell et al., 2012). This has also been observed among indigenous populations living in remote locations of Canada, Australia, and New Zealand (Marrone, 2007).

Sociocultural environment: community norms

People living in areas surrounded by others who share their heritage in coethnic communities are regularly exposed to the group's values and practices through social structures supporting use of culturally tailored facilities (e.g. professionals that serve clients in their native languages), as well as social and cultural opportunities maintaining ties to the cultural group or home country (in the case of immigrants). Protective effects of community coethnic density were observed in studies that examined alcohol consumption among Caribbean Blacks and Pakistani populations living in the U.K. (Bécares, Nazroo, & Stafford, 2011), substance use problems among Hispanics, Caribbean Blacks, and Asians living in the U.S. (Molina, Alegría, & Chen, 2012), and psychiatric disorders among Iraqi immigrants in Sweden (Mezuk et al., 2015). Alternatively, norms within coethnic communities may facilitate risky behaviors such as gambling or smoking, or may stigmatize help/treatment engagement, as well.

Health care system: availability of services

Even when treatment for SUD is affordable or covered by insurance or government bene-fits, service availability and accessibility are other barriers to overcome (Verissimo & Grella, 2017). In some low-income and less populated areas in the U.S., the number of persons who need treatment surpasses the number of available clinicians or program openings. If a treat-ment program is available, treatment accessibility issues may arise in the form of work or household obligations. These are critical barriers facing individuals with low-income back-grounds or are experiencing disabilities who may not have access to transportation and/ or childcare options. Accessibility barriers also include lack of information about available treatment options and payment options (Verissimo & Grella, 2017).

Societal determinants of substance use and SUD

Finally, the societal level of influence includes policies and laws (behavioral), societal struc-ture (physical/built environment), social norms (sociocultural environment), and quality of care (health care system) determinants.

Behavioral domain: policies and laws

At the societal level, the framework includes policies and laws in the behavioral domain because they are modifiable; however, policies and laws overlap somewhat with the societal structures described next (Alvidrez et al., 2019). One policy particularly relevant to addictive behaviors is the Americans with Disabilities Act (ADA) and similar protective policies in other nations. The ADA defines disability as impairment that substantially limits daily func-tioning. Specifically, this law offers protections from discriminatory practices to individuals who currently experience AUD, previously experienced an SUD, and are receiving or have received treatment ("Americans with Disabilities Act of 1990," 1991). Individuals unaware of this protection may refrain from seeking treatment or certain employment opportunities for fear of discrimination. This information gap, combined with uneven implementation and enforcement of the ADA, as well as difficulties with contesting discrimination events, may foster treatment inequities.

Physical/built environment: societal structure

The framework places societal structures, including the organization of educational and crim-inal justice systems, under the physical/built environment domain because these structures are usually quite stable over time (Alvidrez et al., 2019). Historical policies and social forces in the U.S. and other nations influence where people live, and low-income communities tend to be overburdened by retail alcohol outlets such as bars and liquor stores; they also may be less able to offer resistance to incursion of criminal drug distribution activities. Blacks, Hispanics, and Native Americans in the U.S. are more likely than Whites to live in low-income areas, and residents of disadvantaged areas have increased likelihood of substance use (Karriker-Jaffe, 2011). Unlike higher-income neighborhoods, community members in disadvantaged areas typically do not have the resources to mobilize against liquor store placement in their neighborhoods. As a result, alcohol availability policies (e.g. where stores are located and hours of operation) contribute to an excess of retail alcohol outlets disproportionately affecting racial/ethnic minorities (Chartier et al., 2014). Local communities have experienced some success in promoting resistance. For example, indigenous communities in high-income nations such as the U.S., Australia, Canada, and Greenland led policy efforts to prohibit the sale, importation, or possession of alcohol in their communities. These and other strategies driven by leaders within indigenous communities contributed to reduced rates of health and social harms and some show promise for reducing high rates of alcohol use in these areas (Muhunthan et al., 2017).

Sociocultural environment: social norms

National and local policies play a role in facilitating norms around substance use, although norms may also help shape the policy landscape in democratic societies. The alcohol industry is largely unregulated in parts of Africa, where the most common pattern of consumption is heavy episodic use (60 g or more of pure alcohol on an occasion) (Ferreira-Borges, Parry, & Babor, 2017). In addition to lack of knowledge surrounding the harmful effects of alcohol use, citizens in most countries of Africa perceive there to be more pressing public health problems than alcohol (Ferreira-Borges et al., 2017). Some Latin American and European countries and parts of the U.S. have legalized recreational cannabis use, whereas it is criminalized in most African and Asian countries (Aguilar, Gutierrez, Sanchez, & Nougier, 2018). Cannabis prohibition in Japan, for instance, facilitated a negative public perception of its use despite the plant being an integral part of the country's history (Vaughn, Huang, & Ramirez, 1995).

In addition to the interplay between policies and social norms, a community's degree of societal religiosity can play a role in establishing norms related to substance use. Globally, the WHO reports the lowest prevalence rates of alcohol and other substance use and SUD in Muslim countries (Michalak & Trocki, 2006). The textual sources of Islam caution against use of intoxicants; therefore, the possession, sale, or consumption of alcohol has long been illegal in many Muslim-led countries. In other nations, such as Bahrain and Qatar, alcohol remains legally available; however, public displays of intoxicated behavior or driving after alcohol consumption may be punishable by imprisonment (AlMarri & Oei, 2009). Due to changing demographics and shifts in social and cultural norms, SUD may be an emerging issue in these regions despite religious and legal constraints: there is a hidden subset of the Muslim population engaging in heroin and alcohol use (AlMarri & Oei, 2009). On the whole, religious norms can help protect against substance use, heavy use, and SUD, but these prohibitions may stigmatize people who use substances and are in need of treatment.

Health care system: quality of care

While SUDs often co-occur with mental health problems, treatment approaches may not offer integrated services to effectively address both concerns, thereby compromising quality of care (Guerrero et al., 2013). Persons experiencing disabilities may find their treatment options to be severely limited; persons experiencing intellectual disabilities are less likely than others to receive or to remain in treatment (Chapman & Wu, 2012), and physical barriers may preclude those experiencing physical disabilities from accessing treatment (West, Graham, & Cifu, 2009). Other barriers include stigma and perceived discrimination in accessing and receiving treatment, a lack of recognition of disability status by health care providers, and treatment modalities that preclude persons with certain disabilities from accessing care (Moore, 2001).

What social workers can do

Equipped with an understanding of how different determinants of the framework may influence someone's substance use, development of SUD, and treatment access, social workers and allied health professionals are encouraged to incorporate this framework into their practice with diverse populations. In consideration of the interplay of the domains and levels of influence that contribute to addictive behaviors, it becomes clear there are targeted mechanisms relevant to a person's background for strategies to successfully address heavy substance use and SUD. Doing so will move the field closer to meeting one of social work's core values of achieving social justice and in attaining the grand challenge of closing the health gap related to substance use and SUDs (Walters et al., 2016). This section offers a few strategies at the micro and macro levels of social work practice to reduce disparities across race/ethnicity, gender, and disability status. One that applies across levels is the profession's ethical standard of cultural awareness and diversity (National Association of Social Workers, n.d.), with the recognition and understanding of diverse population groups and cultures, particularly their strengths.

Micro-level practice implications

The micro practitioner works one-on-one with individuals and in group settings, and this can include alcohol and drug screening practices, brief intervention, and referral to a variety of other SUD treatment modalities. Practitioners should screen individuals in all racial/ethnic, gender, and ability groups for substance use without imposing stereotypical assumptions that some groups do not engage in risky substance use. The use of evidence-based screening tools validated for the particular population, administered in the client's preferred language, is necessary to avoid inaccurate results. Further, to facilitate clients' recovery efforts, social workers should practice cultural competence and *humility* by relating to clients' values and identities with respect to their perspectives toward substance use, SUD, and treatment.

It also is critical to consider the intersections of multiple identities and how they influence a client's circumstances. For instance, racial/ethnic minority women may be susceptible to using substances to cope with stress stemming from racism, discrimination, and associated mental distress, but individuals in this group may also have strong community ties that provide support and sources of resilience. For women in general, gender-sensitive treatment strategies that address the comorbidity of substance use with other psychiatric disorders and trauma, as well as activities to foster healthy relationships, may be more efficacious compared to pharmacological modalities alone that do not address social factors (Wilsnack et al., 2018).

At the interpersonal level, parents can employ myriad strategies to prevent substance use by young people. These include enhancing family functioning by establishing clear communication and developing skills to foster family closeness and manage conflicts (Velleman, Templeton, & Copello, 2005). Social workers should be mindful of factors such as intergenerational differences in acculturation that may compromise their traditional family resilience patterns. Social workers may consider linking families to appropriate community resources that address/prevent substance use among children and youth.

A relatively small proportion of individuals diagnosed with SUD seek out formal treatment in the community, although these proportions are higher when considering other forms of care, such as 12-step groups and primary care physicians (Guerrero et al., 2013). While mutual aid and 12-step support groups such as Alcoholics Anonymous may incorporate a spiritual component, there are programs that provide social support without spiritual or religious messaging. Availability of these groups varies globally.

Finally, from a societal perspective, social workers may consider incorporating a trauma-informed approach to treatment for specific populations so that they do not become re-traumatized. For example, forced migration means that individuals had no choice but to relocate to areas where the community and work circumstances, as well as the cultural and linguistic environments, are often completely unfamiliar to them. Social workers may consider immigrant clients' backgrounds when screening for and addressing addictive behaviors, especially if there is a possibility that substance use could be overlooked in efforts to help individuals successfully integrate into their new environments.

Macro-level practice implications

The macro practitioner operates within the realms of intervention development, systems of care, community organizing, and policy advocacy, among others, to reduce substance use and SUD disparities. This includes advocating for more culturally appropriate treatment programming and educational opportunities to achieve prevention and treatment equity across diverse groups. For some people, mandated treatment for SUD through the courts may be the first time they become engaged in recovery efforts (Guerrero et al., 2013). Therefore, systems-level change agents should advocate for more supports for individuals in low-income communities or other disadvantaged groups who experience limited access or great barriers to treatment services. This includes creating wraparound programs (e.g. housing and employment support) that reduce disparities in treatment access or impede successful completion and long-term recovery.

For women experiencing SUD, not only should programming and treatment be gender-responsive in terms of biological differences (such as for pregnant and parenting women), but also account for relevant social and environmental factors. For example, many women presenting for treatment have experienced physical and/or sexual trauma, a consequence of which may be PTSD. This, in turn, may manifest in other mental health issues including SUD (McCauley, Killeen, Gros, Brady, & Back, 2012). Interventions for women should consider incorporating interpersonal social supports, given the integral role of relationships (e.g. with intimate partners and children) in women's addictive behaviors and recovery (Wilsnack et al., 2018).

At the community level, macro practitioners can work with community members and researchers in tandem to integrate diverse perspectives in the development of efficacious, culturally appropriate interventions and health promotion policies. Being culturally relevant at the macro level includes being mindful of traditional healing practices, non-conventional methods of addressing addictive behaviors, and natural/indigenous support systems that incorporate a cultural aspect. Practitioners should consider the histories of trauma among indigenous populations resulting from policy sanctions and discriminatory practices. Early efforts to prevent or delay substance use initiation are necessary to ameliorate disparities (Dickerson, Spear, Marinelli-Casey, Rawson, Li, & Hser, 2010). At the societal level, social workers can advocate for policy changes that affect alcohol availability, legal age limits for use, and advertisements regarding the sale of alcohol and cannabis within their communities (Alcohol and Public Policy Group, 2010), as well as the availability of disability-accessible, gender and culturally appropriate alcohol and drug treatment programs.

Conclusions

Social workers have access to resources that report the epidemiology and prevalence statistics for substance use, heavy use, SUDs, and treatment need/utilization within their countries (e.g. SAMHSA's National Drug Use and Health Survey, NESARC, WHO, and other nation-specific reports). Rather than describing these statistics here, since they may be outdated in short order and do not cover all relevant social groups, this chapter instead provided a framework for interpreting such statistics and informing social work practice at micro-, mezzo-, and macro- levels.

Three major social categories—race/ethnicity, gender, and disability status—were examined. The framework applied to individual and social determinants that contribute to disparities in substance use, development of SUD, and treatment access and completion from a global perspective. Considering different lived experiences, social workers may approach addictive behaviors in a more nuanced manner that incorporates ways individuals interact with and react to their communities, sociocultural influences, and health care systems. Each of these domains intersect with levels of influence, from the individual to societal, that engender risk or resilience mechanisms important to substance use. Taken together, it is important to emphasize that individuals do not develop addictive behaviors in a vacuum devoid of external influences; rather, the interpersonal, community, and societal contexts shape behaviors, consequences, and opportunities.

This chapter was not intended to be an exhaustive discussion of diversity. Rather, social workers are encouraged to approach issues of substance use with clients, client systems, constituencies, and stakeholders in a manner that will ultimately help promote long-term recovery and healthy communities. The first step is recognizing that patterns of addictive behaviors are complex, and a prevention approach or treatment modality that works for one social group may be less relevant for another. Questions that the social worker may consider include: *What is my client's/constituents' socioeconomic background? Do they belong to a historically oppressed minority group? How do their community and cultural group(s) view substance use, heavy use, and treatment engagement? How might these factors affect their risk or protect them against heavy drinking or other substance use? How might these factors affect their readiness for and desired approach to treatment? What barriers might they face in terms of successfully completing treatment?* Examining addictive behaviors from a diversity perspective enables social workers and allied practitioners to identify protective factors, facilitators of recovery, and risks for SUD that inform intervention design to benefit individuals, families, communities, and populations. This ultimately will contribute to reduction of inequities in substance use and related problems for all groups.

Acknowledgments

We gratefully acknowledge Lewis E. Kraus, Erica C. Jones, and Jan Garrett at the Pacific ADA Center in Oakland, CA, for their input on disabilities and substance use. This work was supported by the National Institutes of Health's National Institute on Alcohol Abuse and Alcoholism (grants T32AA007240 and P50AA005595); the perspectives are those of the authors and do not represent the views of the supporting institution.

Notes

1 The American Psychiatric Association's Diagnostic and Statistical Manual of Mental Disorders (DSM-5) and the World Health Organization's International Classification of Disease (ICD-10) detail criteria for an SUD diagnosis, including cravings (strong desire to use), difficulty controlling use, social and physical health problems caused by use, and withdrawal symptoms when stopping or cutting down on use (see Chapter 1).
2 Please refer to the DSM-5 or ICD-10 for AUD diagnostic criteria.

References

Aguilar, S., Gutierrez, V., Sanchez, L., & Nougier, M. (2018). *Medicinal cannabis policies and practices around the world.* Retrieved from London, UK http://fileserver.idpc.net/library/Medicinal%20cannabis%20briefing_ENG_FINAL.PDF

Alcohol and Public Policy Group. (2010). Alcohol: No ordinary commodity—A summary of the second edition. *Addiction, 105*(5), 769–779. doi:10.1111/j.1360-0443.2010.02945.x

AlMarri, T. S., & Oei, T. P. (2009). Alcohol and substance use in the Arabian Gulf region: A review. *International Journal of Psychology, 44*(3), 222–233. doi:10.1080/00207590801888752

Alvidrez, J., Castille, D., Laude-Sharp, M., Rosario, A., & Tabor, D. (2019). The national institute on minority health and health disparities research framework. *American Journal of Public Health, 109*(S1), S16–S20. doi:10.2105/AJPH.2018.304883

Barry, E., Laverty, A. A., Majeed, A., & Millett, C. (2015). Ethnic group variations in alcohol-related hospital admissions in England: Does place matter? *Ethnicity & Health, 20*(6), 557–563. doi:10.1080/13557858.2014.950198

Bécares, L., Nazroo, J., & Stafford, M. (2011). The ethnic density effect on alcohol use among ethnic minority people in the UK. *Journal of Epidemiology & Community Health, 65*(1), 20–25. doi:10.1136/jech.2009.087114

Brondolo, E., Ver Halen, N. B., Pencille, M., Beatty, D., & Contrada, R. J. (2009). Coping with racism: A selective review of the literature and a theoretical and methodological critique. *Journal of Behavioral Medicine, 32*(1), 64–88. doi:10.1007/s10865-008-9193-0

Brooks, P. J., Enoch, M.-A., Goldman, D., Li, T.-K., & Yokoyama, A. (2009). The alcohol flushing response: An unrecognized risk factor for esophageal cancer from alcohol consumption. *PLoS Medicine, 6*(3), e1000050. doi:10.1371/journal.pmed.1000050

Chapman, S. L. C., & Wu, L.-T. (2012). Substance abuse among individuals with intellectual disabilities. *Research in Developmental Disabilities, 33*(4), 1147–1156. doi:10.1016/j.ridd.2012.02.009

Chartier, K. G., Scott, D. M., Wall, T. L., Covault, J., Karriker-Jaffe, K. J., Mills, B. A., . . . Arroyo, J. A. (2014). Framing ethnic variations in alcohol outcomes from biological pathways to neighborhood context. *Alcoholism: Clinical and Experimental Research, 38*(3), 611–618. doi:10.1111/acer.12304

Chartier, K. G., Vaeth, P. A. C., & Caetano, R. (2013). Focus on: Ethnicity and the social and health harms from drinking. *Alcohol Research: Current Reviews, 35*(2), 229–237.

Collins, S. E. (2016). Associations between socioeconomic factors and alcohol outcomes. *Alcohol Research: Current Reviews, 38*(1), 83–94.

Delker, E., Brown, Q., & Hasin, D. (2015). Epidemiological studies of substance dependence and abuse in adults. *Current Behavioral Neuroscience Reports, 2*(1), 15–22. doi:10.1007/s40473-015-0030-9

Delker, E., Brown, Q., & Hasin, D. S. (2016). Alcohol consumption in demographic subpopulations: An epidemiologic overview. *Alcohol Research: Current Reviews, 38*(1), 7–15.

Dickerson, D. L., Spear, S., Marinelli-Casey, P., Rawson, R., Li, L., & Hser, Y.-I. (2010). American Indians/Alaska natives and substance abuse treatment outcomes: Positive signs and continuing challenges. *Journal of Addictive Diseases, 30*(1), 63–74. doi:10.1080/10550887.2010.531665

Enoch, M. A., & Albaugh, B. J. (2017). Genetic and environmental risk factors for alcohol use disorders in American Indians and Alaskan Natives. *The American Journal on Addictions, 26*(5), 461–468. doi:10.1111/ajad.12420

Erol, A., & Karpyak, V. M. (2015). Sex and gender-related differences in alcohol use and its consequences: Contemporary knowledge and future research considerations. *Drug and Alcohol Dependence, 156*, 1–13. doi:10.1016/j.drugalcdep.2015.08.023

Ferreira-Borges, C., Parry, C., & Babor, T. (2017). Harmful use of alcohol: A shadow over sub-Saharan Africa in need of workable solutions. *International Journal of Environmental Research and Public Health, 14*(4), 346. doi:10.3390/ijerph14040346

Fiscella, K., Franks, P., Gold, M. R., & Clancy, C. M. (2000). Inequality in quality: Addressing so-cioeconomic, racial, and ethnic disparities in health care. *JAMA, 283*(19), 2579–2584. doi:10.1001/jama.283.19.2579

Gilbert, P. A., & Zemore, S. E. (2016). Discrimination and drinking: A systematic review of the evidence. *Social Science and Medicine, 161*, 178–194. doi:10.1016/j.socscimed.2016.06.009

Glazier, R. E., & Kling, R. N. (2013). Recent trends in substance abuse among persons with disabilities compared to that of persons without disabilities. *Disability and Health Journal, 6*(2), 107–115. doi:10.1016/j.dhjo.2013.01.007

Guerrero, E. G., Marsh, J. C., Khachikian, T., Amaro, H., & Vega, W. A. (2013). Disparities in Latino substance use, service use, and treatment: Implications for culturally and evidence-based interventions under health care reform. *Drug and Alcohol Dependence, 133*(3), 805–813. doi:10.1016/j.drugalcdep.2013.07.027

Hollar, D., & Moore, D. (2004). Relationship of substance use by students with disabilities to long-term educational, employment, and social outcomes. *Substance Use & Misuse, 39*(6), 931–962. doi:10.1081/JA-120030894

Iezzoni, L. I. (2011). Eliminating health and health care disparities among the growing population of people with disabilities. *Health Affairs, 30*(10), 1947–1954. doi:10.1377/hlthaff.2011.0613

Iwamoto, D. K., Kaya, A., Grivel, M., & Clinton, L. (2016). Under-researched demographics: Heavy episodic drinking and alcohol-related problems among Asian Americans. *Alcohol Research: Current Reviews, 38*(1), 17–25.

Jones, L., Bellis, M. A., Wood, S., Hughes, K., McCoy, E., Eckley, L., . . . Officer, A. (2012). Prevalence and risk of violence against children with disabilities: A systematic review and meta-analysis of observational studies. *The Lancet, 380*(9845), 899–907. doi:10.1016/S0140-6736(12)60692-8

Kane, J. C., Johnson, R. M., Iwamoto, D. K., Jernigan, D. H., Harachi, T. W., & Bass, J. K. (2018). Pathways linking intergenerational cultural dissonance and alcohol use among Asian American youth: The role of family conflict, parental involvement, and peer behavior. *Journal of Ethnicity in Substance Abuse*, 1–21. doi:10.1080/15332640.2018.1428709

Karriker-Jaffe, K. J. (2011). Areas of disadvantage: A systematic review of effects of area-level socioeconomic status on substance use outcomes. *Drug and Alcohol Review, 30*(1), 84–95.

Kerr, W. C., Lui, C. K., Williams, E., Ye, Y., Greenfield, T. K., & Lown, E. A. (2017). Health risk factors associated with lifetime abstinence from alcohol in the 1979 National Longitudinal Survey of Youth Cohort. *Alcoholism: Clinical and Experimental Research, 41*(2), 388–398.

Keyes, K. M., Jager, J., Mal-Sarkar, T., Patrick, M. E., Rutherford, C., Schulenberg, J., & Hasin, D. (2019). Is there a recent epidemic of women's drinking? A critical review of national studies. *Alcoholism: Clinical and Experimental Research, 43*(7), 1344–1359. doi: 10.1111/acer.14082.

Kraus, L., Lauer, E., Coleman, R., & Houtenville, A. (2018). *2017 disability statistics annual report*. Durham, NH: University of New Hampshire. Retrieved from https://eric.ed.gov/?id=ED583258

Leão, T. S., Johansson, L.-M., & Sundquist, K. (2006). Hospitalization due to alcohol and drug abuse in first-and second-generation immigrants: A follow-up study in Sweden. *Substance Use & Misuse, 41*(3), 283–296. doi:10.1080/10826080500409100

Lui, P. P. (2015). Intergenerational cultural conflict, mental health, and educational outcomes among Asian and Latino/a Americans: Qualitative and meta-analytic review. *Psychological Bulletin, 141*(2), 404. doi:10.1037/a0038449

Lui, P. P., & Zamboanga, B. L. (2018a). Acculturation and alcohol use among Asian Americans: A meta-analytic review. *Psychology of Addictive Behaviors, 32*(2), 173. doi:10.1037/adb0000340

Lui, P. P., & Zamboanga, B. L. (2018b). A critical review and meta-analysis of the associations between acculturation and alcohol use outcomes among Hispanic Americans. *Alcoholism: Clinical and Experimental Research, 42*(10), 1841–1862.

Luitel, N. P., Jordans, M., Murphy, A., Roberts, B., & McCambridge, J. (2013). Prevalence and patterns of hazardous and harmful alcohol consumption assessed using the AUDIT among Bhutanese refugees in Nepal. *Alcohol and Alcoholism, 48*(3), 349–355. doi:10.1093/alcalc/agt009

Mahli, A., & Hellerbrand, C. (2016). Alcohol and obesity: A dangerous association for fatty liver disease. *Digestive Diseases, 34*(Suppl 1), 32–39. doi:10.1159/000447279

Marrone, S. (2007). Understanding barriers to health care: A review of disparities in health care services among indigenous populations. *International Journal of Circumpolar Health, 66*(3), 188–198. doi:10.3402/ijch.v66i3.18254

McCauley, J. L., Killeen, T., Gros, D. F., Brady, K. T., & Back, S. E. (2012). Posttraumatic stress disorder and co-occurring substance use disorders: Advances in assessment and treatment. *Clinical Psychology: Science and Practice, 19*(3), 283–304. doi:10.1111/cpsp.12006

Mckeigue, P. M., & Karmi, G. (1993). Alcohol consumption and alcohol-related problems in Afro-Caribbeans and South Asians in the United Kingdom. *Alcohol and Alcoholism, 28*(1), 1–10.

Mezuk, B., Li, X., Cederin, K., Concha, J., Kendler, K. S., Sundquist, J., & Sundquist, K. (2015). Ethnic enclaves and risk of psychiatric disorders among first-and second-generation immigrants in Sweden. *Social Psychiatry and Psychiatric Epidemiology, 50*(11), 1713–1722. doi:10.1007/s00127-015-1107-1

Michalak, L., & Trocki, K. (2006). Alcohol and Islam: An overview. *Contemporary Drug Problems, 33*(4), 523–562. doi:10.1177/009145090603300401

Mills, B. A., & Caetano, R. (2016). Alcohol use and related problems along the United States–Mexico border. *Alcohol Research: Current Reviews, 38*(1), 79–81.

Molina, K. M., Alegría, M., & Chen, C.-N. (2012). Neighborhood context and substance use disorders: A comparative analysis of racial and ethnic groups in the United States. *Drug and Alcohol Dependence, 125*, S35–S43. doi:10.1016/j.drugalcdep.2012.05.027

Moore, L. L. D. (2001). Disability and illicit drug use: An application of labeling theory. *Deviant Behavior, 22*(1), 1–21. doi:10.1080/016396201750065784

Muhunthan, J., Angell, B., Hackett, M. L., Wilson, A., Latimer, J., Eades, A.-M., & Jan, S. (2017). Global systematic review of Indigenous community-led legal interventions to control alcohol. *BMJ Open, 7*(3), e013932. doi:10.1136/bmjopen-2016-013932

Mukamal, K. J., Mittleman, M. A., Longstreth, W., Jr., Newman, A. B., Fried, L. P., & Siscovick, D. S. (2004). Self-reported alcohol consumption and falls in older adults: Cross-sectional and longitudinal analyses of the cardiovascular health study. *Journal of the American Geriatrics Society, 52*(7), 1174–1179. doi:10.1111/j.1532-5415.2004.52318.x

Mulia, N., Ye, Y., Greenfield, T. K., & Zemore, S. E. (2009). Disparities in alcohol-related problems among white, black, and Hispanic Americans. *Alcoholism: Clinical and Experimental Research, 33*(4), 654–662. doi:10.1111/j.1530-0277.2008.00880.x

National Association of Social Workers. (n.d.). *NASW code of ethics.* Washington, DC. Retrieved from https://www.socialworkers.org/About/Ethics/Code-of-Ethics/Code-of-Ethics-English

Nolen-Hoeksema, S. (2004). Gender differences in risk factors and consequences for alcohol use and problems. *Clinical Psychology Review, 24*(8), 981–1010. doi:10.1016/j.cpr.2004.08.003

Oslin, D. W. (2000). Alcohol use in late life: Disability and comorbidity. *Journal of Geriatric Psychiatry and Neurology, 13*(3), 134–140. doi:10.1177/089198870001300307

Probst, C., Roerecke, M., Behrendt, S., & Rehm, J. (2014). Socioeconomic differences in alcohol-attributable mortality compared with all-cause mortality: A systematic review and meta-analysis. *International Journal of Epidemiology, 43*(4), 1314–1327. doi:10.1093/ije/dyu043

Reinert, D. F., & Allen, J. P. (2007). The alcohol use disorders identification test: An update of research findings. *Alcoholism: Clinical and Experimental Research, 31*(2), 185–199. doi:10.1111/j.1530-0277.2006.00295.x

Renzaho, A. M. (2016). *Globalisation, migration and health: Challenges and opportunities.* World Scientific. doi:10.1142/p1063

Room, R., Callinan, S., Greenfield, T. K., Rekve, D., Waleewong, O., Stanesby, O., . . . Laslett, A.-M. (2019). The social location of harm from others' drinking in ten societies. *Addiction, 114*(3), 425–433. doi:10.1111/add.14447

Simoni-Wastila, L., & Yang, H. K. (2006). Psychoactive drug abuse in older adults. *The American Journal of Geriatric Pharmacotherapy, 4*(4), 380–394. doi:10.1016/j.amjopharm.2006.10.002

Spillane, N. S., & Smith, G. T. (2007). A theory of reservation-dwelling American Indian alcohol use risk. *Psychological Bulletin, 133*(3), 395. doi:10.1037/0033-2909.133.3.395

Stone, J., & Moskowitz, G. B. (2011). Non-conscious bias in medical decision making: What can be done to reduce it? *Medical Education, 45*(8), 768–776. doi:10.1111/j.1365-2923.2011.04026.x

Substance Abuse and Mental Health Services Administration. (2014). *Results from the 2013 national survey on drug use and health: Summary of national findings.* NSDUH Series, H-48, HHS Publication No. (SMA) 14-4863. Rockville, MD: Substance Abuse and mental Health Services Administration. Retrieved from https://www.samhsa.gov/data/sites/default/files/NSDUHresultsPDFWHTML2013/Web/NSDUHresults2013.pdf.

Tuchman, E. (2010). Women and addiction: The importance of gender issues in substance abuse research. *Journal of Addictive Diseases, 29*(2), 127–138. doi:10.1080/10550881003684582

US Department of Health and Human Services. (2016, November). *Facing addiction in America: The surgeon general's report on alcohol, drugs, and health*. Washington, DC: HHS. Retrieved from https://store.samhsa.gov/system/files/surgeon-generals-report.pdf.

US Department of Health and Human Services. (2018, March 28). Profile: American Indian/Alaska Native. Retrieved from https://minorityhealth.hhs.gov/omh/browse.aspx?lvl=3&lvlid=62

Vaughn, M. S., Huang, F. F., & Ramirez, C. R. (1995). Drug abuse and anti-drug policy in Japan: Past history and future directions. *The British Journal of Criminology, 35*(4), 491–524.

Velleman, R. D., Templeton, L. J., & Copello, A. G. (2005). The role of the family in preventing and intervening with substance use and misuse: A comprehensive review of family interventions, with a focus on young people. *Drug and Alcohol Review, 24*(2), 93–109. doi:10.1080/09595230500167478

Verissimo, A. D. O., & Grella, C. E. (2017). Influence of gender and race/ethnicity on perceived barriers to help-seeking for alcohol or drug problems. *Journal of Substance Abuse Treatment, 75*, 54–61. doi:10.1016/j.jsat.2016.12.013

Wall, T. L., Luczak, S. E., & Hiller-Sturmhöfel, S. (2016). Biology, genetics, and environment: Underlying factors influencing alcohol metabolism. *Alcohol Research: Current Reviews, 38*(1), 59–68.

Walters, K., Spencer, M., Smukler, M., Allen, H., Andrews, C., Browne, T., & Uehara, D. (2016). *Health equity: Eradicating health inequalities for future generations*. Baltimore, MD: American Academy of Social Work & Social Welfare.

West, S. L., Graham, C. W., & Cifu, D. X. (2009). Rates of alcohol/other drug treatment denials to persons with physical disabilities: Accessibility concerns. *Alcoholism Treatment Quarterly, 27*(3), 305–316. doi:10.1080/07347320903008190

Whitesell, N. R., Beals, J., Crow, C. B., Mitchell, C. M., & Novins, D. K. (2012). Epidemiology and etiology of substance use among American Indians and Alaska Natives: Risk, protection, and implications for prevention. *The American Journal of Drug and Alcohol Abuse, 38*(5), 376–382.

Wilsnack, R. W., Wilsnack, S. C., Gmel, G., & Kantor, L. W. (2018). Gender differences in binge drinking: Prevalence, predictors, and consequences. *Alcohol Research: Current Reviews, 39*(1), 57–76.

Wright, E. M., Van Voorhis, P., Salisbury, E. J., & Bauman, A. (2012). Gender-responsive lessons learned and policy implications for women in prison: A review. *Criminal Justice and Behavior, 39*(12), 1612–1632. doi:10.1177/0093854812451088

Wu, L.-T., & Blazer, D. (2015). Substance use disorders and co-morbidities among Asian Americans and Native Hawaiians/Pacific Islanders. *Psychological Medicine, 45*(3), 481–494. doi:10.1017/S0033291714001330

Yap, M. B., Cheong, T. W., Zaravinos-Tsakos, F., Lubman, D. I., & Jorm, A. F. (2017). Modifiable parenting factors associated with adolescent alcohol misuse: A systematic review and meta-analysis of longitudinal studies. *Addiction, 112*(7), 1142–1162.

Zapolski, T. C. B., Pedersen, S. L., McCarthy, D. M., & Smith, G. T. (2014). Less drinking, yet more problems: Understanding African American drinking and related problems. *Psychological Bulletin, 140*(1), 188–223. doi:10.1037/a0032113

Zaso, M. J., Goodhines, P. A., Wall, T. L., & Park, A. (2019). Meta-analysis on associations of alcohol metabolism genes with alcohol use disorder in East Asians. *Alcohol and Alcoholism*. doi:10.1093/alcalc/agz011

Zemore, S. E., Karriker-Jaffe, K. J., Mulia, N., Kerr, W. C., Ehlers, C. L., Cook, W. K., . . . Greenfield, T. K. (2018). The future of research on alcohol-related disparities across U.S. racial/ethnic groups: A plan of attack. *Journal of Studies on Alcohol and Drugs, 79*(1), 7–21. doi:10.15288/jsad.2018.79.7

Zemore, S. E., Murphy, R. D., Mulia, N., Gilbert, P. A., Martinez, P., Bond, J., & Polcin, D. L. (2014). A moderating role for gender in racial/ethnic disparities in alcohol services utilization: Results from the 2000 to 2010 national alcohol surveys. *Alcoholism: Clinical and Experimental Research, 38*(8), 2286–2296. doi:10.1111/acer.12500

17

Substance use across the lifespan of the LGBTQ+ population

Jacob Goffnett and Jeremy Goldbach

Background

Lesbian, gay, bisexual, transgender, and queer/questioning (LGBTQ+) individuals experience higher rates of substance misuse across the lifespan compared to heterosexual and cisgender individuals. LGB adolescents are 90% more likely than their heterosexual peers to misuse substances including alcohol, illicit drugs, and tobacco (Marshal et al., 2008); while LGB adults are more than twice as likely as heterosexual adults to use illicit drugs (Medley et al., 2016), and to have higher rates of alcohol use and binge drinking (Ward, Dahlhamer, Galinsky, & Joestl, 2014). The impact of substance misuse among this population is severe, as these behaviors contribute to morbidity and mortality (Rehm et al., 2009). Thus, it is vital for social work practitioners to understand reasons LGBTQ+ individuals use substances at higher rates than heterosexual and cisgender individuals and methods that exist to help reduce use.

Several behavioral health disparities exist between LGBTQ+ individuals and their heterosexual and cisgender counterparts in addition to substance misuse. These include increased prevalence of suicide (Haas et al., 2010), mood and anxiety disorders (Meyer, 2003). Substance use patterns may differ by sexual orientation, as well as intersecting identities of gender, race, and socioeconomic status. For example, bisexual individuals report more substance misuse than other sexual orientations (McCabe, Hughes, Bostwick, West, & Boyd, 2009; Trocki, Drabble, & Midanik, 2009; Wilsnack et al., 2008), with bisexual women reporting the highest rates of substance misuse (Conron, Mimiaga, & Landers, 2010; Corliss et al., 2010). Moreover, some research suggests having multiple marginalized identities (i.e. race, gender, and sexual orientation) contributes to higher rates of substance misuse (Mereish & Bradford, 2014).

This chapter provides an overview of substance use among the LGBTQ+ population across the lifespan. Relevant terminology is highlighted at the start to help readers conceptualize the LGBTQ+ community. The chapter then introduces minority stress theory as a framework for understanding high rates of substance misuse among the LGBT population. The impact of minority stressors on substance misuse across the lifespan of the LGBT population is discussed within four developmental periods: adolescence, emerging adulthood, middle adulthood, and older adulthood. Finally, the chapter summarizes the state of research on interventions for addressing substance misuse and substance use disorders (SUDs) among this population.

Defining the LGBTQ+ community

The "alphabet soup" of identity labels associated with the LGBTQ+ community often seems daunting, especially when social workers want to use appropriate labels to understand the clients they serve (see University of California Davis Lesbian Gay Bisexual Transgender Queer Intersex Asexual Resource Center, 2013 for a glossary of labels). Here, we use LGBTQ+ as an umbrella term that encompasses individuals identifying as non-heterosexual or non-cisgender. First, it is acceptable for social workers not to know every identity label—it would be a laborious undertaking to know and understand every sexual and gender identity label in use around the world today, and there is no reason to do so. However, it helps to have some working knowledge of foundational concepts. It is important to remember that every person constructs and defines appropriate identity labels for themselves, and that sexual and gender identities and labels may change as individuals evolve, grow, and mature (e.g. see Russell, Clarke, & Clary, 2009).

The LGBT community represents approximately 4.5% of the general population in the United States (Newport, 2018). Challenges exist in the systematic collection of sexual and gender identity information in international contexts (Gates, 2011), in part because of differences in how identities and behaviors are defined or classified, and in part because of stigma and risk in self-identification experienced by LGBTQ+ individuals in many areas. There exists great diversity within the "LGBT" community, coalescing around two primary constructs that fall outside traditional heterosexual norms or sex-defined gender: sexual orientation (attractions, identities, and behaviors) and gender identity (male, female, third gender). This section examines a variety of constructs that should be considered in social work practice with LGBTQ+ individuals.

Sexual orientation

Individuals engaging in same-sex sexual behaviors or reporting same-sex attractions have been documented across a wide range of historical periods and cultural experiences (Blackwood, 1986). More recently, sophistication in defining sexual orientation has grown to include dimensions of attraction (i.e. who a person finds attractive) (Janssen, Everaerd, Spiering, & Janssen, 2000), romantic beliefs (i.e. who a person is romantically interested in) (Diamond, 2004), and identity (i.e. how an individual identifies; Kauth & Kalichman, 1995). Thus, sexual orientation reflects an "enduring emotional, romantic, sexual or affection, attraction or non-attraction to other people; sexual orientation is fluid, and people use a variety of labels to describe their sexual orientation" (University of California Davis Lesbian Gay Bisexual Transgender Queer Intersex Asexual Resource Center, 2013).

Although "gay" often is used generally to describe sexual attraction toward a person of the same gender, this term is commonly associated with male gender as opposed to female gender. Lesbian, however, is commonly used to describe a woman who is attracted to or has affection toward someone of the same gender. Bisexual is a term that is used to describe attraction and/or affection for people of the same or other genders. However, these definitions are not inclusive of all language used to describe sexual orientation. For example, individuals may describe themselves as pansexual, or as having an attraction toward and/or affection for all genders and sexes. Others may define themselves as asexual or not having an attraction to any gender. It should be noted that this does not mean that people who are asexual do not have sex, as many do.

Jacob Goffnett and Jeremy Goldbach

Recognizing that individuals' sexual orientation or sexual identity does not define their sexual behavior is a critical component of social work practice with this population and has important implications for substance use. Thus, a female client's disclosure that all past sexual partners have been male does not necessarily mean that she identifies with a heterosexual orientation or identity. Table 17.1 offers a brief list of common self-labels and definitions.

Table 17.1. Common terminology and definitions

Terminology	Definition
Asexual	A sexual orientation of those who are not sexually attracted to others or do not feel a desire for partnered sexuality
Bisexual	A term to describe the sexual orientation and affectionate attraction for people of the same gender or other gender
Cisgender	Gender identity or gender role that society considers to be aligned with assigned sex at birth
Gay	An umbrella term that can be used for both men and women. It describes the emotional and/or physical attraction or sex orientation toward people of the same gender
Gender	Different from sex assigned at birth. A social and personal construct that is used to categorize people and self as man, woman, or another identity.
Gender expression	Expressing self either in dress or behavior that is socially considered to be feminine, masculine, or somewhere in between
Gender non-conforming	Not subscribing to socially constructed gender expression or roles
Gender queer	Gender role or identity outside the dominant societal expectations for one's assigned sex; can be beyond genders or a combination of genders
Heterosexuality	A sexual orientation of those who are physically and emotionally attracted to people of a gender that is not their own
Intersex	Those who develop (without medical or pharmaceutical intervention) the primary and secondary sexual characteristics that do not fit exactly into societal and medical classification of male or female
Lesbian	One who identifies as a woman who is physically and emotionally attracted to others of the same gender
LGBT	An acronym used for Lesbian, Gay, Bisexual, and Transgender
Pansexual	Used to describe people who are emotionally and sexually attracted to all genders and sexes
Queer	A term that is and can be used by anyone regardless of sexual and gender orientation for many different sexual or gender-related reasons. Some still do consider this offensive due to historical use of this term as derogatory. Recently reclaimed as an umbrella term
Sex	A characterization as male, female, or intersex based on genitalia at birth
Transman	Can be used to describe a female-to-male transgender person. Can capture the gender identification or lived experience as a transperson
Transgender	A person whose gender identity, expression, or role is outside the male/female binary or whose gender does not fit with the dominant societal expectations of assigned sex at birth
Transwoman	Can be used to describe a male-to-female transgender person. Can capture the gender identification or lived experience as a transperson

Gender identity

Gender and sex can be related (although do not have to be) but are not synonymous. *Sex* is a biological term that designates a certain combination of gonads, chromosomes, external gender organs, secondary sex characteristics, and hormonal balances. *Gender* is a socially constructed classification system that ascribes qualities of masculinity and femininity to individuals. Gender can include expression, identity, behavior, role, and feelings. Toomey, Ryan, Diaz, Card, and Russell (2010) state that gender-non-conforming individuals, such as boys who are more feminine than other boys or girls who are more masculine than other girls, can be described as transgressing social gender norms. These social norms are often dominant societal expectations passed down over time and can oppress individuals who may not ascribe to such expectations. Often, gender is used to describe the sex of an individual (e.g. "it's a boy!"). However, since gender is a socially constructed and personal experience, it is more accurate to refer to the sex of a baby as opposed to its gender, assuming that babies lack awareness of their own gender. Of note, Germany was the first European country to offer a third category for biological sex, beginning in 2013 families have the option of "M" (male), "F" (female) or "blank" (Hudson, 2013).

By preschool, most children have a concept of gender and are able to label their own and others' gender (Toomey et al., 2010). Those who conform to socially constructed gender roles are often reinforced by the social environment for maintaining those gendered roles, while those who do not conform may experience criticism, or worse, within various community and familial settings. Egan and Perry (2001) suggested that

> by middle childhood, a strong concept has developed regarding the degree to which they typify their gender category; degree of connection with gender assignment; whether they are free to explore cross-sex options or are compelled to conform to gender stereotypes; and whether their own sex is superior to another.
>
> *(p. 459)*

Pressures to conform often create oppressive experiences for younger and older people alike who are gender non-conforming, are exploring their gender, or whose gender identity is not consistent with their assigned sex.

Cisgender is defined as having a gender identity or gender role that society considers aligned with the sex assigned at birth. *Gender non-conformity* is defined as not conforming to society's expectations of gender expression based on the gender binary expectations of masculinity and femininity, or how individuals should identify their gender (University of California Davis Lesbian Gay Bisexual Transgender Queer Intersex Asexual Resource Center Resource Center, 2014). *Transgender*, on the other hand, can be defined as a psychological self (i.e. gender identity) differing from social expectations based on the physical sex an individual was born with, or a gender identity that does not fit within dominant-group social constructs of assigned sex and gender: or having no gender or multiple genders. It is important to highlight that gender identity and sexual identity can be related but are not always. A transgender female (i.e. an individual assigned male at birth, but who identifies along the female or feminine spectrum) attracted to a male may identify as heterosexual, lesbian, queer, or another sexual identity. Regardless of a client's outward presentation or gender identity, it is always helpful to ask them how they describe their sexual orientation.

Assessing sexual orientation or gender/sexual identity can arouse anxiety for both clients and practitioners. Engagement processes and therapeutic relationships, however, may be the only places that an individual feels safe to talk about sexuality, particularly components of gender and sexuality traditionally viewed as taboo or inappropriate by the dominant culture. Using labels that reflect client preferences, and being open to adjusting language as clients develop, can strengthen engagement and enhance the therapeutic relationship. Creating a non-judgmental space is essential for developing and maintaining engagement and therapeutic relationships, particularly with individuals who have experienced or are fearful of stigma.

Minority stress theory

Minority stress theory (MST) proposes that the LGBTQ+ population experiences higher rates of adverse health problems due to social stigmatization of their sexual orientations and gender identities (Hendricks & Testa, 2012; Meyer, 2003). LGBTQ+ individuals may use substances to cope with experiences of discrimination and victimization attributed to their identities. Minority stressors may manifest in unique ways across the lifespan depending on the LGBTQ+ individual's developmental period.

Poor behavioral outcomes are commonly attributed to the presence of intensely stressful circumstances. As MST explains, there exists an array of social and psychological stressors related to membership in the LGBTQ+ community (Meyer, 2003). MST suggests that the substance use behavior of LGBTQ+ individuals is impacted by a number of distal and proximal stressors, each of which could be the focus of intervention. Distal stressors occur in the environment in the form of negative experiences of discrimination and anti-LGBT victimization. Proximal stressors are situated near the individual and include internalized negative attitudes toward homosexuality, internalization of discomfort with sexuality, and distress related to concealment, rejection, and acceptance by others (Rosario, Rotheram-Borus, & Reid, 1996).

Proximal and distal stressors are interrelated. For example, when internalized, minority stress can encourage negative societal attitudes in an individual, pressure to hide same-sex attractions, and adopting strongly discordant belief systems (e.g. having strong religious convictions against homosexuality; DiPlacido, 1998). Numerous studies describe the theoretical utility of a minority stress framework applied to LGBT adults (e.g. Meyer, 2003; Testa et al., 2015), as well as its applicability to young adults (e.g. Holloway et al., 2012; Traube et al., 2012). However, understanding of these stressors among adolescents or older LGBT adults (50+ years old) is poorly developed, as is how these stressors may be unique in consideration of substance use patterns.

LGBT individuals and substance use across the lifespan

Minority stressor experiences during adolescence may have an enduring impact on substance misuse and other health/mental health problems into adulthood (Marshal, Friedman, Stall, & Thompson, 2009; Needham, 2012). Furthermore, disparities in substance misuse between LGBTQ+ individuals and heterosexual/cisgender individuals exist across the lifespan. In this section, we examine salient conditions of four developmental periods—adolescence, emerging adulthood, middle adulthood, and older adulthood—that interact with minority stressors to facilitate substance misuse among LGBTQ+ individuals.

Adolescence (13–18 years old)

A growing body of evidence identifies high rates of substance use among LGB adolescents, almost three times the rate of their heterosexual peers (Marshal et al., 2008). LGBTQ+ adolescents report higher consumption of cigarettes, alcohol, and marijuana

(Bontempo & D'Augelli, 2002; Russell, Driscoll, & Truong, 2002), as well as less commonly used substances such as cocaine and ecstasy (Corliss et al., 2010). LGBTQ+ adolescents may be more likely to use multiple substances concurrently (Garofalo, Wolf, Kessel, Palfrey, & DuRant, 1998) and more rapidly increase substance use as they age (Marshal et al., 2009). Substance use by LGBTQ+ adolescents is a serious public health concern. Early age of initial use increases the chances of developing a substance use disorder later in life, impairs decision-making, and is associated with other problem behaviors such as poor school performance (Kandel, Johnson, Bird, & Camino, 1997), risky sexual practices (Herrick, Matthews, & Garofalo, 2010), and HIV exposure (Solorio, Swendeman, & Rotheram-Borus, 2003).

Although studies support the applicability of the MST to adolescents, scholars have noted a reliance on adult or young adult samples (e.g. Kelleher, 2009; Shilo & Savaya, 2012), and lack of attention to other non-LGBTQ+ related factors that are common during adolescence: natural developmental influences, emotional dysregulation, cognitive processes (e.g. Herts et al., 2012). In social work, understanding minority stress from an adolescent perspective is necessary. In particular, it is important to consider: (a) identity developmental processes during adolescence; (b) adolescents' social environment experiences; and (c) contemporary experiences of coping and social support among sexual minority adolescents.

Identity development

In a developmental framework, adolescence is a critical period during which individuals establish long-term health trajectories and are still solidifying their sexual identities. Although some sexual identity fluidity during adulthood has been documented, identity development, including gender and sexuality, is a central task of adolescence (Erikson, 1968), and the articulation of attractions, labels, behaviors, and expressions are noteworthy (Goldbach & Gibbs, 2015). Because many LGBTQ+ adolescents "try on" various identity labels as they seek congruence with their sexual identity (e.g. identify as bisexual or pansexual, then gay or lesbian; Rusow et al., 2015), this identification process may itself be a proximal stressor. As described in the original MST, how individuals perceive their membership in a minority community can influence their interpretation of minority stressors (i.e. characteristics of minority identity) as being more or less relevant. Thus, if adolescents are unsure of their identity, or that self-applied label changes, the impact that anti-LGBTQ+ experiences have on substance use patterns may change.

Social environment

The exact distal and proximal minority stressors that LGBTQ+ adolescents encounter may differ from adult experiences. For example, LGBTQ+ adolescents often report disclosure-related stress in the context of two compulsory social environments that adults do not: living at home with family and attending school (D'Augelli, 2006; Goldbach, Tanner-Smith, Bagwell, & Dunlap, 2014; Russell, Franz, & Driscoll, 2001). Negative parental reactions to adolescents' disclosure can create stress in the family home, with significant consequences including adolescent homelessness and substance use (Clatts, Goldsamt, Yi, & Gwadz, 2005; Rosario, Schrimshaw, & Hunter, 2004). This is particularly salient because most adolescents rely on their family's financial support to ensure stability and safety. Transgender adolescents may encounter additional stress within their families regarding their ability to transition socially or medically. Research has also reported a concerning prevalence of school victimization and bullying by peers, staff, and teachers, and many LGBTQ+ adolescents attend schools in which homophobic bullying is common and teachers and other staff do not readily intervene (Kosciw, Greytak, Zongrone, Clark, & Truong, 2018). Transgender adolescents may face additional barriers in schools, such as policies dictating which bathrooms and locker rooms they may or may not use, and their ability to formally (paperwork) and informally (interpersonally) transition to their preferred names and pronouns. Similarly, structural factors out of an adolescent's control (e.g. legal requirements to attend school, inability to secure emancipation from parents) may contribute to behavioral health concerns among sexual minority adolescents (Goldbach & Gibbs, 2015; Hatzenbuehler, 2011).

Coping and social support

Finally, coping processes may differ for youth today compared to just 5 years ago. The United States is a different place for LGBTQ+ individuals than it was a decade ago, due to passage of hate crime legislation in 2009, which applies harsher punishments for crimes motivated by hate toward LGBTQ+ individuals (Matthew Sheppard and James Byrd Jr. Hate Crime Act of 2009); the repeal of Don't Ask, Don't Tell in 2010 allows LGB service members to serve openly in the U.S. Military (of note, recent policies have banned transgender military personnel on the unsubstantiated belief that these individuals finically burden the military and disrupt comradery among troops); the passage of federal marriage equality in 2015 across the United States (*Obergefell v. Hodges*, 2015); and the passage of more than 30 state employment-based LGBT protection laws in the United States (Hunt, 2012). U.S. LGBTQ+ adolescents are maturing in a society that views their identities very differently. For example, general public opinion concerning same-sex couples has changed dramatically in the past 12 years: in 2003, an estimated 31% of the U.S. population supported marriage equality, compared to 61% in 2015 (Gallup, 2016). Although the social climate toward LGBTQ+ individuals has progressed in American and other countries (e.g. Argentina, Australia, Canada, Germany, and Uruguay), some countries still maintain oppressive laws. For example, Brunei recently made international headlines by instituting a law that makes being gay punishable by death. Furthermore, Russian laws prohibit "homosexuality," while being gay carries a prison sentence of up to 14 years in multiple African countries. Thus, it is important to consider national and local laws when conceptualizing social support and coping for LGBTQ+ adolescents.

It is conceivable that LGBTQ+ adolescents around the world now mature in social environments in which their identities are not perceived negatively, or in some cases even seen as a positive. It is particularly important for health providers to not only focus on negative experiences that contribute to substance misuse, but also find protective resources for the LGBTQ+ community. Further, although LGBTQ+ adolescents in many parts of the world, including the United States, may experience minority stressors, they also benefit from access to coping resources (i.e. social or personal tools in the social environment that can be used to cope; Compas, Connor-Smith, Saltzman, Thomsen, & Wadsworth, 2001) not readily available to previous generations nor in some communities around the world. These coping resources may include supportive teachers, a supportive parent, a school gay–straight alliance, and supportive straight peers; social workers and other providers should be mindful of these as they work with young people in the prevention and treatment of substance misuse and substance use disorders.

Emerging adulthood (18–29 years old)

Emerging adulthood is the developmental period of 18–29-year-olds. This is a feature of industrialized nations where shifts in social norms delineate a transitional period between adolescence and adulthood (Arnett, 2000). Emerging adulthood provides individuals with time to explore and develop their sexual and gender identities (Torkelson, 2012). LGBTQ+ adults 18 years of age and older are nearly two times more likely to misuse substances (Medley et al., 2016), with substance use steadily increasing among LGBTQ+ individuals during the transition from adolescence into emerging adulthood and into the early 20s (Halkitis et al., 2014; Newcomb, Heinz, & Mustanski, 2012). Transgender emerging adults report more frequent alcohol misuse and more frequent blackouts due to alcohol than their cisgender peers (Tupler et al., 2017). Substance misuse also varies by race and socioeconomic status during this developmental period. One study found White LGBT emerging adults to report higher alcohol use compared to other races (Newcomb et al., 2012), while another study reported marijuana use to be higher among Hispanic LGBT emerging adults (Halkitis et al., 2014). Furthermore, lower socioeconomic status also correlates with more frequent substance misuse among this population (Halkitis et al., 2014).

Emerging adulthood has been ill-defined for the LGBTQ+ population; they are typically classified as either youth or adults which may curb knowledge of pathways to substance misuse among LGBTQ+ emerging adults, since conditions unique to this developmental period may contribute to substance misuse (Arnett, 2005). In particular, instability and identity exploration salient during emerging adulthood may be important to understanding substance use among LGBTQ+ emerging adults because these conditions are related to distal and proximal minority stressors.

Instability

Changes in life, especially those that are abrupt and harsh, can cause instability that may be coped with through substance use (Arnett, 2005). LGBTQ+ individuals experience higher levels of discrimination in occupation and housing, leaving them vulnerable to instability (Kattari, Whitfield, Walls, Langenderfer-Magruder, & Ramos, 2016; Sears & Mallory, 2011). Moreover, LGBTQ+ individuals are at a higher risk of unstably entering emerging adulthood due to minority stressors experienced during adolescence; stressors leading to homelessness and involvement with child welfare or juvenile justice systems. Experiences of discrimination and subsequent instability may collectively increase substance use among LGBTQ+ emerging adults.

Identity exploration

During emerging adulthood, individuals work to develop an understanding of who they are and what they want out of life (Arnett, 2000). For LGBTQ+ emerging adults, identity exploration includes understanding what it means to have a non-normative sexuality and/or gender and related identity exploration activities. Emerging adulthood provides the LGBTQ+ population latitude to explore and develop their identities in ways restricted during adolescence, such as increasing engagement with the LGBTQ+ community. These connections can reduce the impact of minority stressors on mental health outcomes such as depression and anxiety, but may increase substance misuse (Demant, Hides, White, & Kavanagh, 2018). Increased substance misuse related to engagement with the LGBTQ+ community is likely the result of bars being a common place for LGBTQ+ individuals to connect and develop their identities (Emslie, Lennox, & Ireland, 2017). Engagement with the LGBTQ+ community and culture broadens for LGBTQ+ individuals during emerging adulthood, providing new social environments to navigate, including environments where substance use is prominent. Similarly, LGBTQ+ emerging adults may have to re-negotiate their identities in new social environments, such as college/university or workplace settings. Stress associated with exploring and understanding identity in new ways or contexts may contribute to substance misuse during this period.

Middle adulthood (30–50 years old)

LGBTQ+ adults exhibit higher substance misuse rates than heterosexual and cisgender adults (McCabe et al., 2009). In 2011, The Institute of Medicine released a report outlining health disparities comparing substance misuse between LGBTQ+ and heterosexual/cisgender adults. LGB adults were more likely to smoke tobacco and marijuana, with particularly high use of these substances among bisexual women and individuals identifying as not exclusively heterosexual. Additionally, LGB adults consumed alcohol more frequently and in higher quantities than heterosexuals; however, differences in alcohol use were less pronounced for male-identified individuals. Women identifying as heterosexual but who self-report same-sex behaviors had the highest risk of excessive alcohol consumption. Finally, LGB men were at a higher risk of recreational drug use, which is connected to sexual risk taking (Institute of Medicine, 2011). Substance use may help LGBTQ+ adults manage the emotional impact of minority stressors (McNair et al., 2016). The profound impact of minority stressors on the current generation of LGBTQ+ middle adulthood individuals may be the reason that little attention has been directed to how developmental conditions contribute to substance misuse during this period. Additionally, this could be due to traditional markers of middle adulthood being commonly reserved for heterosexual adults (e.g. marriage and family).

A key feature of middle adulthood that has received some attention in the LGBTQ+ literature concerns the development and sustainment of an occupation. The workplace environment may create additional stress for LGBTQ+ adults that contribute to increased substance use. Between 7% and 41% of LGBTQ+ employees were estimated to have been victimized in the workplace (Badgett, Lau, Sears, & Ho, 2007). Moreover, LGBTQ+ adults may be less likely to be contacted for interviews if their identities could become known to current and potential employers, and LGBTQ+ individuals are often overlooked for promotions (Holman, 2018). Consuming too much alcohol is one method for coping with workplace-related stress (Frone, 2008). Experiences of minority stress in the work place negatively impact mental health outcome, decrease job satisfaction and commitment, and contribute to substance misuse among LGBTQ+ adults.

Older adulthood (50 years and older)

Although little research examines substance misuse among LGBTQ+ older adults, preliminary evidence suggests this age group also has high-risk substance use patterns compared to peers. For example, older LGB adults are almost two times more likely than their heterosexual peers to report excessive drinking (Fredriksen-Goldsen, Kim, Barkan, Muraco, & Hoy-Ellis, 2013). Health disparities among LGBTQ+ older adults may be attributed to both cumulative and contemporary experiences of minority stressors. For example, among older LGB men, excessive drinking was related to daily experiences of discrimination (Bryan, Kim, & Fredriksen-Goldsen, 2017). Moreover, minority stressors relate to substance misuse comorbidities such as poor chronic health outcomes, depression, and sexual risk taking (Emlet, Fredriksen-Goldsen, & Kim, 2013; Hoy-Ellis & Fredriksen-Goldsen, 2016, 2017).

Older LGBTQ+ individuals may be dealing with psychological residue from years of minority stressors that may contribute to subsequent substance misuse during this period.

For example, the current cohort of older LGBTQ+ adults in the United States is 16 times more likely to conceal their identities than younger generations including those in middle adulthood and emerging adulthood (Institute of Medicine, 2011). Furthermore, internalized stigma has a stronger impact on mental health as age increases (Newcomb & Mustanski, 2010). The current generation of LGBTQ+ older adults lived through the HIV/AIDs epidemic, which may have a direct impact through personal infection or loss of friends and loved ones. Historical circumstances such as these serve as context for the health of LGBTQ+ older adults.

LGBTQ+ older adults also experience natural declines in health that may be exacerbated by an inept or intolerant health care system (Brennan-Ing, Seidel, Larson, & Karpiak, 2014). The stress associated with poor quality health care may contribute to LGBTQ+ older adults neglecting their own care or use substances. Aging-related declines in health also mean LGBTQ+ individuals may lose their partners, other close-knit ties, and members of their family or origin or family of choice. Finally, LGBTQ+ older adults may enter retirement or assisted living homes that are ill-equipped to adequately support their needs and identities. These developmental conditions may contribute to minority stressors for LGBTQ+ older adults leading to high rates of substance misuse.

Intervention considerations

Substance use intervention research lacks evidence specific to use with LGBTQ+ populations. Experiences of LGBTQ+ individuals in substance use treatment settings are not well understood. Research has indicated that many lesbian women never seek help for substance use problems (Corliss, Grella, Mays, & Cochran, 2006). One study explored differences at treatment entry between non-heterosexual and heterosexual women (Cochran & Cauce, 2006). This study reported that non-heterosexual women were more likely than heterosexual women to seek treatment for heroin dependence, use at higher frequencies, and experience more mental health hospitalizations and homelessness, report higher rates of domestic violence, and use medical services less frequently. Another study found gay and bisexual men who enter substance abuse treatment were less likely to complete treatment than heterosexual men and women (Senreich, 2009).

Generally, authors have suggested that these disparate treatment outcomes can be attributed to treatment environments that are unsupportive of LGBTQ+ individuals (Hellman, Stanton, Lee, Tytun, & Vachon, 1989; McDermott, Tyndall, & Lichtenberg, 1989; Senreich, 2009) or social workers and other clinicians assuming heterosexuality in their clients (Willging, Salvador, & Kano, 2006). Treatment success and client/professional rapport are linked (Leach, 2005). Indeed, Senreich (2009) found that lesbian women in treatment felt less connected and satisfied with treatment than heterosexual women and reported that their sexual orientation negatively impacted their treatment experience because of clinician bias. With regard to social worker competence, Eliason and Hughes (2004) reported finding no differences between urban or rural practitioners' comfort in treating LGBTQ+ clients or knowledge about pertinent issues such as internalized homophobia, legal problems, the coming out process, or prevalence of substance use.

Only a handful of older studies have examined whether "gay specific" treatment settings are better for LGBT clients (Paul, Barrett, Crosby, & Stall, 1996; Driscoll, 1982). Further, the differences that may exist in these treatment facilities also remain unclear, as a recent national survey of these specialized facilities found few differences from those provided through general programs (Cochran, Peavy, & Robohm, 2007). Taken together, the available literature seems to hypothesize (while perhaps not with a substantial evidence base) that ensuring cultural and linguistic competency in the treatment of LGBT clients is an important factor in predicting treatment outcomes. A thorough assessment of frequency, duration, and longevity of minority stress experiences, coupled with an assessment of social and family support systems available within the client's life, help practitioners to develop an overall picture of emotional symptoms impacting the client and will subsequently inform appropriate treatment options. As always, social workers and other clinicians are advised to match their intervention approach to the specific client, their clinical diagnosis, available evidence, and the client's culture and personal characteristics.

Conclusions

LGBT individuals have significantly higher rates of substance misuse behavior over the course of their lifespans than heterosexual and cisgender individuals. Distal and proximal minority stressors unique to LGBT individuals due to social stigmatization of their identities contribute to adverse substance use outcomes for this population. Minority stressors may be shaped by developmental conditions unique to adolescence, emerging adulthood, middle adulthood, and older adulthood. Furthermore, substance use behaviors may vary based on the intersection of other identities such as gender, race, and socioeconomic status. Social work practitioners need to be aware of the impact minority stressors have on the LGBT population during different developmental periods and tailor their interventions appropriately. Research is needed concerning the way developmental conditions contribute to substance misuse, particularly within the frame of MST.

References

Arnett, J. J. (2000). Emerging adulthood: A theory of development from the late teens through the twenties. *American Psychologist, 55*, 469–480. doi:10.1037/0003-066X.55.5.469

Arnett, J. J. (2005). The developmental context of substance use in emerging adulthood. *Journal of Drug Issues, 35*, 235–254. doi:10.1177/002204260503500202

Badgett, M. V., Lau, H., Sears, B., & Ho, D. (2007). Bias in the workplace: Consistent evidence of sexual orientation and gender identity discrimination. *Chicago-Kent Law Review, 84*, 559–595.

Blackwood, E. (1986). Breaking the mirror: The construction of lesbianism and the anthropological discourse on homosexuality. *Journal of Homosexuality, 11*, 1–18. doi:10.1300/J082v11n03_01

Bontempo, D. E., & D'Augelli, A. R. (2002). Effects of at-school victimization and sexual orientation on lesbian, gay, or bisexual youths' health risk behavior. *Journal of Adolescent Health, 30*, 364–374. doi:10.1016/S1054-139X(01)00415-3

Brennan-Ing, M., Seidel, L., Larson, B., & Karpiak, S. E. (2014). Social care networks and older LGBT adults: Challenges for the future. *Journal of Homosexuality, 61*, 21–52. doi:10.1080/00918369.2013.835235

Bryan, A. E., Kim, H. J., & Fredriksen-Goldsen, K. I. (2017). Factors associated with high-risk alcohol consumption among LGB older adults: The roles of gender, social support, perceived stress, discrimination, and stigma. *The Gerontologist, 57*, 95–104. doi:10.1093/geront/gnw100

Clatts, M. C., Goldsamt, L., Yi, H., & Gwadz, M. V. (2005). Homelessness and drug abuse among young men who have sex with men in New York City: A preliminary epidemiological trajectory. *Journal of Adolescence, 28*, 201–214. doi:10.1016/j.adolescence.2005.02.003

Cochran, B. N., & Cauce, A. M. (2006). Characteristics of lesbian, gay, bisexual, and transgender individuals entering substance abuse treatment. *Journal of Substance Abuse Treatment, 30*, 135–146. doi:10.1016/j.jsat.2005.11.009

Cochran, B. N., Peavy, K. M., & Robohm, J. S. (2007). Do specialized services exist for LGBT individuals seeking treatment for substance misuse? A study of available treatment programs. *Substance Use & Misuse, 42*, 161–176. doi:10.1080/10826080601094207

Compas, B. E., Connor-Smith, J. K., Saltzman, H., Thomsen, A. H., & Wadsworth, M. E. (2001). Coping with stress during childhood and adolescence: Problems, progress, and potential in theory and research. *Psychological Bulletin, 127,* 87–127. doi:10.1037/0033-2909.127.1.87

Conron, K. J., Mimiaga, M. J., & Landers, S. J. (2010). A population-based study of sexual orientation identity and gender differences in adult health. *American Journal of Public Health, 100,* 1953–1960. doi:10.2105/AJPH.2009.174169

Corliss, H. L., Grella, C. E., Mays, V. M., & Cochran, S. D. (2006). Drug use, drug severity, and help-seeking behaviors of lesbian and bisexual women. *Journal of Women's Health, 15,* 556–568. doi:10.1089/jwh.2006.15.556

Corliss, H. L., Rosario, M., Wypij, D., Wylie, S. A., Frazier, A. L., & Austin, S. B. (2010). Sexual orientation and drug use in a longitudinal cohort study of US adolescents. *Addictive Behaviors, 35,* 517–521. doi:10.1016/j.addbeh.2009.12.019

D'Augelli, A. R. (2006). Developmental and contextual factors and mental health among lesbian, gay, and bisexual youths. In A. M. Omoto & H. S. Kurtzman (Eds.), *Contemporary perspectives on lesbian, gay, and bisexual psychology. Sexual orientation and mental health: Examining identity and development in lesbian, gay, and bisexual people* (pp. 37–53). Washington, DC: American Psychological Association. doi:10.1037/11261-002

DiPlacido, J. (1998). Minority stress among lesbians, gay men, and bisexuals: A consequence of heterosexism, homophobia, and stigmatization. In G. M. Herek (Ed.), *Psychological perspectives on lesbian and gay issues, Vol. 4. Stigma and sexual orientation: Understanding prejudice against lesbians, gay men, and bisexuals* (pp. 138–159). Thousand Oaks, CA: Sage Publications, Inc. doi:10.4135/9781452243818.n7

Demant, D., Hides, L., White, K. M., & Kavanagh, D. J. (2018). Effects of participation in and connectedness to the LGBT community on substance use involvement of sexual minority young people. *Addictive Behaviors, 81,* 167–174. doi:10.1016/j.addbeh.2018.01.028

Diamond, L. M. (2004). Emerging perspectives on distinctions between romantic love and sexual desire. *Current Directions in Psychological Science, 13,* 116–119. doi:10.1111/j.0963-7214.2004.00287.x

Driscoll, R. (1982). A gay-identified alcohol treatment program: A follow-up study. *Journal of Homosexuality, 7,* 71–80. doi:10.1300/J082v07n04_08

Egan, S. K., & Perry, D. G. (2001). Gender identity: A multidimensional analysis with implications for psychosocial adjustment. *Developmental Psychology, 37,* 451–463. doi:10.1037/0012-I649.37.4.45I

Eliason, M. J., & Hughes, T. (2004). Treatment counselor's attitudes about lesbian, gay, bisexual, and transgendered clients: Urban vs. rural settings. *Substance Use & Misuse, 39,* 625–644. doi:10.1081/JA-120030063

Emlet, C. A., Fredriksen-Goldsen, K. I., & Kim, H. J. (2013). Risk and protective factors associated with health-related quality of life among older gay and bisexual men living with HIV disease. *The Gerontologist, 53,* 963–972. doi:10.1093/geront/gns191

Emslie, C., Lennox, J., & Ireland, L. (2017). The role of alcohol in identity construction among LGBT people: A qualitative study. *Sociology of Health & Illness, 39,* 1465–1479. doi:10.1111/1467-9566.12605Erikson, E. (1968). *Youth: Identity and crisis.* New York, NY: W.W. Norton.

Fredriksen-Goldsen, K. I., Kim, H.-J., Barkan, S. E., Muraco, A., & Hoy-Ellis, C. P. (2013). Health disparities among lesbian, gay, and bisexual older adults: Results from a population-based study. *American Journal of Public Health, 103,* 1802–1809. doi:10.2105/AJPH.2012.301110

Frone, M. R. (2008). Are work stressors related to employee substance use? The importance of temporal context assessments of alcohol and illicit drug use. *Journal of Applied Psychology, 93,* 199–206. doi:10.1037/0021-9010.93.1.199

Garofalo, R., Wolf, R. C., Kessel, S., Palfrey, J., & DuRant, R. H. (1998). The association between health risk behaviors and sexual orientation among a school-based sample of adolescents. *Pediatrics, 101,* 895–902. doi:10.1542/peds.101.5.895

Gates, G. J. (2011). *How many people are lesbian, gay, bisexual, and transgender?* Los Angeles, CA: The Williams Institute. Retrieved from https://williamsinstitute.law.ucla.edu/wp-content/uploads/Gates-How-Many-People-LGBT-Apr-2011.pdf

Goldbach, J. T., & Gibbs, J. (2015). Strategies employed by sexual minority adolescents to cope with minority stress. *Psychology of Sexual Orientation and Gender Diversity, 2,* 297–306. doi:10.1037/sgd0000124

Goldbach, J. T., Tanner-Smith, E. E., Bagwell, M., & Dunlap, S. (2014). Minority stress and substance use in sexual minority adolescents: A meta-analysis. *Prevention Science, 15,* 350–363. doi:10.1007/s11121-013-0393-7

Haas, A. P., Eliason, M., Mays, V. M., Mathy, R. M., Cochran, S. D., D'Augelli, A. R., . . . Clayton, P. J. (2010). Suicide and suicide risk in lesbian, gay, bisexual, and transgender populations: Review and recommendations. *Journal of Homosexuality, 58*, 10–51. doi:10.1080/00918369.2011.534038

Halkitis, P. N., Siconolfi, D. E., Stults, C. B., Barton, S., Bub, K., & Kapadia, F. (2014). Modeling substance use in emerging adult gay, bisexual, and other YMSM across time: The P18 cohort study. *Drug and Alcohol Dependence, 145*, 209–216. doi:10.1016/j.drugalcdep.2014.10.016

Hatzenbuehler, M. L. (2011). The social environment and suicide attempts in lesbian, gay, and bisexual youth. *Pediatrics, 127*, 896–903. doi:10.1542/peds.2010-3020

Hellman, R. E., Stanton, M., Lee, J., Tytun, A., & Vachon, R. (1989). Treatment of homosexual alcoholics in government-funded agencies: Provider training and attitudes. *Hospital and Community Psychiatry, 40*, 1163–1168. doi:10.1176/ps.40.11.1163

Hendricks, M. L., & Testa, R. J. (2012). A conceptual framework for clinical work with transgender and gender nonconforming clients: An adaptation of the minority stress model. *Professional psychology: Research and Practice, 43*, 460–467. doi:10.1037/a0029597

Herrick, A. L., Matthews, A. K., & Garofalo, R. (2010). Health risk behaviors in an urban sample of young women who have sex with women. *Journal of Lesbian Studies, 14*, 80–92. doi:10.1080/10894160903060440.

Herts, K. L., McLaughlin, K. A., & Hatzenbuehler, M. L. (2012). Emotion dysregulation as a mechanism linking stress exposure to adolescent aggressive behavior. *Journal of Abnormal Child Psychology, 40*, 1111–1122. doi: 10.1007/s10802-012-9629-4

Holloway, I. W., Traube, D. E., Rice, E., Schrager, S. M., Palinkas, L. A., Richardson, J., & Kipke, M. D. (2012). Community and individual factors associated with cigarette smoking among young men who have sex with men. *Journal of Research on Adolescence, 22*, 199–205. doi: 10.1111/j.1532-7795.2011.00774.x

Holman, E. G. (2018). Theoretical extensions of minority stress theory for sexual minority individuals in the workplace: A cross-contextual understanding of minority stress processes. *Journal of Family Theory & Review, 10*, 165–180. doi:10.1111/jftr.12246

Hoy-Ellis, C. P., & Fredriksen-Goldsen, K. I. (2016). Lesbian, gay, & bisexual older adults: Linking internal minority stressors, chronic health conditions, and depression. *Aging & Mental Health, 20*, 1119–1130. doi:10.1080/13607863.2016.1168362

Hoy-Ellis, C. P., & Fredriksen-Goldsen, K. I. (2017). Depression among transgender older adults: General and minority stress. *American Journal of Community Psychology, 52*, 295–305. doi:10.1002/ajcp.12138

Hudson, A. (2013, August 21). Germany allows indeterminate gender on birth register. *Reuters World News*. Retrieved from https://uk.reuters.com/article/uk-germany-gender/germany-allows-indeterminate-gender-on-birth-register-idUKBRE97K0OK20130821

Hunt, J. (2012). A state-by-state examination of nondiscrimination laws and policies. *Center for American Progress*. Retrieved from https://cdn.americanprogress.org/wp-content/uploads/issues/2012/06/pdf/state_nondiscrimination.pdf

Institute of Medicine. (2011). *The health of lesbian, gay, bisexual, and transgender people: Building a foundation for better understanding*. Washington, DC: National Academies Press. doi:10.17226/13128

Janssen, E., Everaerd, W., Spiering, M., & Janssen, J. (2000). Automatic processes and the appraisal of sexual stimuli: Toward an information processing model of sexual arousal. *Journal of Sex Research, 37*, 8–23. doi:10.1080/00224490009552016

Kandel, D., Johnson, J., Bird, H., & Camino, G. (1997). Psychiatric disorders associated with substance use among children and adolescents: Findings from the methods for epidemiology of child and adolescent mental disorders (MECA) study. *Journal of Abnormal Child Psychology, 25*, 121–132. doi:10.1023/A:1025779412167.

Kattari, S. K., Whitfield, D. L., Walls, N. E., Langenderfer-Magruder, L., & Ramos, D. (2016). Policing gender through housing and employment discrimination: Comparison of discrimination experiences of transgender and cisgender LGBQ individuals. *Journal of the Society for Social Work and Research, 7*, 427–447. doi:10.1086/686920

Kauth, M. R., & Kalichman, S. C. (1995). Sexual orientation and development: An interactive approach. In R. D. McAnulty & L. Diamant (Eds.), *The psychology of sexual orientation, behavior, and identity* (pp. 81–103). Westport, CT: Greenwood Press.

Kelleher, C. (2009). Minority stress and health: Implications for lesbian, gay, bisexual, transgender, and questioning (LGBTQ) young people. *Counselling Psychology Quarterly, 22*, 373–379. doi:10.1080/09515070903334995

Kosciw, J. G., Greytak, E. A., Zongrone, A. D., Clark, C. M., & Truong, N. L. (2018). *The 2017 National School Climate Survey: The experiences of lesbian, gay, bisexual, transgender, and queer youth in our nation's schools*. New York: GLSEN.

Leach, M. J. (2005). Rapport: A key to treatment success. *Complementary Therapies in Clinical Practice, 11*, 262–265. doi:10.1016/j.ctcp.2005.05.005

Lewes, K. (1988). *The psychoanalytic theory of male homosexuality*. New York, NY: Simon and Schuster

McCabe, S. E., Hughes, T. L., Bostwick, W. B., West, B. T., & Boyd, C. J. (2009). Sexual orientation, substance use behaviors and substance dependence in the United States. *Addiction, 104*, 1333–1345. doi:10.1111/j.1360-0443.2009.02596.x

McDermott, D., Tyndall, L., & Lichtenberg, J. W. (1989). Factors related to counselor preference among gays and lesbians. *Journal of Counseling & Development, 68*, 31–35. doi:10.1002/j.1556-6676.1989.tb02488.x

McNair, R., Pennay, A., Hughes, T., Brown, R., Leonard, W., & Lubman, D. I. (2016). A model for lesbian, bisexual and queer-related influences on alcohol consumption and implications for policy and practice. *Culture, Health & Sexuality, 18*, 405–421. doi:10.1080/13691058.2015.1089602

Marshal, M. P., Friedman, M. S., Stall, R., King, K. M., Miles, J., Gold, M. A., . . . Morse, J. Q. (2008). Sexual orientation and adolescent substance use: A meta-analysis and methodological review. *Addiction, 103*, 546–556. doi:10.1111/j.1360-0443.2008.02149.x

Marshal, M. P., Friedman, M. S., Stall, R., & Thompson, A. L. (2009). Individual trajectories of substance use in lesbian, gay and bisexual youth and heterosexual youth. *Addiction, 104*, 974–981. doi:10.1111/j.1360-0443.2009.02531.x

Medley, G., Lipari, R. N., Bose, J., Cribb, D. S., Kroutil, L. A., & McHenry, G. (2016). *Sexual orientation and estimates of adult substance use and mental health: Results from the 2015 national survey on drug use and health*. NSDUH Data Review. Retrieved from https://www.samhsa.gov/data/sites/default/files/NSDUH-SexualOrientation-2015/NSDUH-SexualOrientation-2015/NSDUH-SexualOrientation-2015.htm

Mereish, E. H., & Bradford, J. B. (2014). Intersecting identities and substance use problems: Sexual orientation, gender, race, and lifetime substance use problems. *Journal of Studies on Alcohol and Drugs, 75*, 179–188. doi:10.15288/jsad.2014.75.179

Meyer, I. H. (2003). Prejudice, social stress, and mental health in lesbian, gay, and bisexual populations: Conceptual issues and research evidence. *Psychological Bulletin, 129*, 674–697. doi:10.1037/0033-2909.129.5.674

Needham, B. L. (2012). Sexual attraction and trajectories of mental health and substance use during the transition from adolescence to adulthood. *Journal of Youth and Adolescence, 41*, 179–190. doi:10.1007/s10964-011-9729-4

Newcomb, M. E., Heinz, A. J., & Mustanski, B. (2012). Examining risk and protective factors for alcohol use in lesbian, gay, bisexual, and transgender youth: A longitudinal multilevel analysis. *Journal of Studies on Alcohol and Drugs, 73*, 783–793. doi:10.15288/jsad.2012.73.783

Newcomb, M. E., & Mustanski, B. (2010). Internalized homophobia and internalizing mental health problems: A meta-analytic review. *Clinical Psychology Review, 30*, 1019–1029. doi:10.1016/j.cpr.2010.07.003

Newport, F. (2018, May, 22). In U.S., estimate of LGBT population rises to 4.5%. *Gallup*. Retrieved from https://news.gallup.com/poll/234863/estimate-lgbt-population-rises.aspx

Paul, J. P., Barrett, D. C., Crosby, G. M., & Stall, R. D. (1996). Longitudinal changes in alcohol and drug use among men seen at a gay-specific substance abuse treatment agency. *Journal of Studies on Alcohol, 57*, 475–485. doi:10.15288/jsa.1996.57.475

Rehm, J., Mathers, C., Popova, S., Thavorncharoensap, M., Teerawattananon, Y., & Patra, J. (2009). Global burden of disease and injury and economic cost attributable to alcohol use and alcohol-use disorders. *The Lancet, 373*, 2223–2233. doi:10.1016/S0140-6736(09)60746-7

Rosario, M., Rotheram-Borus, M. J., & Reid, H. (1996). Gay-related stress and its correlates among gay and bisexual male adolescents of predominantly Black and Hispanic background. *Journal of Community Psychology, 24*, 136–159. doi:10.1002/(SICI)1520-6629(199604)24:2<136::AID-JCOP5>3.0.CO;2-X

Rosario, M., Schrimshaw, E. W., & Hunter, J. (2004). Predictors of substance use over time among gay, lesbian, and bisexual youths: An examination of three hypotheses. *Addictive Behaviors, 29*, 1623–1631. doi:10.1016/j.addbeh.2004.02.032

Rusow, J., Burgess, C., Klemmer, C., Weskamp, G., Gibbs, J., & Goldbach, J. (2015, May 27). *The implications of self-labels and label changing among sexual minority adolescents*. Washington, DC: Paper presented at the 23rd Annual Meeting of the Society for Prevention Research.

Russell, S. T., Clarke, T. J., & Clary, J. (2009). Are teens "post-gay"? Contemporary adolescents' sexual identity labels. *Journal of Youth and Adolescence, 38*, 884–890. doi:10.1007/s10964-008-9388-2

Russell, S. T., Driscoll, A. K., & Truong, N. (2002). Adolescent same-sex romantic attractions and relationships: Implications for substance use and abuse. *American Journal of Public Health, 92*, 198–202. doi:10.2105/AJPH.92.2.198

Russell, S. T., Franz, B. T., & Driscoll, A. K. (2001). Same-sex romantic attraction and experiences of violence in adolescence. *American Journal of Public Health, 91*, 903–906. doi:10.2105/AJPH.91.6.903

Sears, B., & Mallory, C. (2011). *Documented evidence of employment discrimination & its effects on LGBT people.* Retrieved from the Williams Institute website https://williamsinstitute.law.ucla.edu/wp-content/uploads/Sears-Mallory-Discrimination-July-20111.pdf

Senreich, E. (2009). A comparison of perceptions, reported abstinence, and completion rates of gay, lesbian, bisexual, and heterosexual clients in substance abuse treatment. *Journal of Gay & Lesbian Mental Health, 13*, 145–169. doi:10.1080/19359700902870072

Shilo, G., & Savaya, R. (2012). Mental health of lesbian, gay, and bisexual youth and young adults: Differential effects of age, gender, religiosity, and sexual orientation. *Journal of Research on Adolescence, 22*, 310–325. doi: 10.1111/j.1532-7795.2011.00772.x

Solorio, R., Swendeman, D., & Rotheram-Borus, M. J. (2003). Risks among young gay and bisexual men living with HIV. *AIDS Education and Prevention, 15*, 80–90. doi:10.1521/aeap.15.1.5.80.23610

Testa, R. J., Habarth, J., Peta, J., Balsam, K., & Bockting, W. (2015). Development of the gender minority stress and resilience measure. *Psychology of Sexual Orientation and Gender Diversity, 2*, 65–77. doi: 10.1037/sgd0000081

Toomey, R. B., Ryan, C., Diaz, R. M., Card, N. A., & Russell, S. T. (2013). Gender-nonconforming lesbian, gay, bisexual, and transgender youth: School victimization and young adult psychosocial adjustment. *Psychology of Sexual Orientation and Gender Diversity, 1*, 71–80. doi:10.1037/2329-0382.1.S.71

Torkelson, J. (2012). A queer vision of emerging adulthood: Seeing sexuality in the transition to adulthood. *Sexuality Research and Social Policy, 9*, 132–142. doi:10.1007/s13178-011-0078-6

Traube, D. E., Holloway, I. W., Schrager, S. M., & Kipke, M. D. (2012). Utilizing Social Action Theory as a framework to determine correlates of illicit drug use among young men who have sex with men. *Psychology of Addictive Behaviors, 26*, 78–88. doi: 10.1037/a0024191.

Trocki, K. F., Drabble, L. A., & Midanik, L. T. (2009). Tobacco, marijuana, and sensation seeking: Comparisons across gay, lesbian, bisexual, and heterosexual groups. *Psychology of Addictive Behaviors, 23*, 620–631. doi:10.1037/a0017334

Tupler, L. A., Zapp, D., DeJong, W., Ali, M., O'Rourke, S., Looney, J., & Swartzwelder, H. S. (2017). Alcohol-related blackouts, negative alcohol-related consequences, and motivations for drinking reported by newly matriculating transgender college students. *Alcoholism: Clinical and Experimental Research, 41*, 1012–1023. doi:10.1111/acer.13358

University of California Davis Lesbian Gay Bisexual Transgender Queer Intersex Asexual Resource Center. (2013). Safe zone resource manual. Retrieved from http://lgbtqia.ucdavis.edu.

University of California Davis Lesbian Gay Bisexual Transgender Queer Intersex Asexual Resource Center. (2014). LGBTQIA Resource Center Glossary. Retrieved from http://lgbtqia.ucdavis.edu/lgbt-education/lgbtqia-glossary.

Ward, B. W., Dahlhamer, J. M., Galinsky, A. M., & Joestl, S. S. (2014). *Sexual orientation and health among U.S. adults: National health interview survey, 2013.* Hyattsville, MD: National Center for Health Statistics. Retrieved from https://www.cdc.gov/nchs/data/nhsr/nhsr077.pdf

Willging, C. E., Salvador, M., & Kano, M. (2006). Pragmatic help seeking: How sexual and gender minority groups access mental health care in a rural state. *Psychiatric Services, 57*, 871–874. doi:10.1176/ps.2006.57.6.871

Wilsnack, S. C., Hughes, T. L., Johnson, T. P., Bostwick, W. B., Szalacha, L. A., Benson, P., . . . Kinnison, K. E. (2008). Drinking and drinking-related problems among heterosexual and sexual minority women. *Journal of Studies on Alcohol and Drugs, 69*, 129–139. doi:10.15288/jsad.2008.69.129

Introduction to Section III

Interventions to prevent and address addictive behavior and related problems

Building on the contents from Sections I and II, Section III includes 15 chapters examining evidence-informed, evidenced-supported, and evidence-based intervention strategies for preventing and treating addictive behaviors and their related problems. These chapters discuss strategies at individual, family, community, and service delivery system/policy levels; they are not designed to teach specific practice skills. Relevant to this section's contents is the framework proposed by the Institute of Medicine (1994) for classifying the full range of intervention strategies available for addressing mental health concerns (see Figure III.1). The Section III chapters include aspects across this range of prevention, treatment, and recovery support (maintenance).

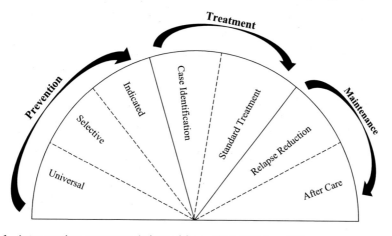

Figure III.1   Intervention spectrum (adapted from IOM, 1994, p. 23)

Reference

Institute of Medicine (IOM). (1994). The mental health intervention spectrum for mental disorders (Figure 2.1). In P. J. Mrazek & R. J. Haggerty (Eds.), *Reducing risks for mental disorders: Frontiers for preventive intervention research* (p. 23). Committee on Prevention of Mental Disorders, Division of Biobehavioral Sciences and Mental Disorders. Washington, DC: National Academy press.

18

Intervening around addictive behaviors

Allen Zweben and Brooke S. West

Background

Global data concerning the percent of persons experiencing alcohol dependence who are engaged with treatment services varied widely from very limited (1–10%) to high (more than 40%), but a large number of nations (40%) did not know the level of treatment coverage (WHO, 2018). In 2016, only one in six individuals around the world who experienced drug use disorders received treatment for them (UNODC, 2018). Therefore, it is important to consider how evidence-supported interventions can be effectively delivered more widely, including their integration into everyday practice settings serving a broad range of individuals.

This chapter is focused on innovative interventions with the strongest evidence of efficacy for addressing substance misuse, substance use disorder (SUD), and related problems. These interventions are considered state-of-the-art methods for helping a broad range of individuals. With respect to scientific evidence, we discuss what is and is not known about these approaches, and we examine how they are applied with individuals at different points along the severity continuum. We discuss how these methods are employed to treat different aspects of or accompanying addictive behaviors, such as motivation, cravings, life style changes, coping capacities, recovery resources, and general, overall client needs. We also explore how a particular approach can be adapted and combined with other treatments to improve outcomes and consider how the combined approach may be used concurrently or sequentially to produce lasting effects. We begin with considering three assessment tasks—screening, evaluation, and diagnosis. These three assessment tasks are interrelated and provide information on how to proceed helping the person. We then explore eight intervention approaches with demonstrated evidence for treating addictive behaviors: motivational interviewing, case management, working with significant others, mutual help, brief interventions, contingency management, cognitive behavioral coping skills training, and medication-assisted treatment.

Strategies to screen for, evaluate, and diagnose substance misuse

Screening

The purpose of routine screening for substance misuse is to identify individuals who may be at risk of or already experiencing problematic substance use, including but not limited to substance use disorder (see Chapters 20 and 27). In asking about alcohol and drug use, a simple screening measure can be intermixed with other questions about health and social issues to reduce defensiveness about drinking or drug use (Miller, Forcehimes, & Zweben, 2019): "*How many times in the past year have you had five or more drinks (men) or four or more drinks (women) in a day?*" And "*How many times in the past year have you used illegal drugs or prescription medications for non-medical reasons?*" A response of 1 or more times indicates that the individual is potentially at-risk for unhealthy alcohol or drug use.

Biological measures are used as additional tools for detecting heavy alcohol use or drug use. These biomarker measures include gamma-glutamyl transferase (GGT), carbohydrate-deficient transferrin (CDT) and ethyl glucuronide (ETG) for alcohol use, or tests for detecting the presence of other drugs (e.g. cocaine, opiates, and amphetamines). Advantages of these measures include: (1) reducing social desirability and denial bias (Babor & Higgins-Biddle, 2000), and (2) individuals are less likely to provide inaccurate data if the information is validated by laboratory tests.

Evaluating

Screening can provide a wide net for identifying individuals potentially experiencing substance use problems. However, just knowing about drug and alcohol use provides little information about which treatment options might be most suitable. In order to determine what is likely to help, several multidimensional evaluation questions deserve consideration (Miller et al., 2019):

1   "*How much have you been drinking and how often?*" (problem severity); similar questions can be asked about drugs.
2   "*How does substance use impact areas of your life such as employment, marriage, interpersonal relationships, emotional concerns, stressors, and health issues?*" (life events).
3   "*How motivated are you to change the circumstances or conditions that may impact on your recovery?*" (level of motivation).
4   "*How much support do you have from family, friends, and significant others to accompany you on your road to recovery?*" (level of social support).
5   "*What do you have going that can help in changing?*" (strengths and capabilities).

Numerous state-of-the-art measures can provide more detail on the questions covered above. Data derived from these evidence-supported measures can be incorporated in a feedback session to raise client awareness of alcohol or drug use problems, to identify and link clients with appropriate treatments and to increase readiness to change.

Problem severity

The Form 90 interview surveys alcohol and drug use patterns (heavy and steady use and periodic binge use) over a 90-day period (Miller, 1996; Tonigan, Miller, & Brown, 1994).

Life events and conditions

The Addiction Severity Index (ASI) (McLellan et al., 1992, 1990) is a psychometrically sound, multidimensional public domain interview examining severity of problems in five different areas potentially affected by alcohol or drug misuse: (1) medical, (2) employment, (3) legal, (4) family relations, and (5) psychiatric. Client and interviewer perceptions of problem severity are rated in each area.

Social support

Support systems play a valuable role in enhancing treatment engagement and adherence, buttressing motivation and offering lifestyle alternatives supporting recovery. The Important People and Activities (IPA) instrument (Longabaugh, Beattie, Noel, Stout, & Malloy, 1993) was constructed specifically to measure network support for drinking and abstinence (in contrast to general social support).

Motivation

Motivation is a consistent predictor of client engagement and outcomes. Two questions dealing with importance and confidence (self-efficacy) help determine client readiness for change and can be incorporated into the clinical interview (Miller et al., 2019).

- *"On a 0–10 scale, how <u>important</u> would you say it is for you to make a change in your use?"*
- *"On a 0–10 scale, how <u>confident</u> would you say you are to make a change in your use?"*

Higher scores on these two dimensions (importance and confidence/self-efficacy) suggest the client is ready to enter, participate in, and benefit from treatment.

CLIENT STRENGTHS

Mobilizing clients' strengths is important in facilitating change. Two strengths-based instruments are the Client Assessment of Strengths, Interest, and Goals (CASIG) and the Strengths Assessment Worksheet (SAW) (Bird et al., 2012; Wallace, Lecomte, Wilde, & Liberman, 2001). These instruments include an array of items pertaining to personal attributes and relationship skills, resilience, and spirituality.

Diagnosing

If screening and evaluation indicate that undergoing a diagnostic process is warranted, a DSM or ICD substance use diagnosis (see Chapter 1) can be determined in a clinical interview. As a general rule, individuals diagnosed as severe or moderately severe on the DSM-5 require more intensive treatment for recovery (Rinker & Neighbors, 2015; Suitt, Castro, Caetano, & Field, 2015). However, a multidimensional evaluation should be conducted along with a diagnostic interview to inform treatment planning.

Expanding the boundaries of treatment with brief intervention

Most individuals experiencing substance use problems never enter specialty treatment settings, but instead might be seen in non-specialty settings for other problems related to or accompanying their substance use. Brief intervention (BI) has been employed opportunistically with individuals who were not initially seeking help concerning substance misuse to redress problems or mitigate problems before they become more serious. Such an approach reflects the expansion of interventions with individuals experiencing varied substance use severity levels encountered in non-specialty settings: primary care clinics, social service programs, emergency and trauma units, employee assistance programs, public schools, child protection services, criminal justice facilities, and college health services (McCambridge & Cunningham, 2014; Miller & Weisner, 2002; Moyer, Finney, Swearingen, & Vergun, 2002; Rollnick, Miller, & Butler, 2008).

BI is used differentially in non-specialty settings, depending upon clients' problem severity, coping capacities, social resources, and state of readiness for change (i.e. precontemplation, contemplation, or action). For some clients, a single brief counseling and advice session offered in an emergency department/trauma setting may suffice to produce behavior change (Barnett et al., 2010). In confirming a connection between injury and substance use, BI may trigger a desire to address substance misuse and contribute to improved treatment outcomes (Barnett et al., 2010).

For individuals seen in non-specialty settings and falling on the high end of the severity continuum, BI serves as a referral adherence strategy to deal with substance use problems (Glass et al., 2015; National Institute on Alcohol Abuse and Alcoholism, 2005). Recognizing the importance of BI, in 2003, the Substance Abuse and Mental Health Services Administration (SAMSHA) added referral adherence to the components of BI to improve the interconnection between specialist and non-specialist services (Bray, Del Boca, McRee, Hayashi, & Babor, 2017; Jonas et al., 2012). Social workers and other practitioners play an important role in facilitating entry, participation, and retention in specialty addiction treatment (Turner et al., 2017). Based on assessment results, a menu of options comprised of intensive case management, medication assistance, and coping skills therapy may be offered. This may involve: (1) orienting the individual to the reasons for referral, (2) arranging same-day appointments, (3) using repeated reminders, and (4) in some cases, conducting escorted visits. Motivational interviewing can play a critical role in reducing referral adherence barriers, such as lack of problem recognition, stigma, and low confidence about following through on the referral options, as well as bolstering commitment to change (Glass et al., 2017).

BI delivered in specialty addiction treatment settings may serve as the entry point for a stepped-care approach where low-intensive treatment is initially provided with the provision that additional help is offered as needed (Miller et al., 2019). BI allows for a greater opportunity to see wait-listed clients, many of whom might drop out if immediate care is not available. BI may also help in improving motivation, which, in turn, may facilitate positive treatment engagement and retention. In short, BI can play a critical role in the continuum of care for alcohol and drug misuse in these settings.

For individuals seen in non-specialty settings, a single advice and feedback session may be insufficient to produce behavior change (Aldridge, Dowd, & Bray, 2017), particularly for individuals who have not as yet experienced potential harms and risks associated with their substance misuse. Individuals seen in non-specialty settings are focused on other concerns and have not yet discovered how substance misuse may be creating or exacerbating problems which initially brought them to the non-specialty setting. Low recognition of substance-related problems renders individuals less amenable, responsive, or reactive to information-sharing/advice about changing their substance use patterns and could create discord in the social worker-client relationship. Motivational interviewing may be incorporated into BI to enhance client awareness and acceptance of problem recognition and explore commitment to change (Zweben & Piepmeier, in press).

Computer-delivered brief intervention

Recent developments in BI involve computer-delivered modules (Bertholet et al., 2015; Blow et al., 2017; Gryczynski et al., 2015; Nilsen, 2010; Ondersma, Svikis, Thacker, Beatty, & Lockhart, 2014; Pemberton et al., 2011; Riordan, Conner, Flett, & Scarf, 2015; Schwartz et al., 2014). Using a touchscreen and audio headphones for privacy, a detailed, tailor-made feedback report addresses quantity/frequency of substance use and related economic, medical, and social consequences, followed by readiness and self-efficacy for change measures. A comparative analysis compares the individual's alcohol consumption with others' of the same gender and age. Interactions between narrator and client emphasize the client's decision-making and empowerment. Essential motivational interviewing skills (i.e. reflecting, affirming, and collaborating) are incorporated throughout. Skill-building and booster sessions are provided if warranted/needed. Most recently, text messaging has been added to computer-delivered brief intervention (CBI) following termination to improve outcomes (Riordan et al., 2015). CBI can be equally effective as counselor-delivered brief intervention, but not in all cases (Blow et al., 2017; Ondersma et al., 2014; Riordan et al., 2015). Nonetheless, despite equivocal results, advantages of CBI exist with respect to managing resources, requiring less training, maintaining standards of quality and integrity, and reducing stigma.

Sustaining the benefits of behavioral treatment with case management

Individuals engaged in substance misuse regularly face medical, psychosocial, economic, and legal problems. At one time, there was the belief that improving drinking and drug use behaviors would naturally produce changes in the social and family arenas; however, this has not been the case (Siegal et al., 1995). Failure to address unemployment, financial, and other problems over the course of treatment places individuals experiencing substance use disorders at increased risk for continuing or recurring substance misuse (Kuerbis, Neighbors, & Morgenstern, 2011; Rapp, Van Den Noortgate, Broekaert, & Vanderplasschen, 2014; Robles et al., 2004). Case management (CM) is not an alternative or replacement intervention but rather a complement to treatment, dealing with issues not routinely addressed in behavioral treatment (Hesse, Vanderplasschen, Rapp, Broekaert, & Fridell, 2007).

Case manager roles and functions

Case managers play a valuable role in helping individuals address issues that interfere with recovery during the course of treatment and follow-up. The kinds and levels of activity associated with case management depend on problem severity, coping capacities, social resources, and motivation of clients seen in community and residential settings. On the low end of the severity continuum, case managers may engage to detect "early warning signs" that can precipitate a return to alcohol or drug use (Zweben, Rose, Stout, & Zywiak, 2003) and help problem-solve solutions. This may involve supporting a client in finding a less stressful job rather than linking the client with resources.

Individuals experiencing more serious substance-related problems (e.g. medical and psychiatric symptoms), and experiencing severe hardships, typically require more intensive case management involvement. In such situations, case managers play an active role in goal setting, case monitoring, and service coordination. Client advocacy may also be necessary—where/when needed services are not available or accessible to clients. The amount of time spent in these core functions is associated with successful outcomes (Alexander, Pollack, Nahra, Wells, & Lemak, 2007; Morgenstern et al., 2008; Noel, 2006).

The most important consideration in CM services concerns establishing a strong case manager-client working relationship (Morgenstern et al., 2008). Conducting an intensive, time-consuming formal assessment using standardized measures mentioned earlier, could be counterproductive; asking too many questions can interfere with listening, understanding, and engaging with clients, and may also engender defensiveness and discord in the relationship. Rather, it may be better to explore reasons for coming, listen reflectively, and affirm client strengths and capacities.

Once the relationship is established, the case manager and client clarify needed services (i.e. finances, childcare, housing, employment, medical care, and behavioral health care) and assess level of commitment toward seeking and participating in particular services. A services request form can be used to assess need for specific services essential for recovery (Miller et al., 2019). Clients identify and assign a priority rating (1–10) for each needed service. For example, a client may rate mental health problems as "10" and score employment as "5" revealing the need to first address psychiatric problems to enable participation in job training. Completing the service request form may enable the individual to assume ownership of goals and objectives, increase readiness for steps necessary to facilitate change, and develop a high-quality change plan.

In contrast, clients who continue to remain uncertain or ambivalent about referral assistance may require additional outreach efforts, such as escorting them to the service, sending out reminders and prompts, and employing motivational interviewing (MI) strategies to facilitate health behavior change (Glass et al., 2015). MI can provide a safe space for a client to reveal underlying uncertainties and ambivalence about carrying out the proposed plan. MI strategies could be useful by asking the client to delay decision-making about a particular task and revisiting it at later time; additional time to contemplate the matter is often a good way of softening resistance to change (Miller, Zweben, DiClimente, & Rychtarik, 1992).

In MI, "failure" to comply with a proposed plan is viewed as a learning opportunity to obtain a better understanding of the issues or barriers interfering with the plan (Tiderington, Stanhope, & Henwood, 2013). Reluctance about following through on a change plan may stem from the client's perceived consequences of change rather than a lack of acceptance of need (Zweben & Zuckoff, 2002). For example, accepting a job that requires living away from family could interfere with maintaining a stable marital relationship, an important factor in facilitating change. Disagreements or differences between the client and case manager about a proposed plan should be accepted, normalized, and affirmed.

Finally, it is not always clear whether the case manager should be embedded in a treatment team or provide stand-alone services. In hospital or health care settings, case managers may be included in the medical care team to address ancillary issues associated with alcohol and drug use. In other situations, case managers serve as referral sources for other practitioners jointly involved (e.g. medication and behavioral treatment) in managing the care of individuals having substance use problems.

Retooling with cognitive behavioral therapy/ coping skills training (CBCST)

Individuals often encounter recovery difficulties due to lack of skills in dealing with stressors of daily life (e.g. relationship or work challenges) and/or symptoms associated with mental health conditions (e.g. depression, anxiety). These stressors and symptoms act as triggers standing in the way of long-lasting recovery. Developing strong, positive coping skills is one tool for supporting individuals' recovery (Hendershot, Witkiewitz, George, & Marlatt, 2011). CBCST is primarily concerned with helping individuals modify their cognitive processes to develop and implement skills necessary for managing life stressors (e.g. avoiding or coping with high-risk situations), cravings (e.g. drink refusal skills), and mental health symptoms (e.g. managing negative moods or depression) without resorting to substance use (see Chapter 6). CBCST is sometimes called Cognitive Behavioral Therapy (CBT) in the clinical and research literature.

The addition of CBCST to other evidence-based interventions, including 12-step facilitation and motivational enhancement therapy, is useful for enhancing treatment effectiveness (Kiluk, Nich, Babuscio, & Carroll, 2010; Miller, Zweben, & Johnson, 2005). Case management, mutual help groups, or individual and group counseling are also beneficial adjuncts to CBCST. CBCST can be offered in group or individual settings and works well with technology-based approaches (i.e. web or mobile phone platforms focused on skills building) making it more widely accessible. However, since different clients may need different skills, CBCST approaches must be client-centered and flexible. Although a range of skill-building opportunities should be offered, common needs include coping with urges and cravings, social skills, emotional regulation, behavioral self-control, and general life skills related to employment and housing. These skills often work synergistically to prevent relapse and build recovery self-efficacy.

Who benefits from CBCST?

CBCST works best with individuals in need of specific emotional and behavioral techniques to support recovery. For instance, clients struggling with cravings and urges (Elwafi, Witkiewitz, Mallik, Thornhill IV, & Brewer, 2013; Navidian, Kermansaravi, Tabas, & Saeedinezhad, 2016) may need skills around avoiding high-risk situations (especially during early recovery), escape from situations where urges are triggered, distraction when alternatives are not available, and endurance strategies when all of the above fail (Miller, 2004a). Establishing strong substance-free social networks is also important, but clients who lack skills in developing and/or maintaining positive social relationships (Hunter-Reel, McCrady, & Hildebrandt, 2009; Owens & McCrady, 2014) may need to learn new social skills to help effectively navigate and develop meaningful social relationships (e.g. listening, nonverbal communication, and assertive rather than passive or aggressive communication). These skills should develop alongside efforts to build new networks through mutual self-help groups or religious communities.

Similarly, clients with limited emotional and behavioral regulation to manage moods (e.g. depression, anger) may benefit from CBCST interventions. CBCST can support client understanding of emotional response patterns (e.g. the STORC model of situation, thoughts, organism, response, consequences) and learning how to alter situations, interpretations, and reactions to challenging emotions, as well as ways to better deal with consequences (Miller & Mee-Lee, 2012). Self-regulation interventions focus on behavioral self-control to manage impulsive behaviors related to substance misuse through goal setting, self-monitoring of use, strategies for reducing consumption, and dealing with high-risk situations and cravings (Hester, 2003).

Many challenges associated with recovery extend beyond personal and emotional skills, however, making coping skills interventions ideal for clients who need assistance with managing life practicalities, like securing housing, managing finances, cooking meals, and finding a job. Employment, in particular, is a strong indicator of recovery success, and job skills can be incorporated into treatment (Hamdi, Levy, Jaffee, Chisholm, & Weiss, 2011; Liu, Huang, & Wang, 2014; Svikis et al., 2012). Through individual or group counseling, or through case management, building skills in preparation of resumes, job-hunting, networking, completing applications, and job interviewing help support recovering clients in a holistic and sustainable manner.

Given the wide range of skills clients may need, one challenge is to help clients identify skills they lack and motivate them to build new skills that will aid with recovery. Not all clients need to develop skills in all areas; therefore, offering a range of skill-building options can help meet diverse client needs. Overall, developing a range of coping skills (e.g. social skills training, and emotional and behavioral regulation), in combination with other evidence-based treatments, can be useful for enhancing self-managing aspects of life that may facilitate recovery.

Setting the stage for behavior change with motivational interviewing (MI)

Individuals often enter treatment struggling with feelings of ambivalence about changing their substance use behaviors. Many are uncertain about whether current difficulties link to their substance use. Some may fear entering and remaining in treatment despite their substance use seriously interfering with their employability, marital relationships, and mental health (e.g. symptoms of anxiety, depression, and sleep disorders; see Chapter 33). Others may be concerned about potential consequences of sustained sobriety, such as increased marital or family demands. Thus, attempts to engage individuals in a collaborative therapeutic relationship may be met with defensiveness, which may create conflict in the practitioner-client relationship.

Motivational Interviewing (MI) sets the stage for resolving a client's underlying ambivalence toward change. MI focuses on benefits of change (e.g. enhanced quality of life) rather than risks of substance misuse. Efforts are devoted to evoking clients' own reasons, capacities, and social resources for change while fostering optimism about efficacy for change. Instead of confronting clients' misperceptions about their substance misuse, MI encourages clients to voice their own perspectives about these harmful practices with the expectation that their views will be genuinely accepted, and not judged harshly by practitioners.

Clinical utility of MI

Several MI strategies are used to enhance motivation for change.

Open-ended questioning

Open-ended questioning is used to gain an understanding of a client's readiness to change. Clients are asked about their perceptions of their current condition (e.g. severity level) and expected benefits they might derive from changing their situation. This helps determine the level of importance to the client of changing. The client also is asked about confidence around changing current substance use patterns (e.g. on a 1–10 scale) and willingness to undertake the necessary steps to move ahead. Strategies to facilitate attitudinal and behavioral change can then be adapted to client readiness and self-efficacy for change (Miller et al., 2019; Miller & Rollnick, 2013).

Reflecting

Information derived from the open-ended questions is used to formulate accurate reflections of "where the client is" about initiating change. This demonstrates understanding and acceptance of the client's perspectives, which is essential in fostering a strong therapeutic relationship.

Affirming

Affirmations are used to underscore personal strengths, abilities, and coping capacities, which reinforce client self-efficacy for change.

Supporting autonomy

Client autonomy is honored throughout the working relationship. Client responsibility and choice are encouraged, disagreements are acknowledged, and authentic apologies offered if the client is hurt or offended by what is being said. All options for change are considered during the sessions.

Promoting optimism

Wherever appropriate, optimism is promoted to soften or reduce talk about not changing or maintaining status quo and to bolster a commitment to health-promoting behavior change.

Summarizing

This entails collecting comments and thoughts in a series or sequence of reflections about what the client has shared during the session. Summarizing helps increase clients' situational understanding and confirms the positive message about change. Once agreement about change is achieved, planning for next steps can begin.

MI is employed both as a stand-alone intervention and in combination with many kinds of treatment, including pharmacotherapy, coping skills therapy, and contingency management (Miller, 2004b; Naar & Safren, 2017). However, the ultimate value has been to integrate spirit of MI principles in many treatment approaches—principles such as respect for autonomy, collaboration, acceptance, compassion, and empathetic reflection. These foundational elements are incorporated into both in-person and computer-delivered interventions (Miller et al., 2019). The results have been impressive. In studies combining MI with another active treatment, benefits of the combination were sustained beyond what the active treatment produced (Hettema, Steele, & Miller, 2005).

Working with significant others (SOs) as active ingredients in behavioral change

The impact of substance misuse extends beyond the individual, making the inclusion of significant others (SOs) in treatment an important tool (see Chapter 24). SOs can influence a person, facilitating entry into treatment, but their involvement also yields higher rates of retention, adherence, abstinence, and maintaining change after treatment is completed (Hunter-Reel et al., 2009; McCrady, Epstein, Hallgren, Cook, & Jensen, 2016; McPherson, Boyne, & Willis, 2017; Meyers & Wolfe, 2004). The benefits of engaging SOs in addiction treatment, in conjunction with addressing relationship issues, extend to both the person engaged in substance misuse and the SO. Numerous evidence-based approaches have been developed to work with SOs.

Community reinforcement and family training (CRAFT)

CRAFT is a technique targeted toward SOs that involves developing skills related to motivation, functional analysis, contingency management, communication, treatment entry, and safety (Meyers & Wolfe, 2004; Smith & Meyers, 2007). Through a series of (about) seven-hour-long sessions, CRAFT builds SOs' confidence to move their partners toward reduced substance use and entering treatment through positive reinforcement for sobriety and identifying opportunities to encourage them to seek help. Across diverse contexts, CRAFT has been effective at getting initially unmotivated individuals into treatment and engaging them in care (Bischof, Iwen, Freyer-Adam, & Rumpf, 2016; Brigham et al., 2014; Meyers, Miller, Smith, & Tonigan, 2002; Miller, Meyers, & Tonigan, 1999). SOs also benefit in terms of improved happiness and reduced depression, anger, and family conflict (Miller et al., 1999). Tools for implementing CRAFT are available for counselors (Smith & Meyers, 2007), as is a self-help guide for family members to use independently (Meyers & Wolfe, 2004); in many geographic areas, practitioners trained in CRAFT may be limited.

Behavioral couples therapy

Behavioral Couples Therapy (BCT) engages SOs in treatment as a means to improve the couple's relationship and support behaviors that encourage sustained abstinence. BCT is designed primarily for married or cohabiting couples, including those experiencing substantial relationship distress, or even a history of violence (O'Farrell, Murphy, Stephan, Fals-Stewart, & Murphy, 2004; Schumm et al., 2009); however, an acute risk of severe violence may exclude couples from BCT (Fals-Stewart & Kennedy, 2005).

BCT involves behaviorally oriented couples sessions, often (but not always) in conjunction with psychosocial and medication-assisted clinical services, delivered over 12–20 weekly 50–60 minutes sessions; a six-session brief BCT also exists (Fals-Stewart & Lam, 2008). The primary components of BCT include establishing goals related to supporting sobriety, improving the positivity of the relationship, strengthening communication skills, and reducing conflicts and negative interactions. BCT has demonstrated success in treating addiction in adults with overall better outcomes than individual treatment (Powers, Vedel, & Emmelkamp, 2008), resulting in increased abstinence, adherence to medications (e.g. disulfiram, naltrexone), and relationship functioning (Kelley, Bravo, Braitman, Lawless, & Lawrence, 2016; Schumm, O'Farrell, Murphy, & Fals-Stewart, 2009). To deliver high-quality and effective care, BCT requires specialized training and ongoing practice (Miller, Sorensen, Selzer, & Brigham, 2006).

Family-involved treatment

Family-involved treatment is especially important for adolescents engaged in substance mis-use since family dynamics and home environment play a huge role in supporting or under-mining their treatment engagement (Stormshak et al., 2011). Effective family-based options tend to use a cognitive behavioral family therapy approach and integrate services to pro-mote protective behaviors and address multiple family, community, and peer risk factors (Kaminer, 2001). Family-involved treatment approaches focus on behavior change related to improved decision-making, problem solving, communication skills, and relationship build-ing (e.g. multisystemic therapy, brief strategic family therapy, multidimensional family ther-apy, adolescent community reinforcement approach, and functional family therapy).

These interventions show promise for reducing adolescent substance use, re-arrest, out-of-home placement (Henggeler, Schoenwald, Liao, Letourneau, & Edwards, 2002), and behavioral problems, while also increasing family involvement (Santisteban et al., 2003; Szapocznik & Williams, 2000) and positive family and peer relationships (Liddle, Rowe, Dakof, Henderson, & Greenbaum, 2009). Effectiveness of family-based approaches has been demonstrated cross-culturally (Santisteban et al., 2003) and as lasting into adulthood (Datchi & Sexton, 2013; Sawyer & Borduin, 2011).

A few considerations should be kept in mind when selecting an approach for work with SOs. First, adding one or more family members into treatment sessions means managing the individual client, significant others, and relationship or family dynamics simultaneously. To do this well requires training that many practitioners never receive, so clients who may bene-fit greatly from these approaches may never even learn of them. Additionally, not all relation-ships are suited for couple or family-based approaches, particularly when safety/relationship violence is a concern (see Chapter 34). Finally, the approaches discussed here may be out of reach for many individuals, in terms of time commitment or financial resources. Despite these potential challenges, working with couples and families has a strong evidence base for supporting treatment and recovery and, in many circumstances, may surpass individual treat-ment in terms of entry into care, engagement, and long-term recovery success.

Increasing network support for behavioral change through mutual help

Mutual help groups are one way to meet the need for support from peer recovery networks. Although mutual help takes many forms, the focus on reciprocal support and active group engagement promotes abstinence or moderation in substance use. Peer networks offer the opportunity to develop both personal and social resources, or "recovery capital," which can be utilized in a flexible way without the potential constraints of formal therapy (Kelly & Hoeppner, 2015). Broadly, the goal of mutual help groups is to build substance-free social networks and lasting support structures that aid with long-term recovery.

Despite not being a formal therapy, a 12-step approach like Alcoholics Anonymous (AA) or Narcotics Anonymous (NA) is widely incorporated into treatment plans. The combi-nation of formal treatment (e.g. cognitive behavioral therapy, motivational enhancement therapy) and mutual help networks can lead to better outcomes (Dawson, Grant, Stinson, & Chou, 2006; Pagano, White, Kelly, Stout, & Tonigan, 2013). Periods of active treatment are the ideal time to encourage clients to try out mutual help groups (Tonigan, Connors, & Miller, 2003). Systematic encouragement such as 12-step facilitation (TSF) therapy, which promotes active engagement in mutual help groups (but is not a 12-step approach itself), rather than passively sharing information, is more likely to result in positive treatment outcomes (Bogenschutz et al., 2014; Sisson & Mallams, 1981).

Mutual help supporting evidence

Many individuals connected with mutual help groups may never receive formal treatment, but evidence demonstrates that participation in such groups alone may have an impact on substance misuse outcomes. Research focused on AA concluded that meeting attendance and especially engagement predict long-term sobriety (Humphreys, Blodgett, & Wagner, 2014; Majer, Jason, Ferrari, & Miller, 2011; Moos & Moos, 2005). Recent work suggests the effectiveness of mutual help groups may stem from their impact on coping skills, motivation-building, self-efficacy, and the formation of new networks (Kelly, 2017; Kelly, Hoeppner, Stout, & Pagano, 2012).

Mutual help groups excel in their ability to help individuals form social support networks, which makes this method advantageous for individuals lacking support for moderation or abstinence (Toumbourou, Hamilton, U'ren, Stevens-Jones, & Storey, 2002). Mutual help networks also tend to be free, be offered at flexible times, and operate outside of professional treatment settings, making them more accessible than other forms of treatment. For instance, mutual support groups may be one of few feasible options for clients with limited or no health insurance coverage or those who need greater scheduling flexibility. However, mutual help groups are not ideal for all clients, especially those experiencing co-occurring substance use and mental health disorders. For some individuals, group interactions may be intimidating or even stigmatizing, making either professionally facilitated support groups or individual treatment better options.

Despite widespread availability and utilization of mutual health groups, especially in North America, one major challenge is that success, in large part, depends on client fit. There exists substantial variation across mutual health groups; individuals may need to try numerous different meetings or groups in order to find one that works for them. For instance, some groups are explicitly religious (e.g. Overcomers Outreach), while others are spiritual (e.g. 12-step programs) or secular (e.g. Secular Organizations for Sobriety, Life Ring Secular Recovery). Individuals also may be interested in specialized groups, like those for women (e.g. Women for Sobriety), adolescents, or LGBTQIA+ individuals; specialized groups may provide safer spaces for vulnerable or marginalized individuals. Mutual help groups also vary in how strongly abstinence is emphasized. AA and NA focus heavily on abstinence, but individuals experiencing less severe alcohol problems may be interested in groups that promote moderation either as a final step or as a step along the way to abstinence (Lembke & Humphreys, 2012). Moderation Management programs are intended for individuals interested in reducing excessive or harmful drinking practices and may help meet diverse needs.

Increasing incentives for change with contingency management (COM)

Contingency management (COM), which is incentive-based, involves positive and tangible reinforcement for progress toward behavior change. These interventions typically involve reward in the form of vouchers for goods or services, prize drawings, or cash that may increase in value over time with sustained behavior change or based on the magnitude of the goal. Behaviors that warrant a reward can vary but should be based on specified targets that are successive and/or scaled from low to high impact, including things like a negative drug screen, taking medication, making or coming to appointments, attending treatment or mutual help meetings, or scheduling a job interview. The goal is to provide immediate and continued opportunities for success that encourage self-efficacy and build motivation to maintain progress (McDonell et al., 2017; Reback et al., 2010). This is offered as a bridging process in light of the contrast between the immediate reinforcing nature of substance use compared to the considerable time-lag before recovery becomes rewarding.

Benefits of COM

COM is best applied in combination with other evidence-based treatments and has been shown to improve short-term outcomes across a range of substances, populations, and settings, such as outpatient care, methadone clinics, shelters, and group treatment (Benishek et al., 2014). For instance, COM combined with cognitive behavioral therapy and motivational interviewing is highly effective (Budney, Roffman, Stephens, & Walker, 2007), as is the integration of COM with medication-assisted treatments (Gray et al., 2011). The impact of COM can also extend beyond substance use to the reduction of HIV risk behaviors and psychological symptoms, as well as improved quality of life (Petry, Alessi, & Rash, 2013; Petry, Weinstock, Alessi, Lewis, & Dieckhaus, 2010). Overall, COM provides a window of opportunity for clients to have positive experiences early in the recovery process, paving the way for future successes with longer-term treatment options.

COM works as a form of motivation early on; therefore, individuals already showing success at abstaining may not be good candidates for this approach (Herrmann et al., 2017; Petry, Barry, Alessi, Rounsaville, & Carroll, 2012). Clients struggling to remain drug-free early during treatment are most likely to benefit from the extra incentives offered through COM (Herrmann et al., 2017). Clients with limited social and economic resources may also find that the tangible resources of COM make behavior change possible, but they may require ongoing case management to create sustained change (Montgomery, Carroll, & Petry, 2015). For other clients, the demands of COM may be overwhelming, as it involves continued, intense monitoring that may compete with meeting their other basic life demands (Petry et al., 2012).

Although efficacious, COM is not without challenges, especially as it relates to cost and misconceptions, both of which stand in the way of its widespread implementation. For instance, COM can be expensive to implement as it involves additional practitioner training, frequent substance use monitoring (e.g. biosensors, urine toxicology), staff time, and the cost of participant incentives. Focusing on clients most likely to benefit from COM helps limit expenses (Cunningham et al., 2017; Rash, Stitzer, & Weinstock, 2017). The other major challenge with COM is practitioner resistance stemming from hesitation around providing monetary rewards. This can be addressed through training or the use of non-monetary or intangible rewards (e.g. certificates of achievement) for behavioral change. COM is potentially an important tool for many clients as it provides an intermediate reward to motivate change.

Offering medication-assisted treatment (MAT)

Pharmacotherapies, or prescribed use of medications, have increasingly become an important component in managing the care of individuals experiencing substance use problems. For alcohol, as a first step, medications such as benzodiazepine, chlordiazepoxide, and lorazepam are effective in helping to stabilize the alcohol withdrawal process. Pharmacotherapy should be accompanied by behavioral intervention to clarify and set expectations of the benefits, side effects management, and potential barriers to compliance with the medication protocol (Weiss et al., 2014; Wilcox & Bogenschutz, 2013). The behavioral intervention also provides the requisite support to facilitate the recovery process. Once alcohol withdrawal symptoms are alleviated, other medications may help maintain gains derived from the initial intervention and set/achieve new intervention goals. Numerous medications effectively facilitate a stable period of abstinence or non-problem drinking (see Chapter 19).

Medications supporting drinking abstinence or reduction

Disulfiram (Antabuse®) has proven useful in helping some individuals achieve sustained abstinence, particularly for clients who are older, more socially stable, and committed to taking the medication daily (Barber & O'Brien, 1999; Fuller & Gordis, 2004). Disulfiram helps clients refrain from alcohol use to avoid aversive reactions (i.e. nausea, vomiting, racing heart, lowering of blood pressure, and shortness of breath) produced by the drug's combination with alcohol.

Naltrexone (Revia®) has been useful in reducing alcohol's euphoric effects, blocking the reward aspects of drinking mediated through the brain's opiate receptors. This helps in returning to abstinence more quickly if a person does engage in drinking, thereby preventing a slip from turning into a full-blown relapse (Kranzler & Van Kirk, 2001). Individuals who experience comorbid psychiatric or other substance use disorders are less likely to benefit from naltrexone (Garbutt, West, Carey, Lohr, & Crews, 1999; Oslin et al., 2008). An injectable form of naltrexone (Vivitrol®) helps manage alcohol use disorders (AUD) and opioid use disorders (OUD); its monthly dosing has the advantage over daily pills for increasing medication adherence. Naltrexone can be employed effectively in managing AUD in primary care settings (Lee et al., 2010).

Medications for opioid use disorders

Extended-release naltrexone has been used effectively with diverse outpatient groups, including individuals with criminal justice involvement, to reduce the rewarding effects of opioid use (Lee et al., 2018). The main drawback is that clients must be opioid-free at least three or more days before being considered for this medication, which places limitations on eligible referrals. Two medications treat opioid withdrawal and promote maintenance among individuals experiencing OUD (Hser, Evans, Grella, Ling, & Anglin, 2015; McKeganey, Russell, & Cockayne, 2013; O'Malley & Kosten, 2006): methadone and buprenorphine (Subutex®).

Methadone relieves opioid withdrawal symptoms while reducing the euphoria associated with opioid use (CSAT, 2005). It has been used effectively in clinical settings where clients receive their daily dose and other support services (McLellan et al., 1999). Buprenorphine also helps alleviate opioid withdrawal symptoms and facilitate recovery by reducing the need for negative reinforcement in continued opioid use. Buprenorphine has advantages over methadone, including less frequent dosing, self-administration at home, and ease of tapering down if a client's goal is to become completely drug-free rather than maintaining medication (methadone). Individuals receiving methadone may fare better than those prescribed buprenorphine (Carroll & Weiss, 2016), primarily due to higher rates of dropout from buprenorphine treatment. The structured support and close monitoring required with methadone maintenance programs might account for the differences between the two approaches (Pinto et al., 2010).

Combining pharmacotherapy and behavioral treatments

It is often difficult to achieve satisfactory treatment outcomes without combining a pharmacotherapy with behavioral treatment approaches. A major consideration to consider in combining medication and behavioral intervention is the severity level of the substance use problems (Miller et al., 2019). Individuals experiencing more severe substance use problems typically require more intensive behavioral intervention in conjunction with an effective medication (Carroll & Weiss, 2016). Problems include failure to attend treatment appointments, inability to produce negative urine tests, not adhering to the medication regimen, and experiencing serious medical, social, and/or interpersonal problems. Lacking the requisite social support and social stability to sustain treatment gains increases the risk of treatment failure. Adequate exposure to a more intensive behavioral approach is often necessary to attend to treatment needs (Nielsen, Hillhouse, Mooney, Ang, & Ling, 2015).

In contrast, for individuals experiencing less severe substance-related problems, a less intensive medical management (MM) approach combined with an effective medication might suffice to produce positive change. MM typically involves a medical practitioner reviewing the regimen, medication side effects, and withdrawal symptoms, providing supports for abstinence or reduced use (harm reduction), attending to medication adherence, and providing relevant information on risk reduction strategies (Anton et al., 2006; Carroll & Kiluk, 2012; Schwartz, Kelly, O'Grady, Gandhi, & Jaffe, 2011). Adding a motivational interviewing component could provide an added benefit to MM (Heffner et al., 2010; Zweben, Piepmeier, Fucito, & O'Malley, 2017).

Another consideration pertains to problems accompanying or associated with continued substance misuse. Some issues may have predated the substance misuse; others may have contributed to the substance misuse or developed after the individual has engaged in recovery. Behavioral intervention supports recovery by addressing these sorts of complicating issues, improving social and coping resources and needed lifestyle changes to sustain the gains derived from medications. In summary, pharmacotherapy may help reduce withdrawal symptoms and craving during recovery, but behavioral interventions are needed to resolve accompanying or associated social, economic, interpersonal, and intrapersonal problems. Not attending to these issues can present a major impediment to recovery.

In some areas, MAT has come to mean substance use disorder treatment managed through medications without the addition of one or more previously discussed evidence-supported interventions. In such situations the behavioral intervention (termed "minimal care") is mainly focused on managing side effects and facilitating medication compliance without addressing the aforementioned social, motivational, and individual coping resources accompanying the substance misuse. The inability to provide an evidenced-based intervention and MAT should not stand in the way of employing pharmacotherapy for substance use problems. MAT along with "minimal care" can have a substantial impact on an individual's functioning. The challenge is to identify and link a particular behavioral intervention with medication that would produce effects beyond what might be achieved with the medication and minimal care alone.

Conclusions

As research and clinical standards have improved, the treatment of addictive behavior has undergone a dramatic transformation, moving away from pessimistic ("difficult to treat") and limited ("one-size fits all") perspectives to recognizing that individuals experiencing substance use problems represent a heterogeneous population with diverse capabilities, coping, social, and motivational resources. Additionally, intervention can be delivered in an array of specialty and non-specialty settings, and recovery can be supported with a variety of options.

A critical component of this changing perspective is an emphasis on client strengths rather than deficiencies. In accordance with this framework, practitioners place greater focus on the benefits of change rather than on the risks of not changing. Much effort is devoted to establishing and maintaining a collaborative client-practitioner partnership, recognized as a major active ingredient of change. Another component involves recognizing the need to make connections between substance misuse and concerns that initially brought them to seek help. Furthermore, practitioners recognize that the intervention(s) provided need to be continually monitored and adapted to clients' changing conditions (e.g. readiness to change) and circumstances (e.g. degree of social support).

In the future, further consideration needs to be given to determining how to combine and sequence interventions so they complement one another to optimize the benefits of addiction treatment. To illustrate, medications and behavioral treatments focus on different aspects of the problem and form an integrative, synergistic approach to promote behavior change: mutual help can provide needed abstinence support, supportive SO involvement can reengage family members and friends who became estranged, and motivational interviewing can enhance and support clients' motivations and efforts to change. Evidence-supported assessment approaches, combined with brief, couples/family, coping skills, contingency management, and other strategies provide clients and practitioners with an array of options to maximize success in establishing and meeting recovery goals.

References

Aldridge, A., Dowd, W., & Bray, J. (2017). The relative impact of brief treatment versus brief intervention in primary health-care screening programs for substance use disorders. *Addiction, 112*, 54–64. doi:10.1111/add.13653

Alexander, J. A., Pollack, H., Nahra, T., Wells, R., & Lemak, C. H. (2007). Case management and client access to health and social services in outpatient substance abuse treatment. *The Journal of Behavioral Health Services & Research, 34*(3), 221–236. doi:10.1007/s11414-007-9072-4

Anton, R. F., O'Malley, S. S., Ciraulo, D. A., Cisler, R. A., Couper, D., Donovan, D. M., . . . LoCastro, J. S. (2006). Combined pharmacotherapies and behavioral interventions for alcohol dependence: the COMBINE study: A randomized controlled trial. *JAMA, 295*(17), 2003–2017. doi:10.1001/jama.295.17.2003

Babor, T. F., & Higgins-Biddle, J. C. (2000). Alcohol screening and brief intervention: Dissemination strategies for medical practice and public health. *Addiction, 95*(5), 677–686. doi:10.1046/j.1360-0443.2000.9556773.x

Barber, W., & O'Brien, C. (1999). Pharmacotheraphies. In B. S. McCrady & E. Epstein (Eds.), *Addictions: A comprehensive guidebook*. New York: Oxford University Press.

Barnett, N. P., Apodaca, T. R., Magill, M., Colby, S. M., Gwaltney, C., Rohsenow, D. J., & Monti, P. M. (2010). Moderators and mediators of two brief interventions for alcohol in the emergency department. *Addiction, 105*(3), 452–465. doi:10.1111/j.1360-0443.2009.02814.x

Benishek, L. A., Dugosh, K. L., Kirby, K. C., Matejkowski, J., Clements, N. T., Seymour, B. L., & Festinger, D. S. (2014). Prize-based contingency management for the treatment of substance abusers: A meta-analysis. *Addiction, 109*(9), 1426–1436. doi:10.1111/add.12589

Bertholet, N., Cunningham, J. A., Faouzi, M., Gaume, J., Gmel, G., Burnand, B., & Daeppen, J. B. (2015). Internet-based brief intervention for young men with unhealthy alcohol use: A randomized controlled trial in a general population sample. *Addiction, 110*(11), 1735–1743. doi:10.1111/add.13051

Bird, V. J., Le Boutillier, C., Leamy, M., Larsen, J., Oades, L. G., Williams, J., & Slade, M. (2012). Assessing the strengths of mental health consumers: A systematic review. *Psychological Assessment, 24*(4), 1024. doi:10.1037/a0028983

Bischof, G., Iwen, J., Freyer-Adam, J., & Rumpf, H.-J. (2016). Efficacy of the community reinforcement and family training for concerned significant others of treatment-refusing individuals with alcohol dependence: A randomized controlled trial. *Drug and Alcohol Dependence, 163*, 179–185. doi:10.1016/j.drugalcdep.2016.04.015

Blow, F. C., Walton, M. A., Bohnert, A. S., Ignacio, R. V., Chermack, S., Cunningham, R. M. . . Barry, K. L. (2017). A randomized controlled trial of brief interventions to reduce drug use among adults in a low-income urban emergency department: The HealthiER You study. *Addiction, 112*(8), 1395–1405. doi:10.1111/add.13773

Bogenschutz, M. P., Rice, S. L., Tonigan, J. S., Vogel, H. S., Nowinski, J., Hume, D., & Arenella, P. B. (2014). 12-step facilitation for the dually diagnosed: A randomized clinical trial. *Journal of Substance Abuse Treatment, 46*(4), 403–411. doi:10.1016/j.jsat.2013.12.009

Bray, J. W., Del Boca, F. K., McRee, B. G., Hayashi, S. W., & Babor, T. F. (2017). Screening, Brief Intervention and Referral to Treatment (SBIRT): Rationale, program overview and cross-site evaluation. *Addiction, 112*, 3–11. doi:10.1111/add.13676

Brigham, G. S., Slesnick, N., Winhusen, T. M., Lewis, D. F., Guo, X., & Somoza, E. (2014). A randomized pilot clinical trial to evaluate the efficacy of Community Reinforcement and Family Training for Treatment Retention (CRAFT-T) for improving outcomes for patients completing opioid detoxification. *Drug and Alcohol Dependence, 138*, 240–243. doi:10.1016/j.drugalcdep.2014.02.013

Budney, A. J., Roffman, R., Stephens, R. S., & Walker, D. (2007). Marijuana dependence and its treatment. *Addiction Science & Clinical Practice, 4*(1), 4. doi:10.1151/ASCP07414

Carroll, K. M., & Kiluk, B. D. (2012). Integrating psychotherapy and pharmacotherapy in substance abuse treatment. In S. Walters & F. Rotgers (Eds.), *Treating substance abuse: Theory and technique* (3rd ed., pp. 320–354). New York, NY: Guilford Press.

Carroll, K. M., & Weiss, R. D. (2016). The role of behavioral interventions in buprenorphine maintenance treatment: A review. *American Journal of Psychiatry, 174*(8), 738–747. doi:10.1176/appi.ajp.2016.16070792

Center for Substance Abuse Treatment (CSAT). (2005). Medication-assisted treatment for opioid addiction in opioid treatment programs. Treatment Improvement Protocol (TIP) Series 43. DHHS Publication No. (SMA)05–4048. Rockville, MD: Substance Abuse and Mental Health Services Administration.

Cunningham, C., Stitzer, M., Campbell, A. N., Pavlicova, M., Hu, M.-C., & Nunes, E. V. (2017). Contingency management abstinence incentives: Cost and implications for treatment tailoring. *Journal of Substance Abuse Treatment, 72*, 134–139. doi:10.1016/j.jsat.2015.08.010

Datchi, C. C., & Sexton, T. L. (2013). Can family therapy have an effect on adult criminal conduct? Initial evaluation of functional family therapy. *Couple and Family Psychology: Research and Practice, 2*(4), 278. doi:10.1037/a0034166

Dawson, D. A., Grant, B. F., Stinson, F. S., & Chou, P. S. (2006). Estimating the effect of help-seeking on achieving recovery from alcohol dependence. *Addiction, 101*(6), 824–834. doi:10.1111/j.1360-0443.2006.01413.x

Elwafi, H. M., Witkiewitz, K., Mallik, S., Thornhill IV, T. A., & Brewer, J. A. (2013). Mindfulness training for smoking cessation: Moderation of the relationship between craving and cigarette use. *Drug and Alcohol Dependence, 130*(1–3), 222–229. doi:10.1016/j.drugalcdep.2012.11.015

Fals-Stewart, W., & Kennedy, C. (2005). Addressing intimate partner violence in substance-abuse treatment. *Journal of Substance Abuse Treatment, 29*(1), 5–17. doi:10.1016/j.jsat.2005.03.001

Fals-Stewart, W., & Lam, W. K. (2008). Brief behavioral couples therapy for drug abuse: A randomized clinical trial examining clinical efficacy and cost-effectiveness. *Families, Systems, & Health, 26*(4), 377. doi:10.1037/1091-7527.26.4.377

Fuller, R. K., & Gordis, E. (2004). Does disulfiram have a role in alcoholism treatment today? *Addiction, 99*(1), 21–24. doi:10.1111/j.1360-0443.2004.00597.x

Garbutt, J. C., West, S. L., Carey, T. S., Lohr, K. N., & Crews, F. T. (1999). Pharmacological treatment of alcohol dependence: A review of the evidence. *JAMA, 281*(14), 1318–1325. doi:10.1001/jama.281.14.1318

Glass, J. E., Andréasson, S., Bradley, K. A., Finn, S. W., Williams, E. C., Bakshi, A.-S. . . . Benegal, V. (2017). Rethinking alcohol interventions in health care: A thematic meeting of the International Network on Brief Interventions for Alcohol & Other Drugs (INEBRIA): BioMed Central. *Addiction Science & Clinical Practice, 12*, 14. doi:10.1186/s13722-017-0079-8

Glass, J. E., Hamilton, A. M., Powell, B. J., Perron, B. E., Brown, R. T., & Ilgen, M. A. (2015). Revisiting our review of Screening, Brief Intervention and Referral to Treatment (SBIRT): Meta-analytical results still point to no efficacy in increasing the use of substance use disorder services. *Addiction, 111*(1), 181–183. doi:10.1111/add.13146

Gray, K. M., Carpenter, M. J., Baker, N. L., Hartwell, K. J., Lewis, A. L., Hiott, D. W., . . . Upadhyaya, H. P. (2011). Bupropion SR and contingency management for adolescent smoking cessation. *Journal of Substance Abuse Treatment, 40*(1), 77–86. doi:10.1016/j.jsat.2010.08.010

Gryczynski, J., Mitchell, S. G., Gonzales, A., Moseley, A., Peterson, T. R., Ondersma, S. J . . . Schwartz, R. P. (2015). A randomized trial of computerized vs. in-person brief intervention for illicit drug use in primary care: outcomes through 12 months. *Journal of Substance Abuse Treatment, 50*, 3–10. doi:10.1016/j.jsat.2014.09.002

Hamdi, N. R., Levy, M., Jaffee, W. B., Chisholm, S. M., & Weiss, R. D. (2011). Implementing an adapted version of the job seekers' workshop in a residential program for patients with substance use disorders. *Journal of Addiction Medicine, 5*(2), 148. doi:10.1097/ADM.0b013e3181e95eb2

Heffner, J. L., Tran, G. Q., Johnson, C. S., Barrett, S. W., Blom, T. J., Thompson, R. D., & Anthenelli, R. M. (2010). Combining motivational interviewing with compliance enhancement therapy (MI-CET): Development and preliminary evaluation of a new, manual-guided psychosocial adjunct to alcohol-dependence pharmacotherapy. *Journal of Studies on Alcohol and Drugs, 71*(1), 61–70. doi:10.15288/jsad.2010.71.61

Hendershot, C. S., Witkiewitz, K., George, W. H., & Marlatt, G. A. (2011). Relapse prevention for addictive behaviors. *Substance Abuse Treatment, Prevention, and Policy, 6*(17). doi:10.1186/1747-597X-6-17

Henggeler, S. W., Schoenwald, S. K., Liao, J. G., Letourneau, E. J., & Edwards, D. L. (2002). Transporting efficacious treatments to field settings: The link between supervisory practices and therapist fidelity in MST programs. *Journal of Clinical Child and Adolescent Psychology, 31*(2), 155–167. doi:10.1207/S15374424JCCP3102_02

Herrmann, E. S., Matusiewicz, A. K., Stitzer, M. L., Higgins, S. T., Sigmon, S. C., & Heil, S. H. (2017). Contingency management interventions for HIV, tuberculosis, and hepatitis control among individuals with substance use disorders: A systematized review. *Journal of Substance Abuse Treatment, 72*, 117–125. doi:10.1016/j.jsat.2016.06.009

Hesse, M., Vanderplasschen, W., Rapp, R., Broekaert, E., & Fridell, M. (2007). Case management for persons with substance use disorders. *Cochrane Database of Systematic Reviews* (4). doi:10.1002/14651858.CD006265.pub2

Hester, R. K. (2003). Behavioral self-control training. In R. K. Hester & W. R. Miller (Eds.), *Handbook of alcoholism treatment approaches: Effective alternatives* (3rd ed., pp. 152–164). Boston: Allyn and Bacon.

Hettema, J., Steele, J., & Miller, W. R. (2005). Motivational interviewing. *Annual Review of Clinical Psychology, 1*, 91–111. doi:10.1146/annurev.clinpsy.1.102803.143833

Hser, Y.-I., Evans, E., Grella, C., Ling, W., & Anglin, D. (2015). Long-term course of opioid addiction. *Harvard Review of Psychiatry, 23*(2), 76–89. doi:10.1097/HRP.0000000000000052

Humphreys, K., Blodgett, J. C., & Wagner, T. H. (2014). Estimating the efficacy of Alcoholics Anonymous without self-selection bias: An instrumental variables re-analysis of randomized clinical trials. *Alcoholism: Clinical and Experimental Research, 38*(11), 2688–2694. doi:10.1111/acer.12557

Hunter-Reel, D., McCrady, B., & Hildebrandt, T. (2009). Emphasizing interpersonal factors: An extension of the Witkiewitz and Marlatt relapse model. *Addiction, 104*(8), 1281–1290. doi:10.1111/j.1360-0443.2009.02611.x

Jonas, D. E., Garbutt, J. C., Amick, H. R., Brown, J. M., Brownley, K. A., Council, C. L., . . . Richmond, E. M. (2012). Behavioral counseling after screening for alcohol misuse in primary care: A systematic review and meta-analysis for the US Preventive Services Task Force. *Annals of Internal Medicine, 157*(9), 645–654. doi:10.7326/0003-4819-157-9-201211060-00544

Kaminer, Y. (2001). Alcohol & drug abuse: Adolescent substance abuse treatment: Where do we go from here? *Psychiatric Services, 52*(2), 147–149. doi:10.1176/appi.ps.52.2.147

Kelley, M. L., Bravo, A. J., Braitman, A. L., Lawless, A. K., & Lawrence, H. R. (2016). Behavioral couples treatment for substance use disorder: Secondary effects on the reduction of risk for child abuse. *Journal of Substance Abuse Treatment, 62*, 10–19. doi:10.1016/j.jsat.2015.11.008

Kelly, J. F. (2017). Is Alcoholics Anonymous religious, spiritual, neither? Findings from 25 years of mechanisms of behavior change research. *Addiction, 112*(6), 929–936. doi:10.1111/add.13590

Kelly, J. F., & Hoeppner, B. (2015). A biaxial formulation of the recovery construct. *Addiction Research & Theory, 23*(1), 5–9. doi:10.3109/16066359.2014.930132

Kelly, J. F., Hoeppner, B., Stout, R. L., & Pagano, M. (2012). Determining the relative importance of the mechanisms of behavior change within Alcoholics Anonymous: A multiple mediator analysis. *Addiction, 107*(2), 289–299. doi:10.1111/j.1360-0443.2011.03593.x

Kiluk, B. D., Nich, C., Babuscio, T., & Carroll, K. M. (2010). Quality versus quantity: Acquisition of coping skills following computerized cognitive–behavioral therapy for substance use disorders. *Addiction, 105*(12), 2120–2127. doi:10.1111/j.1360-0443.2010.03076.x

Kranzler, H. R., & Van Kirk, J. (2001). Efficacy of naltrexone and acamprosate for alcoholism treatment: A meta-analysis. *Alcoholism: Clinical and Experimental Research, 25*(9), 1335–1341. doi:10.1097/00000374-200109000-00014

Kuerbis, A. N., Neighbors, C. J., & Morgenstern, J. (2011). Depression's moderation of the effectiveness of intensive case management with substance-dependent women on temporary assistance for needy families: Outpatient substance use disorder treatment utilization and outcomes. *Journal of Studies on Alcohol and Drugs, 72*(2), 297–307. doi:10.15288/jsad.2011.72.297

Lee, J. D., Grossman, E., DiRocco, D., Truncali, A., Hanley, K., Stevens, D., . . . Gourevitch, M. N. (2010). Extended-release naltrexone for treatment of alcohol dependence in primary care. *Journal of Substance Abuse Treatment, 39*(1), 14–21. doi:10.1016/j.jsat.2010.03.005

Lee, J. D., Nunes Jr, E. V., Novo, P., Bachrach, K., Bailey, G. L., Bhatt, S., . . . Hodgkins, C. C. (2018). Comparative effectiveness of extended-release naltrexone versus buprenorphine-naloxone for opioid relapse prevention (X:BOT): A multicentre, open-label, randomised controlled trial. *The Lancet, 391*(10118), 309–318. doi:10.1016/S0140-6736(17)32812-X

Lembke, A., & Humphreys, K. (2012). Moderation management: A mutual-help organization for problem drinkers who are not alcohol-dependent. *Journal of Groups in Addiction & Recovery, 7*(2–4), 130–141. doi:10.1080/1556035X.2012.705657

Liddle, H. A., Rowe, C. L., Dakof, G. A., Henderson, C. E., & Greenbaum, P. E. (2009). Multidimensional family therapy for young adolescent substance abuse: Twelve-month outcomes of a randomized controlled trial. *Journal of Consulting and Clinical Psychology, 77*(1), 12. doi:10.1037/a0014160

Liu, S., Huang, J. L., & Wang, M. (2014). Effectiveness of job search interventions: A meta-analytic review. *Psychological Bulletin, 140*(4), 1009. doi:10.1037/a0035923

Longabaugh, R., Beattie, M., Noel, N., Stout, R. L., & Malloy, P. (1993). The effect of social investment on treatment outcome. *Journal of Studies on Alcohol, 54*, 465–478. doi:10.15288/jsa.1993.54.465

Majer, J. M., Jason, L. A., Ferrari, J. R., & Miller, S. A. (2011). A longitudinal analysis of categorical twelve-step involvement among a U.S. national sample of recovering substance abusers in residential treatment. *Journal of Substance Abuse Treatment, 41*(1), 37–44. doi:10.1016/j.jsat.2011.01.010

McCambridge, J., & Cunningham, J. A. (2014). The early history of ideas on brief interventions for alcohol. *Addiction, 109*(4), 538–546. doi:10.1111/add.12458

McCrady, B. S., Epstein, E. E., Hallgren, K. A., Cook, S., & Jensen, N. K. (2016). Women with alcohol dependence: A randomized trial of couple versus individual plus couple therapy. *Psychology of Addictive Behaviors, 30*(3), 287. doi:10.1037/adb0000158

McDonell, M. G., Leickly, E., McPherson, S., Skalisky, J., Srebnik, D., Angelo, F., . . . Ries, R. K. (2017). A randomized controlled trial of ethyl glucuronide-based contingency management for outpatients with co-occurring alcohol use disorders and serious mental illness. *American Journal of Psychiatry, 174*(4), 370–377. doi:10.1176/appi.ajp.2016.16050627

McKeganey, N., Russell, C., & Cockayne, L. (2013). Medically assisted recovery from opiate dependence within the context of the UK drug strategy: Methadone and Suboxone (buprenorphine–naloxone) patients compared. *Journal of Substance Abuse Treatment, 44*(1), 97–102. doi:10.1016/j.jsat.2012.04.003

McLellan, A. T., Hagan, T. A., Levine, M., Meyers, K., Gould, F., Bencivengo, M., . . . Jaffe, J. (1999). Does clinical case management improve outpatient addiction treatment. *Drug and Alcohol Dependence, 55*(1), 91–103. doi:10.1016/S0376-8716(98)00183-5

McLellan, A. T., Kushner, H., Metzger, D., Peters, R., Smith, I., Grissom, G., . . . Argeriou, M. (1992). The fifth edition of the Addiction Severity Index. *Journal of Substance Abuse Treatment, 9*(3), 199–213. doi:10.1016/0740-5472(92)90062-S

McLellan, A. T., Parikh, G., Bragg, A., Cacciola, J. S., Fureman, B., & InCOMikofki, R. (1990). *Addiction Severity Index administration manual*. Philadelphia, PA: VA Center for Studies of Addiction.

McPherson, C., Boyne, H., & Willis, R. (2017). The role of family in residential treatment patient retention. *International Journal of Mental Health and Addiction, 15*(4), 933–941. doi:10.1007/s11469-016-9712-0

Meyers, R. J., Miller, W. R., Smith, J. E., & Tonigan, J. S. (2002). A randomized trial of two methods for engaging treatment-refusing drug users through concerned significant others. *Journal of Consulting and Clinical Psychology, 70*(5), 1182. doi:10.1037/0022-006X.70.5.1182

Meyers, R. J., & Wolfe, B. L. (2004). *Get your loved one sober: Alternatives to nagging, pleading, and threatening*. Center City, MN: Hazelden Publishing and Educational Services.

Miller, W. R. (1996). *Form 90: A structured assessment interview for drinking and related behaviors (Vol. 5)*. Bethesda, MD: National Institute on Alcohol Abuse and Alcoholism. doi:10.1037/e563242012-001

Miller, W. R. (2004a). *Combined behavioral intervention manual: A clinical research guide for therapists treating people with alcohol abuse and dependence*. Bethesda, MD: National Institute on Alcohol Abuse and Alcoholism.

Miller, W. R. (Ed.) (2004b). *Combined behavioral intervention manual: A clinical research guide for therapists treating people with alcohol abuse and dependence (Vol. 1)*. Bethesda, MD: National Institute on Alcohol Abuse and Alcoholism.

Miller, W. R., Forcehimes, A. A., & Zweben, A. (2019). *Treating addiction: A guide for professionals* (2nd ed.). New York, NY: Guilford Press.

Miller, W. R., & Mee-Lee, D. (2012). *Self-management: A guide to your feelings, motivations, and positive mental health*. Carson City, NV: The Change Companies.

Miller, W. R., Meyers, R. J., & Tonigan, J. S. (1999). Engaging the unmotivated in treatment for alcohol problems: A comparison of three strategies for intervention through family members. *Journal of Consulting and Clinical Psychology, 67*(5), 688. doi:10.1037/0022-006X.67.5.688

Miller, W. R., & Rollnick, S. (2013). *Motivational interviewing: Helping people change* (3rd ed.). New York, NY: Guilford Press.

Miller, W. R., Sorensen, J. L., Selzer, J. A., & Brigham, G. S. (2006). Disseminating evidence-based practices in substance abuse treatment: A review with suggestions. *Journal of Substance Abuse Treatment, 31*(1), 25–39. doi:10.1016/j.jsat.2006.03.005

Miller, W. R., & Weisner, C. (2002). Integrated Care. In W. R. Miller, C. Miller, & C. Weisner (Eds.), *Changing substance abuse through health and social systems*. New York, NY: Springer Science and Business Media. doi:10.1007/978-1-4615-0669-0

Miller, W. R., Zweben, A., DiClemente, C., & Rychtarik, R. (1992). *Motivational enhancement therapy manual: A clinical research guide for therapists treating individuals with alcohol abuse and dependence (Vol. 2)*. Rockville, MD: National Institute on Alcohol Abuse and Alcoholism.

Miller, W. R., Zweben, J., & Johnson, W. R. (2005). Evidence-based treatment: Why, what, where, when, and how? *Journal of Substance Abuse Treatment, 29*(4), 267–276. doi:10.1016/j.jsat.2005.08.003

Montgomery, L., Carroll, K. M., & Petry, N. M. (2015). Initial abstinence status and contingency management treatment outcomes: Does race matter? *Journal of Consulting and Clinical Psychology, 83*(3), 473. doi:10.1037/a0039021

Moos, R. H., & Moos, B. S. (2005). Paths of entry into Alcoholics Anonymous: Consequences for participation and remission. *Alcoholism: Clinical and Experimental Research, 29*(10), 1858–1868. doi:10.1097/01.alc.0000183006.76551.5a

Morgenstern, J., Blanchard, K. A., Kahler, C., Barbosa, K. M., McCrady, B. S., & McVeigh, K. H. (2008). Testing mechanisms of action for intensive case management. *Addiction, 103*(3), 469–477. doi:10.1111/j.1360-0443.2007.02100.x

Moyer, A., Finney, J. W., Swearingen, C. E., & Vergun, P. (2002). Brief interventions for alcohol problems: A meta-analytic review of controlled investigations in treatment-seeking and non-treatment-seeking populations. *Addiction, 97*(3), 279–292. doi:10.1046/j.1360-0443.2002.00018.x

Moyers, T. B., & Miller, W. R. (2013). Is low therapist empathy toxic? *Psychology of Addictive Behaviors, 27*(3), 878. doi:10.1037/a0030274

Naar, S., & Safren, S. A. (2017). *Motivational interviewing and CBT: Combining strategies for maximum effectiveness*. New York: Guilford Publications.

National Institute on Alcohol Abuse and Alcoholism. (2005). *Helping patients who drink too much: A clinician's guide. Updated 2005 edition*. Retrieved from https://pubs.niaaa.nih.gov/publications/Practitioner/CliniciansGuide2005/clinicians_guide.htm

Navidian, A., Kermansaravi, F., Tabas, E. E., & Saeedinezhad, F. (2016). Efficacy of group motivational interviewing in the degree of drug craving in the addicts under the methadone maintenance treatment (MMT) in South East of Iran. *Archives of Psychiatric Nursing, 30*(2), 144–149. doi:10.1016/j.apnu.2015.08.002

Nielsen, S., Hillhouse, M., Mooney, L., Ang, A., & Ling, W. (2015). Buprenorphine pharmacotherapy and behavioral treatment: Comparison of outcomes among prescription opioid users, heroin users and combination users. *Journal of Substance Abuse Treatment, 48*(1), 70–76. doi:10.1016/j.jsat.2014.06.006

Nilsen, P. (2010). Brief alcohol intervention—where to from here? Challenges remain for research and practice. *Addiction, 105*(6), 954–959. doi:10.1111/j.1360-0443.2009.02779.x

Noel, P. E. (2006). The impact of therapeutic case management on participation in adolescent substance abuse treatment. *The American Journal of Drug and Alcohol Abuse, 32*(3), 311–327. doi:10.1080/00952990500328646

Norcross, J. C., & Lambert, M. J. (2011). Psychotherapy relationships that work II. *Psychotherapy Research, 48*(1), 4. doi:10.1037/a0022180

O'Farrell, T. J., Murphy, C. M., Stephan, S. H., Fals-Stewart, W., & Murphy, M. (2004). Partner violence before and after couples-based alcoholism treatment for male alcoholic patients: The role of treatment involvement and abstinence. *Journal of Consulting and Clinical Psychology, 72*(2), 202. doi:10.1037/0022-006X.72.2.202

O'Malley, S., & Kosten, T. (2006). Pharmacotherapy of addictive disorders. In W. R. Miller & K. M. Carroll (Eds.), *Rethinking substance abuse: What the science shows, and what we should do about it* (pp. 240–256). New York, NY: Guilford Press.

Ondersma, S. J., Svikis, D. S., Thacker, L. R., Beatty, J. R., & Lockhart, N. (2014). Computer-delivered screening and brief intervention (e-SBI) for postpartum drug use: A randomized trial. *Journal of Substance Abuse Treatment, 46*(1), 52–59. doi:10.1016/j.jsat.2013.07.013

Oslin, D. W., Lynch, K. G., Pettinati, H. M., Kampman, K. M., Gariti, P., Gelfand, L., . . . Dackis, C. (2008). A placebo-controlled randomized clinical trial of naltrexone in the context of different levels of psychosocial intervention. *Alcoholism: Clinical and Experimental Research, 32*(7), 1299–1308. doi:10.1111/j.1530-0277.2008.00698.x

Owens, M. D., & McCrady, B. S. (2014). The role of the social environment in alcohol or drug relapse of probationers recently released from jail. *Addictive Disorders & Their Treatment, 13*(4), 179. doi:10.1097/ADT.0000000000000039

Pagano, M. E., White, W. L., Kelly, J. F., Stout, R. L., & Tonigan, J. S. (2013). The 10-year course of Alcoholics Anonymous participation and long-term outcomes: A follow-up study of outpatient subjects in Project MATCH. *Substance Abuse, 34*(1), 51–59. doi:10.1080/08897077.2012.691450

Pemberton, M. R., Williams, J., Herman-Stahl, M., Calvin, S. L., Bradshaw, M. R., Bray, R. M., . . . Hester, R. K. (2011). Evaluation of two web-based alcohol interventions in the US military. *Journal of Studies on Alcohol and Drugs, 72*(3), 480–489. doi:10.15288/jsad.2011.72.480

Petry, N. M., Alessi, S. M., & Rash, C. J. (2013). Contingency management treatments decrease psychiatric symptoms. *Journal of Consulting and Clinical Psychology, 81*(5), 926. doi:10.1037/a0032499

Petry, N. M., Barry, D., Alessi, S. M., Rounsaville, B. J., & Carroll, K. M. (2012). A randomized trial adapting contingency management targets based on initial abstinence status of cocaine-dependent patients. *Journal of Consulting and Clinical Psychology, 80*(2), 276. doi:10.1037/a0026883

Petry, N. M., Weinstock, J., Alessi, S. M., Lewis, M. W., & Dieckhaus, K. (2010). Group-based randomized trial of contingencies for health and abstinence in HIV patients. *Journal of Consulting and Clinical Psychology, 78*(1), 89. doi:10.1037/a0016778

Pinto, H., Maskrey, V., Swift, L., Rumball, D., Wagle, A., & Holland, R. (2010). The SUMMIT trial: A field comparison of buprenorphine versus methadone maintenance treatment. *Journal of Substance Abuse Treatment, 39*(4), 340–352. doi:10.1016/j.jsat.2010.07.009

Powers, M. B., Vedel, E., & Emmelkamp, P. M. (2008). Behavioral couples therapy (BCT) for alcohol and drug use disorders: A meta-analysis. *Clinical Psychology Review, 28*(6), 952–962. doi:10.1016/j.cpr.2008.02.002

Rapp, R. C., Van Den Noortgate, W., Broekaert, E., & Vanderplasschen, W. (2014). The efficacy of case management with persons who have substance abuse problems: A three-level meta-analysis of outcomes. *Journal of Consulting and Clinical Psychology, 82*(4), 605. doi:10.1037/a0036750

Rash, C. J., Stitzer, M., & Weinstock, J. (2017). Contingency management: New directions and re-maining challenges for an evidence-based intervention. *Journal of Substance Abuse Treatment, 72,* 10–18. doi:10.1016/j.jsat.2016.09.008

Reback, C. J., Peck, J. A., Dierst-Davies, R., Nuno, M., Kamien, J. B., & Amass, L. (2010). Con-tingency management among homeless, out-of-treatment men who have sex with men. *Journal of Substance Abuse Treatment, 39*(3), 255–263. doi:10.1016/j.jsat.2010.06.007

Rinker, D. V., & Neighbors, C. (2015). Latent class analysis of DSM-5 alcohol use disorder crite-ria among heavy-drinking college students. *Journal of Substance Abuse Treatment, 57,* 81–88. doi:10.1016/j.jsat.2015.05.006

Riordan, B. C., Conner, T. S., Flett, J. A., & Scarf, D. (2015). A brief orientation week ecological mo-mentary intervention to reduce university student alcohol consumption. *Journal of Studies on Alcohol and Drugs, 76*(4), 525–529. doi:10.15288/jsad.2015.76.525

Robles, R. R., Reyes, J. C., Colón, H. M., Sahai, H., Marrero, C. A., Matos, T. D., . . . Shepard, E. W. (2004). Effects of combined counseling and case management to reduce HIV risk behaviors among Hispanic drug injectors in Puerto Rico: A randomized controlled study. *Journal of Substance Abuse Treatment, 27*(2), 145–152. doi:10.1016/j.jsat.2004.06.004

Rollnick, S., Miller, W. R., & Butler, C. C. (2008). *Motivational interviewing in health care: Helping pa-tients change behavior.* New York: The Guilford Press.

Santisteban, D. A., Coatsworth, J. D., Perez-Vidal, A., Kurtines, W. M., Schwartz, S. J., LaPerriere, A., & Szapocznik, J. (2003). Efficacy of brief strategic family therapy in modifying His-panic adolescent behavior problems and substance use. *Journal of Family Psychology, 17*(1), 121. doi:10.1037/0893-3200.17.1.121

Sawyer, A. M., & Borduin, C. M. (2011). Effects of multisystemic therapy through midlife: A 21.9-year follow-up to a randomized clinical trial with serious and violent juvenile offenders. *Journal of Consulting and Clinical Psychology, 79*(5), 643. doi:10.1037/a0024862

Schmidt, L. A., Rieckmann, T., Abraham, A., Molfenter, T., Capoccia, V., Roman, P., . . . McCarty, D. (2012). Advancing recovery: Implementing evidence-based treatment for substance use dis-orders at the systems level. *Journal of Studies on Alcohol and Drugs, 73*(3), 413–422. doi:10.15288/jsad.2012.73.413

Schumm, J. A., O'Farrell, T. J., Murphy, C. M., & Fals-Stewart, W. (2009). Partner violence before and after couples-based alcoholism treatment for female alcoholic patients. *Journal of Consulting and Clinical Psychology, 77*(6), 1136. doi:10.1037/a0017389

Schwartz, R. P., Gryczynski, J., Mitchell, S. G., Gonzales, A., Moseley, A., Peterson, T. R., . . . O'grady, K. E. (2014). Computerized versus in-person brief intervention for drug misuse: A ran-domized clinical trial. *Addiction, 109*(7), 1091–1098. doi:10.1111/add.12502

Schwartz, R. P., Kelly, S. M., O'Grady, K. E., Gandhi, D., & Jaffe, J. H. (2011). Interim methadone treatment compared to standard methadone treatment: 4-month findings. *Journal of Substance Abuse Treatment, 41*(1), 21–29. doi:10.1016/j.jsat.2011.01.008

Siegal, H. A., Rapp, R. C., Kelliher, C. W., Fisher, J. H., Wagner, J. H., & Cole, P. A. (1995). The strengths perspective of case management: A promising inpatient substance abuse treatment en-hancement. *Journal of Psychoactive Drugs, 27*(1), 67–72. doi:10.1080/02791072.1995.10471674

Sisson, R. W., & Mallams, J. H. (1981). The use of systematic encouragement and community access procedures to increase attendance at Alcoholic Anonymous and Al-Anon meetings. *The American Journal of Drug and Alcohol Abuse, 8*(3), 371–376. doi:10.3109/00952998109009560

Smith, J. E., & Meyers, R. J. (2007). *Motivating substance abusers to enter treatment: Working with family members.* New York, NY: Guilford Press.

Stormshak, E. A., Connell, A. M., Véronneau, M. H., Myers, M. W., Dishion, T. J., Kavanagh, K., & Caruthers, A. S. (2011). An ecological approach to promoting early adolescent mental health and social adaptation: Family-centered intervention in public middle schools. *Child Development, 82*(1), 209–225. doi:10.1111/j.1467-8624.2010.01551.x

Suitt, K. G., Castro, Y., Caetano, R., & Field, C. A. (2015). Predictive utility of alcohol use disor-der symptoms across race/ethnicity. *Journal of Substance Abuse Treatment, 56,* 61–67. doi:10.1016/j.jsat.2015.03.001

Svikis, D. S., Keyser-Marcus, L., Stitzer, M., Rieckmann, T., Safford, L., Loeb, P., . . . Cohen, J. (2012). Randomized multi-site trial of the Job Seekers' Workshop in patients with substance use disorders. *Drug and Alcohol Dependence, 120*(1–3), 55–64. doi:10.1016/j.drugalcdep.2011.06.024

319

Szapocznik, J., & Williams, R. A. (2000). Brief strategic family therapy: Twenty-five years of interplay among theory, research and practice in adolescent behavior problems and drug abuse. *Clinical Child and Family Psychology Review, 3*(2), 117–134. doi:10.1023/A:1009512719808

Tiderington, E., Stanhope, V., & Henwood, B. F. (2013). A qualitative analysis of case managers' use of harm reduction in practice. *Journal of Substance Abuse Treatment, 44*(1), 71–77. doi:10.1016/j.jsat.2012.03.007

Tonigan, J. S., Connors, G. J., & Miller, W. R. (2003). Participation and involvement in Alcoholics Anonymous. In T. Babor & F. Boca (Eds.), *Treatment matching in alcoholism* (pp. 184–204). Cambridge: Cambridge University Press.

Tonigan, J. S., Miller, W. R., & Brown, J. M. (1994). The reliability of Form 90: An instrument for assessing alcohol treatment outcome. *Journal of Studies on Alcohol and Drugs, 58*(4), 358–364. doi:10.15288/jsa.1997.58.358

Toumbourou, J. W., Hamilton, M., U'ren, A., Stevens-Jones, P., & Storey, G. (2002). Narcotics Anonymous participation and changes in substance use and social support. *Journal of Substance Abuse Treatment, 23*(1), 61–66. doi:10.1016/S0740-5472(02)00243-X

Turner, B. J., McCann, B. S., Dunn, C. W., Darnell, D. A., Beam, C. R., Kleiber, B., . . . Fukunaga, R. (2017). Examining the reach of a brief alcohol intervention service in routine practice at a level 1 trauma center. *Journal of Substance Abuse Treatment, 79*, 29–33. doi:10.1016/j.jsat.2017.05.011

United Nations Office on Drugs and Crime (UNODC, 2018). *World Drug Report 2018*. Retrieved from https://www.unodc.org/wdr2018/

Wallace, C. J., Lecomte, T., Wilde, J., & Liberman, R. P. (2001). CASIG: A consumer-centered assessment for planning individualized treatment and evaluating program outcomes. *Schizophrenia Research, 50*, 105–119. doi:10.1016/S0920-9964(00)00068-2

Weiss, R. D., Griffin, M. L., Potter, J. S., Dodd, D. R., Dreifuss, J. A., Connery, H. S., & Carroll, K. M. (2014). Who benefits from additional drug counseling among prescription opioid-dependent patients receiving buprenorphine–naloxone and standard medical management? *Drug and Alcohol Dependence, 140*, 118–122. doi:10.1016/j.drugalcdep.2014.04.005

Wilcox, C., & Bogenschutz, M. (2013). Pharmacotherapies for alcohol and drug use disorders. In B. S. McCrady & E. Epstein (Eds.), *Addiction: A comprehensive guidebook for practitioners* (2nd ed.) (pp. 526–550). New York, NY: Guilford Press.

World Health Organization (WHO). Global status report on alcohol and health 2018. Geneva: Author. Retrieved from https://www.who.int/substance_abuse/publications/global_alcohol_report/gsr_2018/en/

Zweben, A., & Piepmeier, M. (in press). Motivational Interviewing and SBIRT. In J. L. Martin & D. Cimini (Eds.), *Screening, brief intervention and referral to treatment for substance use: A practitioner's guide*. Washington, DC: American Psychological Association.

Zweben, A., Piepmeier, M., Fucito, L., & O'Malley, S. (2017). The clinical utility of the Medication Adherence Questionnaire (MAQ) in an alcohol pharmacotherapy trial. *Journal of Substance Abuse Treatment, 77*, 72–78. doi:10.1016/j.jsat.2017.04.001

Zweben, A., Rose, S., Stout, R. L., & Zywiak, W. H. (2003). Case monitoring and motivational style brief interventions. In R. K. Hester & W. R. Miller (Eds.), *Handbook of alcoholism treatment approaches: Effective alternatives* (3rd ed., pp. 113–130). Boston, MA: Allyn & Bacon.

Zweben, A., & Zuckoff, A. (2002). Motivational interviewing and treatment adherence. In W. R. Miller & S. Rollnick (Eds.), *Motivational interviewing: Preparing people for change* (Vol. 2, pp. 299–319).

19

Current and emerging pharmacotherapies for addiction treatment

Jeanelle Portelli, Vikas Munjal and Lorenzo Leggio

Background

Addiction pharmacotherapy aims to aid individuals who meet criteria for a substance use disorder by diminishing cravings and relapse risk, as well as limiting symptoms arising from drug abstinence, together with achieving pre-drug functioning of physiological processes for these individuals. Addictions are complex in nature, requiring multidisciplinary approaches that often combine pharmacotherapy with psychotherapy and counseling to achieve stable sobriety or, in some cases, reducing substance use below harmful levels. Many advances have been achieved in recent decades, resulting in treatments approved by the Food and Drug Administration (FDA) in the United States, and similar bodies in other countries, for treating different addictive disorders. The concept of medication-assisted treatment (MAT) is promoted because of its proven efficacy in different addiction treatments (Lee, Kresina, Campopiano, Lubran, & Clark, 2015; Ma et al., 2018; Ziedonis, Das, & Larkin, 2017). MAT involves the use of pharmacotherapy in combination with behavioral therapies and/ or counseling.

The addiction scene is constantly changing, with different and novel substances continually entering the market. This situation has kept the scientific research world and practitioners on their toes, constantly reevaluating currently known therapies, as well as identifying new possibilities. Most emerging addiction pharmacotherapy medications are already on the market, approved for other uses (such as topiramate, baclofen, gabapentin) and currently being investigated to be re-purposed for alcohol use disorder or substance use disorders; others are novel compounds not yet in the market for any indication.

Additionally, individuals may experience simultaneous substance use disorders, polydrug use, or comorbidity (when two or more illnesses or disorders are present in the same person) leading practitioners to rely on comprehensive approaches such as combination pharmacological treatments or combined pharmacological and behavioral therapies. Combined treatment strategies may also be preferable for individuals experiencing a single substance use disorder, without other comorbidities. Due to the complexity surrounding each different type of substance use disorder, adopting a personalized approach to treatment is ideal. Unfortunately, this approach is currently more the exception than the rule.

In this chapter, we focus on U.S. FDA-approved pharmacological treatments, as well as promising medications still in the pipeline, for treating the following types of substance use disorders: alcohol, opioid, tobacco, cocaine, and cannabis use disorders. The World Health Organization (WHO, 2010) website provides a listing of medications approved in different countries for use in treating alcohol and opioid use disorders. This chapter describes, in general, how the FDA-approved drugs act in the brain, as well as their overall efficacy and safety profile. These descriptions refer to drugs that may act as *agonists* or *antagonists* to relay their effects on the brain and behavior. Agonist drugs work by binding to a particular type of receptor site in the brain, leading to a specified process in the brain cell (neuron) becoming more active. By contrast, when antagonist drugs bind to a brain cell receptor they block or dampen the biological response or specific process. These agonist and antagonist actions direct the neurochemical processes resulting in changes of experience and behavior for individuals using the drugs involved.

Alcohol use disorder (AUD): first-line treatments

Alcohol acts as a central nervous system depressant, reducing brain activity and slowing other body system functions. In the 2018 American Psychiatric Association (APA) clinical practice guidelines for the treatment of AUD, pharmacotherapy is recommended for treating moderate-to-severe AUD experienced by individuals motivated to reduce their alcohol consumption or achieve complete abstinence but have failed to achieve this through non-pharmacological treatment. Systematic review of randomized controlled trials involving patients with alcohol use disorder who attempt controlled drinking (i.e., non-abstinence) led investigators to conclude that no high-grade evidence currently exists that these pharmacological treatments have efficacy with this population (Palpacuer et al., 2018). Three medications have been approved for first-line treatment in the United States by the FDA: disulfiram, acamprosate, and naltrexone. Other medications may be used off-label, or as second-line treatments, when initial treatment is not successful.

Of the three, naltrexone and acamprosate are normally used as first-line pharmacological treatment options, though in reality these available medications are often underused to treat AUD. The APA recommends the use of disulfiram should the person fail to respond to naltrexone or acamprosate, or else prefers disulfiram treatment. Each of these first-line treatment medications for AUD is described in greater detail below.

Disulfiram

Mechanism of action

Disulfiram acts by increasing levels of acetaldehyde, a toxic metabolite of alcohol when it is broken down in the body, if alcohol is ingested. This disulfiram-ethanol reaction, which can occur even when small amounts of alcohol are consumed, is characterized by flushing, nausea, vomiting, sweating, weakness, hypotension, palpitations, vertigo, and, rarely, serious reactions such as respiratory depression. Anticipation of these unpleasant symptoms, rather than a direct pharmacological action, is what is believed to make this drug effective (Kranzler & Soyka, 2018; see Chapter 6). Individuals initiating treatment with disulfiram should fully comprehend the physiological consequences of consuming alcohol while taking disulfiram. Compared to some other pharmacological treatment approaches, disulfiram has a favorable safety profile (Skinner, Lahmek, Pham, & Aubin, 2014).

Drug indications and duration

After its approval in 1951, for more than four decades, disulfiram remained the only medication approved in the United States to treat AUD. Disulfiram is indicated as an aid to manage and maintain sobriety for individuals experiencing chronic AUD. Indeed, it is important to note that disulfiram is normally prescribed to individuals who exhibit motivation to change and have the necessary supportive therapy and supervision to remain sober. This approach is important in reducing the risk for disulfiram-ethanol reactions. Treatment with this drug is on a strict daily basis, until the individual no longer experiences alcohol cravings and has demonstrated self-control over alcohol consumption (Table 19.1). There is no set timeline for maintenance therapy duration which may range from months to years.

Efficacy and clinical safety

A meta-analysis of 22 randomized controlled trials (RCTs) found a significant success rate for disulfiram compared to no medication in maintaining abstinence and preventing relapse. However, the efficacy of disulfiram in treating AUD remains a controversial topic, despite it being an FDA-approved treatment for many decades (Blanco-Gandia & Rodriguez-Arias, 2018). Disulfiram at the recommended dose is typically well tolerated, with common adverse effects including fatigue and drowsiness. Due to possible direct changes in liver enzyme function, patients prescribed disulfiram are counseled about potential signs and symptoms of hepatotoxicity. Individuals should abstain from alcohol 12 hours before taking disulfiram and understand that disulfiram-ethanol reactions may take place up to 14 days after taking the medication. Moreover, patients should be advised not to use alcohol-containing or alcohol-based products, such as certain cold remedies, other medications, mouthwashes, hand sanitizers, and foods/beverages.

Naltrexone

Mechanism of action

Naltrexone is a full opioid receptor antagonist, having minimal to no agonist activity. In other words, by binding to opioid receptor sites, naltrexone blocks or dampens the brains' response to opioid—and apparently, alcohol—exposure. This drug helps diminish alcohol craving and the rewarding effects of alcohol if it is consumed.

Table 19.1 First-line treatment medications for alcohol use disorder

Medication	Routine Dosage	Administration
Disulfiram	Tablet: 125 mg to 500 mg/day	Initial and average maintenance dose: 250 mg tablet, adjusted based on side effects
Naltrexone hydrochloride	Tablet: 50 mg/day	1 tablet daily
	Injection (slow release): 380 mg/ month	1 intramuscular injection per month
Acamprosate	Tablet: 1998 mg/day	333 mg tablet taken twice per dose; three doses daily

Drug indications and duration

Naltrexone is a long-acting opiate antagonist first synthesized in 1963 for the treatment of opioid addiction, approved by the FDA in 1984 for the treatment of heroin, oxycodone, and morphine addiction. A decade later, the FDA approved the use of oral naltrexone for treating AUD. There is minimal risk that a person will become addicted to naltrexone. Individuals who are also taking opioid medication for chronic pain are cautioned against the use of naltrexone, since as an antagonist it blocks pain relief effect of opioids. Similarly, to avoid symptoms of instant opioid withdrawal, an individual in treatment for AUD should be free of other opioids for 7–10 days prior to naltrexone initiation. Unlike disulfiram, alcohol ingestion while taking naltrexone does not lead to severe adverse reactions and may even lead to reduced feelings of intoxication.

Naltrexone is currently available in three different forms: the most commonly used daily oral tablet, a once monthly depot injection (given as an intramuscular injection), and subcutaneous implants that must be surgically implanted (Table 19.1). The subcutaneous implants consist of small, slow-release drug pellets inserted beneath the skin, allowing release of small, consistent amounts of naltrexone over two to six months. It is important to note that the subcutaneous implants of naltrexone are not currently approved by the FDA for use in the United States. Duration of naltrexone use is dependent on the individual being treated. Since naltrexone is metabolized almost exclusively in the liver, and given reports of potential hepatotoxicity, it is not recommended for patients suffering from clinically significant liver disease, since cases of naltrexone-induced liver toxicity have been rarely reported at the dose approved for AUD (50 mg per day). Oral naltrexone is typically recommended as the first-line treatment for individuals experiencing moderate-to-severe AUD, with the long-acting injectable version to be used should they fail to adhere to daily pill regimen.

Efficacy and clinical safety

Both the oral and depot injection formulations appear to be significantly effective compared to placebo. To date there are no direct comparisons on the efficacy of the oral versus the injectable form of naltrexone in treatment of AUD, making it difficult to conclude whether the injectable version is superior to the oral form (Beatty & Stock, 2017). Naltrexone is normally well-tolerated, with a low incidence of adverse effects, which may include gastrointestinal effects.

Acamprosate

Mechanism of action

Although its mechanism of action is not fully understood, acamprosate seems to act by stabilizing the excitatory neurotransmitter glutamate during alcohol withdrawal by modulating the excitatory N-methyl-D-aspartate (NMDA) and the inhibitory $GABA_A$ receptor transmission in the brain. Additionally, acamprosate is known to enhance the levels of β-endorphins in individuals who have severe alcohol use disorders, and possibly also regulates the hypothalamo-pituitary-adrenal axis. While acute alcohol intake has been found to augment the effect of GABA on the $GABA_A$ receptor, together with lowering the excitatory levels of NMDA, AMPA, and kainate receptors, chronic alcohol consumption normally results in the opposite effect (Kalk & Lingford-Hughes, 2014). These neurotransmitter alterations can result in a hyperglutamatergic, and possibly an excitotoxic, state during the process of alcohol withdrawal. Acamprosate is believed to provide regulation of this transmitter imbalance, thus acting subclinically to limit withdrawal symptoms, together with offering a level of neuroprotection.

Drug indications and duration

Acamprosate has been used in Europe to treat alcohol dependence since 1989; however, it was only approved by the FDA for treatment of AUD in the United States in 2004. It is available as an oral delayed release tablet and is recommended for individuals who have been abstinent from alcohol for at least 5 days at treatment initiation (Table 19.1). Oral ingestion of acamprosate has a very low bioavailability, around 11%, and stable plasma concentrations are reached only after 5 days of daily treatment. It is recommended that treatment be continued even if the person relapses to alcohol use. Treatment duration is determined according to the individual under treatment. Discontinuation of acamprosate may be considered if the person being treated is not adhering to the regimen or has achieved stable abstinence from alcohol.

Efficacy and clinical safety

Numerous RCTs have shown the efficacy of acamprosate when compared to placebo. Many of these positive studies are European-based, where significant effects of acamprosate on increasing complete abstinence, decreasing drinking days, and increased time to relapse compared to placebos have been reported.

Overall, acamprosate has a good safety profile. Long-term treatment of AUD with this drug was not found to lead to dependence or abuse, and individuals were not found to develop tolerance to the medication. It is not known to interact with other psychotropic agents. Very high doses of acamprosate (i.e. 56 g—the normal daily dose is 2 g) remain well tolerated by individuals in treatment, virtually eliminating risk of overdose. Adverse effects, which are mild and transient (diarrhea being the most common), improve over the course of treatment. One advantage of acamprosate is that it can be administered to individuals being treated for alcohol use disorder who also have severe liver disease, since unlike naltrexone and disulfiram it does not involve liver metabolization and there are no known reports of acamprosate-related liver injury.

Alcohol use disorder: second-line and promising treatments

If first-line treatment is not effective, for example, individuals cannot tolerate naltrexone or acamprosate, or simply do not prefer to take these medications, recent APA guidelines suggest the use of anticonvulsant medications like topiramate or gabapentin for which several, yet not all, clinical trials have suggested efficacy in treating AUD.

Efficacy in AUD treatment has also been reported with both nalmefene and baclofen. Nalmefene, which acts on opioid receptors and has FDA approval for treating opioid use disorder (OUD), is approved in Europe for AUD treatment. Three European multicenters found that nalmefene significantly reduced overall alcohol consumption in persons experiencing AUD compared to placebo and meta-analytic review concluded that moderate evidence supports nalmefene's association with improvement in heavy drinking days per month and drinks per drinking day (Jonas et al., 2014). Nalmefene is well tolerated, with nausea being the most frequently reported adverse effect. Interest in baclofen, a $GABA_B$ receptor agonist, has been steadily increasing; however, clinical trials of baclofen for the treatment of AUD have resulted in mixed findings (Agabio et al., 2018). France is currently the only country that has approved this medication for AUD treatment. Despite a lack of consistent evidence, baclofen is used off-label for treatment of AUD in Australia and certain European countries. A potential off-label application of baclofen is as a second-line treatment of AUD for individuals with clinically significant liver disease. To date, no studies assess use of baclofen in conjunction with currently approved FDA treatments for AUD in the United States.

The smoking cessation medication varenicline is also a promising medication for treatment of AUD, and its efficacy appears stronger among individuals experiencing AUD who also smoke. Numerous additional drugs and compounds are currently undergoing preclinical and clinical investigation to assess their potential as AUD treatments, including the antipsychotic aripiprazole; the NMDA receptor antagonist ifenprodil; the α1 adrenergic receptor agents prazosin and doxazosin; agents acting on neuroendocrine pathways such as oxytocin, PF-5190457 (a ghrelin receptor inverse agonist) and ABT-436 (a vasopressin 1b receptor antagonist); the opioid antagonist samidorphan; the anti-emetic serotonin antagonist ondansetron; and the progesterone blocker mifepristone, among others (Litten, Falk, Ryan, Fertig, & Leggio, 2018).

Many individuals experiencing AUD are fearful of symptoms caused by alcohol withdrawal, which can range from minor to serious, such as delirium, seizures, and psychosis. Medications directed to minimize AUD withdrawal include the use of benzodiazepines, barbiturates, and propofol, among others (Mirijello et al., 2015). Benzodiazepines are considered the "gold-standard" of treatment due to their proven efficacy in limiting withdrawal symptoms, together with significantly reducing the incidence of seizures, delirium tremens (a complicated form of alcohol withdrawal syndrome characterized by severe confusion, agitation, and hallucinations, among other symptoms), and risk of death.

Tobacco use disorder (TUD): first-line treatments

The nicotine in tobacco products acts as a central nervous system stimulant and has a high addictive potential. The chances of successfully treating TUD increase when pharmacotherapy is combined with behavioral therapies/counseling (Ziedonis et al., 2017). Combination therapy is often recommended when the person in treatment has only a partial response to the initial medication. This pharmacotherapy typically includes combining a long-acting form of nicotine replacement therapy (NRT) (such as the patch) with a short-acting form (such as gum or lozenge), or a combination of different medications (such as varenicline and NRTs).

Nicotine replacement therapy

Nicotine replacement therapy (NRT) was the first therapy approved by the FDA and is often the first line of treatment used by individuals seeking to quit smoking tobacco. The various forms of NRT include the transdermal patch, gum, sublingual tablet/lozenge, nasal spray, and inhaler. Nasal spray and inhaler NRTs are for prescription-use only in the United States, whereas transdermal patches, gum, and lozenge formulations can be bought over the counter. NRTs contain controlled amounts of nicotine, which allows users to gradually withdraw from a smoking habit (Molyneux, 2004). Moreover, the FDA also approved two non-nicotine smoking cessation products, varenicline tartrate and bupropion hydrochloride, which are available in tablet form by prescription only. Recommendations include counseling in combination with NRT pharmacological treatment (Le Foll, Melihan-Chinin, Rostoker, & Lagrue, 2005).

Mechanism of action

NRT works by stimulating nicotinic receptors in the ventral tegmental area of the brain and, in conjunction with other peripheral effects of nicotine, leading to a reduction in withdrawal symptoms associated with smoking cessation. NRT accomplishes this effect by delivering nicotine at a varying range of doses over an acute or longer period. The various forms of NRT enter through different routes within the human body; however, they all eventually end up in the bloodstream to deliver the desired effect.

Drug indications and duration

Many guidelines advise clinicians to offer NRT as the first line of treatment for individuals seeking pharmacological assistance in tobacco cessation efforts. Withdrawal symptoms may persist, as NRTs are unable to mimic the rapid and high concentrations of arterial nicotine reached through cigarette smoking. These formulations, in theory, contain amounts of nicotine high enough to avoid withdrawal effects and reduce cravings for smoking, while low enough to avoid nicotine dependence themselves (Beard, Shahab, Cummings, Michie, & West, 2016; Foulds, Burke, Steinberg, Williams, & Ziedonis, 2004). Since the development of the chewing gum formulation in 1978, several other controlled nicotine dose formulations have been developed (Table 19.2).

- Nicotine gum: nicotine gum has been available for the longest time, compared to other NRTs. The gum is chewed intermittently to release nicotine into the system. The gum is chewed frequently at first and then tapered down over time.
- Nicotine transdermal patch: the nicotine patch can be applied on the body to deliver the substance at a moderately steady rate over a longer period compared to other nicotine replacement therapies. The patch is available in various doses that can be matched to an individual's previous level of nicotine use.
- Nicotine sublingual tablet/lozenge: lozenges and sublingual tablets are designed to dissolve in the mouth over a period of time, and travel through the buccal mucosa to be delivered to the body's circulatory system (Henningfield, 1995).
- Nicotine inhaler: available in cartridges of several sizes, inhalers deliver nicotine at a pre-determined dose per puff, designed to provide nicotine in a similar fashion to typical cigarette smoking.
- Nicotine oral/nasal spray: the oral spray delivers 1 mg nicotine per spray and enables rapid nicotine absorption.

Efficacy and clinical safety

There exists robust evidence of the efficacy of NRTs in aiding smoking cessation. Systematic reviews reported clear efficacy of NRTs over placebo (Akanbi et al., 2018; Dahne et al., 2018; Gomez-Coronado, Walker, Berk, & Dodd, 2018), further confirmed by the recent Evaluating Adverse Events in a Global Smoking Cessation Study (EAGLES)—a double-blind, randomized trial which included more than 8,000 patients over a roughly three-year period. NRT use was almost twice as likely to result in abstinence at six months compared to placebo (West et al., 2018). The EAGLES trial determined that NRT therapy for TUD was similarly effective for patients with or without psychiatric history. NRT has a very safe clinical profile with adverse effects most often including gastrointestinal symptoms, headache, and localized

Table 19.2 First-line medications for tobacco use disorder

Medication	Routine Dosage	Administration
Nicotine gum (NRT)	2 mg/piece (1st cigarette > 30 minutes after waking up) 4 mg/piece (1st cigarette < 30 minutes after waking up)	Weeks 1–6: 1 piece every 1–2 hours Weeks 7–9: 1 piece every 2–4 hours Weeks 10–12: 1 piece every 4–8 hours
Nicotine inhaler (NRT)	6–16 cartridges/day	Maintained treatment up to 12 weeks, gradual reduction in use weeks 12–24
Nicotine lozenge (NRT)	2 mg/piece (1st cigarette > 30 minutes after waking up) 4 mg/piece (1st cigarette < 30 minutes after waking up)	Weeks 1–6: 1 lozenge every 1–2 hours Weeks 7–9: 1 lozenge every 2–4 hours Weeks 10–12: 1 lozenge every 4–8 hours
Nicotine nasal spray (NRT)	1 mg dose = 1 spray each nostril	1–2 doses/hour up to maximum 40 doses per day
Nicotine transdermal patch (NRT)	7 mg, 14 mg, or 21 mg/24 hours	If > 10 cigarettes/day: Weeks 1–4, one 21 mg patch/day Weeks 5 and 6, one 14 mg patch/day Weeks 7 and 8, one 7 mg patch/day If < 10 cigarettes/day: Weeks 1–6, one 14 mg patch/day Weeks 7–8, one 7 mg patch/day
Bupropion hydrochloride	Tablet: 300 mg/day; smoking quit date set 1-2 weeks after starting medication	150 mg tablet daily for 3 days, then 150 mg twice a day for 7-12 weeks
Varenicline tartrate	Tablet: 0.5 mg to 2 mg/day; begins 1 week before date to stop smoking or quit smoking between days 8 and 35 of treatment	0.5 mg/day for days 1–3, then 0.5 mg twice daily for days 4–7, then 1 mg twice daily for a total of 12 weeks (additional 12 weeks recommended after); treatment for a total of 24 weeks

irritation, depending on the method of nicotine delivery. Additionally, a study focused on critically ill patients in the ICU reported no increase in mortality or serious adverse effects after NRT treatment for TUD compared to placebo (de Jong et al., 2018).

Bupropion hydrochloride

Mechanism of action

The mechanism of action for bupropion is not completely understood; however, studies show bupropion acts both as an inhibitor of the neuronal reuptake of norepinephrine and dopamine and as a stimulator of their release (Stahl et al., 2004). By blocking reuptake, bupropion attenuates the effects of nicotine withdrawal.

Drug indications and duration

Although originally approved in the United States as an antidepressant, bupropion was later approved in 1997 as the first non-nicotinic pharmacotherapy for smoking cessation.

Treatment with bupropion should commence while nicotine is being used to first achieve a steady-state blood level of bupropion (Table 19.2).

Efficacy and clinical safety

Monotherapy with bupropion appears comparable to NRT in its efficacy to attenuate smoking, with twice as many individuals reaching abstinence in a six-month period compared to placebo (West et al., 2018). Bupropion is widely used in clinical settings. The benefits of proposing bupropion to individuals in treatment for TUD include the fact that it is a non-nicotine treatment, it decreases risk of gaining weight following smoking cessation, and it can be used in patients suffering from depression, stable cardiovascular disease, or COPD. In the past, as with varenicline, there were neuropsychiatric and cardiovascular concerns following bupropion treatment; concerns which have been quelled by more recent trials (Anthenelli et al., 2016; Benowitz et al., 2018; Evins et al., 2019; Kress, Obi, & Prochazka, 2017). Bupropion is not recommended for individuals who have a predisposition to seizures.

Varenicline tartrate

Mechanism of action

Nicotine use stimulates the brain's $\alpha_4\beta_2$ nicotinic acetylcholine receptors, leading to release of dopamine into the brain, which is responsible for the reinforcing properties of nicotine use (Benowitz, Porchet, & Jacob, 1989; Fenster, Rains, Noerager, Quick, & Lester, 1997; Rose, 2008). Varenicline is a partial agonist/antagonist of these receptors and mildly stimulates them; however, it does not reach the same level of dopamine-release stimulation as nicotine (Rollema et al., 2007). Due to its antagonistic properties, varenicline also blocks the ability of nicotine to activate dopamine release, thus interfering with the reinforcing nature of nicotine use.

Drug indications and duration

Varenicline was approved for use in the United States by the FDA in 2006 and since has been used as a non-nicotinic pharmacotherapy for TUD. Varenicline should be started one week prior to the date of nicotine cessation. The FDA recommends an additional 12 weeks of treatment for successful quit attempts, increasing the likelihood of long-term abstinence. For individuals unable to quit nicotine use abruptly, varenicline should be taken at the recommended dosage weekly, as explained in Table 19.2.

Efficacy and clinical safety

According to the EAGLES trial, varenicline appeared superior to NRTs and bupropion in the odds of smoking cessation (West et al., 2018). Common adverse effects include sleep disturbances and nausea. In 2008, concerns were raised over possible neuropsychiatric effects following varenicline (and bupropion) treatment; concerns refuted following meta-analyses, prompting the FDA to withdraw their black box warning for both medications in 2016 (Cahill, Stevens, Perera, & Lancaster, 2013; Evins et al., 2019; Gomez-Coronado et al., 2018; Kotz et al., 2015; West et al., 2018). Concerns about cardiovascular effects were also raised (Singh, Loke, Spangler, & Furberg, 2011); however, subsequent trials did not find a clinically meaningful increase of cardiovascular events following varenicline treatment (Benowitz et al., 2018; Gomez-Coronado et al., 2018; Kotz et al., 2015). This finding was further asserted by the FDA in a 2018 labeling update, stating that the benefits of varenicline as a TUD medication outweigh potential harm to individuals suffering from cardiovascular disease.

TUD: second-line and promising treatments

When first-line therapy is not successful, second-line medications that are not FDA approved for this purpose, such as nortriptyline and clonidine, are sometimes considered in the United States. The mechanism of action of nortriptyline, a tricyclic antidepressant, is thought to be due to its mimicking the noradrenergic actions of nicotine, together with nicotine receptor antagonism. A meta-analysis comparing trials found that nortriptyline showed significant benefit over placebo (Gomez-Coronado et al., 2018; Hughes, Stead, Hartmann-Boyce, Cahill, & Lancaster, 2014). The antihypertensive clonidine, a selective α-adrenergic receptor agonist, has been shown to be effective compared to placebo; however, its role in smoking cessation is still undetermined (Gomez-Coronado et al., 2018). Neither of these second-line treatments were shown to be superior than first-line medications in trials.

Cytisine, a partial agonist to the $\alpha_4\beta_2$ subtype of the nicotine acetylcholine receptor, has been used as a smoking cessation medication in Eastern Europe since the 1960s. Its effectiveness is still under investigation, including an ongoing randomized controlled, non-inferiority trial in a population living in Australia comparing the effectiveness, safety, and cost-effectiveness of cysteine versus varenicline (Thomas et al., 2018). Several emerging pharmacotherapies are under development or study, including acetylcholinesterase inhibitors (galantamine, rivastigmine), agents affecting γ-aminobutyric acid (GABA) receptors (baclofen, topiramate, gabapentin, vigabatrin), N-methyl-D-aspartate (NMDA) receptor modulators (memantine, cycloserine, N-acetylcysteine), and dopamine enhancers/receptor modulators (bromocriptine). Nicotine vaccines also are under development, but it is too early to know whether they will be efficacious in TUD (Chen et al., 2019; Gomez-Coronado et al., 2018; Zeigler, Roque, & Clegg, 2019).

One controversial treatment is the use of electronic cigarettes (e-cigarettes/electronic nicotine delivery systems (ENDS)/vapes/vape pens/e-hookahs/mods). E-cigarettes are most often composed of a device which heats up a vapor, transforming it into an aerosol, which is then inhaled by the user. Aerosol substances include nicotine, flavoring, marijuana, or other illicit drugs, among others. Researchers are starting to investigate the concept of "vaping" as a strategy to facilitate smoking cessation. A recently published study by Hajek and colleagues compared the one-year abstinence rate in a group undergoing NRT versus a group using e-cigarettes with nicotine. They found that patients experiencing TUD were twice as likely to cease smoking when tapering down with refillable nicotine e-cigarettes (Hajek et al., 2019). Previous studies reported similar results (Bullen et al., 2013; Caponnetto et al., 2013), though it is generally acknowledged that additional trials should be performed to clearly establish the benefits and safety of e-cigarettes as a smoking cessation treatment, since certain aerosol substances may have addictive properties.

Opioid use disorder (OUD): first-line treatments

The past decade has witnessed a sharp, unprecedented increase in rates of OUD and related deaths. This opioid crisis has been most notable in the United States, declared there a nationwide Public Health Emergency in October 2017. Abused opioids include prescription drugs such as oxycodone, synthetic opioids such as fentanyl, and illegal drugs such as heroin. Opioid misuse remains an unsolved public health issue, with the medical, social work, and health services fields, among others, working to identify ways to address this epidemic. Three medications have been approved by the FDA for OUD treatment in the United States: buprenorphine, methadone, and naltrexone. Unfortunately, OUD medications remain grossly underused (Volkow & Koroshetz, 2019). Despite acting as opioid agonists, the dosages of buprenorphine and methadone used for OUD treatment are not sufficient for a person to experience a "high." The aims of OUD pharmacotherapy are to help reduce opioid cravings and assist in managing opioid withdrawal with the long-term goal of achieving and maintaining abstinence. Choice of treatment depends on different factors, including cost-effectiveness, safety, and efficacy. It is notable to mention that even though methadone is recommended as a first-line treatment, it has the potential to be abused or misused, is potentially addictive itself, and is normally only administered to patients in specialized clinics where dosing and regimen compliance are regulated. For moderate-to-severe OUD, an opioid agonist (methadone or buprenorphine) is normally prescribed, whereas naltrexone is normally reserved for milder cases of OUD.

Methadone

Mechanism of action

Developed as a synthetic, long-acting opiate, methadone displays longer persisting pharmacological actions and effects similar to abused opioids: heroin, morphine, and opioid pain medications (Mattick, Breen, Kimber, & Davoli, 2009).

Drug indications and duration

Approved by the FDA in 1972, methadone is the oldest pharmacotherapy for OUD (Kreek, Borg, Ducat, & Ray, 2010). The drug helps individuals experiencing OUD reduce withdrawal symptoms and craving for opioids by delivering the desired drug effect over a longer period than the abuse substances. It is available orally in liquid or tablet form. Monitoring of the individual being treated during the first weeks of methadone initiation is pivotal to avoid toxicity (Dematteis et al., 2017). Methadone maintenance therapy (MMT) is the primary, and most researched, method of OUD treatment using methadone. In the United States, MMT requires individuals to receive methadone sublingually at specialty clinics, and individuals can be tapered off methadone to achieve opioid abstinence (Table 19.3).

Efficacy and clinical safety

Various studies over the years have established the efficacy of methadone as an OUD treatment medication. In addition to maintaining abstinence, methadone treatment has been shown to reduce overdose death risk, increase treatment retention, and reduce use of illicit drugs when compared to placebo (Calcaterra et al., 2019). Nevertheless, to achieve optimal treatment effects, methadone treatment requires expert skill and extensive monitoring by appropriate specialized clinicians.

Due to methadone's high potential for addiction, it must be used strictly as prescribed. Doses are tailored according to individual case and profile, and clinicians are advised to administer methadone in a controlled specialized clinic. Unsupervised administration of

Table 19.3 First-line treatment medications for opioid use disorder[b]

Medication	Dosage	Administration
Methadone		
Oral concentrate	Variable	Initial dose to reduce withdrawal symptoms: 20–30 mg maintenance—80–120 mg/day; adjusted based on opioid dependency state individualized to obtain estimated dose; titrate slowly with dose increases no more frequent than every 3–5 days; initiation of detoxification and maintenance treatment: single dose of 20–30 mg to suppress withdrawal
Tablet	5 mg and 10 mg	
Buprenorphine		
Implant	74.2 mg (equivalent to 80 mg buprenorphine HCl)	Subdermal implant in upper arm for 6 months of treatment; removed after 6 months
Injection	300 mg or 100 mg/month	300 mg for first 2 months, then 100 mg monthly; injection in abdominal area
Sublingual	Tablet: 2 mg or 8 mg/day	Individualized and titrated for clinical effectiveness; preferred for use only during induction for unsupervised administration of patients who cannot tolerate buprenorphine + naloxone. administered as one single daily dose
Buprenorphine + naloxone		
Buccal	Film: Buprenorphine 2.1 mg/ naloxone 0.3 mg; buprenorphine 4.2 mg/naloxone 0.7 mg buprenorphine 6.3 mg/naloxone 1 mg	The film should be administered in divided doses when used as initial treatment, depending on the patient for maintenance treatment, the recommended target dosage of 8.4 mg/1.4 mg as a single daily dose
Sublingual	Film: 16 mg buprenorphine/ naloxone 4 mg	Film: single daily dose under the tongue after induction, stabilization, and titration to a dose of 16 mg buprenorphine
	Tablet: buprenorphine 0.7 mg/ naloxone 0.18 mg; buprenorphine 1.4 mg/naloxone 0.36 mg; buprenorphine 2 mg/naloxone 0.5 mg[a]; buprenorphine 2.9 mg/ naloxone 0.71 mg; buprenorphine 5.7 mg/naloxone 1.4 mg; buprenorphine 8 mg/naloxone 2 mg[a]; buprenorphine 8.6 mg/ naloxone 2.1 mg; buprenorphine 11.4 mg/naloxone 2.9 mg	Tablet: administered as a single daily dose after initial treatment with divided doses Short-acting opioid dependence: day 1—up to 5.7 mg/1.4 mg dose (divided), day 2—total of 11.4 mg/2.9 mg dose as a single dose Maintenance treatment: 11.4 mg/2.9 mg as a single daily dose
Naltrexone	Injection (slow release): 380 mg	Intramuscular gluteal injection delivered every 4 weeks or once a month

Notes

a Separate formulation administered as a single daily dose and adjusted to a level that holds patient in treatment and suppresses opioid withdrawal signs and symptoms.

b Opioid medication follows strict clinical guidelines to ensure proper maintenance and reduction in withdrawal symptoms. Consult formulation-specific dosing and administration requirements.

methadone is only advised if the individual is clinically responding to the treatment and can be trusted to self-administer methadone in a consistent and appropriate manner. Due to risk of interactions, which can be lethal, persons in methadone treatment are advised to strictly avoid alcohol and sedating drugs. Should the individual show intolerance or lack of improvement with methadone, a switch to buprenorphine is typically recommended. Treatment initiation is typically more complex for buprenorphine, but maintenance efficacy is similar to methadone (Dematteis et al., 2017).

Buprenorphine

Mechanism of action

Initially introduced as an opioid medication for pain management, buprenorphine is now widely used for the treatment of OUD and, in some instances, chronic pain (Malinoff, Barkin, & Wilson, 2005). Buprenorphine displaces or blocks of other drugs acting at the opioid receptors, such as morphine, codeine, fentanyl, or methadone (Walsh, Preston, Bigelow, & Stitzer, 1995). However, since it is a partial agonist, it presents the same effects that other full agonist opioids do, but only to a certain limit. Pharmacological studies have shown a ceiling effect in buprenorphine use that limits the physiological effects at a certain point. This means that once the ceiling has been reached, increasing dosage does not lead to increased levels of euphoria, analgesia, or respiratory depression (Umbricht, Huestis, Cone, & Preston, 2004). Buprenorphine is also available as a fixed-dose combination with naloxone (see the "About naloxone" section).

Drug indications and duration

Buprenorphine was approved by the FDA in 2002 for use in the United States, and since then its efficacy in treatment of OUD has evolved into a maintenance model. In buprenorphine maintenance, buprenorphine is prescribed to reduce risk of relapse caused by withdrawal symptoms. Currently, buprenorphine is available in a variety of forms of administration (buccal/inside cheek, sublingual/under the tongue, subdermal/under the skin, or subcutaneous injection) and sometimes in combination with naloxone (Kumar & Saadabadi, 2018). Duration of buprenorphine treatment is dependent on the individual, and they are advised not to discontinue treatment abruptly. Tapering down gradually is recommended to avoid withdrawal symptoms and opioid relapse. Opioid abstinence (12–24 hours) is also recommended prior to buprenorphine initiation, and buprenorphine was found to ameliorate withdrawal symptoms shortly following opioid discontinuation (Haight et al., 2019).

About naloxone

In 2015, the FDA approved a naloxone nasal spray that has been widely used to reverse overdoses (Wermeling, 2015). In terms of long-term pharmacotherapy, naloxone can be found in formulations with buprenorphine to prevent misuse of opioids by persons seeking OUD treatment. Research has shown that formulations of buprenorphine and naloxone in a 4:1 ratio, respectively, provide an optimal combination that preserves the therapeutic effects of buprenorphine and minimizes opiate antagonist effects of naloxone when administered sublingually. However, this 4:1 ratio of medication taken through a non-oral route (such as injection) negates the therapeutic effects and leads to significant opiate withdrawal symptoms (Mendelson & Jones, 2003; Orman & Keating, 2009; Yokell, Zaller, Green, & Rich, 2011).

Efficacy and clinical safety

Buprenorphine does not require the observed dosage management that methadone does, due to its lower risk of abuse. A constraint with buprenorphine is that there is limited access to this prescribed medication, since clinicians need to complete special training to obtain a waiver that allows them to prescribe it. Different trials have shown significantly improved OUD treatment outcomes under different buprenorphine formulations compared to placebo (Rosenthal et al., 2016; Thomas et al., 2014; Volkow & Koroshetz, 2019). A recently published phase 3 trial involving 36 treatment centers in the United States reported significantly higher abstinence with monthly subcutaneously injected buprenorphine treatment compared to placebo (Haight et al., 2019).

When used in recommended dosages, buprenorphine has a good safety profile, with the possibility of some patients experiencing adverse effects such as sedation. Buprenorphine-related deaths have been reported, occurring primarily when the drug is taken with other substances such as alcohol and benzodiazepines. Intravenously administered high doses of buprenorphine have resulted in deaths due to respiratory depression and hypoxia. There is, however, a lower risk for lethal overdose with buprenorphine than with methadone. Compared to methadone, buprenorphine/naloxone are better at improving social life status and diminishing illicit drug use (Dematteis et al., 2017).

Naltrexone

Mechanism of action

Naltrexone is a full opioid antagonist, blocking the effects of exogenous opioids through competitive binding at receptor sites (Sullivan et al., 2013). It has a similar action to the opioid overdose reversal drug naloxone; however, it is longer acting and available in oral form. By minimizing the rewarding effects of exogenous opiates, naltrexone reduces drug desire and promotes abstinence (Comer et al., 2006; Krupitsky et al., 2011).

Drug indications and duration

Naltrexone is available orally in tablet form; however, lack of adherence to the prescription is a major barrier to ensuring abstinence. To help maintain adherence and improve overall effectiveness, it is also available as a monthly injectable, sustained-release formulation. See the section on "Naltrexone" in the AUD section for more comprehensive information.

Efficacy and clinical safety

Both oral and injectable forms of naltrexone were found to be superior to placebo in treating OUD (Lee et al., 2018; Schuckit, 2016). A recently published RCT comparing oral to extended-release injectable suspension of naltrexone reported that the injectable form of naltrexone showed twice the rate of treatment retention at six months compared to oral naltrexone (Sullivan et al., 2019). A comparative effectiveness trial investigating differences between the extended release naltrexone formulation versus buprenorphine/naloxone showed that both treatments showed a similar safety profile, as well as similar efficacy in preventing relapse (Lee et al., 2018).

Naltrexone is usually well tolerated, and occasional side effects include nausea and headache. To avoid withdrawal precipitated by naltrexone it is important that, prior to initiation, the individual is free from opioids for at least a week. The naloxone challenge test is sometimes performed before treatment initiation to ensure that they have completed withdrawal from opioids: small doses of naltrexone are administered, and the person is then observed for up to one hour to assess whether there are signs of withdrawal.

OUD: second-line and promising treatments

Lofexidine was recently approved by the FDA for treatment of OUD withdrawal in the United States Lofexidine is a selective receptor agonist that minimizes stress-related opioid craving and the production of norepinephrine, which has been implicated in many symptoms of opioid withdrawal. Although long available in Europe, lofexidine was approved by the FDA in 2018 as the first non-opioid treatment for the mitigation of opioid withdrawal and facilitation of opioid discontinuation in adults.

A range of medications may be used off-label for addressing symptomatic relief in the management of opioid withdrawal symptoms. These include clonidine, and supportive medications such as sleep aids for insomnia (zolpidem, eszopiclone, doxepin, trazadone), pain (non-steroidal anti-inflammatory drugs, acetaminophen), muscle spasms (anti-spasmodics), nausea (ondansetron, prochlorperazine, metoclopramide), diarrhea (loperamide, bismuth), and anxiety (diphenhydramine, hydroxyzine) (Kosten & Baxter, 2019).

OUD: opioid overdose reversal with naloxone

As a highly competitive opioid antagonist, naloxone hydrochloride has primarily been used to reverse opiate overdose. Naloxone has an extremely high affinity for the μ-opioid receptor and reverses agonist activity and physiological effects at a rapid rate (Wang, Sun, & Sadee, 2007). It acts rapidly to restore breathing difficulties following opioid overdosing. To limit the lives lost during the still ongoing opioid epidemic in the United States, the FDA approved the hand-held autoinjector in 2014, which can be easily carried and administered by family members or caregivers, and the nasal spray in 2015. Both are normally packed in a carton consisting of two doses should a repeat dose be necessary. Naloxone is an extremely safe drug to use and though withdrawal symptoms following administration may be uncomfortable, they are not fatal.

Cocaine use disorder

Cocaine and crack addiction fall under the category of cocaine use disorder. Cocaine is a central nervous system stimulant with considerable, though variable, addictive potential. Neurotransmitters, such as dopamine and serotonin, among others, are thought to be involved in CUD. According to the National Institute of Drug Abuse (NIDA), part of the U.S. National Institutes of Health, the method of administration of cocaine affects the intensity and duration of the "high" effect (National Institute on Drug Abuse, 2018). Snorted cocaine takes longer than injected cocaine to reach peak effects, though the duration of the "high" lasts longer. Effects are instantaneous when crack is smoked, with a lasting influence of 5–10 min. Due to this action, crack holds more potent addictive properties compared to cocaine.

Currently there are no FDA-approved medications for the treatment of CUD in the United States, though a number of RCTs have been examining potential pharmacological treatments (Anderson et al., 2009; Kosten et al., 2014; Martell et al., 2009; Mello et al., 1993; Shorter et al., 2013; Somoza et al., 2013; Susukida, Crum, Hong, Stuart, & Mojtabai, 2018). Due to the strong correlation between cognitive impairment and meager treatment outcomes, ameliorating cognition effects with cognition enhancing medications such as modafinil, rivastigmine and galantamine are sometimes used as off-label strategies for individuals in treatment for CUD. Other investigated medicines for CUD treatment include baclofen, tiagabine, disulfiram, the antidepressant desipramine, and the anticonvulsant topiramate (Susukida et al., 2018). Vaccinations which would serve as an immunotherapy against cocaine effects are also under investigation (Kimishima, Olson, & Janda, 2018; Kimishima, Olson, Natori, & Janda, 2018; Kosten et al., 2014; Yang & Kosten, 2019).

Clinical use and efficacy of off-label CUD treatments

Despite numerous RCTs, there exists a lack of convincing evidence of a pharmacological agent efficacious in treating CUD. Meta-analysis indicated that the stimulant modafinil, the antihypertensive reserpine, the anxiolytic buspirone, and the anti-emetic ondansetron appear to show promise (Susukida et al., 2018). Disulfiram, which is approved by the FDA for AUD treatment, is sometimes clinically used in combination with behavioral CUD therapies. Despite this, efficacy of disulfiram with this patient cohort is debatable (Carroll et al., 2016; DeVito, Babuscio, Nich, Ball, & Carroll, 2014). To date, behavioral therapies, such as cognitive behavioral therapy (Carroll et al., 2016), appear the most efficacious for CUD treatment.

Cannabis use disorder

In the United States, according to the 2017 National Survey on Drug Use and Health, cannabis (also known as marijuana) tops the list as the most commonly used illicit drug, with an estimated 49 million individuals reporting use in the past year (SAMHSA, 2018). Cannabis use is a double-edged sword: while misuse can lead to addiction and negative consequences, there is heightened interest among researchers in its benefits and potential medical uses. It is unclear how many individuals currently use or misuse cannabidiol-based products medicinally or recreationally.

There are currently no FDA-approved pharmacotherapy treatments for cannabis use disorder in the United States. Pharmacological interventions, which are often used in combination with psychotherapy, are normally directed to relapse prevention, cannabis withdrawal symptoms, and comorbid cannabis use with other psychiatric disorders. Moreover, marijuana and alcohol are often used in conjunction (Subbaraman, Barnett, & Karriker-Jaffe, 2019), leading to enhanced psychoactive effects of cannabis (Hartman, Brown, Milavetz, Spurgin, Gorelick, et al., 2015; Hartman et al., 2016), as well as impairment in performing certain operations such as driving (Hartman, Brown, Milavetz, Spurgin, Pierce, et al., 2015). There is also ongoing research to better understand the effects and treatment of combined alcohol and cannabis use.

Clinical use and efficacy of off-label cannabis use disorder treatments

The most prominent feature of cannabis use withdrawal is disrupted sleep. Promising medications in alleviating this symptom include zolpidem, buspirone, and gabapentin; however, poor efficacy has been shown in combatting the disorder itself (Sherman & McRae-Clark, 2016). To date, identifying efficacious medications for this disorder is proving to be quite challenging, and while many clinical trials have been performed with different medications (Sherman & McRae-Clark, 2016), at present psychotherapeutic therapies remain the main option to treat patients with cannabis use disorder.

Conclusion

This chapter highlights advances made in recent years in trying to curb the rising phenomenon of alcohol and substance addiction. Numerous medications are being investigated for their potential role in treating AUDs and other substance use disorders, though it is proving to be a daunting task, as noted from the restricted selection of FDA-approved medications. There exists a crucial need for more research in medication development for treating addictive behaviors, especially for those which have as yet no approved pharmacotherapies. Personalized medication, where medicines are matched according to the needs of the patient, is slowly gaining traction in treatment of substance use disorders. Nonetheless, we still face both the underdiagnosis of substance use disorders, as well as underutilization of approved addiction treatment medications, hence an immense need for increased education and training of healthcare personnel in addiction pharmacotherapies. Social workers may not be the prescribing providers but can play a significant role in supporting access to medications for substance use disorder treatment, patient adherence to prescribed pharmacotherapy regimens, and behavioral treatment as companion to or in combination with pharmacotherapy.

Acknowledgments

This work was supported by NIH intramural funding ZIA-AA000218 (Section on Clinical Psychoneuroendocrinology and Neuropsychopharmacology; PI: Dr. Lorenzo Leggio), jointly supported by the National Institute on Alcohol Abuse and Alcoholism (NIAAA) Division of Intramural Clinical and Biological Research and the National Institute on Drug Abuse (NIDA) Intramural Research Program.

References

Agabio, R., Sinclair, J. M., Addolorato, G., Aubin, H. J., Beraha, E. M., Caputo, F., . . . Leggio, L. (2018). Baclofen for the treatment of alcohol use disorder: The Cagliari statement. *Lancet Psychiatry, 5*(12), 957–960. doi:10.1016/S2215-0366(18)30303-1

Akanbi, M. O., Carroll, A. J., Achenbach, C., O'Dwyer, L. C., Jordan, N., Hitsman, B., . . . Murphy, R. (2018). The efficacy of smoking cessation interventions in low- and middle-income countries: A systematic review and meta-analysis. *Addiction, 114*(4), 620–635. doi:10.1111/add.14518

Anderson, A. L., Reid, M. S., Li, S.-H., Holmes, T., Shemanski, L., Slee, A., . . . Elkashef, A. M. (2009). Modafinil for the treatment of cocaine dependence. *Drug and Alcohol Dependence, 104*(1–2), 133–139. doi:10.1016/j.drugalcdep.2009.04.015

Anthenelli, R. M., Benowitz, N. L., West, R., St Aubin, L., McRae, T., Lawrence, D., . . . Evins, A. E. (2016). Neuropsychiatric safety and efficacy of varenicline, bupropion, and nicotine patch in smokers with and without psychiatric disorders (EAGLES): A double-blind, randomised, placebo–controlled clinical trial. *Lancet, 387*(10037), 2507–2520. doi:10.1016/S0140-6736(16)30272-0

Beard, E., Shahab, L., Cummings, D. M., Michie, S., & West, R. (2016). New pharmacological agents to aid smoking cessation and tobacco harm reduction: What has been investigated, and what is in the pipeline? *CNS Drugs, 30*(10), 951–983. doi:10.1007/s40263-016-0362-3

Beatty, A., & Stock, C. (2017). Efficacy of long-acting, injectable versus oral naltrexone for preventing admissions for alcohol use disorder. *Mental Health Clinician, 7*(3), 106–110. doi:10.9740/mhc.2017.05.106

Benowitz, N. L., Pipe, A., West, R., Hays, J. T., Tonstad, S., McRae, T., . . . Anthenelli, R. M. (2018). Cardiovascular safety of varenicline, bupropion, and nicotine patch in smokers: A randomized clinical trial. *JAMA Internal Medicine, 178*(5), 622–631. doi:10.1001/jamainternmed.2018.0397

Benowitz, N. L., Porchet, H., & Jacob, P., 3rd. (1989). Nicotine dependence and tolerance in man: Pharmacokinetic and pharmacodynamic investigations. *Progress in Brain Research, 79*, 279–287. doi:10.1001/jamainternmed.2018.0397

Blanco-Gandia, M. C., & Rodriguez-Arias, M. (2018). Pharmacological treatments for opiate and alcohol addiction: A historical perspective of the last 50 years. *European Journal of Pharmacology, 836*, 89–101. doi:10.1016/j.ejphar.2018.08.007

Bullen, C., Howe, C., Laugesen, M., McRobbie, H., Parag, V., Williman, J., & Walker, N. (2013). Electronic cigarettes for smoking cessation: A randomised controlled trial. *Lancet, 382*(9905), 1629–1637. doi:10.1016/S0140-6736(13)61842-5

Cahill, K., Stevens, S., Perera, R., & Lancaster, T. (2013). Pharmacological interventions for smoking cessation: An overview and network meta-analysis. *Cochrane Database of Systematic Reviews, 5*, CD009329. doi:10.1002/14651858.CD009329.pub2

Calcaterra, S. L., Bach, P., Chadi, A., Chadi, N., Kimmel, S. D., Morford, K. L., . . . Samet, J. H. (2019). Methadone matters: What the United States can learn from the global effort to treat opioid addiction. *Journal of General Internal Medicine.* doi:10.1007/s11606-018-4801-3

Caponnetto, P., Campagna, D., Cibella, F., Morjaria, J. B., Caruso, M., Russo, C., & Polosa, R. (2013). EffiCiency and Safety of an eLectronic cigAreTte (ECLAT) as tobacco cigarettes substitute: A prospective 12-month randomized control design study. *PLoS One, 8*(6), e66317. doi:10.1371/journal.pone.0066317

Carroll, K. M., Nich, C., Petry, N. M., Eagan, D. A., Shi, J. M., & Ball, S. A. (2016). A randomized factorial trial of disulfiram and contingency management to enhance cognitive behavioral therapy for cocaine dependence. *Drug and Alcohol Dependence, 160*, 135–142. doi:10.1016/j.drugalcdep.2015.12.036

Chen, X. Z., Zhang, R. Y., Wang, X. F., Yin, X. G., Wang, J., Wang, Y. C., . . . Guo, J. (2019). Peptide-free synthetic nicotine vaccine candidates with alpha-galactosylceramide as adjuvant. *Molecular Pharmaceutics.* doi:10.1021/acs.molpharmaceut.8b01095

Comer, S. D., Sullivan, M. A., Yu, E., Rothenberg, J. L., Kleber, H. D., Kampman, K., . . . O'Brien, C. P. (2006). Injectable, sustained-release naltrexone for the treatment of opioid dependence: A randomized, placebo-controlled trial. *Archives of General Psychiatry, 63*(2), 210–218. doi:10.1001/archpsyc.63.2.210

Dahne, J., Wahlquist, A. E., Boatright, A. S., Garrett-Mayer, E., Fleming, D. O., Davis, R., . . . Carpenter, M. J. (2018). Nicotine replacement therapy sampling via primary care: Methods from a pragmatic cluster randomized clinical trial. *Contemporary Clinical Trials, 72*, 1–7. doi:10.1016/j.cct.2018.07.008

de Jong, B., Schuppers, A. S., Kruisdijk-Gerritsen, A., Arbouw, M. E. L., van den Oever, H. L. A., & van Zanten, A. R. H. (2018). The safety and efficacy of nicotine replacement therapy in the intensive care unit: A randomised controlled pilot study. *Annals of Intensive Care, 8*(1), 70. doi:10.1186/s13613-018-0399-1

Dematteis, M., Auriacombe, M., D'Agnone, O., Somaini, L., Szerman, N., Littlewood, R., . . . Soyka, M. (2017). Recommendations for buprenorphine and methadone therapy in opioid use disorder: A European consensus. *Expert Opinion on Pharmacotherapy, 18*(18), 1987–1999. doi:10.1080/14656566.2017.1409722

DeVito, E. E., Babuscio, T. A., Nich, C., Ball, S. A., & Carroll, K. M. (2014). Gender differences in clinical outcomes for cocaine dependence: Randomized clinical trials of behavioral therapy and disulfiram. *Drug and Alcohol Dependence, 145*, 156–167. doi:10.1016/j.drugalcdep.2014.10.007

Evins, A. E., Benowitz, N. L., West, R., Russ, C., McRae, T., Lawrence, D., . . . Anthenelli, R. M. (2019). Neuropsychiatric safety and efficacy of varenicline, bupropion, and nicotine patch in smokers with psychotic, anxiety, and mood disorders in the EAGLES trial. *Journal of Clinical Psychopharmacology, 39*(2), 108–116. doi:10.1097/JCP.0000000000001015

Fenster, C. P., Rains, M. F., Noerager, B., Quick, M. W., & Lester, R. A. (1997). Influence of subunit composition on desensitization of neuronal acetylcholine receptors at low concentrations of nicotine. *Journal of Neuroscience, 17*(15), 5747–5759. doi:10.1523/JNEUROSCI.17-15-05747.1997

Foulds, J., Burke, M., Steinberg, M., Williams, J. M., & Ziedonis, D. M. (2004). Advances in pharmacotherapy for tobacco dependence. *Expert Opinion on Emerging Drugs, 9*(1), 39–53. doi:10.1517/eoed.9.1.39.32951

Gomez-Coronado, N., Walker, A. J., Berk, M., & Dodd, S. (2018). Current and emerging pharmacotherapies for cessation of tobacco smoking. *Pharmacotherapy, 38*(2), 235–258. doi:10.1002/phar.2073

Haight, B. R., Learned, S. M., Laffont, C. M., Fudala, P. J., Zhao, Y., Garofalo, A. S., . . . RB-US-13-0001 Study Investigators. (2019). Efficacy and safety of a monthly buprenorphine depot injection for opioid use disorder: A multicentre, randomised, double-blind, placebo-controlled, phase 3 trial. *Lancet, 393*(10173), 778–790. doi:10.1016/S0140-6736(18)32259-1

Hajek, P., Phillips-Waller, A., Przulj, D., Pesola, F., Myers Smith, K., Bisal, N., . . . McRobbie, H. J. (2019). A randomized trial of e-cigarettes versus nicotine-replacement therapy. *New England Journal of Medicine, 380*(7), 629–637. doi:10.1056/NEJMoa1808779

Hartman, R. L., Brown, T. L., Milavetz, G., Spurgin, A., Gorelick, D. A., Gaffney, G., & Huestis, M. A. (2015). Controlled cannabis vaporizer administration: Blood and plasma cannabinoids with and without alcohol. *Clinical Chemistry, 61*(6), 850–869. doi:10.1373/clinchem.2015.238287

Hartman, R. L., Brown, T. L., Milavetz, G., Spurgin, A., Gorelick, D. A., Gaffney, G., & Huestis, M. A. (2016). Controlled vaporized cannabis, with and without alcohol: Subjective effects and oral fluid-blood cannabinoid relationships. *Drug Testing and Analysis, 8*(7), 690–701. doi:10.1002/dta.1839

Hartman, R. L., Brown, T. L., Milavetz, G., Spurgin, A., Pierce, R. S., Gorelick, D. A., . . . Huestis, M. A. (2015). Cannabis effects on driving lateral control with and without alcohol. *Drug and Alcohol Dependence, 154*, 25–37. doi:10.1016/j.drugalcdep.2015.06.015

Henningfield, J. E. (1995). Nicotine medications for smoking cessation. *New England Journal of Medicine, 333*(18), 1196–1203. doi:10.1056/nejm199511023331807

Hughes, J. R., Stead, L. F., Hartmann-Boyce, J., Cahill, K., & Lancaster, T. (2014). Antidepressants for smoking cessation. *Cochrane Database of Systematic Reviews, 1*, CD000031. doi:10.1002/14651858.CD000031.pub4

Jonas, D. E., Amick, H. R., Feltner, C., Bobashev, G., Thomas, K., Wines, R., . . . Garbutt, J. C. (2014). Pharmacotherapy for adults with alcohol use disorders in outpatient settings: A systematic review and meta-analysis. *JAMA, 311*(18), 1889–1900. doi:10.1001/jama.2014.3628

Kalk, N. J., & Lingford-Hughes, A. R. (2014). The clinical pharmacology of acamprosate. *British Journal of Clinical Pharmacology, 77*(2), 315–323. doi:10.1111/bcp.12070

Kimishima, A., Olson, M. E., & Janda, K. D. (2018). Investigations into the efficacy of multi-component cocaine vaccines. *Bioorganic Medical Chemistry Letters, 28*(16), 2779–2783. doi:10.1016/j.bmcl.2017.12.043

Kimishima, A., Olson, M. E., Natori, Y., & Janda, K. D. (2018). Efficient syntheses of cocaine vaccines and their in vivo evaluation. *ACS Medical Chemistry Letters, 9*(5), 411–416. doi:10.1021/acsmedchemlett.8b00051

Kosten, T. R., & Baxter, L. E. (2019). Review article: Effective management of opioid withdrawal symptoms: A gateway to opioid dependence treatment. *American Journal of Addiction, 28*(2), 55–62. doi:10.1111/ajad.12862

Kosten, T. R., Domingo, C. B., Shorter, D., Orson, F., Green, C., Somoza, E., . . . Kampman, K. (2014). Vaccine for cocaine dependence: A randomized double-blind placebo-controlled efficacy trial. *Drug and Alcohol Dependence, 140*, 42–47. doi:10.1016/j.drugalcdep.2014.04.003

Kotz, D., Viechtbauer, W., Simpson, C., van Schayck, O. C., West, R., & Sheikh, A. (2015). Cardiovascular and neuropsychiatric risks of varenicline: A retrospective cohort study. *Lancet Respiratory Medicine, 3*(10), 761–768. doi:10.1016/S2213-2600(15)00320-3

Kranzler, H. R., & Soyka, M. (2018). Diagnosis and pharmacotherapy of alcohol use disorder: A review. *JAMA, 320*(8), 815–824. doi:10.1001/jama.2018.11406

Kreek, M. J., Borg, L., Ducat, E., & Ray, B. (2010). Pharmacotherapy in the treatment of addiction: Methadone. *Journal of Addictive Diseases, 29*(2), 200–216. doi:10.1080/10550881003684798

Kress, C. M., Obi, N. U., & Prochazka, A. V. (2017). In smokers with COPD, neither varenicline nor bupropion was linked to increased CV or neuropsychiatric risk vs NRT. *Annals of Internal Medicine, 167*(6), JC31. doi:10.7326/ACPJC-2017-167-6-031

Krupitsky, E., Nunes, E. V., Ling, W., Illeperuma, A., Gastfriend, D. R., & Silverman, B. L. (2011). Injectable extended-release naltrexone for opioid dependence: A double-blind, placebo-controlled, multicentre randomised trial. *Lancet, 377*(9776), 1506–1513. doi:10.1016/s0140-6736(11)60358-9

Kumar, R., & Saadabadi, A. (2018). *Buprenorphine. StatPearls*. Treasure Island, FL: StatPearls Publishing. Retrieved from https://www.ncbi.nlm.nih.gov/books/NBK459126/

Lee, J., Kresina, T. F., Campopiano, M., Lubran, R., & Clark, H. W. (2015). Use of pharmacotherapies in the treatment of alcohol use disorders and opioid dependence in primary care. *BioMed Research International, 2015*, 137020. doi:10.1155/2015/137020

Lee, J. D., Nunes, E. V., Jr., Novo, P., Bachrach, K., Bailey, G. L., Bhatt, S., . . . Rotrosen, J. (2018). Comparative effectiveness of extended-release naltrexone versus buprenorphine-naloxone for opioid relapse prevention (X:BOT): A multicentre, open-label, randomised controlled trial. *The Lancet, 391*(10118), 309–318. doi:10.1016/S0140-6736(17)32812-X

Le Foll, B., Melihan-Cheinin, P., Rostoker, G., & Lagrue, G. (2005). Smoking cessation guidelines: Evidence-based recommendations of the French health products safety agency. *European Psychiatry, 20*(5–6), 431–441. doi:10.1016/j.eurpsy.2004.12.008

Litten, R. Z., Falk, D. E., Ryan, M. L., Fertig, J., & Leggio, L. (2018). Advances in pharmacotherapy development: Human clinical studies. *Handbook of Experimental Pharmacology, 248*, 579–613. doi:10.1007/164_2017_79

Ma, J., Bao, Y. P., Wang, R. J., Su, M. F., Liu, M. X., Li, J. Q., . . . Lu, L. (2018, June 22). Effects of medication-assisted treatment on mortality among opioids users: A systematic review and meta-analysis. *Molecular Psychiatry*, epub. doi:10.1038/s41380-018-0094-5

Malinoff, H. L., Barkin, R. L., & Wilson, G. (2005). Sublingual buprenorphine is effective in the treatment of chronic pain syndrome. *American Journal of Therapeutics, 12*(5), 379–384. doi:10.1097/01.mjt.0000160935.62883.ff

Martell, B. A., Orson, F. M., Poling, J., Mitchell, E., Rossen, R. D., Gardner, T., & Kosten, T. R. (2009). Cocaine vaccine for the treatment of cocaine dependence in methadone-maintained patients: A randomized, double-blind, placebo-controlled efficacy trial. *Archives of General Psychiatry, 66*(10), 1116–1123. doi:10.1001/archgenpsychiatry.2009.128

Mattick, R. P., Breen, C., Kimber, J., & Davoli, M. (2009). Methadone maintenance therapy versus no opioid replacement therapy for opioid dependence. *Cochrane Database of Systematic Reviews, 3*, Cd002209. doi:10.1002/14651858.CD002209.pub2

Mello, N. K., Mendelson, J. H., Lukas, S. E., Gastfriend, D. R., Teoh, S. K., & Holman, B. L. (1993). Buprenorphine treatment of opiate and cocaine abuse: Clinical and preclinical studies. *Harvard Review of Psychiatry, 1*(3), 168–183. doi:10.3109/10673229309017075

Mendelson, J., & Jones, R. T. (2003). Clinical and pharmacological evaluation of buprenorphine and naloxone combinations: Why the 4:1 ratio for treatment? *Drug and Alcohol Dependence, 70*(2 Suppl), S29–S37. doi:10.1016/S0376-8716(03)00057-7

Mirijello, A., D'Angelo, C., Ferrulli, A., Vassallo, G., Antonelli, M., Caputo, F., . . . Addolorato, G. (2015). Identification and management of alcohol withdrawal syndrome. *Drugs, 75*(4), 353–365. doi:10.1007/s40265-015-0358-1

Molyneux, A. (2004). Nicotine replacement therapy. *BMJ (Clinical Research Edition), 328*(7437), 454–456. doi:10.1136/bmj.328.7437.454

National Institute of Drug Abuse (NIDA). (2018) *Cocaine*. Retrieved from https://www.drugabuse.gov/publications/drugfacts/cocaine

Orman, J. S., & Keating, G. M. (2009). Buprenorphine/naloxone. *Drugs, 69*(5), 577–607. doi:10.2165/00003495-200969050-00006

Palpacuer, C., Duprez, R., Huneau, A., Locher, C., Boussageon, R., Laviolle, B., & Naudet, F. (2018). Pharmacologically controlled drinking in the treatment of alcohol dependence or alcohol use disorders: A systematic review with direct and network meta-analyses on nalmefene, naltrexone, acamprosate, baclofen and topiramate. *Addiction, 113*(2), 220–237. doi:10.1111/add.13974

Rollema, H., Chambers, L. K., Coe, J. W., Glowa, J., Hurst, R. S., Lebel, L. A., . . . Williams, K. E. (2007). Pharmacological profile of the alpha4beta2 nicotinic acetylcholine receptor partial agonist varenicline, an effective smoking cessation aid. *Neuropharmacology, 52*(3), 985–994. doi:10.1016/j.neuropharm.2006.10.016

Rose, J. E. (2008). Disrupting nicotine reinforcement: From cigarette to brain. *Annals of the New York Academy of Science, 1141*, 233–256. doi:10.1196/annals.1441.019

Rosenthal, R. N., Lofwall, M. R., Kim, S., Chen, M., Beebe, K. L., Vocci, F. J., & PRO-814 Study Group. (2016). Effect of buprenorphine implants on illicit opioid use among abstinent adults with opioid dependence treated with sublingual buprenorphine: A randomized clinical trial. *JAMA, 316*(3), 282–290. doi:10.1001/jama.2016.9382

Schuckit, M. A. (2016). Treatment of opioid-use disorders. *New England Journal of Medicine, 375*(4), 357–368. doi:10.1056/NEJMra1604339

Sherman, B. J., & McRae-Clark, A. L. (2016). Treatment of cannabis use disorder: Current science and future outlook. *Pharmacotherapy, 36*(5), 511–535. doi:10.1002/phar.1747

Shorter, D., Nielsen, D. A., Huang, W., Harding, M. J., Hamon, S. C., & Kosten, T. R. (2013). Pharmacogenetic randomized trial for cocaine abuse: Disulfiram and α1A-adrenoceptor gene variation. *European Neuropsychopharmacology, 23*(11), 1401–1407. doi:10.1016/j.euroneuro.2013.05.014

Singh, S., Loke, Y. K., Spangler, J. G., & Furberg, C. D. (2011). Risk of serious adverse cardiovascular events associated with varenicline: A systematic review and meta-analysis. *CMAJ, 183*(12), 1359–1366. doi:10.1503/cmaj.110218

Skinner, M. D., Lahmek, P., Pham, H., & Aubin, H. J. (2014). Disulfiram efficacy in the treatment of alcohol dependence: A meta-analysis. *PLoS One, 9*(2), e87366. doi:10.1371/journal.pone.0087366

Somoza, E. C., Winship, D., Gorodetzky, C. W., Lewis, D., Ciraulo, D. A., Galloway, G. P., . . . Winhusen, T. (2013). A multisite, double-blind, placebo-controlled clinical trial to evaluate the safety and efficacy of vigabatrin for treating cocaine dependence. *JAMA Psychiatry, 70*(6), 630–637. doi:10.1001/jamapsychiatry.2013.872

Stahl, S. M., Pradko, J. F., Haight, B. R., Modell, J. G., Rockett, C. B., & Learned-Coughlin, S. (2004). A review of the neuropharmacology of bupropion, a dual norepinephrine and dopamine reuptake inhibitor. *Primary Care companion to the Journal of Clinical Psychiatry, 6*(4), 159–166. Retrieved from https://www.ncbi.nlm.nih.gov/pmc/PMC514842/. https://doi.org/10.4088/PCC.v06n0403

Subbaraman, M. S., Barnett, S. B., & Karriker-Jaffe, K. J. (2019). Risks associated with mid level cannabis use among people treated for alcohol use disorder. *Alcohol: Clinical & Experimental Research*, epub. doi:10.1111/acer.13973

Substance Abuse and Mental Health Services Administration (SAMHSA). (2018). *Results from the 2017 national survey on drug use and health; detailed tables.* Retrieved from https://www.samhsa.gov/data/sites/default/files/cbhsq-reports/NSDUHDetailedTabs2017/NSDUHDetailedTabs2017.pdf

Sullivan, M. A., Bisaga, A., Mariani, J. J., Glass, A., Levin, F. R., Comer, S. D., & Nunes, E. V. (2013). Naltrexone treatment for opioid dependence: Does its effectiveness depend on testing the blockade? *Drug and Alcohol Dependence, 133*(1), 80–85. doi:10.1016/j.drugalcdep.2013.05.030

Sullivan, M. A., Bisaga, A., Pavlicova, M., Carpenter, K. M., Choi, C. J., Mishlen, K., . . . Nunes, E. V. (2019). A randomized trial comparing extended-release injectable suspension and oral naltrexone, both combined with behavioral therapy, for the treatment of opioid use disorder. *American Journal of Psychiatry, 176*(2), 129–137. doi:10.1176/appi.ajp.2018.17070732

Susukida, R., Crum, R. M., Hong, H., Stuart, E. A., & Mojtabai, R. (2018). Comparing pharmacological treatments for cocaine dependence: Incorporation of methods for enhancing generalizability in meta-analytic studies. *International Journal of Methods in Psychiatric Research, 27*(4), e1609. doi:10.1002/mpr.1609

Thomas, C. P., Fullerton, C. A., Kim, M., Montejano, L., Lyman, D. R., Dougherty, R. H., . . . Delphin-Rittmon, M. E. (2014). Medication-assisted treatment with buprenorphine: Assessing the evidence. *Psychiatric Services, 65*(2), 158–170. doi:10.1176/appi.ps.201300256

Thomas, D., Farrell, M., McRobbie, H., Tutka, P., Petrie, D., West, R., . . . Courtney, R. J. (2018). The effectiveness, safety and cost-effectiveness of cytisine versus varenicline for smoking cessation in an Australian population: A study protocol for a randomized controlled non-inferiority trial. *Addiction*, epub. doi:10.1111/add.14541

Umbricht, A., Huestis, M. A., Cone, E. J., & Preston, K. L. (2004). Effects of high-dose intravenous buprenorphine in experienced opioid abusers. *Journal of Clinical Psychopharmacology, 24*(5), 479–487. doi:10.1097/01.jcp.0000138766.15858.c6

Volkow, N. D., & Koroshetz, W. J. (2019). The role of neurologists in tackling the opioid epidemic. *Nature Reviews Neurology*, epub. doi:10.1038/s41582-019-0146-8

Walsh, S. L., Preston, K. L., Bigelow, G. E., & Stitzer, M. L. (1995). Acute administration of buprenorphine in humans: Partial agonist and blockade effects. *Journal of Pharmacology and Experimental Therapeutics, 274*(1), 361–372.

Wang, D., Sun, X., & Sadee, W. (2007). Different effects of opioid antagonists on mu-, delta-, and kappa-opioid receptors with and without agonist pretreatment. *Journal of Pharmacology and Experimental Therapeutics, 321*(2), 544–552. doi:10.1124/jpet.106.118810

Wermeling, D. P. (2015). Review of naloxone safety for opioid overdose: Practical considerations for new technology and expanded public access. *Therapeutic Advances in Drug Safety, 6*(1), 20–31. doi:10.1177/2042098614564776

West, R., Evins, A. E., Benowitz, N. L., Russ, C., McRae, T., Lawrence, D., . . . Anthenelli, R. M. (2018). Factors associated with the efficacy of smoking cessation treatments and predictors of smoking abstinence in EAGLES. *Addiction, 113*(8), 1507–1516. doi:10.1111/add.14208

World Health Organization (WHO). (2010) *Management of substance abuse.* Retrieved from https://www.who.int/substance_abuse/publications/atlas_report/profiles/en/

Yang, F., & Kosten, T. R. (2019). Psychopharmacology: Neuroimmune signaling in psychiatric disease-developing vaccines against abused drugs using toll-like receptor agonists. *Psychopharmacology.* doi:10.1007/s00213-019-5176-9

Yokell, M. A., Zaller, N. D., Green, T. C., & Rich, J. D. (2011). Buprenorphine and buprenorphine/naloxone diversion, misuse, and illicit use: An international review. *Current Drug Abuse Reviews, 4*(1), 28–41. Retrieved from https://www.ncbi.nlm.nih.gov/pmc/PMC3154701/

Zeigler, D. F., Roque, R., & Clegg, C. H. (2019). Optimization of a multivalent peptide vaccine for nicotine addiction. *Vaccine.* doi:10.1016/j.vaccine.2019.02.003

Ziedonis, D., Das, S., & Larkin, C. (2017). Tobacco use disorder and treatment: New challenges and opportunities. *Dialogues in Clinical Neuroscience, 19*(3), 271–280. Retrieved from http://www.ncbi.nlm.nih.gov/pubmed/29302224

Screening, brief intervention, and referral to treatment (SBIRT) in the substance use system of care

Corey Campbell, Douglas Smith, Kelly Lynn Clary and Lori Egizio

Background

The development of Screening, Brief Intervention, and Referral to Treatment (SBIRT) models represents a seismic change in addressing substance misuse in non-traditional settings. That is, substance use treatment has long existed outside of mainstream health care, requiring individuals to receive care at specialized rehabilitation centers. However, the 2017 *National Survey of Drug Use and Health* (NSDUH) estimates that only 12.2% of individuals aged 12 or older in the United States needing substance use treatment received it at a specialty facility in the past year (Substance Abuse and Mental Health Services Administration [SAMHSA], 2018. Globally, drug and alcohol use problems are major risk factors for premature death and years of living with a disability (Whiteford et al., 2013). The World Drug Report 2018 executive summary states that 450,000 deaths globally resulted from drug use (in 2015), that 167,750 deaths were associated with a drug use disorder, and that 31 million individuals engage in drug use "harmful to the point where they may need treatment" (UNDOC, 2018, p. 7). Unmet treatment need, in turn, results in poorer health internationally. The protocol's emphasis on universal screening, brief advice, and referral makes it possible to reach more individuals in more settings.

The standing of SBIRT in the substance use treatment system of care has been solidified by a very promising evidence base, supported by substantial funding from the United States' federal government. For example, SAMHSA funded numerous large demonstration projects, including one national multi-site demonstration project between 2004 and 2010 implementing SBIRT in clinical settings (Aldridge, Linford, & Bray, 2017). This project screened over 700,000 individuals nationally, mostly in healthcare facilities. Another was a massive curriculum development project, targeting medicine, nursing, and social work. Over 60 training programs were funded from 2015 to 2018 to provide training for students entering clinical practice (SAMHSA, 2019). This national training initiative alone invested approximately 60 million dollars to disseminate the SBIRT model.

This chapter begins by discussing complexities involved with defining SBIRT. Then, it provides a brief description of the clinical model. Next, it reviews the research surrounding SBIRT. Finally, it concludes with discussion of best practices for training students and other professionals, as well as new horizons for implementing SBIRT.

SBIRT: definition and place in system of care

As defined by SAMHSA (2015), a brief intervention is an evidence-based practice designed to increase motivation in individuals exhibiting risky substance use. During a brief intervention, the counselor provides feedback on the risk associated with specific behaviors, emphasizes autonomy, delivers personalized advice and options for change, and encourages support through empathic responses (Babor et al., 2007). Brief interventions for substance use are prominent in the professional literature (Zorland et al., 2018). SBIRT is a brief adaptation of Motivational Interviewing (MI; Miller & Rollnick, 2012) for application in situations where opportunistic screening and brief advice are appropriate (i.e. health care visits, emergency room visits, brief incarceration). In MI, clinicians are non-confrontational, offer empathy, emphasize client autonomy, create a partnership with the client, and listen for and reinforce client language favoring change (Miller & Rollnick, 2009; Miller & Rose, 2015). MI is a well-established method of counseling individuals engaged in high-risk behaviors and ambivalent about change (Rubak, Sandbaek, Lauritzen & Christensen, 2005).

In this chapter, we define SBIRT in its purest form as an intervention that involves: (1) brief screening in an opportunistic setting, (2) followed by one or more short sessions, together lasting no more than approximately two hours in a single month, but may be repeated over time at widely spaced intervals, and (3) not being combined with other counseling approaches, such as cognitive behavioral therapy. This definition is consistent with authors advocating for scalable, recurring brief interventions appropriate for use in health care or other opportunistic settings, and requires only 10–15 minutes to administer (Babor et al., 2007). This definition, however, contrasts with definitions applied in some meta-analyses, which we believe used higher session thresholds to have enough studies to review: up to three total sessions (Mitchell, Gryczynski, O'Grady, & Schwartz, 2013) and up to four or five hours (Tanner-Smith & Lipsey, 2015). Although we agree that combining SBIRT with other modalities may be beneficial for individuals engaged in substance misuse, shorter versions of SBIRT may more easily be diffused throughout settings where established treatment options for substance use treatment are not available.

Because substance misuse at any level may influence and exacerbate an individual's health problems (Dawson, Grant, & Li, 2005), the U.S. Prevention Task Force and the United States Surgeon General strongly recommended the practice of screening, brief intervention, and referral to treatment (SBIRT) for implementation in health care settings (O'Connor et al., 2018; Office of the Surgeon General, 2016). Health providers only have limited time with patients and cannot apply lengthy intervention models (Van Hook et al., 2007). Because this is also the case in other settings where substance misuse is not the primary focus and SBIRT implementation would be beneficial (i.e. criminal justice, intimate partner violence shelters, generalist mental health practice), we focus on very time-limited forms of SBIRT.

SBIRT intervention model: description

The main steps of the SBIRT model are screening, brief intervention, and referral to treatment. What follows is a brief review of each of these steps.

Screening

The first step in the SBIRT model involves systematically screening individuals using evidence-supported rapid screening tools. Screening for substance misuse and related problems should assess all risk levels. Notably, SBIRT is not a system of diagnosis, but rather employs rapid screening to identify individuals at risk for substance use problems, not necessarily experiencing a substance use disorder. Two common evidence-supported tools used during the screening step are the Alcohol Use Disorders Identification Test (AUDIT; Saunders, Aasland, Babor, De la Fuente, & Grant, 1993) and the Alcohol, Smoking and Substance Involvement Screening Test (ASSIST) (Barbosa et al., 2017). Other quick-screen tools include the CAGE (Cut down, Annoyed, Guilty, Eye-Opener), CRAFFT (Care, Relax, Alone, Forget, Friends, Trouble), Michigan Alcohol Screening Tool (MAST), and Drug Abuse Screening Tool (DAST) (Agerwala & McCance-Katz, 2012). Practitioners and programs are strongly discouraged from implementing untested screening tools, because there exist many that are free and demonstrate high efficiency in identifying potentially problematic substance use/misuse.

Screening tool selection considerations include whether it can be systematically implemented in the organization/setting (i.e. time, space, cost, and staffing constraints) and its relative sensitivity and specificity. Screening tools range in length from one item (i.e. "How many times in the past year have you had 5 or more drinks in one sitting?" for men, four or more for women) to several items (i.e. AUDIT, CRAFFT, ASSIST) intended to be implemented and scored in a very brief period (Caviness et al., 2009; Pilowsky & Wu, 2012). Screening tool sensitivity refers to the percent of individuals meeting some criteria (i.e. "screening positive" for potentially experiencing a substance use disorder) who actually experience the problem. Specificity refers to the percent of individuals not meeting the criterion of interest (i.e. "screening negative" for substance use disorder) who actually do not experience the problem (Smith, Bennett, Dennis, & Funk, 2017). Sensitivity and specificity relate to reducing the rate of false positive and false negative results.

Brief intervention

If screening results identify the presence of high-risk substance misuse behaviors, the brief intervention follows (Agerwala & McCance-Katz, 2012). The delivery of brief intervention varies depending on the client's identified risk level. This step includes sharing with clients their screening results, building motivation, and setting a goal. Clients are informed of their risk level based on established normative data. For example, with alcohol-focused SBIRT, the National Institute of Alcohol Abuse and Alcoholism (NIAAA) established gender-specific guidelines for low-risk drinking. Specifically, NIAAA defines low-risk drinking for women as no more than three standard drinks on any single day (i.e. daily limit) and no more than seven drinks per week (i.e. weekly limit). For men, low-risk drinking is defined as consuming no more than four drinks in any single day and no more than 14 drinks per week (NIAAA, 2018). The Dietary Guidelines for Americans (2015–2020) defined moderate drinking as up to one standard drink per day for women and up to two standard drinks per day for men (NIAAA, 2018). Recent research aligns with the lower Dietary Guidelines for Americans 2015–2020 (Wood et al., 2018). That is, only 2% of individuals who drink within the suggested limits experience a diagnosable alcohol use disorder, and risks for other health problems such as cancer or heart disease are substantially lower at these drinking levels. Higher drinking levels are associated with greater probability of an alcohol use disorder being present or developing. Feedback may include information linking the person's drinking behavior and problems experienced.

Less is known about safe use limits for substances other than alcohol. For example, it will be important in the next several years to determine if a "healthy cannabis use level" exists, which would facilitate professionals' ability to share accurate screening feedback information.

Compared to alcohol, cannabis screening is problematic due to wide variation in THC content and myriad routes of administration. Nevertheless, the principle in SBIRT is to find out how much a person uses on a typical week (e.g. daily use at three joints per day) as an anchor for negotiating a specific substance use reduction plan (i.e. no more than one joint per day) or treatment referral goal.

Enhancing motivation

Brief methods for enhancing motivation for behavior change are applied in most SBIRT models and vary depending on the duration. Most are based on Motivational Interviewing (Miller & Rollnick, 2012). Compared to many other substance use interventions, MI does not utilize direct persuasion, coercion, or confrontation (Rollnick & Miller, 1995). Key characteristics of MI include expressing empathy, eliciting change language, avoiding confrontation or coercion, and supporting autonomous decision making (Satre, Manuel, Larios, Steiger, & Satterfield, 2015). MI's four main goals include cultivating change talk, softening sustain talk, building a partnership, and expressing empathy (Moyers, Manuel, & Ernst, 2014). Recently, there is heavy emphasis on clients speaking aloud about their own reasons for change, called "change talk." The proportion of change talk relative to sustain talk (i.e. client verbalization about not changing) predicts reduced substance use and related consequences (Magill et al., 2018).

SBIRT represents a truncated version of MI. Thus, discussion of motivation to change substance misuse behavior may be limited in the briefest versions of SBIRT. Furthermore, SBIRT models sometimes encourage clinicians to discuss both the pros (i.e. sustain talk) and cons (i.e. change talk) of substance use, sometimes referred to as a decisional balance activity. However, these are contraindicated in MI, as its theory of change focuses on privileging change talk to resolve client ambivalence (Miller & Rose, 2015).

Setting goals

Typical goals in SBIRT include substance use reduction or treatment engagement. The decision to refer a client to treatment should be determined during the screening step, with referrals for those screened at moderate to high-risk levels of substance use. Substance use reduction goals are typically set for lower risk use and involve reducing the amount used in a typical week and following up at the next appointment (i.e. reducing from three joints a day per day to one joint per day).

Empirical support for SBIRT

In this section we first summarize findings surrounding brief interventions for substance misuse. We note, however, that some reviews include models that differ from how we defined SBIRT, usually by exceeding the specified length we suggest for maximum portability to non-traditional settings. Finally, we explored factors that may moderate SBIRT effectiveness, focusing on gender, socioeconomic status, population, and type of drug (i.e. alcohol or other substances).

Overall effectiveness of brief interventions

Multiple meta-analyses indicated that brief interventions resulted in clinically relevant effect sizes for reducing alcohol and other substance use. By 2012, there were six published meta-analyses and one systematic review on SBIRT's effects on problematic drinking (Alvarez-Bueno,

Rodriguez-Martin, Garicia-Ortiz, Gomez-Marcos, & Martinez-Vizcaino, 2015). Five studies reported a moderate decrease in alcohol consumption and four showed a decrease in the number of participants who consumed alcohol above the established risk level. Additionally, studies concluded that brief SBIRT models, only lasting up to 15 minutes, resulted in decreased alcohol use through six months. Yet, two key gaps in the literature were noted, including the need for more research concerning brief interventions with diverse populations (e.g. women, older and younger drinkers, minority ethnic groups, individuals experiencing alcohol use disorder and/or co-morbid conditions, and individuals living in developing countries), and the optimum brief intervention length and frequency to maintain long-term effectiveness.

More recently, three reviews addressed the lack of SBIRT research involving adolescents and young adults. Yuma-Guerrero and colleagues (2012) reviewed seven adolescent SBIRT studies completed in acute health care settings. The majority reported positive effects for SBIRT on alcohol consumption. Mitchell et al. (2013) reviewed 15 studies evaluating adolescents' SBIRT outcomes. Six of the larger randomized controlled trials detected no differences on alcohol use between SBIRT and control conditions. However, two primary care-based studies showed that SBIRT reduced marijuana use. Finally, results for school-based SBIRT were also promising. Tanner-Smith and Lipsey (2015) reviewed 185 studies of brief interventions, defined as lasting up to four hours. They reported small, but clinically relevant, effect sizes. Furthermore, they concluded that intervention length did not moderate effect sizes. In other words, shorter interventions were just as effective as longer ones.

Treatment initiation outcomes

Although individuals screened at high risk during SBIRT are supposed to be referred to additional assessment and treatment, it appears that initiation in specialized treatment following SBIRT is rare. For example, Glass and colleagues' (2015) meta-analysis of nine studies of alcohol-focused SBIRT revealed no significant increases in post-SBIRT treatment initiation relative to control group participants. This finding is both encouraging and perplexing. It indicates that alcohol use reductions may occur without further treatment beyond SBIRT, supporting the important role of SBIRT in the system of care. However, it also raises important questions about why individuals screened at high risk rarely initiate treatment.

Cost effectiveness and quality-of-life outcomes

Although brief motivational interventions appear efficacious at reducing alcohol use, studies on other benefits such as health care cost savings and quality of life years produce mixed findings. Horn, Crandall, Forcehimes, French, and Bogenschutz (2017) identified no cost savings ($n = 1285$) associated with providing SBIRT in emergency rooms. These results, however, were from a single trial with null findings where drug use was the outcome. Barbosa, Cowell, Bray, and Aldridge (2015) estimated both cost savings and quality of life years gained from delivering SBIRT ($n = 9835$), with higher gains among individuals seen in emergency department settings.

Moderators of treatment effectiveness

Evidence suggests that several factors moderate SBIRT treatment outcomes, including substance type and human diversity characteristics (socioeconomic status, gender, and special populations).

Substance type

We know less about SBIRT outcomes for substances other than alcohol, and the limited research produces mixed findings. That is, although large, multi-site observational studies support the use of SBIRT for substances other than alcohol (Aldridge et al., 2017; Madras et al., 2009), some experimental trials failed to detect reductions in use of substances other than alcohol (Bogenschutz et al., 2014, Saitz, 2014). A recent trial reported promising results for SBIRT to reduce opioid use. D'Onofrio and colleagues (2017) randomized individuals experiencing opioid use disorders to receive either SBIRT, SBIRT plus buprenorphine, or referral only. The combination of SBIRT and buprenorphine resulted in higher treatment initiation (74% vs. 53% for referral only) and fewer days of opioid use at two months.

Socioeconomic status

Although early studies critiqued the lack of economic diversity in SBIRT outcome trials, recent research has shown that SBIRT can work across multiple strata. Yet, additional research is needed, because mixed findings have emerged. For example, Sahker, Lancianese, Jones, and Arndt (2018) observed pre-post reductions in risky alcohol use among patients served at federally qualified health centers. Conversely, Davis, Smith, and Briley's meta-analysis (2017) concluded that brief interventions were less effective if samples included a high proportion of non-college attending young adults. Additionally, studies including large proportions of participants earning lower incomes (63% earned $0–15,000) reported null findings (Bogenschutz et al., 2014). However, Bogenschutz et al. (2014) studied drug use as a primary outcome, so it is unclear if null findings are due to SES, substance type, or the interaction between these two variables.

Gender

Whether gender moderates SBIRT outcomes remains debatable. While some studies reported males benefited more than females (Kaner et al., 2007), other meta-analyses (Ballesteros, Gonzalez-Pinto, Querejeta, & Arino, 2004; Kaner et al., 2018; Whitlock, Polen, Green, Orleans, & Klein, 2004) concluded that gender was not a moderator of treatment effectiveness. In another study (Reinhardt et al., 2008), women experienced a more significant reduction in alcohol use then men. All studies were limited to alcohol use outcomes.

Several studies exclusively focused on women. Velasquez and colleagues' (2017) randomized trial demonstrated that SBIRT models can reduce the number of both alcohol and tobacco exposed pregnancies. This same team also reported that SBIRT can increase rates of testing for sexually transmitted infection among adolescent females (Chacko et al., 2010). Begun, Rose, and Lebel (2011) reported greater reductions in women's risky alcohol use two months after incarceration when screening and brief intervention were provided during preparation for community reentry compared to no such intervention. Further, and consistent with Glass et al.'s meta-analysis (2015), these results were not due to receiving further specialized treatment after getting SBIRT. Thus, tailored SBIRT approaches, designed specifically for females, have been developed and implemented in a variety of settings, addressing multiple target behaviors.

Special populations

Although much of the initial evidence for SBIRT comes from studies in healthcare settings, there is a small but growing literature on its application in other settings. For example, specialized interventions have been designed for combat veterans returning home from active duty (Harris & Yu, 2019), individuals in the criminal justice system (Begun et al., 2011; Lerch, Walters, Tang, & Taxman, 2017; Prendergast, McCollister, & Warda, 2017), adolescents (Mitchell et al., 2013; Ozechowski, Becker, & Hogue, 2016), and youth identifying as transgender (Dentato et al., 2019). Although SBIRT's effectiveness is well-established, ample room exist for generalizing findings to special populations.

Summary

Voluminous research exists on the effectiveness of SBIRT. In the coming years, greater attention needs directing to answer whether SBIRT will work effectively as a stand-alone treatment of drug misuse other than alcohol, what the optimal length of SBIRT interventions may be, and whether SBIRT will be effective in settings where individuals from low-socioeconomic backgrounds seek treatment.

Training social workers on SBIRT

Social workers will likely assume increasing roles in disseminating SBIRT practices. As previously mentioned, one large SAMHSA initiative funded multiple curriculum development projects targeting social work students. Furthermore, some advocate increased use of SBIRT by social workers as part of the Social Work Grand Challenges initiative (Begun & Clapp, 2016). Increased SBIRT training in social work training programs is evident, with a full special issue dedicated to this theme in a 2019 special issue of the *Journal of Social Work Practice in the Addictions* (Volume 19, issues 1–2).

Unlike large randomized training studies for Motivational Interviewing, to our knowledge there are no randomized trials testing SBIRT training outcomes among social work students. Studies of MI skills development among practitioners have primarily focused on the extent to which coaching, and supervision is needed after initial workshop training (Miller & Mount, 2001; Miller, Yahne, Moyers, Martinez, & Pirritano, 2004). Notably, these studies find that coaching and feedback enhance outcomes, and that students of MI typically overrate their skills compared to neutral observers (Miller et al., 2004). This implies that corrective feedback from individuals well-versed in SBIRT may be required for trainees to master the intervention.

Major issues in designing SBIRT training programs for social work students include: whether it is important to engage outside actors as standardized patients (Sacco et al., 2017), the effective use of computer simulations in training (Hitchcock, King, Johnson, Cohen, & Mcpherson, 2019; Smith, Egizio, Bennett, Windsor, & Clary, 2018), and establishing continuity between coursework and field practice experiences (Egizio, Smith, Bennett, Campbell, & Windsor, 2019). Training outcome studies inform these issues and offer recommendations for training program design and future research.

SBIRT training outcome studies in social work

We identified only two studies of SBIRT learning outcomes for social work students. This review exclusively focused on studies reporting observed skills rather than self-reported knowledge gains, because individuals tend to overestimate their skill level (Miller et al., 2004) at delivering interventions. Sacco et al. (2017) delivered a 15-hour, one-credit course to 83 MSW students that included didactic sessions, role plays, and pre–post videotaped standardized patient (SP) interactions. They evaluated SBIRT knowledge, self-reported practice behaviors, and confidence at pretest, 30 days, and six months post training. MSW students demonstrated increased adherence to SBIRT behaviors measured by standardized patient interviews. Self-reported knowledge, skills, and confidence also increased.

Smith and colleagues (2018) reported pre-post findings for both BSW and MSW students. SBIRT training was implemented with 55 BSW and MSW students in three different courses, with content hours varying in each course. Unlike the Sacco et al. study (2017), student outcomes were measured by in-class role plays with other students evaluated by coders blinded to pretest or post-test status. Both BSW MSW students showed pre-post gains in SBIRT skills in increasing amounts as contact hours increased.

Summary and training recommendations

Although these studies report positive findings, they did not implement randomized control designs; Smith et al. (2018) reported interim results from a randomized controlled trial without reporting results by condition assignment. Additionally, student learning outcomes are measured in role plays with standardized patients or other students. A major methodological advance in this research would involve measuring SBIRT performance with real clients. Nevertheless, these studies show positive results that appear robust to different student populations (BSW vs. MSW), teaching methods (e.g. integration of simulations), and training course length.

It is premature to know what factors drive student learning outcomes, given the very small set of SBIRT training studies. Based on this small narrative review, some areas deserve future attention. First, it is important to know to what degree coaching and feedback will enhance student learning outcomes. Providing coaching and feedback require instructors with SBIRT expertise and may be time-consuming for larger classrooms. Pringle, Kowalchuk, Meyers, and Seale (2012) discussed the need for trained faculty to verify students' SBIRT competency in a medical resident training program. Along similar lines, it is important to know if computer simulation training could be a viable, economical, effective substitute for in-person coaching and feedback. It would be interesting to know what combinations of simulation training and live training might produce the best and most cost-efficient student learning outcomes. Smith and colleagues (2018) described a randomized controlled trial protocol where they will compare SBIRT training-as-usual to training-as-usual plus computer simulation training to inform the value added from simulation trainings, since commercially available simulations incur a per capita cost. Finally, more attention could focus on how to best combine field experiences with initial SBIRT coursework training. Egizio and colleagues (2019) discussed a SBIRT certificate program that combines coursework training with completion of fieldwork at an SBIRT-approved site (e.g. SBIRT trained supervisor, number of required SBIRT practice hours, case presentation).

Conclusions

SBIRT has come of age in integrated care facilities, mainly located in primary health care organizations (see Chapter 27). Less is known about its use in non-medical settings where social workers are employed. Social workers practice in settings where the base rates of substance use are higher than in the general population (e.g. criminal justice, intimate partner violence services, child welfare): implementing routine screening and systematic feedback could have a large public health impact. This chapter provided an overview of the development of

SBIRT as a viable brief treatment option for addressing substance misuse and early identification of risky substance use or substance use disorders. SBIRT has universal applications for settings outside of traditional substance use treatment programs. SBIRT has demonstrated effectiveness in a variety of settings with diverse populations; the future appears bright for continued expansion of SBIRT into more settings with even more diverse populations. Social workers and social work training programs may play a critical role in its dissemination, particularly to organizations outside of healthcare settings.

References

Agerwala, S. M., & McCance-Katz, E. F. (2012). Integrating screening, brief intervention, and referral to treatment (SBIRT) into clinical practice settings: A brief review. *Journal of Psychoactive Drugs, 44*(4), 307–317. doi:10.1080/02791072.2012.720169

Aldridge, A., Linford, R., & Bray, J. (2017). Substance use outcomes of patients served by a large US implementation of screening, brief intervention and treatment (SBIRT). *Addiction, 112*(supp. 2), 43–53.

Alvarez-Bueno, C., Rodriguez-Martin, B., Garicia-Ortiz, L., Gomez-Marcos, M. A., & Martinez-Vizcaino, V. (2015). Effectiveness of brief interventions in primary health care settings to decrease alcohol consumption by adult non-dependent drinkers: A systematic review of systematic reviews. *Preventive Medicine, 76*, 533–538. doi:10.1016/j.ypmed.2014.12.010

Babor, T. F., McRee, B. G., Kassebaum, P. A., Grimaldi, P. L., Ahmed, K., & Bray, J. (2007). Screening, brief intervention, and referral to treatment (SBIRT): Toward a public health approach to the management of substance abuse. *Substance Abuse, 28*(3), 7–30. doi:10.1300/J465v28n03_03

Barbosa, C., Cowell, A., Bray, J., & Aldridge, A. (2015). The cost-effectiveness of alcohol screening, brief intervention, and referral to treatment (SBIRT) in emergency and outpatient medical settings. *Journal of Substance Abuse Treatment, 53*, 1–8. doi:10.1016/j.jsat.2015.01.003

Barbosa, C., Cowell, A., Dowd, W., Landwehr, J., Aldridge, A., & Bray, J. (2017). The cost-effectiveness of brief intervention versus brief treatment of Screening, Brief Intervention and Referral to Treatment (SBIRT) in the United States. *Addiction, 112*(supp.2), 73–81. doi:10.1111/add.13658

Ballesteros, J., Gonzalez-Pinto, A., Querejeta, I., & Arino, J. (2004). Brief interventions for hazardous drinkers delivered in primary care are equally effective in men and women. *Addiction, 99*(1), 103–108. doi:10.1111/j.1360-0443.2004.00499.x

Begun, A. L., & Clapp, J. D. (2016). Reducing and preventing alcohol misuse and its consequences: A Grand Challenge for social work. *The International Journal of Alcohol and Drug Research, 5*(2), 73–83. doi:10.7895/ijadr.v5i2.223

Begun, A. L., Rose, S. J., & Lebel, T. P. (2011). Intervening with women in jail around alcohol and substance abuse during preparation for community reentry. *Alcoholism Treatment Quarterly, 29*(4), 453–478. doi:10.1080/07347324.2011.608333

Bogenschutz, M. P., Donovan, D. M., Mandler, R. N., Perl, H. I., Forcehimes, A. A., Crandall, C., . . . Lyons, M. S. (2014). Brief intervention for patients with problematic drug use presenting in emergency departments: A randomized clinical trial. *JAMA Internal Medicine, 174*(11), 1736–1745. doi:10.1001/jamainternmed.2014.4052

Caviness, C. M., Hatgis, C., Anderson, B. J., Rosengard, C., Kiene, S. M., Friedman, P. D., & Stein, M. D. (2009). Three brief alcohol screens for detecting hazardous drinking in incarcerated women. *Journal of Studies on Alcohol and Drugs, 70*(1), 50–54. doi:10.15288/jsad.2009.70.50

Chacko, M. R., Wiemann, C. M., Kozinetz, C. A., von Sternberg, K., Velasquez, M. M., Smith, P. B., & DiClemente, R. (2010). Efficacy of a motivational behavioral intervention to promote chlamydia and gonorrhea screening in young women: A randomized controlled trial. *Journal of Adolescent Health, 46*(2), 152–161. doi:10.1016/j.jadohealth.2009.06.012

Davis, J. P., Smith, D. C., & Briley, D. A. (2017). Substance use prevention and treatment outcomes for emerging adults in non-college settings: A meta-analysis. *Psychology of Addictive Behaviors, 31*(3), 242–254. doi:10.1037/adb0000267

Dawson, D. A., Grant, B. F., & Li, T. K. (2005). Quantifying the risks associated with exceeding recommended drinking limits. *Alcoholism: Clinical and Experimental Research, 29*(5), 902–908. doi:10.1097/01.ALC.0000164544.45746.A7

Dentato, M. P., Ortiz, R., Orwat, J., Kelly, B. L., Gates, T. G., Propper, E. (2019) Peer-based education and use of the SBIRT model in unique settings with transgender young adults. *Journal of Social Work Practice in the Addictions, 19*(1–2), 139–157. doi:10.1080/1533256X.2019.1589884

D'Onofrio, G., Chawarski, M. C., O'Connor, P. G., Pantalon, M. V., Busch, S. H., Owens, P. H., . . . Fiellin, D. A. (2017). Emergency department-initiated buprenorphine for opioid dependence with continuation in primary care: Outcomes during and after intervention. *Journal of General Internal Medicine, 32*(6), 660–666. doi:10.1007/s11606-017-3993-2

Egizio, L. L., Smith, D. C., Bennett, K., Campbell, C., & Windsor, L. (2019). Field supervision training for a Screening Brief Intervention and Referral to Treatment (SBIRT) implementation project. *Clinical Social Work Journal, 47*, 53–60. doi:10.1007/s10615-018-0686-1

Glass, J. E., Hamilton, A. M., Powell, B. J., Perron, B. E., Brown, R. T., & Ilgen, M. A. (2015). Specialty substance use disorder services following brief alcohol intervention: A meta-analysis of randomized controlled trials. *Addiction, 110*(9), 1404–1415. doi:10.1111/add.12950

Harris, B. R., & Yu, J. (2019). Service access and self-reporting: Tailoring SBIRT to active duty military in civilian health care settings. *Journal of Social Work Practice in the Addictions, 19*(1–2), 177–187. doi:10.1080/1533256x.2019.1589886

Hitchcock, L. I., King, D. M., Johnson, K., Cohen, H., & Mcpherson, T. L. (2019). Learning outcomes for adolescent SBIRT simulation training in social work and nursing education. *Journal of Social Work Practice in the Addictions, 1–2*, 47–56. doi:10.1080/1533256X.2019.1591781

Horn, B. P., Crandall, C., Forcehimes, A., French, M. T., & Bogenschutz, M. (2017). Benefit-cost analysis of SBIRT interventions for substance using patients in emergency departments. *Journal of Substance Abuse Treatment, 79*, 6–11. doi:10.1016/j.jsat.2017.05.003

Kaner, E. F. S., Beyer, F., Dickinson, H. O., Pienaar, E., Campbell, F., Schlesinger, C., . . . Burnand, B. (2007). Effectiveness of brief alcohol interventions in primary care populations. *Cochrane Database of Systematic Reviews, 2*, 4–96. Art. No.: CD004148. doi:10.1002/14651858.CD004148.pub3.

Kaner, E. F., Beyer, F., Muirhead, C., Campbell, F., Pienaar, E. D., . . . Burnand, B. (2018). Effectiveness of brief alcohol interventions in primary care populations. *Cochrane Database of Systematic Reviews, 2*. Art. No.: CD004148. doi:10.1002/14651858.CD004148.pub4

Lerch, J., Walters, S., Tang, L., & Taxman, F. (2017). Effectiveness of a computerized motivational intervention on treatment initiation and substance use: Results from a randomized trial. *Journal of Substance Abuse Treatment, 80*, 59–66. doi:10.1016/j.jsat.2017.07.002

Madras, B. K., Compton, W. M., Avula, D., Stegbauer, T., Stein, J. B., & Clark, H. W. (2009). Screening, brief interventions, referral to treatment (SBIRT) for illicit drug and alcohol use at multiple healthcare sites: Comparison at intake and 6 months later. *Drug and Alcohol Dependence, 99*(1–3), 280–295. doi:10.1016/j.drugalcdep.2008.08.003

Magill, M., Apodaca, T. R., Borsari, B., Gaume, J., Hoadley, A., Gordon, R. E., . . . Moyers, T. (2018). A meta-analysis of motivational interviewing process: Technical, relational, and conditional process models of change. *Journal of Consulting and Clinical Psychology, 86*(2), 140–157. doi:10.1037/ccp0000250

Miller, W. R., & Mount, K. A. (2001). A small study of training in motivational interviewing: Does one workshop change clinician and client behavior? *Behavioural and Cognitive Psychotherapy, 29*(4), 457–471. doi:10.1017/S1352465801004064

Miller, W. R., & Moyers, T. B. (2006). Eight stages in learning motivational interviewing. *Journal of Teaching in the Addictions, 5*(1), 3–17. doi:10.1300/J188v05n01_02

Miller, W. R., & Rollnick, S. (2009). Ten things that motivational interviewing is not. *Behavioural and Cognitive Psychotherapy, 37*(2), 129–140. doi:10.1017/S1352465809005128

Miller, W. R., & Rollnick, S. (2012). *Motivational interviewing: Helping people change.* London: Guilford Press.

Miller, W. R., & Rose, G. S. (2015). Motivational interviewing and decisional balance: Contrasting responses to client ambivalence. *Behavioural and Cognitive Psychotherapy, 43*(2), 129–141. doi:10.1017/S1352465813000878

Miller, W. R., Yahne, C. E., Moyers, T. B., Martinez, J., & Pirritano, M. (2004). A randomized trial of methods to help clinicians learn motivational interviewing. *Journal of Consulting and Clinical Psychology, 72*(6), 1050. doi:10.1037/0022-006X.72.6.1050

Mitchell, S. G., Gryczynski, J., O'Grady, K. E., & Schwartz, R. P. (2013). SBIRT for adolescent drug and alcohol use: Current status and future directions. *Journal of Substance Abuse Treatment, 44*(5), 463–472. doi:10.1016/j.jsat.2012.11.005

Moyers, T. B., Manuel, J. K., & Ernst, D. (2015). *Motivational interviewing treatment integrity coding manual 4.1.2.* Retrieved from http://www.motivationalinterviewing.org/sites/default/files/miti4_2.pdf

O'Connor, E. A., Perdue, L. A., Senger, C. A., Rushkin, M., Patnode, C. D., Bean, S. I., & Jonas, D. E. (2018). Screening and behavioral counseling interventions to reduce unhealthy alcohol use in adolescents and adults: Updated evidence report and systematic review for the US Preventive Services Task Force. *JAMA, 320*(18), 1910–1928. doi:10.1001/jama.2018.12086

Office of the Surgeon General. (2016). *Facing addiction in America: The surgeon general's report on alcohol, drugs, and health.* Washington, DC: U.S. Department of Health and Human Services (HHS). Retrieved from https://addiction.surgeongeneral.gov/sites/default/files/surgeon-generals-report.pdf

Ozechowski, T., Becker, S., & Hogue, A. (2016). SBIRT-A: Adapting SBIRT to maximize developmental fit for adolescents in primary care. *Journal of Substance Abuse Treatment, 62,* 28–37. doi:10.1016/j.jsat.2015.10.006

Pilowsky, D. J., & Wu, L. T. (2012). Screening for alcohol and drug use disorders among adults in primary care: A review. *Substance Abuse and Rehabilitation, 3,* 25–34. doi:10.2147/SAR.S30057

Prendergast, M. L., McCollister, K., & Warda, U. (2017). A randomized study of the use of screening, brief intervention, and referral to treatment (SBIRT) for drug and alcohol use with jail inmates. *Journal of Substance Abuse Treatment, 74,* 54–64. doi: 10.1016/j.jsat.2016.12.011

Pringle, J. L., Kowalchuk, A., Meyers, J. A., & Seale, J. P. (2012). Equipping residents to address alcohol and drug abuse: The national SBIRT residency training project. *Journal of Graduate Medical Education, 4*(1), 58–63. doi:10.4300/JGME-D-11-00019.1

Reinhardt, S., Bischof, G., Grothues, J., John, U., Meyer, C., & Rumpf, H. J. (2008). Gender differences in the efficacy of brief interventions with a stepped care approach in general practice patients with alcohol-related disorders. *Alcohol and Alcoholism, 43*(3), 334–340. doi:10.1093/alcalc/agn004

Rubak, S., Sandbæk, A., Lauritzen, T., & Christensen, B. (2005). Motivational interviewing: A systematic review and meta-analysis. *British Journal of General Practice, 55*(513), 305–312.

Sacco, P., Ting, L., Crouch, T. B., Emery, L., Moreland, M., Bright, C., . . . DiClemente, C. (2017). SBIRT training in social work education: Evaluating change using standardized patient simulation. *Journal of Social Work Practice in the Addictions, 17*(1–2), 150–168. doi:10.1080/1533256X.2017.1302886

Sahker, E., Lancianese, D. A., Jones, D., & Arndt, S. (2018). Screening, brief intervention, and referral to treatment demonstrates effectiveness in reducing drinking in a Midwest American service sample. *International Journal of Mental Health and Addiction, 13*(1), 1–11. doi:10.1007/s11469-018-9953-1

Saitz, R. (2014). Screening and brief intervention for unhealthy drug use: Little or no efficacy. *Frontiers in Psychiatry, 5,* 121–126. doi:10.3389/fpsyt.2014.00121

Satre, D. D., Manuel, J. K., Larios, S., Steiger, S., & Satterfield, J. (2015). Cultural adaptation of Screening, Brief Intervention and Referral to Treatment using motivational interviewing. *Journal of Addiction Medicine, 9*(5), 352–357. doi:10.1097/ADM.0000000000000149

Saunders, J. B., Aasland, O. G., Babor, T. F., De la Fuente, J. R., & Grant, M. (1993). Development of the alcohol use disorders identification test (AUDIT): WHO collaborative project on early detection of persons with harmful alcohol consumption-II. *Addiction, 88*(6), 791–804. doi:10.1111/j.1360-0443.1993.tb02093.x

Smith, D. C., Bennett, K. M., Dennis, M. L., & Funk, R. R. (2017). Sensitivity and specificity of the gain short screener for predicting substance use disorders in a large national sample of emerging adults. *Addictive Behaviors, 68,* 14–17. doi:10.1016/j.addbeh.2017.01.013

Smith, D. C., Egizio, L. L., Bennett, K., Windsor, L. C., & Clary, K. (2018). Teaching empirically supported substance use interventions in social work: Navigating instructional methods and accreditation standards. *Journal of Social Work Education, 54*(suppl. 1), S90–S102. doi:10.1080/10437797.2018.1434438

Tanner-Smith, E. E., & Lipsey, M. W. (2015). Brief alcohol interventions for adolescents and young adults: A systematic review and meta-analysis. *Journal of Substance Abuse Treatment, 51,* 1–18. doi:10.1016/j.jsat.2014.09.001

Substance Abuse and Mental Health Services Administration (SAMHSA). (2018). *Key substance use and mental health indicators in the United States: Results from the 2017 National survey on drug use and health (HHS Publication No. SMA 18–5068, NSDUH Series H-53).* Rockville, MD: Center for Behavioral Health Statistics and Quality, Substance Abuse and Mental Health Services Administration. Retrieved from https://www.samhsa.gov/data/

Substance Abuse and Mental Health Services Administration. (2019). *TI-15-001 Individual Grant Awards.* Retrieved from https://www.samhsa.gov/grants/awards/2015/TI-15-001.

United Nations Office on Drugs and Crime (UNODC). (2018). *World drug report 2018.* Retrieved from https://www.unodc.org/wdr2018/

Van Hook, S., Harris, S. K., Brooks, T., Carey, P., Kossack, R., Kulig, J., . . . New England Partnership for Substance Abuse Research. (2007). The "Six T's": Barriers to screening teens for substance abuse in primary care. *Journal of Adolescent Health, 40*(5), 456–461. doi:10.1016/j.jadohealth.2006.12.007

Velasquez, M. M., von Sternberg, K. L., Floyd, R. L., Parrish, D., Kowalchuk, A., Stephens, N. S., . . . Mullen, P. D. (2017). Preventing alcohol and tobacco exposed pregnancies: CHOICES plus in primary care. *American Journal of Preventive Medicine, 53*(1), 85–95. doi:10.1016/j.amepre.2017.02.012

Whiteford, H. A., Degenhardt, L., Rehm, J., Baxter, A. J., Ferrari, A. J., Erskine, H. E., . . . Burstein, R. (2013). Global burden of disease attributable to mental and substance use disorders: Findings from the Global Burden of Disease Study 2010. *The Lancet, 382*(9904), 1575–1586. doi:10.1016/S0140-6736(13)61611-6

Whitlock, E., Polen, M., Green, C., Orleans, T., & Klein, J. (2004). Behavioral counseling interventions in primary care to reduce risky/harmful alcohol use by adults: A summary of the evidence for the U.S. Preventive Services Task Force. *Annals of Internal Medicine, 140,* 557–568. doi:10.7326/0003-4819-140-7-200404060-00017

Wood, A. M., Kaptoge, S., Butterworth, A. S., Willeit, P., Warnakula, S., Bolton, T., . . . Bell, S. (2018). Risk thresholds for alcohol consumption: Combined analysis of individual-participant data of 599 912 current drinkers in 83 prospective studies. *The Lancet, 391*(10129), 1513–1523. doi:10.1016/S0140-6736(18)30134-X

Yuma-Guerrero, P. J., Lawson, K. A., Velasquez, M. M., Von Sternberg, K., Maxson, T., & Garcia, N. (2012). Screening, brief intervention, and referral for alcohol use in adolescents: A systematic review. *Pediatrics, 130*(1), 115–122. doi:10.1542/peds.2011-1589

Zorland, J. L., Gilmore, D., Johnson, J. A., Borgman, R., Emshoff, J., Akin, J., . . . Kuperminc, G. P. (2018). Effects of substance use screening and brief intervention on health-related quality of life. *Quality of Life Research, 27,* 2329–2336. doi:10.1007/s11136-018-1899-z

Mindfulness practices in addictive behavior prevention, treatment, and recovery

Marjorie N. Edguer and Leigh Taylor

Background

Mindfulness techniques, such as meditation and yoga, have long-standing associations with numerous spiritual practices, among them Buddhism, Jainism, Hinduism, Sikhism, Taoism, Judaism, Christianity, and Islam. These centuries-old practices have evolved to inform modern-day secular frameworks and scientific intervention models (Kabat-Zinn & Hanh, 2009; Marlatt & Gordon, 1985). Mindfulness and its associated techniques have been incorporated into therapeutic interventions and applied to a range of biopsychosocial problems (Burke, 2010; Chiesa & Serretti, 2014; Roos, Bowen, Witkiewitz, 2017).

Studied worldwide, the popularity of mindfulness has grown rapidly in the decades since its identification as a psychological and medical tool (Chiesa & Serretti, 2014; Garland, Roberts-Lewis, Tronnier, Graves, & Kelley, 2016; Imani, Vahid, Gharraee, Noroozi, Habibi, & Bowen, 2015; Lee, Bowen & An-Fu, 2011; Roos, Bowen & Witkiewitz, 2017). Research supporting mindfulness-based interventions (MBIs) has shown significant benefits in reducing cravings, post-traumatic symptoms, and negative affect with individuals experiencing addictive behaviors (Cavicchioli, Movalli, & Maffei, 2018; Chiesa & Serretti, 2014). MBIs are routinely applied in settings such as outpatient and residential/inpatient treatment programs, schools, as well as in jails and/or prisons (Chiesa & Serretti, 2014); and MBIs have been crafted for populations spanning the life-course, with curriculum protocols combining techniques of mindfulness with other proven forms of medical and behavioral treatment, including medicinal and medical interventions, individual, group ,and family therapy (Priddy et al., 2018; Zullig et al., 2018).

This chapter recognizes and explores models and methods of MBI as applied to substance use disorders (SUDs) and addictive behaviors, the research regarding their efficacy, resources for social workers, and future directions for research and practice. While mindfulness refers to a wide variety of practices, this chapter focuses on the more structured mindfulness practices, such as Mindfulness-Based Stress Reduction (MBSR) and Mindfulness-Based Relapse Prevention (MBRP).

Marjorie N. Edguer and Leigh Taylor

Defining relevant terms

Meditation

While meditation has various meanings, here we refer to focused attention. Attention may be focused on a specific aspect of experience (e.g. breath or sensation), or an object, thought, visualization, or mantra (Marlatt, 2002). The goal is training attention and awareness to achieve a calm state. Meditation may also refer to a formal seated practice of focusing attention.

Mindfulness

There are two primary components to mindfulness: (1) being present in and attending to the moment, and (2) being accepting and non-judgmental of that experience (Kabat-Zinn, 1982). This includes social workers being present and focused on the clients with whom they are working, actively attending to clients, and awareness of how clients are responding to them and how they are responding to their clients.

Yoga

Yoga is a meditation practice involving physical activity and postures, breathing techniques, and concentration. Stemming from Hindu philosophical principles, yoga has developed multiple forms over time (e.g. Bikram, Ashtanga, Hatha, etc.) becoming a more secular practice, but one still rooted in attending to the mind-body connection (De Michelis, 2008).

Mindfulness-based interventions (MBIs)

MBIs are mindfulness-based interventions. Structured, manualized mindfulness-based psychotherapeutic interventions include Mindfulness-Based Stress Reduction (MBSR), Mindfulness-Based Cognitive Therapy (MBCT), and Mindfulness-Based Relapse Prevention (MBRP); a range of non-manualized and non-standardized MBI variants exist, as well.

History of mindfulness and addictive behavior

Mindfulness as a therapeutic modality or theoretical approach for social work has multiple roots beginning during the latter half of the 20th century. During the 1970s, multiple pioneers explored the use of meditation and mindfulness to support individuals struggling with a range of psychological issues (Benson & Wallace, 1972; Carrington & Ephron, 1975; Marlatt, Pagano, Rose, & Marques, 1984). These early studies included examining the effects of transcendental meditation (TM) on the drinking habits of individuals over time. Results indicated that when compared with a control group, individuals who routinely utilized TM experienced a significant reduction in alcohol consumption (Benson & Wallace, 1972; Shafii, Levy, & Jaffe, 1975). A significant by-product was that participants engaging in TM also reported less anxiety and stress (Marlatt, 1976). Researchers hypothesized that mindfulness practices, like meditation, were acting as positive coping mechanisms in the face of environmental and internal stressors, and that these techniques were contributing to a reduction in substance use (Marlatt, et al., 1984).

Building on these early evaluations, and often acknowledged as being among the first to develop manualized MBIs, were Jon Kabat-Zinn and Alan Marlatt, whose research has informed multiple present-day substance use recovery and relapse prevention models (Chiesa & Serretti, 2014). Dr. Kabat-Zinn, trained in the ways of Buddhism, focused on stress and mindfulness (Kabat-Zinn & Hanh, 2009), while Dr. Marlatt focused on mindfulness as a means of treatment and relapse prevention for addictive behaviors (Marlatt & Gordon, 1985). Their work presented an opportunity for social workers and other mental health care providers to incorporate mindfulness practices in supporting client recovery.

As the evidence base supporting the use of mindfulness has grown, practitioners have increasingly incorporated structured approaches to mindfulness, such as MBSR, MBCT, and MBRP, as well as other practices without the requisite consistency, full range of practices/ skills, or ongoing development of practices/skills. Online resources have emerged, including YouTube videos, and smartphone "apps" have been developed using mindfulness techniques.

Mindfulness-based interventions and addictive behavior

Numerous manualized treatment protocols exist for MBIs and their application as programs of prevention, early intervention, and treatment for individuals managing addictive behaviors (Chiesa & Serretti, 2014; Garland et al., 2016; Imani et al., 2015; Lee et al., 2011; Ross et al., 2017). Manualized interventions have distinct benefits, including more consistent implementation and clearer replicability, as well as wider dissemination and support for the use of empirically tested interventions by a broader range of providers.

Prevention and early intervention

Mindfulness approaches for children, adolescents, and emerging adults are described.

Childhood

Various pre-school and elementary school-based prevention programs embed mindfulness techniques focused on increasing emotional regulation, positive coping skills, and proactive decision making (Campbell, Lanthier, Weiss, & Shaine, 2019; Raes, Griffith, Van der Gucht, & Williams, 2014; Rempel, 2012; Semple & Burke, 2012). These curricula foster development of a generic skill set attending to the "present" lived experience as a means of improving current (proximal) academic, social, and psychological functioning. Prevention programs with preschool and elementary age children apply a range of mindfulness activities: yoga (Galantino, Galbavy, & Quinn, 2008; Mendelson, Greenberg, Dariotis, Gould, Rhoades, & Leaf, 2010), tai chi (Wall, 2005), breathing exercises, and guided meditation (Rempel, 2012). The prevention premise assumes that using mindfulness to regulate emotions not only improves present functioning but decreases future (distal) risky health behaviors).

Research demonstrated that youth who are better able to regulate emotions are less likely to develop substance use disorders during adolescence and/or adulthood (Broderick & Jennings, 2012; Rempel, 2012; Willis, Walker, Mendoza, & Ainette, 2006). While studies demonstrated benefits of mindfulness with general populations of children and short-term improvements in emotional regulation, attention, social skills, externalizing behaviors, anxiety, and depression (Campbell et al., 2019; Raes et al., 2014; Rempel, 2012; Semple & Burke, 2012), there exists a lack of longitudinal research concerning mindfulness program outcomes and their utility as a means of substance use or substance use disorder prevention.

Adolescence and early adulthood

MBI programs focused on middle or high school-aged youth are often part of an early intervention program, with a focus on at-risk adolescents engaged in substance use/misuse and/or other risky health behaviors, but who may not yet have a clinical SUD diagnosis (Davis et al., 2019; Himelstein & Saul 2015; Russell, Gillis, & Heppner, 2016). MBI curricula for adolescents and young adults broadly address impulsivity and decision making—encouraging the development of abstinence self-efficacy and an ability to decline substance use when facing specific stressor scenarios (Davis et al., 2019; Riggs, Greenberg, & Devorka, 2019).

Treatment and relapse prevention models

Mindfulness provides tools to address the cravings and ruminating thoughts often associated with addictive behaviors, directed at delaying or allaying impulsive and/or conditioned actions (Bowen et al., 2006). Bowen and Marlatt (2009) referred to using mindfulness to manage cravings as "surfing the urge," or being able to follow the ebb and flow of craving, seeing it as a temporary sensation that changes and does not have to be acted on (p. 666). Attending to moment of craving by employing a variety of mindfulness techniques is the basis for many of the MBIs developed for addictive behaviors: changing the experience to being aware of a passing thought, emotion, or sensation, rather than a precursor of future action/relapse (Bowen & Marlatt, 2009; Rempel, 2012; Roos, Stein, Bowen, & Witkiewitz, 2019). Several models warrant closer examination.

Mindfulness-based stress reduction (MBSR)

MBSR has been utilized for both SUD and addictive behavior treatment and subsequent relapse prevention (Black, 2014; Davis et al., 2019; Vallejo & Amaro, 2009). MBSR is derived from Buddhist meditation, and includes aspects of meditation and yoga, but specifically applies a mindfulness emphasis: observing and being aware of thoughts and sensations in the moment (Kabat-Zinn, 1982). MBSR is an eight-week psychoeducational program with weekly group training and daily homework, and a full-day retreat between weeks 6 and 7. While originally developed for addressing chronic physical and psychological problems, it has been standardized for use with populations dealing with addictive behaviors (Black, 2014; Davis et al., 2019; Vallejo & Amaro, 2009). MBSR includes formal mindfulness meditations, like body scans, yoga, sitting and walking meditation, as well as informal mindfulness activities, like breath awareness and awareness of daily activities (e.g. toothbrushing or eating).

Mindfulness-based cognitive therapy (MBCT)

MBCT is another 8-week program with weekly group meetings and a full-day retreat, involving extensive homework completed by clients outside of group meetings. MBCT grew out of MBSR, incorporating elements of cognitive behavioral therapy (CBT) for application with individuals diagnosed with depressive disorders (Teasdale, Segal, & Willams, 1995). MBCT is most commonly utilized for addictive behaviors among individuals dually diagnosed with depression, anxiety, or other mood disorders (Fortuna & Vallejo, 2015; Song & Park, 2019). An example of how CBT combines with mindfulness attends to how an individual can disengage from negative self-talk, which is often associated with substance use rumination (Fortuna & Vallejo, 2015). Benefits of MBCT indicate that participants experienced increased awareness about thoughts and emotions surrounding their substance use which leads to increased self-regulation and coping skills, as well as ability to manage cravings (Chiesa & Serretti, 2014). The Center for Mindfulness in Medicine, Health Care, and Society at UMass Medical School (https://www.umassmed.edu/cfm/mindfulness-based-programs/) provides training and resources related to both MBSR and MCBT, including global trainers in both models.

Acceptance and commitment therapy (ACT)

ACT is a contextual behavioral model that uses acceptance and values-directed strategies to encourage development of a participant's abstinence self-efficacy (Hayes, Luoma, Bond, Masudo, & Lillis, 2006). ACT asserts that only after mindfully acknowledging thoughts and "fully feeling" ones' emotions can participants focus on making choices congruent with their goals and values (Luoma, Kohlenberg, Hayes, Bunting, & Rye, 2008). Research has supported ACT as a promising treatment approach contributing to decreased substance use, with additional value as a means of reducing self-stigma and shame (Hayes et al., 2004; Luoma et al., 2008). ACT manuals and protocols are available from the Contextual Science website: (https://contextualscience.org/treatment_protocol_and_manuals).

Mindfulness-oriented recovery enhancement (MORE)

MORE combines mindfulness and cognitive behavioral therapy with the positive psychology principles of reappraisal, and savoring (Garland et al., 2016). Similar to other evidence-based interventions, MORE consists of ten weekly group sessions and homework. MORE has a specific focus on co-occurring trauma, common among individuals engaging in addictive behaviors, and specifically SUDs (Garland et al., 2016). Recent studies evaluating the effectiveness of MORE have shown decreased cravings and emotional distress (Garland, Gaylord, Boettiger, & Howard, 2010; Garland, Schwartz, Kelly, Whitt & Howard, 2012; Garland et al., 2016). MORE protocols and information are available on Dr. Garland's website (https://drericgarland.com/m-o-r-e/).

Mindfulness-based relapse prevention (MBRP)

MBRP, developed and manualized by Marlatt and colleagues (2004), is an eight-week standardized meditation program with group training and at-home practice. Marlatt and colleagues reported reduced cravings (Bowen et al., 2009, 2014), decreased suffering (Witkiewitz & Bowen, 2010), increased ability to cope with cravings despite experiencing a lot of emotional pain (Roos et al., 2017), and decreased substance use (Bowen et al., 2014). Researchers suggested that consistent, ongoing post-intervention support may be important to sustain benefits derived from treatment (Bowen et al., 2009). MBRP can be used in combination with other treatment programs, such as medically assisted treatment (MAT) to improve outcomes, decrease craving severity and negative mood, and increase abstinence (Zgierska et al., 2008). Resources for learning MBRP are available from the website and include recordings as well as a clinician manual (https://www.mindfulrp.com).

Additional options

Non-manualized approaches using mindfulness abound, but their benefits are difficult to confirm. These approaches include the use of brief mindful attention and gratitude exercises by practitioners, some of which have been tested in experimental conditions (Papies, Pronk, Keesman, & Barsalou, 2015). Papies and colleagues (2015) concluded that brief mindful activities modulate how individuals think and act in response to external cues. Study results concerning the impact of mindful attention on cravings are mixed, some showing no effect on cravings (Bowen & Marlatt, 2009) while others showed a decrease (Westbrook et al., 2013).

Emerging approaches in mindfulness and addictive behaviors

In addition to approaches supported by evidence, several are considered to still be emerging as evidence develops.

Pilot studies

Pilot studies of mindfulness-based interventions and their impact on long-term recovery or relapse prevention outcomes have demonstrated encouraging results. Davis and colleagues (2019) indicated that participation in an MBI lead to better outcomes over time, with individuals reporting lower substance use, stress, and craving six months after participating in MBRP (Davis et al., 2019). MBI was associated with fewer days of substance use, and fewer legal and medical problems at 15-week follow-up among a group of women involved in the criminal justice system (Witkiewitz et al., 2014).

Trauma-sensitive mindfulness practice (TSMP)

TSMP recognizes that many current MBIs are lacking trauma-informed practices, potentially exacerbating associated trauma symptomatology and often associated addictive behaviors (Treleaven, 2018). While mindfulness can be a powerful tool, there exists the potential for it to generate problems for individuals who have experienced trauma. Of special concern is the potential for individuals with traumatic experiences to dissociate while practicing meditation (Treleaven, 2018). TSMP has not been researched in populations experiencing addiction, but TSMP principles are important to keep in mind: staying within the window of tolerance (and helping clients gauge what that window is), supporting stability, keeping the body in mind (tuning in to potential dissociation), practicing in relationship, and being aware of the social context (Treleaven, 2018). TSMP fits with making mindfulness-based interventions for addiction trauma-informed.

Technology-based mindfulness interventions

Mindfulness-based interventions using the internet and smartphone applications have increased rapidly and are continuing to grow, presenting both opportunities and concerns (Ly et al., 2014; Spijkerman, Pots, & Bohlmeijer, 2016). Opportunities include their accessibility, portability, and use by individuals who otherwise find it difficult to access other mindfulness-based treatment and recovery options. Moreover, many are free or inexpensive, only needing access to the internet. Concerns include that they are offered by a range of providers, some of whom are untrained or self-trained, with the result being a lack of quality control or guidance regarding their safety or efficacy (Boettcher et al., 2014). While initial studies examining technology-based mindfulness interventions show promising results (Boettcher et al., 2014; Ly et al., 2014; Spijkerman et al., 2016), further empirical assessment of their effectiveness for addictive behaviors needs to be conducted.

Current and future approaches to the study of mindfulness-based interventions

Mindfulness-based interventions have been studied across disciplines, including neuroscience, medicine, psychology, addictions, counseling, and social work. For example, neuroscience has explored the effects of mindfulness on the brain using neuro-imaging to better understand the mechanisms through which mindfulness techniques produce change. Westbrook et al. (2013) identified reductions in neural craving, as well as self-reported craving, among individuals who smoked cigarettes. It is theorized that MBIs may affect neural systems, potentially repairing, reversing, or repairing addiction-related changes (Witkiewitz, Lustyk & Bowen, 2013).

International research has reported similar positive results with MBI. In Iran, MBI showed positive results compared to standard opioid treatment, with participants reporting increased non-judging and non-reacting, and decreased alcohol and opium use (Imani et al., 2015). In Taiwan, a study using an adapted version of MBRP with incarcerated persons who engaged in substance misuse reported decreases in negative mood (depression) and increases in negative expectancies regarding substance use (Lee et al., 2011). It is important to continue exploring the effectiveness of manualized interventions internationally and with non-English-speaking populations to evaluate the generalizability of study results.

There exist a range of research considerations regarding MBIs for addictive behaviors as the field moves forward. Manualized MBI evaluations should begin to account for implementation fidelity, including consistency in moderator training, curriculum modifications, adherence to timelines, number of group members, and more. It is also important to examine effectiveness of the varied MBIs with diverse populations, attending to age, culture, gender identification, setting, and specific addictive behaviors (e.g. substance of preference)—all factors impacting the generalizability of intervention research results.

Previous evaluations need to be supported through replication, and new studies could be expanded to include a variety of methodologies and designs. For example, preliminary quasi-experimental research suggests that MBI might work better for women, so while most randomized controlled trials (RCTs) have not found significant gender differences, these discrepancies would be important to explore further (Katz & Toner, 2013). Additionally, it will be vital to explore whether MBIs or singular mindfulness-based techniques, and online MBIs, delivered outside of the previously studied manualized group interventions are also effective. Finally, research about MBIs applied to addictive behaviors needs to include longitudinal studies, particularly testing the durability of outcomes over time.

Conclusions

Mindfulness-based Interventions have much to offer in preventing and addressing substance use disorders and other addictive behaviors. Research has demonstrated promising results of MBIs as models for early intervention, treatment, and relapse prevention, including lower rates of substance use, decreased craving, increased acceptance and awareness, and increased coping options. MBIs have proven effective when applied in conjunction with additional treatment modalities and with individuals managing co-morbid diagnoses, supporting the likelihood of long-term recovery. Although MBIs appear safe, it is important to assess participants for trauma and apply a trauma-informed lens when appropriate.

References

Benson, H., & Wallace, R. K. (1972). Decreased drug abuse with transcendental meditation: A study of 1,862 subjects. *Drug Abuse: Proceedings of the International Conference* (pp. 369–376). Philadelphia, PA: Lea & Febiger.

Black, D. S. (2014). Mindfulness-based interventions: An antidote to suffering in the context of substance use, misuse, and addiction. *Substance Use & Misuse, 49*(5), 487–491. doi:10.3109/10826084. 2014.860749

Boettcher, J., Åström, V., Påhlsson, D., Schenström, O., Andersson, G., & Carlbring, P. (2014). Internet-based mindfulness treatment for anxiety disorders: A randomized controlled trial. *Behavior Therapy, 45*(2), 241–253. doi:10.1016/j.beth.2013.11.003

Bowen, S., Chawla, N., Collins, S. E., Witkiewitz, K., Hsu, S., Grow, J., . . . Marlatt, A. (2009). Mindfulness-based relapse prevention for substance use disorders: A pilot efficacy trial. *Substance Abuse, 30*(4), 295–305. doi:10.1080/08897070903250084

Bowen, S., Witkiewitz, K., Clifasefi, S. L., Grow, J., Chawla, N., Hsu, S. H., . . . Larimer, M. E. (2014). Relative efficacy of mindfulness-based relapse prevention, standard relapse prevention, and treatment as usual for substance use disorders: A randomized clinical trial. *JAMA Psychiatry, 71*(5), 547–556. doi:10.1001/jamapsychiatry.2013.4546

Bowen, S., Witkiewitz, K., Dillworth, T. M., Chawla, N., Simpson, T. L., Ostafin, B. D., . . . Marlatt, G. A. (2006). Mindfulness meditation and substance use in an incarcerated population. *Psychology of Addictive Behaviors, 20*(3), 343. doi:10.1037/0893-164X.20.3.343

Broderick, P. C., & Jennings, P. A. (2012). Mindfulness for adolescents: A promising approach to supporting emotion regulation and preventing risky behavior. *New Directions for Youth Development, 136*, 111–126. doi:10.1002/yd.20042

Burke, C. A. (2010). Mindfulness-based approaches with children and adolescents: A preliminary review of current research in an emergent field. *Journal of Child and Family Studies, 19,* 133–144. doi:10.1007/s10826-009-9282-x.

Campbell, A. J., Lanthier, R. P., Weiss, B. A., & Shaine, M. D. (2019). The impact of a schoolwide mindfulness program on adolescent well-being, stress, and emotion regulation: A nonrandomized controlled study in a naturalistic setting. *Journal of Child and Adolescent Counseling*, 1–17. doi:10.108 0/23727810.2018.1556989

Carrington, P., & Ephron, H. S. (1975). Meditation and psychoanalysis. *Journal of the American Academy of Psychoanalysis, 3*(1), 43–57. doi:10.1521/jaap.1.1975.3.1.43

Cavicchioli, M., Movalli, M., & Maffei, C. (2018). The clinical efficacy of mindfulness-based treatments for alcohol and drug use disorders: A meta-analytic review of randomized and nonrandomized controlled trials. *European Addiction Research, 24*(3), 137–162.

Chiesa, A., & Serretti, A. (2014). Are mindfulness-based interventions effective for substance use disorders? A systematic review of the evidence. *Substance Use & Misuse, 49*(5), 492–512. doi:10.3109/ 10826084.2013.770027

Davis, J. P., Barr, N., Dworkin, E. R., Dumas, T. M., Berey, B., DiGuiseppi, G., & Cahn, B. R. (2019). Effect of mindfulness-based relapse prevention on impulsivity trajectories among young adults in residential substance use disorder treatment. *Mindfulness*, 1–13. doi:10.1007/ s12671-019-01164-0

De Michelis, E. (2008). Modern yoga: History and forms. In M. Singleton & J. Byrne (Eds.), *Yoga in the modern world: Contemporary perspectives* (pp. 29–47). London, UK: Routledge.

Fortuna, L. R., & Vallejo, Z. (2015). *Treating co-occurring adolescent PTSD and addiction: Mindfulness-based cognitive therapy for adolescents with trauma and substance-abuse disorders.* Oakland, CA: New Harbinger Publications.

Galantino, M. L., Galbavy, R., & Quinn, L. (2008). Therapeutic effects of yoga for children: A systematic review of the literature. *Pediatric Physical Therapy, 20*(1), 66–80. doi:10.1097/ PEP.0b013e31815f1208

Garland, E. L., Gaylord, S. A., Boettiger, C. A., & Howard, M. O. (2010). Mindfulness training modifies cognitive, affective, and physiological mechanisms implicated in alcohol dependence: Results of a randomized controlled pilot trial. *Journal of Psychoactive Drugs, 42*(2), 177–192. doi:10.1080/02 791072.2010.10400690

Garland, E. L., Manusov, E. G., Froeliger, B., Kelly, A., Williams, J. M., & Howard, M. O. (2014). Mindfulness-oriented recovery enhancement for chronic pain and prescription opioid misuse:

Results from an early-stage randomized controlled trial. *Journal of Consulting and Clinical Psychology, 82*(3), 448–459.

Garland, E. L., Roberts-Lewis, A., Tronnier, C. D., Graves, R., & Kelley, K. (2016). Mindfulness-oriented recovery enhancement versus CBT for co-occurring substance dependence, traumatic stress, and psychiatric disorders: Proximal outcomes from a pragmatic randomized trial. *Behaviour Research and Therapy, 77*, 7–16. doi:10.1037/a0035798

Garland, E. L., Schwarz, N. R., Kelly, A., Whitt, A., & Howard, M. O. (2012). Mindfulness-oriented recovery enhancement for alcohol dependence: Therapeutic mechanisms and intervention acceptability. *Journal of Social Work Practice in the Addictions, 12*(3), 242–263. doi:10.1016/j.brat.2015.11.012

Hayes, S. C., Luoma, J. B., Bond, F. W., Masuda, A., & Lillis, J. (2006). Acceptance and commitment therapy: Model, processes and outcomes. *Behaviour Research and Therapy, 44*(1), 1–25. doi:10.1016/j.brat.2005.06.006

Hayes, S. C., Wilson, K. G., Gifford, E. V., Bissett, R., Piasecki, M., Batten, S. V., . . . Gregg, J. (2004). A preliminary trial of twelve-step facilitation and acceptance and commitment therapy with polysubstance-abusing methadone-maintained opiate addicts. *Behavior Therapy, 35*(4), 667–688. doi:10.1016/S0005-7894(04)80014-5

Himelstein, S., & Saul, S. (2015). *Mindfulness-based substance abuse treatment for adolescents: A 12-session curriculum.* London, UK: Routledge. doi:10.4324/9781317607052

Imani, S., Vahid, M. K. A., Gharraee, B., Noroozi, A., Habibi, M., & Bowen, S. (2015). Effectiveness of mindfulness-based group therapy compared to the usual opioid dependence treatment. *Iranian Journal of Psychiatry, 10*(3), 175–184.

Kabat-Zinn, J. (1982). An outpatient program in behavioral medicine for chronic pain patients based on the practice of mindfulness meditation: Theoretical considerations and preliminary results. *General Hospital Psychiatry, 4*(1), 33–47. doi:10.1016/0163-8343(82)90026-3

Katz, D., & Toner, B. (2013). A systematic review of gender differences in the effectiveness of mindfulness-based treatments for substance use disorders. *Mindfulness, 4*(4), 318–331.

Lee, K. H., Bowen, S., & An-Fu, B. A. I. (2011). Psychosocial outcomes of mindfulness-based relapse prevention in incarcerated substance abusers in Taiwan: A preliminary study. *Journal of Substance Use, 16*(6), 476–483. doi:10.3109/14659891.2010.505999

Luoma, J. B., Kohlenberg, B. S., Hayes, S. C., Bunting, K., & Rye, A. K. (2008). Reducing self-stigma in substance abuse through acceptance and commitment therapy: Model, manual development, and pilot outcomes. *Addiction Research & Theory, 16*(2), 149–165. doi:10.1080/16066350701850295

Ly, K. H., Trüschel, A., Jarl, L., Magnusson, S., Windahl, T., Johansson, R., . . . Andersson, G. (2014). Behavioural activation versus mindfulness-based guided self-help treatment administered through a smartphone application: A randomised controlled trial. *BMJ Open, 4*(1), e003440. doi:10.1136/bmjopen-2013-003440

Marcus, M. T., Schmitz, J., Moeller, G., Liehr, P., Cron, S. G., Swank, P., . . . Granmayeh, L. K. (2009). Mindfulness-based stress reduction in therapeutic community treatment: A stage 1 trial. *The American Journal of Drug and Alcohol Abuse, 35*(2), 103–108. doi:10.1080/00952990902823079

Marlatt, G. A. (1976). Alcohol, stress, and cognitive control. In I. G. Sarason, & C.D. Spielberger, (Eds.), *Stress and anxiety* (Vol. 3, pp. 271–296). Washington, DC: Hemisphere Publishing Corp.

Marlatt, G. A. (2002). Buddhist philosophy and the treatment of addictive behavior. *Cognitive and Behavioral Practice, 9*(1), 44–50. doi:10.1016/S1077-7229(02)80039-6

Marlatt, G. A., & Gordon, J. R. (1985). *Relapse prevention.* New York, NY: Guilford Press.

Marlatt, G. A., Pagano, R. R., Rose, R. M., & Marques, J. K. (1984). Effects of meditation and relaxation training upon alcohol use in male social drinkers. In D. H. Shapiro & R. N. Walsh (Eds.), *Meditation: Classic and contemporary perspectives* (pp. 105–120). New York, NY: Aldine. doi:10.4324/9780203785843-16

Marlatt, G. A., Witkiewitz, K., Dillworth, T. M., Bowen, S. W., Parks, G. A., Macpherson, L. M., . . . Crutcher, R. (2004). Vipassana meditation as a treatment for alcohol and drug use disorders. In S. C. Hayes, V. M. Follette, & M. M. Linehan (Eds.), *Mindfulness and acceptance: Expanding the cognitive-behavioral tradition* (pp. 261–287). New York, NY: Guilford Press.

Mendelson, T., Greenberg, M. T., Dariotis, J. K., Gould, L. F., Rhoades, B. L., & Leaf, P. J. (2010). Feasibility and preliminary outcomes of a school-based mindfulness intervention for urban youth. *Journal of Abnormal Child Psychology, 38*(7), 985–994. doi:10.1007/s10802-010-9418-x

Papies, E. K., Pronk, T. M., Keesman, M., & Barsalou, L. W. (2015). The benefits of simply observing: Mindful attention modulates the link between motivation and behavior. *Journal of Personality and Social Psychology, 108*(1), 148–170. doi:10.1037/a0038032

Priddy, S. E., Howard, M. O., Hanley, A. W., Riquino, M. R., Friberg-Felsted, K., & Garland, E. L. (2018). Mindfulness meditation in the treatment of substance use disorders and preventing future relapse: Neurocognitive mechanisms and clinical implications. *Substance Abuse and Rehabilitation, 9*, 103. doi:10.2147/SAR.S145201

Raes, F., Griffith, J. W., Van der Gucht, K., & Williams, J. M. G. (2014). School-based prevention and reduction of depression in adolescents: A cluster-randomized controlled trial of a mindfulness group program. *Mindfulness, 5*(5), 477–486. doi:10.1007/s12671-013-0202-1

Rempel, K. (2012). Mindfulness for children and youth: A review of the literature with an argument for school-based implementation. *Canadian Journal of Counselling and Psychotherapy/Revue Canadienne de Counseling et de Psychothérapie, 46*(3), 1923–6182.

Riggs, N. R., Greenberg, M. T., & Dvorakova, K. (2019). A role for mindfulness and mindfulness training in substance use prevention. In Z. Sloboda, H. Petras, E. Robertson, & R. Hingson (Eds.), *Prevention of substance use* (pp. 335–346). New York, NY: Springer. doi:10.1007/978-3-030-00627-3_21

Roos, C. R., Bowen, S., & Witkiewitz, K. (2017). Baseline patterns of substance use disorder severity and depression and anxiety symptoms moderate the efficacy of mindfulness-based relapse prevention. *Journal of Consulting and Clinical Psychology, 85*(11), 1041-1051. doi:10.1037/ccp0000249

Roos, C. R., Stein, E., Bowen, S., & Witkiewitz, K. (2019). Individual gender and group gender composition as predictors of differential benefit from mindfulness-based relapse prevention for substance use disorders. *Mindfulness*, 1–8. doi:10.1007/s12671-019-01112-y

Russell, K. C., Gillis, H. L., & Heppner, W. (2016). An examination of mindfulness-based experiences through adventure in substance use disorder treatment for young adult males: A pilot study. *Mindfulness, 7*(2), 320–328. doi:10.1007/s12671-015-0441-4

Semple, R. J., & Burke, C. A. (2012). Mindfulness-based treatment for children and adolescents. In P. C. Kendall (Ed.), *Child and adolescent therapy: Cognitive-behavioral procedures* (4th ed., pp. 411–428). New York, NY: Guilford Press.

Shafii, M., Lavely, R., & Jaffe, R. (1976). Meditation and the prevention of alcohol abuse. *Alcohol Health & Research World, 1976*, 18–21.

Song, W. J., & Park, J. W. (2019). The influence of stress on Internet addiction: Mediating effects of self-control and mindfulness. *International Journal of Mental Health and Addiction*, 1–13. doi:10.1007/s11469-019-0051-9

Spijkerman, M. P. J., Pots, W. T. M., & Bohlmeijer, E. T. (2016). Effectiveness of online mindfulness-based interventions in improving mental health: A review and meta-analysis of randomised controlled trials. *Clinical Psychology Review, 45*, 102–114. doi:10.1016/j.cpr.2016.03.009

Teasdale, J. D., Segal, Z., & Williams, J. M. G. (1995). How does cognitive therapy prevent depressive relapse and why should attentional control (mindfulness) training help? *Behaviour Research and Therapy, 33*(1), 25–39. doi:10.1016/0005-7967(94)E0011-7

Treleaven, D. A. (2018). *Trauma-sensitive mindfulness: Practices for safe and transformative healing.* New York, NY: W.W. Norton & Company.

Vallejo, Z., & Amaro, H. (2009). Adaptation of mindfulness-based stress reduction program for addiction relapse prevention. *The Humanistic Psychologist, 37*(2), 192–206. doi:10.1080/08873260902892287

Wall, R. B. (2005). Tai chi and mindfulness-based stress reduction in a Boston public middle school. *Journal of Pediatric Health Care, 19*(4), 230–237. doi:10.1016/j.pedhc.2005.02.006

Westbrook, C., Creswell, J. D., Tabibnia, G., Julson, E., Kober, H., & Tindle, H. A. (2013). Mindful attention reduces neural and self-reported cue-induced craving in smokers. *Social Cognitive and Affective Neuroscience, 8*(1), 73–84. doi:10.1093/scan/nsr076

Witkiewitz, K., & Bowen, S. (2010). Depression, craving, and substance use following a randomized trial of mindfulness-based relapse prevention. *Journal of Consulting and Clinical Psychology, 78*(3), 362. doi:10.1037/a0019172

Witkiewitz, K., Lustyk, M. K. B., & Bowen, S. (2013). Retraining the addicted brain: A review of hypothesized neurobiological mechanisms of mindfulness-based relapse prevention. *Psychology of Addictive Behaviors, 27*(2), 351. doi:10.1037/a0029258

Witkiewitz, K., Warner, K., Sully, B., Barricks, A., Stauffer, C., Thompson, B. L., & Luoma, J. B. (2014). Randomized trial comparing mindfulness-based relapse prevention with relapse prevention for women offenders at a residential addiction treatment center. *Substance Use & Misuse, 49*(5), 536–546. doi:10.3109/10826084.2013.856922

Zgierska, A., Rabago, D., Zuelsdorff, M., Coe, C., Miller, M., & Fleming, M. (2008). Mindfulness meditation for alcohol relapse prevention: A feasibility pilot study. *Journal of Addiction Medicine, 2*(3), 165. doi:10.1097/ADM.0b013e31816f8546

Zullig, K. J., Lander, L. R., Sloan, S., Brumage, M. R., Hobbs, G. R., & Faulkenberry, L. (2018). Mindfulness-based relapse prevention with individuals receiving medication-assisted outpatient treatment for opioid use disorder. *Mindfulness, 9*(2), 423–429. doi:10.1007/s12671-017-0784-0

Working with children whose parents engage in substance misuse

Shulamith Lala Ashenberg Straussner and Christine H. Fewell

Background

The misuse of alcohol and other psychoactive drugs is a worldwide phenomenon whose impact on families and children is widely felt. According to the United Nations, about 275 million people worldwide, roughly 5.6% of the global population aged 15–64 years, used drugs at least once during 2016, while an estimated 31 million people experience drug use disorders, meaning their drug use is harmful to the point where they may need treatment (United Nations Office on Drugs and Crime, 2018). Many of these individuals are parents of young children. In the United States, data from the combined 2009 to 2014 National Surveys on Drug Use and Health indicated that about 12.3% of children aged 17 or younger resided with at least one parent experiencing a substance use disorder (SUD). More specifically, about 1 in 8 children (8.7 million) lived in households with at least one parent experiencing past-year alcohol, other drug, or both disorders, about 1 in 10 children (7.5 million) lived in households with at least one parent experiencing a past-year alcohol use disorder, and an estimated 1 in 35 children (2.1 million) lived in households with at least one parent experiencing a past-year illicit drug use disorder (Lipari & Van Horn, 2017). When examining the ages of children who lived with at least one parent experiencing a SUD, on average 1.5 million were aged 0–2 (12.8% of this age group), 1.4 million were aged 3–5 (12.1% of this age group), 2.8 million were aged 6–11 (11.8%), and the largest group, 3.0 million, were aged 12–17 (12.5%) (Lipari & Van Horn, 2017).

Numerous research studies consistently found that children whose parents experience SUD are at great risk for myriad problems which vary depending on numerous factors, in-cluding the child's age. These children are found in every socioeconomic, ethnic, religious, and racial group in the United States and abroad (Lander, Howsare, & Byrne, 2013; Messina, Calhoun, Conner, & Miller, 2015; Substance Abuse Mental Health Service Administration [SAMHSA], 2008, 2017). They can be found in every setting ranging from preschools to colleges and universities, and from community agencies to mental health facilities. While keeping in mind the global context and multi-dimensions of problems related to alcohol and other drug misuse, this chapter focuses on the impact of parental misuse of substances such as alcohol, heroin and other opiates, cocaine and methamphetamines, tobacco, and marijuana on their children. Because these children exhibit not only problematic behaviors but also strengths or resilience, careful individual assessment is warranted. This chapter provides an overview of the dynamics of families with parents engaged in substance misuse, the impact on their children at different ages, and effective treatment approaches for such children and their parents.

Terminology

The latest edition of the *Diagnostic and Statistical Manual of Mental Disorders* (DSM-5; American Psychiatric Association, 2013) applies the overall category of "substance use disorder" (SUD) when referring to individuals meeting criteria for this disorder with an indication of severity such as *mild, moderate,* or *severe* (see Appendix A). Thus, the degree of parental dysfunction can vary widely depending on the SUD severity. Moreover, many parents do not fully meet criteria for SUD and are commonly referred to as individuals who "misuse" substances. When talking about their children, past literature referred to them variously as "children of substance abusing parents" (COSAPs), "children of alcoholics" (COAs), "adult children of alcoholics" (ACOAs), and "children of addicted parents." To avoid perpetuating such labeling language (see Begun, 2016), throughout this chapter parents are described in terms of their substance misuse behavior and children in terms of their relationship to the parents.

Impact of substance use disorders on families

Although the effects of alcohol and other drug misuse by a parent (or caretaker) vary considerably from family to family, common patterns of problematic familial interaction and behavior have been described in the literature (Gruber & Taylor, 2006; Lam & O'Farrell, 2011). Dysfunctional patterns may include "communication problems, conflict, chaos and unpredictability, inconsistent messages to children, breakdown in rituals and traditional family rules and boundaries and emotional, physical and sexual abuse" (Straussner, 2011, p. 5). In sum, substance misuse can reduce a parent's ability to provide a safe and nurturing home for his or her children (Straussner & Donath, 2015). Recent neurological and psychological studies reveal that children growing up in violent and otherwise traumatizing households suffer from not just the psychological impact, such as emotional dysregulation and difficulties in social relationships (Eiden, Colder, Edwards, & Leonard, 2009; Fewell, 2011), but may also experience permanent neurological changes affecting them for the rest of their lives (Dayton, 2011).

In addition, the legal status of a substance has a differential impact on parents and their children. For example, alcohol, commonly misused prescription medications, and tobacco can be legally obtained. Consequently, the lifestyles and socioeconomic and ethnic backgrounds of individuals using these substances vary widely, reflecting diversity in the population at large. Moreover, alcohol use disorders develop slowly and thus the insidious impact of a parent's problematic alcohol use is commonly seen after adult independence has been achieved. Nonetheless, paternal alcohol abuse often is correlated with domestic violence, child abuse, and incest (Gruber & Taylor, 2006).

Unlike the use of alcohol, the nonprescription use of opiates is illegal, and many engaged in their use grew up in dysfunctional and physically abusive families with parents and even grandparents who engaged in alcohol and/or opiate misuse (Pederson et al., 2008; Straussner, 2011). Since opiates are generally highly addictive, individuals engaged in their misuse tend to become affected at a younger age, often before completing their education and being able to function as self-supporting adults. Consequently, they may have difficulties in forming and/or maintaining their own stable family of procreation.

Since the time and effort necessary to obtain and pay for drugs are considerable, the life-style associated with opiate addiction is highly unstructured and generally characterized by poverty and illegal activities. Despite a growing use of opiates in the United States among white, middle-class individuals (Cicero, Ellis, Surratt, & Kurtz, 2014), the misuse of opi-ates is more frequent among members of minority or disenfranchised low-income groups throughout the world. A series of live-in partners, prostitution, and incarcerations are com-mon and have a severe negative impact on family life (Mazza, 2017). Individuals engaged in intravenous opiate use and their partners may be infected with HIV/AIDS, hepatitis C, and other sexually transmitted diseases, as well as experiencing other chronic medical conditions. Parental use of stimulants, such as methamphetamines and cocaine (including crack), can also lead to various medical complications, severe financial and legal repercussions, nega-tive psychological effects, such as increased paranoia and suicidal ideation, and even sudden death—all of which wreak havoc on family life. The growing legalization of marijuana is likely to lead to increased use among some individuals (Palamar, Ompad, & Petkova, 2014). While little is known about the impact of parental marijuana use on family life, individuals misusing marijuana appear more inner-focused and less socially interactive, making them less physically and emotionally available to their families.

Based on clinical observations, it appears that many women, whether or not they expe-rience a substance use problem, choose to remain in relationships with men who engage in substance misuse, while men, in general, tend to leave relationships with women experienc-ing a substance use problem, leaving the women with limited resources, making it difficult for the women to care for themselves, much less their children. Many such women are re-ported to child welfare services, perhaps losing custody of their children.

Family-system dynamics

In recent years, with increasing numbers of women experiencing substance use (Cotto et al, 2010), the potential that both parents experience substance use problems is more common. In such instances, children are often functionally parentless and needing to take care of them-selves. Depending on a child's age, he or she may become a "parentified child" (Fitzgerald et al., 2008), functioning as a caretaker for parents and siblings at the cost of his or her own development. It is not unusual for the entire family to organize itself around the parent engaging in substance misuse, resulting in dysfunctional dynamics such as role confusion and unclear boundaries, secrecy, and shame (Lam & O'Farrell, 2011). The individual's use of denial is often reinforced by family members engaging in denial, with family members viewing the parent's erratic behavior as normative. Unfortunately, while there exists a large body of literature concerning gay and lesbian individuals experiencing SUD (Senreich & Vairo, 2014), the literature about gay/lesbian or other non-traditional families with a parent engaging in substance misuse is sparse.

Family trauma

Recently, attention has focused on two significant areas relating to children whose parents misuse substances: the impact of early trauma and problematic emotional attachment. The Adverse Childhood Experiences (ACE) study provided epidemiological evidence of the cumulative negative effects of childhood trauma (Anda et al., 2006). The currently large set of ACE studies involving different populations show consistent correlations between childhood experiences of abuse, neglect, domestic violence, and parental substance abuse with negative physical health throughout the lifespan (Centers for Disease Control and Prevention [CDC], 2016). As the number of adverse childhood experiences increases, so does the magnitude of severe health problems. One of the strongest relationships found was between the number of adverse childhood experiences and early initiation of alcohol use, or marrying a partner experiencing an alcohol use disorder (Anda et al., 2006), showing the transgenerational impact of cumulative childhood stressors, including parental substance misuse, that manifest later in life.

Parent-child relationships

The issue of attachment and the related concept of mentalization—the ability of a parent to understand and accurately reflect on a child's behavior—are helpful in providing a context for assessing relationships between parents/caregivers engaged in substance misuse and their children. Mentalizing by a parent contributes to attachment security and is very important to developing psychological health in young children (Fonagy, Gergely, Jurist, & Target, 2002). Parental substance misuse impedes mentalizing. In addition, the dysregulated behaviors demonstrated by a parent engaged in substance misuse, as well as by the other parent who becomes preoccupied with a partner's substance misuse, may render them unable to accurately mentalize about their child's inner world (Fewell, 2010; Jordan, 2019).

Unfortunately, addiction treatment programs rarely address their clients' parenting problems. Recent developments in neuroscience highlight a significant relationship between the neural circuitry involved with chronic drug use and parenting (Rutherford, Williams, Moy, Mayes, & Johns, 2011), recognizing that chronic drug use activates the same dopaminergic pathways as caregiving. Programs supporting parents' skills and capacities to manage the challenges of parenthood, together with addiction treatment, may promote both better parenting and relapse prevention (Suchman et al., 2017). In addition, increasing attention is paid to the role of insecure attachment in alcohol and other drug use to self-regulate distressing emotional states; this further impairs a parent's emotional availability (Jordan, 2019; Padykula & Conklin, 2010).

Impact on children at different ages

The following sections explore the impact of parental substance misuse on children of various ages, applying a developmental lens and identifying best interventions for children and their families.

Newborns and infants

Biological, environmental, and systemic risk factors commence in pregnancy and are compounded by the postnatal caregiving environment (Tsantefski, Humphreys, & Jackson, 2014). While indications that *paternal* substance use is detrimental to the fetus and newborn child exist, research in this area remains limited (Kandel, 2013). However, there exists a great deal of knowledge about the consequences of maternal substance abuse during pregnancy (see Chapters 10, 11, 12, and 26). It is worth noting that for many women, pregnancy and motherhood function as a motivating factor in seeking treatment for a substance use disorder; conversely, fear of losing custody of their children or the lack of childcare are frequent treatment obstacles.

While some newborns appear to suffer no ill effects, others prenatally exposed to various substances (alcohol, tobacco, opiates, and others) may be premature or small for gestational age and experience various health and developmental complications as a result. They may be at greater risk for sudden infant death syndrome (SIDS), as well (Floyd et al., 2008). As the prenatally exposed child develops, other physiological effects may become evident, including developmental delays of various kinds, such as failure to thrive, cognitive deficits, neurobehavioral problems, and speech, language, and motor delays. During the school years, learning disabilities and behavioral problems such as attention deficit disorder with or without hyperactivity (ADD/ADHD) and conduct disorder may become evident (Azmitia, 2001; Floyd et al., 2008). All of these consequences compound the challenges associated with parenting, a situation worsened when the parent's abilities are also compromised through continued substance misuse.

School-aged children

School-aged children of parents engaged in substance misuse range from those known as "resilient children" who do very well in school and are rarely recognized as having any problems at home to those exhibiting severe emotional and behavioral problems. In a well-known longitudinal study, Werner and Johnson (2004) followed children of parents experiencing alcohol disorders for a 30-year period beginning at age two. They observed that the availability of support systems within the extended family or in the community significantly and positively affected the children's development into adulthood. Strong extended family support and maintenance of family routines represented important mediating factors for positive child development outcomes. A systematic review of research on protective mental health factors for children whose parents misuse substances identified four main components (Wlodarczyk, Schwarze, Rumpf, Metzner, & Pawlis, 2017):

• bonding, which included emotional attachment to caregivers;
• competence, which included cognitive abilities and self-regulation;
• optimism, which included a positive identity; and
• environment, which included an organized home and socioeconomic advantages.

Other studies of children whose parents engage in substance misuse focused on "externalizing behavior problems" (Eiden, Edwards, & Leonard, 2007). Such children, particularly boys, not only exhibited attention deficits, hyperactivity, conduct disorders, and academic problems, but also caused difficulties for teachers and other students, at times leading them to become scapegoated by their peers. Consequently, not only do these children lack the basic supports at home, but they also may not obtain the support from peers and school personnel that could ameliorate some of the difficulties experienced through a parent's substance misuse. Other children, particularly girls, are more likely to exhibit *internalizing* behaviors and feelings, such as social withdrawal, low self-esteem, and feelings of loneliness. These behaviors and feelings can predispose children toward depression, suicidality, and addictive behavior, which become more noticeable during adolescence.

Adolescents

An estimated 10% of adolescent children in the United States live with a parent's substance misuse (SAMHSA, 2008). While less susceptible than younger children to being physically harmed by their parents, these adolescents are at high risk for suffering other negative physical, emotional, and behavioral health consequences. Compared with younger children, adolescents may experience greater risk because, on average, they have had more prolonged exposure to their parents' substance abuse and its consequences (Fenster, 2011; Peleg-Oren & Teichman, 2006).

There exists great variability between early, mid, and late adolescence periods, as well as individual differences among adolescents. For example, a 14-year-old can be as physically developed as another 18-year-old but have the cognitive and emotional development of a 12-year-old. Generally, younger adolescents are more dependent on peers for a sense of identity, loyal to their family, and more concrete in their thinking (Freshman, 2014). In contrast, older adolescents' abstract reasoning abilities render them better able to understand their parents' SUD and recovery.

At times, the physical and psychological changes faced by adolescents may play a more critical role in their lives than parental substance misuse. Therefore, understanding adolescents' developmental issues is crucial to effective interventions (Fenster, 2011). For example, because the prefrontal cortex of the adolescent brain is not fully developed (see Chapter 13), they lack a well-developed capacity to control emotions and make good judgments. Hormonal changes during adolescence affect the amygdala, the part of the brain that controls emotions, causing emotions to be intensified. Thus, adolescents may experience everything as a crisis; have mood swings; be impulsive, self-absorbed, and overly sensitive; and be unable to plan or understand cause and effect (Corzolino, 2006).

In addition to emotional lability, adolescents likely confront a constellation of stress factors within and outside their families. Pre-existing internalizing and externalizing problems become more evident, placing these children at an increased risk for encountering emotional, familial, social, academic, and legal problems. Of particular concern is the increased risk of intergenerational transmission of substance-use problems during the adolescent years: more than half of all children exposed to parental SUDs during adolescence developed their own substance-use disorders, compared with 15% who were not so exposed (Rothman, Edwards, Heeren, & Hingson, 2008).

Intervention approaches

Available interventions and treatments range from the removal of children from homes where parents engage in substance misuse (with foster care placement) to individual and group treatment of children and/or their parents, as well as family-based interventions. Specific interventions may include the use of medications, psychoeducation and behavioral therapy, play therapy, pediatric occupational therapy, use of bibliotherapy, and Internet-based supports (Pomeroy & Parrish, 2011; Straussner, 2011; Straussner & Donath, 2015).

Removing children from the family home

Physical abuse and/or neglect by a parent engaged in substance misuse is a major cause for removing a child from the family of origin to enter the child welfare system (Kahn & Greenberg, 2017). However, this intervention is just the beginning of the helping process. Using age-appropriate approaches, both the children and their caregivers need to be educated about parental substance misuse—the impacts of the different substances on the brain and body and that it is never the child's fault or responsibility to address parents' issues. Special attention needs to be paid to children placed in kinship care, particularly grandparents, some of whom may experience their own substance misuse problems. Others may be engaged in

S. L. Ashenberg Straussner and C. H. Fewell

on-going conflict with the child's parents, putting the child in the middle of the conflict (Kelley, Whitley, & Campos, 2011; see Chapter 25).

For parents who enter substance abuse treatment, it is important that they learn parenting skills and maintain contact with their children if family reunification is a possibility. Parenting skills should not be limited to mothers, but also need to be offered to the fathers. This is particularly important for the many incarcerated fathers (Mazza, 2017).

Services for young children

Interventions for children born with neonatal abstinence syndrome (NAS) or fetal alcohol syndrome disorders (FASD) vary depending on the severity of their problems. These may include medication to help with behavioral symptoms, educational and behavioral therapy (for both children and their caregivers) play therapy, and interdisciplinary team interventions involving nutrition, speech/language, physical, and occupational therapies. Older children may need help with self-image, depression, and suicidality (Straussner & Fewell, 2015).

Services for school-aged children

For the school-aged child, peer groups are critically important and can serve as the basis for both diagnostic comparison and treatment. It is important to assess the child's relationship with peers, including bullying dynamics and other antisocial behaviors; group intervention can provide a critical source of support and an arena for developing appropriate social skills. In addition, changes and/or difficulties in school performance need to be assessed and appropriate services offered (Johnson, Gryczynski, & Moe, 2011; Morehouse, 2011).

Psychoeducation for both parents needs to focus on understanding what to expect from their child at various developmental phases and developing appropriate parenting skills aimed at establishing and enforcing limits, as well as how to reward and discipline children (Johnson et al., 2011). Moreover, as adolescent children whose parents engage in substance misuse are particularly susceptible to developing their own substance use problems, preadolescence is a prime period to deliver family-systems interventions; at this stage, youth are more open to parenting influences. Additionally, opportunities to engage extended family members should be encouraged, as these natural supports provide protections against some deleterious effects of a parent's substance misuse (Werner & Johnson, 2004).

Assessment and services for adolescents

Assessment of adolescents should focus on psychological, behavioral, cognitive, social, and physical aspects, as well as family dynamics. The clinician also needs to attend to the adolescent's strengths, attitudes, aspirations, and resources. Although standardized instruments for assessing children whose parents engage in substance misuse need to be developed, one screening tool appropriate for use with adolescents is the Family Drinking Survey (Whitfield, 1991), assessing effects of a parent's drinking on an adolescent's physical, emotional, and social health. Another instrument that can help to screen for adolescent's own substance misuse is the CRAFFT, a mnemonic acronym of the first letters of key words in each of six screening questions (Knight et al., 1999). Moreover, making adolescents aware of their increased genetic risks for developing a substance use disorder, and helping them come to terms with such risks, is an essential part of clinical work with adolescents whose parents engage in substance misuse.

Insight-oriented treatment and cognitive-behavioral therapies are frequently used with this age group (David-Ferdon & Kaslow, 2008). Regardless of approach, the overarching treatment goal is to enhance adolescents' abilities to care for themselves emotionally, physically, socially, and, where appropriate, spiritually. Adolescents also need to be helped to develop coping strategies to deal with negative affect, develop awareness of their own thinking processes, and build skills in problem-solving, interpersonal communication, conflict resolution, and negotiation. Relaxation techniques, exercises, and other strategies for self-soothing can diminish anxiety or other negative mood states. Helping adolescents set and follow through with educational and vocational goals is also important: adolescents with clear goals are less likely to engage in drug use (Fletcher, Harden, Brunton, Oakley, & Bonell, 2008).

Group treatment is a common format for intervention with adolescents living with a parent engaging in substance misuse (Fenster, 2011). Treatment typically is short-term and helpful in teaching adolescents that they are not alone and reducing feelings of guilt and shame, as well as sharing helpful strategies for daily life. Finally, because adolescents who associate with peers exhibiting deviant behaviors are more likely to engage in substance misuse and other deviant behaviors themselves, therapeutic groups provide opportunities to interact with peers engaged in more prosocial behaviors (Fenster, 2011).

School- and community-based individual, group, and family counseling approaches, as well as self-help group participation, are all helpful for this population. One of the most widely available, free, community-based programs for adolescent children of parents experiencing alcohol use disorders are Alateen self-help groups offered under the auspices of Al-Anon Family Groups. Utilizing principles from Alcoholics Anonymous and Al-Anon, Alateen teaches youth about the progressive nature of alcohol and other substance use disorders, as well as the importance of detaching from the parent's pathological behavior and focusing on their own functioning. Another free resource is a web-based discussion board run by the National Association for Children of Alcoholics (www.nacoa.org), where teens can discuss online their experiences of living with parental substance misuse. In addition, a variety of books, booklets, and movies about children whose parents misuse substances are readily available for use in conjunction with other interventions.

Parents of adolescents may need help establishing developmentally appropriate expectations and effective discipline. Of particular value is help in reinstituting or creating such family routines and rituals as family meals, holiday and religious celebrations, and school events, as these help strengthen bonds and restore a sense of normalcy to the family. Parents should be referred for SUD treatment as appropriate. As discussed below, a number of empirically based family programs are increasingly being used in different settings.

Regardless of the treatment methods selected, clinicians working with adolescents should exhibit good engagement skills and the ability to tune-in to indirect and nonverbal signals often expressed by adolescents. Additionally, it is essential to clearly address issues of confidentiality: adolescent clients need to be informed early on of their rights—as well as any limits—to confidentiality.

Finally, it is critically important to help adolescents whose parents engage in substance misuse develop relationships with at least one caring adult who can model healthy behaviors. Community supports, including extended family members, teachers, and religious leaders can provide positive role models and growth experiences.

Family treatment

SUD often is referred to as a "family disease." Consequently, it is important to include the whole family in treatment and be cognizant of the importance of cultural considerations when determining appropriate family interventions (Straussner, 2011; see Chapter 24). Recent randomized controlled trials of interventions for children whose parents engage in substance misuse indicated that focusing on improved parenting practices and family functioning might be effective in reducing negative consequences for these children (Calhoun, Conner, Miller, & Messina, 2015). Among a number of evidence-based family interventions are:

Focus on families (FOF)

FOF is a Seattle, Washington-based intervention (Catalano, Haggerty, Fleming, Brewer, & Gainey, 2002) helping parents develop particular skills. FOF combines clinic- and home-based work with parents and their children, a combination more effective than either service alone, particularly among higher-risk families. FOF consisted of a five-hour family retreat and 90-minute parent training sessions conducted twice weekly over 16 weeks. Children attend 12 of the sessions. Topics include family goal setting, family communication skills, family management skills, creating family expectations about drugs and alcohol, teaching children skills, and helping children succeed in school. Parents and children practice the newly acquired skills together in family sessions at home, with a home-based case manager.

Strengthening families program (SFP)

SFP (www.strengtheningfamiliesprogram.org) is an evidence-based family preventive intervention adapted for use to accommodate cultural diversity; effectiveness has been demonstrated in 16 different countries (Kumpfer, Pinyuchon, Teixeira de Melo, & Whiteside, 2008). SFP is designed for parents in the early stages of recovery. It aims to reduce risk factors for behavioral, emotional, academic, and social problems in high-risk families with both young children (aged 3–5) and adolescents (aged 12–16) by teaching parents and children skills in problem-solving, interpersonal communication, and conflict resolution. SFP is comprised of 14-sessions, each week beginning with a multi-family group dinner followed by separate group meetings for parents and youth and ending with a family session. Studies showed positive changes in parenting, family relationships, and children's mental health and behavioral outcomes (Kumpfer, Whiteside, Greene, & Allen, 2010).

Celebrating families!

This intervention (www.celebratingfamilies.net/CFmodel.htm) applies a holistic model to treat the whole family. Originally developed for parents involved in drug court proceedings, it was later adapted for use with families in which there is a high risk for domestic violence, child abuse, or neglect due to a parent's alcohol misuse. Celebrating Families! consists of a cognitive-behavioral, support-group model that works with every member of the family, from ages three through adult.

Multidimensional family therapy (MDFT)

MDFT is an empirically based, family-oriented treatment model, particularly when the adolescent engages in substance misuse (Liddle, 2002). Its primary goals are to improve adolescent, parental, and overall family functioning, in turn, reducing intergenerational alcohol misuse and other problematic behavior. MDFT views adolescent substance abuse as resulting from multiple interacting factors, including failure to meet developmental challenges, and different forms of abuse or trauma, including parental substance misuse. MDFT is a highly flexible approach; treatment length is determined by the treatment provider, setting, and family, and may include a combination of individual and family sessions. The assessment and intervention modules include five distinct intervention components: with the adolescent; with the parent; with parent(s) and the adolescent; with other family members; and with systems external to the family (e.g. educational and legal systems).

Mentalization-based therapy

Mentalization parenting programs assist parents engaged in substance misuse by combining an attachment-based psychodynamic understanding of behavior with elements of cognitive-behavioral therapy, including psychoeducation. Helping parents develop the ability to mentalize about their children aids in stopping child maltreatment and the intergenerational transfer of insecure attachment, thereby decreasing the development of substance misuse in the next generation (Fewell, 2011). One example is offered by The Yale Child Study Center, which has implemented a program aimed at mothers with young children (birth to three years) attending an outpatient drug treatment program (Suchman, Decoste, Rosenberger, & McMahon, 2012). The goal is to help mothers increase their maternal reflective or mentalizing function so they understand their own and their children's intentions within a developmental framework. Techniques such as demonstrating curiosity about the baby's mind ("What is the baby thinking?") or giving the baby a voice (demonstrate another point of view) are part of the manual-guided, 12-session, weekly individual therapy protocol. Based on the same principles, a program in Finland called *Holding Tight*, works with mothers experiencing severe substance use disorders and their babies in residential treatment. In addition to group meetings on parenting themes, intensive work is conducted in individual therapy sessions to enhance the mothers' reflective functioning about her baby's mind and strengthen her capacity for "previewing," to be aware and supportive of the child's next developmental steps. Two randomized control trials evaluated an outpatient mentalization-based program based on the same principles in the United States called *Mothering from the Inside Out* (MIO): a 12-week intervention for mothers and their children between birth and age 3. MIO resulted in improvements in parental reflective functioning and reduction of substance use (Suchman et al., 2017). A third trial is underway in the United States in a community-based addiction treatment center (Suchman, Borelli, & DeCoste, 2018).

Community reinforcement and family training (CRAFT)

CRAFT is a behavioral, skills-based approach teaching family members effective strategies for helping change the way the family interacts with a member engaged in substance misuse without using detachment and confrontational approaches (Meyers, Miller, Hill, & Tonigan, 1999; Smith & Meyers, 2004). Participants learn the power of positive reinforcement for desirable behavior and withdrawing it for undesirable behavior, as well as how to use positive communication skills to improve interactions and maximize their influence. CRAFT teaches several skills, including understanding a loved one's triggers to use substances, positive communication strategies, positive reinforcement strategies—rewarding non-using behaviors, problem-solving, self-care, domestic violence precautions, and getting a loved one to accept help (see http://motivationandchange.com/outpatient-treatment/for-families/craft-overview/).

No single approach works for everyone, but all are aimed at recognizing the impact of substance misuse on all members of the family and addressing them directly.

Clinician issues

Helping children of parents engaged in substance misuse often evokes difficult emotional reactions on the part of the clinician. Some may want to side with the child against the parent, not realizing that the child loves and identifies with this parent. Others may desire to protect the child, thus may be reluctant to initiate the painful topic of parental substance use and its impact on the family. Alternatively, clinicians may identify with the parent's denial, even those in recovery, either wanting to believe that the child did not suffer as a result of the addictive behavior or not accurately remembering the effects of their parental behavior while using substances. Finally, clinicians may themselves come from families where substances were misused, and thus be uncomfortable in addressing the issues with either parents or their children. These counter-transference feelings may interfere with providing needed services to children whose parents misuse substances.

Conclusions

An increasing body of neurobiological, epidemiological, and attachment-and trauma-related research makes a strong case for the need to intervene early with families and children in order to prevent intergenerational recurrence of substance misuse and other costly and life-threatening disorders. Numerous studies demonstrated that for healthy development children needs safe and stable environments and a caring family that provides acceptance, trust, a sense of autonomy, and security. When parents engage in substance misuse, their children are often unable to experience such an environment and are at increased risk of lifelong problems, including a relatively high level of depressive symptoms and anxiety, low self-esteem, feelings of guilt and loneliness, and their own misuse of substances or connecting with a partner who does.

However, each child is unique and has strengths serving as protective factors that need to be acknowledged and reinforced. This assessment of strengths, the child's age, and details of their particular family situation are critical in determining what kind of intervention should be offered. Increasingly, attention is directed to intervening prenatally and during early childhood, including efforts to mitigate mentalizing deficits that may result from parental substance misuse (Jordan, 2019). Programs aimed at increasing problem-solving skills in elementary and secondary schools may enhance children's resilience and provide primary and secondary prevention. For children in need of treatment, providing services in school-based programs can overcome barriers to access.

Programs aimed at assisting the entire family with cohesion and problem-solving skills can provide relief simultaneously for both parents experiencing a SUD and their children. Helping both children and parents engaged in substance misuse has the potential to interrupt the intergenerational transfer of emotional distress and insecure attachment that leads to a myriad of related health problems. Finally, even the minimal intervention of providing children and adolescents with the opportunity to speak about what they have experienced in relation to their parents' substance misuse and reassure them that it is not their fault or responsibility can be a powerful healing force.

References

American Psychiatric Association. (2013). *Diagnostic and statistical manual of mental disorders* (DSM-5). Washington, DC: American Psychiatric Association. doi:10.1176/appi.books.9780890425596

Anda, R., Felitti, V., Bremner, J., Walker, J., Whitfield, C., Perry, B., . . . Giles, W. H. (2006). The enduring effects of abuse and related adverse experiences in childhood. *European Archives of Psychiatry and Clinical Neuroscience, 256*(3), 174–186. doi:10.1007/s00406-005-0624-4

Azmitia, E. C. (2001). Impact of drugs and alcohol on the brain through the life cycle: Knowledge for social workers. *Journal of Social Work Practice in the Addictions, 1*(3), 41–64. doi:10.1300/J160v01n03_04

Begun, A. L. (2016). Considering the language we use: Well worth the effort. *Journal of Social Work Practice in the Addictions, 16*(3), 332–336. doi:10.1080/1533256X.2016.1201372

Calhoun, S., Conner, E., Miller, M., & Messina, N. (2015). Improving the outcomes of children affected by parental substance abuse: A review of randomized controlled trials. *Substance Abuse Rehabilitation, 6*, 15–24. doi:10.2147/SAR.S46439

Catalano, R. F. Haggerty, K. P., Fleming, C. B., Brewer, D. D., & Gainey, R. R. (2002). Children of substance-abusing parents: Current findings from the focus on families project. In R. J. McMahon & R. D. Peters (Eds.), *The effects of parental dysfunction on children* (pp. 179–204). New York, NY: Kluwer Academic/Plenum Publishers. doi:10.1007/978-1-4615-1739-9_9

Centers for Disease Control and Prevention (CDC). (2016). *Adverse childhood experiences journal articles by topic area.* Retrieved from https://www.cdc.gov/violenceprevention/childabuseandneglect/acestudy/journal.html

Cicero, T. J., Ellis, M. S., Surratt, H. L., & Kurtz, S. P. (2014). The changing face of heroin use in the United States: A retrospective analysis of the past 50 years. *JAMA Psychiatry, 71*(7), 821–826. doi:10.1001/jamapsychiatry.2014.366

Corzolino, L. (2006). *The neuroscience of human relationships.* New York, NY: W.W. Norton Co.

Cotto, J. H., Davis, E., Dowling, G. J., Elcano, J. C., Staton, A. B., & Weiss, S. R. (2010). Gender effects on drug use, abuse, and dependence: A special analysis of results from the national survey on drug use and health. *Gender Medicine, 7*(5), 402–413.

David-Ferdon, C., & Kaslow, N. (2008). Evidence-based psychosocial treatments for child and adolescent depression. *Journal of Clinical Child and Adolescent Psychology, 37*(1), 62–104. doi:10.1080/15374410701817865

Dayton, T. (2011). Treatment issues and psychodrama interventions with adults who grew up with substance abusing parents. In S. L. A. Straussner & C. H. Fewell (Eds.), *Children of substance-abusing parents: Dynamics and treatment* (pp. 143–160). New York, NY: Springer.

Eiden, R. D., Colder, C., Edwards, E. P., & Leonard, K. E. (2009). A longitudinal study of social competence among children of alcoholic and nonalcoholic parents: Role of parental psychopathology, parental warmth, and self-regulation. *Psychology of Addictive Behaviors, 23*(1), 36–46. doi:10.1037/a0014839

Eiden, R. D., Edwards, E. P., & Leonard, K. E. (2007). A conceptual model for the development of externalizing behavior problems among kindergarten children of alcoholic families: Role of parenting and children's self-regulation. *Developmental Psychology, 43*(5), 1187–1201. doi:10.1037/0012-1649.43.5.1187

Fenster, J. (2011). Treatment issues and interventions with adolescents from substance-abusing families. In S. L. A. Straussner & C. H. Fewell (Eds.), *Children of substance abusing parents: Dynamics and treatment* (pp. 127–152). New York, NY: Springer. doi:10.1891/9780826165084.0006

Fewell, C. H. (2010). Using a mentalization-based framework to assist hard-to-reach clients in individual treatment. In S. Bennett and J. K. Nelson (Eds.), *Adult attachment in clinical social work* (pp. 113–126). New York, NY: Springer. doi:10.1007/978-1-4419-6241-6_7

Fewell, C. H. (2011). An attachment and mentalizing perspective on children of substance abusing parents. In S. L. A. Straussner & C. H. Fewell (Eds.), *Children of substance abusing parents: Dynamics and treatment* (pp. 29–47). New York, NY: Springer. doi:10.1891/9780826165084.0002

Fitzgerald, M. M., Schneider, R. A., Salstrom, S., Zinzow, H. M., Jackson, J., & Fossel, R. V. (2008). Child sexual abuse, early family risk, and childhood parentification: Pathways to current psychosocial adjustment. *Journal of Family Psychology, 22*(2), 320–324. doi:10.1037/0893-3200.22.2.320

Fletcher, A., Harden, A., Brunton, G., Oakley, A., & Bonell, C. (2008). Interventions addressing the social determinants of teenage pregnancy. *Health Education, 108*, 29–39. doi:10.1108/09654280810842111

Floyd, R. L., Jack, B. W., Cefalo, R., Atrash, H., Mahoney, J., Herron, A., . . . Sokol, R. J. (2008). The clinical content of preconception care: Alcohol, tobacco, and illicit drug exposures. *American Journal of Obstetrics & Gynecology, 199*(6), S333–S339. doi:10.1016/j.ajog.2008.09.018

Fonagy, P., Gergely, G., Jurist, E., & Target, M. (2002). *Affect regulation, mentalization, and the development of the self.* New York, NY: Other Press.

Freshman, A. (2014). Assessment and treatment adolescent substance abusers. In S. L. A. Straussner (Ed.), *Clinical work with substance-abusing clients* (3rd ed., pp. 305–420). New York, NY: Guilford.

Gruber, K. J., & Taylor, M. F. (2006). A family perspective for substance abuse: Implications from the literature. *Journal of Social Work Practice in the Addictions, 6*(1/2), 1–29. doi:10.1300/J160v06n01_01

Johnson, J. L., Gryczynski, M. S., & Moe, J. (2011). Treatment issues and intervention with young children and their substance abusing parents. In S. L. A. Straussner & C. H. Fewell (Eds.), *Children of substance abusing parents: Dynamics and treatment* (pp. 101–120). New York, NY: Springer. doi:10.1891/9780826165084.0005

Jordan, J. (2019). Alcoholics anonymous: A vehicle for achieving capacity for secure attachment relationships and adaptive affect regulation. *Journal of Social Work Practice in the Addictions, 19*(3). doi:10.1080/1533256X.2019.1638180

Kahn, J. M. & Greenberg, J. P. (2017). Urban children in foster care placement. In N. K. Phillips & S. L. A. Straussner (Eds.), *Children in the urban environment: Linking social policy and clinical practice* (3rd ed., pp. 253–277). Springfield, IL: Charles C. Thomas, Publisher, Ltd.

Kandel, R. R. (2013, September 6). The new science of mind. *New York Times.* Retrieved from https://www.nytimes.com/2013/09/08/opinion/sunday/the-new-science-of-mind.html

Kelley, S. J., Whitley, D. M., & Campos, P. E. (2011). Behavior problems in children raised by grandmothers: The role of caregiver distress, family resources, and the home environment. *Children and Youth Services Review, 33*(11), 2138–2145. doi:10.1016/j.childyouth.2011.06.021

Knight, J. R., Shrier, L. A., Bravender, T. D., Farrell, M., Vander Bilt, J., & Shaffer, H. J. (1999). A new brief screen for adolescent substance abuse. *Archives of Pediatric Adolescent Medicine, 153,* 591–596. doi:10.1001/archpedi.153.6.591

Kumpfer, K. L., Pinyuchon, M., Teixeira de Melo, A., & Whiteside, H. O. (2008). *Cultural adaptation process for international dissemination of the strengthening families program.* Retrieved from http://ehp.sagepub.com/cgi/content/abstract/31/2/226, doi:10.1177/0163278708315926

Kumpfer, K. L., Whiteside, H. O., Greene, J. A., & Allen, K. C. (2010). Effectiveness outcomes of four age versions of the strengthening families program in statewide field sites. *Group Dynamics: Theory, Research, and Practice, 14*(3), 211–219. doi:10.1037/a0020602

Lam, W. K. K., & O'Farrell, T. J. (2011). Dynamics of substance abusing parents and implications for treatment. In S. L. A. Straussner & C. H. Fewell (Eds.), *Children of substance abusing parents: Dynamics and treatment* (pp. 49–75). New York, NY: Springer. doi:10.1891/9780826165084.0003

Lander, L., Howsare, J. K., & Byrne, M. (2013). The impact of substance use disorders on families and children: From theory to practice. *Substance Abuse, 23*(1), 133–141. doi:10.1080/08897070209511511

Lipari, R. N., & Van Horn, S. L. (2017, August 24). *Children living with parents who have a substance use disorder.* The CBHSQ report. Rockville, MD: Center for Behavioral Health Statistics and Quality, SAMHSA. Retrieved from https://www.samhsa.gov/data/sites/default/files/report_3223/ShortReport-3223.html

Liddle, H. A. (2002). *Multidimensional family therapy for adolescent cannabis users, cannabis youth treatment series* (DHHS Publication Number 02-3660, Vol. 5). Rockville, MD: Center for Substance Abuse Treatment, Substance Abuse and Mental Health Services Administration.

Mazza, C. (2017). Children of incarcerated parents. In N. K. Phillips & S. L. A. Straussner (Eds.), *Children in the urban environment: Linking social policy and clinical practice* (3rd ed., pp. 308–334). Springfield, IL: Charles C. Thomas, Publisher, Ltd.

Messina, N., Calhoun, S., Conner, E., & Miller, M. (2015). Improving the outcomes of children affected by parental substance abuse: A review of randomized controlled trials. *Substance Abuse and Rehabilitation, 15.* doi:10.2147/SAR.S46439

Meyers, R. J., Miller, W. R., Hill, D. E., & Tonigan, J. S., (1999). Community reinforcement and family training (CRAFT): Engaging unmotivated drug users in treatment. *Journal of Substance Abuse, 10,* 1–18. doi:10.1016/S0899-3289(99)00003-6

Morehouse, E. R. (2011). Programs for adolescent children of substance-abusing parents in school and residential settings. In S. L. A. Straussner & C. H. Fewell (Eds.), *Children of substance abusing parents: Dynamics and treatment* (pp. 207–222). New York, NY: Springer. doi:10.1891/9780826165084.0010

Padykula, N. L. & Conklin, P. (2010). The self-regulation model of attachment trauma and addiction. *Clinical Social Work Journal, 38*, 351–360. doi:10.1007/s10615-009-0204-6

Palamar, J. J., Ompad, D. C., & Petkova, E. (2014). Correlates of intentions to use cannabis among U.S. high school seniors in the case of cannabis legalization. *International Journal of Drug Policy, 25*(3), 424–435. doi:10.1016/j.drugpo.2014.01.017

Pederson, C. L., Vanhorn, D. R., Wilson, J. F., Martorano, L. M., Venema, J. M., & Kennedy, S. M. (2008). Childhood abuse related to nicotine, illicit and prescription drug use by women: Pilot study. *Psychological Reports, 103*(2), 459–466. doi:10.2466/pr0.103.2.459-466

Peleg-Oren, N., & Teichman, M. (2006). Young children of parents with substance use disorders (SUD): A review of the literature and implication for social work practice. *Journal of Social Work Practice in the Addictions, 6*(1/2), 49–61. doi:10.1300/J160v06n01_03

Pomeroy, E. C., & Parrish, D. E. (2011). Prenatal impact of alcohol and drugs on young children: Implications for intervention with children and parents. In S. L. A. Straussner & C. H. Fewell (Eds.), *Children of substance abusing parents: Dynamics and treatment* (pp. 77–100). New York, NY: Springer. doi:10.1891/9780826165084.0004

Rothman, E. F., Edwards, E. M., Heeren, T., & Hingson, R. W. (2008). Adverse childhood experiences predict earlier age drinking onset: Results from a representative US sample of current or former drinkers. *Pediatrics, 122*(2), e298–e304. doi:10.1542/peds.2007-3412

Rutherford, H. J. V., Williams, S. K., Moy, S., Mayes, L. C., & Johns, J. M. (2011). Disruption of maternal parenting circuitry by addictive process: Rewiring of reward and stress symptoms. *Frontiers in Psychiatry, 2*, 37. doi:10.3389/fpsyt.2011.00037

Senreich, E., & Vairo, E. (2014). Assessment and treatment of lesbian, gay and bisexual substance abusers. In S. L. A. Straussner (Ed.), *Clinical work with substance-abusing clients* (3rd ed., pp. 466–494). New York, NY: Guilford Press.

Smith, J. E., & Meyers, R. J. (2004). *Motivating substance abusers to enter treatment: Working with family members.* New York, NY: Guilford Press.

Straussner, S. L. A. (2011). Children of substance abusing parents: An overview. In S. L. A. Straussner & C. H. Fewell (Eds.), *Children of substance abusing parents: Dynamics and treatment* (pp. 1–27). New York, NY: Springer. doi:10.1891/9780826165084

Straussner, S. L. A., & Donath, R. (2015). Children and teens with substance-abusing parents. In N. B. Webb (Ed.), *Play therapy with children and adolescents in crisis* (4th ed., 78–99): New York, NY: Guilford Press.

Straussner, S. L. A., & Fewell, C. H. (2015). Children of parents who abuse alcohol and other drugs. In A. Reupert, D. Mayberry, J. Nicholson, M. Gopfert, & M. V. Seeman (Eds.), *Parental psychiatric disorders: Distressed parents and their families* (3rd ed., pp.138–153). Cambridge, UK: Cambridge University Press. doi:10.1017/CBO9781107707559.015

Substance Abuse and Mental Health Services Administration (SAMHSA). (2008). *The NSDUH report: Children living with substance-dependent or substance-abusing parents: 2002 to 2007.* Rockville, MD: Office of Applied Studies.

Substance Abuse and Mental Health Services Administration (SAMHSA). (2017). *National survey on drug use and health.* Retrieved from https://www.samhsa.gov/data/nsduh/reports-detailed-tables-2017-NSDUH

Suchman, N., Borelli, J., & DeCoste, C. (2018). Can addiction counselors be trained to deliver mothering from the inside out, a mentalization-based parenting therapy, with fidelity? Results from a community-based randomized efficacy trial. *Attachment and Human Development.* Published online: 26 December 2018. doi:10.1080/14616734.2018.1559210.

Suchman, N., DeCoste, C., McMahon, T., Dalton, R., Mayes, L., & Borelli, J. (2017). Mothering from the inside out: Results of a second randomized clinical trial testing a mentalization-based intervention for mothers in addiction treatment. *Development and Psychopathology, 29*, 617–636. doi:10.1017/S0954579417000220

Suchman, N., DeCoste, C., Rosenberger, P., & McMahon, T. (2012). Attachment-based intervention for substance-abusing mothers: A preliminary test of the proposed mechanism of change. *Infant Mental Health Journal, 33*(4), 360–371. doi:10.1002/imhj.21311

Suchman, N., Pajulo, M., Kalland, M., DeCoste, C., & Mayes, L. (2012). In A. Bateman & P. Fonagy (Eds.), *Handbook of mentalizing in mental health practice* (pp. 309–346). Arlington, VA: American Psychiatric Publishing.

Tsantefski, M., Humphreys, C., & Jackson, A. C. (2014). Infant risk and safety in the context of maternal substance use. *Children and Youth Services Review, 47,* 10–17. doi:10.1016/j.childyouth.2013.10.021

United Nations Office on Drugs and Crime (2018). *World drug report: Executive summary conclusions and policy implications.* Retrieved from https://www.unodc.org/wdr2018/prelaunch/WDR18_Booklet_1_EXSUM.pdf, doi:10.18356/a1062695-en

Werner, E. E., & Johnson, J. L. (2004). The role of caring adults in the lives of children of alcoholics. *Substance Use and Misuse, 39*(5), 699–720. doi:10.1081/JA-120034012

Whitfield, C. (1991). *Co-dependence: Healing the human condition.* Deerfield Beach, FL: Health Communications, Inc.

Wlodarczyk, O., Schwarze, M., Rumpf, H., Metzner, F., & Pawlis, S. (2017). Protective mental health factors in children of parents with alcohol and drug use disorders: A systematic review. *PLOS One, 12*(6), e0179140. doi:10.137/journal.pone.0179140

23

All drugs aren't created equal

Exploring the general and specific effects of psychoactive substances to understand child maltreatment risk by drug type

Nancy Jo Kepple and Bridget Freisthler

Background

Addictive behaviors often arise as a central concern when working with families at risk for child harm (Smith & Wilson, 2016). Internationally, 12–30% of children aged 17 years or younger are estimated to live with at least one parent who engaged in substance misuse (Laslett, Ferris, Dietze, & Room, 2012; Lipari & Van Horn, 2017; Manning, Best, Faulkner, & Titherington, 2009). The proportion of children exposed to parental substance misuse increases within high-risk populations. Approximately 46–67% of individuals receiving substance use disorder (SUD) treatment identified as a parent (Lipari & Van Horn, 2017; Grella, Hser, & Huang, 2006; Stewart, Gossop, & Trakada, 2007), and an estimated 34–78% of child welfare cases within industrialized nations indicated parental substance misuse (De Bortoli, Coles, & Dolan, 2013; Forrester, 2000; Young, Boles, & Otero, 2007).

These estimates are concerning given associated substance-related harms range from affecting a parent's ability to function to exposing a child to environmental hazards (Smith & Wilson, 2016). For example, parental substance use increases risk for a child's direct physical exposure to substances through prenatal exposure (see Chapters 10, 11, and 12), accidental poisoning, or manufacturing within the home (Smith & Wilson, 2016). Alternatively, a child's exposure to parental substance use can shape expectancies related to their own future substance use behaviors (see Chapter 6). Parental substance misuse may also create unsafe environments through increased exposure to related crime and/or violence (see Chapter 7) or create unstable home environments through the loss of access to one's parent due to incarceration (refer to Chapter 32) or overdose and possible death (Radel, Baldwin, Crouse, Ghertner, & Waters, 2018).

While we acknowledge that no single risk factor or system can explain any complex human behavior (Cicchetti & Toth, 2005), this chapter focuses on child maltreatment as one facet of substance-related child harm. *Child maltreatment* refers to a constellation of harmful, interrelated behaviors directed toward a child, having the ability to cause or contribute to imminent physical, cognitive, and emotional harm to the child (Leeb, Paulozzi, Melanson, Simon, & Arias, 2008).

Psychoactive substances are defined by their ability to alter brain structures and functions when consumed or administered into one's system (Koob & Volkow, 2010), directly affecting how parents perceive, think about, feel about, understand, and interact with the world around them. As a result, we explored how substance use may directly affect parental functioning and how substance-specific impairments create unique risks for child maltreatment behaviors.

Identifying key mechanisms in models of parenting behavior

Several parenting models identify how parental functioning contribute to a parent's response to his/her child. Table 23.1 summarizes and compares core components of neuropsychological, cognitive, and attachment models of parenting.

Human models of parental brain circuits

Recent innovations in neuroscience allow us to understand brain structures and functions that are critical for parenting behaviors (Rutherford, Potenza, & Mayes, 2013; Swain et al., 2014). First, parents engage in *salience appraisal* arising from sensory, autonomic, and neuroendocrine assessments that interact with memory and motivation/reward structures in response to child stimuli or behaviors (Rutherford et al., 2013; Swain et al., 2014). If successful, this information passes through other *cortico-limbic modules* that help parents evaluate and integrate perceived information through: (1) reflexive caring; (2) complex cognitions that allow the parent to understand the child's internal state (i.e. mentalization and empathy) and plan responses; and (3) emotion regulation that helps to manage parental worries, stress reactivity, and habitual responses (Swain et al., 2014). Disruption of these mechanisms can contribute to parental failure to respond (Rutherford et al., 2013). For example, high reactivity to stress can impede associated executive functions and motivation critical for appropriate parental responding (Rutherford et al., 2013). Alternatively, addictive behaviors can adversely affect neuropsychological processes critical to parental responding, including: reward and motivation; memory; executive functions; and stress reactivity (Koob & Volkow, 2010). Associated substance-related impairments in attention, emotion processing, and mentalization also likely play a role in being able to appraise a child's behavior or cues and to understand a child's internal state, associated needs, or intentions (Rutherford et al., 2013; see Chapter 22).

Social information processing models of abuse and neglect

Social information processing (SIP) models help us identify potential cognitive and behavior correlates of the neuropsychological processes detailed in the prior section. Milner (2000) detailed the SIP model for abuse, whereby an incongruent perspective/response of a child's behavior may result if parents experience impairments in any of the following: (1) perceptions of child behavior, (2) interpretation and evaluation of child behavior, (3) integration of information and response selection activities, or (4) response implementation and monitoring processes. Crittenden (1993) parallels this approach when applying SIP to neglect. Parents may: (1) fail to perceive a child's communication for help, (2) interpret or evaluate the signal as not severe enough to require a response, (3) have limited response options and/or believe he or she is not responsible for or incapable of implementing any given response, or (4) be distracted before being able to implement a decision by a competing need.

Additionally, how parents attend to and process emotion information (nonverbal or verbal) conveyed by children is likely to play a critical role (De Paul & Guibert, 2008). For example, when a parent interprets a child's behavior as threatening or misinterprets emotional cues,

Table 23.1 Comparing models of parenting behaviors

Neuropsychological Model	Cognitive Model	Attachment & Empathy Model
Child enacts behavior/signals for help ↓	Child enacts behavior/signals for help ↓	Child enacts behavior/signals for help ↓
Salience appraisal Sensory cortical regions appraise information from the child and interacts with subcortical memory, and motivation/reward structures ↓	**Perceive** Attend to and encode situational cues or child behavior ↓	**Underlying attachment to child** Closeness and trust between parent and child based on interpersonal interactions for regular physical and emotional care ↓
Other cortico-limbic modules *Reflexive caring* / *Automatic caring impulses* — *Complex cognitions*: Mentalization, empathy, & cognitive flexibility — *Stress reactivity & emotion regulation*: Arousal and top-down regulation ↓	**Evaluate** Interprets perceived behavior/signal based on pre-existing cognitive schemata (i.e. beliefs about child ability, child intent, and child rearing practices) and environmental cues ↓	**Parental empathy** Parent's ability to understand and share the child's internal reality and feelings ↓
Modules interact Resulting in parental love and attachment formation ↓	**Integrate** Selecting responses based on behavioral response options (or related self-efficacy), beliefs about child rearing and child ability, and mitigating contextual factors ↓	**Motivation & reward** Parent perception of whether meeting child's need will be low/high cost based on personal reward — **Personal distress**: Parent experience self-efficacy or control over child behavior/signal ↓
Output Hormonal, autonomic, and behavioral output required for parental responding to occur. *Executive functions* in the prefrontal cortex are important in addition to functions of the sensorimotor cortices	**Respond** Ability to implement planned parental response and modify behavioral responses in real time	**Respond** Parent implement response to child behavior/signal when empathy pathways are not disrupted. This includes resulting levels of parental warmth, sensitivity, & emotion expression
<u>Sources:</u> Rutherford et al. (2013), Swain et al. (2014)	<u>Sources:</u> Crittenden (1993), Milner (2000)	<u>Source:</u> Bowlby (1982), De Paul and Guibert (2008)

this interpretation can trigger an automatic behavioral response, resulting in an extreme response to the child's behavior (e.g. disengagement or assault) (De Paul & Guibert, 2008).

Attachment models rooted in parental warmth and empathy

Attachment and empathy models of parenting focus on how these processes may be disrupted once attachment is adequate or inadequately established (Bowlby, 1982; De Paul & Guibert, 2008). In relation to prior models, impairments in mentalization are key to understanding disruption in attachment processes (Swain et al., 2014). In addition, the first three phases of SIP likely contribute to compromised parental empathy and impaired parental responding (De Paul & Guibert, 2008). When information processing is not compromised, other factors influencing parental motivation and reward, self-efficacy and control, and experiences of distress around responding to a child may also disrupt attachment and empathy pathways (De Paul & Guibert, 2008). For example, a parent may prioritize seeking a euphoric high from stimulant use in lieu of responding to a clearly identified child need; in this case, substance use is perceived as more rewarding than the satisfaction of meeting the child's need (Rutherford et al., 2013).

Summary of individual-level mechanisms critical for parental functioning

When key neuropsychological, cognitive, and affective processes are significantly impaired for any reason, an increased risk for child maltreatment behaviors is likely. Mechanisms associated with attention, memory, executive functions, reward and motivation structures, mentalization and empathy, and emotion processing and regulation are critical to parental functioning. The following section explores the empirical evidence for substance-specific impairments to mechanisms identified as critical for parental functioning and how these impairments may contribute to substance-specific child maltreatment risks.

Substance-specific psychoactive effects contribute to abusive & neglectful behaviors

Among populations at high risk for parenting problems, substance use behaviors ranging from light drinking to meeting criteria for an SUD have been associated with abusive be-haviors (Kepple, 2018; Leonard, 2002). In contrast, most studies have observed only meeting criteria for an SUD as significantly related to neglectful behaviors (Ondersma, 2002; Sedlak et al., 2010). However, we know less about how specific types of substances may result in differential child maltreatment risk (Testa & Smith, 2009). Thus, this section concentrates on the substance-specific effects that may directly impair parental functioning and how these impairments may affect create variable risk for abusive and neglectful parenting behaviors. Tables 23.2 and 23.3 summarize these relationships by substance type.

Alcohol

Substance-specific effects

Alcohol is a central nervous system (CNS) depressant and classified as a sedative hypnotic (Kuhn, Swartzwelder, & Wilson, 2014; see Chapter 3). At low doses (i.e. one to two drinks), alcohol can moderately impair attention and vigilance for external stimuli (Oscar-Berman & Marinković, 2007). Acute alcohol intoxication (i.e. based on blood alcohol content;

Table 23.2 Alcohol and cannabis-specific correlates with child maltreatment behaviors and individual functioning

Drug Type	Examples	Neuropsychological Impairments	Cognitive/ Behavioral Impairments	Affective Processes	Hypothesized Relationship to Child Maltreatment Risk
Alcohol	Beer Wine Spirits	*Acute (0–48 hours)* Attention Executive functions Working memory Inhibition Decision making Planning Emotion processing *Chronic (48 hours–6 weeks)* Attention Executive functions Cognitive flexibility Problem solving Emotion processing Reward & motivation	*Intoxication* Alertness Memory (blackout) Inhibition Decision making *Withdrawal* Concentration Exhaustion	*Intoxication* Euphoria Relaxation Changes in mood *Withdrawal* Anxiety Irritability Depression	*Light to moderate drink* Low to moderate risk for abuse *Frequent intoxication/problematic use* High risk for abuse *Recurring, heavy use/alcohol use disorder* High risk for abuse or neglect
Cannabis	Marijuana Hashish	*Acute (0–48 hours)* Attention Memory Executive function Inhibition *Chronic (48 hours–6 weeks)* Attention Memory	*Intoxication* Memory Inhibition Decision making *Withdrawal* Attention Concentration	*Intoxication* Euphoria Relaxation Derealization Anxiety Paranoia *Withdrawal* Negative mood Irritability Anxiety	*Light cannabis use* Low to moderate risk for abuse or neglect *Heavy cannabis use/cannabis use disorder* Moderate to high risk for abuse or neglect

385

Table 23.3 Opioid- and stimulant-specific correlates with child maltreatment behaviors and individual functioning

Drug Type	Examples	Neuropsychological Impairments	Cognitive/Behavioral Impairments	Affective Processes	Hypothesized Relationship to Child Maltreatment
Opioids	Codeine Morphine Heroin	*Acute (0–48 hours)* Attention Executive function Cognitive flexibility Decision making Planning *Chronic (48 hours–1 month)* Attention Executive function Working memory Cognitive flexibility Inhibition Emotion processing Reward & motivation	*Intoxication* Consciousness Orientation Alertness Concentration Decision making *Withdrawal* Delirium Hallucinations	*Intoxication* Euphoria Calmness Restlessness Agitation *Withdrawal* Anxiety Lethargy Paranoia	*Opioid use* Low risk for abuse Moderate risk for neglect *Opioid misuse* Moderate risk for abuse High risk for neglect *Opioid use disorder* High risk for abuse or neglect
Stimulants (excluding caffeine & nicotine)	Cocaine Crack Meth	*Acute (0–48 hours)* Memory Executive function Working memory Cognitive flexibility Planning *Chronic (48 hours to 1+ years)* Attention Executive function Working memory Cognitive flexibility Inhibition Decision making Emotion processing	*Intoxication* Decision making *Withdrawal* Concentration Attention	*Intoxication* Euphoria Irritability *Withdrawal* Dysphoria Anxiety Agitation Anhedonia Hypersomnia	*Light stimulant use* Low risk for abuse or neglect *Binge or heavy stimulant use* High risk for abuse or neglect *Stimulant use disorder* High risk for abuse or neglect

about three to four drinks for women and four to five drinks for men) is associated with time-limited disinhibition and associated impulsive actions (Fernández-Serrano, Pérez-García, & Verdejo-García, 2011; Oscar-Berman & Marinković, 2007). Higher doses are associated with impairments in reward and motivation, attention, executive functions, and emotion processing (Fernández-Serrano et al., 2011). Impairments associated with alcohol use disorder (AUD) are similar to those described above but may be more severe and persisting. However, these negative effects may be partially reversed within a month of stable abstinence (Oscar-Berman & Marinković, 2007). Withdrawal after intoxication can include side effects that impair parents' ability to engage with their children, including exhaustion, difficulty concentrating, and symptoms of anxiety, irritability, or depression (Oscar-Berman & Marinković, 2007). These effects differ across baseline cognitive functioning and health status (Oscar-Berman & Marinković, 2007). For example, alcohol intoxication likely contributes to aggressive actions; however, it may contribute more when exacerbating existing emotion dysregulation and impulsivity (Giancola, Godlaski, & Roth, 2012).

Empirical evidence concerning alcohol and child maltreatment

Clear associations exist between any problematic alcohol use and physically abusive behaviors toward a child (Leonard, 2002; Stith et al., 2009). In addition, parental AUD was a predominant issue among families where children were being emotionally abused (Sedlak et al., 2010). A higher frequency of physically or emotionally abusive behaviors may be present for parents reporting even light to moderate levels of drinking when compared to parents reporting lifetime abstinence or no past-year alcohol use (Freisthler, Holmes, & Wolf, 2014; Kepple, 2018). In contrast, only parental AUD or frequent heavy drinking are associated with higher likelihood of neglectful behaviors toward a child (Freisthler, Johnson-Motoyama, & Kepple, 2014; Kepple, 2018).

Mechanisms for abusive and neglectful behaviors

Impaired attention and disinhibition associated with even low levels of drinking may explain empirical findings as to why light to moderate levels of drinking would correspond to an increased frequency of abusive behaviors. Parenting models suggest heavier and more frequent alcohol use align with impairment of multiple executive functions, heightening risk for abusive behaviors. Given the importance of emotion processing for mentalization and development of empathy, persisting impairments in emotion processing for individuals with recurring, heavy use may disrupt attachment processes and explain why frequent heavy drinking and/or AUD are primarily associated with neglectful behaviors.

Cannabis

Substance-specific effects

Cannabis is a plant-based, psychoactive substance that has variable effects depending on strain, potency, and ingestion methods (Kuhn et al., 2014; see Chapters 3 and 31). Strongest evidence for acute cannabis-related impairments exists for attention, verbal learning and memory, and executive functions related to inhibition (Broyd, van Hell, Beale, Yücel, & Solowij, 2016; Fernández-Serrano et al., 2011). Intoxication effects are related to cognitive impairments in decision-making, memory and learning, and inhibition paired with withdrawal effects associated with attention deficits and poor concentration (Vik, Cellucci, Jarchow, & Hedt, 2014). Affective changes during intoxication are variable and can include experiences of euphoria, relaxation, derealization, anxiety, and paranoia paired with withdrawal effects of negative mood, irritability, and anxiety (Vik et al., 2014). Recurring, heavy cannabis use was primarily associated with impairments in attention and memory (Broyd et al., 2016). Evidence for persisting effects beyond 48 hours after cannabis use are mixed; however, there is some evidence for impairment in verbal memory and attention after prolonged abstinence (Broyd et al., 2016). If present, persisting effects post-abstinence are most likely for individuals engaging in heavy, long-term cannabis use, particularly those with early initiation of use during adolescence (Meier et al., 2012).

Empirical evidence concerning the association between cannabis and child maltreatment

Freisthler, Gruenewald, and Wolf (2015) observed parents reporting past-year cannabis use were associated with a higher frequency of physically abusive behaviors toward their children (aged 0–12 years) compared to those reporting lifetime abstinence and no past-year use of cannabis. Thornberry et al. (2014) observed parental lifetime cannabis use was not associated with maltreatment of adolescents. Within the broader literature on violence, contradictory findings were observed for the relationship between cannabis use and violent behaviors (Ostrowsky, 2011), possibly due to the variable nature of cannabis-specific effects and differential effects associated with frequency, dosage, and age of initiation of cannabis use.

Mechanism for abusive and neglectful behaviors

Acute intoxication and withdrawal from cannabis use may decrease attention and increase inhibition; however, these periods must align with a parent's exposure to a child to present a maltreatment risk. It is more likely that persisting impairments due to recurring, heavy use will impair parental attention in ways that may moderately increase risk for abuse or neglect; however, even these impairments would likely resolve shortly after stable abstinence.

Opioids

Substance-specific effects

Opioids are CNS depressants that include both plant-based and synthetic substances; they alleviate experiences of pain, with varying degrees of potency (Kuhn et al., 2014; see Chapter 3). Intoxication effects from acute administration of opioids include decreased consciousness, drowsiness, or impaired communication; impaired thinking processes, decreased attention span, disorientation to time, delirium, or hallucinations; and feelings of restlessness or agitation (Kuhn et al., 2014). Immediate to short-term opioid use effects that can affect parenting include impairments in attention, memory, and executive functions specific to cognitive flexibility, planning, and decision-making (Fernández-Serrano et al., 2011). For example, decreased attention (aligning with decreased consciousness or drowsiness) increases the likelihood that a child's signal for help will go unnoticed by a parent. The most robust impairments associated with recurring opioid use were observed for executive functions related to working memory, inhibition, and cognitive flexibility

(Gruber, Silveri, & Yurgelun-Todd, 2007). Opioid use disorder (OUD) is associated with similar impairments in addition to impairments in attention, memory, emotion processing, and reward and motivation (Arias et al., 2016; Fernández-Serrano et al., 2011; Koob & Volkow, 2010).

Empirical evidence concerning the association between opioids and child maltreatment

Limited information exists about the specific relationship between parental opioid use and child maltreatment behaviors. Mothers in drug treatment who primarily used heroin or other opiates were less likely to reunify with their children compared to mothers who primarily used alcohol (Grella, Needell, Shi, & Hser, 2009). Yet, one study with mothers engaged in outpatient treatment directly observed less negative parent-child interaction and less negative self-reported parenting behaviors among mothers diagnosed with OUD compared to mothers diagnosed with alcohol use disorder (Slesnick, Feng, Brakenhoff, & Bringham, 2014). Vulnerable mothers may experience poor maternal attachment due to OUD, as well as lower levels of maternal sensitivity to the child cues and of maternal involvement (Romanowicz et al., 2019). Child abandonment or neglect due to parental overdose and/or death has increased attention to opioid use in the child welfare system (Radel et al., 2018).

Mechanisms for abusive and neglectful behaviors

The sedating effects of opioids can impair parental abilities to attend to child signals for help, increasing risk for neglect (particularly for young children) but only during windows of time that align with intoxication. Impairments in attention and memory can interfere with information encoding (Arias et al., 2016), which may moderately increase risk for abuse or neglect when parents are engaging in chronic, regular misuse of opioid. Any misuse of opioids can place all individuals at risk for overdose, resulting in unintentional neglect of children due to parental incapacitation and possible death. The most severe impairments and highest risks align with parental OUD; however, risks likely decrease after a period of protracted abstinence.

Stimulants

Substance-specific effects

Stimulants are aptly named due to their stimulating effects on the central and sympathetic nervous systems (Kuhn et al., 2014), and include cocaine, methamphetamine, and some prescription drugs (see Chapter 3). Acute administration of stimulants typically results in experiences that may not be deleterious to parental functioning, such as heightened energy, increased alertness, increased productivity, and short-term enhancements in attention (Scott et al., 2007). However, heavy doses and/or binge use of stimulants can result in short-term impairments in memory and executive functions related to working memory, cognitive flexibility, and planning (Fernández-Serrano et al., 2011). Individuals may also experience anxiety, irritability, insomnia, and confusion that counter initial euphoric effects, followed by withdrawal symptoms that can last a week or longer (Zweben et al., 2004). Detrimental effects for chronic stimulant use include impairments in attention, memory and learning, and executive functions related to cognitive flexibility, decision-making, inhibition, and working memory; all of which can hinder a parent's ability to process complex social information (Fernández-Serrano et al., 2011; Scott et al., 2007). Chronic methamphetamine use showed moderate effect sizes for a range of functions while chronic cocaine use showed small effect sizes for similar functions (Scott et al., 2007). Recurring, heavy stimulant use (both cocaine and methamphetamines) was associated with impaired emotion processing, particularly around accurate recognition of anger or fear (Fernández-Serrano, Pérez-García, Perales, & Verdejo-García, 2010; Payer et al., 2008). Stable abstinence over a year or more from stimulant use can result in improvements in functioning (Iudicello et al., 2010).

Empirical evidence concerning the association between stimulants and child maltreatment

Parents reporting cocaine and methamphetamine use are at an increased risk for child maltreatment. In a sample of mothers, those with a history of cocaine use showed significantly lower levels of attentiveness and responsive toward their infants at three months post-partum (compared to mothers reporting no cocaine use and those reporting no drug use; Mayes et al., 1997). Mothers with a history of cocaine use disorder self-reported difficulties specific to providing daily structure for their children, inability to supervise children when withdrawing from binge use, and experiencing impatience and anger toward children that often escalated into violence (Coyer, 2001). Chronic methamphetamine use and methamphetamine use disorder may also contribute to extreme feelings of anger or apathy toward a child and relational violence in the home (Brown & Hohman, 2006). Within a U.S. child welfare setting, cases where children were removed children due to parental methamphetamine use were associated with lower rates of reunification and higher rates of adoption compared to removal for non-drug reasons (Akin, Brook, & Lloyd, 2015).

Mechanisms for abusive and neglectful behaviors

Acute intoxication due to low doses and/or infrequent use may only pose low risk for child maltreatment, given increased alertness and euphoric effects often counter possible impairments. However, intoxication and withdrawal symptoms associated with heavy and/or binge use of methamphetamine or cocaine align with higher risk for child harm due to parental experiences of agitation, dysphoria, and hypersomnia that can last up to a week or longer. Due to pervasive impairments in information and emotion processing, we hypothesize that parents meeting criteria for a stimulant use disorder have the highest risk for maltreatment behaviors; however, a period of stable abstinence can ameliorate these effects.

Polysubstance use

Substance-specific effects

Polysubstance use is defined by two patterns of use behavior: *concurrent*, where different types of substances are used over a period of time, and *simultaneous*, where different types of substances are used together (Ives & Ghelani, 2006). Polysubstance use is associated with the highest likelihood of impaired learning and memory, which affects an individual's ability to engage in treatment-oriented tasks demanding new skill development, in addition to impaired executive function, leading to difficulty engaging in goal-oriented behavior and difficulty managing complex tasks (Arias et al., 2016). In addition, individuals diagnosed with an SUD and reporting polysubstance use experience deficits in emotion processing, with poorer recognition of negative emotions (i.e. anger, disgust, fear, and sadness; Fernández-Serrano et al., 2010).

Empirical evidence concerning the association between polysubstance use and child maltreatment

In a clinic-based sample of mothers seeking SUD treatment, 57.2% reported polysubstance use (Grella et al., 2006). In a sample of families at risk for child welfare involvement, 87% of individuals meeting past-year criteria for an SUD reported polysubstance use, and polysubstance use was associated with a higher average frequency of child maltreatment compared to non-use (Kepple, 2017). In addition, parents in the general population who used two or more substances (particularly concurrent past-year cannabis and alcohol use) were associated with a higher average frequency of physically aggressive parenting behaviors (Freisthler & Kepple, 2019). Finally, Brook and McDonald (2009) observed in a child welfare sample that child removal due to alcohol and drug use resulted in a higher likelihood of children reentering foster care over time compared to reasons for removal due to alcohol only, drug only, or neither alcohol or drugs.

Mechanisms for abusive and neglectful behaviors

Robust impairments in information and emotion processing associated with parental polysubstance use create a high risk for both abuse and neglect behaviors. Three parenting populations showed heightened risk for child maltreatment among parents reporting polysubstance use compared to single substance or non-substance use. Future work should continue to explore how these relationships may vary by concurrent and simultaneous polysubstance use (Ives & Ghelani, 2006).

Application to current screening, prevention, and intervention practices

These complex relationships suggest a range of strategies across children and family, child welfare, and SUD services are needed to best serve these families. Child removal is necessary only in the most extreme of cases where both the presence of a SUD fully compromises a parent's ability to care for a child and the parent has not established an alternative care plan to keep the child safe. Beyond removal, social workers can implement screening, prevention, and interventions that reduce risk of substance-related harm to the child and the family system.

Screening, prevention, and harm reduction

Medical settings increasingly implement screenings for alcohol and other drug use as a part of screening, brief intervention, and referral to treatment (SBIRT) processes (U.S. Department of Health and Human Services, 2011; see Chapter 20). Screening for use and high-risk behaviors is essential to prevent escalation of behaviors to an SUD and to engage in early identification of underlying concerns contributing to child maltreatment risk. Brief interventions can also incorporate education and support for parents (who do not meet criteria for SUD) in ways that help them consider ways to minimize substance-specific harms to the child. Strategies could utilize harm reduction philosophies. For example, parents could benefit from education around responsible use (e.g. limiting alcohol consumption to one drink around children), refraining from substance use when caring for a child, or planning for safe and appropriate care with a trustworthy provider for times when use may occur.

Assessment

Understanding drug-specific effects can guide assessment practices. For example, maltreatment risks should be assessed based on actual substance-specific effects rather than perceptions of harm or legality of a substance (Wolf, Kepple, & Freisthler, 2019). In addition, neuropsychological assessments of parental cognitive functioning may be important to understand underlying issues that could impede successful engagement and participation in treatment and case management activities, particularly when polysubstance use and/or heavy and chronic use of alcohol or stimulants have been identified. Information about neuropsychological functioning can help social workers determine if cognitive remediation and functional supports are necessary in addition to other case plan activities (Arias et al., 2016).

Intervention

Parenting interventions can incorporate current knowledge about underlying processes correlated with parental substance use. For example, chronic effects of heavy alcohol or stimulant use are associated with notable impairments in emotion processing, increasing risk of interfering with parental interpretation of child cues, mentalization, and attachment processes. Intervention strategies focused on improving parental reflective functioning, or mentalization, can ameliorate some concerns, particularly for parents with a recent history of heavy alcohol use or frequent stimulant use (Camoirano, 2017). In addition, family-centered strategies, such as the Sobriety Treatment and Recovery Team (START) program, allow children to remain safe while remaining in their parents' care through tailoring case management, providing therapeutic supports around parents' substance-specific needs, and using peer recovery mentors; all of which help parents engage in recovery and improve parenting skills (Huebner, Willauer, & Posze, 2012).

Finally, social workers should tailor case plan activities to the severity of drug-related risk. For example, social workers should address parental alcohol use with the seriousness that the extant literature suggests: alcohol misuse has the most evidence for impaired information and emotion processing and is consistently and strongly associated with child abuse and neglect behaviors. In addition, neuropsychological impairments are more severe and longer lasting when parents have recently misused methamphetamines compared to cannabis. Thus, more structured, supportive processes are required to help these parents with a history of recurring, heavy methamphetamine use to navigate persistent challenges in working memory, learning, and executing complex actions required to manage childcare, extensive treatment plans, and court proceedings.

Regarding opioid misuse, social work treatments protocols should incorporate best practices to help parents achieve and maintain recovery and reduce likelihood of relapse, such as medication-assisted treatment (MAT; Radel et al., 2018; see Chapters 18 and 19).

Next steps

Future work should continue to integrate measures of substance type, neuropsychological functioning, and associated parenting behaviors. Beyond this, we must navigate further methodological challenges that arise when incorporating dimensions of severity, frequency, route of administration, drug purity, and drug potency. Given parental substance use is just one of many prevailing child maltreatment risk factors (e.g. Stith et al., 2009), substance-specific effects are likely moderated by other factors (Milner, 2000). Confounding risk factors, such as baseline cognitive functioning, parental depression, and limited social connections providing resource, may better explain observed associations between child maltreatment and SUDs involving alcohol and illicit drugs (Testa & Smith, 2009). Social stressors also appear to be particularly important in models of addiction and parental functioning (Rutherford et al., 2013). It is plausible that social conditions exist where substance use is buffered or controlled in a way that protects children from substance-related harms (Cicchetti & Toth, 2005).

Conclusions

As a first step, this chapter provided a deep dive into understanding individual-level mechanisms that may directly compromise parental functioning. Future work will need to address ways that social and environmental factors bolster parental functioning and/or compensate for existing challenges, so social workers can tailor services better to minimize substance-related harms.

Social workers will need to collaborate with other disciplines to overcome methodological challenges associated with measuring the relative contribution of biological, psychological, social, and environmental mechanisms.

Glossary of selected terms

Term	Definition
Attention	Ability to either respond to multiple tasks/demands, maintain focus in the face of distracting or competing stimuli, or maintain a consistent behavioral response
Empathy	Ability to accurately interpret, understand, and share the feelings of another
Executive functions:	Integrated functions that generate, supervise, and monitor behaviors directed toward the execution of a goal
Working memory	Temporary storage and management of information necessary to carry out complex cognitive tasks
Cognitive flexibility	Ability to shift or switch between different tasks or mental operations
Inhibition	Ability to stop or lessen automatic or impulsive responses when necessary
Decision making	Ability to select the best course of action among a set of possible choices
Planning	Ability to set goals, develop strategies, and outline a clear plan to achieve these goals
Emotion processing	Ability to recognize, experience, and express the range of emotions (i.e. negative, neutral, and positive)
Emotion regulation	Ability to manage and respond to an emotional experience in a way that helps one modulate his/her response
Memory	Acquisition, retention, and recollection of knowledge in addition to the ability to perform an intended action in the future.
Mentalization	Ability to understand another's underlying mental state, which is viewed as critical for empathic responding

Sources: Fernández et al. (2011), Giancola et al. (2012), Swain et al. (2014).

References

Akin, B. A., Brook, J., & Lloyd, M. H. (2015). Examining the role of methamphetamine in permanency: A competing risks analysis of reunification, guardianship, and adoption. *American Journal of Orthopsychiatry, 85*(2), 119–130. doi:10.1037/ort0000052

Arias, F., Arnsten, J. H., Cunningham, C. O., Coulehan, K., Batchelder, A., Brisbane, M., . . . Rivera-Mindt, M. (2016). Neurocognitive, psychiatric, and substance use characteristics in opioid dependent adults. *Addictive Behaviors, 60*, 137–143. doi:10.1016/j.addbeh.2016.03.018

Bowlby, J. (1982). Attachment and loss: Retrospect and prospect. *American Journal of Orthopsychiatry, 52*(4), 664–678. doi:10.1111/j.1939-0025.1982.tb01456.x

Brook, J., & McDonald, T. (2009). The impact of parental substance abuse on the stability of family reunifications from foster care. *Children and Youth Services Review, 31*(2), 193–198. doi:10.1016/j.childyouth.2008.07.010

Brown, J. A., & Hohman, M. (2006). The impact of methamphetamine use on parenting. *Journal of Social Work Practice in the Addictions, 6*(1–2), 63–88. doi:10.1300/j160v06n01_04

Broyd, S. J., van Hell, H. H., Beale, C., Yücel, M., & Solowij, N. (2016). Acute and chronic effects of cannabinoids on human cognition—A systematic review. *Biological Psychiatry, 79*(7), 557–567. doi:10.1016/j.biopsych.2015.12.002

Camoirano, A. (2017). Mentalizing makes parenting work: A review about parental reflective functioning and clinical interventions to improve it. *Frontiers in Psychology, 8*, 14. doi:10.3389/fpsyg.2017.00014

Cicchetti, D., & Toth, S. L. (2005). Child maltreatment. *Annual Review of Clinical Psychology, 1*, 409–438. doi:10.1146/annurev.clinpsy.1.102803.144029

Coyer, S. M. (2001). Mothers recovering from cocaine addiction: Factors affecting parenting skills. *Journal of Obstetric, Gynecologic, & Neonatal Nursing, 30*(1), 71–79. doi:10.1111/j.1552-6909.2001.tb01523.x

Crittenden, P. M. (1993). An information-processing perspective on the behavior of neglectful parents. *Criminal Justice and Behavior, 20*(1), 27–48. doi:10.1177/0093854893020001004

De Bortoli, L., Coles, J., & Dolan, M. (2013). Parental substance misuse and compliance as factors determining child removal: A sample from the Victorian children's court in Australia. *Children and Youth Services Review, 35*(9), 1319–1326. doi:10.1016/j.childyouth.2013.05.002

De Paul, J., & Guibert, M. (2008). Empathy and child neglect: A theoretical model. *Child Abuse & Neglect, 32*(11), 1063–1071. doi:10.1016/j.chiabu.2008.03.003

Fernández-Serrano, M. J., Pérez-García, M., Perales, J. C., & Verdejo-García, A. (2010). Prevalence of executive dysfunction in cocaine, heroin and alcohol users enrolled in therapeutic communities. *European Journal of Pharmacology, 626*(1), 104–112. doi:10.1016/j.ejphar.2009.10.019

Fernández-Serrano, M. J., Pérez-García, M., & Verdejo-García, A. (2011). What are the specific vs. generalized effects of drugs of abuse on neuropsychological performance? *Neuroscience & Biobehavioral Reviews, 35*(3), 377–406. doi:10.1016/j.neubiorev.2010.04.008

Forrester, D. (2000). Parental substance misuse and child protection in a British sample. A survey of children on the child protection register in an inner London district office. *Child Abuse Review, 9*(4), 235–246. doi:10.1002/1099-0852(200007/08)9:4<235::AID-CAR626>3.0.CO;2-4

Freisthler, B., Gruenewald, P. J., & Wolf, J. P. (2015). Examining the relationship between marijuana use, medical marijuana dispensaries, and abusive and neglectful parenting. *Child Abuse & Neglect, 48*, 170–178. doi:10.1016/j.chiabu.2015.07.008

Freisthler, B., Holmes, M. R., & Wolf, J. P. (2014). The dark side of social support: Understanding the role of social support, drinking behaviors and alcohol outlets for child physical abuse. *Child Abuse & Neglect, 38*(6), 1106–1119. doi:10.1016/j.chiabu.2014.03.011

Freisthler, B., Johnson-Motoyama, M., & Kepple, N. J. (2014). Inadequate child supervision: The role of alcohol outlet density, parent drinking behaviors, and social support. *Children and Youth Services Review, 43*, 75–84. doi:10.1016/j.chiabu.2014.04.001

Freisthler, B. & Kepple, N.J. (2019). Types of substance use and punitive parenting: A preliminary exploration. *Journal of Social Work Practice in Addictions, 19*(3), 262–283. doi: 10.1080/1533256X.2019.1640019

Giancola, P. R., Godlaski, A. J., & Roth, R. M. (2012). Identifying component-processes of executive functioning that serve as risk factors for the alcohol-aggression relation. *Psychology of Addictive Behaviors, 26*(2), 201–211. doi:10.1037/a0025207

Grella, C. E., Hser, Y. I., & Huang, Y. C. (2006). Mothers in substance abuse treatment: Differences in characteristics based on involvement with child welfare services. *Child Abuse & Neglect, 30*(1), 55–73. doi:10.1016/j.chiabu.2005.07.005

Grella, C. E., Needell, B., Shi, Y., & Hser, Y. I. (2009). Do drug treatment services predict reunification outcomes of mothers and their children in child welfare? *Journal of Substance Abuse Treatment, 36*(3), 278–293. doi:10.1016/j.jsat.2008.06.010

Gruber, S. A., Silveri, M. M., & Yurgelun-Todd, D. A. (2007). Neuropsychological consequences of opiate use. *Neuropsychology Review, 17*(3), 299–315. doi:10.1007/s11065-007-9041-y

Huebner, R. A., Willauer, T., & Posze, L. (2012). The impact of sobriety treatment and recovery teams (START) on family outcomes. *Families in Society, 93*(3), 196–203. doi:10.1606/1044-3894.4223

Iudicello, J. E., Woods, S. P., Vigil, O., Cobb Scott, J., Cherner, M., Heaton, R. K., . . . HIV Neurobehavioral Research Center (HNRC) Group. (2010). Longer term improvement in neurocognitive functioning and affective distress among methamphetamine users who achieve stable abstinence. *Journal of Clinical and Experimental Neuropsychology, 32*(7), 704–718. doi:10.1080/13803390903512637

Ives, R., & Ghelani, P. (2006). Polydrug use (the use of drugs in combination): A brief review. *Drugs: Education, Prevention and Policy, 13*(3), 225–232. doi:10.1080/09687630600655596

Kepple, N. J. (2017). The complex nature of parental substance use: Examining past year and prior use patterns as correlates of child maltreatment frequency. *Substance Use & Misuse, 52*(6), 811–821. doi:10.1080/10826084.2016.1253747

Kepple, N. J. (2018). Does parental substance use always engender risk for children? Comparing incidence rate ratios of abusive and neglectful behaviors across substance use behavior patterns. *Child Abuse & Neglect, 76*, 44–55. doi:10.1016/j.chiabu.2017.09.015

Koob, G. F., & Volkow, N. D. (2010). Neurocircuitry of addiction. *Neuropsychopharmacology, 35*(1), 217–238. doi:10.1038/npp.2009.110

Kuhn, C., Swartzwelder, S., & Wilson, W. (2014). *Buzzed: The straight facts about the most used and abused drugs from alcohol to ecstasy* (4th ed.). New York, NY: W.W. Norton & Company.

Laslett, A. M., Ferris, J., Dietze, P., & Room, R. (2012). Social demography of alcohol-related harm to children in Australia. *Addiction, 107*(6), 1082–1089. doi:10.1111/j.1360-0443.2012.03789.x

Leeb, R., Paulozzi, L., Melanson, C., Simon, T., & Arias, I. (2008). *Child maltreatment surveillance: Uniform definitions for public health and recommended data elements.* Atlanta, GA: Centers for Disease Control and Prevention (CDC). doi:10.1037/e587022010-001

Leonard, K.E. (2002). Alcohol and substance abuse in marital violence and child maltreatment. In C. Wekerle & A. Wall (Eds.), *The violence and addiction equation: Theoretical and clinical issues in substance abuse and relationship violence* (pp. 194–219). Philadelphia PA: Brunner/Mazel.

Lipari, R. N., & Van Horn, S. L. (2017, August). *Children living with parents who have a substance use disorder* [The CBHSQ report]. Rockville, MD: Center for Behavioral Health Statistics and Quality, Substance Abuse and Mental Health Services Administration.

Manning, V., Best, D. W., Faulkner, N., & Titherington, E. (2009). New estimates of the number of children living with substance misusing parents: Results from UK national household surveys. *BMC Public Health, 9*(1), 377. doi:10.1186/1471-2458-9-377

Mayes, L. C., Feldman, R., Granger, R. H., Haynes, O. M., Bornstein, M. H., & Schottenfeld, R. (1997). The effects of polydrug use with and without cocaine on mother-infant interaction at 3 and 6 months. *Infant Behavior and Development, 20*(4), 489–502. doi:10.1016/S0163-6383(97)90038-2

Meier, M. H., Caspi, A., Ambler, A., Harrington, H., Houts, R., Keefe, R. S., . . . Moffitt, T. E. (2012). Persistent cannabis users show neuropsychological decline from childhood to midlife. *Proceedings of the National Academy of Sciences, 109*(40), E2657–E2664. doi:10.1073/pnas.1206820109

Milner, J. S. (2000). Social information processing and child physical abuse: Theory and research. In D. J. Hansen (Ed.), *Nebraska symposium on motivation, Vol. 46, 1998: Motivation and child maltreatment* (pp. 39–84). Lincoln: University of Nebraska.

Ondersma, S. J. (2002). Predictors of neglect within low-SES families: The importance of substance abuse. *American Journal of Orthopsychiatry, 72*(3), 383–391. doi:10.1037/0002-9432.72.3.383

Oscar-Berman, M., & Marinković, K. (2007). Alcohol: Effects on neurobehavioral functions and the brain. *Neuropsychology Review, 17*(3), 239–257. doi:10.1007/s11065-007-9038-6

Ostrowsky, M. K. (2011). Does marijuana use lead to aggression and violent behavior? *Journal of Drug Education, 41*(4), 369–389. doi:10.2190/DE.41.4.c

Payer, D. E., Lieberman, M. D., Monterosso, J. R., Xu, J., Fong, T. W., & London, E. D. (2008). Differences in cortical activity between methamphetamine-dependent and healthy individuals performing a facial affect matching task. *Drug and Alcohol Dependence, 93*(1–2), 93–102. doi:10.1016/j.drugalcdep.2007.09.009

Radel, L., Baldwin, M., Crouse, G., Ghertner, R., & Waters, A. (2018). *Substance use, the opioid epidemic, and the child welfare system: Key findings from a mixed methods study* (ASPE research brief). Washington, DC: U.S. Department of Health and Human Services, Office of the Assistant Secretary for Planning and Evaluation. Retrieved from https://bettercarenetwork.org/sites/default/files/SubstanceUseChildWelfareOverview.pdf

Romanowicz, M., Voort, J. L. V., Shekunov, J., Oesterle, T. S., Thusius, N. J., Rummans, T. A., . . . Schak, K. M. (2019). The effects of parental opioid use on the parent–child relationship and children's developmental and behavioral outcomes: A systematic review of published reports. *Child and Adolescent Psychiatry and Mental Health, 13*, 5. doi:10.1186/s13034-019-0266-3

Rutherford, H. J. V., Potenza, M. N., & Mayes, L. C. (2013). The neurobiology of addiction and attachment. In N. E. Suchman, M. Pajulo, & L. C. Mayes (Eds.), *Parenting and substance abuse: Developmental approaches to intervention* (pp. 3–23). New York, NY: Oxford University Press. doi:10.1093/med:psych/9780199743100.003.0001

Scott, J. C., Woods, S. P., Matt, G. E., Meyer, R. A., Heaton, R. K., Atkinson, J. H., & Grant, I. (2007). Neurocognitive effects of methamphetamine: A critical review and meta-analysis. *Neuropsychology Review, 17*(3), 275–297. doi:10.1007/s11065-007-9031-0

Sedlak, A. J., Mettenburg, J., Basena, M., Peta, I., McPherson, K., & Greene, A. (2010). *Fourth national incidence study of child abuse and neglect (NIS-4)*. Washington, DC: U.S. Department of Health and Human Services. doi:10.1037/e565022012-001

Slesnick, N., Feng, X., Brakenhoff, B., & Brigham, G. S. (2014). Parenting under the influence: The effects of opioids, alcohol and cocaine on mother–child interaction. *Addictive Behaviors, 39*(5), 897–900. doi:10.1016/j.addbeh.2014.02.003

Smith, V. C., & Wilson, C. R. (2016). Families affected by parental substance use. *Pediatrics, 138*(2), e20161575. doi:10.1542/peds.2016-1575

Stewart, D., Gossop, M., & Trakada, K. (2007). Drug dependent parents: Childcare responsibilities, involvement with treatment services, and treatment outcomes. *Addictive Behaviors, 32*(8), 1657–1668. doi:10.1016/j.addbeh.2006.11.019

Stith, S. M., Liu, T., Davies, L. C., Boykin, E. L., Alder, M. C., Harris, J. M., . . . Dees, J. E. M. E. G. (2009). Risk factors in child maltreatment: A meta-analytic review of the literature. *Aggression and Violent Behavior, 14*(1), 13–29. doi:10.1016/j.avb.2006.03.006

Swain, J. E., Kim, P., Spicer, J., Ho, S. S., Dayton, C. J., Elmadih, A., & Abel, K. M. (2014). Approaching the biology of human parental attachment: Brain imaging, oxytocin and coordinated assessments of mothers and fathers. *Brain Research, 1580*, 78–101. doi:10.1016/j.brainres.2014.03.007

Testa, M., & Smith, B. (2009). Prevention and drug treatment. *The Future of Children, 19*, 147–168. doi:10.1353/foc.0.0033

Thornberry, T. P., Matsuda, M., Greenman, S. J., Augustyn, M. B., Henry, K. L., Smith, C. A., & Ireland, T. O. (2014). Adolescent risk factors for child maltreatment. *Child Abuse & Neglect, 38*(4), 706–722. doi:10.1016/j.chiabu.2013.08.009

U.S. Department of Health and Human Services, Centers for Medicare & Medicaid Services. (2011, October). *Fact sheet: Substance (other than tobacco) abuse structured assessment and brief intervention (SBIRT) services* (ICN 904084). Retrieved from http://www.integration.samhsa.gov/clinical-practice/sbirt

Vik, P. W., Cellucci, T., Jarchow, A., & Hedt, J. (2004). Cognitive impairment in substance abuse. *Psychiatric Clinics of North America, 27*, 97–109. doi:10.1016/S0193-953X(03)00110-2

Wolf, J. P., Kepple, N. J., & Freisthler, B. (2019). Understanding the role of parental opiate or marijuana use in child welfare substantiation decisions. *Journal of Social Work Practice in Addictions, 19*(3), 238–261.

Young, N. K., Boles, S. M., & Otero, C. (2007). Parental substance use disorders and child maltreatment: Overlap, gaps, and opportunities. *Child Maltreatment, 12*(2), 137–149. doi:10.1177/1077559507300322

Zweben, J. E., Cohen, J. B., Christian, D., Galloway, G. P., Salinardi, M., Parent, D., & Iguchi, M. (2004). Psychiatric symptoms in methamphetamine users. *American Journal on Addictions, 13*(2), 181–190. doi:10.1080/10550490490436055

Working with families affected by a member's addictive behavior

Megan Petra and Toula Kourgiantakis

Background

Researchers estimate that more than 100 million family members worldwide are affected by someone's addictive behavior (Orford, Velleman, Natera, & Copello, 2013). This is a conservative estimate when considering that 5.1% of the worldwide population are coping with alcohol use disorder, 0.6% with drug use disorders, and between 0.1% and 5.8% are coping with gambling disorder (Calado & Griffiths, 2016; Carrà, Bartoli, Brambilla, Crocamo, & Clerici, 2015; United Nations, 2018; World Health Organization [WHO], 2018; see Chapter 8). The negative effects of a member's addictive behavior on families are extensive, including harm to physical and mental health, relationships, finances, and overall well-being (Orford et al., 2005). Although some evidence-informed family interventions have been developed (Kourgiantakis, Saint-Jacques, & Tremblay, 2013), little help is available to support families, as treatment tends to be individually focused (Ventura & Bagley, 2017). Service provisions need to be more family-centered for two main reasons. First, families affected by a member's addictive behavior deserve quality support when needed. Second, family involvement in addiction treatment not only benefits the family, but also the individual experiencing problematic addictive behavior (Center for Substance Abuse Treatment [CSAT], 2005).

Social workers are well-positioned to apply family-centered approaches when working with families affected by a member's addictive behavior. Social workers are the largest group of professionals in the mental health workforce (Heisler, 2018), and almost all social workers encounter individuals experiencing substance use disorders, regardless of practice sector (Whitaker, Weismiller, & Clark, 2006).

This chapter reviews current evidence about families affected by a member's substance misuse. It opens with an overview addictive behavior effects on families, then explores explanatory theories (family systems theory, stress and coping theory, and codependency theory) and assesses theory suitability for social work. Next addressed are each of four main categories of interventions for families affected by a member's substance misuse (conjoint treatment of the individual and family members, direct services to family members, interventions to build family members' skills as supportive significant others, and mutual aid interventions). For each category of family interventions, we review evidence surrounding key interventions and offer suggestions for their use and further development. The chapter concludes with a discussion of implications for social work education, practice with families affected by a member's addictive behavior, and research.

Families and addictive behavior

Here we define families as individuals linked biologically, legally, or through bonds of affection, with a shared commitment, and define themselves as family. Family members may be related by blood, marriage, legal action, kinship network, custom, or choice (CSAT, 2005). This definition of family is inclusive of concerned/supportive significant others (CSOs or SSOs) who are close friends, roommates, honorary kin, and so forth, in addition to those who fit more traditional definitions of family. This chapter focuses on families affected by an adult member's addictive behavior; different family interventions and systems of care apply when the addictive behavior problem is experienced by an adolescent.

Substance use disorders (SUDs) and gambling disorder cause significant family stress and affect many biopsychosocial, spiritual, and cultural spheres of family life. Problematic addictive behavior can create a chaotic, unpredictable family life, as well as increased family isolation and legal, employment, and financial difficulties (Dowling, Rodda, Lubman, & Jackson, 2014; Orford et al., 2005). As a result, family members may suffer significant mental health (Karriker-Jaffe, Li, & Greenfield, 2018) and physical health issues (Ray, Meriens, & Weisner, 2007). CSOs typically shoulder additional family responsibilities, including providing care for the person engaged in addictive behavior (Jiang, Callinan, Laslett, & Room, 2017). Furthermore, these families experience an elevated risk for family violence and/or family transitions such as separation/divorce (Choenni, Hammink, & van de Mheen, 2017; Dowling et al., 2014; Petra, 2014).

Both intrafamilial and contextual factors are important to families' experience of a member's addictive behavior. Not only do addiction-related problems add to the burden CSOs experience, they also complicate the family's task of coping with the member's addictive behavior. Poverty and other additional burdens also impact CSOs' ability to cope effectively (Orford, 2017). Cultural factors such as strong extended family systems or reluctance about sharing family problems with non-family members may either facilitate or constrain social support opportunities, coping options, and/or help-seeking (Church et al., 2018; Holdsworth, Breen, Hing, & Gordon, 2013). Finally, families living in regions where treatment is unavailable may simply be unable to engage formal assistance (Orford et al., 2013; WHO, 2010).

CSOs often deal with the challenging situation for years before seeking help (Sakiyama, Padin, Canfield, Laranjeira, & Mitsuhiro, 2015). Yet evidence-informed family-centered addiction interventions have been developed and may be a way for social workers to assist this potentially underserved population.

Theories explaining family effects of addictive behavior

This section provides an overview of three theories concerning families affected by a member's addictive behavior: family systems theory, stress and coping theory, and codependency theory. Each theory is examined in terms of social work tenets, perspectives, and/or values.

Family systems theory

According to family systems theory, families are complex, interconnected systems made up of individual members (CSAT, 2005; Steinglass, 2009). Each family member both contributes to the system and is influenced by it (circular influence). Thus, addictive behavior exhibited by one family member affects the entire system; conversely, the family context influences the functioning of each member (Cunha & Relvas, 2013; see Chapter 7). Family systems strive to achieve and maintain a stable status quo (the homeostasis principle), even in the face of a problem such as addiction. For instance, a family system affected by a member's addictive behavior may reach stability by becoming organized around the problem (Steinglass, 2009). Alternately, the addictive behavior may be self-reinforcing in a family system if it serves a family function: for instance, allowing members to bond over gambling or shifting focus away from another problem that the family does not wish to address (Rohrbaugh, 2014).

A family system at homeostasis may be difficult to change via any single member's unilateral efforts. For this reason, family systems' interventions view the entire family, or at least the main couple, as the identified "client" (CSAT, 2005). The goal of family systems therapy is to interrupt harmful behavior patterns, change relationships or interactions between members and within subsystems, and help the family achieve and maintain more functional homeostasis. This involves supporting the family and drawing on strengths of the family system and its members.

Family systems theory is consistent with social work's person-in-environment focus. It also recognizes the value in supporting CSOs, as well as persons engaging in efforts to change their addictive behavior. Family system mechanisms explain multiple ways one member's addictive behavior affects the family as a whole. Some have critiqued family systems theory for being a deficit-oriented model that places blame on families and views addictive behavior as a symptom of pathology or dysfunction within the family system (Calderwood & Rajesparam, 2014; Orford, Copello, Velleman, & Templeton, 2010). Others have argued that this is an inaccurate perception of systems theory: that using a systems lens does not include families as part of the problem, but recognizes the (healthy) interdependence and interactivity within families (CSAT, 2005). Family systems theory is important in providing a framework for social work practice with families seeking help to address individual distress, family relationships, and other consequences related to a member's addictive behavior.

Stress and coping theory

The transactional theory of stress and coping applies to families affected by a member's addictive behavior (Folkman, 2011). According to Folkman, when individuals face significant stressors—events or situations beyond their ability to easily handle—they apply coping strategies. Problem-focused coping strategies address the problem by attempting to solve or avert it. Emotion-focused coping strategies reduce distress about a stressor through meaning-making or temporary avoidance. Problem-focused coping is considered more beneficial with solvable problems, but emotion-focused coping may be more adaptive with intractable problems.

Orford et al. (2010) adapted stress and coping theory to families affected by a member's addiction. According to their Stress-Strain-Coping-Support (SSCS) model, the behavior of a person experiencing addiction is a stressor on CSOs, who then experience strain (exhibited in poor physical or emotional health, low quality of life, and so forth). However, beneficial coping strategies and receiving support may lessen CSOs' strain. The SSCS model recognizes three types of coping: engaged (attempting to get the loved one to quit or cut down via emotional or active strategies), tolerant-inactive (putting up with the addictive behavior), and withdrawal (removing oneself from the effects of the addictive behavior and/or that family member). SSCS theorists recommend withdrawal coping as being associated with lower distress levels among CSOs (Orford et al., 2017).

The SSCS model offers a unique contribution to social work with CSOs, as it is among few models focusing on family members' experiences without blaming or pathologizing them. According to the SSCS model (Orford et al., 2010), CSOs are viewed as individuals coping as best as they can with the chronic stress created by a family member's addictive behavior. With support, CSOs can learn to cope effectively and reduce their stress. This is congruent with social work's strengths perspective, which acknowledges families' strengths that contribute to wellness and recovery. The SSCS model also recognizes self-determination concerning decisions regarding treatment options and goal-setting.

A limitation of the SSCS model is that it does not directly acknowledge the importance of interactive, familial, contextual, or cultural factors in CSOs' lives and experiences. Early SSCS publications (e.g. Orford et al., 2010) considered the experience of dealing with a family member's addictive behavior to be largely universal. However, more recent work acknowledges the role of contextual elements (e.g. poverty, family violence, or culture) in shaping CSOs' experiences (Orford, 2017). This aspect of the SSCS model—the importance of familial and extra-familial environments to CSOs' experiences—must be strengthened before the SSCS model is fully consistent with social work's emphasis on person-in-environment fit.

Codependency theory

Codependency theory posits that, just as a person experiencing a substance use disorder may develop a dependence on the substance, so too CSOs may develop a dependence (codependence) on the disorder's presence within the family (Cutland, 1998). Primarily applied to women, criteria for codependency include a focus on others to the point of self-sacrifice, lack or loss of sense of self, difficulty in experiencing or expressing emotions, inflexibility, a need to control others, and a tendency to sabotage their family member's attempts at recovery despite an expressed desire for change (Dear, Roberts, & Lange, 2005; Harkness & Cotrell, 1997). Proponents of codependency theory consider codependency unhealthy, with codependent family members being blame-worthy as "enablers" for impeding the individual's recovery, and thus needing help for their own problematic behavior. Codependency theory was popularized by Beattie (1986), and has resonated with some practitioners and CSOs.

Critics of codependency theory have noted that the concept of codependency is both overly broad and ill-defined, and that the concept has little empirical validation (Orford et al., 2005). Codependency theory pathologizes CSOs, and relies considerably on criteria resembling women's traditional gender roles (Cunha & Relvas, 2013). Furthermore, codependency theory implies that collective or interdependent family structures are harmful or maladaptive; as such, it is not culturally sensitive, does not support strengths-based social work practice, and is inconsistent with the value social work places on the importance and centrality of human relationships.

Family-centered intervention options

Ample evidence indicates that family-centered interventions are important and beneficial for CSOs, families, and individuals engaged in addictive behaviors. Family involvement enhances addiction treatment engagement, retention, and outcomes (McCrady et al., 2016; McPherson, Boyne, & Willis, 2017; Roozen, de Waart, & van der Kroft, 2010). Family-centered interventions also result in decreased distress and better coping skills among CSOs, and improved family functioning (Kourgiantakis et al., 2013). These approaches may reduce the overall healthcare system costs of addiction treatment (Meads, Ting, Dretzke, & Bayliss, 2007).

Despite the indicated potential benefits of engaging family members in addiction treatment interventions, services and policies continue to be individually focused, neglecting families (Csiernik, 2002; Orford et al., 2010; Ventura & Bagley, 2017). This may be due to macro-level barriers. In a study of systemic barriers to family-centered treatment, Selbekk and Sagvaag (2016) noted that health care systems typically consider the person experiencing addiction to be the client/patient, introducing added complexity and potentially reduced reimbursement for providers intervening to help the entire family. In addition, traditional cultural narratives about families may impede family involvement in addiction interventions. Orr, Barbour, and Elliott (2014) observed that many clinicians and policymakers held assumptions and misconceptions about families being "part of the problem," viewing engaged, helpful families as the exception rather than the rule (p. 412).

Evidence-informed interventions do exist for families coping with a member's addictive behavior. Much research has focused on family interventions for substance use disorders; however, research on interventions for families affected by gambling has increased (Kourgiantakis et al., 2013; see Chapter 8). Family-centered interventions involve CSOs, but techniques and ultimate goals may vary. This section reviews four categories of family-centered interventions (conjoint treatment, direct services to family members, interventions to build CSO skills to promote treatment engagement, and mutual aid).

Conjoint treatment

Conjoint treatments acknowledge the effects of individuals' addictive behaviors on their families and view the family or couple as an appropriate focus of treatment. While the treatment focus remains the addictive behavior, these approaches also promote family/couple functioning and engage CSOs in supporting their family member's recovery.

Behavioral couples therapy (BCT)

BCT is an evidence-informed treatment for couples, originally developed to address SUDs (Fletcher, 2013; Meis et al., 2013). Based on cognitive-behavioral techniques, BCT acknowledges that couples' interactions can reinforce either the addictive behavior or sobriety, and that stressful relationships can increase the risk of relapse. BCT engages CSOs in helping their partners identify risks and consequences for their addictive behaviors. It also enlists CSOs in supporting their partners' attempts to cut down or quit, and focuses on improving couples' communication and relationship functioning (Fletcher, 2013).

BCT is a manualized treatment, typically involving 12–20 couple sessions in addition to individual treatment for the person experiencing an addictive disorder. A meta-analysis of 16 BCT studies (Meis et al., 2013) reported that BCT is more effective at decreasing addictive behavior and improving relationship functioning than individual treatment alone, with small to medium effect sizes that persist through follow-up. Preliminary evidence suggests that BCT may have ancillary benefits for children's adjustment, as well, and may also decrease intimate partner violence (Fletcher, 2013).

BCT variations are also effective: short-term versions, BCT plus additional modules, or Alcohol Focused Behavioral Couples Therapy (Meis et al., 2013). While BCT effectiveness evidence is strongest with SUDs, an initial study of internet-delivered BCT to address gambling disorder reported reductions in gambling behavior and both CSO depression and anxiety (Nilsson, Magnusson, Carlbring, Andersson, & Gumpert, 2018).

Family systems interventions

Family systems therapy is a conjoint treatment approach applying structural-strategic family therapy techniques. Family systems interventions involve CSOs for support to the individual and because the family itself is a focus of treatment. Family systems interventions are more common in work with families affected by an adolescent's rather than an adult's addictive behavior. Only one intervention has undergone development across multiple studies: Congruence Couple Therapy (CCT; Lee & Awosoga, 2015), a couple treatment to address addictive gambling behavior. CCT treats gambling addiction by helping couples improve their alignment (congruence) with each other. Preliminary evidence suggests that CCT reduces gambling, lowers overall distress, and improves family system functioning. CCT is promising, as it is the only family systems-based intervention for CSOs affected by an adult's addictive behavior. There exists preliminary evidence for its effectiveness with families affected by gambling, although more research is needed. As there are relatively few evidence-informed interventions for families affected by gambling (see Chapter 8), more focus is needed on this population.

Conjoint treatment summary

In summary, both BCT and family systems therapy consider the effects of addictive behavior on CSOs and include them in the addiction treatment process. As such, CSOs have an opportunity to benefit directly from the intervention, in addition to indirect benefits resulting from reductions in addictive behavior. However, conjoint interventions are only possible if CSOs and the family member engaged in addictive behavior agree to be involved in treatment; this simultaneous readiness may be difficult to achieve, especially in families where more than one member experiences a problem with addictive behavior. The effectiveness evidence supporting BCT is currently stronger than that for other couple interventions (Fletcher, 2013). Due to the strong evidence base for BCT and its variants, it is recommended for families where a SUD is involved; BCT's effectiveness is less certain with gambling or diverse populations. Moreover, as most research on BCT has been carried out in the United States, its applicability in other countries is not clear. Also, because BCT focuses largely on the addiction, CSO needs for psychoeducation, coping skills, self-care, and peer support may be insufficiently addressed.

Direct services to family members

This category of family interventions focuses on supporting family members and offering services focused on their specific needs. Primary goals of these interventions are to reduce the harm of a member's addictive behaviors on the rest of the family, address CSOs' needs, and empower them to make choices that will improve their well-being. Despite the widespread consensus that CSOs are greatly impacted by someone's addictive behavior, less research examines this category than other categories of family interventions (Rane et al., 2017). Two direct services interventions for CSOs are reviewed.

The 5-Step Method

The 5-Step Method is based on the SSCS model (Copello, Templeton, Orford & Velleman, 2010), consisting of listening to CSOs' experiences, providing information, exploring coping behaviors, exploring social support, and planning for additional support. This intervention is flexible in that it can be delivered in individual, group, or self-help formats (e.g. online or via workbooks). Results of uncontrolled studies and one randomized controlled trial are promising, suggesting that this intervention reduces CSO experiences of physical and psychological strain, improves coping, and increases their received support. The 5-Step Method has been implemented with promising results in England, Italy, and Mexico (Rey, Aguilar, Pérez, Juárez, & Tiburcio, 2011; Velleman et al., 2008, 2011), but did not have the same results in India (Nadkarni et al., 2017). Researchers attributed observed difference to inadequate adaptation of the intervention to the cultural context. This intervention strategy needs more systematic evaluation, particularly with diverse groups and contexts.

Family psychoeducation

Family psychoeducation is an evidence-informed approach originally developed for families affected by a member's mental illness. It educates CSOs about the problem and addresses their personal coping skills, problem solving, support, and crisis management (Substance Abuse and Mental Health Services Administration, 2009). Research on family psychoeducation with addictive behaviors is limited; some studies examined family psychoeducation with dual disorders (Lucksted, McFarlane, Downing, Dixon, & Adams, 2012). A recent study of family psychoeducation for dual disorders found that CSOs experienced reduced stress and enhanced coping skills after participating in the program (Denomme & Benhanoh, 2017).

Direct services summary

Interventions in this category support and empower CSOs and are focused on helping them improve their own coping and overall well-being. These interventions are relatively brief, with a flexible delivery format. An advantage of these interventions is that CSOs can participate in these interventions regardless of whether their family member seeks treatment for a problematic addictive behavior. However, CSOs entirely focused on engaging their family member in addiction treatment may find these interventions do not fulfill their needs. The 5-Step Method is perhaps the most internationally implemented intervention reviewed, with studies conducted in multiple countries. However, the approach may need significant adaptation to be appropriate for specific cultural contexts.

Interventions to build CSO skills to promote treatment engagement

A third category of interventions focuses on CSOs whose primary goal is to promote a family member's entry into treatment. These family interventions may have dual goals, including improved functioning of the CSO.

Community reinforcement and family training (CRAFT)

CRAFT has the strongest evidence base among treatment engagement interventions (Miller, Meyers, & Tonigan, 1999; Roozen et al., 2010). In CRAFT, CSOs learn to encourage a family member's abstinence through behavioral techniques (such as scheduling enjoyable activities at times that conflict with addictive behaviors), rewarding abstinence behavior, and allowing their family member to experience negative consequences of addictive behavior. CRAFT also includes communication training and promotes self-care activities. A meta-analysis of CRAFT studies reported that 67% of CRAFT participants' family members entered treatment, with CSOs reporting lower distress, greater family cohesion, and improved relationship functioning (Roozen et al., 2010).

Initially developed for addressing a family member's SUD, CRAFT has also been tested in studies involving a family member's gambling (Hodgins, Toneatto, Makarchuk, Skinner, & Vincent, 2007; Nayoski & Hodgins, 2016). Outcomes were mixed, with CRAFT consistently producing lower levels of gambling but having no significant effects on treatment engagement. Researchers attributed the lack of treatment engagement to minimal availability of gambling treatment.

Confrontational interventions

Interventions exist that intend to promote treatment engagement by encouraging CSOs to be confrontational with family members engaged in addictive behavior. (For instance, the television show *Intervention* features CSOs undergoing such an intervention; see Kosovski & Smith, 2011.) In general, confrontational family interventions do not have a strong supporting evidence base. A study examining the Johnson Intervention observed a 30% treatment engagement rate for family members of participants who completed the intervention; however, many dropped out before completing the Johnson Intervention (Miller et al., 1999). In a meta-analysis, Roozen and colleagues (2010) concluded that CRAFT performed better than the Johnson Intervention.

Promoting treatment engagement summary

CRAFT is the only intervention in this category with enough empirical evidence to support its effectiveness. It is appropriate for CSOs whose family member engages in problematic substance use but does not wish to seek treatment. An advantage is that CRAFT is skill-based and teaches techniques that CSOs can apply unilaterally; as such, it is empowering for CSOs. However, CRAFT may not be as effective in coping with gambling disorders, and there is no systematic evidence available concerning its effectiveness with diverse populations.

Mutual aid

Twelve-step groups are the primary form of mutual aid available to CSOs affected by a family member's alcohol (Al-Anon, Ala-Teen, and Adult Children of Alcoholics), drugs (Nar-Anon), or gambling (Gam-Anon) disorder. Meeting in over 130 countries (Al-Anon Family Groups, 2019), groups adapt the 12 steps of Alcoholics Anonymous as a structure for family members' personal recovery from their presumed codependency. CSOs are encouraged to admit powerlessness over their family member's addictive behavior, rely on their "higher power" for help, and detach from the addictive behavior in order to reduce their own suffering and experience recovery (Al-Anon Family Groups, 2008).

Empirical research on 12-step groups is limited, with most published studies being descriptive and uncontrolled, or testing clinician-led groups rather than directly examining the effectiveness of common 12-step groups. One six-month longitudinal study compared outcomes for new Al-Anon members who continued versus stopped attending (Timko, Halvorson, Kong, & Moos, 2015; Timko, Laudet, & Moos, 2016). Al-Anon attendance was associated with improved quality of life, self-esteem, and confidence, as well as lower stress, anxiety, anger and depression. Social processes (support and bonding between members, and group norms and expectations) mediated the relationship between Al-Anon attendance and outcomes.

Although strong efficacy evidence for CSO 12-step mutual aid groups is lacking, these programs are widely available, free of charge, and considered helpful by long-time members (Al-Anon Family Group Headquarters, 2018). However, the spiritual nature of the 12 steps may not be a good fit for some CSOs, and others may find the emphasis on powerlessness unhelpful. Other mutual aid programs may be available (c.f. Kelly, Fallah-Sohy, Cristello, & Bergman, 2017; Kondo & Wada, 2009), though none are currently considered evidence-informed practices.

Summary of family interventions

In examining family interventions overall, it is evident that they result in many positive outcomes for families coping with a member's addictive behaviors. The available research on BCT and CRAFT is more robust and rigorous than for most other interventions (Meis et al., 2013) and emerging evidence supporting the 5-Step Method exists (Roozen et al., 2010). To advance the evidence base for existing family interventions in addictions, more replication studies, greater diversity in populations and contexts studied, and more randomized controlled trials and comparison studies are needed (Meis et al., 2013). It is also important to develop and evaluate family psychoeducation interventions for specific addictive behaviors, so that families affected by a member's addictive behaviors can benefit in the same way as families affected by serious mental illness (Lucksted et al., 2012).

Implications for social work education and practice

Important implications for social work (and other professional) education, practice, and research can be gleaned from this overview. First, the absence of family-centered addictions practice in clinical settings may be "a consequence of the lack of a family orientation in professional training and practice" (Orford et al., 2005, p. 231). To prepare practitioners to work effectively with families affected by a member's addictive behaviors, up-to-date knowledge and research must be included in social work curricula and in professional continuing education (Begun, Clapp, and The Alcohol Misuse Grand Challenge Collective, 2016). Training content should include the impact of addictions on CSOs, the benefits of family involvement in addiction treatment, and evidence-informed interventions that social workers and other professionals can apply when working with families.

As practitioners in one of five core mental health professions, social workers are often the first point of contact for families affected by a member's addictive behavior (Kean, 2009). They may encounter CSOs needing medical, mental health, child welfare, or domestic violence services, also coping with addictive behavior problems, or supporting someone coping with addictive behavior problems. Brief screenings for issues common to these CSOs may identify families who would benefit from additional assistance and/or referral.

When choosing evidence-informed interventions for families affected by a member's addictive behavior, social workers should consider feasibility. For instance, BCT is a lengthy, manualized treatment, requiring extensive clinician training (Meis et al., 2013); schedules and resources would have to accommodate the 12–20 session course of treatment for each couple, and reimbursement for services may not be available. Other interventions may be more feasible. Direct interventions for CSOs, such as the 5-Step Method (Velleman et al., 2011), are briefer and more flexible to administer (in person, online, or via workbook/self-administered), so they may be a better fit for agencies and clinicians with heavy caseloads. An agency or government unit with an online presence may be able to provide online interventions at minimal cost. Another advantage to online interventions is that agencies could serve clients unable to travel for services.

Macro-level healthcare policy can influence the availability of assistance for families affected by a member's addictive behaviors. For instance, in countries with universal health care, services are likely to be affordable but may not be available or may have long waitlists. Conversely, in countries without single-payer systems, health insurance companies may control access to care: CSOs may be unable to access services in systems that consider the individual to be the primary client (not the family) and/or require a DSM/ICD diagnosis in order to receive services (Selbekk & Sagvaag, 2016). These system-level barriers to caring for CSOs and families represent areas where social workers can advocate for more equitable policies around access to best-practice care.

The salient points highlighted in this chapter also have implications for social work research. First, though evidence-informed psychoeducation interventions are helpful for families affected by mental health problems (Lucksted et al., 2012), they are not yet developed for CSOs of adults engaged in addictive behaviors. Research to fill this service gap is needed. Second, involving practitioners and CSOs in designing and conducting research would enhance studies' applicability. This could be achieved through collaborative community-research partnerships and advisory committees. Finally, few family-centered interventions have been created, adapted, and tested for application with diverse populations and contexts (Gainsbury, 2017). Further research is needed on the ways existing evidence-informed programs can be culturally and situationally adapted.

Conclusions

Many families are greatly affected by a member's addictive behaviors, and it is important to have services available to those who need them. It is critical that these families have choices: some may not seek support, while for others it may be essential. For families seeking services, a wide range of needs may exist, and service providers should recognize that one "size" does not fit all. It behooves social workers and other practitioners to be nonjudgmental and accepting of the services families choose (if any), and the areas they wish to address while receiving services.

Social workers play important roles in engaging, screening, assessing, and involving families in addiction treatment. Evidence-informed interventions exist to support CSOs and strengthen their coping and well-being and involve them in their family member's treatment and recovery. Yet family-centered interventions are not uniformly available, due in part to policy-level barriers. Social workers can and should apply their micro, mezzo, and macro-level skills to facilitate the availability and implementation of evidence-informed family-centered interventions across settings.

References

Al-Anon Family Groups. (2008). Detachment, love, and forgiveness. In *How Al-Anon works for families & friends of alcoholics* (pp. 83–87). Virginia Beach, VA: Author.
Al-Anon Family Groups. (2019). *Media kit*. Retrieved from https://al-anon.org/media-kit/
Al-Anon Family Group Headquarters. (2018). *2018 Membership survey: Results and longitudinal comparison*. Retrieved from https://al-anon.org/pdf/2018MembershipSurvey.pdf
Beattie, M. (1986). *Codependent no more: How to stop controlling others and start caring for yourself*. Center City, MN: Hazelden Publishing.
Begun, A. L., Clapp, J. D., & The Alcohol Misuse Grand Challenge Collective. (2016). Reducing and preventing alcohol misuse and its consequences. *International Journal of Alcohol and Drug Research, 5*(2), 73–83. doi:10.7895/ijadr.v5i2.223

Calado, F., & Griffiths, M. D. (2016). Problem gambling worldwide: An update and systematic review of empirical research (2000–2015). *Journal of Behavioral Addictions, 5*(4), 592–613. doi:10.1556/2006.5.2016073

Calderwood, K. A., & Rajesparam, A. (2014). Applying the codependency concept to concerned significant others of problem gamblers: Words of caution. *Journal of Gambling Issues, 29*, 1–16. doi:10.4309/jgi.2014.29.11

Center for Substance Abuse Treatment. (2005). *Substance abuse treatment and family therapy: Treatment improvement protocol (TIP) 39*. DHHS Publication No. (SMA) 05–4006. Rockville, MD: Substance Abuse and Mental Health Services Administration.

Choenni, V., Hammink, A., & van de Mheen, D. (2017). Association between substance use and the perpetration of family violence in industrialized countries: A systematic review. *Trauma, Violence, & Abuse, 18*(1), 37–50. doi:10.1177/1524838015589253

Church, S., Bhatia, U., Velleman, R., Velleman, G., Orford, J., Rane, A., & Nadkarni, A. (2018). Coping strategies and support structures of addiction affected families: A qualitative study from Goa, India. *Families, Systems, & Health, 36*(2), 216–224. doi:10.1037/fsh0000339

Copello, A., Templeton, L., Orford, J., & Velleman, R. (2010). The 5-Step Method: Evidence of gains for affected family members. *Drugs: Education, Prevention and Policy, 17*(S1), 100–112. doi:10.3109/09687637.2010.514234

Csiernik, R. (2002). Counseling for the family: The neglected aspect of addiction treatment in Canada. *Journal of Social Work Practice in the Addictions, 2*(1), 79–91. doi:10.1300/J160v02n01_05

Cunha, D., & Relvas, A. P. (2013). Pathological gambling and couple: Towards an integrative systemic model. *Journal of Gambling Studies, 30*(2), 213–228. doi:10.1007/s10899-013-9366-9

Cutland, L. (1998). A codependency perspective. In R. Velleman, A. Copello, & J. Maslin (Eds.), *Living with drink: Women who live with problem drinkers* (pp. 89–98). New York, NY: Addison Wesley Longman.

Dear, G. E., Roberts, C. M., & Lange, L. (2005). Defining codependency: A thematic analysis of published definitions. In S. P. Shohov (Ed.), *Advances in psychology research, Vol. 34*. Hauppauge, NY: Nova Science Publishers, Inc., 189–205.

Denomme, W. J., & Benhanoh, O. (2017). Helping concerned family members of individuals with substance use and concurrent disorders: An evaluation of a family member-oriented treatment program. *Journal of Substance Abuse Treatment, 79*, 34–45. doi:10.1016/j.sat.2017.05.012

Dowling, N. A., Rodda, S. N., Lubman, D. I., & Jackson, A. C. (2014). The impacts of problem gambling on concerned significant others accessing web-based counselling. *Addictive Behaviors, 39*, 1253–1257. doi:10.1016/j.addbeh.2014.04.011

Fletcher, K. (2013). Couple therapy treatments for substance use disorders: A systematic review. *Journal of Social Work Practice in the Addictions, 13*, 327–352. doi:10.1080/1533256X.2013.840213

Folkman, S. (2011). Stress, health, and coping: Synthesis, commentary, and future directions. In S. Folkman (Ed.), *The Oxford handbook of stress, health, and coping* (pp. 3–11). New York, NY: Oxford University Press. doi:10.1093/oxfordhb/9780195375343.013.0022

Gainsbury, S. M. (2017). Cultural competence in the treatment of addictions: Theory, practice and evidence. *Clinical Psychology and Psychotherapy, 24*, 987–1001. doi:10.1002/cpp.2062

Harkness, D., & Cotrell, G. (1997). The social construction of co-dependency in the treatment of substance abuse. *Journal of Substance Abuse Treatment, 14*(5), 473–479. doi:10.1016/S0740-5472(97)00121-9

Heisler, E. J. (2018). *The mental health workforce: A primer*. (R43255). Washington, DC: Congressional Research Service.

Hodgins, D. C., Toneatto, T., Makarchuk, K., Skinner, W., & Vincent, S. (2007). Minimal treatment approaches for concerned significant others of problem gamblers: A randomized controlled trial. *Journal of Gambling Studies, 23*, 215–230. doi:10.1007/s10899-006-9052-2

Holdsworth, L., Breen, H., Hing, N., & Gordon, A. (2013). One size doesn't fit all: Experiences of family members of Indigenous gamblers. *Australian Aboriginal Studies, 2013*(1), 73–84.

Jiang, H., Callinan, S., Laslett, A-M., & Room, R. (2017). Measuring time spent caring for drinkers and their dependents. *Alcohol and Alcoholism, 52*(1), 112–118. doi:10.1093/alcalc/agw070

Karriker-Jaffe, K. J., Li, L., & Greenfield, T. K. (2018). Estimating mental health impacts of alcohol's harms from other drinkers: Using propensity scoring methods with national cross-sectional data from the United States. *Addiction, 113*, 1826–1839. doi:10.1111/add.14283

Kean, J. (2009). Mental illness and addictions: Our responsibility to support the family. *Aotearoa New Zealand Social Work, 3*, 26–32. doi:10.11157/anzswj-vol21iss3id272

Kelly, J. F., Fallah-Sohy, N., Cristello, J., & Bergman, B. (2017). Coping with the enduring unpredictability of opioid addiction: An investigation of a novel family-focused peer-support organization. *Journal of Substance Abuse Treatment, 77,* 193–200. doi:10.1016/j.sat.2017.02.010

Kondo, A., & Wada, K. (2009). The effectiveness of a mutual-help group activity for drug users and family members in Japan. *Substance Use & Misuse, 44,* 472–489. doi:10.1080/10826080701801501

Kosovski, J. R., & Smith, D. C. (2011). Everybody hurts: Addiction, drama, and the family in the reality television show. *Intervention. Substance Use & Misuse, 46,* 852–858. doi:10.3109/10826084.2011.470610

Kourgiantakis, T., Saint-Jacques, M-C., & Tremblay, J. (2013). Problem gambling and families: A systematic review. *Journal of Social Work Practice in the Addictions, 13*(4), 353–372. doi:10.1080/1533 256X.2013.838130

Lee, B. K., & Awosoga, O. (2015). Congruence couple therapy for pathological gambling: A pilot randomized controlled trial. *Journal of Gambling Studies, 31*(3), 1047–1068. doi:10.1007/s10899-014-9464-3

Lucksted, A., McFarlane, W., Downing, D., Dixon, L., & Adams, C. (2012). Recent developments in family psychoeducation as an evidence-based practice. *Journal of Marital and Family Therapy, 38*(1), 101–121. doi:10.1111/j.1752-0606.2011.00256.x

McCrady, B. S., Wilson, A. D., Muñoz, R. E., Fink, B. C., Fokas, K., & Borders, A. (2016). Alcohol-focused behavioral couple therapy. *Family Process, 55*(3), 443–459. doi:10.1111/famp.12231

McPherson, C., Boyne, H., & Willis, R. (2017). The role of family in residential treatment patient retention. *International Journal of Mental Health and Addiction, 15,* 933–941. doi:10.1007/s11469-016-9712-0

Meads, C., Ting, S., Dretzke, J., & Bayliss, S. (2007). *A systematic review of the clinical and cost-effectiveness of psychological therapy involving family and friends in alcohol misuse or dependence.* (DPHE report number 65). Birmingham, England: Department of Public Health and Epidemiology.

Meis, L. A., Griffin, J. M., Greer, N., Jensen, A. C., MacDonald, R., Carlyle, M.,… Wilt, T. J. (2013). Couple and family involvement in adult mental health treatment: A systematic review. *Clinical Psychology Review, 33,* 275–286. doi:10.1016/j.cpr.2012.12.003

Miller, W. R., Meyers, R. J., & Tonigan, J. S. (1999). Engaging the unmotivated in treatment for alcohol problems: A comparison of three strategies for intervention through family members. *Journal of Consulting and Clinical Psychology, 67,* 688–697. doi:10.1037/0022-006X.67.5.688

Nadkarni, A., Bhatia, U., Velleman, R., Orford, J., Velleman, G., Church, S., . . . Pednekar, S. (2017). Supporting addictions affected families effectively (SAFE): A mixed methods exploratory study of the 5-Step Method delivered in Goa, India, by lay counsellors. *Drugs: Education, Prevention, and Policy, 26*(2), 195–204. doi:10.1080/09687637.2017.1394983

Nayoski, N., & Hodgins, D. C. (2016). The efficacy of individual Community reinforcement and family training (CRAFT) for concerned significant others of problem gamblers. *Journal of Gambling Issues, 33,* 189–212. doi:10.4309/jgi.2016.33.11

Nilsson, A., Magnusson, K., Carlbring, P., Andersson, G., & Gumpert, C. H. (2018). The development of an internet-based treatment for problem gamblers and concerned significant others: A pilot randomized controlled trial. *Journal of Gambling Studies, 34,* 539–559. doi:10.1007/s10899-017-9704-4

Orford, J. (2017). How does the common core to the harm experienced by affected family members vary by relationship, social and cultural factors? *Drugs: Education, Prevention, and Policy, 24*(1), 9–16. doi:10.1080/09687637.2016.1189876

Orford, J., Natera, G., Copello, A., Atkinson, C., Mora, J., Velleman, R., . . . Walley, G. (2005). *Coping with alcohol and drug problems: The experiences of family members in three contrasting cultures.* East Sussex, England: Routledge.

Orford, J., Copello, A., Velleman, R., & Templeton, L. (2010). Family members affected by a close relative's addiction: The stress-strain-coping-support model. *Drugs: Education, Prevention and Policy, 17*(S1), 36–43. doi:10.3109/09687637.2010.514801

Orford, J., Cousins, J., Smith, N., & Bowden-Jones, H. (2017). Stress, strain, coping, and social support for affected family members attending the National Problem Gambling Clinic, London. *International Gambling Studies, 17*(2), 259–275. doi:10.1080/14459795.2017.1331251

Orford, J., Velleman, R., Natera, G., Templeton, L., & Copello, A. (2013). Addiction in the family is a major but neglected contributor to the global burden of adult ill-health. *Social Science & Medicine, 78,* 70–77. doi:10/1016/j.soc.scimed.2012.11.036

Orr, L., C., Barbour, R. S., & Elliott, L. (2014). Involving families and carers in drug services: Are families 'part of the problem'? *Families, Relationships and Societies, 3*(3), 405–424. doi:10.1332/204674313X669900

Petra, M. M. (2014). Coping with intimate partners' substance use and gambling problems: The role of intimate partner violence (IPV). *Unpublished dissertation*. Retrieved from https://openscholarship. wustl.edu/cgi/viewcontent.cgi?article=2334&context=etd

Rane, A., Church, S., Bhatia, U., Orford, J., Velleman, R., & Nadkarni, A. (2017). Psychosocial interventions for addiction-affected families in low and middle income countries: A systematic review. *Addictive Behaviors, 74*, 1–8. doi:10.1016/j.addbeh.2017.05.015

Ray, G. T., Meriens, J. R., & Weisner, C. (2007). The excess medical cost and health problems of family members of persons diagnosed with alcohol or drug problems. *Medical Care, 45*, 116–122. doi:10.1097/01.mlr.0000241109.55054.04

Rey, G. N., Aguilar, P. S. M., Pérez, F. C., Juárez, F., & Tiburcio, M. (2011). Efectos de una intervención a familiars de consumidores de alcohol en una region indigena en México. *Salud Mental, 34*(3), 195–201.

Rohrbaugh, M. J. (2014). Old wine in new bottles: Decanting systemic family process research in the era of evidence-based practice. *Family Process, 53*, 434–444. doi:10.1111/famp.12079

Roozen, H. G., de Waart, R., & van der Kroft, P. (2010). Community reinforcement and family training: An effective option to engage treatment-resistant substance-abusing individuals in treatment. *Addiction, 105*, 1729–1738. doi:10.1111/j.1360-0443.2010.03016.x

Rychtarik, R. G., McGillicuddy, N. B., & Barrick, C. (2015). Web-based coping skills training for women whose partner has a drinking problem. *Psychology of Addictive Behaviors, 29*(1), 26–33. doi:10.1037/adb0000032

Sakiyama, H. M. T., Padin, M. F. R., Canfield, M., Laranjeira, R., & Mitsuhiro, S. S. (2015). Family members affected by a relative's substance misuse looking for social support: Who are they? *Drug and Alcohol Dependence, 147*(2015), 276–279. doi:10.1016/j.drugalcdep.2014.11.030

Selbekk, A. S., & Sagvaag, H. (2016). Troubled families and individualized solutions: An institutional discourse analysis of alcohol and drug treatment practices involving affected others. *Sociology of Health & Illness, 38*(7), 1058–1073. doi:10.1111/1467-9566.12432

Steinglass, P. (2009). Systemic-motivational therapy for substance abuse disordres: An integrative model. *Journal of Family Therapy, 31*, 155–174. doi:10.1111/j.1467-6427.2009.00460.x

Substance and Mental Health Services Administration. (2009). *Family psychoeducation: Building your program* (HHS Pub. No. SMA-09–4422). Rockville, MD: Author.

Timko, C., Halvorson, M., Kong, C., & Moos, R. H. (2015). Social processes explaining the benefits of Al-Anon participation. *Psychology of Addictive Behaviors, 29*(4), 856–863. doi:10.1037/adb0000067

Timko, C., Laudet, A., & Moos, R. H. (2016). Al-Anon newcomers: Benefits of continuing attendance for six months. *The American Journal of Drug and Alcohol Abuse, 42*(4), 441–449. doi:10.3109/00952 990.2016.1148702

United Nations. (2018). *World drug report 2018*. (Sales No. E.18.XI.9). Vienna, Austria: Author.

U.S. Department of Health and Human Services, Office of the Surgeon General. (2016). *Facing addiction in America: The surgeon general's report on alcohol, drugs, and health*. Washington, DC: Author.

Velleman, R., Arcidiacono, C., Procentese, F., Copello, A., & Sarnacchiaro, P. (2008). A 5-step intervention to help family members in Italy who live with substance misusers. *Journal of Mental Health, 17*(6), 643–655. doi:10.1080/09638230701677761

Velleman, R., Orford, J., Templeton, L., Copello, A. Patel, A. Moore, L., . . . Godfrey, C. (2011). 12-month follow-up after brief interventions in primary care for family members affected by the substance misuse problem of a close relative. *Addiction Research and Theory, 19*(4), 362–374. doi:10.3 109/16066359.2011.564691

Ventura, A. S., & Bagley, S. M. (2017). To improve substance use disorder prevention, treatment and recovery: Engage the family. *Journal of Addiction Medicine, 11*(5), 339–341. doi:10.1097/ ADM.0000000000000331

Whitaker, T., Weismiller, T., & Clark, E. (2006). *Assuring the sufficiency of a frontline workforce: A national study of licensed social workers*. Washington, DC: National Association of Social Workers & Center for Health Workforce Studies.

World Health Organization. (2018). *Global status report on alcohol and health, 2018*. Geneva: Author.

25

The impact of addictive behavior on grandfamilies

Nancy Mendoza, Christine Fruhauf and Bert Hayslip, Jr.

Background

Understanding and helping individuals experiencing substance use disorders (SUDs) involves not only the person, but the entire family. As Daley, Smith, Balogh, and Toscolani (2018) stated, "...these disorders often create ripple effects through the family. Countless lives are irrevocably altered in the 'collateral damage' caused by a SUD" (p. 98). Unfortunately, limited attention has been directed to supporting children, parents, and relatives impacted by an individual's addictive behavior (Daley et al., 2018). Significance of attending to family-wide impact is underscored by large numbers of children in the United States living with a grandparent or other relative during the opioid epidemic because middle-generation parents are unable or unavailable to care for their children (Generations United, 2018). It is estimated that 7.7 million children in the United States live with a grandparent or other relative, and over a third of all children placed in foster care due to parental drug use are placed with relatives (Generations United, 2018). Furthermore, for every child placed with a grandparent or other relative in the foster care system, there are 19 children living with a grandparent or other relative outside of the foster care system (Generations United, 2018). In Canada families missing the middle generation are referred to as skipped-generation families. According to the 2011 National Household Survey by Statistics Canada an estimated 12.4% of grandparents were in a skipped-generation family (Milan, Laflamme, & Wong, 2015).

The impact of parental SUD on grandfamilies (i.e. families in which grandparents or other relatives are raising children) is not a new challenge as grandparents and other relatives have historically provided safe havens for grandchildren whose parents engage in substance misuse (Hayslip, Fruhauf, & Dolbin-MacNab, 2017). Prevalence of these families continues to increase over time. For example, from 1970 to 1997 the number of children living in a home maintained by a grandparent nearly doubled from 2.2 million to 4 million (Bryson & Casper, 1999). The rate of removal of children from their homes due to parental substance use almost doubled from 2000 (18.5%) to 2015 (34.4%) (Daley et al., 2018). Grandfamilies impacted by a parent's substance misuse face numerous challenges. These growing numbers substantiate the need to understand and support these types of families.

Grandparents as caregivers to their grandchildren: the big picture

The need for grandparents or other relatives to raise a child due to a parent's inability or unavailability cuts across all races, ethnicities, geographical areas, education levels, and SES levels (Hayslip et al., 2017); grandfamilies are quite diverse in these respects. While grandparent caregiving is most frequent in the United States among Caucasian families, African Americans and Latinos have a higher probability of becoming a grandparent caregiver (U.S. Census Bureau, 2017). African American and Latino grandparent caregivers are also more likely to be single, have lower levels of education, keep their children in their care longer, and live in poverty (Fuller-Thomson, Minkler, & Driver, 1997; Hayslip & Kaminski, 2005). Generally speaking, grandparent caregivers are more likely to be women (Fuller-Thomson et al., 1997), and nearly one in five grandfamilies lives in poverty (U.S. Census Bureau, 2017). Among Mexican American grandparents, grandparents living below the poverty level were twice as likely to become grandparent caregivers (Fuller-Thomson & Minkler, 2007).

Grandfamilies are diverse

Grandparent caregivers are diverse in age, ranging from 30 to over 80 years (Engstrom, 2008), with 41% being older than 60 (U.S. Census Bureau, 2017). This variation in age suggests that some grandparents (57%) are still active in the workforce (U.S. Census Bureau, 2017), while others may be retired or are forced to retire due to caregiving responsibilities (Lent & Otto, 2019). Underscoring the diversity of grandparent caregiving experiences is an observation that the traditional grandmother role in many African American families is to serve as kin-keeper; this tradition may result in less perceived burden among these grandmothers (Engstrom, 2008). Pruchno (1999) reported that Black grandmother caregivers compared to white grandmother caregivers were more likely to co-reside with peers, live in multigenerational homes, and receive formal social services. Black or African American and Latino grandparent caregivers are also more likely to co-parent with one of the child's parents than are white grandparent caregivers (Hayslip & Kaminski, 2005). Latino grandparent caregivers are more likely than other races/ethnicities to co-parent with an adult child who is not a parent of the grandchild they are raising (Burnette, 1999); they are also more likely to experience language barriers to services (Mendoza, Fruhauf, Bundy-Fazioli, & Weil, 2017). Diversity across multiple parameters suggests that each grandfamily's experiences are likely to differ.

Impact of grandfamily experiences on grandparents

Grandfamilies affected by a parent's substance misuse experience unique social, financial, physical, and mental health challenges. The majority of grandparents or other family members who assume caregiving roles do so unexpectedly (Lent & Otto, 2019), during a time in their life when they did not anticipate raising children (Engstrom, 2008). This "off-time" event can disrupt life plans, and result in competing responsibilities and demands, role confusion, and role overload (Hayslip & Kaminski, 2005). Complicating matters, grandparents may experience guilt over their adult child's inability to parent, perceiving themselves as responsible for the situation (Hayslip et al., 2017); it is common for family members of individuals experiencing SUD's to feel ashamed, guilty, hopeless, anxious, and cheated (Daley et al., 2018). Simultaneously, grandparents may grieve loss of normalcy from being traditional grandparents, uncertainty about the future, and threats to financial security (Lent & Otto, 2019). Grandparents may also grieve their loss of freedom, social relationships, and feeling accepted by others due to associated stigma (Hayslip & Kaminski, 2005). Caregiving grandparents often report experiencing loneliness and isolation from peers (Hayslip & Kaminski, 2005).

Grandparents may struggle in coping with an adult child's substance misuse and finding help (Generations United, 2018; Hirshorn, Van Meter, and Brown, 2000; Mignon & Holmes, 2013). Indeed, the lived experience of many grandparent caregivers reflects sadness, grief, and frustration with an adult child who engages in substance misuse (Hayslip, 2010). They may experience complicated, unresolved, under-recognized, or unsupported grief over the death of an adult child due to drug overdose or substance-related health issues (Miltenberger, Hayslip, Harris, & Kaminski, 2003–2004). In addition to their own grief, grandparents must help their grandchildren cope with the loss of a parent (Hayslip & Kaminski, 2005).

Health and mental health

These emotions, coupled with the challenges of raising a grandchild, can negatively affect the physical and mental health of grandparent caregivers (Smith, Palmieri, Hancock, & Richardson, 2008). Over a 20-year period, grandparent caregivers were more likely to experience poorer physical and mental health than non-caregivers (Strawbridge, Wallhagen, Shema, & Kaplan, 1997) and experience higher incidences of hypertension, diabetes, insomnia, depression, and chronic stress (Lent & Otto, 2019). Many grandparents prioritize their grandchildren's needs over their own, thus ignoring their own health needs (Baker & Silverstein, 2008b; Minkler, Roe, & Price, 1992; Lent & Otto, 2019). Health problems may also cause grandparents to worry about what could happen to their grandchildren if something were to happen to them (Hayslip & Kaminski, 2005).

Relationships

While raising grandchildren can have a negative impact on grandparents' friendships (Kirby, 2015), marriages, relationships with other adult children, other grandchildren, and their own parents and siblings (Lent & Otto, 2019), caregiving grandparents often report enjoying a close relationship with the grandchild/ren they are raising (Hayslip et al., 2017). Caregiving can provide a grandparent with satisfaction, pride, and enjoyment (Engstrom, 2008). They often feel they have been given a second chance at parenting (Kirby, 2015); if asked again to raise their grandchildren they would do so (Hayslip et al., 2017).

Impact of grandfamily experience on grandchildren

There exists growing attention toward understanding the negative and positive developmental impact on grandchildren of living in a grandfamily (Dunifon, 2018). For example, grandchildren may experience difficulty with social networking and developing friendships with peers as they often feel out of place or shame when their grandparents serve as their parents (Edwards, 2003). They may find that friends do not understand their family situation, thus they withdraw from each other (Edwards, 2003). Children in grandfamilies may be at risk for behavior problems (Jooste, Hayslip, & Smith, 2008), as well as mental health difficulties (Edwards, 2006). In some cases, their problems emerge later in adulthood (Carpenter & Clyman, 2004). These difficulties may be due to parental absence (i.e. death, deployment, or incarceration) or abuse and neglect while in the care of biological parents (Strong, Bean, & Feinauer, 2010); the difficulties may be exacerbated by grandchildren feeling abandoned by their parents.

Evidence suggests that grandchildren experience learning difficulties (Edwards, 2006), developmental delays that impact school performance (Mauderer, 2008), or truancy, school suspension, and fighting in school that prevents them from on-time graduation (Musil, Warner, McNamara, Rokoff, & Turek, 2008; Ryan, Hong, Herz, & Hernandez, 2010). Negative impacts such as these may be further exacerbated if grandchildren have little support from service providers (Fruhauf, Pevney, & Bundy-Fazioli, 2015). Among youth in the juvenile justice system, custodial grandchildren have higher rates of reoffending when compared to youth in parent-headed homes (Campbell, Hu, & Oberle, 2006).

Positive impact

Despite challenges, being raised by grandmothers can "build competency in youth, protecting them from engaging in delinquent behavior or substance abuse" (Goulette, Evans, & King, 2016, p. 354). A strengths perspective of grandfamily-raised children is evidenced when compared to children raised in foster care: children in grandfamily homes experience greater stability, are less likely to run away, experience fewer school changes, and have better behavioral and mental health outcomes (Lent & Otto, 2019). Moreover, feeling loved and cared for by grandparents lays the groundwork for better future life trajectories (Dolbin-MacNab & Keiley, 2009; Dolbin-MacNab, Rodgers, & Traylor, 2009; Dunifon, 2018). Indeed, it is not surprising that grandchildren's relationships with their grandparents is described as strong and emotionally close (Messing, 2006), and they emphasize gratitude and respect toward their grandparents (Dolbin-MacNab & Keiley, 2009). While practitioners should be cognizant of the challenges children may experience when parental substance misuse leads to grandparents raising them, we also need to recognize the potential for building resilience offered by their grandfamilies.

Strengths perspective of grandparents raising grandchildren

One of the most important and impactful new developments in the literature on grandparent caregiving has been the reformulation of our ideas about grandparents' strengths (Hayslip et al., 2017). Strengths indices include resilience and resourcefulness (Hayslip & Smith, 2013; Musil et al., 2019), finding benefit (Castillo, Henderson, & North, 2013), empowerment (Cox, 2014; Tang, Jang, & Copeland, 2015), and positive caregiving appraisal (Smith & Dolbin-MacNab, 2013). Emphasizing resilience also focuses on protective factors such as social support (Dolbin-MacNab, Roberto, & Finney, 2013; Hayslip, Blumenthal, & Garner, 2015; Whitley, Kelley, & Lamis, 2016) and good health (Hayslip, Blumenthal, & Garner, 2014; Roberto, Dolbin-MacNab, & Finney, 2008).

Many custodial grandparents face multiple challenges (poverty, poor health/disability, raising multiple grandchildren, substance abuse, caring for an older parent, a grandchild with a physical disability or mental illness, a dysfunctional adult child), underscoring the importance of their being resilient. Being personally resilient is especially important in coping with an adult child's substance misuse (Generations United, 2018). Grandparent resilience, defined as positive adaptation and positive outcomes despite adversity (Rutter, 2007), can counteract the negative effects of personal (e.g. depression), interpersonal (feeling rejected and stigmatized, social isolation/loneliness), parenting (setting limits, discipline, communication), and systemic (accessing legal, mental health, social, and medical care services) stressors on grand-parents' physical and mental health (Lee & Blitz, 2014).

Resilient grandparent caregivers are both proactive and reactive. Resilient grandparents realign their goals in light of parenting demands, create opportunities to learn and grow from their interactions with a grandchild, and are personally resourceful (see Musil et al., 2019). They are hopeful yet realistic in setting goals for themselves and in anticipating the changing nature of what lies ahead for them and their grandchildren (e.g. coping with the drug addiction of the adult child, a grandchild's health difficulties or adjustment problems (Mendoza, 2018; Strom & Strom, 2011).

As the demands on many grandparents are real, *how* they deal with stressful caregiving (i.e. emotion-focused or problem-focused coping, information seeking, meaning-making, proactive coping, religious coping, or asking for help from others) is important (see Bjorkland, 2015). Thus, effective efforts at coping may grow out of existing resilience, where Bonnano (2004) suggests that resilience can be viewed as a form of psychological immunity. This immunity may protect one from further health-related and/or psychosocial damage (Almedon, 2005; Smith & Hayslip, 2013). In this respect, Hayslip et al. (2013) concluded that grandparents' resilience mediated the relationship between stress and psycho-social functioning. Reflecting resilience is the ability to set boundaries with adult children while not losing hope for their growth and healing (Hirshorn et al., 2000). Support from others also may be uncertain, complicated by the stigma of raising a child whose parent is coping with substance misuse (Hirshorn et al., 2000). Resilient grandparent caregivers *can* emerge from uncertainty feeling empowered, being committed to improving the life of the grandchild, and being able to set boundaries, reducing the uncertainties of coping with an adult child's substance misuse.

Resilience skills can be learned. Clinicians can facilitate resilience among grandparent caregivers by enhancing protective factors such as social support, health management, and self-care (Fruhauf & Bundy-Fazioli, 2013), as well as empowering grandparents' proactive decision-making, choices, and assertive expression of their needs (Cox, 2014). Grandparents' resilience can also be enhanced by reducing risk factors leading to feeling overwhelmed by stress and distress, such as social isolation, depression, or neglecting one's physical and mental health (Baker & Silverstein, 2008a, 2008b). That resilience can grow out of what life hands out is consistent with it also being a learned behavior. In finding solutions to problems, grandparents can become more self-efficacious (Bandura, 1989) and resourceful (Musil et al., 2019).

Resilience can also be intergenerational in nature. For example, grandparents' ability to "weather the storm" in raising grandchildren could increase their ability to parent grandchildren. Thus, better parenting might foster better behavior in the child in allowing the child to be more securely attached to the grandparent. In turn, such attachment can positively impact the well-being of the grandparent, further enhancing his/her resilience skills. This dualistic perspective is consistent with the bidirectionality of a grandchild's behavior and a grandparent's mental health (Goodman & Hayslip, 2008).

Despite the many challenges faced by grandparent caregivers, most are dedicated to the welfare of their grandchildren and are resilient and resourceful in coping with the challenges of raising a grandchild. Grandparent caregiver resilience can be seen as an internal personal attribute or as a skill or behavior(s) growing out of the need to solve problems and meet challenges linked to what may be the overwhelming task of raising a grandchild. Being resilient also can enable one to successfully negotiate a new relationship with/get help for an adult child engaged in substance misuse. Resilient grandparents are able to meet these challenges and are able to care for themselves physically, mentally, socially, and spiritually. Resilient grandparent caregivers not only persevere in the face of barriers, but they also find ways to grow beyond such challenges and fashion a fulfilling life for themselves and their grandchildren.

Interventions for grandfamilies

The importance attached to interventions with grandfamilies is underscored by the fact that grandparents are often asked to raise their grandchildren with little warning, at inopportune times, and under stigmatizing and stressful conditions (Hayslip et al., 2017). There exists increasing interest among scholars and practitioners in developing and testing interventions to intervene with grandparents and grandchildren to reduce or prevent problems (McLaughlin, Ryder, & Taylor, 2017). At present, focus is on community programs and services for grandparent caregivers (McLaughlin et al., 2017). Individual and interdisciplinary case management, support groups, psychoeducational programs, and cognitive-behavioral or skills-based interventions are at the forefront of interventions for grandparent caregivers (see McLaughlin et al., 2017; Smith, Hayslip, Hancock, Strieder, & Montoro-Rodriguez, 2018).

Interest in formal, structured interventions and programs with grandchildren is growing (Kolomer, McCallion, & Van Voorbis, 2008; Yancura, Fruhauf, Riggs, Mendoza, & Greenwood-Junkermeier, 2017). Additionally, family-based interventions may be useful, yet few scholars have tested these approaches with grandfamilies (McLaughlin et al., 2017). Finally, individual counseling and family therapy are valuable strategies for working with grandparents (Dolbin-MacNab & Targ, 2003; Maiden & Zuckerman, 2008), grandchildren (Kaminski & Murrell, 2008; Strong et al., 2010), and parents (Edwards & Ray, 2010). Each approach may be beneficial when a parent's substance misuse becomes a family concern.

Case management

Social workers are trained to assess and evaluate strengths and needs of individuals and families while linking them to resources and services that best meet their needs, including financial support. In addition to generic case management training, some practitioners believe they need more education and support when working with grandfamilies (Fruhauf et al., 2015). Both individual and interdisciplinary case management are useful in meeting the needs of grandparent caregivers, especially as it relates to grandparents' health and wellness (Hrostowski & Forster, 2010; Kelley, Whitley, & Campos, 2013). Several states responded to the unique needs of grandfamilies by hiring providers to serve as kinship navigators who provide information, referral, and follow-up services to grandparents. Kinship navigators may be situated within public, private, or community-based agencies (Child Welfare Information Gateway, 2018). When dedicated case managers or kinship navigators are not available or their caseloads are too high, communities may benefit from grandparent and grandchildren mentoring programs (James & Ferrante, 2013; Weinberger, 2014).

Practitioners should encourage grandparents to seek such support and remove as many barriers to doing so as possible. Grandparent caregivers may not seek services because they are unfamiliar with the system or they are reluctant to share their experiences due to the stigma surrounding their child's substance misuse (Coleman & Wu, 2016). Grandparent caregivers may also have experienced stigma or microaggression that lessens their willingness to seek help (Yancura, Fruhauf, & Greenwood-Junkermeier, 2016).

Support groups

In addition to case management or counseling, grandparent caregivers may choose to participate in support groups (Roe, 2000; Smith, 2003). Support groups offer social support for individuals experiencing similar phenomena social support, as well as providing opportunities for exchanging information and resource sharing (Brown, Tang, & Hollman, 2014). Sometimes, humor is utilized during the group setting and friendships between attendees may develop from support group attendance (Brown et al., 2014). Thus, support groups potentially reduce isolation and loneliness grandparents may experience as their previous peer networks decrease (Mendoza, 2018). In one study grandparent caregivers reported some emotional support benefit after attending a support group; fewer reported receiving instrumental support in the form of help with child rearing, finances, or navigating the legal/social services system (Leder, Grinstead, & Torres, 2007).

Despite these potential benefits, some research suggested that support groups might be harmful (Brown et al., 2014; Smith, 2003). For example, Smith's (2003) exploratory study with 42 grandparents raising grandchildren discovered that support groups characterized by a lack of structure and clear objectives foster self-pity and complaining among grandparents. Further, support group participants in another study reported unwanted behaviors and hostility among group members (Brown et al., 2014). Poor-quality support groups are ineffective long-term strategies or stand-alone approaches for intervening with grandparent caregivers. However, support groups for grandparent caregivers vary in facilitator leadership, content delivered, and evidence base (Hayslip et al., 2013; Littlewood, 2014). To enhance participation in support groups, leaders should consider providing meals, transportation, childcare, and attendance incentives (Roe, 2000). Practitioners and support group facilitators may also encourage combining support group attendance with psychoeducational or cognitive-behavioral interventions and/or case management when working with grandfamilies (McCallion, Janicki, & Kolomer, 2004).

Psychoeducation and cognitive-behavioral interventions

Psychoeducation includes providing resources and information about specific topics and is often delivered in group format programs or workshops (Furman, Rowan, & Bender, 2009). For example, psychoeducational interventions for grandfamilies may focus on parenting skills, well-being/stress and coping, financial management, and exploring legal issues (Vacha-hasse, Ness, Dannison, & Smith, 2000). Additionally, psychoeducational programs have addressed these issues along with contemporary concerns including technology and social media, and communication skills when texting is common (Dunn & Wamsley, 2018). Many grandparents provide excellent parenting to grandchildren, yet they can learn additional skills when necessary to help them and their grandchildren and learn new ways of thinking and coping to assist them in life (see Dolbin-MacNab, 2006). Parenting skills training and cognitive-behavioral interventions both are successful in improving grandparent caregivers' well-being (Smith et al., 2018).

Although such programs exist, few are rigorously tested (McLaughlin et al., 2017; Smith, Strieder, Greenberg, Hayslip, & Montoro-Rodriguez, 2016). Smith et al. (2016) completed a randomized clinical trial with 343 grandmothers raising grandchildren assigned either to a parenting program, a cognitive-behavioral coping program, or an information-only condition. They discovered higher treatment satisfaction and compliance rates among grandparents receiving the parenting training and the cognitive-behavioral coping program.

Thus, service providers should consider expanding the types of interventions they offer grandparents (Fruhauf & Hayslip, 2013).

Cognitive-behavioral interventions teach grandparent caregivers skills and strategies that result in behavior changes as they cope with the mental, physical, and social challenges of rearing grandchildren (McLaughlin et al., 2017). For example, interventions addressing resourcefulness (Zauszniewski, Au, & Musil, 2012), stress and depression (Zauszniewski, Musil, Burant, & Au, 2014), chronic disease self-management (McCallion, Ferretti, & Kim, 2013), and self-care practices (Yancura, Greenwood-Junkermeier, & Fruhauf, 2017) have been developed, implemented, and evaluated with positive results for grandparent caregivers.

Family system interventions

Family systems theory and research utilizing this theoretical framework suggests families share routines (e.g. mealtime, grooming patterns, bedtimes) and traditions (e.g. celebrations, religious observations), and are shaped by family values (e.g. perceptions about smoking or substance use), which contribute to individual health behaviors (e.g. food choices, physical activity) (Hamburger, Mayberry, Savin, & Jaser, 2018). As a result, intervening with the family system is an option for promoting healthy behaviors (Hamburger et al., 2018). Unfortunately, few tested interventions targeted to grandparent caregivers or their grandchildren utilized family-based or family-level approaches (McLaughlin et al., 2017), thus evidence that family system interventions with grandfamilies have positive outcomes is sorely lacking.

Future directions

There exist many opportunities for future research addressing grandfamilies. To date, little attention documents the possibility of grandparents' own misuse of alcohol and other substances while caring for their grandchildren (Hayslip et al., 2017). Other research questions relate to the experiences of grandfather caregivers, grandparents' grief, and cultural differences among grandfamilies applying a global and contextual lens (Hayslip et al., 2017). More research is needed focusing on changes that occur in a grandparents' convoy of support as a result of becoming a caregiver; this would help social workers gain a better understanding of the challenges these families face and the resources that are useful and needed (Hayslip et al., 2017; Mendoza, 2018). Another area in need of further research, as previously discussed, is the development and rigorous evaluation of interventions for grandfamilies.

Conclusion

Grandfamilies impacted by a parent's substance misuse face numerous challenges. Their family social interactions and responsibilities are more complex than usual (Generations United, 2018). As a grandfamily they experience a unique set of social, mental, and physical health challenges. As caregivers, grandparents not only assume a challenging and unexpected role for which they likely are under-prepared, they are also vulnerable to experiencing negative physical and mental health outcomes (Hayslip & Kaminski, 2005). The children of grandfamilies have likely experienced trauma, are struggling with not having their parent(s) present, may feel insecure about their future, may exhibit behavioral or mental health difficulties, and may be at risk for developing unhealthy habits (Dunifon, 2018; Generations United, 2018). Despite the challenges faced by many grandfamilies, grandparents are resilient

(Hayslip & Smith, 2013) and decades of research demonstrated that many children who cannot remain with their parents thrive when they are raised by grandparents (Generations United, 2018). Thus, supporting grandfamilies is crucial for both generations, and research demonstrates that when grandfamilies receive adequate support and services the children experience better social and mental outcomes (Generations United, 2018). Researchers and practitioners must continue striving to understand the experiences of grandfamilies, offer culturally and developmentally appropriate services, and work to develop improved interventions for grandfamilies.

References

Almedon, A. M. (2005). Resilience, hardiness, sense of coherence, and post-traumatic growth: All paths leading to "The light at the end of the tunnel"? *Journal of Loss and Trauma, 10*, 253–265. doi:10.1080/15325020590928216

Baker, L. A., & Silverstein, M. (2008a). Preventative health behaviors among grandmothers raising grandchildren. *The Journals of Gerontology, Series B: Psychological Sciences and Social Sciences, 63*, S304–S311.

Baker, L. A., & Silverstein, M. (2008b). Depressive symptoms among grandparents raising grandchildren: The impact of participation in multiple roles. *Journal of Intergenerational Relationships, 6*, 285–304. doi:10.1080/15350770802157802

Bandura, A. (1989). Regulation of cognitive processes through self-efficacy. *Developmental Psychology, 25*, 729–735. doi:10.1037/0012-1649.25.5.729

Bjorkland, B. (2015). *The Journey of Adulthood* (Updated 8th Edition). New York, NY: Pearson.

Bonnano, G. (2004). Loss, trauma, and human resilience: Have we underestimated the human capacity to thrive after extremely aversive events? *American Psychologist, 39*, 20–28. doi:10.1037/0003-066X.59.1.20

Brown, L. D., Tang, X., & Hollman, R. L. (2014). The structure of social exchange in self-help support groups: Development of a measure. *American Journal of Community Psychology, 53*, 83–95. doi:10.1007/s10464-013-9621-3.

Bryson, K. & Casper, L. M. (1999). *Coresident grandparents and grandchildren*. U.S. Census Bureau. Retrieved from https://books.google.com/books?hl=en&lr=&id=1zNHAAAAMAAJ&oi=fnd&pg=PA1&dq=Bryson+%26+Casper,+1999&ots=zMz8AhcuPw&sig=yq1zy1QrjW_uoWIb81KxgY0E3Pg#v=onepage&q=Bryson%20%26%20Casper%2C%201999&f=false

Burnette, D. (1999). Physical and emotional well-being of custodial grandparents in Latino families. *American Journal of Orthopsychiatry, 69*, 305–317. doi:10.1037/h0080405

Campbell, L. R., Hu, J., & Oberle, S. (2006). Factors associated with future offending: Comparing youth in grandparent-headed homes with those in parent-headed homes. *Archives of Psychiatric Nursing, 20*, 258–267. doi:10.1016/j.apnu.2006.07.003

Carpenter, S., & Clyman, R. (2004). The long-term emotional and physical wellbeing of women who have lived in kinship care. *Children and Youth Services Review, 26*(7), 673–686). doi: 10.1016/j.childyouth.2004.02.015

Castillo, K., Henderson, C., & North, L. (2013). The relation between caregiving style, coping, benefit finding, grandchild symptoms, and caregiver adjustment among custodial grandparents. In B. Hayslip Jr. & G. Smith (Eds.), *Resilient grandparent caregivers: A strengths-based perspective* (pp. 25–37). New York, NY: Routledge.

Child Welfare Information Gateway. (2018, June). *Working with kinship caregivers*. Retried from: https://www.childwelfare.gov/pubPDFs/kinship.pdf

Coleman, K. L., & Wu, Q. (2016). Kinship care and service utilization: A review of predisposing, enabling, and need factors. *Children and Youth Services Review, 61*, 291–210. doi:10.1016/j.childyouth.2015.12.014

Cox, C. (2014). Personal and community empowerment for grandparent caregivers. *Journal of Family Social Work, 17*, 162–164. doi:10.1080/10522158.2014.880824

Daley, D. C., Smith, E., Balogh, D., & Toscolani, J. (2018). Forgotten but not gone: The impact of the opioid epidemic and other substance use disorders on families and children. *Commonwealth: A Journal of Pennsylvania Politics and Policy, 20*(2–3). doi:10.15367/v2012-3.189

Dolbin-MacNab, M. L. (2006). Just like raising your own? Grandmothers' perceptions of parenting a second time around. *Family Relations, 55*, 564–575. doi:10.1111/j.1741-3729.2006.00426.x

Dolbin-MacNab, M. L., & Keiley, M. K. (2009). Navigating interdependence: How adolescents raised solely by grandparents experience their family relationships. *Family Relations, 58*, 162–175. doi:10.1111/j.1741-3729.2008.00544.x

Dolbin-MacNab, M., Roberto, K., & Finney, J. (2013). Formal social support: Promoting resilience in grandparents parenting grandchildren. In B. Hayslip Jr. & G. C. Smith (Eds.), *Resilient grandparent caregivers: A strengths-based perspective* (pp. 134–151). New York, NY: Routledge.

Dolbin-MacNab, M. L., Rodgers, B. E., & Traylor, R. M. (2009). Bridging the generations: A retrospective examination of adults' relationships with their kinship caregivers. *Journal of Intergenerational Relationships, 7*, 159–176. doi:10.1080/15350770902851197

Dolbin-MacNab, M. L., & Targ, D. B. (2003). Grandparents raising grandchildren: Guidelines for family life educators and other family professionals. In B. Hayslip, Jr. & J. H. Patrick (Eds.), *Working with custodial grandparents* (pp. 213–228). New York, NY: Springer.

Dunifon, R. E. (2018). *You've always been there for me: Understanding the lives of grandchildren raised by grandparents*. New Brunswick, NJ: Rutgers University Press.

Dunn, B., & Wamsley, B. (2018). Grandfamilies: Characteristics and needs of grandparents raising grandchildren. *Journal of Extension, 56*(5), 5RIB2.

Edwards, O. W. (2003). Living with grandma: A grandfamily study. *School Psychology International, 24*, 204–217. doi:10.1177/0143034303024002005

Edwards, O. W. (2006). Teacher's perceptions of the emotional and behavioral functioning of children raised by grandparents. *Psychology in the Schools, 43*(5), 565–572. doi:10.1002/pits.20170

Edwards, O. W., & Ray, S. L. (2010). Value of family and group counseling models where grandparents function as parents to their grandchildren. *International Journal for the Advancement of Counselling, 32*, 178–190. doi:10.1007/s10447-010-9098-9

Engstrom, E. (2008). Involving caregiving grandmothers in family interventions when mothers with substance abuse use problems are incarcerated. *Family Process, 47*(3), 357–371. doi:10.1111/j.1545-5300.2008.00258.x

Fruhauf, C. A., & Fazioli-Bundy (2013). Grandparent caregivers' self-care practice: Moving toward a strengths-based approach. In B. Hayslip Jr. & G. Smith (Eds.), *Resilient grandparent caregivers: A strengths-based perspective* (pp. 88–102). New York, NY: Routledge.

Fruhauf, C. A., & Hayslip, B., Jr. (2013). Understanding collaborative efforts to assist grandparent caregivers: A multileveled perspective. *Journal of Family Social Work, 16*, 382–391. doi:10.1080/105 22158.2013.832462

Fruhauf, C. A., Pevney, B., & Bundy-Fazioli, K. (2015). The needs and use of programs by service providers working with grandparents raising grandchildren. *Journal of Applied Gerontology, 34*(2), 138–157. doi:10.1177/0733464812463983

Fuller-Thomson, E., & Minkler, M. (2007). Mexican American grandparents raising grandchildren: Findings from the Census 2000 American Community Survey. *Families in Society, 88*, 567–574. doi:10.1606/1044-3894.3679

Fuller-Thomson, E., Minkler, M., & Driver, D. (1997). A profile of grandparents raising grandchildren in the United States. *The Gerontologist, 37*, 406–411.

Furman, R., Rowan, D., & Bender, K. (2009). *An experiential approach to group work*. Chicago, IL: Lyceum.

Generations United (2018, updated). *The state of grandfamilies in America: Raising the children of the opioid epidemic: Solutions and support for grandfamilies*. Washington, DC.

Goodman, C.C., & Hayslip, B. (2008). Mentally healthy grandparents' impact on their grandchildren's behavior. In B. Hayslip & P. Kaminiski (Eds.), *Parenting the custodial grandchild: Implications for clinical practice* (pp. 41–52). New York, NY: Springer.

Goulette, N. W., Evans, S. Z., & King, D. (2016). Exploring the behavior of juveniles and young adults raised by custodial grandmothers. *Children and Youth Services Review, 70*, 349–356. doi:10.1016/j.childyouth.2016.10.004

Hamburger, E. R., Mayberry, L. S., Savin, K. L., & Jaser, S. S. (2018). Interventions with the family system. In M. E., Hilliard, K. A., Riekert, J. K. Ockene, & L. Pbert (Eds.). *The handbook of health behavior change* (pp. 406–420). New York, NY: Springer. doi:10.1891/9780826180148.0019

Hayslip, B. (2010). *A focus group approach to grandparent caregivers' needs*. Final Report to North Central Texas Area Agency on Aging.

Hayslip, B., Jr., Blumenthal, H., & Garner, A. (2014). Health and grandparent-grandchild well-being: One-year longitudinal findings for custodial grandfamilies. *Journal of Aging and Health, 26*, 558–581. doi:10.1177/0898264314525664

Hayslip, B., Jr., Blumenthal, H., & Garner, A. (2015). Social support and grandparent caregiver health: One-year longitudinal findings for custodial grandparents. *The Journals of Gerontology, Series B: Psychological Sciences and Social Sciences, 70*, 804–812.

Hayslip, B., Jr., Davis, S., Goodman, C., Smith, G. C., Neumann, C., Maiden, R., & Carr, G. (2013). The role of resilience in understanding grandparents raising their grandchildren. In B. Hayslip Jr. & G. Smith (Eds.), *Resilient grandparent caregivers: A strengths-based perspective* (pp. 48–67). New York, NY: Routledge. doi:10.4324/9780203803905

Hayslip, B. Jr., Fruhauf, C., & Dolbin-MacNab, M. (2017). Grandparents raising grandchildren: What have we learned over the past decade? *The Gerontologist*, gnx124, doi:10.1093/geront/gnx124

Hayslip, B., Jr., & Kaminski, P. (2005). Grandparents raising their grandchildren: A review of the literature and suggestions for practice. *The Gerontologist, 45*, 262–269. doi:10.1093/geront/45.2.262

Hayslip, B., Montoro-Rodriguez, J., Smith, G., & Strieder, F. (2015). Group leaders' perceptions of interventions with grandparent caregivers: Content and process. *Grandfamilies, 2*, 1–33.

Hayslip, B., Jr., & Smith, G. (2013). *Resilient grandparent caregivers: A strengths-based perspective.* New York, NY: Routledge. doi:10.4324/9780203803905

Hirshorn, B. A., Van Meter, M., & Brown, D. R. (2000). When grandparents raise grandchildren due to substance abuse: Responding to a uniquely destabilizing factor. In B. Hayslip & R. Goldberg-Glen (Eds.), *Grandparents raising grandchildren: Theoretical, empirical, and clinical perspectives* (pp. 269–288). New York, NY: Springer.

Hrostowski, S., & Forster, S. (2010). Grandfamilies health watchers program. *Journal of Intergenerational Relationships, 8*, 369–385. doi:10.1080/15350770.2010.520622

James, L. C., & Ferrante, C. R. (2013). Skip generations: A strengths-based mentoring program for resilient grandparent caregivers. In B. Hayslip Jr., & G. C. Smithe (Eds.) *Resilient grandparent caregivers: A strengths-based perspective* (pp. 184–194). New York, NY: Routledge.

Jooste, J. L., Hayslip, B. Jr., & Smith, G. C. (2008). The adjustment of children and grandparent caregivers in grandparent-headed families. In B. Hayslip Jr., & P. L. Kaminski (Eds), *Parenting the custodial grandchild: Implications for clinical practice* (pp 17–39). New York, NY: Springer.

Kaminski, P. L., & Murrell, A. R. (2008). Counseling custodial grandchildren. In B. Hayslip Jr., & P. L. Kaminski (Eds.), *Parenting the custodial grandchild: Implications for clinical practice* (pp 215–236). New York, NY: Springer.

Kelley, S. J., Whitley, D. M., & Campos, P. E. (2013). African American caregiving grandmothers: Results of an intervention to improve health indicators and health promotion behaviors. *Journal of Family Nursing, 19*, 53–73. doi:10.1177/1074840712462135

Kirby, J. M. (2015). The potential benefits of parenting programs for grandparents: Recommendations and clinical implications. *Journal of Child & Family Studies, 24*, 3200–3212. doi:10.1007/s10826-015-0123-9

Kolomer, S., McCallion, P., & Van Voorbis, C. (2008). School-based support group intervention for children in the care of their grandparents. In B. Hayslip Jr., & P. L. Kaminski (Eds.), *Parenting the custodial grandchild: Implications for clinical practice* (pp. 251–263). New York, NY: Springer.

Leder, S., Grinstead, L. N. & Torres, E. (2007). Grandparents raising grandchildren: Stressors, social support, and health outcomes. *Journal of Family Nursing, 13*(3), 333–352. doi:10.1177/1074840707303841

Lee, Y., & Blitz, L. V. (2014). We're GRAND: A qualitative design and development pilot project addressing the needs and strengths of grandparents raising grandchildren. *Child & Family Social Work, 21*, 381–390. doi:10.1111/cfs.12153

Lent, J. P., & Otto, A. (2019). Grandparents, grandchildren, and caregiving: The impacts of America's substance use crisis. *American Society on Aging.* Retrieved February 14, 2019 from https://www.asaging.org/blog/grandparents-grandchildren-and-caregiving-impacts-americas-substance-use-crisis

Littlewood, K. A. (2014). Grandfamilies outcome workgroup's (GrOW) review of grandfamilies support groups: An examination of concepts, goals, outcomes and measures. *Grandfamilies: The Contemporary Journal of Research, Practice and Policy, 1*(1), Article 3.

Maiden, R. J., & Zuckerman, C. (2008). Counseling grandparents parenting their grandchildren: Case studies. In B. Hayslip Jr., & P. L. Kaminski (Eds.), *Parenting the custodial grandchild: Implications for clinical practice* (pp. 197–214). New York, NY: Springer.

Mauderer, R. (2008). Adjusting and succeeding in school: Helping grandparent caregivers and their grandchildren. In B. Hayslip Jr. & P. Kaminiski (Eds.), *Parenting the custodial grandchild: Implications for clinical practice* (pp. 265–283). New York, NY: Springer.

McCallion, P., Ferretti, L. A., & Kim, J. (2013). Challenges in translating an evidence-based health self-management intervention for grandparent caregivers. In B. Hayslip Jr., & G. C. Smithe (Eds.). *Resilient grandparent caregivers: A strengths-based perspective* (pp. 195–208). New York, NY: Routledge.

McCallion, P., Janicki, M. P., & Kolomer, S. R. (2004) Controlled evaluation of support groups for grandparent caregivers of children with developmental disabilities and delays. *American Journal on Mental Retardation, 109*(5), 352–361.

McLaughlin, B., Ryder, D., & Taylor, M. F. (2017). Effectiveness of interventions for grandparent caregivers: A systematic review. *Marriage & Family Review, 53*, 509–531. doi:10.1080/01494929.2016.1177631

Mendoza, A. N. (2018). A social network analysis of the relation between social support and resilience in grandparents raising their grandchildren. *Dissertation Abstracts International Section A: Humanities and Social Sciences, 70*(10-A)(E), 2018.

Mendoza, A. N., Fruhauf, C. A., & Weil, J. (2018). Understanding Latino grandparents raising grandchildren through a bioecological lens. *International Journal of Aging & Human Development, (3)*, 281. doi:10.1177/0091415017702907

Messing, J. T. (2006). From the child's perspective: A qualitative analysis of kinship care placements. *Children and Youth Services Review, 28*, 1415–1434. doi:10.1016/j.childyouth.2006.03.001

Mignon, S. L., & Holmes, W.M. (2013). Substance abuse and mental health issues within Native American grandparenting families. *Journal of Ethnicity in Substance Abuse, 12*, 210–227. doi:10.1080/15332640.2013.798751

Milan, A., Laflamme, N., & Wong I. (April, 2015). Diversity of grandparents living with their grandchildren. *Insights on Canadian Society*. Statistics Canada Catalogue no. 75–006-X.

Miltenberger, P., Hayslip, B., Harris, B., & Kaminski, P. (2003–2004). Perceptions of the losses experienced by custodial grandmothers. *Omega: Journal of Death and Dying, 48*, 245–262.

Minkler, M., Roe, K. M., & Price, M. (1992). The physical and emotional health of grandmothers raising grandchildren in the crack cocaine epidemic. *The Gerontologist, 32*(6), 752–761. doi:10.1093/geront/32.6.752

Musil, C. M., Warner, C. B., McNamara, M., Rokoff, S., & Turek, D. (2008). Parenting concerns of grandparents raising grandchildren: An insider's picture. In B. Hayslip, Jr. & P. Kaminiski (Eds.), *Parenting the custodial grandchild: Implications for clinical practice* (pp. 101–114). New York, NY: Springer.

Musil, C., Zauszniewski, J., Givens, S., Henrich, C., Wallace, M., Jeanblanc, A., & Burant, C. (2019). Resilience, resourcefulness, and grandparenting. In B. Hayslip & C. Fruhauf (Eds.), *Grandparenting: Influences on the dynamics of family relationships*. New York, NY: Springer.

Roberto, K., Dolbin-MacNab, M. L., & Finney, J. (2008). Promoting health for grandmothers parenting young children. In B. Hayslip Jr. & P. Kaminiski (Eds.), *Parenting the custodial grandchild: Implications for clinical practice* (pp. 75–92). New York, NY: Springer.

Roe, K. M. (2000). Community interventions to support grandparent caregivers: Lessons learned from the field. In C. B. Cox (Ed.), *To grandmother's house we go and stay: Perspectives on custodial grandparents* (pp. 283–303). New York, NY: Springer.

Rutter, M. (2007). Resilience, competence, and coping. *Journal of Child Abuse and Neglect, 31*, 205–209. doi:10.1016/j.chiabu.2007.02.001

Ryan, J. P., Hong, J. S., Herz, D., & Hernandez, P. M. (2010). Kinship foster care and the risk of juvenile delinquency. *Children and Youth Services, 32*, 1823–1830.

Smith, G. C., & Dolbin-MacNab, M. L. (2013). The role of negative and positive caregiving appraisals in key outcomes for custodial grandmothers and grandchildren. In B. Hayslip Jr. & G. C. Smith (Eds.), *Resilient grandparent caregivers: A strengths-based perspective* (pp. 3–24). New York, NY: Routledge.

Smith, G. C., Hayslip, B., Hancock, G., Strieder, F., & Montoro-Rodriguez, J. (2018). A randomized clinical trial of interventions for improving well-being in custodial grandfamilies. *Journal of Family Psychology, 32*, 816–827.

Smith, G. C., Palmieri, P. A., Hancock, G. R., & Richardson, R. A. (2008). Custodial grandmothers' psychological distress, dysfunctional parenting, and grandchildren's adjustment. *International Journal of Aging and Human Development, 67*, 327–357. doi:10.2190/AG.67.4.c

Smith, G. C., Strieder, F., Greenberg, P., Hayslip, B. Jr., & Montoro-Rodriguez, J. (2016). Patterns of enrollment and engagement of custodial grandmothers in a randomized clinical trial of psychoeducational interventions. *Family Relations, 65*, 369–386. doi:10.1111/fare.12194

Strawbridge, W. J., Wallhagen, M. I., Shema, S. J., & Kaplan, G. A. (1997). New burdens or more of the same? Comparing grandparent, spouse, and adult-child caregivers. *The Gerontologist, 37*, 505–510. doi:10.1093/geront/37.4.505

Strom, P., & Strom, R. (2011). Grandparent education: Raising grandchildren. *Educational Gerontology, 37*, 910–923. doi:10.1080/03601277.2011.595345

Strong, D. D., Bean, R. A., Feinauer, L. L. (2010). Trauma, attachment, and family therapy with grandfamilies: A model for treatment. *Children and Youth Services Review, 32*, 44–50. doi:10.1016/j.childyouth.2009.06.015

Tang, F., Jang, F., & Copeland, V. C. (2015). Challenges and resilience in African American grandparents raising grandchildren: A review of the literature and practice implications. *Grandfamilies: The Contemporary Journal of Research, Practice, and Policy, 2*(2). Retrieved from http://scholarworks.wmich.edu/grandfamilies/vol2/iss2/2/

U.S. Census Bureau. (2017). *American community survey 1-year estimates.* Retrieved January 6, 2019 from tinyurl.com/jkwl6l4

Vacha-hasse, T., Ness, C. M., Dannison, L., & Smith, A. (2000) Grandparents raising grandchildren: A psychoeducational group approach. *The Journal for Specialists in Group Work, 25*, 67–78. doi:10.1080/01933920008411452

Weinberger, S. G. (2014). Mentors support grandfamilies raising grandchildren. *Grandfamilies: The Contemporary Journal of Research, Practice and Policy, 1*, 72–84.

Whitley, D. M., Kelley, S. J., & Lamis, D. A. (2016). Depression, social support, and mental health: A longitudinal mediation analysis in African American custodial grandmothers. *International Journal of Aging and Human Development, 82*, 166–187. doi:10.1177/0091415015626550

Yancura, L., Fruhauf, C. A., & Greenwood-Junkermeier, H. (2016). Recognizing microaggressions: A framework for helping grandfamilies. *Grandfamilies: The Contemporary Journal of Research, Practice and Policy, 3*(1), 106–121.

Yancura, L., Fruhauf, C. A., Riggs, N., Mendoza, A. N., & Greenwood-Junkermeier, H. (2017, November). *Development of a curriculum for children in grandparent-headed families.* Paper presented at the National Council on Family Relations, Orlando, FL.

Yancura, L., Greenwood-Junkermeier, H., & Fruhauf, C. A. (2017). "These classes have been my happy place": Feasibility study of a self-care program in Native Hawaiian custodial grandparents. *Asian/Pacific Island Nursing Journal, 2*(3), 103–109. doi:10.9741/23736658.1062

Zauszniewski, J. A., Au, T. Y., & Musil, C. M. (2012). Resourcefulness training for grandmothers raising grandchildren: Is there a need? *Issues in Mental Health Nursing, 33*, 680–686. doi:10.3109/01612840.2012.684424

Zauszniewski, J. A., Musil, C. M., & Au, T. (2013). Resourcefulness training for grandmothers: Feasibility and acceptability of two methods. *Issues in Mental Health Nursing, 34*, 435–441. doi:10.3109/01612840.2012.758208

Zauszniewski, J. A., Musil, C. M., Burant, C. J., & Au, T. (2014). Resourcefulness training for grandmothers: Preliminary evidence of effectiveness. *Research in Nursing & Health, 37*, 42–52. doi:10.1002/nur.21574

26

Planning health promotion programs to prevent substance use disorders and their consequences

Sylvia Roozen, Gerjo Kok and Leopold Curfs

Background

Substance misuse and substance use disorders (SUDs) belong to the category of serious health problems. The misuse of alcohol or other substances can have serious consequences not only for one's own health (e.g. diseases, self-harm, addiction) but also to the lives of others (e.g. road traffic injuries, interpersonal violence, fetal alcohol spectrum disorders) (World Health Organization, 2018). Measures that effectively work to reduce harms, health risks, and societal disruption are needed.

Developing evidence-based health promotion programs to prevent substance misuse and substance use disorders, as well as their negative consequences, is imperative. This should be a priority for professionals working in a variety of health and mental health fields, including social workers engaged with individuals, families, communities, and policy. This chapter's focus is on planning effective health promotion programs to prevent substance use disorders. Alcohol consumption during pregnancy was chosen as a substance abuse problem to illustrate concepts, as the authors have experience in this area. First, the topic of alcohol consumption during pregnancy, which can result in Fetal Alcohol Spectrum Disorders (FASD), is introduced. Next described is the process from problem identification to problem solving, essential for developing a successful health promotion program. Attention is directed to preventing substance use disorders more generally and health promotion programs at various levels of prevention. Substance use disorders do not usually occur in isolation but are influenced by various contextual factors which should be taken into account. These are also attended to as a means of increasing the intervention effectiveness. Applying a systematic framework to develop evidence-based health promotion programs can increase the effectiveness of such programs is demonstrated. Lastly, conclusions and recommendations are provided.

Alcohol and pregnancy: example for prevention planning

Children, young adults, and adults are vulnerable to alcohol effects that can have lifelong consequences. Adverse health consequences of alcohol misuse may be especially harmful when consumed by women during pregnancy. Alcohol use during pregnancy has been determined by medical research to cause the most serious health consequences in fetal development among common psychoactive substances (Abel & Sokol, 1987; Hoyme et al., 2016). These adverse outcomes are referred to as Fetal Alcohol Spectrum Disorders (FASD) (Hoyme et al., 2016). FASD is a spectrum of disorders ranging from mild to severe birth defects as a consequence of prenatal alcohol exposure. Individuals diagnosed within the spectrum experience lifelong physical, behavioral, and cognitive disabilities (British Medical Association, 2016; Hoyme et al., 2016; Popova et al., 2016; see Chapters 11 and 12 for more information).

The financial, human, and societal costs of particular health and social problems are important to discuss in the context of prevention, as they are relevant to policy makers and others responsible for funding prevention programs. The costs of FASD for society and a healthcare system are significant (Ericson, Magnusson, & Hovstadius, 2017; Mäkelä, 2010; Popova et al., 2013; Popova, Lange, Burd, Shield, & Rehm, 2014; Thanh & Jonsson, 2009). In a systematic literature review, significant annual costs (health care, residential care, education, social services) and lifetime costs were reported (Popova, Stade, Bekmuradov, Lange, & Rehm, 2011). Estimating the financial toll of any substance use problem is not simple, given the complexity of types of impact and differences in cost calculation techniques. For example, Stade and colleagues (2009) estimated annual costs for FASD at a population level in Canada as high as 5.3 billion CAD. Popova et al. (2011) also pointed out the high inter-sectoral costs (i.e. costs between different sectors such as school systems, healthcare, and policy interventions). In addition, some costs cannot be expressed in terms of numbers or are difficult to calculate reliably; for instance, suffering of affected individuals and their families. Given this tremendous (preventable) burden for individuals and society, it is important to pay close attention to the topic of prevention.

To prevent the negative health and social consequences of drinking alcohol during pregnancy, a strategy underpinned by a systematic, evidence-based approach is needed. First, it is necessary to identify which specific prenatal alcohol drinking behavior(s) are most in need of intervention (Roozen et al., 2018). Because little is known to date about dose-response relationships between prenatal alcohol exposure and the risk of FASD, not all alcohol consumption by pregnant women places their babies at risk for lifelong negative health effects. For example, the amount, pattern, and timing of prenatal alcohol exposure are thought by child development experts and researchers to play a role in determining outcomes. Other confounding factors influence the outcome of FASD, such as maternal nutrition and lifestyle, body profile, age, and genetic disposition (Ehrhart et al., 2018). The conclusion derived by most pediatric health advocates is that the best message for pregnant women is that there is no proven safe amount of drinking.

Developing effective intervention programs in all areas of alcohol and other substance misuse is a complex process, mainly because there exist gaps in our knowledge of what is most effective, and there are complicated contextual factors (Bartholomew Eldredge, Markham, Ruiter, Fernandez, & Kok, 2016). For alcohol, these are: (1) an alcohol industry primarily concerned with profit using marketing strategies to promote drinking of alcoholic beverages, and (2) alcohol tax systems enforced by governments. Social and policy responses to the issue of heavy drinking differ between countries. Some countries, for religious reasons, discourage or prohibit alcohol consumption and apply punitive measures within their law system. Other nations have an entirely different focus and attempt to implement supportive programs and measures. Differences in alcohol consumption patterns attributed to sociodemographic factors, level of economic development, religion and cultural norms, and preferred alcohol drinks were described by the World Health Organization (World Health Organization, 2018). When developing intervention programs, it is important to take these contextual factors into consideration.

Other factors contribute to the complexity of designing effective prevention intervention programs. For example, stigmatization of parents having a child with FASD is a crucial aspect (Roozen, 2019). If key factors such as stigmatization are overlooked, resulting interventions may be ineffective or counterproductive. In the next section, we introduce an approach to develop effective intervention programs (Bartholomew Eldredge et al., 2016; Roozen, Black et al., 2016). It is recommended to follow approaches like this because they offer a methodology for systematically developing, implementing, and evaluating health promotion programs.

Preventing substance use disorders and their consequences

On a national level, many countries have implemented policies to discourage substance misuse. In 2018, the Dutch Ministry of Health Welfare and Sport launched the national prevention agreement. Alcohol-related issues in this prevention agreement included communication campaigns for awareness of harmful alcohol use, reducing alcohol points of sale, limiting alcohol advertisements, and implementing alcoholic beverage price policies. In preventing drinking during pregnancy, these activities will be more effective when tailored to different subgroups of pregnant woman and based on evidence concerning why these subgroups consume alcohol during pregnancy. For understanding FASD-related risk behaviors and determinants, it is also necessary to account for commercial business models and other possible factors that impeded effective prevention. Analyzing interactions between science, practice, and policy is of utmost importance for substance use disorder prevention programs.

Currently FASD prevention campaigns and implemented preventive measures are missing evaluation data concerning effectiveness (Schölin, 2016; Symons, Pedruzzi, Bruce, & Milne, 2018). Systematic evidence-based evaluation approaches are necessary to avoid problems of inconclusive data. Comparison with programs that attempt to influence tobacco smoking behavior may be illustrative. For years, ineffective attempts to reduce smoking existed and persisted. In one example, graphic, frightening images and text depicting the serious health consequences of smoking appeared on packs of cigarettes in Taiwan. However, research into the effectiveness of this strategy has shown, time and again, that such an approach is not effective in changing behavior (Kok, Peters, Kessels, ten Hoor, & Ruiter, 2018). Risk perception theories predict that if people will experience a threat, they want to counter that threat. However, how they do so is determined by their coping efficacy level: if efficacy is high, they may change their behavior in the suggested direction; if efficacy is low, they react defensively. There is evidence that messages that provide coping information to increase self-efficacy can be effective, for example, in interventions to promote smoking cessation. In developing preventive measures for at-risk alcohol consumption, it is important to learn from intervention studies of smoking and other unhealthy behaviors. In short, the use of evidence-supported strategies is essential. For alcohol abuse, as well as abuse of other substances, taking into account aspects of stigmatization, stereotyping, and ethical complications are complex, yet extremely important.

Influencing change

Prevention can be divided into three general categories: primary, secondary, and tertiary prevention (Kirch, 2008). Primary prevention activities occur prior to the target problem emerging or occurring. Secondary prevention efforts occur when the problem appears with the goal of reducing its potential for producing negative consequences or harms. Tertiary prevention includes efforts to manage or treat negative consequences and harms. For FASD, primary prevention implies developing strategies aimed at preventing alcohol-exposed pregnancies.

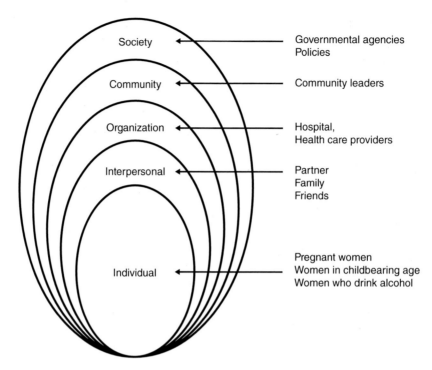

Figure 26.1   The socio-ecological approach (derived from Bartholomew Eldredge et al., 2016 with permission)

Secondary and tertiary prevention refer to minimizing alcohol-related harm (e.g. early screening, optimizing management and care) and providing early intervention programs for affected children. In prevention, it is important to apply an ecological approach to the health problem under study, such as the micro-, meso-, exo-, macro-system ecological model originally developed by Bronfenbrenner (1979; see Figure 26.1).

Health promotion interventions are situated within a social or physical ecosystem. When the target individual is, for example, a pregnant woman, she is embedded in the surrounding social structures: including her partner, relatives, workplace, neighborhood, healthcare providers, and workers at government agencies. These external agents influence individual behavior at various levels: interpersonal (e.g. partner, family, friends); organizational (e.g. hospital, healthcare providers); community (e.g. community leaders, neighborhood); and societal (e.g. government agencies, lifestyle policies, alcohol marketing, insurance/health care coverage). Health promotion interventions too often focus only on individual behavior change without addressing the behavior of environmental decision makers or agents. It is important when developing health promotion interventions, to target these environmental agents, as well. Examples of prevention interventions related to alcohol consumption during pregnancy at various levels; individual, interpersonal, organizational, and societal are described below.

Brief intervention

Brief intervention, including motivational interviewing, is an individual-level method (Miller & Rollnick, 2012). The CHOICES program, for example, applies motivational interviewing techniques (Velasquez et al., 2010). The program is based on four individual counseling sessions and a contraception-counseling visit. The sessions consist of face-to-face counseling based on providing personal feedback on drinking behavior(s), as well as contraception options.

An example of a prevention intervention targeted to interpersonal and organizational levels involves enhanced linkage networks. The Canadian Prevention Network Action Team on FASD Prevention (CanFASD) built a multidisciplinary FASD network aimed at advancing national prevention activities. In Australia, for instance, community-led approaches are used to make FASD history (Fitzpatrick et al., 2017). The CANFASD network consists of individuals in different roles—such as researchers, service providers, health system planners, policy analysts, community-based advocates, and (where possible) birth mothers. To achieve this comprehensive participation, the network employed a virtual community of inquiry (vCoI) model (Garrison, 2011), supplemented by face-to-face meetings often held in conjunction with national and international conferences. Through the vCoI, participants were able to voluntarily attend monthly web meetings providing opportunities to share updates on their work, learn of recent additions to the evidence on FASD prevention, and discuss research, service provision, and advocacy developments undertaken by members and others in Canada, as well as discuss/plan collective ongoing action. In this way, participants learned together about FASD prevention and were able to better align their own work within the field. A virtual research network involving multisectoral participants, focused on co-learning and collective action, proved to be a useful model guiding FASD prevention efforts in Canada. Over a decade, participants have voluntarily participated in the opportunity for co-learning, networking, and collaboration. Collective engagement has produced varied and strong knowledge products that support critical thinking and action on multiple levels of prevention for varied audiences. Such transdisciplinary, participatory, appreciative, and dialogic approaches appear to be important to understanding and facilitating the uptake of FASD prevention practices, such as brief intervention, on the part of professionals and systems of care (Schmidt et al., 2019).

Prevention activities can also be based on multilevel approaches, such as the Healthy Mother Healthy Baby© Program (Olivier, 2017). This program addressed a multitude of aspects related to FASD prevention and intervention through community participation. Through this program, pregnant women in different areas across South Africa were invited to enroll in project activities, striving to decrease stigma and focus on healthy pregnancies and healthy babies, rather than telling women what not to do during pregnancy. Babies born to participants received full pediatric and neurodevelopmental assessments at nine months of age. This information was reported back to the mothers and pediatricians, and used to assess the program's impact, especially in terms of behavior change and support. The projects were implemented in partnership with local government services, other NGO's/CBO's and community members, thereby striving to facilitate optimum participation and capacity development (Olivier, 2017).

FASD prevention intervention effectiveness

For FASD, primary, secondary, and tertiary prevention goals are all important. A wide variety of FASD prevention and management activities have been carried out in different countries. Examples include:

- implementing large-scale (inter)national campaigns, such as the "Too Young To Drink" media campaign (Bazzo et al., 2017);

- forming research networks, such as the international FASD prevention interest group and the Collaborative Initiative on Fetal Alcohol Spectrum Disorders (CIFASD);
- mobilizing advocacy, such as International FASD Awareness Day on the 9th of September each year;
- strengthening maternal and child health through brief interventions, such as Healthy Mother Healthy Baby© (Olivier, 2017);
- engaging in motivational interviewing, such as the CHOICES program (Ingersoll et al., 2018); and
- screening and improving management and care, such as with the Alert Program (Wagner et al., 2018).

However, little is known about the effectiveness of these prevention activities (Symons et al., 2018), or what would be involved in implementing them more widely (see Chapter 36 on implementation science). Up to now, systematically developed evidence-based prevention programs are scarce.

The need for a systematic, stepwise approach

In prevention planning, a systematic, stepwise, approach is indispensable. First, as for all substance misuse and use disorders, it is essential to have a good understanding of what is known and what is still unknown about the addictive behavior. Evidence-informed prevention practice entails integrating scientific evidence and clinical expertise to form the basis for problem prevention and management. As described in Roozen et al. (2016), an iterative approach can be applied in the process of problem identification and problem solving. Pre-existing protocols and strategies are helpful, such as Intervention Mapping (IM) (Bartholomew Eldredge et al., 2016). Intervention Mapping is a planning approach based on using theory and evidence as foundations for an ecological approach to assessing and intervening in health problems and engendering community participation. IM offers a methodology to systematically develop, implement, and evaluate health promotion programs, including substance abuse disorders as illustrated in Figure 26.2.

Each step of Intervention Mapping comprises several tasks, the completion of which creates a product guiding subsequent steps. Completion of all steps creates a blueprint for designing, implementing, and evaluating an intervention based on a foundation of theoretical, empirical, and practical information. Although Intervention Mapping comprises six steps, the process is iterative rather than linear. Program developers move back and forth between tasks and steps as they gain new information and perspective. However, the process is also cumulative; planners base each step on previous steps, and inattention to one step can jeopardize the potential effectiveness of later steps. These six IM steps could be applied to the prevention of prenatal alcohol exposure, FASD, or other substance use disorders as follows (Roozen, Black et al., 2016).

Step 1. Develop a logic model

The first step in development of a systematic evidence-based health promotion program is to conduct a needs assessment or problem analysis by identifying what, if anything, needs to be changed and for whom. Planners need to develop a good understanding of the nature, extent, and causes of the preventable problem before starting to develop a prevention program. The following questions may apply to the FASD example:

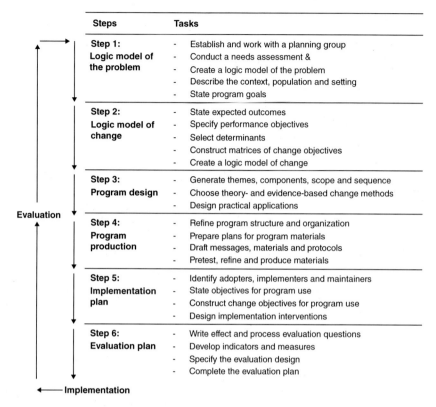

Steps	Tasks
Step 1: **Logic model of the problem**	- Establish and work with a planning group - Conduct a needs assessment & - Create a logic model of the problem - Describe the context, population and setting - State program goals
Step 2: **Logic model of change**	- State expected outcomes - Specify performance objectives - Select determinants - Construct matrices of change objectives - Create a logic model of change
Step 3: **Program design**	- Generate themes, components, scope and sequence - Choose theory- and evidence-based change methods - Design practical applications
Step 4: **Program production**	- Refine program structure and organization - Prepare plans for program materials - Draft messages, materials and protocols - Pretest, refine and produce materials
Step 5: **Implementation plan**	- Identify adopters, implementers and maintainers - State objectives for program use - Construct change objectives for program use - Design implementation interventions
Step 6: **Evaluation plan**	- Write effect and process evaluation questions - Develop indicators and measures - Specify the evaluation design - Complete the evaluation plan

Evaluation

◀——— Implementation

Figure 26.2 Intervention Mapping step and tasks (adapted from Bartholomew Eldredge et al., 2016 with permission)

Is FASD a significant world-wide problem?

The meta-analyses of global FASD prevalence estimates can inform this question's answer (Roozen, Peters et al., 2016). Data were available for a limited number of countries, with FASD prevalence estimates ranging from 0 to 176.77 per 1,000 live births. Prevalence studies varied considerably in terms of their methodology, so caution is warranted in interpreting the results. However, one can conclude that FASD is indeed a world-wide problem that merits attention (see Chapters 2 and 11).

What maternal behaviors are related to FASD?

There is no consensus on what should be identified under harmful and desired behaviors among pregnant women regarding alcohol consumption. Some studies report that heavy (binge) drinking by pregnant women increases the risk of having a child born with FASD. Other studies report that mild to moderate amounts of alcohol consumption during pregnancy have adverse effects on important health and developmental outcomes for the unborn child. Therefore, various international organizations, such as the World Health Organization (WHO), the American Academy of Pediatrics (AAP), the U.S. National Institute on Alcohol Abuse and Alcoholism (NIAAA), and the British Medical Association (BMA), concluded that there is no known safe amount of alcohol to consume while pregnant.

What are the determinants and environmental influences on these behaviors?

To elicit behavior change, it is important to provide insight into the exact behaviors under consideration, as well as into the determinants and environmental factors which influence these behaviors. Determinants include risk perceptions, attitudes, perceived norms, perceived skills, but also impulsivity and habits (Bartholomew Eldredge et al., 2016). Once this has been established, it is essential to determine the highest at-risk target group. For FASD, this could be pregnant women, women planning a pregnancy, or women who potentially might get pregnant and who experience an alcohol use disorder or engage in risky drinking behavior.

Who are the stakeholders involved?

This question concerns who can likely contribute to the development and implementation of the program. Their selection is not straightforward, but stakeholders potentially concerned with FASD include: biological and adoptive parents, persons affected by FASD, the alcohol industry, government (various departments from health agencies to education, and even criminal justice agencies), healthcare professionals, researchers, and policy makers.

What role is played by stigma?

This question concerns the different types of stigma that may play a role and need to be considered while developing a program.

What ethical considerations need to be addressed?

Based on results of this first problem analysis step, planners then continue onto Step 2 to determine the program outcomes and objectives that should lead to a decrease of the health problem.

Step 2. Develop a logic model of change: program outcomes and objectives

The second step is to create what are known as "change objectives" by combining health promoting (sub)behaviors with their determinants to identify which determinants and underlying beliefs should be targeted by the intervention. Here, the focus shifts from unhealthy behaviors to health promoting behaviors. This step is not only conducted for the behaviors of the at-risk target group but repeated for behaviors required by relevant stakeholders (e.g. midwives, general practitioners, social workers). The analyses and selection of relevant determinants and environmental factors (both of which become desired intervention outcomes) are based on both theory and empirical evidence. Moreover, relevant stakeholders are consulted and involved.

Step 3. Develop the program plan

The third step is to select theory-based behavior change methods, strategies, or techniques that align with the broader determinants into which the elements identified in Step 2 aggregate, and then translate these into practical applications that satisfy the parameters for effectiveness of the selected methods (Kok et al., 2016). A strong program plan includes scope, sequence, change methods, and practical applications.

For example, France and colleagues (2014) developed messages to increase women's intention to abstain from alcohol while pregnant. They combined risk information and self-efficacy messages to achieve the goal. While risk information alone may be effective in increasing intention not to drink, theory and evidence suggests that threatening messages by themselves do not change actual behavior (Kok et al., 2018). The capacity to change behavior often depends on perceived skills, or self-efficacy (one's belief in own ability to succeed) for change. Risk can be a motivator for changing behavior when the message is combined with messages increasing or improving self-efficacy.

Mollen, Rimal, Ruiter, Jang, and Kok (2013) focused on motivation to engage in intervening or non-intervening behaviors among friends in risky alcohol consumption contexts: in this case telling them to either stop drinking or not drive home. They provided participants with descriptive social norm messages or injunctive social norm messages, either positive or negative. Descriptive norms convey what (most) others do/not do, while injunctive norms convey approval or disapproval of (most) others for the behavior. For example, one positive descriptive norm message stated: "When students are at a party, the majority makes sure their friends don't drink too much." One positive injunctive norm stated: "According to students, when you are at a party, you should make sure your friends don't drink too much" (Mollen et al., 2013, p. 6). The investigators identified positive norms as stronger motivators for intervening and negative norms as motivating non-intervening behavior. Moreover, they found that injunctive norms had a stronger effect on intervening behavior than descriptive norms. The investigators concluded that to increase individuals' motivation to intervene in others' drinking behavior, in this case telling them to stop drinking, intervention messages should focus on the high prevalence of intervening behavior and the approval thereof among friends. They also warn against messages conveying high prevalence of negative behavior, not intervening when your friends drink too much, because those messages enforce the notion that such behavior is in fact normative (Mollen, Rimal, & Lapinski, 2010).

Step 4. Produce the intervention, including program materials and messages

Once all program components have been developed, they can be integrated into one coherent program. One example is the brochure corresponding with the publication by France and colleagues. The fourth step is based on pre-testing program materials together with the planning group (including members of the target population) and refining the program elements as necessary.

Step 5. Plan for program sustainability

The fifth step is to plan for adoption, implementation, and sustainability of the program. Program development alone does not guarantee effectiveness. Program participants and implementers need to be identified. The most obvious and important implementers for FASD prevention are healthcare professionals in fields related to pregnancy. Analysis of the stakeholders from the first step can assist in the choice of implementers, as not all relevant stakeholders are motivated, qualified, or in a position to deliver a program. The process and considerations for adoption, implementation, and sustainability of programs are often not reported in the description of prevention programs, but, they are essential for effectiveness (see Chapter 36).

Step 6. Develop and implement an evaluation plan

The sixth step is to generate an evaluation plan to measure program effectiveness (outcome evaluation) and implementation (process evaluation). For each of the objectives from step 2, a measurable outcome should be determined. Then, the planners specify the evaluation design to conduct outcome and process evaluations, making sure that question of adherence to the original intervention plan is addressed (intervention fidelity) and that variations from the plan are identified and analyzed for their possible impact on outcomes.

Example of IM in action

Brendryen, Johansen, Nesvåg, Kok, and Duckert (2013) provided an example of an online alcohol intervention, Balance, using Intervention Mapping. Based on the needs assessment (IM Step 1), they estimated the prevalence of at risk drinking as 18% for men and 5% for women. Their overall goal was to reduce at-risk drinking. The health promoting sub-behaviors (IM Step 2) were formulated in terms of self-regulation—self-observation and self-evaluation, implementation of the change attempt, and change maintenance. Relevant determinants included awareness, attitudes, and self-efficacy, resulting in performance objectives such as: expressing positive feelings for receiving help to drink less (positive attitude/belief related to implementation of the change attempt); expressing confidence in ability to cope with urges and temptation (self-efficacy belief related to change maintenance); and avoiding lapse by coping adequately with the antecedents of drinking.

Brendryen at al. continued with finding theory-based methods for change (IM Step 3), based on cognitive behavior therapy and social cognitive theory (see Chapter 18).

- Consciousness raising: providing information, guidelines, assignments, examples, and tips to increase self-awareness. Parameters: feedback and confrontation should be followed by an increase in problem-solving ability and self-efficacy.
- Modeling or vicarious experience for self-efficacy: presenting potential role models and how they coped with difficulties to increase self-efficacy. Parameters: requires identification with the model and the model to be reinforced.

The resulting e-intervention (IM Step 4) started with substance use screening and then two complementary strategies for delivering intervention content: tunnel design and just-in-time therapy. In a tunnel design, clients followed a predetermined sequence of curriculum units. The advantage was that the user engages in activities and sees content that otherwise would not be encountered; the disadvantage is that reduced autonomy may lead to frustration and drop-out. By applying just-in-time therapy, giving immediate feedback, and making clients set their own targets, autonomy is restored. The program focused on emotion regulation, as well as drinking lapse and relapse prevention.

The authors did not provide information on anticipating implementation of their program (IM Step 5), besides arguing that the success criterion in e-health should not be keeping participants until the end of the program but keeping them long enough to achieve a clinically significant effect on the relevant health behavior (IM Step 6). Brendryen et al. (2014) described that their intervention significantly affected alcohol consumption in the desired direction at six months.

Conclusions

In conclusion, we presented prenatal alcohol exposure as an example illustrating use of systematic evidence-based tools for prevention. These tools are applicable to social workers and other health professionals working in a variety of settings with different populations at risk for substance misuse and substance use disorders. In planning systematic health promotion programs, the use of a theoretical framework has been strongly recommended. Intervention Mapping as a strategy was discussed and explained as a tool for such a framework. For the prevention of FASD and other problems associated with substance misuse, this framework can be very helpful. Globally, these problems are embedded in different environmental contexts. For this reason, using an ecological approach has been recommended. For professionals working together on multidisciplinary teams, remaining aware of the problems of the particular substance under study is of utmost importance. Never forget the old African proverb: "If you want to go fast, go alone. If you want to go far, go together."

The FASD example, like many of the other problems stemming from substance misuse and substance use disorders, is an important health problem which affects individuals, their families, and communities world-wide. FASD is theoretically entirely preventable. The development of effective intervention programs is a complex process; substance misuse and substance use disorders are seldom stand-alone problems. If interfering key factors are overlooked, ineffective or counterproductive prevention programs may be the result. Social workers and allied health professionals are often in position to carry out the recommendations presented here.

References

Abel, E. L., & Sokol, R. J. (1987). Incidence of fetal alcohol syndrome and economic impact of FAS-related anomalies. *Drug and Alcohol Dependence, 19*(1), 51–70. doi:10.1016/0376-8716(87)90087-1

Bartholomew Eldredge, L. K., Markham, C., Ruiter, R. A. C., Fernandez, M., & Kok, G. (2016). *Planning health promotion programs: An intervention mapping approach.* New York, NY: John Wiley & Sons.

Bazzo, S., Black, D., Mitchell, K., Marini, F., Moino, G., Riscica, P., & Fattori, G. (2017). 'Too young to drink'. An international communication campaign to raise public awareness of fetal alcohol spectrum disorders. *Public Health, 142,* 111–115. doi:10.1016/j.puhe.2016.08.001

Brendryen, H., Johansen, A., Nesvåg, S., Kok, G., & Duckert, F. (2013). Constructing a theory-and evidence-based treatment rationale for complex eHealth interventions: Development of an online alcohol intervention using an intervention mapping approach. *JMIR Research Protocols, 2*(1). doi:10.2196/resprot.2371

Brendryen, H., Lund, I. O., Johansen, A. B., Riksheim, M., Nesvåg, S., & Duckert, F. (2014). Balance-a pragmatic randomized controlled trial of an online intensive self-help alcohol intervention. *Addiction, 109*(2), 218–226. doi:10.1111/add.12383

British Medical Association. (2016). *Alcohol and pregnancy: Preventing and managing fetal alcohol spectrum disorders* (June 2007, updated February 2016). Retrieved from https://www.bma.org.uk/collective-voice/policy-and-research/public-and-population-health/alcohol/alcohol-and-pregnancy

Bronfenbrenner, U. (1979). *The ecology of human development: Experiments by nature and design.* Cambridge, MA: Harvard University Press.

Ehrhart, F., Roozen, S., Verbeek, J., Koek, G., Kok, G., van Kranen, H., . . . Curfs, L. M. G. (2018). Review and gap analysis: Molecular pathways leading to fetal alcohol spectrum disorders. *Molecular Psychiatry, 24,* 10–17. doi:10.1038/s41380-018-0095-4

Ericson, L., Magnusson, L., & Hovstadius, B. (2017). Societal costs of fetal alcohol syndrome in Sweden. *European Journal of Health Economics, 18*(5), 575–585. doi:10.1007/s10198-016-0811-4

Fitzpatrick, J. P., Oscar, J., Carter, M., Elliott, E. J., Latimer, J., Wright, E., & Boulton, J. (2017). The Marulu Strategy 2008-2012: Overcoming fetal alcohol spectrum disorder (FASD) in the Fitzroy Valley. *Australian and New Zealand Journal of Public Health, 41*(5), 467-473.

France, K. E., Donovan, R. J., Bower, C., Elliott, E. J., Payne, J. M., D'Antoine, H., & Bartu, A. E. (2014). Messages that increase women's intentions to abstain from alcohol during pregnancy: Results from quantitative testing of advertising concepts. *BMC Public Health, 14*(30), 1–13. doi:10.1186/1471-2458-14-30

Garrison, D. R. (2011). *E-learning in the 21st century: A framework for research and practice.* New York, NY: Routledge. doi:10.4324/9780203838761

Hoyme, H. E., Kalberg, W. O., Elliott, A. J., Blankenship, J., Buckley, D., Marais, A. S., . . . Jewett, T. (2016). Updated clinical guidelines for diagnosing fetal alcohol spectrum disorders. *Pediatrics, 138*(2), e20154256–e20154256. doi:10.1542/peds.2015-4256

Ingersoll, K., Frederick, C., MacDonnell, K., Ritterband, L., Lord, H., Jones, B., & Truwit, L. (2018). A pilot RCT of an Internet intervention to reduce the risk of alcohol-exposed pregnancy. *Alcoholism: Clinical and Experimental Research, 42*(6), 1132–1144. doi:10.1111/acer.13635

Kirch, W. (Ed.). (2008). *Encyclopedia of public health: Volume 1: A-H volume 2: I-Z.* Springer Science & Business Media. Retrieved from https://link.springer.com/referencework/10.1007/978-1-4020-5614-7

Kok, G., Gottlieb, N. H., Peters, G.-J. Y., Mullen, P. D., Parcel, G. S., Ruiter, R. A. C., . . . Bartholomew-Eldredge, L. K. (2016). A taxonomy of behavior change methods: An intervention mapping approach. *Health Psychology Review, 10*(3). doi:10.1080/17437199.2015.1077155

Kok, G., Peters, G. J. Y., Kessels, L. T. E., ten Hoor, G. A., & Ruiter, R. A. C. (2018). Ignoring theory and misinterpreting evidence: The false belief in fear appeals. *Health Psychology Review, 12*(2), 111–125. doi:10.1080/17437199.2017.1415767

Mäkelä, K. (2010). The cost of fetal alcohol spectrum disorder. *NAT Nordisk Alkohol & Narkotikatidskrift, 27*(4), 327–333. Retrieved from http://search.ebscohost.com/login.aspx?direct=true&db=psyh&AN=2011-00295-004&site=ehost-live. https://doi.org/10.1177/145507251002700409

Miller, W. R., & Rollnick, S. (2012). *Motivational interviewing: Helping people change.* New York, NY: Guilford Press.

Mollen, S., Rimal, R. N., & Lapinski, M. K. (2010). What is normative in health communication research on norms? A review and recommendations for future scholarship. *Health Communication, 25*(6), 544–547. doi:10.1080/10410236.2010.496704

Mollen, S., Rimal, R. N., Ruiter, R. A. C., Jang, S. A., & Kok, G. (2013). Intervening or interfering? The influence of injunctive and descriptive norms on intervention behaviours in alcohol consumption contexts. *Psychology and Health, 28*(5), 561–578. doi:10.1080/08870446.2012.752827

Olivier, L. (2017). *Fetal alcohol spectrum disorders in South Africa: A 20-year journey.* (Doctoral dissertation). Maastricht University. Retrieved from https://cris.maastrichtuniversity.nl/portal/en/publications/fetal-alcohol-spectrum-disorders-in-south-africa(cb29facb-96ab-432f-9f93-3619e43540f6).html

Popova, S., Lange, S., Burd, L., Chudley, A. E., Clarren, S. K., & Rehm, J. (2013). Cost of fetal alcohol spectrum disorder diagnosis in Canada. *PLoS One, 8*(4). doi:10.1371/journal.pone.0060434

Popova, S., Lange, S., Burd, L., Shield, K., & Rehm, J. (2014). Cost of speech-language interventions for children and youth with foetal alcohol spectrum disorder in Canada. *International Journal of Speech-Language Pathology, 16*(6), 571–581. doi:10.3109/17549507.2013.862858

Popova, S., Lange, S., Shield, K., Mihic, A., Chudley, A. E., Mukherjee, R. A. S., . . . Rehm, J. (2016). Comorbidity of fetal alcohol spectrum disorder: A systematic review and meta-analysis. *Lancet (London, England), 387*(10022), 978–987. doi:10.1016/S0140-6736(15)01345-8

Popova, S., Stade, B., Bekmuradov, D., Lange, S., & Rehm, J. (2011). What do we know about the economic impact of fetal alcohol spectrum disorder? A systematic literature review. *Alcohol and Alcoholism, 46*(4), 490–497. doi:10.1093/alcalc/agr029

Roozen, S. (2019). *Fetal alcohol spectrum disorders: An important health problem in need of prevention.* Maastricht, Netherlands: Gildeprint Drukkerijen.

Roozen, S., Black, D., Peters, G.-J. Y., Kok, G., Townend, D., Nijhuis, J. G., . . . Curfs, L. M. G. (2016). Fetal alcohol spectrum disorders (FASD): An approach to effective prevention. *Current Developmental Disorders Reports, 3*(4), 229–234. doi:10.1007/s40474-016-0101-y

Roozen, S., Peters, G.-J. Y., Kok, G., Townend, D., Nijhuis, J., & Curfs, L. (2016). Worldwide prevalence of fetal alcohol spectrum disorders: A systematic literature review including meta-analysis. *Alcoholism, Clinical and Experimental Research, 40*(1), 18–32. doi:10.1111/acer.12939

Roozen, S., Peters, G.-J. Y., Kok, G., Townend, D., Nijhuis, J., Koek, G., & Curfs, L. (2018). Systematic literature review on which maternal alcohol behaviours are related to fetal alcohol spectrum disorders (FASD). *BMJ Open, 8*(12). doi:10.1136/bmjopen-2018-022578

Schmidt, R., Harding, K., Talbot, C., Poole, N., Centre of Excellence for Women's Health, & CanFASD Research Network. (2019). *FASD PREVENTION: An annotated bibliography of articles published in 2017.* Retrieved from https://canfasd.ca/wp-content/uploads/sites/35/2019/03/FASD-Prevention-Literature-2018.pdf

Schölin, L. (2016). *Prevention of harm caused by alcohol exposure in pregnancy.* Copenhagen, Denmark: WHO Regional Office for Europe.

Stade, B., Ali, A., Bennett, D., Campbell, D., Johnston, M., Lens, C., . . . Koren, G. (2009). The burden of prenatal exposure to alcohol: Revised measurement of cost. *The Canadian Journal of Clinical Pharmacology = Journal Canadien de Pharmacologie Clinique, 16*(1), e91–e102. Retrieved from http://www.ncbi.nlm.nih.gov/pubmed/19168935

Symons, M., Pedruzzi, R. A., Bruce, K., & Milne, E. (2018). A systematic review of prevention interventions to reduce prenatal alcohol exposure and fetal alcohol spectrum disorder in indigenous communities. *BMC Public Health, 18*(1), 1–18. doi:10.1186/s12889-018-6139-5

Thanh, N. X., & Jonsson, E. (2009). Costs of fetal alcohol spectrum disorder in Alberta, Canada. *The Canadian Journal of Clinical Pharmacology = Journal Canadien de Pharmacologie Clinique, 16*(1), e80–e90.

Velasquez, M. M., Ingersoll, K. S., Sobell, M. B., Floyd, R. L., Sobell, L. C., & von Sternberg, K. (2010). A dual-focus motivational intervention to reduce the risk of alcohol-exposed pregnancy. *Cognitive and Behavioral Practice, 17*(2), 203–212. doi:10.1016/j.cbpra.2009.02.004

Wagner, B., Jirikowic, T., Symons, M., Latimer, J., Carter, M., Wright, E., . . . Mazzucchelli, T. G. (2018). Study protocol for a self-controlled cluster randomised trial of the alert program to improve self-regulation and executive function in Australian aboriginal children with fetal alcohol spectrum disorder. *BMJ Open, 8*(3), e021462. doi:10.1136/bmjopen-2017-021462

World Health Organization. (2018). *Global status report on alcohol and health 2018.* Geneva. Retrieved from https://www.who.int/substance_abuse/publications/global_alcohol_report/en/

27

Integrated care

Identifying and intervening with substance misuse in primary healthcare

Stacey Saunders-Adams, Catherine Hechmer,
Adriane Peck and Margaret M. Murray

Background

According to the 2017 Substance Abuse and Mental Health Administration's (SAMHSA) National Survey on Drug Use and Health (NSDUH), 7.2% of persons in the United States over the age of 12 (19.7 million) experienced a substance use disorder (SUD) involving alcohol and/or other psychoactive substances (SAMHSA, 2018). Worldwide, 16% of individuals over age 15 who drink engage in "heavy episodic drinking" (World Health Organization, 2018). An estimated 7.6% of individuals in the United States aged 12 or older experienced a need for substance use treatment in 2017; only 0.9% received it at a specialty facility (SAMHSA, 2018). In a cross-sectional study of primary care patients in Europe, over half of the study sample experiencing an alcohol use disorder had not received treatment within the previous 12 months (Probst, Manthey, Martinez, & Rehm, 2015). By comparison, according to Hill, Miller, and Sing (2011), only 2.4% of individuals diagnosed with diabetes in the United States were untreated. The vast majority of persons experiencing substance use disorders are under- or untreated.

Most medical associations in the United States consider addiction a complex disease of the brain and body, often chronic in nature, caused by a combination of behavioral, environmental, and biological factors (Center on Addiction, 2017). This perspective suggests that substance misuse and SUD should be managed and treated in the same manner as other chronic health conditions that require ongoing monitoring and intervention (such as diabetes and hypertension). One probable reason SUD is undertreated in the United States is the separation between medical and mental health/substance use treatment (Barry & Sindelar, 2007). Given the many negative consequences of substance misuse, increased capacity for prevention, early identification, and treatment access is essential. Primary healthcare settings providing integrated physical and behavioral healthcare are well-suited to provide these services.

The term "Integrated Care" has been broadly interpreted, but in most instances, it specifically refers to the practice of providing behavioral healthcare in a primary healthcare setting. Thus, the phrase "primary care behavioral health" (PCBH) is gaining popularity, as it more accurately describes the service delivery model. Integrated care means: "integrated, on-site teamwork with a unified care plan as a standard approach to care for designated populations. Connotes organizational integration as well, often involving social and other community services" (Peek & The National Integration Academy Council, 2013, p. 44).

This chapter presents an overview of why integrating care offers an important opportunity for screening and intervention for problematic substance use. Contents include the current state of substance misuse screening in primary care settings, evidence for the effectiveness of screening and intervention for improving outcomes, an overview of integrated care as applied to intervening around substance misuse, health risks associated with substance misuse of which integrated care professionals need to be aware, and challenges to implementing integrated physical and behavioral healthcare in both privately and publicly funded healthcare systems.

The importance of early identification and intervention

Individuals engaged in substance misuse are often introduced to treatment systems during late rather than early stages of the problem, often through involvement in the legal system or crisis/emergency medical care. Late engagement is impactful for several reasons (Dennis & Scott, 2007): individuals whose first treatment occurred within 10 years of initiating substance use engaged in an average 15 years of use before achieving one year of abstinence; if treatment commenced 20 or more years after initiating use, an average 35 years of use occurred before one year of abstinence was achieved. Later onset of intervention concurrently increased the burden of co-morbid complications, as well. One critical strategy for increasing early identification and decreasing the negative impact of substance misuse is to promote universal screening of all adults and adolescents, irrespective of whether they present with known risk factors.

Although primary healthcare settings and other healthcare system points of entry (urgent care, emergency department) provide optimal opportunities to increase universal screening for substance misuse and use disorders, screening is currently underutilized in these settings. In one study, although the majority of primary care physicians screened for alcohol misuse, only 38% utilized a tool capable of capturing the full range of alcohol misuse (Tan, Hungerford, & Denny, 2018). Integrated primary care and behavioral healthcare (Integrated Care) settings provide opportunity for improved screening practices and increased assessment and intervention. Intervention in integrated physical and behavioral health settings can lead to significant reduction in substance misuse across all demographics (Padwa, Urada, Antonini, Ober, Crevecoer-MacPhail, & Rawson, 2012). Integration of social workers within primary care systems has potential to improve outcomes significantly (Zerden, Lombardi, & Jones, 2018).

Substance misuse and primary healthcare settings

Without formal means of identifying substance misuse or substance use disorders in primary care, management of chronic health conditions may become complicated and individuals may experience negative health consequences of substance use. Not only do patients fail to experience relief from symptoms, without consideration of substance use or relevant information, providers may not be able to identify treatment strategies to effectively manage health conditions.

In the United States, private and public insurance companies encourage individuals to have a primary care provider, and through implementation of the Affordable Care Act, all individuals were required to carry health insurance so that, whenever possible, chronic illnesses can be prevented, slowed, or optimally managed to prevent more expensive or restrictive levels of care, such as inpatient hospitalization. SUD responds better to treatment the earlier that diagnosis and intervention is accomplished (Dennis & Scott, 2007). Of course, prevention is always a goal. In one study (John, Zhu, Mannelli, Schwartz, & Subramaniam, 2018), 75% of patients in primary care settings reported substance use during the previous 12 months and 1/3 experienced at least one SUD (alcohol, tobacco, or other drug); approximately 48% of individuals reporting some substance use met criteria for a SUD (applying Diagnostic and Statistics Manual version 5, criteria). Specifically, approximately 25% of patients met criteria for nicotine use disorder, 13.8% for alcohol use disorder, and 3.3% for opioid use disorder (primarily heroin, but 2.4% met criteria through prescription opioids). These high rates suggest that primary care providers frequently see patients engaging in substance misuse or experiencing SUD, diagnosed or not. Thus, primary care appointments provide valuable opportunities for prevention, screening, early identification, and intervention around substance misuse and SUD.

Health complications associated with substance misuse

The importance of addressing substance use in primary care extends beyond focusing on intervention with patients engaging in substance misuse or experiencing a diagnosable SUD. Studies have determined that substance misuse, in addition to its acute negative effects, contributes to the risk of developing or complicating other illnesses, as well as the substances interacting negatively with medications used to treat medical conditions. For example, alcohol use at any level can impact the metabolism of various medications, making either more or less of the drug available with concomitant effects, and chronic alcohol misuse can result in certain medications being processed in the body as toxic rather than curative substances (National Institute on Alcohol Abuse and Alcoholism, 2014). Opioids interact harmfully with medications treating HIV and seizure disorder (McCance-Katz, Sullivan, & Nallani, 2010). Even with prescribed, monitored opioid use, nearly 6% of individuals with chronic pain in one study had a potential for major drug interaction between their opioid pain prescription and another medication (Pergolizzi, et al., 2014). Components of cannabis may impact the metabolizing of various medications, as well, including the anti-coagulant warfarin (Yamaori et al., 2012). Thus, when medical providers suspect noncompliance with prescription medication protocols, an alternative explanation to explore is the possibility of drug interactions with alcohol or other psychoactive substances. Additionally, substance misuser may also impact medication adherence (Vaughn & Williams, n.d.).

Individuals experiencing substance use disorders often experience physical health problems that negatively affect quality of life and life expectancy, including lung disease (including pneumonia), cardiovascular disease, liver disease, hepatitis, HIV/AIDS, and cancer (Vaughn & Williams, n.d.). Infection and infectious disease exposure associated with substance misuse occurs with, but is not limited to, injection use. Specific health risks associated with mode of administration and substance type are discussed in Chapter 2. Because alcohol use and misuse are so frequently encountered in medical (and other) settings, related health concerns that appear in primary care settings are discussed here in greater detail.

Health concerns associated with alcohol

From the multiple possible harms that come from alcohol exposure to the developing human in utero, to the devastating effects of liver and pancreatic diseases and a number of specific cancers, the misuse of alcohol is an important contributor to the global burden of disease, representing the seventh leading cause of mortality and Disability Adjusted Life Years (DALYs) in 2016 (GBD 2016 Alcohol Collaborators, 2018; see Chapter 3). Specific concerns which may arise in primary care settings include:

- fetal alcohol exposure (see Chapters 3, 11, 12, and 26);
- hypertension, such that more than two drinks per day increases hypertension in men and women, and no evidence persists for a hypertension protective effect of light drinking for men or women (Roerecke et al., 2018), and alcohol-induced hypertension appears reversible with abstinence (Roerecke et al., 2017);
- cardiac arrhythmias (atrial);
- ischemic heart disease (IHD) occurs in a J-shaped relationship with alcohol use by men and women—risk of IHD decreased with low-risk drinking levels compared to both never or heavy alcohol use, and a detrimental IHD risk was enhanced at heavier drinking levels—the relative benefit was slightly more pronounced and speed of the detrimental upturn were more pronounced for women (Roerecke & Rehm, 2014);
- cardiomyopathy is associated with alcohol consumption beyond moderate levels—moderation being one to two standard drinks for men, one for women (Maisch, 2016);
- ischemic and hemorrhagic stroke occurs at a higher-than-normal incidence among individuals who consume more than four drinks per day (O'Keefe, DiNicolantorio, O'Keefe, & Lavie, 2018);
- gastrointestinal problems (heartburn/reflux, esophagitis, esophageal cancer, chronic diarrhea) and malabsorption of nutrients associated with heavy chronic drinking (Bode & Bode, 1997);
- acute or chronic pancreatitis;
- liver disease is strongly linked to heavy drinking, but it is important for social workers and other health professionals to recognize that many other causes of liver disease exist, as well—not all liver disease is caused by heavy drinking, just as not all heavy drinkers will develop liver disease; hematologic disorders may arise when liver functions are impaired, as well;
- cancers may be caused by alcohol misuse, particularly esophageal and gastric cancers (Choi et al., 2017), liver cancer (occurring in 15–20% of individuals with alcohol-induced cirrhosis), pancreatic cancer, head and neck cancers, colorectal cancer, breast cancer—and cancer risk is potentiated when nicotine is involved, as well (Schulte & Hser, 2014);
- sexual dysfunction is a not uncommon experience associated with alcohol consumption by men and women, despite the potential for enhanced sexual activity explained through disinhibition and expectancies (see Chapter 6)—chronic, heavy alcohol use can lead to male impotence, testicular atrophy, and decreased fertility, and to decreased libido, decreased vaginal lubrication, menstrual cycle abnormalities, early menopause, lower fertility, and spontaneous abortion among women; alcohol use by pre-adolescents may delay sexual maturation (Dees, Hiney, & Srivastava, 1990);
- eating disorders and alcohol problems frequently co-occur with estimates varying widely depending on the type of eating disorder and sub-population characteristics (Grilo, Sinha, & O'Malley, 2002);
- dementia, Wernicke-Korsakoff's psychosis, cognitive deficits, and cerebellar degeneration represent organic brain diseases recognized as clinical problems associated with chronic heavy drinking;

- migraine and other headaches are sometimes triggered by alcohol consumption (Panconesi, 2016);
- sleep disorders potentially contribute to alcohol use disorders (self-medicating insomnia) and alcohol misuse, as well as alcohol withdrawal following AUD, contribute to disordered sleep (Arnedt, Conroy, & Brower, 2007);
- alcohol-induced peripheral neuropathy, closely resembling diabetic neuropathy, occurs in some individuals experiencing AUD and may resolve with abstinence accompanied by adequate nutrition; and,
- infections, including HIV and tuberculosis, may be associated with alcohol (and other substance) misuse, in part because of weakened immune system and slowed ability to ward off infection, and in part because alcohol misuse contributes to risk-taking behavior (e.g. unsafe sex practices) that can lead to infectious disease exposure.

Pain management in primary care settings

The prevalence of chronic pain among primary care patients is another reason to address substance misuse in primary care. For example, joint, osteoarthritis, and back pain represent 57.5% of chief complaints presenting to primary care providers, which makes them the most prevalent presenting problem (St. Sauver et al., 2013). According to SAMHSA (2011), 32% of individuals who present with chronic pain may experience SUD and 19% of persons aged 12 years or older report that their illegal drug use started with opioid pain relievers. Further, 29–60% of individuals who experience opioid use disorder report also having chronic pain. Individuals may self-medicate pain with alcohol and marijuana-based products as well (Alford et al., 2016; Campbell et al., 2018).

Mental health concerns

Mental health concerns, including depression, anxiety, and bipolar disorder, are among the top 10 most prevalent reasons adults choose to see their primary care providers (St. Sauver et al., 2013). Between 2012 and 2014, primary care providers comprised almost 1/3 of the average of 30 million office visits for mental health issues (Cherry, Albert, & McCaig, 2018). Data suggest that up to half of individuals experiencing a serious mental illness will develop a SUD at some time during their lives, and half of all persons experiencing SUD develop a mental illness (NIDA, 2018).

In summary

There exists substantial need for screening, identification, and intervention for substance misuse and use disorder in primary care settings. Individuals often present to their primary care providers with a diagnosable SUD, conditions or medications impacted by substance misuse, and conditions that put them at higher risk for developing SUDs. Therefore, the primary care provider visit is an important point of access for trained screening and education about substance misuse.

Trends in alcohol and other drug screening in primary care settings

Although data suggest that the primary care setting has tremendous potential for positive impacts on patients' substance misuse, surveys and studies indicate this opportunity is often missed. By one study estimate, 88% of primary care providers ask patients about alcohol use, suggesting that there is general awareness of the issue (Fleming, 2004). However, of the 88% of primary care providers who ask, only about 13% use a standardized screening tool. Additionally, 50% of patients reported that even when their provider became aware of substance use issues, the provider took no action to address the problem. Further, another study reported that 94% of primary care physicians (excluding pediatricians) failed to diagnose SUD when presented with early symptoms of alcohol use disorder (mild) and 41% of pediatricians failed to recognize a possible SUD when presented with a classic description of an adolescent using illicit substances (Friedmann, McCullough, Chin, & Saitz, 2000). Similarly, in Sweden, primary care providers were less likely to discuss alcohol use than lifestyle changes (e.g. diet and exercise) with patients, and providers often failed to detect alcohol use disorders until lab work revealed abnormal liver function which reflects relatively late problem identification (Probst et al., 2015).

Friedmann et al. (2000) identified the following reasons that screening and intervention are not routine in primary healthcare settings:

- lack of adequate training in medical school, residency, and continuing medical education courses
- skepticism about treatment effectiveness
- discomfort discussing substance use
- time constraints
- perceived patient resistance.

Specifically, 58% of physicians said they did not discuss substance misuse with their patients because they believe their patients are not honest about it; nearly 85% of patients admitted to lying to their physicians (Friedmann et al., 2000). More than one-third of physicians cited time constraints, and nearly 11% were concerned that they would not be reimbursed for the time necessary to screen and treat a patient experiencing addiction (CASA, 2000). Worldwide, physicians received half as much substance use disorder education compared to any other chronic condition, and graduating students reported less confidence treating SUD compared to other chronic conditions (Ayu, Schellekens, Iskander, Pinxten, & Jong, 2015). Compared to attitudes toward patients with diseases such as diabetes and depression, "regard" for patients experiencing SUD was lower in all European countries, with lower scores among primary care providers compared to general psychiatry and addiction specialists (Gilchrist et al., 2011). Integrating behavioral health into primary care settings provides opportunity to overcome many of these barriers.

Social workers in integrated care settings

Experts, organizations, and policies have called for the integration of services to address substance misuse and substance use disorder into primary care (Padwa et al., 2012). Models that integrate behavioral health and substance use screening and intervention into primary care settings can address concerns expressed by primary care providers: lack of adequate training in medical school, residency, and continuing medical education courses; skepticism about treatment effectiveness; discomfort with discussing substance misuse; time constraints; and perceived patient resistance. Social workers trained in identification and treatment of substance use disorders are especially well-suited to provide integrated behavioral healthcare services in primary care settings.

Heath, Wise, and Reynolds (2013) proposed a continuum of behavioral health integration adapted by Vogel, Malcore, Illes, and Kirkpatrick (2014). Their continuum identified three types of behavioral health integration—coordinated, co-located, and integrated. At one end of the continuum, coordinated care refers to models similar to traditional models of behavioral healthcare and medical treatment characterized by minimal communication between systems located in separate facilities, and where communication occurs only periodically, driven only by specific patient needs. Co-located care refers to models where behavioral healthcare and primary care are located in the same facility; the two may share health records and other system resources, but care is separate. Patients may be referred from one provider to the other and the systems may collaborate to meet specific patient needs. Integrated care models are at the opposite end of the continuum. In these models, primary care and behavioral health providers are co-located and share practice space, health records, and other resources. Care is fully integrated with a shared concept of team-based care for patients, and both primary care and behavioral health needs can be addressed in one office visit.

The social work profession has a long history of providing services across a wide range of settings while working concurrently with other disciplines/professions, including medicine and allied health. However, this work typically lacks shared information, decision-making, and intervention planning processes. Social work is poised to assume an integral position in the context of healthcare reform and integrated care (Andrews, Darnell, McBride, & Gehlert, 2013). The social work profession also relies on a comprehensive understanding of health, one that includes both physical and mental health as part of the wellness equation. Though it is often unavoidable to separate "mental" and "physical" health for assessment and treatment purposes, social workers make conscious efforts to remember that mental and physical well-being are interconnected and deeply influence each other.

Compared to medical students, social workers may have more education in mental health disorders, though not necessarily in substance use disorders; their education includes familiarity with multiple modes of intervention and treatment (Zerden et al., 2018). Social workers are guided by values and an ethical code that reflect respect for patient autonomy and shared decision making (Zerden et al., 2018). Integrating behavioral healthcare into primary care settings allows licensed social workers with specialized training to screen, educate, and, when necessary, provide intervention and referral for patients along a continuum of substance use—from "nonproblematic" to "at-risk" to "dependent." Additionally, social workers can educate primary care providers, helping them become more comfortable and skilled in addressing substance use with patients. And, critical in terms of making integrated care viable and sustainable, the model is designed to enable licensed social workers to bill directly for screening and intervention services, which further addresses concerns regarding physician time constraints and reimbursement.

Social work practice in an integrated care setting

Social work practice in an integrated care setting is quite different than social work in traditional community-based behavioral health facilities. Vogel et al. (2014) outlined several key implications for behavioral health professionals in integrated care settings:

- Provide culturally tailored practices. Social workers and other behavioral health clinicians must understand the unique needs of the communities they serve.
- Understand the pace and structure of working in integrated care settings. Providing services in a primary care setting is fast-paced and requires a team-based approach.

- Change scheduling and service delivery strategy. Social workers and other behavioral health clinicians must be immediately available when a provider identifies a need and also must have time to schedule follow-up appointments with patients who need additional intervention. The traditional "50-minute hour" model of behavioral health counseling is not a good fit in integrated care.

Central to fully integrated care models is the concept of a "same-day" access to behavioral healthcare (Vogel et al., 2014). In practice, this approach looks very different than the traditional community behavioral health approach. Once screening has identified a potential problem, there is immediate access to a behavioral health provider in the same physical space. The primary care provider can introduce the behavioral health provider to the patient—a practice known to increase referral success. In many cases, patients have history with their providers in integrated care settings and social workers or other behavioral health practitioners can build on these established relationships. Following screening and assessment, intervention recommendations are presented where appropriate. In integrated care settings, social workers may conduct assessments in patient exam rooms during the same appointment in which the screening occurred; if this is not possible, the social worker can schedule an assessment appointment as soon as possible. At the conclusion of the patient visit, the primary care provider and the social worker collaborate in treatment planning and follow-up recommendations. Treatment options can include continued care from the primary care provider and/or appropriately trained social worker, or possibly referral to specialist. Both the primary care provider and the social worker document their contacts in the health record.

Necessary social worker competencies

In their Integrated and Culturally Relevant Care Curriculum, Davis et al. (2015) identified multiple required areas of social work competence in providing integrated care. These include knowledge and understanding of each of the following:

- integrated care models and structures;
- basic healthcare information and medical terminology;
- working with diverse populations;
- healthcare documentation standards and practices;
- screening, assessment and diagnosis tools and approaches (substance use and common mental health concerns);
- care coordination and intervention planning;
- evidence-based behavioral health interventions; and,
- motivational interviewing, trauma-informed care, and health education.

Levels of care continuum

The American Society for Addiction Medicine (ASAM) outlined five levels of care to guide treatment of high-risk substance use and SUD, with sub-levels in between (https://www.asam.org/resources/the-asam-criteria/about). The zero (0) point is no intervention necessary and the half-point (0.5) is early intervention. More intrusive/intensive care is reflected in outpatient services (1), intensive outpatient (2.1) or partial hospitalization (2.5), residential or inpatient care (3), and medically managed intensive inpatient care (4). While all five levels of care are necessary to address the full spectrum of substance use, substance misuse, and SUD, levels of care 0 through 1 are particularly well-suited to be provided within integrated care settings.

Early identification in integrated care settings

The goal of ASAM Level.05 Early Intervention services is educating about the risks of substance misuse and avoiding risky substance use behaviors (Medicaid Innovation Accelerator Program from Medicaid.gov, 2017). Services provided at this level of care include individual counseling, group counseling, motivation interventions, and screening, brief intervention, and referral to treatment (SBIRT). Social workers in integrated care settings must be skilled in providing these early intervention services.

SBIRT is a model for addressing alcohol use, particularly at-risk alcohol use, in a variety of settings and with a variety of populations (see Chapter 20). The choice of screening tool, how brief intervention is conducted, and treatment referral options vary depending on the setting, patient circumstances, and individual providers' decisions. SBIRT in primary care settings is about preventing alcohol misuse, alcohol use disorder, and negative consequences of alcohol misuse, as well as education about the risks of substance use. Primary care clinics are excellent places to identify patients who may lack education regarding safe levels of alcohol use, or to identify individuals experiencing a SUD. SBIRT in integrated care settings can result in early identification of at-risk substance use or SUD, thus allowing for earlier intervention. Also, time constraints, whether real or perceived, are one reason for under-utilization of substance use screening in primary care settings; SBIRT may be less time-intensive than other screening protocols and more directive in providing helpful feedback of screening results.

Although the SBIRT protocol addresses alcohol and tobacco problems, the protocol is not supported by evidence for other drugs. Screening for other substance misuse can be completed in integrated care settings, but evidence-supported tools and procedures need to be employed. Brief screening is not intended to diagnose SUD, only to help identify at-risk behaviors and areas for further assessment. Multiple validated brief screening tools exist that may be utilized in primary care settings (see Table 27.1).

Table 27.1 Examples of validated brief screening tools

Screen	Brief Description
NIDA Quick Screen (NIDA, 2012)	The NIDA quick screen contains four questions about the frequency of use of alcohol, tobacco, prescription drugs used other than as prescribed, and illicit or illegal drugs in the past 12 months
AUDIT (Babor, Higgins-Biddle, Saunders, & Montiero, 2001)	The AUDIT contains ten questions to screen for high-risk alcohol use. The AUDIT was developed by the World Health Organization and is available in many languages
AUDIT-C (Bradley et al., 2003)	The AUDIT-C is a three-item screen derived from the AUDIT
DAST-10 (Skinner, 1982)	The DAST-10 contains ten questions to screen for problem use of drugs other than alcohol within the previous 12 months. The DAST-10 was derived from the 28-item DAST. The DAST-10 is designed to be completed in eight minutes or less
CAGE-AID (Brown & Rounds, 1995)	The CAGE-AID contains five questions to screen concurrently for at-risk alcohol and drug use

Substance use assessment in primary care settings

Social workers in integrated care settings access patient health records. Access to this information can decrease time and irritation spent redundantly gathering information from the patient. Access can also increase assessment accuracy relative to biomedical conditions and complications, patient support systems, challenges to service access, living environments, and other emotional, behavioral, and cognitive conditions the patient may experience. Robust access to patient information allows assessment to be completed efficiently and comprehensively.

Trained social workers in integrated care settings conduct multi-dimensional substance use assessments that address all six dimensions outlined in the ASAM Multi-Dimensional Assessment (Mee-Lee, 2013). The goal is a complete biopsychosocial assessment that informs treatment planning and level of care decisions. The six dimensions involve exploring:

- past and current history of substance use, intoxication, and withdrawal;
- physical health history and current conditions;
- emotional, behavioral, and mental health conditions;
- readiness to change problematic substance-involved behaviors;
- relapse experiences, continued substance use, and problems related to substance use; and
- environment and context hazards and support for recovery.

Several SUD assessment tools address many or all six ASAM recommended domains. These include the Global Appraisal of Individual Needs (GAIN) (Chestnut Health System, 2002–2016), the Addiction Severity Index (ASI) (McLellan, Carise, & Coyne, 1998), and the Dual Diagnosis Capability in Addiction Treatment (DDCAT) Index (McGovern, Matzkin, & Giard, 2007). For example, across Sweden, the ASI is routinely used at intake to National Board of Health and Welfare programs (Padyab et al., 2018). Social workers practicing in integrated care settings need to be skilled at conducting comprehensive substance use assessments.

Outpatient substance use services in primary care settings

Trained social workers can provide many outpatient behavioral health services in integrated care settings: all services outlined in Level 1 of the ASAM Levels of Care Continuum (Mee-Lee, 2013) are appropriate to deliver in integrated care settings. Level 1 Outpatient Services are intended for patients experiencing less severe SUD, those early in the stages of change process, or those who may be stepping down from more intensive services (Medicaid. gov, 2017). In integrated care settings, social workers trained, licensed, and certified to deliver substance abuse treatment can provide outpatient services such as individual counseling, group counseling, motivational enhancement, family therapy, psychotherapy, or other relevant interventions. Medication-assisted treatment (MAT) for SUD, prescribed by the primary care provider, can be supported by social workers; there exists great need for behavioral health support when MAT is prescribed (see Chapters 18 and 19). In 2018, 48% of community health centers provided MAT (Zur, Tolbert, Sharac, & Markus, 2018). Although the very nature of the term "Medication-Assisted Treatment" indicates the use of medication in addition to psychosocial and other treatment methods, in practice, medication is often prescribed without these behavioral health components. Evidence supports MAT for reducing relapse and other negative outcomes related to substance misuse, and supports the practice of combining medication with psychosocial interventions (Barry et al., 2019; Minozzi et al., 2011; Pashaei et al., 2013). Trained social workers in integrated care settings can assist with accurate assessment and diagnosis to warrant MAT prescriptions, and provide the appropriate psychosocial interventions such as relapse prevention, contingency management, and cognitive behavioral therapy.

Withdrawal management in primary care

Ambulatory withdrawal, both Level 1 and Level 2 on the ASAM Withdrawal Management Levels of Care, may be conducted in primary care settings (Medicaid.gov, 2017; Mee-Lee, 2013). Social workers in integrated care settings who have been trained in withdrawal management can support Level 1 Ambulatory Withdrawal Management care without Extended On-site Monitoring services.

During this process, social workers can:

- meet with the patient for regularly scheduled sessions to assess withdrawal symptoms;
- serve as a conduit between patient and physician to assure medical care is provided when needed;
- conduct SUD assessments;
- provide education about withdrawal processes and symptoms;
- provide clinical support during the process;
- refer for more intensive services if necessary; and,
- plan for patient discharge.

In addition, social workers can meet daily with patients and coordinate outpatient services either in the current setting or with other providers.

Wrap-around services in primary care settings

Patients often experience barriers to accessing SUD intervention (Office of the Surgeon General, 2016). There exists an important case management role for social workers in addressing these barriers. Social workers in integrated care settings help patients problem-solve and overcome barriers to recovery. Social workers may assist clients with arranging transportation, coordinating appointments, managing the impact on employment, arranging childcare, maintaining suitable housing, attending to legal and financial problems, and securing coverage for health and substance-related care. Without addressing situational issues, services to reduce substance misuse or treat SUD are likely to be ineffective. A significant challenge to providing wrap-around and case management services is unavailability of needed services, including services where need exceeds capacity. Resource insufficiency is a tremendous barrier to implementation and maintenance of integrated care.

Challenges to integrating substance misuse services in primary care settings

Although integrated care approaches provide a natural fit for addressing substance misuse and substance use disorder in primary care settings, several implementation challenges exist. The greatest challenges are lack of healthcare and coverage for behavioral health services; coverage for behavioral health services varies by region and provider. Additional barriers include stigma, resources, commitment.

Stigma

Stigma about substance use problems exists systemically and culturally, and among patients and providers, as well. Labeling and shame may prevent patients from accessing treatment (Rosenbaum, Turton, & Williams, 2015). In one European study, among patients not re-ceiving treatment for an alcohol use disorder, 28% identified stigma or shame as the reason compared to 22.8% identifying barriers to treatment itself (Probst et al., 2015). One benefit of integrated care is that patients receive treatment for behavioral health issues within the same system where they receive less stigmatized medical care, reducing the experience of being labeled or judged by others (Ernst, Miller, & Rollnick, 2007). Stigma may also impede acceptance of substance abuse treatment or treatment referral. Additionally, stigma held by medical providers regarding substance misuse and SUD can impede motivation to conduct screening: they may believe that individuals engaging in substance use cannot recover, so "why bother?" (O'Donnell, Wallace, & Kaner, 2014; Rosenbaum et al., 2015). For SUD treatment to be successful in integrated care settings, stigma must be addressed at an agency level. Social workers have an important role in reducing stigma through education and ad-vocacy within the organization.

Cost reimbursement

As with any service, SBIRT and SUD treatment creates cost for providers. In a fee-for-service healthcare system, if a service cannot be reimbursed, it can be difficult, if not impossi-ble, for primary care practices to provide, and cost is frequently cited as a reason for providers' reluctance to provide integrated care (Ernst et al., 2007; O'Donnell et al., 2014; Rosenbaum et al., 2015; World Health Organization, 2008). Insurers may provide some reimbursement for SBIRT and other SUD treatment services; without that, social workers must be paid from practice profits, which can be unsustainable. In the United States, Medicaid has authorized the provision of early intervention, outpatient services, and withdrawal management services as billable (Medicaid.gov, 2017); however, the billing structure for a primary care medical facility differs from that of a specialized treatment facility. Additionally, even if a practice can pay for clinicians or clinicians can bill for services, it can be challenging to find trained cli-nicians certified in providing the spectrum of substance use services in primary care settings (Office of the Surgeon General, 2016).

Infrastructure issues

Space, patient records, and agency process issues also serve as potential barriers to integrated care. Space is a critical resource in busy primary care practices; remaining financially viable may mean seeing many patients every day. While SBIRT or screening can be completed in relatively short time, it can also take as long as the primary care provider visits itself (Ernst et al., 2007; O'Donnell et al., 2014; Rosenbaum et al., 2015). Assessment and outpatient services increase the required time that space is utilized. In primary care settings, the ex-amination room often needs to be quickly available for the next patient, so the practice must have adequate space to preserve patient confidentiality, provide the spectrum of desired services, and still maintain the fast-paced schedule. The practice must have work space for social workers that is easily accessed by providers and other care team members to facilitate collaboration. Having to call, page, or walk to another part of the facility to contact the social worker impacts the likelihood that SBIRT and other SUD services will be provided (Ernst et al., 2007; Rosenbaum et al., 2015).

Patient records and information sharing pose another potential infrastructure barrier. In technology-supported integrated care settings, social workers and medical providers may use the electronic health records (EHR) to document patient services. To effectively document SBIRT, assessment, and other services, the EHR must include fields necessary to document screening, assessment, and intervention. Because the EHR can be viewed by all members of the medical team, it is necessary to consider patient confidentiality relative to clinical contacts. This may require the social worker to keep clinical documentation outside of the EHR in order to maintain compliance with confidentiality and record-sharing policies.

Team member commitment

A lack of commitment to the integrated care model threatens implementation success even if other barriers are addressed. Services become disconnected when consistent communication and commitment to substance use services is lacking. Team members may not be equally convinced of the value of integrated behavioral health, or some may believe they already adequately address substance use issues without involving behavioral health specialists (Ernst et al., 2007; Gilchrist et al., 2011; Probst et al., 2015; Rosenbaum et al., 2015). For successful implementation of integrated care, every person in contact with a patient needs to be aware of the process for identifying those who need services and how to access the social worker to provide those services.

Additional challenges to implementing SUD treatment in integrated care settings were identified in by the Surgeon General (Office of the Surgeon General, 2016). Specifically, SUD treatment systems may be unprepared to coordinate with primary care settings. For example, social workers in a primary care setting who identify that Level 2 or greater services are needed refer individuals for services from a community provider. Insurance and billing restrictions related to reimbursement for SUD assessments may require the community provider to rely on the assessment previously completed at the primary care office; relying on another professional's assessment requires a level of trust and collaborative relationship that may not naturally exist across systems of care and between treatment providers.

Conclusions

Although there exist challenges to integrating substance use services into primary care settings, there also exists potential for successful identification, assessment, prevention, and treatment of at-risk substance use and SUD in these settings. Trained social workers in integrated care settings have the potential to effectively support and provide services to address substance misuse and substance use disorders in primary care through screening, assessment, individual counseling, group counseling, motivational interventions, psychotherapy, wrap-around services, withdrawal support, care coordination, and service referral. Because of the Affordable Care Act and Medicaid expansion in the United States, integrated primary care and behavioral health models are gaining traction as an effective service model. Unfortunately, this model only works if individuals seek treatment from a primary care provider and behavioral health represents reimbursed or covered services. Expanding access to screening, identification, and treatment requires exploration of similar models in urgent care centers, emergency departments, and other points of access to the healthcare system.

References

Alford, D. P., German, J. S., Samet, J. H., Cheng, D. M., Lloyd-Travaglini, C. A., & Saitz, R. (2016). Primary care patients with drug use report chronic pain and self-medicate with alcohol and other drugs. *Journal of General Internal Medicine, 31*(5), 486–491. doi:10.1007/s11606-016-3586-5

Andrews, C. M., Darnell, J. S., McBride, T. D., & Gehlert, S. (2013). Social work and implementation of the affordable care act. *Health & Social Work, 2*(1), 67–71. doi:10.1093/hsw/hlt002

Arncdt, J. T., Conroy, D. A., & Brower, K. J. (2007). Treatment options for sleep disturbances during alcohol recovery. *Journal of Addictive Diseases, 26*(4), 41–54. doi:10.1300/J069v26n04_06

Ayu, A. P., Schellekens, A. F., Iskander, S., Pinxten, L., & Jong, C. A. (2015). Effectiveness and organization of addiction medicine training across the globe. *European Addiction Research, 21*(5), 223–239. doi:10.1159/000381671

Babor, T. F., Higgins-Biddle, J. C., Saunders, J. B., & Montiero, M. G. (2001). *The alcohol use disorders identification test guidelines for use in primary care* (second ed.). Vienna, Austria: World Health Organization, General Department of Mental Health and Substance Dependence.

Barry, C. L., & Sindelar, J. L. (2007). Equity in private insurance coverage for substance abuse: A perspective on parity. The many commonalities between substance abuse and mental health disorders call for a consistent regulatory approach. *Health Affairs, 26*(suppl 2), 706–716. doi: 10.1377/hlthaff.26.6.w706

Barry, D. T., Beitel, M., Cutter, C. J., Fiellin, D. A., Kerns, R. D., Moore, B. A., . . . Schottenfeld, R. S. (2019). An evaluation of the feasibility, acceptability, and preliminary efficacy of cognitive-behavioral therapy for opioid use disorder and chronic pain. *Drug and Alcohol Dependence, 194*, 460–467.

Bode, C., & Bode, J. C. (1997). Alcohol's role in gastrointestinal tract disorders. *Alcohol Health and Research World, 21*(1), 76–83.

Bradley, K. A., Bush, K. R., Epler, A. J., Dobie, D. J., Davis, T. M., Sporleder, J. L., . . . Kivlahan, D. R. (2003). Two brief alcohol-screening tests from the alcohol use disorders identification test (AUDIT): Validation in a female veterans affairs patient population. *Archives of Internal Medicine American Medical Association, 163*, 821–829. doi:10.1001/archinte.163.7.821

Brown, R. L., & Rounds, L. A. (1995). Conjoint screening questionnaires for alcohol and other drug abuse: Criterion validity in a primary care practice. *Wisconsin Medical Journal, 94*(3), 135–140.

Campbell, G., Hall, W. D., Peacock, A., Lintzeris, N., Bruno, R., Larance, B., . . . Degenhardt, L. (2018). Effect of cannabis use in people with chronic non-cancer pain prescribed opioids: Findings from a 4-year prospective cohort study. *The Lancet Public Health, 3*(7), E341–E350. doi:10.1016/s2468-2667(18)30110-5

CASA. (2000). *Missed opportunity: National survey of primary care physicians and patients on substance abuse.* New York, NY: The National Center on Addiction and Substance Abuse at Columbia University.

Center on Addiction. (2017). *Is addiction a disease?* Retrieved from https://www.centeronaddiction.org/what-addiction/addiction-disease

Cherry, D., Albert, M., & McCaig, L. F. (2018). *Mental health-related physician office visits by adults aged 18 and over: United States, 2012–2014.* Hyattsville, MD: National Center for Health Statistics.

Chestnut Health System. (2002–2016). *Global appraisal of individual needs—Initial measurement instrument.* Retrieved from http://gaincc.org/instruments/

Choi, Y. J., Lee, D. H., Han, K. D., Kim, H. S., Yoon, H., Shin, C. M., Park, Y. S., & Kim, N. (2017). The relationship between drinking alcohol and esophageal, gastric or colorectal cancer: A nationwide population-based cohort study of South Korea, *PloS One, 12*(10), e0185778. doi 10.1371/journal.pone.0185778

Davis, T. S., Guada, J., Reno, R., Peck, A., Evans, S., Moskow Sigal, L., & Swenson, S. (2015). Integrated and culturally relevant care: A field education model for social work in primary care. *Social Work in Health Care, 54*, 909–938. doi:10.1080/00981389.2015.1062456

Dees, W. L., Hiney, J. K., & Srivastava, V. K. (1990). Alcohol and puberty: Mechanisms of delayed development. *Alcohol Research: Current Reviews, 38*(2), 277–282.

Dennis, M., & Scott, C. K. (2007). Managing addiction as a chronic condition. *Addiction Science & Clinical Practice, 4*(1), 45–55. doi:10.1151/ascp074145

Ernst, D., Miller, W. R., & Rollnick, S. (2007). Treating substance abuse in primary care: A demonstration project. *International Journal of Integrated Care, 7*(4). doi:10.5334/ijic.213

Fleming, M. F. (2004). Screening and brief intervention in primary care settings. *Alcohol Research & Health, 28*(2), 57–62.

Friedmann, P. D., McCullough, D., Chin, M. H., & Saitz, R. (2000). Screening and intervention for alcohol problems. A national survey of primary care physicians and psychiatrists. *Journal of General Internal Medicine, 15*(2), 84–91. doi:10.1046/j.1525-1497.2000.03379.x

GBD 2016 Alcohol Collaborators. (2018). Alcohol use and burden for 195 countries and territories, 1990–2016: A systematic analysis for the global burden of disease study 2016. *Lancet, 392*, 115–1035.

Gilchrist, G., Moskalewicz, J., Slezakova, S., Okruhlica, L., Torrens, M., Vaid, R., & Baldacchino, A. (2011). Staff regard towards working with substance users: A European multi-centre study. *Addiction, 106*(6), 1114–1125. doi:10.1111/j.1360-0443.2011.03407.x

Grilo, C. M., Sinha, R., & O'Malley, S. (2002). *Eating disorders and alcohol use disorders*. NIAAA Publications. Retrieved from https://pubs.niaaa.nih.gov/publications/arh26-2/151-160.htm

Heath, B., Wise, R. P., & Reynolds, K. (2013). *A review and proposed standard framework for levels of integrated healthcare*. Washington, DC: SAMHSA-HRSA Center for Integrated Health Solutions.

Hill, S. C., Miller, G. E., & Sing, M. (2011). Adults with diagnosed and untreated diabetes: Who are they? How can we reach them? *Journal of Health Care for the Poor and Underserved, 22*(4), 1221–1238. doi:10.1353/hpu.2011.0149

John, W. S., Zhu, H., Mannelli, P., Schwartz, R. P., & Subramaniam, G. A. (2018). Prevalence, patterns, and correlates of multiple substance use disorder among primary care patients. *Drug and Alcohol Dependence, 187*, 79–87. doi:10.1016/j.drugalcdep.2018.01.035

Maisch, B. (2016). Alcoholic cardiomyopathy: The result of dosage and individual predisposition. *Herz, 41*(6), 484–493 (English translation). doi:10.1007/s00059-016-4469-6

McCance-Katz, E. F., Sullivan, L. E., & Nallani, S. (2010). Drug interactions of clinical importance among the opioids, methadone and buprenorphine, and other frequently prescribed medications: A review. *The American Journal on Addictions, 19*(1), 4–16. doi:10.1111/j.1521-0391.2009.00005.x

McGovern, M., Matzkin, A., & Giard, J. (2007). Assessing the dual diagnosis capability of addiction treatment services. *Journal of Dual Diagnosis, 3*(2), 111–123. doi:10.1300/J374v03n02_13

McLellan, T., Carise, D., & Coyne, T. H. (1998). *Addiction severity index 5th edition*. Philadelphia, PA: Treatment Research Institute.

Medicaid.gov. (2017, April). *Medicaid innovation accelerator program*. Retrieved from Medicaid.gov/state-resources https://www.medicaid.gov/state-resource-center/innovation-accelerator-program/iap-downloads/reducing-substance-use-disorders/asam-resource-guide.pdf

Mee-Lee, D. (Ed.). (2013). *The ASAM criteria: Treatment criteria for addictive substance-related and co-occurring conditions*. Chevy Chase, MD: American Society of Addiction Medicine.

Minozzi, S., Amato, L., Vecchi, S., Davoli, M., Kirchmayer, U. & Verster, A. (2011). Oral naltrexone maintenance treatment for opioid dependence. *Cochrane Database of Systematic Reviews*, 4. doi:10.1002/14651858.CD001333.pub4.

National Institute on Alcohol Abuse and Alcoholism (NIAAA). (2014). *Harmful interactions: Mixing alcohol with medicines*. Retrieved from https://www.niaaa.nih.gov/publications/brochures-and-fact-sheets/harmful-interactions-mixing-alcohol-with-medicines

National Institute of Drug Abuse (NIDA). (2012). *Resource guide: Screening for drug use in general medical settings*. Retrieved from https://www.drugabuse.gove/publications/resource-guide-screening-drug-use-in-general-medial-settings

National Institute on Drug Abuse (NIDA). (2018). *Drug facts. Comorbidity: Substance use disorders and other mental illnesses*. Retrieved from https://d14rmgtrwzf5a.cloudfront.net/sites/default/files/drugfacts-comorbidity.pdf

O'Donnell, A., Wallace, P., & Kaner, E. (2014). From efficacy to effectiveness and beyond: What next for brief interventions in primary care? *Frontiers in Psychiatry, 5*, 113. doi:10.3389/fpsyt.2014.00113

Office of the Surgeon General. (2016). *Facing addiction in America: The surgeon general's report on alcohol, drugs, and health*. Washington, DC: U.S. Department of Health and Human Services (HHS).

O'Keefe, E. L., DiNicolantorio, J. J., O'Keefe, J. H., & Lavie, C. J. (2018). Alcohol and CV health: Jekyll and Hyde J-curves. *Progress in Cardiovascular Disease, 61*(1), 68–75. doi:10.1016/j.pcad.2018.02.001

Padwa, H., Urada, D., Antonini, V. P., Ober, A., Crevecoer-MacPhail, D. A., & Rawson, R. A. (2012). Integrating substance use disorder services with primary care: The experience in California. *Journal of Psychoactive Drugs, 44*(4), 299–306. doi:10.1080/02791072.2012.718643

Padyab, M., Armelius, B. A., Armelius, K., Nysstrom, S., Blom, B., Gronlund, A. S., & Lundgren, L. (2018). Is clinical assessment of addiction severity of individuals with substance use disorder, using the addiction severity index, a predictor of future inpatient mental health hospitalization? A nine-year registry study. *Journal of Dual Diagnosis, 14*(3), 187–191. doi:10.1080/15504263.2018.1466086

Panconesi, A. (2016). Alcohol-induced headaches: Evidence for a central mechanism? *Journal of Neurosciences in Rural Practice, 7*(2), 269–275. doi:10.4103/0976-3147.178654

Pashaei, T., Shojaeizadeh, D., Rahimi Foroushani, A., Ghazitabatabae, M., Moeeni, M., Rajati, F., & Razzaghi, E. M. (2013). Effectiveness of relapse prevention cognitive-behavioral model in opioid-dependent patients participating in methadone maintenance treatment in Iran. *Iranian Journal of Public Health, 42*(8), 896–902.

Peek, C. J., & The National Integration Academy Council. (2013). *Lexicon for behavioral health and primary care integration: Concepts and definitions developed by expert consensus* (AHRQ Publication No. 13-IP001-EF). Rockville, MD: Agency for Healthcare Research and Quality.

Pergolizzi, J. V., Ma, L., Foster, D. R., Overholser, B. R., Sowinski, K. M., . . . Sommers, K. H. (2014, May). The prevalence of opioid-related major potential drug-drug interactions and their impact on health care costs in chronic pain patients. *Journal of Managed Care Pharmacy, 20*(5), 467–476. doi:10.18553/jmcp.2014.20.5.467

Probst, C., Manthey, J., Martinez, A., & Rehm, J. (2015). Alcohol use disorder severity and reported reasons not to seek treatment: A cross-sectional study in European primary care practices. *Substance Abuse Treatment, Prevention, and Policy, 10*(1). doi:10.1186/s13011-015-0028-z

Roerecke, M., Kaczorowski, J., Tobe, S. W., Gmel, G., Hasan, O. S. M., & Rehm, J. (2017). The effect of a reduction in alcohol consumption on blood pressure: A systematic review and meta-analysis. *Lancet Public Health, 2*(2), e108–e120. doi:10.1016/S2468-2667(17)30003-8

Roerecke, M., & Rehm, J. (2014). Alcohol consumption, drinking patterns, and ischemic heart disease: A narrative review of meta-analyses and systematic review and meta-analysis of the impact of heavy drinking occasions on risk for moderate drinkers. *BMC Medicine, 12*(182). doi:10.1186/s12916-014-0182-6

Roerecke, M., Tobe, S. W., Kaczorowski, J., Bacon, S. L., Vafaei, A., Hasan, O. S. M. . . . Rehm, J. (2018). Sex-specific associations between alcohol consumption and incidence of hypertension: A systematic review and meta-analysis of cohort studies. *Journal of the American Heart Association, 7*(13), e008202. doi:10.1161/JAHA.117.008202

Rosenbaum, M., Turton, J. S., & Williams, A. (2015). Implementing SBIRT in health centers: Examples from the field [Webinar]. Retrieved from https://hospitalsbirt.webs.com/health-centers-sbirt

SAMHSA. (2011). Screening tools. Retrieved from https://www.integration.samhsa.gov/clinical-practice/screening-tools#drugs

SAMHSA. (2018). *Key substance use and mental health indicators in the United States: Results from the 2017 National Survey on Drug Use and Health.* Retrieved from https://www.samhsa.gov/data/report/2017-nsduh-annual-national-report

Schulte, M. T., & Hser, Y. I. (2014). Substance use and associated health conditions throughout the life span. *Public Health Reviews, 35*(2). doi:10.1007/BF03391702

Skinner, H. A. (1982). The drug abuse screening test. *Addictive Behaviors, 7*(4), 363–371. doi:10.1016/0306-4603(82)90005-3

St. Sauver, J. L., Warner, D. O., Yawn, B. P., Jacobson, D. J., McGree, M. E, Pankratz, J. J., . . . Rocca, W. A. (2013). Why patients visit their doctors: Assessing the most prevalent conditions in a defined American population. *Mayo Clinic Proceedings, 88*(1), 56–67. doi:10.1016/j.mayocp.2012.08.020

Tan, C. H., Hungerford, D. W., & Denny, C. H. (2018). Screening for alcohol misuse: Practices among primary care providers. *American Journal of Preventative Medicine, 54*(2), 173–180. doi:10.1016/j.amepre.2017.11.008

Vaughn, B., & Williams, A. (n.d.). *Integrating addiction and primary care services.* Retrieved from https://www.integration.samhsa.gov/about-us/esolutions-newsletter/integrating-substance-abuse-and-primary-care-services#A%20Window%20into%20addiction

Vogel, M. E., Malcore, S. A., Illes, R. C., & Kirkpatrick, H. A. (2014). Integrated primary care: Why you should care and how to get started. *Journal of Mental Health Counseling, 36*(2), 130–144. https://doi.org/10.17744/mehc.36.2.5312041n10767k51

World Health Organization (WHO). (2008). *Mental health gap action programme: Scaling up care for mental, neurological and substance use disorders.* Geneva, Switzerland: World Health Organization.

World Health Organization (WHO). (2018). *Global status report on alcohol and health 2018.* Geneva, Switzerland: World Health Organization.

Yamaori, S., Koeda, K., Kushihara, M., Hada, Y., Yamamoto, I., & Watanabe, K. (2012). Comparison in the in vitro inhibitory effects of major phytocannabinoids and polycyclic aromatic hydrocarbons contained in marijuana smoke on cytochrome P450 2C9 activity. *Drug Metabolism and Pharmacokinetics, 27*(3), 294–300. doi:10.2133/dmpk.DMPK-11-RG-107

Zerden, L. D., Lombardi, B. M., & Jones, A. (2018). Social workers in integrated health care: Improving care throughout the life course. *Social Work in Health Care, 58*(1), 142–149. doi:10.1080/00981389.2019.1553934

Zur, J., Tolbert, J., Sharac, J., & Markus, A. (2018). *The role of community health centers in addressing the opioid epidemic.* Retrieved from https://www.kff.org/medicaid/issue-brief/the-role-of-community-health-centers-in-addressing-the-opioid-epidemic/

28

Drug treatment courts

Margaret Lloyd and Michael Fendrich

Background

Beginning in the mid-1970s, the United States witnessed a decades-long trend in tremendous increases in state and federal prison populations, from 96 per 100,000 in 1970 to over 300 per 100,000 in 1990 (Blumstein & Beck, 1999; Bureau of Justice Statistics, 1986). By 2005, the number of individuals serving time in state prisons alone had burgeoned to over 1.2 million people (Harrison & Beck, 2006). Much of the increase in the prison population can be attributed to the sharp increase in drug arrests, which more than doubled during the 20-year period between 1980 and 2000 (Harrison & Beck, 2003; Lurigio, 2008). In 2005, about 20% of state prison inmates were there for a drug crime (Harrison & Beck, 2006).

Scholars point to several factors contributing to this mass incarceration phenomenon, including changes to policing strategies, drug laws, and sentencing policies coinciding with the spread of "crack" cocaine. The inaugural legislative action spurring the new era of mass incarceration was the "War on Drugs" initiated in 1970 with the Comprehensive Drug Abuse Prevention and Control Act (Pub. L. No. 91–513, 84 Stat. 1236). This law included provisions for treatment and rehabilitation for individuals experiencing substance use disorders, but also strengthened law enforcement authority related to drug regulation, representing a mixed approach to drug policy aimed at minimizing both supply and demand (see Chapter 30). In 1984, the Sentencing Reform Act (Pub. L. No. 98–473, 98 Stat. 1987) contributed to sentencing guidelines and mandatory minimum penalties for drug, weapon, and violent crimes. The Anti-Drug Abuse Act of 1986 (Pub. L. No. 99–570, 100 Stat. 3207 1986) and the Omnibus Anti-Drug Abuse Act of 1988 (Pub. L. 100–690, 102 Stat. 4181) mandated substantially longer prison sentences for "crack" cocaine relative to powder cocaine. While these policies occurred at the federal level, mandatory minimum sentences with increased penalties for drug offenses emerged in every state in subsequent years (Hora, Schma, & Rosenthal, 1999).

By the end of the 1980s, these policy changes resulted in an overburdened court system and growing prison population (Blumstein & Beck, 1999). The profile of the incarcerated population had also changed—many individuals had no history of violence; rather, substance use disorders seemed to be the driving force behind their criminal activity (Franco, 2010). Without treatment, individuals experiencing substance use disorders returned to drug use when released from custody and, ultimately to the system.

Drug court

Recognizing the "revolving door" of substance use, crime, and incarceration, in 1989 the Honorable Herbert Klein of Dade County (Florida) "reasoned that investing a year of comprehensive treatment coupled with close surveillance in these typical [drug] cases would pay off in the long run with reduced costs to the police, courts, and jail as more drug users kicked the habit" (Finn & Newlyn, 1993, p. 268). Judge Klein initiated a new court program specifically for drug offenses that differed considerably from traditional processing. Participants in this "drug court" program were offered the opportunity to avoid incarceration by completing substance use treatment. Unlike traditional courts, the drug court utilized a non-adversarial legal framework, a pragmatic problem-solving approach, and an informal milieu (Hora, 2002). For example, instead of the district attorney working against the defendant's counsel, all parties convened before hearings to discuss the case and jointly determine a best course of action. One of the earliest studies of Miami's program reported lower incarceration rates for drug court defendants, less frequent arrests, and longer times to re-arrest compared to defendants served in traditional criminal courts (Goldkamp & Weiland, 1993).

In the United States, 3,100 drug courts were operating in 2018 (National Institute of Justice, Bureau of Justice Assistance, & Office of Juvenile Justice and Delinquency Prevention [OJJDP], 2018). It is estimated that drug courts exist in over half of all U.S. counties, serving approximately 125,000 individuals per year (Marlowe, Hardin, & Fox, 2016). This estimate may also include a growing number of specialty courts such as Veteran's Courts, DWI Courts, Dual Diagnosis Courts, and Mental Health Courts. We note that the nomenclature for the range of specialty courts is evolving. For example, some jurisdictions (and states) have begun referring to "Recovery Courts" as a term encompassing the range of court-based treatment options (North Carolina Judicial Branch, n.d.); other states use the term "Recovery Courts" to refer to what have formerly been called drug courts (Tennessee Department of Mental Health & Substance Abuse Services, n.d.). Specialty courts other than three main types of drug courts (adult, juvenile, and family) are beyond the scope of this chapter. Further, we will continue to refer to these three options as "drug courts" in this chapter as the word "recovery" in the drug treatment field typically focuses on a set of guiding principles and dimensions that do not directly relate to court-based interventions.

Global reach

The U.S. "War on Drugs" coincided with a global increase in interest in drug control. The United Nations adopted three drug control conventions between 1960 and 1990, with financial assistance to lower-income countries for drug control first made available in 1971 (United Nations Office on Drugs and Crime, 2008). With each effort at control in one country or market, "ballooning" in other countries occurred: harsher drug enforcement in one market shifted drug production and trafficking to another. For example, following Turkey's decision to prohibit opium cultivation in 1972, Mexico and Iran became primary producers; after the Islamic Revolution made opium illegal in Iran, production shifted to Afghanistan (United Nations Office on Drugs and Crime, 2008). Despite international efforts to reduce supply, drug manufacturing increased during every decade from 1960 to 2000 (United Nations Office on Drugs and Crime, 2008). Stricter drug control within U.S. borders led to ballooning in nearby Central and South American countries (Puyana et al., 2017) and, ultimately, an increase in global production of certain drugs, including cocaine (United Nations Office on Drugs and Crime, 2008). Increased drug availability in these localities led to expanded control efforts, resulting in rising rates of conviction and incarceration for drug offenses. For example, the proportion of the Argentinian prison population incarcerated for drug offenses increased from 9% in 2005 to nearly 20% in 2009 and one-third of prisoners in Bolivia were incarcerated for drug offenses (Guzman, 2012).

Given the deleterious effects of illicit drugs throughout the world and recognizing that supply-based criminalization results in substantial consequences, including ballooning, incarceration, and drug trafficking-/cartel-related violence (United Nations Office on Drugs and Crime, 2008; Puyana et al., 2017), countries outside the United States also explored instituting drug courts. Drug courts currently exist in at least 16 countries, including Australia, Belgium, Bermuda, Brazil, Canada, Chile, Caymen Islands, Ireland, Jamaica, Mexico, New Zealand, Norway, Scotland, Surinam, the United Kingdom, and the United States (Guzman, 2012). No reliable estimate of the number of drug courts outside the United States exists.

Juvenile and family drug court

Due to their social work relevance, this chapter discusses both juvenile and family drug courts, in addition to the original adult criminal model. The first juvenile drug court was started in 1993 in Key West, Florida, as juvenile court officers witnessed sharp increases in youth and adolescent drug involvement and repeat criminal activity. The juvenile court system originated as a means of facilitating therapeutic processes to rehabilitate criminally involved youth (Bureau of Justice Assistance, 2003). Therefore, juvenile drug courts were implemented within the existing framework of juvenile justice and functioned as enhancements to traditional processes, rather than a therapeutic alternative. According to the National Institute of Justice (2018), there are 409 juvenile drug courts currently operating in the United States.

The year after the first juvenile drug court opened, two family drug courts appeared when judges in Washoe County (Nevada) and Pensacola (Florida) applied the model to their dependency dockets to address cases involving both criminal drug charges and child abuse/neglect due to parents' substance use disorder (McGee, 1997; National Center on Addiction and Substance Abuse at Columbia University [CASA], 1999). Subsequent family drug courts did not require concurrent criminal charges; only that a parent's substance use disorder contributed to child welfare system involvement.

While the criminal drug court sought to reduce incarceration and re-arrest, family drug courts aimed to increase the likelihood that families would achieve reunification in a timely manner, with the parents remaining sober and the children being safe (Center for Substance Abuse Treatment, 2004; Choi, 2012). The first published case studies on family drug courts reported positive findings including high levels of parent compliance, successful exit, and few reports of re-entry into the child welfare system (CASA, 1999). The family drug court model has proliferated in the United States and internationally. Close to 500 family drug courts currently operate in the United States and U.S. territories (Lemus & Richter, 2018). Although no international accounting of family drug courts exists, internet searches revealed their presence in Canada, Australia, Ireland, and the United Kingdom.

Attributes of the drug court model

As the number of drug court programs, and judges interested in starting drug court programs, increased, core features of the model needed to be identified and disseminated. In 1997, national drug court stakeholders convened and developed *The10 Key*

Table 28.1 Ten key components of drug courts (Bureau of Justice Assistance, 1997)

1	Integrate alcohol and other drug treatment services with case processing
2	Use a non-adversarial approach while protecting participants' due process rights
3	Identify eligible participants early for quick placement in the drug court program
4	Provide access to a continuum of alcohol, drug, and other related treatment and rehabilitation services
5	Monitor abstinence with frequent alcohol and other drug testing
6	Govern drug court responses to participant compliance using a coordinated strategy
7	Ensure ongoing judicial interaction with each drug court participant
8	Monitor and evaluate the achievement of program goals and effectiveness
9	Promote effective drug court planning, implementation, and operation through continuing interdisciplinary education
10	To generate local support and enhance drug court program effectiveness, forge partnerships among drug courts, public agencies, and community-based organizations

Components of Drug Courts to crystallize the central features of these courts (Bureau of Justice Assistance, 1997) (see Table 28.1).

Adult drug courts are optimally targeted to "high risk/high need" offenders, where "risk" refers to probability of failure under typical supervision and "need" refers to "functional impairments" or clinical diagnoses, such as substance dependence (Marlowe, 2012). Accordingly, drug courts typically screen eligible participants by assessing substance involvement/dependence and criminal justice history (Fendrich & LeBel, 2019). Once screened into the program, a participant typically progresses through a staged or phased program of treatment and supervision. Positive sanctions and progression through stages and negative sanctions (including longer time within phases) are administered according to successes or failures in meeting program expectations (Marlowe, 2012).

The total time in drug court—across all stages—typically lasts from 9 to 18 months. There typically exist four or more treatment and assessment phases; participants failing any stage are terminated from the program and required to serve their original sentences or receive other criminal justice sanctions. Judged by program completion alone, just over half of all enrolled participants experience successful outcomes (Marlowe et al., 2016; Strong, Rantala, & Kyckelhahn, 2016). Juvenile drug treatment courts report similar rates of completion (Stein, Homan, & DeBerard, 2015). Courts adhering to all 10 Key Components produced significantly and substantially better outcomes compared to those that did not (Carey, Mackin, & Finigan, 2012).

Across court types, variability exists regarding nearly every aspect of drug court process including core team composition, participation eligibility criteria, program phase structure, types of rewards and sanctions, the number of community partnerships, and requirements for graduation (Carey et al., 2012). In addition to the court processes, the timing and length of program participation, and the consequence for failing to successfully complete the program also differ (see Table 28.2). Criminal drug courts frequently require defendants to plead guilty to charges and, if they fail to complete the program within 12–24 months, to serve the length of their original sentence. Family drug court programs, however, begin after a child is placed into foster care and, due to federal child welfare policy, require successful completion within 12–15 months. Parents failing to complete the program successfully are at risk of permanent loss of custody and termination of parental rights. Juvenile drug courts, however, have no time limit unless stipulated by law.

Table 28.2 Drug court similarities and differences

	Adhere to 10 Key Components[a]	Best Practices[a]	Target Population[a]	Client[a]	Timeline[a]	What is Leveraged[a]	Benchmarks of Success[a]	Team Members[a]	Approx. Number of Courts[b]
Criminal	Yes	10 Standards	Charged in criminal court; "high risk/high need"	Defendant	Pre- or post-plea; program lasts 12–24 months	Incarceration	Graduation & no re-arrest or criminal recidivism	Core Drug Court Team plus Law Enforcement	1,558
Family	Yes	10 Recommendations	Open child welfare case; parental substance use disorder	Child, parent, & family	Typically post-removal; program lasts 12 months	Termination of parental rights	Graduation & Reunification/ permanency	Core Drug Court Team plus Child Welfare	312
Juvenile	Yes	7 Objectives	Youth ages 14–18 with substance use disorder and moderate to high risk of re-offense	Youth & family (broadly defined)	As long as legally permitted; Termination is a last resort	Incarceration is last resort	Graduation & no recidivism	Core Drug Court Team plus Juvenile Officers and School Representative	409

a See National Association of Drug Court Professionals (2013, 2015). Adult Drug Court Best Practice Standards Vol. I & II; Young, Breitenbucher, and Pfeifer (2013) Guidance to States: Recommendations for Developing Family Drug Court Guidelines; Office of Juvenile Justice and Delinquency Prevention (2016). Juvenile Drug Court Guidelines; Gurnell, Holmberg, and Yeres (2014). Starting a Juvenile Drug Court: A Planning Guide.
b National Institute of Justice (2018). *Drug Courts*. Retrieved from https://www.nij.gov/topics/courts/drug-courts/pages/welcome.aspx

Drug courts differ not only in their jurisdictional setting (i.e. criminal, juvenile, or family), but also in their day-to-day practices. For example, the Key Components stipulate that drug courts use a non-adversarial approach, but do not dictate which professionals to include on the court's core team. The composition of court teams reflects the purpose and domain of the specific court program (Table 28.2); however, each court may include or exclude various professionals. These and other differences between courts means that natural experiments have identified court characteristics leading to the most desirable outcomes. As a result, best practice standards or guidelines exist for each of the three drug court types (National Association of Drug Court Professionals, 2013, 2015; OJJDP, 2016; Young, Breitenbucher, & Pfeifer, 2013).

Empirical outcomes

The body of research about drug courts has grown considerably over the last two decades and includes rigorous randomized controlled trials and meta-analyses. However, the field has yet to achieve consensus on the model's efficacy for several reasons, including methodological limitations of existing research and varied definitions of "success." The National Institute of Justice (NIJ) published or sponsored 44 research reports since its 1993 evaluation of the first drug court, as well as an adult drug court logic model delineating the relationship between the key components and hypothesized outcomes. Short-term outcomes include that drug court clients will stay in treatment longer than adults served in a traditional setting. Long-term outcomes include all indicators of drug court success, including reductions in recidivism, fewer relapses, successful case closure, and improvements in education, housing, and health.

The 2003–2009 Multi-Site Adult Drug Court Evaluation (MADCE) was a five-year study involving participants from 23 drug courts and 6 non-drug court comparison programs (Rossman, Roman, Zweig, Rempel, & Lindquist, 2011). This study assessed participants on all long-term outcomes described in the NIJ logic model. At 18-month follow-up, MADCE drug court participants reported significantly less substance use and criminal activity than did comparison participants. Study limitations included its reliance on self-report measures, lack of random selection and assignment, and limited follow-up window. Study strengths included its varied sample, representing probationers from rural, suburban, and urban settings in eight states, rigorous comparison group, and array of measures (Rossman et al., 2011).

A relatively short follow-up window is a limitation of most drug court studies. Additionally, most studies report non-generalizable results only about individual programs. Finally, the literature is mixed regarding key outcomes. For example, several meta-analyses suggest that drug court participation is associated with reductions in criminal- and drug-related recidivism, but drug court participants may spend as much time incarcerated as comparison cases. For example, Mitchell, Wilson, Eggers, and MacKenzie (2012) conducted a meta-analysis of 92 independent adult drug court evaluations and reported an average of a 12% reduction in general recidivism for adult drug court participants versus non-participants. However, Sevigny, Fuleihan, and Ferdik (2013) conducted a meta-analysis of 19 studies that calculated and reported effect sizes related to incarceration outcomes and concluded that, while drug court participation was associated with a decreased likelihood of incarceration for the precipitating offense, participants spent similar average lengths of time incarcerated as non-participants. Sevigny et al. (2013) observed that certain drug court practices, such as using a post-plea model and more frequent status hearings in early phases, are associated with less jail use.

To date, one of the most rigorous randomized controlled trials is the three-year investigation of the Baltimore City Drug Treatment Court (BCDTC), a two-track (circuit/felony or district/misdemeanor) post-conviction court with clients entering as a condition of probation (Gottfredson, Najaka, & Kearley, 2003; Gottfredson, Najaka, Kearley, & Rocha, 2006). The study measured several outcomes including days incarcerated and in-program and post-program recidivism. Results revealed that drug court participants had significantly fewer re-arrests and significantly fewer subsequent charges versus control participants up to two years post-randomization. Across the sample, rate of any re-arrest was high, with three-fourths of clients re-arrested regardless of treatment assignment. Additionally, both groups spent approximately the same number of days incarcerated. As reflected in the meta-analyses, differences in program implementation were predictive of variability in outcomes.

While short-term outcomes are mixed, a recent dissertation extended the evaluation of the BCDTC with a long-term 15-year follow-up (Kearley, 2017). Results revealed that drug court participation was associated with significantly fewer arrests, charges, and convictions over 15 years. Circuit/felony court involvement was associated with better long-term outcomes than district/misdemeanor court involvement. This may reflect the fact that the drug court target population is considered "high risk/high need" with misdemeanor clients not meeting the ideal level of criminogenic risk.

Juvenile drug court outcomes

Evaluation studies of juvenile drug court outcomes yield mixed results. Inconsistencies between three recent meta-analyses (Mitchell et al., 2012; Stein et al., 2015; Tanner-Smith, Lipsey, & Wilson, 2016) cast doubt on the efficacy of juvenile drug court. Mitchell et al. (2012) reviewed 34 drug court evaluations, concluding that the average effect of drug court participation was equivalent to a 6.5% reduction in recidivism (from a rate of 50% to a rate of 43.5%). Mitchell et al. (2012) detected a 28% recidivism risk (odds ratio) reduction among juveniles experiencing drug court compared to other youth. Odds ratio comparisons specific to drug-related recidivism were essentially small (6%) and non-significant in the Mitchell et al. (2012) study. Stein et al. (2015) reviewed 31 studies, concluding that the mean effect size for recidivism within the program and for post-program recidivism at follow-up were relatively small (.07 and .11, respectively). These results, coupled with a majority of studies producing effect sizes near 0, underscore the limited impact of juvenile drug courts (Stein et al., 2015). The most recent meta-analysis of juvenile drug courts to date provided by Tanner-Smith et al. (2016) is even less optimistic. Focusing on 46 controlled evaluation studies, their meta-analysis suggested "no clear pattern of evidence" supporting a stance that general or drug recidivism, nor drug use, was better reduced through juvenile drug court programs than in the traditional court processes (Tanner-Smith et al., 2016, p. 509).

Null findings in relation to juvenile drug courts contrasted with results obtained from adult drug courts underscore the differences between traditional juvenile and adult court systems (Tanner-Smith et al., 2016). Adult court systems are traditionally more punitive, while juvenile courts tend to be more problem-solving/therapeutically oriented. Thus, the drug court experience is more different from traditional adult court compared to the difference between the two types of juvenile court. Scholars have argued that the very structure of juvenile courts obviates the need for juvenile drug courts (Butts & Roman, 2004). Tanner-Smith et al. (2016) also note that youth in the drug court programs they studied tended not to meet clinical criteria for substance use disorders, thus substance-focused treatment programming may not have been appropriate. Mismatch between treatment provided and treatment needed may be a generic problem among juvenile drug court programs, given that adolescence is a period characterized by multiple co-occurring problem behaviors that may not be causally linked, such as where delinquency and experimental drug use co-occur (Derzon & Lipsey, 1999; Donovan, 1996).

Family drug court outcomes

Although the body of family drug court literature continues to grow, it is far smaller than for adult criminal drug courts: at the time of this writing, roughly 40 publications about family drug court appeared in peer- and non-peer-reviewed literature, including conceptual articles, case studies, and evaluations. Similar to criminal drug courts, family drug court findings are somewhat mixed. An earlier systematic review of quantitative research comparing family to non-family drug court participants on likelihood of, and time to, reunification identified 18 studies (Lloyd, 2015). Of the nine peer-reviewed studies found, three compared children's time in foster care: family drug court saved 94–213 days. All nine studies reported statistically significant differences in reunification rates: 11–34% more children returned home with family drug court participation than in the comparison group. Program completion was associated with 40% greater likelihood of reunification compared to parents referred who did not enroll, and 49% greater likelihood compared to non-completion (Gifford, Eldred, Vernerey, & Sloan, 2014). Only one peer-reviewed study reported statistically significant differences for re-entry rates: the comparison group was 10% more likely to re-enter the child welfare system (Chuang, Moore, Barrett, & Young, 2012).

Lloyd's (2015) review included eight non-peer-reviewed studies, as well. These studies also reported positive outcomes but with wider ranges. Seven identified significant differences regarding time children spent in foster care, ranging from 94 to 307 fewer days among the family drug court group. Differences in reunification statistics were also significant in seven of eight studies, with the effect of family drug court involvement on reunification ranging from 6% to 54%. Similarly, graduates of family drug court were 64% more likely to reunify than those who did not enter the program and 75% more likely to reunify than those discharged prior to program completion (McMillin, 2007). Only two non-peer-reviewed studies literature reported re-entry statistics. Family drug court participants were 5% more likely to re-enter at three of the family drug courts reviewed by Worcel, Green, Furrer, Burrus, and Finigan (2007). In McMillin (2007), graduates were 52% less likely to re-enter than comparison cases, and 75% less likely to re-enter than those not completing.

Together, these findings are generally consistent with a recently published meta-analysis of family drug court studies. Zhang, Huang, Wu, Li, and Liu (2019) identified 17 studies published between 2000 and 2018 that compared family drug court participation to traditional child welfare services for families experiencing substance use problems. The authors pooled for reunification analysis 3,402 family drug court participants and 3,683 non-participant comparison cases and 842 family drug court and 632 non-family drug court comparison cases for the re-entry to child welfare system analysis from studies meeting specific criteria. Seven studies reported significant differences favoring family drug court-involved families and nine showed no statistically significant effect; the pooled effect showed that family drug court participants were at 75% increased odds of reunification versus non-family drug court cases. Effect sizes were larger if the study used a propensity score-matched comparison group, longer observation period, and children as the unit of analysis (versus parents), as well as being published in peer-reviewed journals in 2011 or later. Regarding repeat maltreatment, of the eight studies, three reported family drug court-involved children were at significantly reduced risk of recurrent maltreatment. The pooled effect showed no significant effect for family drug court involvement on maltreatment recurrence (Zhang et al., 2019).

Findings from earlier family drug court research are promising but hardly conclusive. With no randomized controlled trials or nationally representative studies, existing literature is limited in its generalizability. Moreover, few extant publications examine differences in family drug court practice and relate those differences to outcomes. Finally, although no studies reported statistically significantly worse outcomes for family drug court-involved families, similar to criminal drug court research, certain outcomes appear unaffected by family drug court participation. Future research is needed to address these gaps, including clarifying best practices, identifying a target population, and testing interaction effects for varied combinations of family drug court client and program characteristics, as well as analyzing cost effectiveness.

Two key challenges in drug courts

Despite promising impact and increasingly systematic implementation plans, challenges persist in how drug courts function. Two key challenges surround racial disparities and the use of medication-assisted treatments.

Race disparities

Perhaps the most problematic challenge currently facing U.S. drug courts is the observed disparity in participation and outcomes depending on participants' race/ethnicity. Marlowe (2013) reported that, in 2008, Black representation in drug courts was lower relative to arrests, probation/parole, and incarceration in jails and prisons. In fact, Black participants were 23% less represented in drug courts than in prisons. Latinx individuals were also represented at lower rates in drug courts compared to probation/parole, jail, and prison, with representation 10% lower in drug courts compared to prisons. In contrast, White individuals more often were in community supervision versus jails or prisons. Several studies also detected substantially lower drug court graduation rates among minority participants, with disparities particularly high for young adult Black males (Marlowe, 2013).

An earlier study of ten drug courts in Missouri pointed to the intersecting effects of race and socioeconomic status on drug court outcomes. Dannerbeck, Harris, Sundet, and Lloyd (2006) reported that, across drug courts, 55% of White participants versus 28% of Black participants graduated the program prior to June 2001. The greatest predictors of graduation were employment (243% higher odds of graduating if employed), community socioeconomic status (160% higher odds of graduating if community socioeconomic status was rated as "medium/high" versus "low), and Black persons using cocaine (53% lower odds of graduating if Black and drug of choice was cocaine). Potential race effects in drug court outcomes may be moderated by the type of substance use. These findings may be related to the well-known criminal justice disparities that historically existed with respect to cocaine (especially crack cocaine) and minority offenders.

A more recent Texas study similarly observed disparities depending on race/ethnicity and employment status. Gallagher (2013) evaluated drug court graduation for 100 randomly selected participants between 2007 and 2009, observing that 65% of White participants, 52% of Black participants, and 46% of Latinx participants graduated. Employment status was the strongest predictor of graduation (399% higher odds of graduating if employed/in school) and race/ethnicity produced the second largest effect with White participants at 337% higher odds of graduating compared to Black or Latinx participants. Both these effects were statistically significant, and present after controlling for all other variables identified above. The only other significant predictor was positive drug tests, with each additional positive drug test reducing odds of graduating by 50%; drug of choice was not significantly associated with graduating.

Family drug court research has similarly observed these racial differences. Breitenbucher et al. (2018) reported on disparate enrollment rates and child welfare outcomes for participants in 11 federally funded family drug court programs. Compared to rates in the U.S. child welfare population, White children were over-represented and Black children and Latinx children under-represented in these 11 family drug courts, with the largest disparity present for Black children. While Black children make up close to a quarter of all child welfare-involved children (but only 11% of the general U.S. population), less than 10% of family drug court children were Black. However, over 50% of U.S. children, 41% of the child welfare population, and 46% of family drug court-involved children are White. These disparities were also reflected in time spent in foster care, with Black children spending the most days in care (median = 431) and White children spending the fewest (median = 335). Finally, reunification within 12 months occurred most often for Asian/Pacific Island children, and least often for multi-racial children. Only a slightly higher percentage of White children reunified in 12 months compared to Black children.

Medication-assisted treatment (MAT)

The current well-documented, sustained opioid crisis in the United States has considerable implications for the population entering drug courts. Recognizing that programs in the United States are faced with dramatically increasing numbers of clients experiencing opioid use disorders, the Substance Abuse and Mental Health Services Administration-supported funding expands the use of various medications for opioid treatment in drug courts (Fendrich & LeBel, 2019). Despite their demonstrated efficacy, medication–assisted treatment (MAT) has been particularly challenging and potentially controversial in the drug court setting.

Ideally, MAT includes the use of one or more FDA-approved opioid medications: methadone, buprenorphine, or naltrexone (Fendrich & LeBel, 2019; see Chapter 19) in conjunction with substance use/behavioral health counseling. Criminal justice professionals have shown a long-standing negative bias toward the use of medications such as methadone and buprenorphine, as a result of misperceptions surrounding their potential analgesic effects and related concerns about their addictive potential (Belenko, Hiller, & Hamilton, 2013; Friedmann et al., 2012; Matusow et al., 2013; Mitchell et al., 2016). Consistent with this bias, drug courts have historically conceptualized substance abstinence as the primary goal of treatment and definition of recovery, thus, in order to successfully graduate from many drug court programs participants must prove substance abstinence with numerous consistent negative drug tests (National Association of Drug Court Professionals, 2015). Similarly, the Substance Abuse and Mental Health Services Administration's 2005 recommendations regarding treatment for individuals in the criminal justice system reflected the final action stage as one of sustained abstinence (Center for Substance Abuse Treatment, 2005). Many treatment approaches historically available for this population, such as the Matrix Model, also support client abstinence as the treatment goal. A recent study reported that only 36% of substance use treatment facilities in the United States offer any medication–assisted treatment, and only 6% offer all three FDA-approved medications (Mojtabai, Mauro, Wall, Barry, & Olfson, 2019).

Nevertheless, past practices and standards are rapidly changing in response to the opioid crisis. For example, Fendrich and LeBel (2019) document MAT implementation and associated obstacles in a Milwaukee County drug treatment court. Friedman and Wagner-Goldstein (2016) provided strategies for successful implementation of MAT in drug courts, based on their experience in New York. The CEO of the National Association of Drug Court Professionals (NADCP) stated at the 2018 training conference that drug courts must include, serve, and graduate clients using appropriately prescribed MAT medications (National Drug Court Institute, n.d.). Although no current data on the proportion of drug courts that exclude MAT patients exist, indicators of drug court practice, including the NADCP's stance as well as federal drug court funding mechanisms, are clear that drug courts must include MAT in its treatment offerings.

Social work and drug courts

Several attributes of drug courts align with social work perspectives, and certain realities of the model's implementation rightly raise concerns for social workers. To understand this tension, it is necessary to first consider the philosophical foundation of the drug court model.

Therapeutic jurisprudence

Scholars consider drug courts to reflect the theoretical construct of therapeutic jurisprudence (Hora, 2002): "the use of social science to study the extent to which a legal rule or practice promotes the psychological and physical well-being of the people it affects" (Slobogin, 1995, p. 196). The construct theorizes a relationship between legal rules and procedures, and therapeutic or non-therapeutic outcomes (Wexler, 1997). It recognizes that the courts are a component in the social fabric that contributes to individual social experiences and "regards the law as a social force that produces behaviors and consequences" (Hora, 2002, p. 1471). Therapeutic jurisprudence asserts that the court can function as a setting with the capacity to psychologically and behaviorally affect involved parties. In the case of drug courts, the 10 Key Components and best practices literature describe how a court is to operate in a manner that improves client outcomes (e.g. results in successful treatment completion and reduced recidivism).

Social justice concerns

Although drug courts may theoretically align with therapeutic jurisprudence, the realities of drug court practice have raised concerns for social justice advocates. A case study, reflecting experiences of a social worker in a Midwestern adult drug court, highlighted areas of potential philosophical conflict (Roberts, Phillips, Bordelon, & Seif, 2014). The worker reported being the mediator between the defense council's and treatment provider's leniency recommendations and law enforcement's negative views following a participant's relapse to substance use. The social worker also played a role in implementing each of the 10 Key Components of drug court practice (Roberts et al., 2014). For example, Key Component 4 regarding participant access to treatment is conservatively defined as only drug treatment services. The social worker emphasized the need for services to address barriers to treatment completion, such as co-occurring mental illness and socioeconomic challenges. Additionally, the worker sought to ensure that clients gained access to treatment specific to their gender, age, and ethnicity. Without the social worker's contributions, the drug court clients may have experienced a much different program; one lacking attention to their unique position in the world, previous experiences, and internal motivations.

Social work values also shed light on areas of concern within drug courts. For example, self-determination is of primary importance to our profession (National Association of Social Workers [NASW], 2009). Consistent with this value, drug courts are "opt-in" programs: the client voluntarily enters the program. Nevertheless, the potential for coercion exists if clients perceive limited choice: entering the program occurs during a time of crisis, such as facing incarceration or losing child custody. Preserving self-determination means that courts must take proper precautions to ensure that potential clients are not coerced to enter a drug court program, even if a case worker or attorney believes the person is an appropriate candidate who would benefit from drug court participation. Ultimately, the decision rests with the individual.

Confidentiality is another issue facing drug courts. Judges and court team members have access to client substance abuse treatment records and discuss the progress of the case during pre-hearing meetings and hearings. Legally, confidentiality dilemmas are circumvented when a participant signs an informed consent document (Lu, 2001). However, from a social worker's perspective, this does not relieve the court team from the professional obligation to maintain privacy and confidentiality (NASW, 2009).

Implications for social workers

Social workers serve many roles in drug courts: drug court administrator, admissions screener, treatment professional, case manager, or program evaluator. Specific to juvenile and family drug courts, social workers may be involved as representatives of the child welfare system, office of the guardian ad litem, or children's mental health provider. The drug court team makes joint decisions regarding each case at the time of the hearing (Center for Substance Abuse Treatment, 2004). Because social workers deliver the lion's share of community and social services across the United States and in many other nations, social workers may also be tangentially involved with drug courts as mental health, domestic violence, housing, economic sufficiency, or family training providers who work with drug court clients.

Many aspects of drug court practice align with social work's therapeutic approach. For example, drug courts attend holistically to the person-in-environment. Drug court team members seek to address clients' multiple, complex needs, not just their substance use problem, through intensive case management. Drug courts also are strengths-based. Consistent with the strengths-perspective (Saleebey, 2012), drug courts recognize the goals and desires of the client in case planning, work with the clients using a collaborative framework, and rely on resources in the community (Lloyd & Brook, 2014). For example, in a family drug court setting, parents experiencing substance use disorders are viewed as human beings full of potential for growth, resilience, and strengths. This orientation stands in stark opposition to the perspective in traditional child welfare courts where the parent may be considered "bad," and must correct conditions leading to their child's maltreatment (Ross, 2003).

Drug court involvement does not necessarily guarantee of better criminal justice outcomes for participants. Social workers referring individuals to drug courts must take extreme caution not to pressure a person in crisis to enter a drug court program without providing them with adequate information concerning the intensive approach adopted in drug courts, issues surrounding confidentiality, and the possibility that failure could result in worse outcomes than if they were to enter into the traditional system.

Drug court teams are typically led by a judge who exercises decision making in collaboration with a team consisting of defense attorneys, prosecutors, other stakeholders in the criminal justice system, and a team coordinator. The coordinator role is ideally suited for social workers with micro and macro practice skills. Knowledge of substance abuse treatment, comorbid mental health conditions, other co-occurring problems, the treatment provider network, and community resources than can aid and sustain in recovery would be a considerable asset for a person occupying this role. At the same time, since the coordinator needs to facilitate intra-agency collaborations, develop partnerships between community organizations and the court, and serve as an advocate for policies and funding needed to sustain the program, macro practice social work skills are also essential. The value of social work-trained coordinators for facilitating the implementation of each of the 10 Key Components was demonstrated by Roberts et al. (2014). Given the proliferation of drug court programs throughout the United States and elsewhere, there is a need for social work education programs to more directly tailor training to enhance social work capacity to fulfill critical roles as members of drug court teams (Roberts et al., 2014).

Social work researchers can serve as active, on-site evaluators of drug court processes and outcomes. With their unique person-in environment and social justice perspectives, social workers understand that individual outcomes are impacted by social conditions and systems such as racism, economic disparities, disparities in criminal justice treatment, and the availability of suitable housing, education, and health care in the community. As on-site evaluators, social work evaluation team members can provide critical direct feedback to drug court team members, as well as policy makers, when they observe racial disparities in participation and outcomes. Gallagher and Wahler (2018) illustrated the unique kind of in-depth, qualitative follow-up research social worker evaluators can provide—meeting drug court participants where they are—to both understand and potentially eliminate the persistence of racial disparities in drug court graduation rates and enhance the overall social benefit of drug court interventions.

Conclusions

Drug courts emerged in an era characterized by mass incarceration and growing rates of substance misuse amidst under-resourced and over-loaded substance abuse treatment and criminal justice systems. Increasingly, substance use disorders are viewed as conditions to be addressed by public health measures and rather than punished by courts and incarceration. Supporting this is the large-scale federal HEAL initiative (NIH) launched by the National Institutes of Health, which is funneling billions of dollars into treatment-oriented interventions in community settings (National Institutes of Health, 2018).

Enhanced availability and efficacy of treatment resources may eventually obviate the need for a drug treatment system centered in the justice system, but currently drug courts exist as a major addictions intervention strategy in the United States and other nations. Social workers can play crucial roles in drug court programs, despite encountering inherent challenges. It remains to be seen whether contemporary societal forces will result in a pullback, continuation, or expansion of drug courts, or in their adaptation and emergence in some other future form.

References

Belenko, S., Hiller, M., & Hamilton, L. (2013). Treating substance use disorders in the criminal justice system. *Current Psychiatry Reports, 15*(11), 414. doi:10.1007/s11920-013-0414-z

Blumstein, A., & Beck, A. J. (1999). Population growth in U. S. prisons, 1980–1996. *Crime and Justice, 26,* 17–61. doi:10.2307/1147683

Breitenbucher, P., Young, N. K., Bermejo, R., Duong, L., Killian, C. M., & DeCerchio, K. (2018). Exploring racial and ethnic disproportionalities and disparities in family treatment courts: Findings from the Regional Partnership Grant Program. *Journal for Advancing Justice, 1*(1), 35–51.

Bureau of Justice Assistance. (1997). *Defining drug courts: The key components*. Washington, DC: U.S. Dept. of Justice, Office of Justice Programs, Bureau of Justice Assistance. Retrieved from https://www.ncjrs.gov/pdffiles1/bja/205621.pdf

Bureau of Justice Assistance. (2003). *Juvenile drug courts: Strategies in practice*. Washington, DC: U.S. Dept. of Justice, Office of Justice Programs, Bureau of Justice Assistance.

Bureau of Justice Statistics. (1986). *State and federal prisoners, 1925–1985*. Washington, DC: U.S. Dept. of Justice, Office of Justice Programs, Bureau of Justice Assistance.

Butts, J. A., & Roman, J. (2004). *Juvenile drug courts and teen substance abuse*. Washington, DC: U.S. Dept. of Justice, Office of Justice Programs, Bureau of Justice Assistance.

Carey, S., Mackin, J., & Finigan, M. (2012). What works? The 10 key components of drug courts: Research based best practices. *Drug Court Review, 8*(1), 6–42.

Center for Substance Abuse Treatment. (2004). *Family dependency treatment courts: Addressing child abuse and neglect cases using a drug court model*. Washington, DC: U.S. Dept. of Justice, Office of Justice Programs, Bureau of Justice Assistance.

Center for Substance Abuse Treatment. (2005). *Substance abuse treatment for adults in the criminal justice system*. Treatment Improvement Protocol (TIP) Series 44. HHS Publication No. (SMA) 13–4056. Rockville, MD: Substance Abuse and Mental Health Services Administration.

Choi, S. (2012). Family drug courts in child welfare. *Child & Adolescent Social Work Journal, 29*(6), 447–461. doi:10.1007/s10560-012-0272-2

Chuang, E., Moore, K., Barrett, B., & Young, M. S. (2012). Effect of an integrated family dependency treatment court on child welfare reunification, time to permanency and re-entry rates. *Children and Youth Services Review, 34*(9), 1896–1902. doi:10.1016/j.childyouth.2012.06.001

Dannerbeck, A., Harris, G., Sundet, P., & Lloyd, K. (2006). Understanding and responding to racial differences in drug court outcomes. *Journal of Ethnicity and Substance Abuse, 5*, 2–22. doi:10.1300/J233v05n02_01

Derzon, J. H., & Lipsey, M. W. (1999). A synthesis of the relationship of marijuana use with delinquent and problem behaviors. *School Psychology International, 20*(1), 57–68. doi:10.1177/0143034399201005

Donovan, J. E. (1996). Problem-behavior theory and the explanation of adolescent marijuana use. *Journal of Drug Issues, 26*(2), 379–404. doi:10.1177/002204269602600205

Fendrich, M., & LeBel, T. P. (2019). Implementing access to medication assisted treatment in a drug treatment court: Correlates, consequences, and obstacles. *Journal of Offender Rehabilitation*. doi:10.1080/10509674.2019.1582573

Finn, P., & Newlyn, A. K. (1993). Miami drug court gives drug defendants a second chance. *Judicature, 77*, 268.

Franco, C. (2010). Drug courts: Background, effectiveness, and policy issues for congress. Washington, DC: DIANE Publishing.

Friedman, S., & Wagner-Goldstein, K. (2016). *Medication-assisted treatment in drug courts: Recommended strategies*. Retrieved from https://lac.org/wp-content/uploads/2016/04/MATinDrugCourts.pdf

Friedmann, P. D., Hoskinson, R., Gordon, M., Schwartz, R., Kinlock, T., Knight, K., . . . Frisman, L. K. (2012). Medication-assisted treatment in criminal justice agencies affiliated with the Criminal Justice-Drug Abuse Treatment Studies (CJ-DATS): Availability, barriers, and intentions. *Substance Abuse, 33*(1), 9–18. doi:10.1080/08897077.2011.611460

Gallagher, J. R. (2013). Drug court graduation rates: Implications for policy advocacy and future research. *Alcoholism Treatment Quarterly, 31*(2), 241–253. doi:10.1080/07347324.2013.772019

Gallagher, J. R., & Wahler, E. A. (2018). Racial disparities in drug court graduation rates: The role of recovery support groups and environments. *Journal of Social Work Practice in the Addictions, 18*(2), 113–127. doi:10.1080/1533256X.2018.1448277

Gifford, E. J., Eldred, L. M., Vernerey, A., & Sloan, F. A. (2014). How does family drug treatment court participation affect child welfare outcomes? *Child Abuse & Neglect, 38*(10), 1659–1670. doi:10.1016/j.chiabu.2014.03.010

Goldkamp, J. S., & Weiland, D. (1993). *Assessing the impact of Dade County's felony drug court*. Washington, DC: U.S. Department of Justice, Office of Justice Programs. doi:10.1037/e438202008-001

Gottfredson, D. C., Najaka, S. S., & Kearley, B. (2003). Effectiveness of drug treatment courts: Evidence from a randomized trial. *Criminology & Public Policy, 2*(2), 171–196. doi:10.1111/j.1745-9133.2003.tb00117.x

Gottfredson, D. C., Najaka, S. S., Kearley, B. W., & Rocha, C. M. (2006). Long-term effects of participation in the Baltimore City drug treatment court: Results from an experimental study. *Journal of Experimental Criminology, 2*(1), 67–98. doi:10.1007/s11292-005-5128-8

Gurnell, B., Holmberg, M., & Yeres, S. (2014). Starting a juvenile drug court: A planning guide. Reno, NV: National Council of Juvenile and Family Court Judges (NCJFCJ). Retrieved from http://www.ncjfcj.org/sites/default/files/NCJFCJ_JDC_PlanningGuide_Final.pdf

Guzman, D. E. (2012). *Drug courts: Scope and challenges of an alternative to incarceration*. London: International Drug Policy Consortium.

Harrison, P. M., & Beck, A. J. (2003). *Prisoners in 2002*. Washington, DC: U.S. Dept. of Justice, Office of Justice Programs, Bureau of Justice Assistance.

Harrison, P. M., & Beck, A. J. (2006). *Prisoners in 2005*. Washington, DC: U.S. Dept. of Justice, Office of Justice Programs, Bureau of Justice Assistance. Retrieved from https://www.bjs.gov/content/pub/pdf/p05.pdf

Hora, H. P. F. (2002). A dozen years of drug treatment courts: Uncovering our theoretical foundation and the construction of a mainstream paradigm. *Substance Use & Misuse, 37*(12–13), 1469–1488. doi:10.1081/JA-120014419

Hora, P. F., Schma, W. G., & Rosenthal, J. T. A. (1999). Therapeutic jurisprudence and the drug treatment court movement: Revolutionizing the criminal justice system's response to drug abuse and crime in America. Notre Dame Law Review, 74(2), 439–538.

Kearley, B. W. (2017). Long-term effects of drug court participation: Evidence from a 15-year follow-up of a randomized controlled trial. (Ph.D. Dissertation), University of Maryland, College Park, College Park, MD.

Lemus, T., & Richter, T. (2018). *A new approach – family treatment courts as part of a continuum of care*. Paper presented at the NADCP 2018, Houston, TX.

Lloyd, M. H. (2015). Family drug courts: Conceptual frameworks, empirical evidence and implications for social work. *Families in Society, 96*(1), 49–57. doi:10.1606/1044-3894.2015.96.7

Lloyd, M. H., & Brook, J. (2014). Strengths based approaches to practice and family drug courts: Is there a fit? *Journal of Family Strengths, 14*(1), article 15.

Lu, C. (2001). Family drug court: An alternative answer. *Children's Legal Rights Journal, 21*, 32.

Lurigio, A. J. (2008). The first 20 years of drug treatment courts: Brief description of their history and impact. *Federal Probation, 72*(1), 13–17.

Marlowe, D. B. (2012). Targeting the right participants for adult drug courts: Part one of a two-part series. *Drug Court Practitioner Fact Sheet, 7*(1), 1–11.

Marlowe, D. B. (2013). Achieving racial and ethnic fairness in drug courts. *Court Review, 49*, 40–47.

Marlowe, D. B., Hardin, C. D., & Fox, C. L. (2016). *Painting the current picture: A national report on drug courts and other problem-solving courts in the United States*. Alexandria, VA: National Drug Court Institute. Retrieved from https://www.ndci.org/wp-content/uploads/2016/05/Painting-the-Current-Picture-2016.pdf

Matusow, H., Dickman, S. L., Rich, J. D., Fong, C., Dumont, D. M., Hardin, C., . . . Rosenblum, A. (2013). Medication assisted treatment in U.S.drug courts: Results from a nationwide survey of availability, barriers and attitudes. *Journal of Substance Abuse Treatment, 44*(5), 473–480. doi:10.1016/j.jsat.2012.10.004

McGee, H. C. M. (1997). Another permanency perspective: Family drug court. *Juvenile and Family Court Journal, 48*(4), 65–68. doi:10.1111/j.1755-6988.1997.tb00775.x

McMillin, H. E. (2007). *Process and outcome evaluation of the Spokane County Meth Family Treatment Court*. (Doctor of Philosophy), Washington State University, Spokane, WA.

Mitchell, O., Wilson, D. B., Eggers, A., & MacKenzie, D. L. (2012). Drug courts' effects on criminal offending for juveniles and adults. *Campbell Systematic Reviews, 8*. doi:10.4073/csr.2012.4

Mitchell, S. G., Willet, J., Monico, L. B., James, A., Rudes, D. S., Viglioni, J., . . . Friedmann, P. D. (2016). Community correctional agents' views of medication-assisted treatment: Examining their influence on treatment referrals and community supervision practices. *Substance Abuse, 37*(1), 127–133. doi:10.1080/08897077.2015.1129389

Mojtabai, R., Mauro, C., Wall, M. M., Barry, C. L., & Olfson, M. (2019). Medication treatment for opioid use disorders in substance use treatment facilities. *Health Affairs, 38*(1), 14–23. doi:10.1377/hlthaff.2018.05162

National Association of Drug Court Professionals. (2013). *Adult drug court best practice standards Volume I*. Alexandria, VA: Author.

National Association of Drug Court Professionals. (2015). *Adult drug court best practice standards Volume II*. Alexandria, VA: Author.

National Association of Social Workers. (2009). *Social work speaks: National Association of Social Workers policy statements, 2009–2012*. Washington, DC: NASW Press.

National Center on Addiction and Substance Abuse at Columbia University. (1999). *No safe haven: Children of substance-abusing parents.* New York, NY: Columbia University.

National Drug Court Institute. (n.d.). *Medication-assisted treatment* [web article]. Retrieved April 1, 2019 from https://www.ndci.org/resource/training/medication-assisted-treatment/

National Institutes of Health. (2018, Wednesday April 4, 2018). *NIH Lauches HEAL Initiative, doubles funding to accelerate scientific solutions to stem national opioid epidemic* [press release]. Retrieved from https://www.nih.gov/news-events/news-releases/nih-launches-heal-initiative-doubles-funding-accelerate-scientific-solutions-stem-national-opioid-epidemic

National Institute of Justice. (2018). *Drug courts.* Alexandria, VA: NADCP. Retrieved from https://www.nij.gov/topics/courts/drug-courts/pages/welcome.aspx

National Institute of Justice, Bureau of Justice Assistance, & Office of Juvenile Justice and Delinquency Prevention. (2018). *Drug courts.* Washington, DC: U.S. Dept. of Justice, Office of Justice Programs, Bureau of Justice Assistance.

North Carolina Judicial Branch. (n.d.). *Recovery courts.* Retrieved from https://www.nccourts.gov/courts/recovery-courts

Office of Juvenile Justice and Delinquency Prevention. (2016). *Juvenile drug treatment court guidelines.* Washington, DC: U.S. Dept. of Justice, Office of Justice Programs, Bureau of Justice Assistance. Retrieved from https://www.ojjdp.gov/pubs/250368.pdf

Puyana, J. C., Puyana, J. C. J., Rubiano, A. M., Montenegro, J. H., Estebanez, G. O., Sanchez, A. I., & Vega-Rivera, F. (2017). Drugs, violence, and trauma in Mexico and the USA. *Medical Principles and Practice, 26*(4), 309–315. doi:10.1159/000471853

Roberts, M. R., Phillips, I., Bordelon, T. D., & Seif, L. (2014). A social worker's role in drug court. *SAGE Open, 4*(2). doi:10.1177/2158244014535413

Ross, C. J. (2003). The tyranny of time: Vulnerable children, bad mothers, and statutory deadlines in parental termination proceedings. *Virginia. Journal of Social Policy & the Law, 11*, 176.

Rossman, S. B., Roman, J. K., Zweig, J. M., Rempel, M., & Lindquist, C. (2011). *The multi-site adult drug court evaluation: Study overview and design*: Urban Institute Justice Policy Center. doi:10.1037/e718342011-001

Saleebey, D. (2012). The strengths perspective in social work practice. Boston, MA: Pearson Higher Education.

Sevigny, E. L., Fuleihan, B. K., & Ferdik, F. V. (2013). Do drug courts reduce the use of incarceration?: A meta-analysis. *Journal of Criminal Justice, 41*(6), 416–425. doi:10.1016/j.jcrimjus.2013.06.005

Slobogin, C. (1995). Therapeutic jurisprudence: Five dilemmas to ponder. *Psychology, Public Policy, and Law, 1*(1), 193. doi:10.1037/1076-8971.1.1.193

Stein, D. M., Homan, K. J., & DeBerard, S. (2015). The effectiveness of juvenile treatment drug courts: A meta-analytic review of literature. *Journal of Child & Adolescent Substance Abuse, 24*(2), 80–93. doi:10.1080/1067828X.2013.764371

Strong, S. M., Rantala, R. R., & Kyckelhahn, T. (2016). *Census of problem-solving courts, 2012.* Retrieved from https://www.bjs.gov/content/pub/pdf/cpsc12.pdf

Tanner-Smith, E. E., Lipsey, M. W., & Wilson, D. B. (2016). Juvenile drug court effects on recidivism and drug use: A systematic review and meta-analysis. *Journal of Experimental Criminology, 12*(4), 477–513. doi:10.1007/s11292-016-9274-y

Tennessee Department of Mental Health & Substance Abuse Services. (n.d.). *Recovery/drug court programs in TN: Get into recovery, stay out of jail.* Retrieved from https://preprod.tn.gov/behavioral-health/substance-abuse-services/criminal-justice-services/recovery-drug-court-programs-in-tn.html

United Nations Office on Drugs and Crime. (2008). *A century of international drug control.* Vienna, Austria: United Nations Office of Drug Use and Crime.

Wexler, D. B. (1997). Therapeutic jurisprudence in a comparative law context. *Behavioral Sciences & the Law, 15*(3), 233–246. doi:10.1002/(sici)1099-0798(199722/06)15:3<233::aid-bsl263>3.0.co;2-s

Worcel, S. D., Green, B. L., Furrer, C. J., Burrus, S. W. M., & Finigan, M. W. (2007). *Family treatment dug court evaluation.* Portland, OR: NPC Research.

Young, N. K., Breitenbucher, P., & Pfeifer, J. (2013). *Guidance to states: Recommendations for developing family drug court guidelines.* Retrieved from http://www.cffutures.org/files/publications/FDC-Guidelines.pdf

Zhang, S., Huang, H., Wu, Q., Li, Y., & Liu, M. (2019). The impacts of family treatment drug court on child welfare core outcomes: A meta-analysis. *Child Abuse & Neglect, 88*, 1–14. doi:10.1016/j.chiabu.2018.10.014

29

Roles for social work and other professions in support of recovery-oriented addiction policies and services

Clifford Bersamira

Background

The concept of "recovery" has increasingly become a center of conversation for those involved with the addiction service delivery system. Substance use disorder (SUD) treatment providers, community-based organizations, addiction advocacy groups, and government agencies are utilizing recovery-oriented language and policies and embracing the role of persons in recovery from alcohol and drug problems in many facets of service delivery and policy advocacy. For example, in addiction treatment programs, individuals in long-term recovery from alcohol and drug problems are often hired as paraprofessionals, usually called peers, and provide recovery support services that complement treatment services administered by specially trained and certified professionals.

Recovery community organizations (RCOs) have become important community stakeholders. Their physical spaces provide venues for delivering recovery-oriented services and supports, including mutual aid groups and substance-free activities and events. RCO leaders and members advocate and educate their communities about issues pertaining to addiction, recovery, and stigma. Similarly, at state and national levels in the United States, grassroots advocacy is aggregated through statewide and national coalitions such as Faces and Voices of Recovery (FAVOR), a national recovery advocacy organization that has been influential in reducing stigma associated with addiction and promoting policy reforms in addiction treatment, healthcare, and other sectors. Federal government agencies such as the Substance Abuse and Mental Health Services Administration (SAMHSA) and the Single State Authorities (SSAs—state agencies responsible for administering publicly funded addiction services) have adopted recovery-oriented policies and initiatives, including increased funding for recovery support services such as peer-delivered services (Humphreys & McLellan, 2010; Laudet & Humphreys, 2013). This national movement in the United States is joined by comparable movements across the globe (Humphreys & Lembke, 2014).

This growing adoption of recovery-oriented values and involvement of individuals in recovery as service providers and advocates provides opportunities for social workers and other professionals to support peer service delivery, engage in grassroots community advocacy, and facilitate policy and systems change toward what is being described as a recovery-oriented system of care, or recovery-oriented system of care (ROSC). However, this changing landscape in addiction services requires one to ask several questions: what exactly is addiction recovery and how is it being operationalized through services, policies, and a system of care; what are the origins of this recent addiction recovery movement and how are social workers involved; and, finally, what role and responsibility do social workers and other professionals have in supporting this movement that empowers individuals in recovery from alcohol and drug problems?

This chapter aims to: (1) provide an understanding of addiction recovery as an organizing framework for addiction treatment services, systems, and policies; (2) describe the role of social workers in addressing addiction problems and discuss how social work (and other professions') practices align with addiction recovery values; (3) identify areas where social workers and other professionals can play a role in facilitating recovery-oriented systems of care, including fostering policy advocacy and promoting engagement of peers as collaborators in addiction treatment settings; and (4) critically explore potential tensions and barriers in social workers' contributions to recovery-oriented policy change.

Recovery as an organizing framework for addiction treatment

"Recovery" is certainly not a new concept in addiction treatment. Historically, persons experiencing alcohol and drug problems in the United States and many other countries have turned to self-help and mutual aid groups to address their problems and achieve wellness. These include, but are not limited to, Alcoholics Anonymous (AA), Narcotics Anonymous (NA), Blue Cross in Switzerland, Croix d'Or in France, and the Danshukai movement in Japan. What is notably different between historical use of the term "recovery" and its more contemporary use is the growing advocacy and political participation of persons in recovery. Self-identifying as a person in recovery is a means of increasing the community's political voice. This advocacy addresses perceived shortcomings in addiction treatment, healthcare, and social services, and reduce stigma around experiencing and recovering from substance use disorders (SUDs).

What is addiction recovery?

It is important to clarify what is meant by "recovery." The way recovery is defined has implications for research, service delivery, and policy. Without getting caught up in the term's historical etymology, it is important to understand how recovery is defined within the context of current use.

Recent empirical efforts explored how individuals experiencing SUDs define recovery for themselves. Based on response to the question, "Did you used to have a problem with alcohol or drugs but no longer do?" approximately 9.1% of the U.S. population was estimated to be in recovery, with 46% of them self-identifying as being "in recovery" and 53.9% using an assisted pathway to achieve recovery (Kelly, Bergman, Hoeppner, Vilsaint, & White, 2017). Among persons using assisted pathways, 45.1% engaged mutual aid such as AA or other recovery groups, 27.6% formal addiction treatment, 21.8% recovery support services, and 6.2% recovery support centers. According to the same study, more than half (54%) of individuals deemed "in recovery" did not identify with that terminology, implicating the sustained stigma of affiliating with one's alcohol and drug problems and the recovery label. This has consequences for future prevalence studies, community advocacy, and funding efforts which often have the objective of securing resources based on numbers of individuals needing services.

Few studies have been conducted with the aim of understanding the subjective definition of recovery for both immediate service consumers and persons in long-term recovery (Kaskutas et al., 2014; Laudet, 2007). Even less has been done to understand how recovery-oriented service outcomes should be measured and aligned with personal defini-tions of recovery (Andresen, Caputi, & Oades, 2010). Laudet (2007) attempted to under-stand whether, according to individuals in recovery, total abstinence from alcohol and other substances is required to achieve recovery and whether recovery is defined solely within the context of addiction, or are other factors considered. Laudet concluded that most re-spondents (n = 289) defined recovery as requiring total abstinence from alcohol and drugs but added that recovery's scope goes beyond addiction-related needs. In the more recent "What is Recovery?" study, 9,341 respondents identified as being in recovery, recovered, in medication-assisted recovery, or having had a problem with alcohol or drugs (but no longer do) identified which of 34 elements mattered most (Kaskutas et al., 2014).

The six most endorsed factors were:

- elements of "essential recovery" (being honest with myself, handling negative feelings without using drugs or alcohol, being able to enjoy life without drinking or using drugs like I used to); and
- elements of "enriched recovery" (process of growth and development, reacting to life's ups and downs in a more balanced way than I used to, taking responsibility for the things I can change).

In addition, other recovery factors were identified by a smaller, but still significant, propor-tion of respondents, shedding light on the diversity of defining elements among persons in recovery (Kaskutas et al., 2014).

The New Recovery Advocacy Movement gained momentum across the United States in the early 2000s mutually influencing similar advocacy movements in other countries, including the United Kingdom, Canada, and Australia around the same time and in the subsequent decade (Best, De Alwis, & Burdett, 2017; White, 2014). In 2007, the Betty Ford Institute convened addiction treatment and recovery stakeholders to develop a consen-sus definition of *addiction recovery*. They determined that recovery "from substance depen-dence is a voluntarily maintained lifestyle characterized by sobriety, personal health, and citizenship" (Betty Ford Institute Consensus Panel, 2007, p. 222). In 2012, the Substance Abuse and Mental Health Services Administration (SAMHSA), as the U.S. federal agency charged with administering the national public safety net of addiction services, convened its own workgroup of national stakeholders and mental health service delivery systems. They defined recovery as, "… a process of change through which individuals improve their health and wellness, live a self-directed life, and strive to reach their full potential" (SAMHSA, 2012). These two definitions highlight values important in recovery, including an individual's relationship with substances and maintaining their health and wellness, self-determination, and civic participation.

Notably, "sobriety" is not explicitly defined by SAMHSA in their definition for recovery for two reasons: first, SAMHSA's definition is meant to be applicable to a broad behavioral health audience, inclusive of persons experiencing substance use and/or mental health dis-orders; and second, the recovery community's attitudes about abstinence and sobriety are complex. Previous dominant norms around abstinence, stemming from the Twelve-Step tradition, are in direct conflict with current values and attitudes about addictive behaviors that embrace harm reduction and "multiple pathways to recovery." Attitudes around the use of evidence-based medication treatments for alcohol and other substance use disorders also are evolving beyond previous dominant traditions.

What is a recovery-oriented system of care?

Adequately defining recovery is just a first step among many in improving systems of care. Compared with the number of efforts to define recovery, even fewer definitions and conceptualizations connected with a recovery-oriented system of care (ROSC) have been developed. Some scholarly work addresses how recovery is used as an organizing construct for addiction service delivery systems (Hser & Anglin, 2011; White & Kelly, 2011). Even less addresses service delivery transformations toward ROSC and the necessary elements of system reform that work to ensure improvement in community and individual outcomes. Case studies have been conducted to better understand system transformation efforts undertaken in the U.S. state of Connecticut (Kirk, 2011) and county of Philadelphia (Achara-Abraham, Evans, & King, 2011), but little has been done to identify key elements of transformation that made these system changes successful.

In *Recovery Management and Recovery-oriented Systems of Care: Scientific Rationale and Promising Practices* (2008), addiction recovery scholar and historian William White developed one of the early descriptions of ROSC:

> The phrase *recovery-oriented systems of care* as used in this monograph refers to the complete network of indigenous and professional services and relationships that can support the long-term recovery of individuals and families and the creation of values and policies in the larger cultural and policy environment that are supportive of these recovery processes. The "system" in this phrase is not a federal, state, or local agency, but a macro-level organization of the larger cultural and community environment in which long-term recovery is nested.
>
> *(White, 2008, p. 18)*

Two years later, SAMHSA defined ROSC as:

> A coordinated network of community-based services and supports that is person-centered and builds on the strengths and resiliencies of individuals, families, and communities to achieve abstinence and improved health, wellness, and quality of life for those with or at risk of alcohol and drug problems.
>
> *(SAMHSA, 2010)*

From these definitions, we understand that ROSC is more than coordinated care within an addiction treatment system. ROSC relies on services and supports beyond the professionally delivered treatment system and, as White described, requires the availability of community-based indigenous supports. Its scope extends beyond the formal and informal interventions and supports typically considered for persons experiencing alcohol or drug problems. In other words, the services and supports included in a ROSC should directly address the life domains impacted by alcohol and drug problems: remission and relapse prevention, restoring behavioral and physical health functioning, and addressing other life domains impacted by alcohol and drug problems, such as family and community connectedness and meaningful participation in school or the workforce.

Evolving beyond "treatment-as-usual"

ROSCs differ from addiction treatment service delivery systems as they have existed in the past. In 2007, addiction recovery stakeholders convened at the U.S. National Summit

Table 29.1 Differences between treatment-as-usual and ROSC

Service System	"Treatment-as-Usual"	ROSC[a]
Treatment focus	"Expert"-centered	Person-centered, self-directed, strengths-based
Role of family and allies	Limited involvement	Full involvement
Service provision	Generalized, acute episodes of care	Individualized, comprehensive, across the lifespan
System context	Anchored in treatment	Anchored in the community

a Adapted from Center for Substance Abuse Treatment (2007). *National Summit on Recovery.*

on Recovery, one of the first SAMHSA-implemented meetings to support and promote the National Recovery Advocacy Movement (Center for Substance Abuse Treatment [CSAT], 2007). In developing a conceptual framework to address effective and ineffective elements of existing addiction treatment systems, they highlighted notable differences. Traditional addiction treatment service delivery systems often focus on education, training, and "expertise" of credentialed professional counselors or clinicians (including social workers), while ROSCs centralize the role and perspective of the client: services are person-centered, self-directed, and strengths-based. In traditional addiction treatment systems, family members, friends, and other community allies have limited involvement in an individual's treatment, while in ROSCs full involvement from supportive significant others and allies is expected. In traditional addiction treatment systems, services are typically generalized across all recipients and delivered to address acute episodes, while in ROSCs services are individualized, comprehensive, and delivered as appropriate across the lifespan to address the chronic nature of SUDs. Lastly, from a systems perspective, traditional addiction treatment systems are anchored in treatment facilities while ROSC services are anchored in the broader community, inclusive of both professionally delivered treatment services and indigenous, community-based supports (see Table 29.1).

Brief history of addiction treatment

The history of addiction treatment is longstanding, complex and reflective of how alcohol and other substances were perceived in given historical periods and the perceived culturally and politically appropriate ways to address them. There exist far too many important moments in this history to recount in this chapter; rather, a few themes shed light on the rise of the addiction recovery movement: the rise of mutual aid groups prior to the professionalization of addiction treatment; alcohol use and other substance use disorders being addressed through disparate approaches and systems; perceptions of substance use problems as health disorders, criminal issues, or religious and moral problems shaping interventions; and the shift toward understanding substance use disorders as a chronic disease.

Mutual aid

Early support for individuals experiencing alcohol use disorder came through informal supports with alcohol mutual aid societies developing as early as the 1750s to the early 1800s. From this early tradition of mutual aid, Alcoholics Anonymous (AA) and subsequently Narcotics Anonymous (NA) stemmed forth. AA was founded in 1935 and its principles and policies were articulated in the text, *Alcoholics Anonymous* (known as the Big Book), in 1939 (Borkman, Kaskutas, & Owens, 2007; Kurtz, 1991; White, 2014). Arguably, no mutual aid movement for alcohol use disorder has reached more individuals, has achieved greater geographic/global dispersion, or has been more widely adapted, than the AA model (White, 2014). AA's reach has extended world-wide and, at present, AA exists in over 180 countries with the Big Book translated into 71 languages (Alcoholics Anonymous, 2018). Narcotics Anonymous (NA) derived from the AA tradition with its first meetings taking place in California during the 1950s. At present, NA meetings take place in more than 130 countries with the Narcotics Anonymous book and pamphlets available in 45 languages (Narcotics Anonymous World Services, Inc, 2014).

The relationship between mutual aid groups, such as AA and NA, and professionally directed addiction treatment is a common theme and point of tension in the contemporary history of addiction treatment, critically shaped by the early history and interaction between AA and alcohol use disorder treatment programs (White, 2014). AA is more clearly elaborated than early descriptions of addiction treatment, and AA is influential in its early approaches to addressing alcohol use disorder as well as for its use in the treatment of other drug problems. Treatment and supports for alcohol use disorder had distinctly been provided in separate intervention approaches and systems of care, whereas other drugs had growth in distinct treatment and support programs later, in the 1950s and 1960s.

Disparate approaches

Narcotic addiction had been framed as both criminal deviance and a health disorder. For example, opioid use disorder may be addressed through "narcotic courts" in the criminal justice system (White, 2014; see Chapter 28). In a medical and psychiatric context, the rise of medication treatment for opioid use disorder began with administering methadone as a treatment in 1964 and continues with various forms of pharmacotherapy treatment (see Chapter 19). Moreover, religious interventions saw their rise in the 1950s and 1960s, as did the use of community-based supports (White, 2014).

Chronic disease

Historically, SUDs were treated as an acute illness with few strategies for long-term disease management and monitoring, but the modern addiction treatment community increasingly began viewing SUDs as a chronic disease at the turn of the 21st century (McLellan, Lewis, O'Brien, & Kleber, 2000). Not all addiction problems are chronic in nature—especially because some individuals who meet the diagnostic criteria for a SUD recover completely, often without engaging with the formal addiction treatment system or informal recovery services and supports (see Chapter 1). However, many entering into addiction treatment experience relapse on multiple occasions. For this reason, continuity of care beyond successive doses of acute treatment should be provided through a continuing care approach attractive to patients, recognizing ongoing cooperation and partnership between patients and the service delivery system (McLellan, 2002).

Recovery movement implications

Among these historical highlight, two factors are important to review before further exploring the recovery addiction movement and the role of social workers in addiction treatment.

First, addiction treatment is arguably unique from other health and social service fields given the historical importance of peer support and mutual aid as an early and continued form of intervention. Trained clinical professionals such as social workers are integral to the addiction treatment system in implementing evidence-based interventions but so are peers whose value comes from their lived experience. Second, the shift toward a chronic disease model to address SUDs holds several implications for the kinds of addiction treatment and recovery support services delivered in a ROSC. A chronic disease model suggests the critical importance of ancillary and community-based services in a comprehensive system of care, including peer-based services and supports, housing, education and employment supports, among others. Further discussion on the role of social workers and other professionals in the delivery of these recovery support services and in developing this comprehensive system of care will follow.

New recovery advocacy movement

Recovery as an organizing framework for addiction services and policies has its roots in the history of peer-based movements and mutual aid groups previously described. It has received revitalized attention in recent decades through grassroots advocacy by individuals in recovery from alcohol and drug problems in what recovery advocacy leaders call the New Recovery Advocacy Movement (White, 2005). This advocacy, in many ways, has patterned itself after the social movement within the HIV/AIDS domain, where individuals living with HIV/AIDS voluntarily identified themselves as living with the stigmatized disease to mobilize and advocate for improved healthcare policies and services, and contribute to its de-stigmatization.

The New Recovery Advocacy Movement has roots in the United States and, arguably, the grassroots advocacy and adoption of recovery-oriented policy and systems change in the United States has influenced similar movements in other countries. Examples from the United States appear in this chapter with evidence of burgeoning movements in other countries when available. Beginning in the late 1990s, the U.S. federal government agency, SAMHSA, supported Recovery Community Organizations (RCOs) to develop leadership, promote local advocacy, and engage the community in public education about SUD treatment and recovery through the Recovery Community Service Program (Humphreys & Lembke, 2014). Since then, an array of recovery-oriented policies, programs, and initiatives have been put in place, including, but not limited to:

- the inclusion of recovery as a goal within the U.S. Office of National Drug Control Policy's National Drug Control Strategy (Laudet & Best, 2015);
- the Access to Recovery (ATR) federal grants to states for voucher-supported treatment and recovery support services;
- the Bringing Recovery Supports to Scale Technical Assistance Center Strategy (BRSS TACS) federal initiative to provide technical assistance to community-based recovery organizations, service providers, and government agencies on the development of ROSC and promotion of peer-based services; and,
- the creation of federal, state, and local government agency administrative roles primarily focused on promoting recovery.

Significant strides were made in Scotland, then the rest of the United Kingdom during the late 2000s (Humphreys & Lembke, 2014). For example, SMART Recovery organizations, an alternative to AA and NA self-help groups, were implemented in 2008 using funding from the National Treatment Agency (NTA) for Substance Misuse (Humphreys & Lembke, 2014). The adoption of recovery-oriented policies in the United Kingdom stems from dissatisfaction with pre-existing addiction treatment systems—much like the recovery advocacy movement in the United States—and the influence of recovery advocates in the United States who offered ideas for potential system reforms (Gilman, 2011; Humphreys & Lembke, 2014).

Other significant gains across the globe are worth noting. For example, there have been comparable efforts to understand the experiences of persons in recovery through the Life in Recovery Study, conducted in 2013 in the United States (Laudet, 2013), 2015 in Australia (Turning Point, Easternhealth, & South Pacific Private, 2015) and the United Kingdom (Best et al., 2015), and in 2017 in Canada (McQuaid et al., 2017). The Life in Recovery Study examined demographic traits of persons in recovery, self-identified costs of substance use problems, and self-identified life improvements achieved through recovery, among other characteristics. This was the first international comparison of its kind. Additionally, only in the past few years, recovery advocacy movements have flourished across the globe, including in Ghana (White, 2018b), Japan (White, 2019), and the Philippines (White, 2018a).

Comparing social work practices and addiction recovery values

The history of addiction treatment and the more contemporary New Recovery Advocacy Movement demonstrate the complicated history and legacy of how alcohol and drug problems have been addressed. Two important questions are: How have social workers historically been involved in addressing alcohol and drug problems? And, what role do they potentially play in supporting this movement toward recovery as a conceptual framework for addiction treatment?

Brief history of social workers addressing alcohol and drug problems

The social work profession has played an important role in addressing alcohol and other drug problems, ranging from the organization of public education initiatives to the delivery of prevention interventions, direct practice in addiction treatment, and long-term recovery support. Stemming back to the days of Charity Organization Societies and the settlement house movement, the social work profession—at least to some extent—has addressed alcohol and other drug problems in the community (DiNitto & McNeece, 2007). However, the extent to which the profession focused on SUD problems has historically been, and continues to be, contested given the arguably limited focus on addiction in social work's education and training (Amodeo & Litchfield, 1999; Straussner, 2001). Moreover, little is known about social work's historical role in promoting recovery-oriented services and policies.

Sarah Tracy's historical examination of alcohol problems in the United States affirms that social workers had an early role in addressing alcohol problems (Tracy, 2005). As early as the 1880s through 1910, trained professional men and middle-class women in particular began to address issues of poverty as they visited homes of immigrant and working-class individuals, "where alcohol was often present even if it was not problematic" (Tracy, 2005, p. 70). "Without question," Tracy recounted, "alcohol appeared to pose the greatest threat to civil order within the urban jungle of the Gilded Age and Progressive Era" (Tracy, 2005, p. 10). In these early days of the profession, social workers and settlement reformers addressed alcohol problems through a range of activities, including assessment through social surveys, addiction treatment in health clinics, and English classes and citizenship education to promote long-term recovery, among other activities (Tracy, 2005, p. 11). Currently, social workers practicing primarily within the domains of child welfare, criminal justice, education, and medicine, among others, can provide screening, early interventions, and service referrals to clients who might be at risk for or are diagnosed with SUDs (DiNitto & McNeece, 2007).

Early social workers, like other health professions at the time, presented arguments about the link between alcohol problems and negative social and health outcomes. "Preventive medicine and psychoanalysis gave [the social work] profession specialized bodies of knowledge that furthered its own claims to professional status, and alcoholism fit within both of these sociomedical contexts" (Tracy, 2005, p. 58). Arguably, the social work profession had a strong emphasis on furthering its status as a profession distinct from other health and social service providers. The implications of this professionalization on recovery-oriented services and policies, however, remain largely unstudied. Even prior to the formalization of AA and NA as widely accepted forms of intervention, mutual aid was an important component of how individuals sought and provided help for their substance use disorder problems. The self-help tradition has remained largely separate from the social work profession and, arguably, social workers in the present-day have had a marginal role in recent efforts to promote advocacy in the recovery community to improve service delivery and transform the system of care.

Aligning social work and recovery values and practices

The National Association of Social Workers' Code of Ethics preamble states that

> the primary mission of the social work profession is to enhance human well-being and help meet the basic human needs of all people, with particular attention to the needs and empowerment of people who are vulnerable, oppressed, and living in poverty.
>
> *(NASW, 2017, para. 2)*

The profession's mission is rooted in core values based on service, social justice, dignity and worth of the person, importance of human relationships, integrity, and competence (NASW, 2017). Social work's emphases on enhancing well-being and the empowerment of vulnerable populations, including those experiencing alcohol and drug problems and impacted by the associated stigma, align with the values of addiction recovery, which emphasize the importance of self-direction and wellness.

A recovery-oriented system of care calls for the transformation of addiction service delivery systems beyond the confounds of professionally delivered services to include a re-centering around communities' indigenous services and supports. The social work profession's person-in-environment emphasis on mezzo- and macro-level systems provides an openness to thinking beyond traditional clinical settings for addiction treatment.

Roles for social workers in promoting recovery

There exists disagreement in the field as to whether the social work workforce receives adequate education and training needed address substance use disorders (see Chapter 37). More specifically, social workers who focus on addiction issues may receive adequate training through field instruction and certification programs to address these problems. However, social workers who are not addiction specialists are often inadequately trained to address substance use problems. This matters because, regardless of their fields of practice, these professionals interface with individuals, families, and communities directly impacted by SUDs and should have, at minimum, the capacity to identify SUDs and make effective referrals to appropriate, evidence-based services. Given efforts to shift addiction service delivery systems toward a recovery-oriented framework, now is an opportune time to consider how social workers and other professionals can promote advancement toward a recovery-oriented system of care. Below, recommendations are offered for social workers within the realms of policy advocacy, community empowerment, and service delivery.

Policy advocacy

Social workers hold the potential to serve many policy roles, including providing input to policymakers, involvement in policy implementation, creating effective policies where none currently exist (Powell, Garrow, Woodford, & Perron, 2013), and conducting research to inform and evaluate policy. First, social workers can and do advocate for changes to current behavioral health policies, including the adoption of recovery-oriented policies, through direct advocacy with policy makers. They provide first-hand experiences and evidence-based testimony about individuals and communities impacted by alcohol and drug problems that include stories of recovery. Second, within social service agencies and organizations, social workers with the right knowledge and training have the expertise, as front-line workers, to implement addiction policies and promote recovery-oriented values and practices, such as ensuring that organizational policy decisions are made in partnership with those who have lived experience. Third, in instances where policies do not currently exist, social workers who have adopted recovery-oriented values possess the skills necessary to create recovery-oriented policies for their local agencies and communities, and even at larger system levels.

Community empowerment

In addition to social workers having the ability to directly participate in policy advocacy to influence recovery-oriented policy change, they also have the ability and responsibility for empowering clients and communities to become civic participants and grassroots advocates. Social workers have skills to work with the recovery community to empower the creation or continued maintenance of RCOs, as well as promote public education efforts focused on stigma reduction and recovery-oriented service delivery and policy reforms.

Service delivery

Within social service agencies, social workers can influence the adoption of recovery-oriented values and practices and the delivery of recovery supports and services, including peer-delivered services. Social workers can ensure that services and practices are not driven solely by professional expertise but that client empowerment and lived experience are also valued. Social workers can also work to ensure the inclusion of persons in recovery on decision-making teams, including peers in the case of care plan decision-making, and on leadership teams that drive organizational decision-making.

Potential barriers and tensions for social workers

Recovery-oriented policy and service delivery system changes face challenges and barriers. It is important to identify barriers that might be faced by social workers and other professionals as they promote addiction recovery. One is a tension that originated in the social work profession in its historical advancement toward professionalization, purposefully distancing itself from mutual aid traditions. Professions built on professional education, training, clinical expertise, diagnosis, and evidence-supported interventions can appropriately embrace as service delivery colleagues peer providers whose training and expertise are lived experience; however, this may create tensions as illustrated in the policy structure for peers providing services in the United States. Medicaid-reimbursable settings. For an agency to receive Medicaid insurance reimbursement covering peer-delivered addiction services, the peer must be directly supervised by a licensed clinical professional, such as a social worker. Professional clinicians, such as social workers, must then learn how to work collaboratively in teams with these peers. Inclusion of peers as service providers may pose a perceived threat to professionally trained service providers who might perceive peer providers as placing their own positions at risk. However, the intent of including peers to provide recovery support services is to facilitate and extend the work of professional providers in improving client access to care, engagement, care transitions, long-term follow-up, outreach, and treatment reengagement.

Conclusions

The addiction recovery advocacy movement embraces client-driven decision-making and community-based policy advocacy and support, values and approaches that align with those of the social work profession. However, there exists an underlying tension between embracing a recovery-oriented system valuing lived experience and professionalization. It is important to understand professionals' roles as trained clinical experts and ancillary service providers, to reduce the potential for "turf wars" with addiction recovery peers. The social work profession needs to understand the complexities of its relationship with the addiction recovery community—as service providers, as community organizing partners, and as clinical supervisors for peers with lived experience.

References

Achara-Abraham, I., Evans, A. C., & King, J. K. (2011). Recovery-focused behavioral health system transformation: A framework for change and lessons learned from Philadelphia. In J. F. Kelly & W. L. White (Eds.), *Addiction recovery management: Theory, research and practice* (pp. 187–208). New York, NY: Humana Press. doi:10.1007/978-1-60327-960-4_11

Alcoholics Anonymous. (2018). *Our twelve traditions: A.A.'s future in the modern world, alcoholics anonymous 2th world service meeting (final report).* Retrieved from https://www.aa.org/assets/en_US/f-150_25th_WSM_finalreport_2018.pdf

Amodeo, M., & Litchfield, L. (1999). Integrating substance abuse content into social work courses: Effects of intensive faculty training. *Substance Abuse, 20*(1), 5–16. doi:10.1080/08897079909511390

Andresen, R., Caputi, P., & Oades, L. (2010). Do clinical outcome measures assess consumer defined recovery? *Psychiatry Research, 177*(3), 309–317. doi:10.1016/j.psychres.2010.02.013

Best, D., Albertson, K., Irving, J., Lightowlers, C., Mama-Rudd, A., & Chaggar, A. (2015). *UK life in recovery survey 2015: The first national UK survey of addiction recovery experiences.* Sheffield, UK: Helena Kennedy Centre for International Justice.

Best, D., De Alwis, S. J., & Burdett, D. (2017). The recovery movement and its implications for policy, commissioning and practice. *Nordic Studies on Alcohol and Drugs, 34*(2), 107–111. doi:10.1177/1455072517691058

Betty Ford Institute Consensus Panel. (2007). What is recovery? A working definition from the Betty Ford Institute *Journal of Substance Abuse Treatment, 33*(3), 221–228. doi:10.1016/j.jsat.2007.06.001

Borkman, T., Kaskutas, L. A., & Owen, P. (2007). Contrasting and converging philosophies of three models of alcohol/other drugs treatment: Minnesota model, social model, and addiction therapeutic communities. *Alcoholism Treatment Quarterly, 25*(3), 21–38. doi:10.1300/J020v25n03_03

Center for Substance Abuse Treatment (CSAT). (2007). *National summit on recovery: Conference report* (SMA) 07-4276. Rockville, MD: Substance Abuse and Mental Health Services Administration. Retrieved from https://www.samhsa.gov/sites/default/files/partnersforrecovery/docs/Summit_Rpt_1.pdf

DiNitto, D. M., & McNeece, C. A. (2007). Additions and social work practice. In D. M. DiNitto & C. A. McNeece (Eds.), *Social work: Issues and opportunities in a challenging profession* (pp. 171–192). Chicago, IL: Lyceum Books.

Gilman, M. (2011). Founding fathers of the contemporary UK recovery movement. *Druglink, 26,* 12–13.

Hser, Y. I., & Anglin, M. D. (2011). Addiction treatment and recovery careers. In J. F. Kelly & W. L. White (Eds.), *Addiction recovery management: Theory, research and practice* (pp. 9–29). New York, NY: Humana Press. doi:10.1007/978-1-60327-960-4_2

Humphreys, K., & Lembke, A. (2014). Recovery-oriented policy and care systems in the UK and USA. *Drug and Alcohol Review, 33*(1), 13–18. doi:10.1111/dar.12092

Humphreys, K., & McLellan, A. T. (2010). Brief intervention, treatment, and recovery support services for Americans who have substance use disorders: An overview of policy in the Obama administration. *Psychological Services, 7*(4), 275–284. doi:10.1037/a0020390

Kaskutas, L. A., Borkman, T. J., Laudet, A. B., Ritter, L. A., Witbrodt, J., Subbaraman, M. S., & Bond, J. (2014). Elements that define recovery: The experiential perspective. *Journal of Studies on Alcohol & Drugs, 75*(6), 999–1010. doi:10.15288/jsad.2014.75.999

Kelly, J. F., Bergman, B., Hoeppner, B. B., Vilsaint, C., & White, W. L. (2017). Prevalence and pathways of recovery from drug and alcohol problems in the United States population: Implications for practice, research, and policy. *Drug & Alcohol Dependence, 181,* 162–169. doi:10.1016/j.drugalcdep.2017.09.028

Kirk, T. A. (2011). Connecticut's journey to a statewide recovery-oriented health-care system: Strategies, successes, and challenges. In J. F. Kelly & W. L. White (Eds.), *Addiction recovery management: Theory, research and practice* (pp. 209–234) New York, NY: Humana Press. doi:10.1007/978-1-60327-960-4_12

Kurtz, E. (1991). *Not god: A history of alcoholics anonymous.* Center City, MN: Hazelden Publishing.

Laudet, A. B. (2007). What does recovery mean to you? Lessons from the recovery experience for research and practice. *Journal of substance abuse treatment, 33*(3), 243–256. doi:10.1016/j.jsat.2007.04.014

Laudet, A. B. (2013). *"Life in recovery": Report of the survey findings.* Washington, DC: Faces and Voices of Recovery.

Laudet, A., & Best, D. (2015). Addiction recovery in services and policy: An international overview. In N. el-Guebaly, G. Carrà, & M. Galanter, (Eds.), Textbook of addiction treatment: International perspective, (pp. 1065–1083). New York, NY: Springer.

Laudet, A. B., & Humphreys, K. (2013). Promoting recovery in an evolving policy context: What do we know and what do we need to know about recovery support services? *Journal of Substance Abuse Treatment, 45*(1), 126–133. doi:10.1016/j.jsat.2013.01.009

McLellan, A. T. (2002). Have we evaluated addiction treatment correctly? Implications from a chronic care perspective. *Addiction, 97*(3), 249–252. doi:10.1046/j.1360-0443.2002.00127.x

McLellan, A. T., Lewis, D. C., O'Brien, C. P., & Kleber, H. D. (2000). Drug dependence, a chronic medical illness: Implications for treatment, insurance, and outcomes evaluation. *Journal of the American Medical Association* (JAMA), *284*(13), 1689–1695. doi: 10.1001/jama.284.13.1689

McQuaid, R. J., Malik, A., Moussouni, K., Baydack, N., Stargardter, M., & Morrisey, M. (2017). *Life in recovery from addiction in Canada.* Ottawa, Canada: Canadian Centre on Substance Use and Addiction.

Narcotics Anonymous World Services, Inc. (2014). *Information about NA.* Retrieved from https://www.na.org/admin/include/spaw2/uploads/pdf/PR/Information_about_NA.pdf

National Association of Social Workers. (2017). *Code of ethics of the national association of social workers.* Retrieved from https://www.socialworkers.org/About/Ethics/Code-of-Ethics/Code-of-Ethics-English

Powell, T. J., Garrow, E., Woodford, M. R., & Perron, B. (2013). Policymaking opportunities for direct practice social workers in mental health and addiction services. *Advances in Social Work, 14*(2), 367–378. doi:10.18060/2227

Straussner, S. L. A. (2001). The role of social workers in the treatment of addictions. *Journal of Social Work Practice in the Addictions, 1*(1), 3–9. doi:10.1300/J160v01n01_02

Substance Abuse and Mental Health Services Administration (SAMHSA). (2010). *Recovery-oriented systems of care (ROSC) resource guide.* Retrieved from http://www.samhsa.gov/sites/default/files/rosc_resource_guide_book.pdf

Substance Abuse and Mental Health Services Administration (SAMHSA). (2012, March 23). *SAMHSA's working definition of recovery updated.* Retrieved from http://blog.samhsa.gov/2012/03/23/defintion-of-recovery-updated/

Tracy, S. W. (2005). *Alcoholism in America: From reconstruction to prohibition.* Baltimore, MD: Johns Hopkins University Press.

Turning Point, Easternhealth, & South Pacific Private. (2015). *The Australian life in recovery survey.* Retrieved from https://www.rec-path.co.uk/wp-content/uploads/2017/10/2015_au_life_in_recovery_survey.pdf

White, W. L. (2005). Recovery: Its history and renaissance as an organizing construct concerning alcohol and other drug problems. *Alcoholism Treatment Quarterly, 23*(1), 3–15. doi:10.1300/J020v23n01_02

White, W. L. (2008). *Recovery management and recovery-oriented systems of care: Scientific rationale and promising practices.* Chicago, IL: Great Lakes Addiction Technology Transfer Center, Northeast Addiction Technology Transfer Center, and Philadelphia Department of Behavioral Health and Mental Retardation Services. Retrieved from http://attcnetwork.org/regcenters/productDocs/3/RM_ROSC%20Scientific.pdf

White, W. L. (2014). *Slaying the dragon: The history of addiction treatment and recovery in America.* Bloomington, IL: Chestnut Health Systems.

White, W. L. (2018a, September 28). Recovery advocacy in the Philippines, Bill White and Emily G. Mora [Blog post]. Retrieved from http://www.williamwhitepapers.com/blog/2018/09/recovery-advocacy-in-the-philippines-bill-white-and-emily-g-mora.html

White, W. L. (2018b, November 26). Recovery celebration and advocacy in Ghana, Africa [Blog post]. Retrieved from http://www.williamwhitepapers.com/blog/2018/11/recovery-celebration-and-advocacy-in-ghana-africa.html

White, W. L. (2019, May 23). Recovery advocacy in Japan [Blog post]. Retrieved from http://www.williamwhitepapers.com/blog/2019/05/recovery-advocacy-in-japan.html

White, W. L., & Kelly, J.F. (2011). Introduction: The theory, science, and practice of recovery management. In J. F. Kelly & W. L. White (Eds.), *Addiction recovery management: Theory, research and practice* (pp. 1–6). New York, NY: Humana Press. doi:10.1007/978-1-60327-960-4_1

Policy reforms to reduce harms associated with substance misuse

Sheila P. Vakharia and Jeannie Little

Background

Drug policy is "any targeted effort on the part of governments to minimize or prevent drug use and drug-related harm to both individuals and society" (Babor et al., 2010, p. 97). These policies fall into two major categories: supply reduction and demand reduction (National Research Council, 2001). Supply reduction policies aim to decrease or eliminate availability of certain drugs. Globally, the primary supply reduction policies:

- create restrictions and regulations intended to limit or eliminate access to certain drugs;
- fund law enforcement to target drug supply chains domestically and internationally; and
- fund the eradication of drug crops (i.e. cannabis, coca, and opium) domestically and internationally (Murphy, 1994).

Meanwhile, demand reduction policies aim to decrease or eliminate drug use and related harms. Demand reduction policies support:

- drug prevention programming and messaging;
- drug treatment and rehabilitation; and
- harm reduction interventions (e.g. naloxone access, syringe access, alternatives to impaired driving).

Drug policies in the United States over the past century

The United States has incorporated both supply and demand reduction strategies in a multifaceted approach over the past century (Babor et al., 2010). Law enforcement and incarceration efforts toward supply reduction, aimed to deter the use and availability of drugs deemed "illicit," have led to mixed results. America's current relationship with drugs demonstrates that illicit drug use did not stop with each subsequent prohibitive policy: it has persisted, sometimes with an increase or a shift in the choice of drugs favored. In addition, the fallacy that drug laws were passed to protect public health has been refuted with ample evidence that racist and xenophobic caricatures of people who use drugs (PWUD) often mobilized and motivated increased criminalization.

Before the early 20th century, Americans frequently (and legally) used substances such as cannabis, alcohol, cocaine, and opiates without restriction (Bancroft, 2009). These substances could be purchased in various forms and amounts, often through mail order, chemists, stores, and other establishments. These substances held distinct places within American society for both medicinal and recreational use (Musto, 1973).

Opium and cocaine

Opium was imported into the United States as early as the 1700s, and was subject to no limitation other than a moderate tariff, for many decades (Musto, 1973). Many found opium useful in treating anxiety and nervous disorders, gastrointestinal problems, respiratory problems, menstrual cramps, and other ailments (DeGrandpre, 2006). It was often consumed orally, in the form of tonics, syrups, or lozenges, and sale was heavily targeted to middle- and upper-class women. Opium smoking was associated with Chinese immigrant laborers, though some Americans smoked it recreationally. At the time, Chinese workers were increasingly viewed as a competitive employment threat to Americans, casting a negative shadow over opium smoking. San Francisco passed the first ordinance in the United States against opium smoking in 1875, contending that opium dens (frequented by Chinese immigrants) tempted American men, women, and children into immorality (Davenport-Hines, 2001).

The Opium Exclusion Act of 1909 was the first federal drug prohibition law passed by the U.S. Congress. It made the import and non-medical use of opium illegal. This law specifically applied to processed opium intended for smoking (Davenport-Hines, 2001). Other forms of opium for "medical" use remained legal, such as forms that could be ingested or injected. It should be noted that the legislation targeted the most common route of administration by Chinese immigrants while the average opium consumers at the time—white, middle-aged housewives—continued to legally consume opium in forms they preferred (Degrandpre, 2006; Musto, 1973).

Cocaine shares a similar history: a medically used substance criminalized after being linked to a "dangerous" or threatening minority group (Musto, 1973). Cocaine's popularity beginning in the mid-1800s grew rapidly, and its import reached a peak near the turn of the 20th century, much like opium (Davenport-Hines, 2001). Cocaine was distinct from opiates because of its exhilarating and energizing effects, as well as its promise in increasing worker productivity.

Cocaine was added to beverages and medicinal tonics with the belief that it could heal a plethora of ailments and was even offered as a valid treatment for morphine addiction and alcoholism (Musto, 1973). Habitual cocaine use cocaine was minimized as a problem because it did not create the same physiological withdrawal symptoms as opiates, although anecdotal reports from the time acknowledged that some individuals were prone to overuse cocaine. Cocaine was cheap and readily accessible. However, as its use spread to the Southern United States, concerns grew about its impact on the black community even though the white community more commonly used the substance. "The fear of the cocainized black coincided with the peak of lynchings, legal segregation, and voting laws all designed to remove political and social power from him" (Musto, 1973, p. 7).

Early prohibition

The federal Harrison Narcotics Tax Act of 1914 laid the foundation for American drug prohibition policy up until 1970 (Musto, 1973). Narcotics were defined in the law as any drug derived from opium or coca leaves; however, the medical definition of "narcotic" applied to substances that cause numbness or stupor, such as opiates or alcohol (Narcotic, n.d.). The Harrison Act resulted in narcotics being subject to stringent government controls on distribution, import, production, sales, and use. Possession or use of a narcotic was legal only with a valid medical prescription written by a physician, and physicians were required to keep record of all written prescriptions for at least two years. Individuals who violated the act were not necessarily subject to federal law, but individual states could criminalize the possession of certain drugs (Davenport-Hines, 2001).

The Jones-Miller Narcotic Drugs Import and Export Act of 1922 provided additional restrictions, and explicitly articulated maximum fines and prison terms for import and distribution violations of the Harrison Act. Narcotic possession without a prescription became a federal crime (DeGrandpre, 2006). By 1924, The Heroin Act made manufacture of heroin illegal in the United States. In 1934, the federal Uniform State Narcotic Drug Act was passed to ensure that every state had, at minimum, additional punitive and enforcement clauses for narcotics, because the Harrison Act was viewed as insufficient in deterring their manufacture and distribution (Musto, 1973).

Cannabis

The history of cannabis in the United States is not marked by as much widespread use (or controversy) as opium and cocaine were in the late 1800s and early 1900s (Musto, 1973).

Similarly, cannabis was first valued for its potential medicinal benefits. Yet, cannabis fears grew in the Southwest United States and spread during the late 1920s, largely influenced by racial fears (Musto, 1973). By then, the number of Mexican laborers and immigrants had increased in response to demand from the agricultural sector. They were regarded with growing suspicion by white Americans, and recreational use of cannabis by Mexican immigrants was depicted as contributing to violence and criminality (Davenport-Hines, 2001). In response to pressure from local municipalities and governors, the federal government passed the Marijuana Tax Act in 1937; this act was later ruled unconstitutional. Note that advocates for cannabis criminalization strategically referred to cannabis as "marijuana" with the intent to strengthen xenophobic fears about this supposedly "foreign" substance (DeGrandpre, 2006).

The Boggs Act, passed in 1951, was the first to place cannabis into narcotics policy. This act instituted the first mandatory sentences for violating existing state and federal drug laws. It was passed at a time when fears about young people using drugs were growing, and a time of strong McCarthyism fears, including suspicions of China profiting from American drug money (Musto, 1973). By 1956, the Narcotic Drug Control Act was passed, creating minimum prison terms ranging into years for even first-time drug offenses; multiple convictions could lead to subsequently lengthier sentences. This was, so far, the most punitive federal drug legislation passed in the United States to date and would be for decades to come.

The modern war on drugs

The modern War on Drugs was officially declared in 1970, when the Comprehensive Drug Abuse Prevention and Control Act was passed by the U.S. Congress and signed into law

Table 30.1 Current U.S. drug scheduling system

Schedule	Characteristics	Examples
I	"Substances or chemicals defined as drugs with no currently accepted medical use and a high potential for abuse"	Heroin, lysergic acid diethylamide (LSD), cannabis, ecstasy
II	"Substances or chemicals are defined as drugs with a high potential for abuse, with use potentially leading to severe psychological or physical dependence."	Cocaine, methamphetamine, methadone, fentanyl, Adderall
III	"Substances or chemicals are defined as drugs with a moderate to low potential for physical and psychological dependence."	Ketamine, anabolic steroids
IV	"Substances or chemicals are defined as drugs with a low potential for abuse and a low risk of dependence"	Xanax, Valium, Ativan, Ambien, Tramadol
V	"Substances or chemicals are defined as drugs with lower potential for abuse than Schedule IV and consist of preparations containing limited quantities of certain narcotics."	Lyrica

Note: Updated information can be obtained directly from the Drug Enforcement Agency (n.d.)

by President Nixon who was quoted as saying: "The war on drugs is our second civil war" (Davenport-Hines, 2001, p. 339). The policy focused on both domestic law enforcement and international interdiction, instituting a five-level scheduling system to rank drugs on various criteria, including medicinal use and potential for abuse; see Table 30.1 (Drug Enforcement Agency, n.d.). The intent was to enhance tight controls by the U.S. Drug Enforcement Agency. Ironically, the law has made it extremely difficult for medical researchers studying harms and benefits, to obtain these drugs for their research that has limited such knowledge even today. The Act also lifted the mandatory minimum sentences implemented in the 1954 policy. Finally, unlike any prior federal drug policy, the Act also provided for funding of addiction treatment, research, and prevention efforts (Musto, 1973).

The Reagan-era Anti-Drug Abuse Act passed in 1986 responded to the perception of a growing crack cocaine problem in some parts of the nation (Musto, 1973). Crack cocaine, a relatively cheap version of cocaine, was viewed differently from other drugs on the market (including powder cocaine), although its depiction clearly hearkened back to early drug hysteria driving earlier U.S. drug laws (Davenport-Hines, 2001). The sale and use of crack cocaine in poor, minority neighborhoods was sensationalized in the media, as were births of "crack babies;" white populations used powder cocaine at comparable rates (Reinarman & Levine, 1997). The new anti-drug abuse legislation was intended to address a perceived growing drug use problem in general, but crack use in particular (Beaver, 2010).

Arguably, the most controversial law included as part of this legislation was the Narcotics Penalties and Enforcement Act that created new minimum sentencing laws. Of note was their differential application to powder and crack cocaine (Beaver, 2010; Davenport-Hines, 2001; Reinarman & Levine, 1997). A 100:1 ratio was created in which the penalties for possession of crack cocaine would be equivalent to penalties for 100 times the amount of powder cocaine (i.e. 10 grams of crack cocaine would lead to penalties equivalent for 1,000 grams of powder cocaine). Policy makers justified this disparity based on inflated claims about crack cocaine's addictiveness and harmfulness. However, this disparity was driven by the differential perception of *who* used these substances rather than true pharmacological difference (Beaver, 2010).

Recognizing this and other drivers of the nation's biased mass incarceration problems, the Obama administration reduced the sentencing disparity to 18:1 and eliminated the mandatory minimum for first-time crack offenses when the Fair Sentencing Act was passed in 2010.

Other troubling subtitles included in the 1986 Anti-Drug Abuse Act expanded and militarized the criminalization of drugs, making the pursuit of drug charges more profitable for police departments and communities. These included allowances for the government to seize assets of individuals arrested for drug offenses, penalties for money laundering of illegal drug distribution profits, and even the potential application of the death penalty for certain drug offenses (Library of Congress, n.d.). The second title of the Act focused on international narcotics control, a supply reduction strategy, and the stipulation that countries that do not cooperate with American anti-drug efforts within their own countries could be subject to tariffs. Latin American countries were among those targeted and recruited into greater anti-drug efforts within their borders (Corva, 2008). The Act's third title primarily involved the coordination/cooperation of the Department of Defense, the Drug Enforcement Agency, and U.S. Customs in monitoring and law enforcement. A 1988 amendments to the act revised minimum penalties, established drug-free America as a policy goal, and formalized the Office of National Drug Control Policy (ONDCP).

Budgeting for drug policies

Drug policy enforcement requires substantial federal, state, and local funding. The ONDCP budget for fiscal year 2018 funded supply reduction policies with 56.3% of their total allocation ($15.6 billion), and demand reduction policies with 43.7% ($12.1 billion) (ONDCP, 2017).

Figure 30.1 depicts the proposed allocation of funds from the budget, divided by function. Notably, funds allocated for prevention in fiscal year 2018 decreased by 11.1% and U.S. federal dollars rarely, if ever, support harm reduction interventions, unlike other nations, particularly in Western Europe.

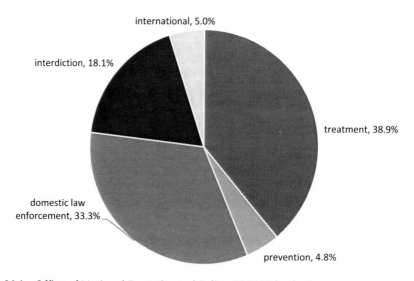

Figure 30.1 Office of National Drug Control Policy FY 2018 budget

Since the late 1800s, the United States has increasingly chosen to prioritize a criminal justice response to illicit drug use, as demonstrated in the laws and spending priorities. Maintaining a criminal justice response is costly for local, state, and federal governments—from hiring police, staffing court and legal proceedings, staffing jails and prisons, and other expenses. A 2010 report suggested that ending drug prohibition and legalizing drugs would save local and state governments $25.6 billion and the federal government could save $15.6 billion per year (Miron & Waldock, 2010). Expenditures on criminalization and punishment often come at the expense of responses to drug use that prioritize prevention, treatment, and health. The U.S. War on Drugs has fundamentally changed the landscape, both domestically and internationally, by expanding the criminal justice system and all systems of surveillance in the name of targeting illicit drug use. The increasing harshness of these policies has been largely responsible for the exponential expansion in the U.S. prison system, which has contributed to the current situation of criminalization and to the United States having the largest prison population in the world (Alexander, 2012). Moving from mass incarceration to smart decarceration requires alternatives to current U.S. drug policy (Pettus-Davis & Epperson, 2015).

Notable drug policy reforms

Reforms have occurred in the United States and internationally in the decades since these initial policies were passed. In the United States, cannabis policies have undergone tremendous state-level revisions since the 1970s although federal prohibition remains intact. The first states passed cannabis decriminalization in the late 1970s; decriminalization policy varies but is passing in increasing numbers of states (NORML, 2019). By the 1990s, states began to pass medicalization laws to allow some patients to consume marijuana as a treatment for some conditions and now over half of all U.S. states allow some form of medicinal access. Recreational use is also becoming increasingly legalized.

In 2001, Portugal became the first country in the world to decriminalize the personal possession of drugs by turning it into an administrative offense and offering treatment on demand to those who may want or need it (Domostawski, 2011). Several Andean countries, including Bolivia and Peru, have adopted national policies that allow for indigenous uses of coca-derived products once again, after decades of prohibition. In recent years, Canada and Uruguay both lifted their own federal prohibition of cannabis as well.

A readily available, unregulated drug supply

The availability of illicit drugs remains high in the United States and abroad. The U.S. Drug Enforcement Agency (DEA), federal, state, and local law enforcement are tasked with implementing and tracking supply-side policies in the United States to reduce access to illicit and controlled drugs. According to the 2018 *National Drug Threat Assessment,* the availability of heroin, fentanyl, cocaine, marijuana, methamphetamine, and controlled medicines continues to increase or remains high in the United States (United States Department of Justice, 2018). The *2018 World Drug Report* compiled by the United Nations Office on Drugs and Crime (UNODC) also indicates that global drug markets are increasing, and drug crops have increased in recent years (UNODC, 2018). These increases occurred despite billions of dollars spent on crop elimination, drug interdiction, and other efforts to restrict drug supplies.

One in nine Americans over the age of 12 (30.5 million) in 2017 reported that they used an illicit drug in the previous month (SAMHSA, 2018a). Cannabis is the most widely used illicit drug in the United States; stimulant drugs (prescription stimulant medications, methamphetamine, and cocaine) are the next most commonly misused class of drugs (SAMHSA, 2018a). Cannabis and stimulant drugs are also the most commonly used drugs globally, with regional variations in rates of use (UNODC, 2018). Illicit drug use and the misuse of prescription drugs (i.e. opioids, stimulants, sedatives, and tranquilizers) are substantially higher in the United States than many other countries. Globally, it is estimated that 5.6% of the population aged 15–64 (275 million) misused drugs in the past year, and 31 million experienced a drug use disorder (UNODC, 2018).

Since illicit drugs are produced and distributed without regulatory oversight, they are of unknown purity and intensity, and may contain a wide array of adulterants; together these factors increase risks for unintentional overdose and other adverse health effects. Increased enforcement and drug seizures (the "iron law of prohibition") disrupt supply chains incentivize suppliers to add adulterants (e.g. fentanyl-enhanced heroin), masking lower quality or diluted drugs (Beletsky & Davis, 2017). Supply-side focus on a single drug (e.g. opioid misuse) can also shift the market to other drugs (e.g. heroin). Although America's current overdose crisis was initially driven by prescription opioids, it has actually occurred in three waves, starting with prescription opioids, shifting to street heroin, and transitioning to a fentanyl-adulterated heroin supply (Ciccarone, 2019).

Mass criminalization and racial disparities

As previously noted, U.S. drug policy has been influenced by racial and ethnic stereotypes of "prototypical drug users," resulting in targeted/disparate policing, enforcement, and sentencing across racial and ethnic lines. During 2016, over 1.25 million people were arrested in the United States on drug-related charges, including roughly 80,000 youth under the age of 18, most commonly for cannabis (Federal Bureau of Investigations [FBI], 2017). Drug offenses constituted the highest number of arrests in the United States, more than all violent crimes combined. Persons of color were disproportionately arrested on drug charges: 20% identified as Latinx/Hispanic and 26.7% as African-American/black. Arrest rates for all classes of illicit drugs were significantly higher within minority than white groups despite comparable rates of drug use in the United States.

Although arrests do not necessarily lead to incarceration, they can lead to pretrial detention when an individual cannot post bail. Pretrial detention accounted for 67,000 of the over 80,000 Americans jailed for drug offenses on any given day of 2015 (Drug Policy Alliance, 2017).

Arrest can also lead to community supervision: an ever-expanding tool of surveillance for individuals convicted of drug charges, whether in lieu of incarceration or post-release. A recent report suggested that almost 1 million individuals on probation in the United States (25% of those on probation) and over 260,000 on parole (1/3 of those on parole) had a drug charge as the most serious offense for which they were under supervision (Drug Policy Alliance, 2017). While individuals on probation or parole are not incarcerated, they experience intensive surveillance, must adhere to strict guidelines, and violation of terms can lead to incarceration. In other words, arrest and sentencing policies contribute to inequities and mass incarceration with no added benefit of protecting society from criminal violence.

In addition, arrest records contribute to collateral consequences and lost opportunities. Collateral consequences are institutionalized in policies such as those dictating eligibility for federal financial aid, public housing residency, voter registration, and opportunities to pursue certain professional licenses and credentials (National Inventory of Collateral Consequences of Conviction, 2019). Other collateral consequences are due to stigma associated with arrest or conviction history appearing on a background check, including those conducted by private landlords, neighbors, potential employers, and others. The history of a drug conviction can also lead to harsher, enhanced sentences for any subsequent charges, particularly in jurisdictions with "third strike" laws and other mandatory minimum policies.

Racial and ethnic disparities in enforcement of drug laws and the harsh impact of incarceration disproportionately affect families and communities of color. Collateral consequences of arrest and a criminal record deny communities of color opportunities for educational and professional advancement, thereby contributing to reduced generational wealth and perpetuating systems of poverty. These harsh consequences drive larger systemic and institutional racial disparities.

Treatment and criminalization

Utilization of specialty substance use treatment remains low in the United States and globally. In the United States, it is estimated that just over 12% of all individuals who meet criteria for a substance use disorder receive treatment through a specialty treatment facility, and it is estimated that one in six people (roughly 15%) needing drug abuse treatment globally received it in the past year (SAMHSA, 2018a; UNODC, 2018). Surveys consistently reveal that barriers to treatment include high thresholds for engagement such as abstinence-only requirements, affordability, and accessibility (SAMHSA, 2018a).

Up to 33% of substance use treatment admissions across the United States in 2017 involved referrals from the criminal justice system, with some programs receiving a majority of their referrals this way (SAMHSA, 2018b). Although individuals experiencing substance use disorders are offered treatment rather than incarceration, the increasing relationship between drug treatment and the criminal justice system can overwhelm the treatment system, especially where treatment providers are inexperienced or ill-equipped to meet the challenge of working with a criminal justice-involved population. Recognizing this and the prevalence of substance use disorders among persons involved in the criminal justice system, policy increasingly supports treatment alternatives to incarceration (see Chapter 28). Individuals may complete substance use treatment in lieu of incarceration, complete substance use treatment while on parole or probation, or have their adjudicated case moved to a drug treatment/recovery court. Treatment court is an option offered to individuals willing to participate in court-prescribed and monitored treatment plans with the possibility of suspended, deferred, or modified sentences at successful completion (Csete & Tomasini-Joshi, 2015). Non-compliance or discharges from treatment may be met with various sanctions, including incarceration.

The potential exists for coercion in these referral systems. Treatment engagement under threat of incarceration becomes less than truly voluntary, and enforcing treatment compliance, including monitoring progress and protected health information, can jeopardize treatment progress and privacy. Involvement of the criminal justice system in treatment decisions potentially presents ethical challenges. For example, evidence-based treatments such as medication-assisted treatments for opioid use disorder may not be encouraged or supported by the directing court. Or, for example, court mandate to attend mutual aid support groups grounded in the 12-steps may violate individual freedom of religion rights.

Another challenge of this nexus is that the majority of jails and prisons do not provide specialty or evidence-based treatment to help individuals address their substance use problems, even though individuals experiencing substance use problems are overrepresented in these settings. This has contributed to exacerbating the overdose crisis as individuals undergo a forced abstinent period during incarceration and may attempt to renew use at pre-arrest doses, leading to overdose if their drug tolerance shifted during abstinence. Recent data collected in New York City demonstrated that individuals experiencing opioid use disorders were eight times more likely than non-incarcerated individuals to die of an overdose within the first two weeks following release from incarceration (Lim et al., 2012).

Medication-assisted treatment

The criminal justice system is not the only system with limited capacity for treating opioid use disorder in the United States and abroad. Although medication-assisted treatments such as buprenorphine and methadone combined with behavioral treatment are known as the gold standard for treating opioid use disorder (see Chapters 18 and 19), access to these treatments remains low in the community. A recent international review reported that only 86 countries provide access to methadone or buprenorphine (Stone & Shirley-Beavan, 2018). Although both medications are available in the United States and utilization rates are increasing, studies show that extensive barriers to access remain, and the majority of individuals experiencing opioid use disorders do not receive either medication. By policy, buprenorphine must be prescribed by a specially trained and waivered medical provider; a recent study showed that over half of all rural counties in the United States do not have a single waivered prescriber (Andrilla, Moore, Patterson, & Larson, 2019). A 2017 review of over 13,000 publicly funded treatment facilities in the United States demonstrated that only 29% made buprenorphine available, and only 10% provide methadone (SAMHSA, 2018c). Only 32% of patients admitted to publicly funded treatment programs for treatment of an opioid use disorder in the United States were going to be initiated onto medication (SAMHSA, 2018b).

Co-occurring disorders

Treating co-occurring substance use and mental health disorders is also limited in current systems; these problems co-occur at high rates in criminal justice-involved populations. In 2017, 92% of substance abuse treatment programs in the United States reported having clients experiencing co-occurring mental health disorders (SAMHSA, 2018c; see Chapter 33). Yet policy does not require programs to address co-occurring mental health disorders: only 74% of programs screened for mental health disorders, 52% offered comprehensive assessment or diagnosis, and 44% offered psychiatric medications. Despite this, and despite the lack of mental health training of substance use counselors, 68% reported that they provided some kind of mental health counseling (SAMHSA, 2018c).

Criminalization and public health

Criminalization of drug use has a negative impact on public health.

Infectious disease exposure

Injecting drugs raises risk for HIV exposure due in large part to limited availability of sterile syringes and injecting equipment. Sharing used equipment allows for blood-borne transmission of between individuals. Criminalization can also encourage high-risk injecting practices such as rushed injection in unsafe environments as means of avoiding police detection, particularly for individuals experiencing homelessness or housing instability. In recent years, Hepatitis C has overtaken HIV as the most common blood-born infection associated with drug injection (Des Jarlais et al., 2018). Both infections are completely preventable through public health and harm reduction measures, such as the provision of sterile syringes injecting equipment, and access to Safer Consumption Spaces for consuming pre-obtained drugs in a sterile setting. However, criminalization of drug use and drug paraphernalia laws limits availability of these public health interventions and makes them politically and economically challenging to implement.

In addition, incarceration carries its own health risks for individuals who use drugs. Drug use does occur within jails and prisons. Due to lack of access to sterile injecting equipment and lack of access to medication-assisted treatments, HIV and Hepatitis C transmission rates are higher among incarcerated populations compared to those not incarcerated (Csete et al., 2016).

Overdose

Globally, it is estimated that over 167,000 individuals died of drug-related overdose during 2015 (UNODC, 2018); over 70,000 in the United States during 2017, and this number has been steadily increasing over the past decade (Scholl, Seth, Kariisa, Wilson, & Baldwin, 2019). The increased all-cause mortality rate among middle-aged non-Hispanic white Americans at least partially can be attributed to the disturbingly high overdose rate among Americans for the first time in generations (Case & Deaton, 2015).

The overdose crisis is exacerbated by the criminalization of drugs: policing and fear of arrest have played a notable role in perpetuating the crisis. The presence of police officers during first responder overdose calls is a perceived barrier to seeking help (Latimore & Bergstein, 2017).

Overdose often occurs in settings where others also use drugs; bystanders may be arrested for drug/paraphernalia possession and probation/parole and although Good Samaritan Laws offer some protections to those calling 911 in good faith, even they do not protect all bystanders at an overdose scene. Recently, jurisdictions are seeing increases in bystander homicide charges or charges against individuals who procured the drugs causing an overdose (Peterson et al., 2019).

Drug policy reform advocacy: a social work opportunity

Social workers are committed to solving societal problems by challenging social injustice and addressing environmental factors that cause or contribute to them (National Association of Social Workers [NASW], 2017). In a diverse range of roles and practice settings, social workers witness the harms of punitive and prohibitionist drug policies; sometimes even being complicit in perpetrating harms. The lasting impact of drug-related arrest, conviction, and/ or incarceration results in family separation, denied opportunity, and access for millions, particularly within the most marginalized communities. At an international level, farmers of drug crops may have few alternative economic opportunities, and individuals living in drug transit countries face violence connected to illicit drug trade. Policy advocacy is one avenue through which social workers can address these problems. Professional values and ethics compel us to think critically about policy paradigms that undermine well-being and ways we can advocate for humane and compassionate alternatives.

The U.S. National Association of Social Workers released a social justice brief entitled *A Social Work Perspective on Drug Policy Reform: A Public Health Approach*, identifying the following drug policy problems: (1) "over-incarceration" (p. 1) and "over-criminalization" (p. 3) of persons convicted of non-violent drug possession, (2) racial disparities in drug arrests, and (3) current approaches maintaining the cycle of poverty among people struggling to reintegrate following release from incarceration (NASW, 2013). NASW supports a criminal justice response for "violent drug crimes and drug trafficking, while simultaneously reducing criminal prosecution and incarceration of low-level drug offenders" (NASW, 2013, p. 5).

The brief provides little detail concerning *how* to reduce drug-related prosecutions or incarceration, but stresses the need for greater access to incarceration alternatives and substance use treatment. Although the brief intended to offer a social work and public health perspective, it retained criminal justice system language (using terms like "offender") and did not challenge assumptions that non-violent drug charges required contact with law enforcement or the criminal justice system at all. Nor were concrete solutions proposed to reduce racial disparities and the lasting impacts of drug convictions.

The social work profession's relative inattention substance use policy is highlighted by a relative lack of training; few social work programs offer even single courses, let alone opportunities for specialization, wherein drug policy would be explored (Bowen & Redmond, 2016; Vakharia, 2014). As a result, social work students and practitioners are provided with little space to explore and question dominant conceptualizations of illicit drug use that drive punitive drug policy: those at the intersection of moralism, racism, sexism, classism, and xenophobia.

Harm reduction as a policy framework

A harm reduction perspective toward drug use acknowledges that individuals will use drugs, and that pragmatic solutions ensure that individuals who do use them can remain as safe and healthy as possible. Such policies promote public health over punishment and can increase access to life-saving treatments for individuals needing them.

Decriminalization

Decriminalization of all drugs is a viable drug policy reform to work toward. For example, the Portuguese experiment in decriminalization is now approaching two decades of implementation. They have found that rates of drug use did not climb, blood-borne infection rates (e.g. HIV and viral hepatitis) have decreased, and individuals who use drugs are connected to harm reduction services and treatment rather than criminalized (Domostawski, 2011). The world has been watching the Portugal experience: in fact, the United Nations Chief Executive Board, representing 31 UN agencies, released a statement in January of 2019 supporting drug decriminalization as a path forward to ensure both the human rights of individuals who use drugs and protection of public health (United Nations Chief Executive Board, 2019).

Although drug decriminalization may be challenging to implement in the short term, policy solutions at the municipal level can reduce harms associated with drug criminalization. For example, Law Enforcement Assisted Diversion (LEAD) programs allow police officers encountering someone using drugs to connect them to case workers who link them to services, diverting them from criminal justice system involvement. Seattle's LEAD program for individuals who use and/or sell drugs showed positive results for participants compared to controls; 60% lower odds of arrest in the six months after beginning the program and 39% lower odds of a future felony charge (Collins, Lonczak, & Clifasefi, 2017). The liberalization of cannabis laws (including decriminalization, medicalization, and legalization) is a feasible policy direction to reduce the role of the criminal justice system in the lives of otherwise law-abiding citizens, given that cannabis is the substance for which the largest number of Americans are arrested (FBI, 2017). The most recent Pew Survey reported that upwards of 60% of the American population now supports cannabis legalization for recreational use by adults (Pew Research Center, 2018). Liberalization of cannabis laws can reduce racial disparities promoted through criminalization harms and legalization states show dramatic reductions in arrest numbers: in Colorado, cannabis-related arrests dropped by 39% among Latinx persons and 51% among black persons between 2012 and 2017 (Colorado Division of Criminal Justice, 2018).

In addition, social workers could advocate for more robust, accessible, affordable, and evidence-based health care, mental health care, and addiction treatment. Part of Portugal's success in implementing decriminalization policy stemmed from its health care and harm reduction infrastructures, capable of meeting the needs of individuals diverted from criminal justice involvement. Expanding insurance coverage of needed treatment should be included in advocacy efforts.

At present, funding for harm reduction programs is not provided by the U.S. federal government, and harm reduction solutions such as free sterile syringe access are not legal in some states.

Allocating appropriate funding and instituting policies to implement harm reduction programs is one of the best ways to ensure individuals and communities are protected from many health risks associated with substance misuse. In addition to preventing and treating substance use and related problems, social workers could support public health program strategies and interventions to prevent or reduce harm, including:

- overdose prevention training and distribution of naloxone, an opioid overdose reversal medication;
- Safer Consumption Spaces (SCS) and syringe access programs;
- fentanyl test strips and other drug testing equipment to monitor one's own drugs; and
- education for safer drug use and safer sex practices.

The public health goals of harm reduction are explicit: to prevent death and disease. Making harm reduction services and programs mobile and accessible is essential, particularly for rural communities having limited access to public transportation and other resources.

Conclusions

Given the current substance use treatment landscape in the United States, significant reforms to ensure voluntary and confidential services for individuals and families are in order. The treatment system must be functionally separate from the criminal justice system's punitive sanctions. In addition, treatment should be trauma-informed, and adequately equipped to treat co-occurring disorders. Access to evidence-informed, evidence-supported, and evidence-based addiction treatment, conducted by staff trained and qualified to treat substance use and co-occurring disorders, should be the standard of care.

In addition, treatment should be aligned with a harm reduction perspective that allows for goals other than abstinence alone. Integration and normalization of substance-related treatment and recovery is essential to ensuring access to care. Harm reduction strategies meet individuals where they are and are aligned with social work ethics: recognizing and supporting client dignity, diversity, and self-determination. Person-centered approaches to reducing harm and facilitating change require collaboration among social workers and other allied health professionals to end arrest, conviction, and incarceration as the primary solution to substance misuse and related problems. In order for individuals to address substance use problems, ambivalence toward substance misuse, and alternatives for the future, they must be living outside of a prohibition culture. Thus, social workers have a responsibility to engage as advocates for social change, reversing the War on Drugs as currently waged and its associated harms.

References

Alexander, M. (2012). *The new Jim Crow: Mass incarceration in the age of colorblindness*. New York, NY: The New Press.

Andrilla, C. H. A., Moore, T. E., Patterson, D. G., & Larson, E. H. (2019). Geographic distribution of providers with a DEA waiver to prescribe buprenorphine for the treatment of opioid use disorder: A 5-year update: Distribution of providers with a DEA waiver. *The Journal of Rural Health, 35*(1), 108–112. doi:10.1111/jrh.12307

Babor, T., Caulkins, J., Edwards, G., Fischer, B., Foxcroft, D., Humphreys, K., . . . Strang, J. (2010). *Drug policy and the public good*. New York, NY: Oxford University Press. doi:10.1093/acprof:oso/9780199557127.001.0001

Bancroft, A. (2009). *Drugs, intoxication & society*. Malden, MA: Polity Press.

Beaver, A. (2010). Getting a fix on cocaine sentencing policy: Reforming the sentencing scheme of the Anti-Drug Abuse Act of 1986. *Fordham Law Review, 78*(5), 2531–2575.

Beletsky, L., & Davis, C. S. (2017). Today's fentanyl crisis: Prohibition's Iron Law, revisited. *International Journal of Drug Policy, 46*, 156–159. doi:10.1016/j.drugpo.2017.05.050

Bowen, E. A., & Redmond, H. (2016). Teaching note—No peace without justice: Addressing the United States' War on Drugs in social work education. *Journal of Social Work Education, 52*(4). 503–508. doi: 10.1080/10437797.2016.1198296

Case, A., & Deaton, A. (2015). Rising morbidity and mortality in midlife among white non–Hispanic Americans in the 21st century. *Proceedings of the National Academy of Sciences, 112*(49), 15078–15083. doi:10.1073/pnas.1518393112

Ciccarone, D. (2019). The triple wave epidemic: Supply and demand drivers of the US opioid overdose crisis. *The International Journal on Drug Policy*. doi:10.1016/j.drugpo.2019.01.010

Collins, S. E., Lonczak, H. S., & Clifasefi, S. L. (2017). Seattle's Law Enforcement Assisted Diversion (LEAD): Program effects on recidivism outcomes. *Evaluation and Program Planning, 64*, 49–56. doi:10.1016/j.evalprogplan.2017.05.008

Colorado Division of Justice, Department of Public Safety. (2018). *Impacts of marijuana legalization in Colorado: A Report Pursuant to Senate Bill 13-283*. Retrieved May 13, 2019 from https://cdpsdocs.state.co.us/ors/docs/reports/2018-SB13-283_Rpt.pdf

Corva, D. (2008). Neoliberal globalization and the war on drugs: Transnationalizing illiberal governance in the Americas. *Political Geography, 27*(2), 176–193. doi:10.1016/j.polgeo.2007.07.008

Csete, J., Kamarulzaman, A., Kazatchkine, M., Altice, F., Balicki, M., Buxton, J., . . . Beyrer, C. (2016). Public health and international drug policy. *The Lancet, 387*(10026), 1427–1480. doi:10.1016/S0140-6736(16)00619-X

Csete, J., & Tomasini-Joshi, D. (2016). Drug courts: Equivocal evidence on a popular intervention. New York, NY: Open Society Foundations.

Davenport-Hines, R. (2001). *The pursuit of oblivion: A global history of narcotics 1500–2000*. London: Weidenfeld & Nicolson.

DeGrandpre, R. (2006). *The cult of pharmacology*. Durham, NC: Duke University Press. doi:10.1215/9780822388197

Des Jarlais, D. C., Arasteh, K., Feelemyer, J., McKnight, C., Barnes, D. M., Perlman, D. C., . . . Tross, S. (2018). Hepatitis C virus prevalence and estimated incidence among new injectors during the opioid epidemic in New York City, 2000–2017: Protective effects of non-injecting drug use. *Drug and Alcohol Dependence, 192*, 74–79. doi:10.1016/j.drugalcdep.2018.07.034

Domostawski, A. (2011). *Drug policy in Portugal: The benefits of decriminalizing drug use*. Retrieved May 13, 2019 from https://www.opensocietyfoundations.org/sites/default/files/drug-policy-in-portugal-english-20120814.pdf

Drug Enforcement Agency. (n.d.) *Drug scheduling*. Retrieved May 12, 2019 from https://www.dea.gov/drug-scheduling

Drug Policy Alliance. (2017). *It's time for the US to decriminalize drug use and possession report.* New York, NY: Drug Policy Alliance.

Federal Bureau of Investigations. (2017). *Uniform crime report: Crime in the United States, 2016.* Retrieved May 13, 2019 from https://ucr.fbi.gov/crime-in-the-u.s/2016/crime-in-the-u.s.-2016/topic-pages/persons-arrested

Latimore, A. D., & Bergstein, R. S. (2017). "Caught with a body" yet protected by law? Calling 911 for opioid overdose in the context of the Good Samaritan Law. *International Journal of Drug Policy, 50,* 82–89. doi:10.1016/j.drugpo.2017.09.010

Library of Congress (n.d.). Bill Summary and Status, 99th Congress (1985–1986), H.R. 5484, CRS Summary. Retrieved May 13, 2019 from https://www.congress.gov/bill/99th-congress/house-bill/05484

Lim, S., Seligson, A. L., Parvez, F. M., Luther, C. W., Mavinkurve, M. P., Binswanger, I. A., & Kerker, B. D. (2012). Risks of drug-related death, suicide, and homicide during the immediate post-release period among people released from New York City jails, 2001–2005. *American Journal of Epidemiology, 175*(6), 519–526. doi:10.1093/aje/kwr327

Miron, J. A., & Waldock, K. (2010). *The budgetary impact of ending drug prohibition.* Washington, DC: Cato Institute. doi:10.2139/ssrn.1710812

Murphy, P. (1994). *Keeping score: The fragilities of the federal drug budget.* Santa Monica, CA: RAND Corporation. Retrieved February 18, 2019 from https://www.rand.org/pubs/issue_papers/IP138.html

Musto, D. F. (1973). *The American disease.* New Haven, CT: Yale University Press.

National Association of Social Workers. (2017). *Code of Ethics of the National Association of Social Workers.* Washington, DC: Author.

National Association of Social Workers. (2013). *Social justice brief: A social work perspective on drug policy reform.* Washington, DC: Author.

National Inventory of Collateral Consequences. (2019). *Collateral consequences inventory.* Retrieved February 20, 2019 from https://niccc.csgjusticecenter.org/database/results/?jurisdiction=&consequence_category=&narrow_category=&triggering_offense_category=&consequence_type=&duration_category=&page_number=1

National Research Council. (2001). *Informing America's policy on illegal drugs: What we don't know keeps hurting us.* Washington, DC: National Academy Press.

Narcotic. (n.d.). Dictionary.com. Retrieved May 12, 2019 from https://www.dictionary.com/browse/narcotic

The National Organization for the Reform of Marijuana Laws (NORML). (2019). *State laws.* Retrieved May 13, 2019 from https://norml.org/laws

Office of National Drug Control Policy. (2017). *National drug control budget: FY 2018 funding highlights.* Retrieved February 18, 2019 from https://www.whitehouse.gov/sites/whitehouse.gov/files/ondcp/Fact_Sheets/FY2018-Budget-Highlights.pdf

Peterson, M., Rich, J., Macmadu, A., Truong, A. Q., Green, T. C., Beletsky, L., . . . Brinkley-Rubinstein, L. (2019). "One guy goes to jail, two people are ready to take his spot": Perspectives on drug-induced homicide laws among incarcerated individuals. *International Journal of Drug Policy, 70,* 47–53. doi:10.1016/j.drugpo.2019.05.001

Pettus-Davis, C., & Epperson, M. W. (2015). From mass incarceration to smart decarceration. American Academy of Social Work & Social Welfare Grand Challenges for Social Work. Retrieved from http://grandchallengesforsocialwork.org/wp-content/uploads/2015/12/WP4-with-cover.pdf

Pew Research Center. (2018). *About six in ten Americans support marijuana legalization.* Retrieved May 13, 2019 from https://www.pewresearch.org/fact-tank/2018/10/08/americans-support-marijuana-legalization/

Reinarman, C. & Levine, H. G. (1997). *Crack in America: Demon drugs and social justice.* Los Angeles, CA: University of California.

Scholl, L., Seth, P., Kariisa, M., Wilson, N., & Baldwin, G. (2019). Drug and opioid-involved overdose deaths – United States, 2013–2017. *Morbidity and Mortality Weekly Report, 67*(51 & 52), 1419–1427. doi:10.15585/mmwr.mm6751521e1

Stone, K., & Shirley-Beavan, S. (2018). *Global state of harm reduction 2018.* London: Harm Reduction International.

Substance Abuse and Mental Health Services Administration (SAMHSA). (2018a). *Key substance use and mental health indicators in the United States: Results from the 2017 National Survey on Drug Use and Health* (HHS Publication No. SMA 18–5068, NSDUH Series H-53). Rockville, MD: Center for Behavioral Health Statistics and Quality, Substance Abuse and Mental Health Services Administration.

Substance Abuse and Mental Health Services Administration (SAMHSA). (2018b). *Treatment episode data set (TEDS): 2016. Admissions to and discharges from publicly funded substance use treatment.* Rockville, MD: Substance Abuse and Mental Health Services Administration, Center for Behavioral Health Statistics and Quality.

Substance Abuse and Mental Health Services Administration (SAMHSA). (2018c). *National survey of substance abuse treatment services (N-SSATS): 2017. Data on substance abuse treatment facilities.* Rockville, MD: Author.

United Nations Chief Executive Board. (2019). *Summary of deliberations of the second regular session of 2018 held on 7 and 8 November 2018.* Retrieved March 1, 2019 from https://www.unsceb.org/CEB PublicFiles/CEB-2018-2-SoD.pdf

United Nations Office on Drugs and Crime. (2018). *World drug report 2018.* Retrieved February 16, 2019 from https://www.unodc.org/wdr2018/prelaunch/WDR18_Booklet_2_GLOBAL.pdf

United States Department of Justice, Drug Enforcement Agency. (2018). *2018 National drug threat assessment.* Retrieved February 16, 2019 from https://www.dea.gov/sites/default/files/2018-11/DIR-032-18%202018%20NDTA%20final%20low%20resolution.pdf

Vakharia, S. P. (2014). Incorporating substance use content into social work curricula: Opioid overdose as a micro, mezzo, and macro problem. *Social Work Education, 33*(5), 692–698. Doi: 10.1080/02615479.2014.919093

31

Decriminalization and medicalization of cannabis

Implications of the Caribbean experience for global social work practice

Barris Malcolm

Background

The primary concern of this chapter is the lack of both research and adequate literature focused on cannabis use and misuse among Caribbean populations, both in the immediate region and as diasporic subpopulations overseas. Given this context, the main purpose of this chapter is to inform a broad audience of social workers and colleagues in allied health professions about nuanced historical backgrounds, etiology, epidemiology, concerns, research, policies, and interventions related to cannabis use and misuse in the Caribbean. Social workers and other health and mental health professionals worldwide can learn valuable policy and practice lessons for their work in substance use, substance misuse, and substance use disorders.

Organizing and integrating the varied etiologic models generated by substance use researchers can be a colossal undertaking (Campbell, 2010), but is nonetheless necessary for research progress; even research conducted in such exotic locations as the Caribbean. The task is made more difficult when examining the Caribbean relationship with cannabis because of complexities compounded by political status, lingering colonial and international relationships, language and dialect differences (i.e. Dutch, English, French, Spanish, Creole, Papiamento, and local/indigenous dialects), religious practices, socio-economic status, cultural traditions, and ongoing and rapid attitudinal changes. Superimposed on these factors is the influence of the Rastafari Movement stemming from Jamaica, a phenomenon which aptly fits Campbell's (2010) argument that drug use represents a form of deviant behavior: Rastafari can be viewed as a deviant group born out of poverty. Consequently, sociological constructs (poverty and urban blight that converged in 1930s Jamaica) are factors in shaping their ideology around cannabis use.

Cannabis: history, prevalence, associated problems

Cannabis is an inclusive term applied to many psychoactive substances derived from plants called *cannabis sativa* and *cannabis indica*. Scientists have identified tetrahydrocannabinol (THC)

497

to be the major psychoactive component of cannabis (NIDA, 2018), and have denoted compounds with structural similarities to THC as cannabinoids (UNODC, 2018). THC directly affects the brain when smoked, by triggering increased activity of the endocannabinoid system causing the release of dopamine (Doweiko & Evans, 2019). Genetically modified or manufactured cannabis products can contain and deliver large amounts of THC that may prove very harmful to some users. The production of cannabis extracts should also be of concern because the process can be very dangerous and pose severe risks to amateur chemists and extraction operators (ONDCP, 2019).

Cannabis was known in India before 1400 B.C.E. and regarded as sacred because it had euphoric and medicinal properties (Gumbiner, 2011). People in India consumed cannabis in a variety of ways, including a potent form called "ganja" made from leaves and flowers of female cannabis plants, and "charas," considered the most potent form, made from blooming cannabis flowers. Ganja and charas were communally smoked using an earthenware pipe called a "chillum" or "chalice."

The term "marijuana" originated in Mexico and refers to cannabis leaves, as well as other plant materials. Marijuana has been used in various cultures for hundreds of years, is immensely popular, and has many nicknames and street names (Sclar, 2019) which vary by country, community, age group, and historical cohorts. Unpollinated female plants are used in the extraction of hashish oil (cannabis oil), highly concentrated with cannabinoids, that can be further processed from plant materials or resins with the application of solvents (UNODC, 2018).

Caribbean scholars and drug researchers prefer the scientific term "cannabis" citing racist and propagandist connotations of the word "marijuana" (Antoine & Douglas, 2018). Nonetheless, "marijuana" and "cannabis" often are used interchangeably. The term "ganja" has religious and cultural significance in Jamaica (notably among Rasta). This chapter and briefly describes the Rastafari movement because of its influence in the Caribbean and beyond. Rastafari are uncomfortable with the terms "Rastafarian" and "Rastafarianism," preferring "Rastafari" "Rasta," or "Dread" (RQS, 2019). Recognizing the complexities and power of such self-identity, these preferred terms are used in this chapter.

Epidemiology

The United Nations Office of Drugs Crime (UNODC) collects, analyzes, and reports annual data on extent, patterns, and trends in drug use and its health consequences through the Annual Reports Questionnaires (ARQ) submitted by Member States. UNODC presents results in its World Drug Report. The 2018 World Drug Report (UNODC, 2018) estimated that 183 million persons worldwide engage in cannabis use, making it the most commonly used psychoactive substance (not including alcohol) on the planet. Globally, cannabis was the most common drug of choice among an estimated 13.8 million young people (aged 15–16 years), mostly in Western countries (UNODC, 2018). The Report also stated that cannabis use had increased 16% during the decade between 2006 and 2016, and that this was equal to the global population growth rate (16%) during that decade. An earlier World Drug Report (UNDOC, 2014) also described rapid growth in cannabis use globally since 1960, and that the most rapid increases occurred in North America, Western Europe and Australia. The ten countries with the highest rates of smoked cannabis were: Iceland (18.3% of the population), Zambia (17.7%), the United States (14.8%), Italy (14.6%), New Zealand (14.6%), Nigeria (14.3%), Canada (12.2%), Spain (10.6%), Australia (10.3%), and Jamaica (9.86%). The report also concluded that cannabis was often used in conjunction with other substances and that the use of other, more dangerous drugs was usually preceded by cannabis use.

The National Survey of Drug Use and Health (NSDUH; SAMHSA, 2018) identified cannabis as the most commonly used drug (other than alcohol) in the United States. Nearly half of adults reported lifetime use of cannabis (47.5%), 12.2% during the past year, and 7.9% during the past month. Cannabis use was most commonly reported among emerging adults (18–25 years old), with 52.7% reporting lifetime use. According to the Monitoring the Future study, 43.6% of U.S. high school seniors (12th graders) in 2018 reported having used cannabis during their lifetime, 34.9% in the past year, 22.2% in the past month, and 5.8% use daily (Johnston et al., 2019).

The 2014 World Drug Report concluded that globally cannabis was the most cultivated and traded illicit drug (UNODC, 2014). According to the 2014 World Drug Report, seizure of cannabis was global, occurring in every member country, and accounted for half of all illicit drug seizures worldwide. According to the 2018 World Drug Report, quantities of cannabis seized globally declined by 27%, to 4,386 tons due in North America to several states' policy changes concerning medical and recreational cannabis (UNODC, 2018).

The United States is situated in close geographic proximity to the Caribbean region. Results from a 2014 Barbados Government survey (population 287,010), reported a 43% past-month cannabis use prevalence (Antoine & Douglas, 2018). Results from a similar study in 2017 in the Bahamas (population 402,095) reported 17% current use. A 2016 Guyana Government survey (population 776,601) reported a 9.8% current use prevalence (Antoine & Douglas, 2018). A 2018 Jamaica survey (population, 2.9 million) conducted by the National Council on Drug Abuse (NCDA) sampled 4,623 households and reported that 5% of females and 27% of males were currently using cannabis, and 70% reported having "easy access to ganja" (Antoine & Douglas, 2018).

Cannabis effects

Cannabis use is associated with a range of adverse health effects. Acute effects include altered senses and sense of time, impaired motor coordination, impaired memory, and problem-solving abilities (see Chapter 3). Recent research suggests that early use of cannabis may impact thinking, memory, and learning. Cannabis use is also associated with other substance use and dependency, respiratory problems, developmental problems related to fetal exposure, and mental health problems including psychotic episodes, depression, and anxiety. Cannabis misuse itself can result in addiction in some individuals, diagnosable cannabis use disorders appear in both the DSM-5 and ICD-11, along with accompanying withdrawal symptoms.

Other effects from cannabis include changes in perceptions and mood, lack of coordination, difficulty with thinking and problem-solving, and disrupted learning and memory (Boyce & McArdle, 2008). Several studies showed associations between cannabis use and psychosis when large doses are consumed over an extended period, with symptoms characteristic of paranoid schizophrenia (Degenhardt & Hall, 2006; D'Souza et al., 2005; Gage, Hickman, & Zammit, 2016). Other studies reported that cannabis use significantly increased the risk of developing mental health problems among young people genetically predisposed with high risk for schizophrenia familial factors (Boyce & McArdle, 2008; Hollis et al., 2008). Heavy marijuana use is linked to a reduction of hippocampus and amygdala volume in the brain (Yucel et al., 2008), potential cognitive deficits (Khamsi, 2013; Mizrahi, Watts, & Tseng, 2017), and suppression of REM sleep cycles (Babson, Sottile, & Morabito, 2017).

Most concerning is evidence that marijuana use changes the brain in ways that make an individual more likely to experiment with other drugs and potentially become addicted to other substances (Martz et al., 2016). One investigator concluded that cannabis use may pose a greater risk to developing brains of teenagers than alcohol (Morin et al., 2019). The conclusion was based on her study of four cognitive functions: problem-solving, long-term memory, short-term memory manipulation, and the ability to stop a habitual behavior when needed. Cannabis had "significant" negative effects on all four, while the study could not tie alcohol to the same negative effects.

Cannabis in the Caribbean

This chapter is presented within the context of Trevithick's (2000) characterization that the context of social work often changes rapidly with time, but one principal element which persists is that the profession is involved with some of the most complex problems and per-plexing areas of human experience. Substance misuse represents one such complex prob-lem, and the use of cannabis for recreational and medical purposes has grown increasingly perplexing for public policy makers, as well as for medical-, mental-, and public health and addiction practitioners. Social workers are well suited for addressing the complexities and perplexities posed by current discourses and developments regarding cannabis avail-ability, preventing its use/misuse, addressing its effects and consequences of its misuse, and developing/implementing treatment and recovery strategies grounded in the substantial and significant body of knowledge produced through objective, peer-reviewed, systematic inves-tigations into cannabis use, and its effects on human beings. In this light we next analyze and discuss cannabis in the Caribbean and global implications of its decriminalization, medical-ization, and commercialization.

Cannabis and the Caribbean

The Caribbean is diverse, layered, and complex, and refers to the archipelago of islands ex-tending over 1,000 miles from the coast of Florida to South America off the coast of Venezuela. The wider Caribbean region, comprised of 32 nations, is estimated to have a population of 35 million, and the total population of the Caribbean Community and Common Market (CARICOM) countries is at 17.7 million (CARICOM, 2019). Commonwealth Caribbean refers to the former British West Indian territories, Antigua and Barbuda, Bahamas, Belize, Dominica, Grenada, Guyana Jamaica, Montserrat, St. Kitts & Nevis, St Lucia, St Vincent and the Grenadines, and Trinidad and Tobago, as well as current British Overseas Territories, Cayman Islands, British Virgin Islands, and Turks and Caicos. They are called Common-wealth because they hold membership in a 53-nation organization that includes the United Kingdom.

Cannabis has deep historical and social significance across the Caribbean where it has been simultaneously reviled, denounced, prohibited, tolerated, and revered. Diverse forces have shaped a multidimensional understanding of, and attitudes toward, the use and conse-quences of cannabis throughout the Caribbean, and among diasporic groups scattered across the globe. Consequently, this chapter sheds light that may be informative and helpful to practice in the Caribbean and with the various diasporic populations around the globe, as well as their descendants (Malcolm, 2014).

Attitudinal changes toward cannabis in the Caribbean resulted from decades of relentless activism mainly by grassroots groups, notably the Rasta of Jamaica, and advocacy by artists, musicians, medical researchers, social organizations, policy makers, media, and public opin-ion. These groups shared abiding concerns not only about the Caribbean "War on Cannabis" and its disparate impact on the poor, including Rasta, but also embraced social justice, human rights, and equity issues, even as regulatory policies were contemplated (Antoine & Douglas, 2018). Changes were largely influenced by rapid development of cannabis policy in Canada and the United States. Canada legalized medical cannabis in 2001 and was treating over 330,000 individuals with it by 2014, including cancer patients registered with licensed producers (Cannabis Act, 2018). The United States saw a proliferation of medical and recreational cannabis legislation beginning with Colorado in 2014 and has since expanded (at the time of this writing) to 33 states allowing medical cannabis and 11 allowing recreational use (Governing the States and Localities, 2019). Canada legalized recreational cannabis throughout the country in 2018 (Bilefsky, 2018).

Social history of cannabis in the Caribbean

The history and use of cannabis in Jamaica and the Caribbean are steeped in culture and folklore, reflecting a complicated interplay between myth, religion, misinformation, ambivalence, and scientific curiosity. The following narrative history comes from investigating primary and secondary sources and oral interviews. *Cannabis indica* was introduced to the Caribbean in the 1840s by indentured people from India, laborers brought to the region by the British after 1834 to replace emancipated slaves (Antoine & Douglas, 2018). As previously mentioned, cannabis was known in India before 1400 B.C.E. and regarded as sacred because it has euphoric and medicinal properties (Gumbiner, 2011). During the 1890s, the British in India grew concerned about heavy cannabis use among laborers, and about its effects on productivity and health. They sought to prohibit cannabis and established the India Hemp Drugs Commission to investigate "cannabis cultivation, drug contents, properties and effects" (Inversen, 2008, p. 19). After a few years of research and analysis, the Commission advised against prohibition and recommended a harm reduction approach, due to the long historic and religious use of cannabis and its relative harmlessness when used in moderation, compared to alcohol (Gumbiner, 2011).

Meanwhile, in the Caribbean, indentured Indians grew and smoked ganja, and soon the habit expanded to settlers and freed Africans throughout many British territories, eventually reaching Spanish, French, and Dutch territories. In the Caribbean, the British again grew concerned about cannabis use by the labor force, and in 1913 outlawed its cultivation and importation under the Opium Law in Jamaica (Antoine & Douglas, 2018). In response to international treaty formation, mainly with the United States, the Dangerous Drug Ordinance of 1937 was passed in the United Kingdom, which classified cannabis as a "dangerous drug," subsequently criminalizing its production and use (Antoine & Douglas, 2018).

This marked the beginning of a turbulent history of cannabis in the Caribbean, abetted by the rapacious eruption, vibrant ferocity, and long career of Harry Jacob Anslinger (1930–1962) who was at the helm of the U.S. Narcotics Bureau (Smith, 2018). According to Smith (2018), during his employ on alcohol prohibition, Anslinger demonstrated little concern about the cannabis trade and its effects on persons who use in the United States. However, post-Prohibition Anslinger turned the Bureau's focus into a campaign on the prohibition of cocaine, heroin, and cannabis (Courtwright, 1992). Anslinger was accused of conflating cannabis use with lifestyles of African Americans, "their music" (Jazz) and "work ethic," contributing to the racialization of drug use (see Chapter 30).

Anslinger remained head of the Bureau until the John F. Kennedy administration, retiring in 1962, but his views still permeate U.S drug policies, reverberating through the War on Drugs that has resulted in the interdiction of millions of tons of illicit drugs, valued in the billions of dollars, and the incarceration of millions of people involved in using and trading illicit drugs. Anslinger polarized the debate between supply reduction and demand reduction policies, international interdiction treaties and strategies, punitive laws, and harsh penalties (Smith, 2018). All CARICOM members and several of other countries in the region are also members of the Organization of American States (OAS). The OAS Charter (Article 53) in 1986 established the Inter-American Drug Abuse Control Commission (CICAD), to promote and facilitate multilateral cooperation to control production, abuse, and traffic in illicit drugs and related crimes in the hemisphere.

The Caribbean's proximity to the south-east U.S. coast allows easy access to transshipment routes and high volumes of recreational vessels, making it attractive and successful for drug trafficking from South America to North America and other international markets. Caribbean coastlines are difficult to patrol (United States Department of State, 2018). As part of the Anslinger legacy, the United States maintains a multi-layered approach for interdicting illicit drugs from the Caribbean, including Drug Enforcement Administration (DEA), Coast Guard, Homeland Security, and the National Drug Control Strategy. The U.S. DEA has authority to enforce laws and regulations over cultivation, manufacture, and distribution of controlled substances, and money laundering of illicit finances derived from drug trafficking in many Caribbean countries (United States Department of State, 2018).

Despites prohibiting laws, cannabis can be found throughout the Caribbean. Enforcement is lax in most countries as regards possession of small amounts. Social attitudes toward recreational cannabis use are also lax, and effects are mostly regarded as benign. Research on cannabis use among Caribbean populations and subpopulations has been difficult to conduct, but what does exist has not been widely disseminated in the United States or elsewhere. It may be surprising to some to learn that extensive, rigorous research on drug use and misuse are conducted in the region. A collection of these research activities and findings are documented in the *Final Report of the CARICOM Regional Commission on Marijuana 2018* (Antoine & Douglas, 2018). Recent legalization of cannabis for medicinal and recreation use in the region and internationally has heightened the need for this analysis. There are expectations that new/ expanded markets for cannabis will emerge, creating new economic potential for the region, but also unforeseen environmental, social, and health risks, to which social work will need to bring attention and advocacy. Social work in the Caribbean must safeguard against injustice and ensure that policies reflect the intended reforms without sending ambiguous, incorrect, or harmful messages about cannabis, particularly to young people of the Caribbean.

The Rasta experience

A history of cannabis use and misuse in the Caribbean after the 1930s is incomplete without a discussion of the Rastafari Movement and its influence on cannabis use and misuse, in Jamaica in particular. Rastafari have a long history of advocating for the recognition and liberalization of cannabis (ganja). Rastafari culture is known internationally but remains misunderstood in the context of the literature on addictive behavior. The Rastafari Movement is best understood as an urban counterculture. Campbell (2010) claims that general models of causation and consequences are shaped by prominent historical events, and to some degree reflect cultural parameters. This model aptly describes the relationship between cannabis and the Rastafari Movement. Rastafari emerged during the1930s in pre-independent Jamaica as a non-violent, protest movement focused on police brutality and incarceration of Rasta for smoking cannabis (BBC, 2009).

The Movement consisted of amorphous unorganized groups of mostly impoverished, disaffected, socially stigmatized, and marginalized citizens living in urban slums. Loosely organized groups banded together for personal safety and residential security, coalescing into substantial "ghettos." One formed under the leadership of Leonard Percival Howell, a Jamaican and a Garveyite deported from the United States in 1932. Howell had been a member of The United Negro Improvement Association (UNIA) founded by Marcus Mosiah Garvey that embraced and preached black nationalism, anti-colonialism, and Pan-Africanism (RQS, 2019). Howell was expelled by Garvey for smoking and selling marijuana.

Howell, referred to as the first Rasta, founded the Ethiopian Salvation Society as a commune of 5,000 people in 1935, and promoted the sale and use of cannabis (BBC, 2009; Hall, 2007). They claimed that cannabis originally sprouted out of the grave of King Solomon, an Israelite renown for great wisdom, and so, by extension, smoking cannabis ("the holy weed") would confer wisdom (RQS, 2019). Howell's followers were called Rastafari or Rasta, after Ras Tafari Makonnen of Ethiopia (BBC, 2009). After Hailie Selassie I's coronation as Emperor on December 2, 1930, Rasta in Jamaica proclaimed and worshipped him the Messiah. Many Rastas flocked to the Ethiopian Orthodox church in Jamaica named for Selassie when it opened, including famous Reggae music artists. However, many developed an uneasy relationship with the Orthodox clergy who scoffed at considering or worshiping Selassie as divine and reviled the use of marijuana as a religious sacrament (RQS, 2019). Subsequently, many Rastas left the Orthodox Church and created the Ethiopian Coptic, and Zion Coptic churches led by Jamaican Rasta clergy who supported their theology and sacramental cannabis use (E. Keith, personal communication, 1980, January 15, The Coptic Tabernacle, Whitehorses, St. Thomas Jamaica, January 15).

Rastas refer to religious meetings as "reasoning sessions" accompanied by ritual communal cannabis smoking (Grant, 2002; E. Keith, personal communication, 1980, January 15, The Coptic Tabernacle, Whitehorses, St. Thomas Jamaica; Lewis, 1993). Rasta claim that smoking cannabis heightens their spirituality (RQS, 2019). Rastas smoke ganja (blunt, reefer) almost daily, both individually and communally shared between family members, including children. Rastas generally oppose cocaine, heroin, alcohol, tobacco and caffeine, and avoid meat and use of salt in their mostly vegetarian diet.

Rastafari beliefs and culture have found acceptance and large followings internationally due to tourism, music (Reggae) concerts, and cannabis (BBC, 2009). Songs are often about love and peace, but also about rebellion and revolution against social injustice, oppressive forces, poverty, and racism. Rastafari subgroups have dispersed across many Caribbean countries and the United States, Canada, Europe, Asia, Africa, and Australia (BBC, 2009; RQS, 2019). According to the British Ministry of Defense, the number of Rastafari followers joining the armed forces has increased by more than any other faith group (Jamaica Gleaner, 2019). In 2019 there were 210 Rastas in the British armed forces, up 40% since 2016 (Jamaica Gleaner, 2019). Rastas vehemently refuse to be counted for any purpose, including government-directed census or research, because of their religious beliefs, thereby complicating data collection efforts (E. Keith, personal communication, 1980, January 15, The Coptic Tabernacle, Whitehorses, St. Thomas Jamaica).

Cannabis decriminalization

Jamaica was first among the CARICOM Members to legalize medical cannabis and decriminalize possession and recreational use in limited amounts, by passage of its Dangerous Drug Amendment Act (DDAA) in 2015 (Miller, 2018). The DDAA created two statutory agencies: the Cannabis Licensing Authority (CLA) and the Medicinal Cannabis Unit (MCU), which operates Under the Jamaican Ministry of Health. The MCU oversees the implementation of medicinal cannabis guidelines, registration and regulation of cannabis and related products (including hemp), medicinal products produced locally or internationally, and all pharmaceutically accepted derivatives (with less than 1% THC) other than plants. The CLA operates independently of the Ministry of Health, and oversees growth, development, and regulation of the legal cannabis and hemp industry for medical, therapeutic, and scientific purposes. The CLA grants permits and licenses for cultivation, transportation, and processing of cannabis and oversees retailing of all cannabis-derived products for medical, scientific, and therapeutic purposes. The CLA has no jurisdiction over ganja for religious use by Rasta, which is under the Jamaican Ministry of Justice (Antoine & Douglas, 2018). The DDAA decriminalizes possession of two ounces or less of cannabis (previously subjected to arrest or detention). Under DDAA, any person found in possession of two ounces or less of cannabis is subjected to a fine of $500 Jamaican, about U.S.$4 (Jamaica Gleaner, 2015). The DDAA also stipulates that any person found in possession of two ounces or less of cannabis, who is under the age of 18 years, or who appears to the police to be dependent on the drug, is required to pay the fine and be referred to the National Council on Drug Abuse for counseling (Antoine & Douglas, 2018; Miller, 2018).

The DDAA allows for possession of cannabis prescribed by a licensed health professional and for scientific research by an institution of higher education. Each household is permitted to grow no more than five cannabis plants. Smoking cannabis is prohibited in or within five meters of a public place; it is legally permitted in licensed places, including places for medical or therapeutic purposes (Antoine & Douglas, 2018). Under DDAA, Rastafari members are permitted to smoke cannabis for sacramental purposes in registered places of worship. The DDAA also stipulates that Rastas 18 years of age or older, or Rastafari organizations, may apply for authorization to cultivate cannabis for religious purposes. Under DDAA, fines for cultivation, possession selling, and trafficking of illegal drugs without license were significantly increased (Antoine & Douglas, 2018; United States Department of State, 2018).

Cannabis medicalization

Medical applications of cannabis are not new, dating to 2727 B.C.E. (Doweiko & Evans, 2019). Chinese physicians practiced using medical cannabis for centuries for treating constipation, malaria, gout, and for surgical anesthesia when mixed with wine (Doweiko & Evans, 2019). In the 1950s, American physicians were trained to prescribe cannabis as a hypnotic, sedative, anticonvulsant, and to treat migraines (Doweiko & Evans, 2019). Cannabis extracts have been extensively studied in use for medical treatments over the 30 years (Buggy et al., 2003). Studies from the 1970s showed that when smoked, marijuana relieved glaucoma symptoms (Elsohly, Harland, Murphy, Wirth, & Waller, 1985). A 1997 review and meta-analysis identified 6,059 cannabis-related articles in the medical literature: 194 on antiemetic properties, 56 on glaucoma, 10 on multiple sclerosis, 23 on appetite, and 11 on palliative or terminal care (Buggy et al. 2003). Jamaican scientist Dr. Henry Lowe is renowned for his long history in medical cannabis research, leading to several cannabis-based drug patents.

A substantial body of work revealed that the cannabis or its derivatives provided relief from pain (Matsuda, Lolait, Brownstein, Young, & Bonner, 1990). Recent interest in analgesic properties of the drug have been renewed due to the prescription opiate and heroin crises in the United States. Because of the addictive qualities of opiates, cannabis may be preferred as an effective remedy for pain (Holdridge & Holdridge, 2015). Legalized cannabis use for managing chronic pain resulted in significantly fewer deaths from prescription painkiller overdoses (Boyette & Wilson, 2015).

In 2015, under the DDAA, the Jamaica Medical Marijuana Program made medical cannabis accessible to patients with conditions including: cancer, HIV/AIDS, Lou Gehrig's disease (ALS), Parkinson's disease, multiple sclerosis, damage to the nervous tissue of the spinal cord (for neurological indication of intractable spasticity, epilepsy, inflammatory bowel disease, neuropathies, and Huntington's disease (Jamaica Gleaner, 2015). By comparison, the United States (NIH) has identified five areas where possible therapeutic values of medical cannabis exist: (1) stimulating appetite or alleviate severe weight loss due to decreased caloric intake among patients with AIDS or cancer; (2) managing nausea and vomiting associated with cancer chemotherapy; (3) treating glaucoma; 4) treating neuropathic pain; and 5) treating neurological and (spastic) movement disorders such as symptoms produced by multiple sclerosis and partial spinal cord injury (Renard et al., 2017; Yadav et al., 2014). However, the American Academy of Neurology (AAN) raised concerns over policies approving medical use of cannabis to treat neurological disorders on the basis of insufficient research evidence substantiating its effectiveness and safety, particularly with long-term use. Furthermore, proper dosing can be difficult (Yadav et al., 2014), and it is not without potential negative side effects, such as disorientation, paranoia, depression, anxiety, memory loss, and lack of motivation (Hampson & Deadwyler, 1999; Rubino & Parolaro, 2008). Not all research results are conclusive or replicable leaving significant questions as to the efficacy of medical cannabis for treating some illnesses or conditions.

Penalties

The United States and now, except for Jamaica, CARICOM and most other Caribbean countries maintain legal authority over cannabis, grounded in prohibition and enveloped by criminal sanctions. The trend in cannabis possession arrests in Trinidad and Tobago remained constant between 2012 and 2017: on average, 3,123 males and 245 females. From 2015 to 2017, Guyana experienced an increase of 53% in cannabis-related arrests. In Jamaica, between January 1 and November 30, 2017, a total of 937 arrests were made for breach of the DDAA (Antoine & Douglas, 2018). Penalties for illegal cultivation, possession, transportation, and trade of cannabis include forfeiture of assets, massive fines, and/or imprisonment, depending on the quantities (Jamaica Gleaner, 2015).

Prevention and treatment

The Caribbean boasts some of the finest "luxury" rehabilitation centers for drug addiction treatment, mainly targeting and serving wealthy foreigners. The regional University of the West Indies in collaboration with Inter-American Drug Abuse Control Commission (CICAD) offers a university-level certificate program in drug addiction and drug prevention. Many Caribbean countries strive to provide their citizens with substance abuse prevention and treatment, provided by trained practitioners through both public and private organizations. Services are located mainly in urban centers with limited access and limited participation, especially for rural populations. In Jamaica, for example, the main detoxification center is located at the University Hospital (UHWI) in Kingston. It is not uncommon for imprisonment to be a first step toward treatment, but persons experiencing substance use disorders are sometimes confined to mental institutions for long periods, despite efforts to deinstitutionalize. In Granada, Jamaica, Barbados, Trinidad, and Tobago governments work through the primary health care system and mental health clinics, and fund non-government organizations (NGOs) to provide substance use assessment, counseling, and treatment services. The National Council on Drug Abuse (NCDA) based in Jamaica provides prevention materials and services for children and adolescents, Narcan for opioid overdose reversal, an emergency hotline and telephone counseling services, assessments, brief treatment, referrals for detoxification and addiction treatment services, and is a partner of The National Alliance of Advocates for Buprenorphine Treatment. Self-help groups such as Narcotics Anonymous (NA) and Alcoholics Anonymous (AA) are scarce in many Caribbean countries, tend to be based in the larger urban centers, and participation is generally low (D. Alexander, personal communication, July 6, 2015, Grenada).

Cannabis commercialization and equity

The global market in illicit cannabis has an estimated value of U.S.$141.80 billion (Havocscope Global Black-Market Information, 2015), and it is also estimated that one metric ton of cannabis can produce 1.17 million cannabis joints (cigars) (Havocscope Global Black-Market Information, 2015). The revenue from one marijuana plant is approximated at U.S.$2,200 in the illicit market (Havocscope Global Black-Market Information, 2015). Cannabis has been cultivated clandestinely in the Caribbean since the 1830s. With the passage of DDAA in Jamaica and legalization in other countries, cannabis agriculture presented enormous new economic opportunities in cultivation, agronomic and medical research, production, administrative regulation, marketing, and distribution, all contributing to financial windfalls.

Given this potential, commercial cannabis production in the region may become rapid and wide scale. According to the University of Berkeley Cannabis Research Center, the potential financial windfalls anticipated, and new economies from legal cannabis, need to be balanced against risks and costs, including: environmental and ecological impact on land degradation; water resources; food crop production; pesticides and fertilizer use; and non-compliance (Butsic & Brenner, 2017; Wang, Brenner, & Butsic, 2017). Henry Lowe, Jamaican scientist and founder of Medicanja Ltd, acclaimed the first Jamaican medical cannabis company in 2013; more are likely to follow. Medicanja now operates in the United States, and Lowe has pledged to maintain independence from control by large pharmaceutical companies (Cannabis Law Report, 2017).

Miller (2018) pointed out that, in the case of Jamaica, government has allowed private cannabis production, and the absence of commercial promotion may reduce costs associated with prohibition without also creating an industry with goals than run counter to public welfare. This policy makes it possible for Rastas to be involved in the new cannabis market. It would be ironic, unjust, and unacceptable for Rastas to be denied the largess resulting from cannabis reform, particularly in Jamaica. Rastas, grassroots groups, and advocates in civil society are mostly pleased with the reforms but not all are convinced that the poor will benefit (BBC, 2014), which should raise social justice concerns for social work.

Research on cannabis use epidemiology in the Caribbean

CICAD, in consultation with experts from CARICOM member countries, has created and implemented numerous mechanisms for conducting cannabis research in the region (Antoine & Douglas, 2018). The Multilateral Evaluation Mechanism (MEM) was developed in 1998 to undertake high-quality, objective multilateral governmental (nations) research involving persons 12–65 years old, to evaluate the drug problem in the region, regional trends and issues, and evidence-based solutions for addressing the problems (Antoine & Douglas, 2018). The MEM has become a cornerstone CICAD activity, undertaking several studies across CARICOM states and other countries, and instrumental in developing and applying research capacity and methodology for investigating illicit drug use in the region. The Inter-American Uniform Drug Use Data System (SIDUC) is one such innovation utilizing uniform, reliable data collection systems and analysis capabilities for comparisons among and across various countries (Antoine & Douglas, 2018). Two demonstrations of this collaborative research methodology are the 2018 National Drug Survey of CARICOM Countries and the 2016 National Student Drug Survey.

2018 National Drug Survey

Results from the 2018 National Drug Survey show much variability in lifetime cannabis use prevalence rates by country, although rates were generally high even in countries with laws prohibiting its use. There were higher rates among males compared to females. Lifetime, past-year, and current cannabis was reported by broad cross-sections of social classes, profession, race, religion, and income. Most respondents reported that cannabis was easily available and accessible throughout the region (Antoine & Douglas, 2018). Respondents, including medical practitioners and lawyers, shared their current or past use and beliefs that cannabis was more helpful than harmful, and that they intend to never stop using the substance (Antoine & Douglas, 2018).

2016 National Student Drug Survey

Information gleaned from this study are contextualized and regarded as a treasure trove for research and policy practitioners. The survey was conducted in 13 CARICOM member countries using the SIDUC system and included a random sample of 21,597 persons 13–17 years of age (Antoine & Douglas, 2018). The sample had a gender distribution of 46.6% male and 52.4% female (Antoine & Douglas, 2018).

The survey identified students "*not having a problem,*" "having *low risk,*" or "*having a high risk*" of cannabis abuse using the Cannabis Abuse Screening Test (CAST) (Antoine & Douglas, 2018).

Overall, average lifetime cannabis use prevalence was reported by 20.6% of Caribbean students surveyed, with 13.7% reporting past-year, and 8.8% past-month cannabis use. Results varied widely in the region with highest rates reported in Dominica (31.4%, 19.6% and 12.5% respectively) and the lowest rates reported in Haiti (3.2%, 2.4% and 1.2% respectively) (Antoine & Douglas, 2018). Prevalence rates were higher among male students compared to females: an average of 28.5% of males and 15.9% of females reported lifetime; 17.5% of males and 10.3% of females for past-year use; and 11.6% of males and 6.2% of females for past-month use (Antoine & Douglas, 2018).

Results varied by country but show that the largest increase in cannabis use prevalence occurred among students in the 15–16 years of age cohort in all countries (Antoine & Douglas, 2018). Study results also demonstrate a positive relationship between both past-year and past-month cannabis use and the number of behavioral problems reported, as well as for the prevalence of school grades repeated by students (Antoine & Douglas, 2018). Students were asked about how easy it would be to obtain marijuana if they wanted it: "easy," "hard," "not able to get any," and "don't know" In 9 of the 13 countries, 40–50% indicated that they could access marijuana easily; only about 13% of students (range 8.5–29%) on average indicated that marijuana was hard to obtain and a surprisingly high proportion in each country (average of 27%) indicated that they did not know how easy it would be to obtain marijuana

(Antoine & Douglas, 2018). Prevalence rates of past-year use were 2½ to 7 times higher among groups with "easy" access compared to the other groups (Antoine & Douglas, 2018).

Among students assessed for possible cannabis abuse, 64% were identified as having some risk for cannabis abuse (37.3% at low risk and 26.6% at high risk); about 20% of students admitted using cannabis once or twice per day. Additionally, the perception of harm associated with cannabis appears to be declining among secondary school students (Antoine & Douglas, 2018).

It is the view of CICAD researchers that cannabis use-related risk among students surveyed was notable in the categories of getting a low grade, problems with family, getting into arguments or fights, memory loss, and trying without success to stop using substances. The researchers further noted the importance of recognizing that a small but notable proportion of students were at risk of self-inflicted violence seriously thinking about suicide and inflicting self-harm. A substantial body of research in the area has also found that higher risks are concentrated in adolescents, which can lead to a spectrum of psychopharmacological illnesses, economic-compulsive behaviors and crimes, systemic crimes and drug law offenses (Antoine & Douglas, 2018).

Implications for social work in the Caribbean and other countries

Jamaica so far is the only Caribbean country to decriminalize recreational marijuana use and permits its use for medical treatments. As in some Caribbean countries, Central and South America, Europe, Asia, Africa, and many states in the United States, cannabis continues to be regulated as an illicit drug with a high abuse potential and no approved therapeutic use. Jamaica's attempt at cannabis decriminalization and development of a medicalized cannabis industry represent bold steps for a small nation within close proximity to the United States and stands to inform policy and practice globally.

Findings reported from 2016 and 2018 CICDAD research in the Caribbean suggest that early use of cannabis may impact thinking, memory, and learning in students from several countries. Other research shows that cannabis use is associated with misuse of and dependency for other more dangerous substances; respiratory problems; child development problems related to use during pregnancy; and mental health problems including psychotic episodes, depression, and anxiety. These results support the crucial need for education, prevention, engagement, and treatment of significant numbers of students in the countries surveyed, and probably others in the region. Regulation does seem to have a relationship to supply and demand sides of the cannabis use equation; however, it does not eliminate use by students or adults. Cannabis has import implications for local and regional economies, as well. Furthermore, much of what is known about cannabis use among persons in the Caribbean applies to cannabis use among persons from the Caribbean: individuals who have emigrated to many parts of the world and with whom social workers and other professionals engage.

Social workers worldwide are neither monolithic nor universal, do not share the same beliefs, and the numbers engaged in practice with substance use and misuse are insufficient to address the problem; in addictions research and policy practice the numbers are even fewer. Consequently, there exist great discrepancies in commitment and effort to innovate around the promotion of cannabis for medical/mental health treatment, decriminalization for recreational purposes, and community/economic development through cannabis production and distribution. Strong advocates view decriminalization as a means for curtailing the disproportionate rates of incarceration for cannabis possession and use among poorer citizens, racial and ethnic minorities groups, and Rastas in some countries (see Chapter 30).

Under the DDAA, Rastafari communities in Jamaica gained the right to cultivate, distribute and use cannabis for sacramental purposes without state intervention. While social work celebrates this as a human rights victory, unrelenting concerns remain about cannabis use during pregnancy and exposure to developing adolescent brains. This remains a major public health concern that must be recognized, discussed, and resolved. Children have human rights under the United Nations Universal Declaration of Human Rights and the Convention on the Rights of the Child (OAS, 2012) and states can invoke *guardian ad litem policies*. Whereas CARICOM nation leaders called for "a mature, intelligent conversation" concerning medical marijuana and decriminalization (Charles, 2014) social workers and allied practitioners should need no further invitation to become more engaged. Whereas many social workers have welcomed the recent changes in policies and practices related to marijuana, they should also be acutely aware that social and economic policies often contribute to negative and unintended consequences. Caribbean social workers can be helpful as they are trained in and have competencies as micro, mezzo, and macro practitioners with a focus in social and economic justice and human rights.

Conclusions

There should be concerns among social workers and other professionals about the implications of cannabis decriminalization and medicalization in the Caribbean and elsewhere. These include availability and easy access to cannabis; increased and relatively high cannabis use prevalence; effects of religious cannabis use; effects of cannabis on developing brains; continued monitoring and research in medical cannabis; equity in the emerging market in cannabis; justice reinvestments in individuals and communities disparately impacted by the "War on Drugs"; policing; risks from corruption; effects from the alternative illegal market; policy advocacy, substance use and misuse prevention; assessment and treatment; and identifying and responding to unintended consequences. Social workers, like all service providers, should be concerned that there is still the danger of licensed agents selling medical marijuana without attention to actual medical need or the risks of resale on substance use disorder. Of concern too should be the potentially easier access to high potency cannabis and production and sale of cannabis edibles and extracts. The recent proliferation of countries, as well as several states in the United States, which have legalized either medical cannabis only or both medical and recreational cannabis use, will provide an abundance of data for future research, the results of which should guide policy and practice on the merits or harms associated with cannabis use and misuse.

References

Antoine, B. R., & Douglas, K. G. (2018). *Final report of the CARICOM regional commission on Marijuana 2018*. Georgetown, Guyana: Caribbean Community.

Babson, K. A., Sottile, J., & Morabito, D. (2017). Cannabis, cannabinoids, and sleep: A review of the literature. *Current Psychiatry Reports, 19*, 23. doi:10.1007/s11920-017-0775-9.

Bilefsky, D. (2018, October 17). Legalizing recreational Marijuana, Canada begins a national experiment. New York, NY: *The New York Times*. Retrieved from http://www.tokeofthetown.com/2013/03/barbados_attorney_general_wants_ganja_laws_reviewed.php

Boyce, A., & McArdle, P. (2008). Long-term effects of cannabis. *Paediatrics and Child Health, 18*(1), 37–41. doi:10.1016/j.paed.2007.10.006.

Boyette, C., & Wilson, J. (2015). It's 2015: Is weed legal in your state? By CNN, updated 8:09 AM ET, Wed January 7, 2015 Marijuana laws vary by state. *CNN.com*. Retrieved from http://www.cnn.com/2015/01/07/us/recreational-marijuana-laws/index.html

British Broadcasting Corporation (BBC). (2009). *Rastafarian history: The origins and history of Rastafari, beginning with the colonisation of Africa by Europeans.* London, UK: *BBC News.* Retrieved from http://www.bbc.co.uk/religion/religions/rastafari/history/history.shtml.

British Broadcasting Corporation (BBC). (2014, March 14). *Jamaica's marijuana growers split on legalization.* London, UK: *BBC News.*

Buggy, D. J., Toogood, L., Maric, S., Sharpe, P., Lambert, D. G., & Rowbotham, D. J. (2003). Lack of analgesic efficacy of oral delta-9-tetrahydrocannabinol in postoperative pain. *Pain, 106,* 169–172. doi:10.1016/S0304-3959(03)00331-2

Butsic, V., & Brenner, J. C. (2017). Cannabis (*cannabis sativa* or *c. indica*) agriculture and the environment: A systematic, spatially explicit survey and potential impacts. In R. B. Standiford & Y. Valachovic (Eds.), *Coast redwood science symposium—2016: Past successes and future direction. Proceedings of a workshop* (pp. 383–393). Gen. Tech. Rep. PSW-GTR-258. Albany, CA: U.S. Department of Agriculture, Forest Service, Pacific Southwest Research Station: 383–393.

Campbell, N. D. (2010). Multiple paths to partial truths: A history of drug use etiology. In L. M. Scheier (Ed.), *Handbook of drug use etiology* (pp. 29–50). Washington, DC: American Psychological Association.

Cannabis Act. (2018). Government of Canada, justice law website. Cannabis Act, S.C. 2018, c.16. Retrieved from https://laws-lois.justice.gc.ca/eng/acts/C-24.5/page-1.html#h-76878

Cannabis Law Report. (2017). FDA approves, chrysoeriol, developed by Jamaican scientist Dr. Henry Lowe. Retrieved from https://cannabislaw.report/fda-approves-chrysoeriol-developed-by-jamaican-scientist-dr-henry-lowe/

CARICOM. (2019). *CARICOM Caribbean community. A community for all.* Retrieved from https://caricom.org/about-caricom/who-we-are/our-governance/about-the-secretariat

Charles, J. (2014, March 29). Caribbean countries consider loosening marijuana laws. *Miami Herald.* Retrieved from https://www.miamiherald.com/news/nation-world/world/americas/haiti/article2087895.html

Courtwright, D. T. (1992). Century of American narcotic policy. In D. R. Gerstein & H. J. Harwood (Eds.), *Treating drug problems* (Vol. 2, pp. 1–63). Washington, DC: National Academy Press.

Degenhardt, L., & Hall, W. (2006). Is cannabis use a contributory cause of psychosis? *Canadian Journal of Psychiatry, 51,* 556–565. doi:10.1177/070674370605100903

D'Souza, D. C., Abi-Saab, W. M., Madonick, S., Forselius-Bielen, K., Doersch, A., Braley, G., & Krystal, J. H. (2005). Delta-9-tetrahydrocannabinol effects in schizophrenia: Implications for cognition, psychosis, and addiction. *Biological Psychiatry, 57,* 594–608. doi:10.1016/j.biopsych.2004.12.006

Doweiko, H. E., & Evans, A. L. (2019). *Concepts of chemical dependency* (10th ed.). Stamford, CT: Cengage Learning.

Elsohly, M. A., Harland, E., Murphy, J. C., Wirth, P., & Waller, C. W. (1985). Cannabinoids in glaucoma: A primary screening procedure. *Journal of Clinical Pharmacology, 21,* 472S–478S. doi:10.1002/j.1552-4604.1981.tb02627.x

Gage, S. H., Hickman, M., & Zammit, S. (2016). Association between cannabis and psychosis: Epidemiologic evidence. *Biological Psychiatry, 79,* 549–556. doi:10.1016/j.biopsych.2015.08.001

Governing the States and Localities. (2019). State marijuana laws in 2019 map. Retrieved from http://www.governing.com/gov-data/safety-justice/state-marijuana-laws-map-medical-recreational.html

Grant, W. (2002). Rastafari culture: The extreme Ethiopian Rasta vs. the mellow Dallas Rasta. Reggae/Speech 214. Retrieved from https://debate.uvm.edu/dreadlibrary/grant02.htm

Gumbiner, J. (2011, June). History of cannabis in India. *Psychology Today.* Retrieved from https://www.psychologytoday.com/us/blog/the-teenage-mind/201106/history-cannabis-in-india

Hall, T. (2007, April 12). *Rastafarianism: Origins and beliefs.* London: *The Telegraph.* Retrieved from https://www.telegraph.co.uk/news/uknews/1548384/Rastafarianism-Origins-and-beliefs.html

Hampson, R. E., & Deadwyler, S. A. (1999). Cannabinoids, hippocampal function and memory. *Life Sciences, 65,* 715–723. doi:10.1016/S0024-3205(99)00294-5

Havocscope Global Black-Market Information. (2015). Marijuana facts and statistics. Retrieved from http://www.havocscope.com/tag/marijuana/

Holdridge, S. L., & Holdridge, D. C. (2015). Cannabis and mental health problems. *InnovAiT, 8*(1), 5–10. doi:10.1177/1755738014558339

Hollis, C., Groom, M. J., Das, D., Calton, T., Bates, A. T., Andrews, H. K., . . . Liddle, P. F. (2014). Different psychological effects of cannabis use in adolescents at genetic risk for schizophrenia and with attention deficit/hyperactivity disorder (ADHD). *Schizophrenia Research, 105*(1–3), 216–223. doi: 10.1016/j.schres.2008.07.010

Inversen, L. L. (2008). *The science of marijuana.* New York, NY: Oxford University Press.

Jamaica Gleaner. (2015, April 15). Ganja amendment law comes into effect today. Retrieved from http://jamaica-gleaner.com/article/news/20150415/ganja-amendment-law-comes-effect-today

Jamaica Gleaner. (2019, March 3). Rastafarianism fastest growing religion among British Army. Retrieved from http://jamaica-gleaner.com/article/news/20190303/rastafarianism-fastest-growing-religion-among-british-army.

Johnston, L. D., Miech, R. A., O'Malley, P. M., Bachman, J. G., Schulenberg, J. E., & Patrick, M. E. (2019). *Monitoring the future national survey results on drug use 1975–2018: Overview, key findings on adolescent drug use.* Ann Arbor, MI: Institute for Social Research, University of Michigan. Retrieved from https://www.drugabuse.gov/related-topics/trends-statistics/monitoring-future, doi:10.3998/2027.42/150621

Khamsi, R. (2013). Going to pot. *Scientific American, 308*(6), 34, 36. doi:10.1038/scientificamerican0613-34

Lewis, W. (1993). *Soul rebels the Rastafari.* Prospect Heights, IL: Waveland Press, Inc.

Malcolm, B. P. (2014). Expanding children's rights in Jamaica through international educational partnership. In K. R. Libal, S. M. Berthold, R. L. Thomas, & L. M. Healy, (Eds.), *Advancing human rights in social work education* (pp. 369–389). Alexandria, VA: CSWE Press.

Martz, M. E., Tracco, E. M., Cope, L. M., Hardee, J. E., Jester, J. M., Zucker, R. A., & Heitzeg, M. M. (2016). Association of marijuana use with blunted nucleus accumbens response to reward anticipation. *JAMA Psychiatry, 73*(8), 838–844. doi:10.1001/jamapsychiatry.2016.1161

Matsuda, L. A., Lolait, S. J., Brownstein, M. J., Young, A. C., & Bonner, T. I. (1990). Structure of a cannabinoid receptor and functional expression of the cloned DNA. *Nature, 346*(6284), 561–564. doi:10.1038/346561a0

Miller, P. (2018, June 13). Laying down the law with cannabis. *Jamaica Observer.* Retrieved from http://www.jamaicaobserver.com/news/laying-down-the-law-with-cannabis_135696?profile=1373

Mizrahi, R., Watts, J. J., Tseng, K. Y. (2017). Mechanisms contributing to cognitive deficits in cannabis users. *Neuropharmacology, 124*, 84–88. doi: 10.1016/j.neuropharm.2017.04.018

Morin, J. G., Afzali, M. H., Bourque, J., Stewart, S. H., Séguin, J. R., O'Leary-Barrett, M., & Conrod, P. J. (2019). A population-based analysis of the relationship between substance use and adolescent cognitive development. *American Journal of Psychiatry, 176*(2), 98–106. doi:10.1176/appi.ajp.2018.18020202

National Institute on Drug Abuse (NIDA). (2019). Marijuana: Facts for teens. Retrieved from https://www.drugabuse.gov/publications/marijuana-facts-teens/want-to-know-more-some-faqs-about-marijuana

Office of National Drug Control Policy (ONDCP). (2019). *National drug control strategy final report.* Washington, DC: The White House. Retrieved from https://www.whitehouse.gov/wp-content/uploads/2019/01/NDCS-Final.pdf.

Organization of American States (OAS). (2012). *Inter-American commission on human rights, 2012 annual report.* Washington, DC: OAS. Retrieved from https://www.oas.org/en/iachr/docs/annual/2012/TOC.asp

Renard, J., Rosen, L. G., Loureiro, M., Oliveira, C. D., Schmid, S., Rushlow, W., & Laviolette, S. R. (2017). Adolescent cannabinoid exposure induces a persistent sub-cortical hyper-dopaminergic state and associated molecular adaptations in the prefrontal cortex. *Cerebral Cortex, 27*(2), 1297–1310. doi:10.1093/cercor/bhv335

Royal Queen Seeds (RQS). (2019). *The history of the Rastafari movement and cannabis.* London, UK: Royal Queen Seeds. Retrieved from https://www.royalqueenseeds.com/blog-the-history-of-the-rastafari-movement-and-cannabis-n1018.

Rubino, T., & Parolaro, D. (2008). Long lasting consequences of cannabis exposure in adolescence. *Molecular and Cellular Endocrinology, 286*, S108–S113. doi:10.1016/j.mce.2008.02.003

Substance Abuse and Mental Health Services Administration (SAMHSA). (2018). Results from the 2017 national survey on drug use and health: Summary of national findings. Retrieved from https://www.samhsa.gov/data/sites/default/files/cbhsq-reports/NSDUHDetailedTabs2017/NSDUHDetailedTabs2017.pdf

Sclar, K., (Ed.). (2019). Marijuana street names and nicknames. Retrieved from https://luxury.rehabs.com/marijuana-rehab/street-names-and-nicknames/

Smith, L. (2018). How a racist hate-monger masterminded America's war on drugs. *Timeline*. Retrieved from https://timeline.com/harry-anslinger-racist-war-on-drugs-prison-industrial-complex-fb5cbc281189

Trevithick, P. (2000). Social work skills: A practice handbook. Philadelphia: Open University Press.

United Nations Office on Drugs and Crime (UNODC). (2014). *World drug report 2014*. Vienna, Austria: United Nations Publication, Sales No. E.14.XI.7. Retrieved from https://www.unodc.org/documents/wdr2014/World_Drug_Report_2014_web.pdf, doi:10.18356/bdf42380-en

United Nations Office on Drugs and Crime (UNODC). (2018). *World drug report 2018*. Vienna, Austria: United Nations Publication, Sales No. E.18.XI.9. Retrieved from https://www.unodc.org/wdr2018

United States Department of State. (2018). *International narcotics control strategy report, Vol. 1: Drug and chemical control* (pp. 1–294). Washington, DC: U.S. Department of State, Bureau for International Narcotics and Law Enforcement Affairs. Retrieved from https://www.hsdl.org/?abstract&did=809034

Wang, I. J., Brenner, J. C., & Butsic, V. (2017). Cannabis, an emerging agricultural crop, leads to deforestation and fragmentation. *Frontiers in Ecology and the Environment, 15*, 495–501. doi:10.1002/fee.1634

Yadav, V., Beaver, C., Bowen, J., Bowling, A., Weinstock-Guttman, B., Cameron, M., . . . Narayanaswami, P. (2014). Summary of evidence-based guideline: Complementary and alternative medicine in multiple sclerosis: Report of the guideline development subcommittee of the American Academy of neurology. *Neurology, 82*, 1083–1092. doi:10.1212/WNL.0000000000000250

Yucel, M., Solowij, N., Respondek, C., Whittie, S., Fornito, A., Pantelis, C., & Lubman, D. I. (2008). Regional brain abnormalities associated with long-term heavy cannabis use. *Archives of General Psychiatry, 65*(5), 694–701. doi:10.1001/archpsyc.65.6.694

32

Emerging policy and practice responses to substance use with currently and formerly incarcerated women

Susan J. Rose and Thomas P. LeBel

Background

Substance use drives high levels of incarceration in the United States, especially among women. The Sentencing Project (2018) reports that the number of incarcerated women in the United States increased by more than 700% between 1980 and 2016, from a total of 26,378 to 213,722 (with 111,422 in prison; 102,300 in jail). Moreover, the number of women and girls in prison worldwide (now estimated at 714,000) has increased by 53% since 2000, while the worldwide male prison population has increased by only 20% during this period. The female prison population has risen in all continents since 2000 and may be increasing at a faster rate than for males (Walmsley, 2018).

Many authors attribute this dramatic rise to consequences of the War on Drugs, a "war" that took many impoverished women "prisoner" with few options for alternatives. These women often were engaged in problematic substance use, commonly introduced through relationships with male partners (UNDOC, 2018). They rarely had connections to larger distribution networks, so their ability to negotiate "a deal" to reduce their sentence was infrequent, and they often were unwilling to turn in a partner, who might also be the father of their children, to obtain an alternative to incarceration (Johnson, Dunlap, & Tourigny, 2000). Prisons and jails have been slow to accommodate these women, as they still represent a minority (about 7%) of the total incarcerated population both in the United States (Carson, 2018) and worldwide (Walmsley, 2018). Policies and macro-practice interventions have not kept up with the needs of incarcerated women, a majority of whom are mothers of minor children, survivors of physical and sexual trauma, underemployed, poorly educated, the sole source of income in their families, living in resource starved neighborhoods, and with multiple undiagnosed physical and mental health conditions (Ney, Ramirez, & Van Dieten, 2012).

The needs of women in our correctional systems who engage in substance misuse are garnering more attention as legislators debate criminal justice reform. This chapter focuses on: (1) our current state of knowledge of issues these women faced before incarceration, while incarcerated, and as they re-enter their communities; (2) current thinking about integrated treatment and interventions for incarcerated women, barriers faced in obtaining care, and some examples of promising programs; and (3) policy and system changes recommended to help these women build healthier and more sustainable lives for themselves and their families.

Incarcerated women and substance misuse

A key distinction must first be made between jails and prisons in the United States. Jails detain persons awaiting disposition of their cases (i.e. pretrial detainees), serving sentences for misdemeanors or low-level felonies, facing revocation from probation or parole, or awaiting a transfer to prison. In the United States, jails are operated by county or city governments and situated either in the community or nearby. In contrast, prisons confine individuals convicted of more serious crimes (primarily felonies) and serving longer sentences. Prisons are operated by either state or federal authorities and are generally located a significant distance from an incarcerated person's community and family. Because incarceration in jails is relatively brief, services are minimal and usually include only basic health care and medication for physical and mental health disorders. Prisons, however, generally provide a broader array of physical health, mental health, educational, vocational, and substance use treatment services based on longer stays. This distinction between jails and prisons is specific to the United States as many countries do not have both local jails and prisons.

The increasing incarceration of women experiencing substance use disorders is an emerging issue in many countries (Hughes, Wilsnack, & Kantor, 2016). In the United States, recent estimates from the Bureau of Justice Statistics show that 25% of females serving time in a state prison at the end of 2015 were convicted of a drug offense, compared to 14% of males (Carson, 2018). The proportion of women in state prisons for a drug offense increased dramatically from 12% in 1986 to 25% in 2016 (The Sentencing Project, 2018), and 56% of female federal prisoners were serving sentences for a drug offense (primarily drug trafficking charges) compared to 47% of males (Carson, 2018). More women than men in state prisons were incarcerated for a property offense often related to substance use, with 27% of incarcerated women versus 17% of incarcerated men having been convicted of a property crime. Further, 29% of women in U.S. jails were incarcerated due to drug-related offenses, excluding crimes related to drug use, such as prostitution, driving without a license, petty theft, or disorderly conduct (Swavola, Riley, & Submaranian, 2016).

Worldwide, the increased incarceration of women for participating in drug trafficking, has largely been attributed to women's lower status, and greater poverty (Emmott, 2007). However, it is also important to understand the level of problem substance use among incarcerated women in addition to any role they may have in international or domestic drug trafficking.

About one in five prisoners worldwide were incarcerated for drug offenses, with approximately 83% serving sentences involving drug possession for personal use (Nougier, 2018; Penal Reform International, 2018). Similar to the United States, about a quarter (28%) of women incarcerated in European countries were in prison for drug offenses (Iakobishvili, 2012). In the 27 countries comprising the European Union, 10–25% of persons were incarcerated for the use, possession, and supply of illicit drugs (Aebi & Del Grande, 2011), with females more likely than males to be incarcerated for offenses related to drug use (Borill et al., 2003). In some South and Central American countries (e.g. Argentina [federal prisons], Brazil, Costa Rica, Ecuador, Honduras, Mexico [federal prisons], Nicaragua, Panama, Venezuela) and Southeast Asian countries (e.g. Thailand), between 50% and 80% of women were in prison for drug offenses (Giacomello, 2013; Nougier, 2018). In Asia, 77% of incarcerated women in Thailand were imprisoned for a drug related offense and in Japan 39% of incarcerated women are reported to have a substance use disorder (UNODC, 2018).

Substance use

In a meta-analysis of 24 studies of substance use disorders among male and female prisoners in ten countries, the 12-month prevalence of alcohol and drug use disorders on reception to prison is high (Fazel, Yoon, & Hayes, 2017). Ten studies determined that an estimated 20% of women (ranging from 10–30%) met criteria for an alcohol use disorder, while 51% (ranging from 30% to 60%) met criteria for a substance use disorder. Overall, women more often experienced a drug use disorder than men (51% vs. 30%). In the United States, analyzing data from the nationally representative 2004 Survey of Inmates in State and Federal Facilities (SISFF), Marotta (2017) concluded that women (58.5%) were statistically significantly more likely than men (52.6%) to meet criteria for a substance use disorder, while rates of alcohol dependence were comparable (23.3% vs. 25.0%). In this sample of incarcerated persons, compared to men, women were also at increased risk of injecting drugs and sharing needles.

Studies focusing exclusively on women in U.S. jails identified even higher rates (see, e.g. Karberg & James, 2005). In a multisite study involving randomly selected women in rural and urban jails, 82% met lifetime criteria for a substance use disorder (SUD) (Lynch et al., 2014). Among 725 inmates in a large Midwestern jail system, women were more likely to report a substance use problem than men, with 71.2% of women reporting a SUD versus 49.1% of men (Fries, Fedock, & Kubiak, 2014). Other studies in Cook County Jail in Chicago and the Milwaukee County jail system reported similar results (Begun, Rose, & LeBel, 2010; Rose & LeBel, 2017; Scott, Grella, Dennis, & Funk, 2014).

Challenges for incarcerated women

Many women are incarcerated for crimes related to substance use (Sabol, West, & Cooper, 2009), and share common pre-incarceration experiences of stressed family and interpersonal relationships, mental health histories (e.g. depression, anxiety), victimization, trauma, interrupted education, lack of vocational experience or training, low income, and physical health problems (Drapalski, Youman, Stuewig, & Tangney, 2009; Lynch, DeHart, Belknap, & Green, 2012; Sered & Norton-Hawk, 2008). When coupled with the presence of current or past trauma and victimization, serious mental illness increases a woman's involvement in criminal activity and the likelihood of incarceration in jail (Lynch et al., 2012).

Co-occurring disorders involving substance use

Comorbid psychiatric and substance use disorders are especially prevalent among women in jail (Abram, Teplin, & McClelland, 2003; James & Glaze, 2006; Lynch et al., 2014; Rose & LeBel, 2017; Swavola et al., 2016). Between 62% and 75% of women in jail with a severe mental health disorder also experience a SUD (Abram et al., 2003; Potter, 2013). Rose and LeBel (2017) observed that co-occurring health conditions were common among the 240 incarcerated mothers of minor children in a Midwestern jail sample. In this study, over two-thirds (68.8%) reported some type of health-related co-occurring condition with more than half (52.5%) self-reporting both a mental health treatment history and a substance use problem, 41.3% both a substance use and a physical health problem history, and one-third (33.8%)

all three conditions: physical health, mental health, and substance use problems. Compared with other incarcerated mothers of minor children, mothers jailed six or more times had nearly three times the odds of reporting all three health conditions. This prevalence level was slightly above that of Mallik-Kane and Visher's (2008) report that roughly six in ten women returning home from state prison reported a combination of physical health, mental health, and substance abuse conditions. Similarly, Lynch et al. (2014) observed that about one-fourth (26%) of jailed women met lifetime criteria for co-occurring serious mental illness, PTSD, and a substance use disorder.

Childhood and adult victimization

Untold numbers of incarcerated women have been exposed to trauma, often beginning in childhood with neglect or physical and sexual abuse, continuing as an adult with intimate partner violence (IPV), and sexual assaults (Clements-Nolle, Wolden, & Bargmann-Losche, 2009; Jones, Worthen, Sharp, & McLeod, 2018; Radatz & Wright, 2017; Sharp, 2014). Myriad studies concluded that childhood and/or adult victimization (IPV) was related to illicit drug use (DeHart, 2008; Friestad, Ase-Bente, & Kjelsberg, 2014; Jones et al., 2018; Radatz & Wright, 2017; Sharp, Peck, & Hartsfield, 2012). In the nationally representative 2004 Survey of Inmates in State and Federal Facilities in the United States (SISFF), Marotta (2017) reported that more than one-fourth (27.3%) of women experienced childhood sexual abuse, and nearly one-third (31.5%) experienced childhood physical abuse. Child victimization experiences were strongly related to women's risk for substance misuse before prison. Moreover, among women, the prevalence of sexual abuse was significantly related to increased risk of alcohol dependence, as well as injection drug use and syringe (needle) sharing. These findings influenced Marotta (2017) to conclude that "childhood adversities play a significant role in the development of substance misuse in an inmate population" (p. 731). Similarly, Kennedy, Tripodi, Pettus-Davis, and Ayers (2016) observed that incarcerated women who experienced multi-victimization (i.e. both childhood physical and sexual abuse) were nearly four times as likely to meet criteria for a substance use disorder. Additionally, the frequency of physical abuse significantly predicted substance misuse (Kennedy et al., 2016; Tripodi & Pettus-Davis, 2013).

While the estimated rate of PTSD in the general population is 9.4% lifetime, 5.3% in the past 12 months, and 4.2% in the past 6 months (Kilpatrick et al., 2013), among incarcerated women it is much higher (Jones et al., 2018; Wolff et al., 2011). High rates of exposure to trauma was related to an earlier age of first drug use and a later diagnosis of PTSD among women entering jail in Chicago (Scott, Lurigio, Dennis, & Funk, 2016). Similarly, Rose and LeBel (2017) noted that 30.0% of women in jail self-reported receiving mental health treatment specifically for physical abuse or trauma. Women in prison who experienced IPV (physical and psychological abuse) were significantly more likely to report engaging in heavy illicit drug use before their most recent incarceration (Jones et al., 2018). Incarcerated women's substance misuse may be a (maladaptive) coping mechanism to deal with the trauma caused by childhood and adult victimization, as well as PTSD (DeHart, 2008; Lynch et al., 2012; Radatz & Wright, 2017).

Substance use before incarceration

Prior to incarceration, a majority of women reported engaging in regular and heavy (more than once a week for at least a month) illicit drug use (Solinas-Saunders & Stacer, 2017; Yule, Pare, & Gartner, 2015). In a study of 200 women jailed in the eastern United States, about half reported being under the influence of drugs or alcohol at the time of arrest (McGee, Williams, Strickland, Dobson-Brown, & Foreman, 2016). Other studies concluded that involvement in drug dealing, prostitution (or trading sex for drugs or money), and having an intimate partner who uses drugs all significantly increase the likelihood women will use drugs (Yule et al., 2015).

An Australian study reported that the presence of a substance use disorder was the strongest risk factor for women offending (Papalia, Ogloff, Cutajar, & Mullen, 2018). Incarcerated women who indicated regular substance use, having been in a drug or alcohol treatment program, and having friends who use drugs, reported a higher number of previous incarcerations (Solinas-Saunders & Stacer, 2017). Interviews with 259 incarcerated women in Ontario, Canada depicted a strong and positive relationship between drug use and earning money illegally, and that drug use was the strongest predictor of income-generating crime (Yule et al., 2015). Similarly, other studies have noted that many incarcerated women experiencing substance use problems reported trading sex for drugs or money (Scott et al., 2016) or committing another type of offense to support their drug use (McGee et al., 2016).

Prisoner reentry and women's substance use

According to the U.S. Bureau of Justice Statistics, 35% of female and 45% of male prisoners were re-arrested during the first year following release, and by nine years post release 77% of women state prisoners were re-arrested as compared to 84% of men (Alper & Durose, 2018). Drug use caused a substantial percentage of women to return to prison (Sharp, 2014; Western, 2018). Among reincarcerated women in Oklahoma, about three-quarters reported remaining drug free as a major difficulty and two-thirds reported staying away from friends/family who engaged in drug use or crime as a major difficulty.

Women who recidivate are more likely to have used drugs before incarceration and again soon after release (Cobbina, 2010; Scott, Dennis, & Lurigio, 2017). Women experiencing more serious substance use problems were three times as likely as other released women to be arrested for committing a new crime or returned to prison for a parole violation (Huebner, DeJong, & Cobbina, 2010). Women returned to prison experienced substance use problems before and after release, while those who desisted from crime received needed treatment and developed support networks to promote abstinence (Sharp & Ortiz, 2016).

One year removed from prison, women were more likely than men to engage in drug use and to experience problems due to drug use (LaVigne, Brooks, & Shollenberger, 2009). Lynch and Heath (2017) identified several factors predicting women's jail post-release substance use problems: experiencing PTSD and depression after release, using maladaptive coping strategies (e.g. disengagement, self-blame, denial), and experiencing interpersonal violence after returning to the community. A study involving formerly incarcerated Black Americans in New York City reported that women returning from prison returned to drug use more quickly than men (median 1 day versus 30 days, respectively) (Rowell-Cunsolo, Szeto, McDonald, & El-Bassel, 2018).

Women in prison often report that to be successful after release they must have will power, but also need to ask for (and receive) help and support (Coalition for Women Prisoners, 2008). Women experiencing substance use disorders released from jail and/or prison who do not receive treatment were at higher risk of returning to substance use and recidivism (Grella & Greenwell, 2007; Oser, Knudsen, Staton-Tindall, & Leukefeld, 2009). For example, Scott and colleagues (2017) identified higher levels of substance use treatment, self-help engagement, and reduced substance use as predicting lower recidivism. Prisoners participating in substance abuse programs while incarcerated and immediately after release were less likely to return to prison (LaVigne, Shollenberger, & Debus, 2009) and reported less frequent drug use (LaVigne, Brooks, & Shollenberger, 2007; Visher & Courtney, 2007). Moreover, receiving treatment for substance use while in prison reduced the risk for all-cause and overdose mortality following release to the community (Binswanger et al., 2016).

Persons experiencing co-occurring problems are more likely to report challenges at community reentry, including housing, employment, family support, and criminal involvement in addition to their substance misuse (Mallik-Kane & Visher, 2008). Women engaged in substance misuse often received less help from families during reentry, intensifying negative outcomes they experienced from their poorer health status (Mallik-Kane & Visher, 2008), and must overcome more issues than their male counterparts (Bloom, Owen, & Covington, 2003; LeBel, 2012; O'Brien, 2001; Richie, 2001; Van Olphen, Eliason, Freudenberg, & Barnes, 2009).

Integrated treatment and intervention

A concerted effort to provide evidence-based, gender-responsive programs for incarcerated women has recently emerged (Smith & Manchak, 2015). Several gender-responsive programs integrated treatment for substance abuse, trauma, and mental health (Bloom, 2015; Covington, 1999, 2003; Najavits, 2002). Although research about the effectiveness of integrated programs to address substance use problems experienced by incarcerated women is fairly limited (Bartlett et al., 2015; Taxman, 2015), there exists preliminary evidence suggesting some effectiveness (Messina & Calhoun, 2014; Najavits & Hien, 2013; Swopes, Davis, & Scholl, 2017; Wolff, Frueh, Shi, & Schumann, 2012). Integrated substance use and trauma-informed interventions with women involved with the justice system have reduced recidivism and improved substance misuse and mental health-related (e.g. PTSD) outcomes (Messina, Grella, Cartier, & Torres, 2010; Zlotnick, Johnson, & Najavits, 2009). Messina and Calhoun (2014) detected significant between-group differences in reduction of PTSD with a couple of programs. Additionally, in a study involving the sequential delivery of *Helping Women Recover* (Covington, 1999) and *Beyond Trauma* (Covington, 2003), Swopes and colleagues (2017) reported that integrating these two approaches produced greater reduction in PTSD symptoms and substance-related self-efficacy compared to women not receiving this treatment protocol.

Treatment barriers

For women, seeking treatment for substance use problems while incarcerated and after release is fraught with challenges different from those facing males re-entering the community. In general, women face perceived and actual barriers that include stigma, questions about the efficacy of treatment that does not address trauma, a lack of family support, and family responsibilities of child care (Taylor, 2010; UNDOC, 2018; Van Olphen & Freudenberg, 2004). Significantly, both men and women reported more barriers to receiving treatment for substance use if released from jail than from prison (Begun, Early, & Hodge, 2016).

The relative dearth of integrated treatment services for incarcerated women as they re-enter the community is a significant barrier to care (Covington, Burke, Keaton, & Norcott, 2008). Among women returning to the community from state prisons, lack of financial resources or health care coverage were cited as the most significant barriers to obtaining treatment for their substance-related problems (Sung, Mellow, & Mahoney, 2010). Women recently released from local jails who experienced substance use problems identified inadequate child care and a lack of protection from sexual harassment as additional barriers to their seeking and remaining in treatment (Richie, 2001). Rose, LeBel, Begun, and Fuhrmann (2014) reported that women in jail perceived lack of financial ability to pay for treatment, treatment sites' distant locations, and a general lack of information about available services as key barriers to engaging in treatment after release (Rose et al., 2014).

Many structural barriers to receiving substance abuse treatment exist (Verissimo & Grella, 2017): despite detecting no differences between men and women in perceptions of structural barriers, women were more likely to hold negative attitudes, such as fear and pessimism, about treatment programs. Women who were pregnant or had young children expressed fear of losing custody or parental rights if they sought treatment (Verissimo & Grella, 2017). Similarly, Medley and Thumath (2018) noted that the prosecution of prenatal drug use in the United States appears to reduce enrollment by pregnant women in evidence-based drug treatment programs.

Promising programs

Gender responsive programs have been developing during the past 20 years, focused specifically on women who misuse substances and have experienced past and current trauma. Bloom (2015) developed a "toolkit" providing a description of best practices and programs for addressing the needs of women involved with the criminal justice system. Gender responsive programs with strong evidence support include *Helping Women Recover: A Program for Treating Addiction* (Covington, 1999), *Beyond Trauma: A Healing Journey for Women* (Covington, 2003), and *Seeking Safety: A Treatment Manual for PTSD and Substance Abuse* (Najavits, 2002). Both the *Beyond Trauma* and *Seeking Safety* programs include cognitive-behavioral treatment components.

Forever free

This program combines 6 months of intensive work with women experiencing substance use problems before release from prison with community-based residential treatment after release (Hall, Prendergast, Wellisch, Patten, & Cao, 2004). While in prison, women were housed in a segregated unit and provided 4 hours of treatment, 5 days a week near their scheduled time of release. Treatment consists of group and individual sessions, with a focus on issues relevant to recovery (i.e. self-esteem, anger management, sexual and personal relationships, interpersonal violence, trauma, sexual health, and parenting). The model's developers reported that women enrolled in the program while in prison were re-arrested and convicted at a significantly lower rate than women not in the program. In addition, after 1-year post release, women who completed the in-prison and residential components were significantly more likely to remain drug free and avoid re-incarceration.

Oxford House

Other interventions for women released from jails or prisons reduce substance use and/or recidivism (Jason, Salina, & Ram, 2016; Lurigio, Stalans, Roque, Seng, & Ritchie, 2007; Scott et al., 2017). For example, in a Chicago metropolitan area study involving women engaged in substance misuse (heroin as major problem) and recently engaged with the criminal justice system, women with longer stays in Oxford House (OH) recovery homes demonstrated better outcomes (Jason et al., 2016). OHs are self-run by peers in recovery rather than professional staff and provide abstinent housing for individuals dealing with substance misuse problems. Women who stayed for 6 months or more had better outcomes in terms of substance use, abstinence self-efficacy, employment, and recidivism than those with shorter stays.

Additional program options

Osher, Steadman, and Barr (2002) developed an integrated framework for persons experiencing co-occurring mental health and substance use problems to help correctional systems direct limited resources to where they can be most effective, but this framework is not in wide use. Several studies reported positive effects for interventions which include specialized probation and recovery management checkups (RMCs) (Lurigio et al., 2007; Scott et al., 2017). A specialized probation program with enhanced referral mechanisms to community-based services for substance use and trauma, as well as motivational interventions to remain engaged in these services, increased rates of participation in substance abuse treatment, lowered rates of weekly substance use, and reduced recidivism (Lurigio et al., 2007; Scott et al., 2017). The RMCs were similarly effective when women were not on probation (Scott et al., 2017). The RMC model used "linkage managers" to connect women experiencing substance use issues to treatment services as soon as possible and interventions to enhance engagement and retention in these services to improve outcomes. In one qualitative study, providing mentoring programs also improved successful transition to the community for formerly incarcerated women (Garcia, 2016).

Policy and system changes to meet challenges

Incarcerated women experience multiple challenges both before their incarceration and as they return to their communities. These women face the impact of incarceration on co-occurring physical health, mental health, and substance use problems, as well as the complexities of their roles as mothers with minor children. Changes in practice policies in jail and prison settings could be implemented that would take advantage of opportunities to address physical health, mental health, and substance use problems early in an incarceration.

- All women entering a correctional facility should be screened and evaluated for physical health issues (including pregnancy testing), mental health history and functioning (including an evaluation of suicidal thinking and intent), substance misuse/substance use disorder, and traumatizing victimization experiences (both childhood and adult). Identification of specific issues through universal screening is important in assessing the need for and targeting specific resources and assisting women in connecting with these resources before their release.
- Women should have easy, non-stigmatized access to services while incarcerated and direct linkages to them after their release. In jails, this access should focus on identifying issues, locating resources, making direct linkages to these resources, identifying barriers to their use, and increasing motivation to use them. In prisons, emphasis should be focused on reducing the stigma attached to using services by both the woman and correctional staff. Trauma-informed care should be the first treatment of choice for incarcerated women experiencing substance misuse. Evidence of incarcerated women's consistent experiences with trauma is robust, strongly suggesting trauma informed care interventions should be considered before other methods.

- Correctional staff in jails should receive training in recognizing symptoms and behavioral manifestations of common mental health problems, including trauma, among women inmates. Women who are depressed, anxious, traumatized, and who experience psychosis are consistent discipline problems for jail staff. Correctional staff should also be trained in positive interpersonal action techniques and good communication skills.
- Female inmates should be protected from further victimization while incarcerated: victimization by other inmates, as well as by correctional staff, through close monitoring and ongoing staff training.
- While incarcerated in prison all women should have access to education and vocational services that would increase their ability to become self-sufficient at release. This includes housing assistance and connection with children in the public child welfare system.
- All incarcerated women should be encouraged to sign up for healthcare and healthcare benefits before their release (in the United States, under the Affordable Care Act/ACA, or other relevant public health programs in the United States and elsewhere). Enrollment should be part of a broader reentry plan including an individualized transition plan for the first 24 hours after release (a period critical to successful reintegration into the community), planning for medication renewals, and connecting women to integrated treatments for medication, individual treatment, group support, illness management techniques, supported employment, affordable housing, and cognitive-behavioral treatments.

Conclusions

In considering the contributions of trauma, substance misuse, mental health histories, physical health problems, poverty, racism, inadequate educational systems, and lack of employment opportunities to women's criminal behaviors and probability of incarceration, clinicians, policy makers, and researchers should consider the locus of concern. Social inequities perceived as individual failings will continue to frustrate the search for effective interventions at all levels. Continuing to blame women, especially poor, non-white women, for engaging in non-violent criminal behavior to assuage ongoing pain from chronic trauma will not produce needed societal and individual changes.

While the field has committed to the need for "gender-sensitive" treatment, what is needed is a new look at occasions of oppression experienced by many incarcerated women. Women, especially mothers of minor children, are viewed as even more deviant than fathers for engaging in addictive behaviors: it seems to the general public a violation of gender norms for a mother to pursue substance misuse and neglect her children (McKim, 2017). Yet, these women also face increased stigma and risk losing custody of their children when they seek treatment for substance use problems (UNDOC, 2018).

Many women are introduced to substance use through a relationship with a male partner, which then becomes a liability; some treatment programs require women to end their relationship with a partner engaged in substance use, echoing old methods of welfare eligibility when women could not receive financial assistance if a man was in the house. But their partners may be reluctant to attend family-based treatment sessions if they are also wary of outstanding warrants for their arrest for other criminal activities. The lack of family cohesion is then considered a function of individual responsibility (or lack of responsibility) rather than of policies that foster barriers to family stability experienced by many women, particularly women in poverty.

The intersections of gender, race, class, and criminal behavior is inherently dangerous for women engaged in substance misuse and calls for an in-depth analysis of the interconnectedness of individual abilities and identities and institutional oppression in the lives of incarcerated women (see Mehrotra, 2010 cited in Willison & O'Brien, 2017). Without this analysis, women will continue to (over)populate correctional institutions for engaging in substance-related behaviors that cover layers of socio-economic, mental health, physical health, and traumatic experiences without providing tools for promoting individual and societal changes.

References

Aebi, M., & Del Grande, N. (2011). *Council of Europe annual penal statistics: SPACE I—2009.* Strasourg, France: Council of Europe.

Abram, K. M., Teplin, L. A., & McClelland, G. M. (2003). Comorbidity of severe psychiatric disorders and substance use disorders among women in jail. *American Journal of Psychiatry, 160*(5), 1007–1010. doi:10.1176/appi.ajp.160.5.1007

Alper, M., & Durose, M. R. (2018). *2018 update on prisoner recidivism: A 9-year follow-up period (2005–2014).* Special report, NCJ 250975. Washington, DC: U.S. Department of Justice, Office of Justice Programs, Bureau of Justice Statistics.

Bartlett, A., Jhanji, E., White, S., Harty, M., Scammell, J., & Allen, S. (2015). Interventions with women offenders: A systematic review and meta-analysis of mental health gain. *The Journal of Forensic Psychiatry & Psychology, 26,* 133–165. doi:10.1080/14789949.2014.981563

Begun, A. L., Early, T. J., & Hodge, A. (2016). Mental health and substance abuse service engagement by men and women during community reentry following incarceration. *Administration and Policy in Mental Health and Mental Health Research, 43,* 207–218.

Begun, A. L., Rose, S. J., & LeBel, T. P. (2010). Helping address women's substance abuse problems in jail and preparing for community reentry. In S. Stojkovic (Ed.), *Managing special populations in jails and prisons* (Vol. 2, pp.1–2, 1–29). Kingston, NJ: Civic Research Institute (CRI).

Binswanger, I. A., Stern, M. F., Yamashita, T. E., Mueller, S. R., Baggett, T. P., & Blatchford, P. J. (2016). Clinical risk factors for death after release from prison in Washington State: A nested case-control study, *Addiction, 111*(3), 499–510. doi:10.1111/add.13200

Bloom, B., Owen, B., & Covington, S. (2003). *Gender-responsive strategies: Research, practice, and guiding principles for women offenders.* Washington, DC: National Institute of Corrections.

Bloom, B. E. (2015). *Meeting the needs of women in California's county justice systems: A toolkit for policymakers and practitioners.* Oakland: Californians for Safety and Justice.

Borrill, J., Maden, A.M., Weaver, T., Stimson, G., Farrell, M., & Barnes, T. (2003). *Differential substance misuse treatment needs of women, ethnic minorities and young offenders in prison:prevalence of substance misuse and treatment needs.* London: The Home Office.

Carson, E. A. (2018). *Prisoners in 2016. NCJ 251149.* Washington, DC: U.S. Department of Justice, Office of Justice Programs, Bureau of Justice.

Clements-Nolle, K., Wolden, M., & Bargmann-Losche, J. (2009). Childhood trauma and risk for past and future suicide attempts among women in prison. *Women's Health Issues, 19*(3), 185–192. doi:10.1016/j.whi.2009.02.002

Coalition for Women Prisoners. (2008). *My sister's keeper: A book for women returning home from prison or jail.* New York: Correctional Association of New York.

Cobbina, J. E. (2010). Reintegration success and failure: Factors impacting reintegration among incarcerated and formerly incarcerated women. *Journal of Offender Rehabilitation, 49,* 210–232. doi:10.1080/10509671003666602

Covington. S. (1999). *Helping women recover: A program for treating substance abuse: Special edition for use in the criminal justice system.* San Francisco, CA: Jossey-Bass.

Covington, S. (2003). *Beyond trauma: A healing journey for women.* Center City, MN: Hazelden.

Covington, S. S., Burke, C., Keaton, S., & Norcott, C. (2008). Evaluation of a trauma-informed and gender-responsive intervention for women in drug treatment. *Journal of Psychoactive Drugs, 5,* 387–398. doi:10.1080/02791072.2008.10400666DeHart, D. D. (2008). Pathways to prison. *Violence Against Women, 14,* 1362–1381. doi:10.1177/1077801208327018

Drapalski, A. L., Youman, K., Stuewig, J., & Tangney, J. (2009). Gender differences in jail inmates' symptoms of mental illness, treatment history and treatment seeking. *Criminal Behaviour and Mental Health, 19*(3), 193–206. doi:10.1002/cbm.733

Emmott, R. (2007, April 4). More women rule, and die, in Mexico's drug gangs. *Reuters*. Retrieved from https://www.reuters.com/article/us-mexico-drugs/more-women-rule-and-die-in-mexicos-drug-gangs-idUSN2028028620070420.

Fazel, S., Yoon, I. A., & Hayes, A. J. (2017). Substance use disorders in prisoners: An updated systematic review and meta-regression analysis in recently incarcerated men and women. *Addiction, 112*(10), 1725–1739. doi:10.1111/add.13877

Fries, L., Fedock, G., & Kubiak, S. P. (2014). Role of gender, substance use, and serious mental illness in anticipated post-jail homelessness. *Social Work, 38*(2), 107–116. doi:10.1093/swr/svu014

Friestad, C., Ase-Bente, R., & Kjelsberg, E. (2014). Adverse childhood experiences among women prisoners: Relationships to suicide attempts and drug abuse. *International Journal of Social Psychiatry, 60*, 40–46. doi:10.1177/0020764012461235

Garcia, J. (2016). The importance of the mentor-mentee relationship in women's desistance from destructive behaviors. *International Journal of Offender Therapy & Comparative Criminology, 60*(7), 808–827. doi:10.1177/0306624X14568257

Giacomello, C. (2013). *Women, drug offenses and penitentiary systems in Latin America* (IDPC briefing paper). London, UK: International Drug Policy Consortium.

Grella, C. E., & Greenwell, L. (2007). Treatment needs and completion of community-based aftercare among substance-abusing women offenders. *Women's Health Issues, 17*, 244–255. doi:10.1016/j.whi.2006.11.005

Hall, E. A., Prendergast, M. L., Wellisch, J., Patten, M., & Cao, Y. (2004). Treating drug-abusing women prisoners: An outcome evaluation of the Forever Free program. *The Prison Journal, 84*(1):81–105. doi:10.1177/0032885503262456

Huebner, B. M., DeJong, C., & Cobbina, J. (2010). Women coming home: Long-term patterns of recidivism. *Justice Quarterly, 27*(2), 225–254. doi:10.1080/07418820902870486

Hughes, T. L., Wilsnack, S. C., & Kantor, L. W. (2016). The influence of gender and sexual orientation on alcohol use and alcohol-related problems: Toward a global perspective. *Alcohol Research: Current Reviews, 38*(1), 121–132.

Iakobishvili, E. (2012). *Cause for alarm: The incarceration of women for drug offences in Europe and Central Asia, and the need for legislative and sentencing reform.* London, UK: Harm Reduction International.

James, D. J., & Glaze, L. E. (2006). *Mental health problems of prison and jail inmates.* Washington, DC: U.S. Department of Justice, Office of Justice Programs, Bureau of Justice Statistics.

Jason, L. A., Salina, D., & Ram, D. (2016). Oxford recovery housing: Length of stay correlated with improved outcomes for women previously involved with the criminal justice system. *Substance Abuse, 37*(1), 248–254. doi:10.1080/08897077.2015.1037946

Johnson, B., Dunlap, E., & Tourigny, S. C. (2000). Crack distribution and abuse in New York. *Crime Prevention Services, 11*, 19–57.

Jones, M. S., Worthen, M. G. F., Sharp, S. F., & McLeod, D. A. (2018). Bruised inside out: The adverse and abusive life histories of incarcerated women as pathways to PTSD and illicit drug use. *Justice Quarterly, 35*(6), 1004–1029. doi:10.1080/07418825.2017.1355009

Karberg, J. C., & James, D. J. (2005). *Substance dependence, abuse, and treatment of jail inmates, 2002.* Bureau of justice statistics special report (NCJ 209588). Washington, DC: US Department of Justice, Bureau of Justice.

Kennedy, S. C., Tripodi, S. J., Pettus-Davis, C., & Ayers, J. (2016). Examining dose–response relationships between childhood victimization, depression, symptoms of psychosis, and substance misuse for incarcerated women. *Women & Criminal Justice, 26*(2), 77–98. doi:10.1080/08974454.2015.1023486

Kilpatrick, D. G., Resnick, H. S., Milanak, M. E., Miller, M. W., Keyes, K. M., & Friedman, M. J. (2013). National estimates of exposure to traumatic events and PTSD prevalence using DSM-IV and DSM-5 criteria. *Journal of Traumatic Stress, 26*(5), 537–547. doi:10.1002/jts.21848

LaVigne, N. G., Brooks, L. E., & Shollenberger, T. L. (2007). *Returning home: Exploring the challenges and successes of recently released Texas prisoners.* Washington, DC: The Urban Institute. doi:10.1037/e719852011-001

LaVigne, N. G., Brooks, L. E., & Shollenberger, T. L. (2009). *Women on the outside: Understanding the experiences of female prisoners returning to Houston, Texas.* Washington, DC: The Urban Institute. doi:10.1037/e719232011-001

LaVigne, N. G., Shollenberger, T. L., & Debus, S.A. (2009). *One year out: Tracking the experiences of male prisoners returning to Houston, Texas.* Washington, DC: The Urban Institute. doi:10.1037/e719212011-001

LeBel, T. P. (2012). "If one doesn't get you another one will": Formerly incarcerated persons' perceptions of discrimination. *The Prison Journal, 92*(1), 63–87. doi:10.1177/0032885511429243

Lurigio, A. J., Stalans, L., Roque, L., Seng, M., & Ritchie, J. (2007). The effects of specialized supervision on women probationers: An evaluation of the POWER program. In R. Muraskin (Ed.), *It's a crime: Women and justice* (4th ed., pp. 127–145). Englewood Cliffs, NJ: Prentice Hall.

Lynch, S. M., DeHart, D. D., Belknap, J., & Green, B. L. (2012). *Women's pathways to jail: The roles & intersections of serious mental illness & trauma.* Washington, DC: U.S. Department of Justice, Office of Justice Programs, Bureau of Justice Assistance. doi:10.1037/e528222013-001

Lynch, S. M., DeHart, D. D., Belknap, J. E., Green, B. L., Dass-Brailsford, P., Johnson, K. A., & Whalley, E. (2014). A multisite study of the prevalence of serious mental illness, PTSD, and substance use disorders of women in jail. *Psychiatric Services, 65,* 670–674. doi:10.1176/appi.ps.201300172

Lynch, S. M., & Heath, N. M. (2017). Predictors of incarcerated women's postrelease PTSD, depression, and substance-use problems. *Journal of Offender Rehabilitation, 56*(3), 157–172. doi:10.1080/10 509674.2017.1290007

Mallik-Kane, K., & Visher, C. A. (2008). *Health and prisoner reentry: How physical, mental, and substance abuse conditions shape the process of reintegration.* Washington, DC: Urban Institute Justice Policy Center. doi:10.1037/e719772011-001

Marotta, P. L. (2017). Childhood adversities and substance misuse among the incarcerated: Implications for treatment and practice in correctional settings. *Substance Use & Misuse, 52*(6), 717–733. doi:10.1080/10826084.2016.1261899

McGee, Z. T., Williams, K., Strickland, N., Dobson-Brown, T., & Foreman, M. (2016). Inequality among female offenders: Racial disparities in substance abuse and medical treatment among mothers in prison. In S. F. Sharp, S. Marcus-Medoza, K. A. Cameron, & E. S. Daniel-Roberson (Eds.), *Across the spectrum of women and crime: Theories, offending and the criminal justice system* (pp. 205–224). Durham, NC: Carolina Academic Press.

McKim, A. (2017). *Addicted to rehab: Race, gender, and drugs in the era of mass incarceration.* New Brunswick, NJ: Rutgers University Press. doi:10.2307/j.ctt1pwtdfw

Medley, B., & Thumath, M. (2018). *Expecting better: Improving health and rights for pregnant women who use drugs.* New York, NY: Open Society Foundations.

Mehrotra, G. (2010). Toward a continuum of intersectionality theorizing for feminist social work scholarship. *Affilia: Journal of Women and Social Work, 25,* 417–430. doi:10.1177/0886109910384190

Messina, N. P., Braithwaite, J., Calhoun, S., & Kubiak, S. (2016). Examination of a violence prevention program for female offenders. *Violence and Gender, 3*(3), 143–149. doi:10.1089/vio.2015.0048

Messina, N. P., & Calhoun, S. (2014). Trauma-informed treatment decreases posttraumatic stress disorder among women offenders. *Journal of Trauma & Dissociation, 15,* 6–23. doi:10.1080/15299732.2 013.818609

Messina, N., Grella, C. E., Cartier, J., & Torres, S. (2010). A randomized experimental study of gender-responsive substance abuse treatment for women in prison. *Journal of Substance Abuse Treatment, 38,* 97–107. doi:10.1016/j.jsat.2009.09.004

Najavits, L. M. (2002). *Seeking safety: A treatment manual for PTSD and substance abuse.* New York, NY: Guilford Press.

Najavits, L. M., & Hien, D. (2013). Helping vulnerable populations: A comprehensive review of the treatment outcome literature on substance use disorder and PTSD. *Journal of Clinical Psychology, 69*(5), 433–79. doi:10.1002/jclp.21980Ney, B., Ramirez, R., & Van Dieten, M. (2012). *Ten truths that matter when working with justice involved women.* New York, NY: National Resource Center on Justice Involved Women.

Nougier, M. (2018). *Taking stock: A decade of drug policy. A civil society shadow report.* International Drug Policy Consortium Publication.

O'Brien, P. (2001). "Just like baking a cake": Women describe the necessary ingredients for successful reentry after incarceration. *Families in Society, 82*(3), 287–295. doi:10.1606/1044-3894.200

Oser, C., Knudsen, H., Staton-Tindall, M., & Leukefeld, C. (2009). The adoption of wraparound services among substance abuse treatment organizations serving criminal offenders: The role of a women-specific program. *Drug and Alcohol Dependence, 103,* S82–S90. doi:10.1016/j.drugalcdep.2008.12.008

Osher, F., Steadman, H. J., & Barr, H. (2002). A best practice approach to community reentry from jails for inmates with co-occurring disorders: The APIC model. *Crime & Delinquency, 49*(1), 79–96. doi:10.1177/0011128702239237

Papalia, N., Ogloff, J. R. P., Cutajar, M., & Mullen, P. E. (2018). Child sexual abuse and criminal offending: Gender-specific effects and the role of abuse characteristics and other adverse outcomes. *Child Maltreatment, 23*(4), 399–416. doi:10.1177/1077559518785779

Penal Reform International. (2018). *Global prison trends 2018. The rehabilitation and reintegration of offenders in the era of sustainable development.* London, UK: Penal Reform International.

Potter, R. H. (2013). Chronic disease and mental health within correctional facilities. In E. Waltermaurer & T. A. Akers (Eds.), *Epidemiological criminology: Theory to practice* (Vol. 11, pp. 155–161). New York, NY: Routledge.

Radatz, D. L., & Wright, E. M. (2017). Does polyvictimization affect incarcerated and non-incarcerated adult women differently? An exploration into internalizing problems. *Journal of Interpersonal Violence, 32*, 1379–1400. doi:10.1177/0886260515588921

Richie, B. (2001). Challenges incarcerated women face as they return to their communities: Findings from life history interviews. *Crime & Delinquency, 47*, 368–389. doi:10.1177/0011128701047003005

Rose, S. J., & LeBel, T. P. (2017). Incarcerated mothers of minor children: Physical health, substance use, and mental health needs. *Women & Criminal Justice, 27*(3), 170–190. doi:10.1080/08974454.2016.1247772

Rose, S. J., LeBel, T. P., Begun, A. L., & Fuhrmann, D. (2014). Looking out from the inside: Incarcerated women's perceived barriers to treatment of substance use. *Journal of Offender Rehabilitation, 53*(4), 300–316. doi:/10.1080/10509674.2014.902006

Rowell-Cunsolo, T. L., Szeto, B., McDonald, C., & El-Bassel, N. (2018). Return to illicit drug use post-incarceration among formerly incarcerated Black Americans. *Drugs: Education, Prevention & Policy, 25*(3), 234–240. doi:10.1080/09687637.2016.1259391

Sabol, W. J., West, H. C., & Cooper, M. (2009). *Prisoners in 2008.* Washington, DC: U.S. Department of Justice, Bureau of Justice Statistics.

Scott, C. K., Dennis, M. L., & Lurigio, A. J. (2017). The effects of specialized probation and recovery management checkups (RMCs) on treatment participation, substance use, HIV risk behaviors, and recidivism among female offenders: Main findings of a 3-year experiment using subject by intervention interaction analysis. *Journal of Experimental Criminology, 13*(1), 53–77. doi:10.1007/s11292-016-9281-z

Scott, C. K., Grella, C. E., Dennis, M. L., & Funk, R. R. (2014). Predictors of recidivism over 3 years among substance-using women released from jail. *Criminal Justice and Behavior, 41*, 1257–1289. doi:10.1177/0093854814546894

Scott, C. K., Lurigio, A. J., Dennis, M. L., & Funk, R. R. (2016). Trauma and morbidities among female detainees in a large urban jail. *The Prison Journal, 96*(1), 102–125. doi:10.1177/0032885515605490

Sered, S., & Norton-Hawk, M. (2008). Disrupted lives, fragmented care: Illness experiences of criminalized women. *Women & Health, 48*, 43–61. doi:10.1080/03630240802131999

Sharp, S.F. (2014). *Mean lives, mean laws: Oklahoma's women prisoners.* New Brunswick, NJ: Rutgers University Press.

Sharp, S. F., Peck, B. M., & Hartsfield, J. (2012). Childhood adversity and substance use of women prisoners: A general strain theory approach. *Journal of Criminal Justice, 40*, 202–211. doi:10.1016/j.jcrimjus.2012.01.003Sharp, S. F., & Ortiz, J. (2016). Staying out or going back? A qualitative study of women prisoners, recidivism, and reintegration. In S. F. Sharp, S. Marcus-Mendoza, K. A. Cameron, & E. S. Daniel-Robinson (Eds.), *Across the spectrum of women and crime: Theories, offending and the criminal justice system* (pp. 243–272). Durham, NC: Carolina Academic Press.

Smith, P., & Manchak, S. M. (2015). A gendered theory of offender rehabilitation. In F. T. Cullen, P. Wilcox, J. L. Lux, & C. L. Jonson (Eds.), *Sisters in crime revisited: Bringing gender into community* (pp. 371–395). New York, NY: Oxford University Press.

Solinas-Saunders, M., & Stacer, M. J. (2017). A retrospective analysis of repeated incarceration using a national sample: What makes female inmates different from male inmates? *Victims & Offenders, 12*(1), 138–173. doi:10.1080/15564886.2015.1101033

Sung, H., Mellow, J., & Mahoney, A. M. (2010). Jail inmates with co-occurring mental health and substance use problems: Correlates and service needs. *Journal of Offender Rehabilitation, 49*, 126–145. doi:10.1080/10509670903534811

Swavola, E., Riley, K., & Subramanian, R. (2016). *Overlooked: Women and jails in an era of reform.* New York, NY: Vera Institute of Justice.

Swopes, R. M., Davis, J. L., & Scholl, J. A. (2017). Treating substance abuse and trauma symptoms in incarcerated women. *Journal of Interpersonal Violence, 32*(7), 1143–1165. doi:10.1177/0886260515587668

Taxman, F. S. (2015). Dual diagnosis: Interventions designed to address substance abuse, mental health, and criminal thinking. In R. L. Trestman, K. L. Appelbaum, & J. L. Metzner (Eds.), *Oxford textbook of correctional psychiatry* (pp. 254–259). New York, NY: Oxford University Press. doi:10.1093/med/9780199360574.003.0045

Taylor, O. D. (2010). Barriers to treatment for women with substance use disorders. *Journal of Human Behavior in the Social Environment, 20,* 393–409. doi:10.1080/10911351003673310

The Sentencing Project. (2018, May 10). *Incarcerated women and girls.* Retrieved from https://www.sentencingproject.org/publications/incarcerated-women-and-girls/

Tripodi, S. J., & Pettus-Davis, C. (2013). Histories of childhood victimization and subsequent mental health problems, substance use, and sexual victimization for a sample of incarcerated women in the US. *International Journal of Law and Psychiatry, 36*(1), 30–40. doi:10.1016/j.ijlp.2012.11.005

United Nations Office on Drugs and Crime (UNDOC). (2018). *World drug report 2018.* Retrieved from https://www.unodc.org/wdr2018/

Van Olphen, J., Eliason, M. J., Freudenberg, N., & Barnes, M. (2009). Nowhere to go: How stigma limits the options of female drug users after release from jail. *Substance Abuse Treatment, Prevention, and Policy, 4,* Article 10, 1–10. doi:10.1186/1747-597X-4-10

Van Olphen, J., & Freudenberg, N. (2004). Harlem service providers' perceptions of the impact of municipal policies on their clients with substance use problems. *Journal of Urban Health, 81,* 222–231. doi:10.1093/jurban/jth109

Verissimo, A. D. O., & Grella, C. E. (2017). Influence of gender and race/ethnicity on perceived barriers to help-seeking for alcohol or drug problems. *Journal of Substance Abuse Treatment, 75,* 54–61. doi:10.1016/j.jsat.2016.12.013

Visher, C. A., & Courtney, S. M. E. (2007). *One year out: Experiences of prisoners returning to Cleveland.* Washington, DC: The Urban Institute. doi:10.1037/e719862011-001

Walmsley, R. (2018). *World female imprisonment list, fourth edition. Women and girls in penal institutions, including pre-trial detainees/remand prisoners. World prison brief.* London, UK: Institute for Criminal Policy Research.

Western, B. (2018). *Homeward: Life in the year after prison.* New York, NY: Russell Sage Foundation. doi:10.7758/9781610448710

Willison, J. S., & O'Brien, P. (2017). A feminist call for transforming the criminal justice system. *Affilia: Journal of Women & Social Work, 32*(1), 37–49. doi:10.1177/0886109916658080

Wolff, N., Frueh, B. C., Shi, J., Gerardi, D., Fabrikant, N., & Schumann, B. E. (2011). Trauma exposure and mental health characteristics of incarcerated females self-referred to specialty PTSD treatment. *Psychiatric Services, 62,* 954–958. doi:10.1176/ps.62.8.pss6208_0954

Wolff, N., Frueh, B. C., Shi, J., & Schumann, B. E. (2012). Effectiveness of cognitive-behavioral trauma treatment for incarcerated women with mental illnesses and substance abuse disorders. *Journal of Anxiety Disorders, 26,* 703–710. doi:10.1016=j.janxdis.2012.06.001

Yule, C., Paré, P.-P., & Gartner, R. (2015). An examination of the local life circumstances of female offenders: Mothering, illegal earnings and drug use. *British Journal of Criminology, 55*(2), 248–269. doi:10.1093/bjc/azu073

Zlotnick, C., Johnson, J., & Najavits, L. M. (2009). Randomized controlled pilot study of cognitive-behavioral therapy in a sample of incarcerated women with substance use disorder and PTSD. *Behavior Therapy, 40*(4), 325–336. doi:10.1016/j.beth.2008.09.004

Introduction to Section IV

Issues frequently co-occurring with addictive behaviors

The three chapters in Section IV examine complex relationships and intersections that occur between addictive behaviors and other major problems. Each chapter includes background context, prevalence data, theories of co-occurrence, and implications for social work practice or intervention. Chapter 33 discusses four models explaining the co-occurrence of substance misuse with diagnosable mental health problems and addictive behaviors: anxiety disorders, mood disorders, post-traumatic stress disorder (PTSD), and severe and persistent mental health disorders (e.g., schizophrenia and other psychosis disorders). Complex relationships between substance misuse and the perpetration of intimate partner violence (IPV), as well as being the target of IPV are analyzed in Chapter 34. Chapter 35 explores substance-involved sexual assault, in terms of perpetrating and being the victim of sexual assault, and offers evidence concerning intervention and prevention. These three topics were selected from among a longer list of possible topics because the prevalence of their co-occurrence is globally significant, strength of the evidence base, and impact on life and social work practices.

33

Understanding addictive behaviors and co-occurring disorders

Amanda R. Reedy

Background

Mental health disorders (MHD) and other significant problems commonly co-occur with addictive behaviors and substance use disorders (SUD) (SAMHSA, 2017). What may be less understood is why individuals have both mental health and substance use disorders. This chapter introduces key terms related to co-occurring disorders, knowledge about co-occurring disorders, perspectives and models that may explain why individuals have two or more co-occurring disorders, and concepts applied in interventions for addressing co-occurring disorders.

Key terms

Terms used to describe individuals who experience two or more health/mental health disorders have evolved over time. Co-morbid and dual diagnosis remain in common use (Morisano, Babor, & Robaina, 2014), though these terms are somewhat limited by being associated specifically with medical diagnoses and implying that only two disorders co-exist. More recent terms include co-occurring and co-existing. Velleman and Baker (2008) suggested co-existing because it addresses the possibility that a person may experience more than one disorder and does not imply which disorder occurred first. While the term co-existing disorder may best describe the true nature of experiencing multiple disorders, it has not caught on in the literature to the same extent as dual diagnosis and co-occurring disorders. Throughout this chapter, the term co-occurring is used.

While SUD and other addictive behaviors may co-occur with health problems, disabilities, and mental health problems in the same individual, this chapter focuses on co-occurring MHDs. MHDs include mood disorders such as depression, bipolar disorder, anxiety disorders; Post Traumatic Stress Disorder (PTSD); and severe and persistent mental disorders such as schizophrenia. While not a formal diagnosis, exposure to trauma is also an important factor to consider when thinking about co-occurring disorders and treatment. Social workers seeking detail about various mental health disorders are encouraged to review the Diagnostic and Statistical Manual, DSM-5 (APA, 2013), the International Classification of Diseases, ICD-11 (WHO, 2018), or related resources.

Challenges associated with co-occurring disorders

Individuals experiencing co-occurring substance use and other disorders present treatment and relapse challenges for social work practice (Aharonovich, Liu, Nunes, & Hasin, 2002; Bradizza, Stasiewicz, & Pass, 2005; Gamble et al., 2010; Greenfield et al., 1998; Grella & Stein, 2006; Hasin et al., 2002; Oliva et al., 2018; Oquendo et al., 2010). Co-occurring substance use and mental health disorders often present with more severe mental health problems, earlier relapse, greater difficulty maintaining abstinence, more mental health hospitalizations, and greater risk for suicide attempts (e.g. Hall, Vaughan-Sarrazin, Reedy, & Huber, 2008; Norman, Haller, Hamblen, Southwick, & Pietrzak, 2018; Painter et al., 2018; Price, Risk, Haden, Lewis, & Spitznagel, 2004; Ritsher, Moos, & Finney, 2002). For example, in a study of 65 participants in an inpatient SUD treatment program, participants experiencing co-occurring PTSD were more likely to use substances in response to feelings of sadness or depression than participants only experiencing a SUD (Ouimette, Coolhart, Funderburk, Wade, & Brown, 2007). A different study reported that veterans in SUD treatment who experienced co-occurring PTSD exhibited a greater risk of relapse in situations involving negative emotions and negative physiological contexts than those who experienced only a SUD (Norman, Tate, Anderson, & Brown, 2007).

Blanco et al. (2013) reported that persons experiencing co-occurring PTSD and alcohol use disorder (AUD) experienced more symptoms of each disorder, more suicide attempts, and higher rates of other mental health disorders than those solely experiencing either PTSD or AUD. Individuals experiencing co-occurring disorders may experience a higher rate of mortality due to suicide, overdose, and related problems (Abroms & Sher, 2016; Adan, Marques-Arrico, & Gilchrist, 2017; Greig, Baker, Lewin, Webster, & Carr, 2006). They may also experience more victimization (e.g. de Waal, Dekker, & Goudriaan, 2017; Gearon, Kaltman, Brown, & Bellack, 2003). Together, these issues present special challenges for individuals and providers.

Gender

Challenges associated with co-occurring disorders may vary based on gender. Mangrum, Spence, and Steinley-Bumgarner (2006) examined gender differences among 128 male and 85 female clients in SUD treatment who experienced a co-occurring MHD. Women were more likely than men to be younger (33.5 vs. 40.6 years), have children (38% vs. 24%), and have legal involvement (33% vs. 18%). The women were also more likely to experience PTSD (40% vs. 23%) and report more days of problems with medical (4.7 vs. 1.8), employment (8.2 vs. 3.0), family (6.9 vs. 2.3), social (5.3 vs. 2.3), and psychological issues (5.6 vs. 2.2). The men reported more problem days with drugs or alcohol and more severe psychiatric problems.

Grunebaum et al. (2006) explored gender differences between 83 women and 63 men in treatment for bipolar disorder. SUD was statistically associated with being male, aggression, and earlier onset of depression or mania symptoms. In a French study of co-occurring bipolar disorder with 1,090 participants, male gender was associated with increased odds (OR-2.68) of experiencing a co-occurring lifetime AUD (Azorin et al., 2017). Combined, the research evidence suggested that, among individuals receiving treatment for substance use problems and co-occurring mental health disorders, women tended to experience more problems in various areas of life while men experienced more problems with substances and mental health.

Prevalence of co-occurring disorders

The co-occurrence of MHDs with SUDs, particularly AUDs, and the associated complications was discussed in the literature as early as the 1940s (Kushner, 2014). More consistent diagnostic criteria established with DSM-III in the 1970s allowed researchers during the 1980s to conduct systematic studies evaluating the co-occurrence of these disorders (Kushner, 2014). During the 1990s and early 2000s, several large-scale studies were conducted to evaluate the general prevalence of co-occurring MHDs and SUDs (Conway, Compton, Stinson, & Grant, 2006; Grant et al., 2004; Kessler et al. 1997, 2006; Kessler, Chiu, Demler, & Walters, 2005; Regier et al., 1990).

The U.S. Epidemiologic Catchment Area (ECA) study (Regier et al., 1990), National Comorbidity Study (NCS) (Kessler et al. 1997), National Comorbidity Survey Replication (NCS-R) (Kessler et al., 2005; Kessler et al., 2006), and the National Epidemiologic Survey on Alcohol and Related Conditions (NESARC) (Conway et al., 2006; Grant et al., 2004) used a variety of methodologies with representative, large sample sizes or methods to adjust for sampling concerns to assess the prevalence of co-occurring disorders in the general population. Results indicated that co-occurring disorders are relatively common. For example, the NCS-R concluded that 45% of those with a SUD or MHD had a second or third co-occurring diagnosis (Kessler et al., 2005, 2006). Applying the research protocols established in the ECA, similar studies were conducted in Canada, Australia, and Puerto Rico (Bland, Newman, & Orn, 1988; Bland, Orn, Newman, 1988; Wells, Bushnell, Hornblow, Joyce, Oakley-Browne, 1989; Canino et al., 1987). Subsequent prevalence studies have reported that co-occurring disorders are common in other global regions, as well; including Europe, Australia, New Zealand, and North America, but less is known about Africa and Asia (Morisano et al., 2014).

More recent prevalence studies reported similar results. The NESARC III evaluated the prevalence and co-occurrence of AUD, SUD, and MHD using DSM-5 criteria (Grant et al., 2015, 2016). Researchers used probability sampling to obtain a representative sample of 36,309 non-institutionalized civilian adults in the United States. The reported lifetime prevalence for AUD was 29.1% and drug use disorder (DUD) was 3.9%. The 12-month prevalence for AUD was 13.9% and DUD was 9.9%. An AUD in the past 12 months was associated with MHDs, including having any mood disorder (AOR = 2.1), any anxiety disorder (AOR = 1.8), and PTSD (AOR = 2.0). Lifetime AUD was also associated with having any mood disorder (AOR = 2.5), any anxiety disorder (AOR = 2.4), and PTSD (AOR = 3.0). Results were similar for DUDs: experiencing a DUD in the past 12 months was significantly associated with any mood disorder (AOR = 1.9) and PTSD (AOR = 1.6). Lifetime DUD was significantly associated with any mood disorder (AOR = 1.2), any anxiety disorder (AOR = 1.3), and PTSD (AOR = 1.5). In most cases, more severe AUD or DUD was associated with greater odds of also having a MHD.

The most recent National Survey on Drug Use and Health (SAMHSA, 2017) used stratified multistage probability sampling to obtain a sample of 63,082 individuals ages 12 and older. Similar to previous studies, results indicated that, among adults who met criteria for a SUD in the past year, 45.6% had a co-occurring MHD. Furthermore, among adults who experienced a past year SUD, 16.5% also had a serious mental illness like schizophrenia.

MHDs that commonly co-occur with SUDs

As previously mentioned, anxiety, depression, bipolar disorder, PTSD, and severe and persistent MHDs like schizophrenia most commonly co-occur with SUDs.

Anxiety disorders

In the United States, results from NESARC III indicated that SUDs were significantly related to anxiety disorders (Grant et al., 2015, 2016). In a systematic review of literature concerning individuals seeking SUD treatment in Australia, 14 studies were identified that included data about co-occurring anxiety disorders (Kingston, Marel, & Mills, 2017). Results indicated that 12-month prevalence rates of co-occurring SUD and any anxiety disorder was between 45% and 68%. A German study analyzed data from the German Addiction Care System which included 822 outpatient and 200 inpatient centers (Dauber, Braun, Pfeiffer-Gerschel, Kraus, & Pogarell, 2018). The analysis focused on 12,956 clients meeting criteria for a co-occurring MHD. Co-occurring anxiety disorders were identified in 19% of outpatient and 20% of inpatient clients. Compared to cannabis and stimulant use, sedatives and alcohol use were associated with anxiety and mood disorders. Individuals who are more sensitive to symptoms of anxiety may also be more likely to use substances (Berenz et al., 2016; Conrod, Pihl, Stewart, & Dongier, 2000; DeHass, Calamari, & Bair, 2002; Forsyth, Parker, & Finlay, 2003; Paulus, Hogan, & Zvolensky, 2018).

Mood disorders

In the United States, results from the NESARC III indicated that SUDs were significantly associated with mood disorders like depression and bipolar disorder (Grant et al., 2015, 2016). In their systematic review, Kingston et al. (2017) identified 18 Australian studies that assessed the co-occurrence of SUDs and depression. In those studies, 27–85% of individuals seeking SUD treatment currently experienced co-occurring depression; 30–55% experienced co-occurring depression during the past 12 months.

Co-occurring bipolar disorder was less common than depression (Kingston et al., 2017). The reviewed studies indicated that the current co-occurrence of SUDs and bipolar disorder was between 4% and 11%, with a 12-month prevalence of 10%. In the Dauber et al. (2018) study of individuals receiving addiction treatment in Germany, 46% of outpatient and 41% of inpatient clients experienced a co-occurring mood disorder like depression or bipolar disorder. Additionally, more severe symptoms of mania and impulsivity, which are common symptoms of bipolar disorder, are associated with SUDs (Nery et al., 2013; Swann et al., 2007).

PTSD

Research also indicated that exposure to trauma may be related to co-occurring depression and SUDs (Norman et al., 2018). In the NESARC III study, PTSD was associated with SUDs (Grant et al., 2015, 2016). Results from a study with a nationally representative sample of U.S. veterans indicated that, among veterans with probable AUD, 20.3% had probable PTSD (Norman et al., 2018). Among veterans with probable PTSD, 16.8% experienced probable AUD. Veterans who met criteria for co-occurring AUD and PTSD were more likely to have depression, anxiety, and suicide ideation. Fewer studies in the Australian review included PTSD (Kingston et al., 2017). The one study identified in the review that focused on PTSD reported that 31% of individuals seeking SUD treatment had co-occurring PTSD in the last 12 months. In a study of cannabis use, PTSD, and depression among 301 veterans receiving services through the U.S. Veterans Health Administration, PTSD was significantly associated with major depressive disorder (r = 0.37) and cannabis use disorder (r = 0.27) (Metrik et al., 2016). Veterans experiencing both PTSD and a SUD is important to consider because lower quality of life, depression, anxiety, suicide ideology, and attempts were more likely among veterans experiencing co-occurring AUD and PTSD (Norman et al., 2018). Substance use may be associated with severity of PTSD symptoms, hyperarousal symptoms, and avoidance symptoms (McCauley, Killeen, Gros, Brady, & Back, 2012).

Severe and persistent MHDs

Kingston et al. (2017) identified eight Australian studies that included schizophrenia and other psychosis disorders. Current prevalence rates were 2–41%, 12-month prevalence was 5%, and lifetime prevalence was 36%. Another Australian study examining the co-occurrence of MHDs among 130 males involved in the criminal justice system identified high lifetime co-occurrence of psychotic or mood disorders with SUDs (Ogloff, Talevski, Lemphers, Wood, & Simmons, 2015). Individuals experiencing co-occurring disorders were more likely to have committed violent offenses and to have used illicit drugs prior to the offense (Ogloff et al., 2015). In the German study, cannabis and stimulant use disorders were associated with disorders like schizophrenia (outpatient 14.8%, inpatient 14.7%) (Dauber et al., 2018). A mental health clinic study compared 9,142 clients with schizophrenia, schizoaffective disorder, or bipolar disorder with psychotic features to 10,311 control participants: substance use was significantly more prevalent among participants with a severe mental illness (Hartz et al., 2014).

Four models of co-occurrence

Several models explain why SUDs and MHDs might co-occur. The four models most commonly addressed in the literature, introduced by Mueser and colleagues in 1998, include: (1) MHDs lead to SUDs, possibly as an effort at self-medication; (2) substance use leads to MHDs; (3) shared underlying factors contribute to both SUDs and MHDs; and (4) a combination of these models apply (see Figure 33.1). While each model contributes to our understanding about what causes co-occurrence in SUDs and MHDs, no single model is sufficient to explain its prevalence. The reasons why a person might experience both SUDs and MHDs vary.

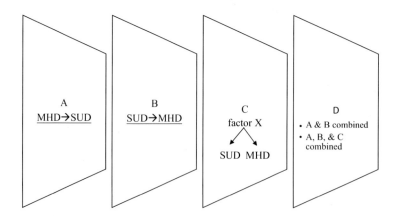

Figure 33.1 Direction of influence models

Mental health disorder leads to substance use disorder

Also called a self-medication model, this model is frequently referenced by practitioners and scholars discussing co-occurring disorders. The idea that a person might treat uncomfortable mental health symptoms with alcohol or other substances makes intuitive sense (Khantzian, 1974, 1985, 1997). Research indicated the onset of anxiety disorders, like phobias, preceded the onset of SUDs (Rosenthal, Nunes, & Le Fauve, 2012). Other researchers proposed that individuals use substances to dampen the effects of anxiety (Conrod et al., 2000; DeHass, Calamari, Bair, & Martin, 2001; DeHass et al., 2002; Forsyth et al., 2003). Like anxiety, the onset of depression may precede the onset of the SUD (Boschloo et al., 2011). The self-medication model is best understood in the context of learning theories, especially traditional and social learning theories (see Chapter 6). According to traditional learning theory, individuals develop behavioral patterns based on reinforcement experiences (Miller, 1993). In terms of co-occurring disorders, negative reinforcement is a key concept: a negative situation or uncomfortable feeling being taken away as a result of a certain behavior becomes reinforcing of that behavior. For example, a person who feels anxious may find that drinking or using marijuana relieves anxiety; eventually, the drinking or marijuana use becomes more frequent because relief, although temporary, was obtained with substance use, the behavior was repeatedly reinforced. Depending on the pattern of use and other factors, the substance use may subsequently develop into an AUD or SUD.

Bandura expanded on traditional learning theory with the theory of social learning (Miller, 1993) with the addition of observational learning or modeling principles (see Chapter 6). New behaviors may be learned through a person's observation of others' behavior and experienced consequences. For example, observing that another person experiences positive or negative reinforcement for using substances (e.g. lifts depressed mood, reduces anxiety, reduces social isolation) may increase the likelihood that the observer imitates that behavior. Bandura also discussed the reciprocal nature of the relationship between a person's behavior and the environment (Sommers-Flanagan & Sommers-Flanagan, 2004): not only does the environment shape a person's behavior, but a person also shapes the environment. For example, alcohol use might negatively reinforce a person's experience of social anxiety; interacting with others in a drinking environment might involve them reinforcing the drinking behavior; this, in turn, may lead to the person seeking out future drinking/socializing contexts. Three aspects of this model whereby MHDs precedes SUDs warrant attention: symptom severity, trauma, and cognitions.

Symptom severity

Research generally supports the idea that individuals who experience more severe or certain types of mental disorder symptoms may be more likely to experience a co-occurring SUD (Petrakis, Rosenheck, & Desai, 2011; Shipherd, Stafford, & Tanner, 2005; Smith, Smith, Cercone, McKee, & Homish, 2016; Swann et al., 2007; Taft et al., 2007; Tull, Gratz, Akin, & Lejuez, 2010; Wu, Woody, Yang, Pan, & Blazer, 2011). Several studies provide support for the self-medication model, where those experiencing more severe mental health symptoms are more likely to use substances to relieve anxiety (Berenz et al., 2016; Conrod et al., 2000; DeHass et al., 2002; Forsyth et al., 2003; McHugh, 2015). This relationship tends to exist for symptoms of anxiety, impulsivity, hyperarousal, avoidance, and mania. Additionally, individuals experiencing co-occurring MHDs tend to experience more severe SUDs (Rosenthal et al., 2012).

Trauma

Trauma exposure and multiple trauma exposures are related to the development of PTSD and depression (Bolton, Litz, Adler, & Roemer, 2001; Washburn, Carr, & Dettlaff, 2018). Some scholars conceptualized substance use as a way to cope with trauma and symptoms of PTSD (Kaysen et al., 2014; Stappenbeck et al., 2015), but the relationship could also be conceptualized as trauma being a third factor contributing to both disorders. Farrugia and colleagues (2011) reported that childhood trauma was associated with a longer duration of PTSD, more lifetime trauma exposure, and more severe SUDs. One possible mechanism relates to how substances might affect the learning theory process called extinction (Cobb, 2016): over time, when expected negative consequences of an anxiety-arousing event/activity repeatedly fail to occur, fear or anxiety surrounding that activity/event should decrease. Research indicates that alcohol and other substance use may affect the extinction process, possibly through effects on the hippocampus area of the brain where memories of fearful events are stored (Bisby et al., 2015; Lacagnina et al., 2019; Tipps, Raybuck, & Lattal, 2014). In the process of extinction, new memories are created that are also stored in the hippocampus; alcohol and other drugs seem to disrupt the storage of the new extinction memories, allowing the fearful memories to persist (Lacagnina et al., 2019; Tipps et al., 2014). This hypothesis may help explain why individuals with co-occurring PTSD and SUD have more severe and longer lasting symptoms than individuals with PTSD only (Petrakis et al., 2011; Shipherd et al., 2005; Smith et al., 2016; Swann et al., 2007; Taft et al., 2007; Tull et al., 2010; Wu et al., 2011).

Substance-related cognitions

Research indicates that substance use and misuse occur when individuals hold expectations that use will decrease negative feelings and enhance positive feelings (Berenz et al., 2016; Bizzarri et al., 2007; Bountress et al., 2019; Cooper, Frone, Russell, & Mudar, 1995; Pedersen, Myers, Browne, & Norman, 2014; Ullman, Filipas, Townsend, & Starzynski, 2005). In other words, positive alcohol or other drug use expectancies may play a role in the self-medication process (see Chapter 6). Since positive expectancies may cover more range than alleviating symptoms of mental disorders, this relationship between positive expectancies and substance us is not limited to individuals experiencing co-occurring MHDs and SUDs.

Substance misuse leads to mental health disorders

This model is challenging to diagnose and study because substance use can precipitate mental symptoms during intoxication and withdrawal without a co-occurring primary MHD being involved. Therefore, it can be difficult to determine whether the substance use or mental health problems started first. This relationship is commonly discussed in four different ways.

Substance use disrupts life

A person's substance use may lead to significant disruptions in life circumstances, disruptions which then lead to MHDs. For example, job loss may result from a person's alcohol misuse, subsequently leading to problems with depression. While this hypothesis may make intuitive sense, research supporting this relationship is limited (Nunes, Liu, Samet, Matseone, & Hasi, 2006; Reedy & Kobayashi, 2012).

Intoxication and withdrawal

The neurobiology of substance use or withdrawal may lead to MHDs (Frank, Boland, Novick, Bizzari, & Rucci, 2007). For example, cannabis use may "trigger" the onset of schizophrenia in some individuals. An Australian retrospective study of 997 individuals who used cannabis prior to the onset of psychosis identified earlier age of cannabis initiation as significantly associated with early onset of psychosis (adjusted $R2 = 0.19$); the time between initiating cannabis use and the onset of psychosis was seven to eight years (Stefanis et al., 2013). A study of 99 participants in London with a diagnosis of schizophrenia or a related disorder also found a linear relationship between initiation of cannabis use and the onset of symptoms of schizophrenia ($r = 0.47$) (Leeson, Harrison, Ron, Barnes, & Joyce, 2012). Another study out of England compared participants who had schizophrenia and had used cannabis to those with schizophrenia and no lifetime cannabis use (Donoghue et al., 2014). Those who had used cannabis had an earlier mean age of first onset of schizophrenia symptoms compared to those who had not used cannabis (25.7 vs. 29.2 years). In a systematic review and meta-analysis of 83 studies that compared the age of psychosis onset for participants using versus not using cannabis, Large, Sharma, Compton, Slade, and Nielssen (2011) concluded there was strong evidence for a relationship between cannabis use and an earlier age of onset of severe MHDs like schizophrenia. Similar results were identified in a systematic review and meta-analysis of 61 tobacco studies: participants who used tobacco daily had an increased risk of developing psychosis and an earlier age of onset of symptoms (Gurillo, Jauhar, Murray, & MacCabe, 2015).

Shared underlying factors

Co-occurring MHD and SUD may share one or more underlying causal factors in common, a variety of which are discussed in the literature. A few of the most common include biology, personality traits, anxiety, and trauma factors previously discussed in this chapter and/or in other chapters of this book. Brain development represents another potential shared factor worthy of examination.

Brain development

Adolescence is a vulnerable period where individuals are at risk of developing both MHDs and SUDs (Cohen-Gilbert, Jensen, & Silveri, 2014; see Chapter 13). This is in part due to the brain's plasticity and its ability to adapt to various situations and environments, particularly during childhood and adolescence (Giedd, 2015). During adolescence, the brain reorganizes to transmit information faster, allowing for more complex brain processes to emerge (Cohen-Gilbert et al., 2014). Additionally, adolescents are particularly susceptible to reinforcers in the environment and sensation seeking (Meyer & Lee, 2019). While brain plasticity is an adaptive process, the adolescent brain is also highly susceptible to both MHDs and SUDs (Giedd, 2015). The changes in the brain, early experimentation with substance use, and vulnerability to the onset of mental health problems, may be related to the development of co-occurring disorders.

Combination models

While each of these models contributes to our understanding of co-occurring SUD and MHD, no single model is sufficient. Various combinations of the models might best explain co-occurring disorders. Kushner, Abrams, and Borchardt (2000) described model combinations in three different ways. First, the causes of onset and continuation of the disorders may differ. For example, a person with genetic predisposition to schizophrenia might experiment with LSD which triggers the first psychotic symptoms. That person then might use cannabis to cope with the psychosis symptoms. This would be an iterative combination of substance use leading to MHD leading to additional/other substance use.

Second, causes of the co-occurring disorders may differ for different individuals. For example, MHDs such as PTSD might lead to substance use disorder for some persons whereas substance use/misuse such as marijuana might lead to MHDs in others, and a third factor like living in a household or neighborhood characterized by a great deal of violence might lead to both a MHD and SUD. Third, the processes or causes of MHD and SUD may interact and overlap. For example, a person may be genetically predisposed to AUD (see Chapter 5). Depending on a host of environmental context factors (e.g. access to alcohol, trauma experiences, stress), alcohol use may or may not occur, thus an AUD may or may not occur (see Chapter 7). Concurrently, the same person also may have a genetic predisposition to an anxiety or depression disorder.

Depending on environmental factors, the disorder may or may not emerge—including substance use/misuse. If these predispositions and environmental factors converge, the likelihood of co-occurring MHD and SUD increases.

Directions for social work practice and research

In addressing the problem of co-occurring SUD and MHD, traditional approaches include sequential and parallel treatment (Mueser, Noordsy, Drake, & Fox, 2003). Integrated treatment and harm reduction are additional important approaches to be considered.

Sequential treatment for co-occurring SUD and MHD

In sequential treatment, a client engages in treatment for one problem, typically the one defined as the highest priority, and then later engages in treatment for the other. Some clinicians believe that by treating the substance use problems first, the mental health problems will diminish; others are prepared to address one problem and then refer the client to address the other. Sequential treatment is favored by practitioners believing that a SUD will interfere with MHD treatment, or vice versa.

Unfortunately, both substance use and mental health disorders contribute to significant problems in daily living. Furthermore, they generally have a synergistic effect and either can impede treatment of the other when traditional unidimensional treatment is provided. Additionally, sequential treatment may mean that the second problem is never treated because the person drops out of primary treatment when not making satisfactory progress or referral to treat the co-occurring problem might be missed when the client is discharged (Mueser et al., 2003). It can also be difficult to establish when one or the other disorder has been effectively treated (Mueser et al., 2003).

Parallel treatment for co-occurring SUD and MHD

In parallel treatment, the SUD and MHD are treated at the same time, by different providers at the same or different agencies (Mueser et al., 2003). In this scenario, the providers may or may not be communicating effectively about client needs and progress. In some cases, providers may be treating the client with interventions that do not complement or even contradict each other (Mueser et al., 2003). While parallel treatment may include elements of treatment co-ordination and integration, this responsibility often falls on the client (Mueser et al., 2003).

Integrated treatment

Because of potential obstacles in sequential and parallel treatment, the Substance Abuse and Mental Health Services Administration (SAMHSA, 2017) and others (e.g. Rizvi & Harned, 2013) recommend integrated treatment for co-occurring disorders. Integrated treatment is de-scribed as "requiring collaboration across disciplines" in order to address "both mental health and substance abuse, each in the context of the other disorder" (SAMHSA, 2017, para. 18). Ideally, the same clinician provides both the substance use and mental health services (Mueser et al., 2003), but integration can include clinicians at the same agency closely collaborating on treatment. Mueser and colleagues (2003) described key components of integrated treatment:

- treatment that comprehensively addresses the range of client needs, such as housing and medical care;
- physically meeting clients "where they are" through outreach or diversion programs;
- using motivation-based interventions to help clients increase their readiness to change;
- reducing negative consequences (harm reduction);
- acknowledging that treatment is likely to be long-term; and
- taking steps to remove barriers and time constraints of treatment.

Additional components of integrated treatment recommended by Substance Abuse and Mental Health Services Administration (2009) include:

- matching treatment approaches to the client's stage of change;
- offering services in a range of formats;
- incorporating services for medication; and
- incorporating a cognitive behavioral approach.

After reviewing the literature on co-occurring disorders, Morisano and colleagues (2014) affirmed that integrative treatment that adopts a holistic approach and is designed to meet the needs of the individual client over months or years is the most promising approach. Mangrum, Spence, and Lopez (2006) reported that participants receiving integrated treat-ment had fewer hospitalizations and arrests than those receiving parallel treatment. In a meta-analysis, Chow, Wieman, Cichocki, Qvicklund, and Hiersteiner (2013) concluded that integrated treatment was more effective than non-integrated treatment for MHDs and AUDs treated in a residential setting. McKee, Harris, & Cormier (2013) determined that SUD and MHD treatment can be integrated in a residential setting and that it is effective for improv-ing mental health. Gobbart (2013) observed that an integrated, multi-modal skill-building group was effective in improving mental health. In another study, an integrated treatment for co-occurring PTSD and SUD first manualized by Lisa Najavits in 2002, *Seeking Safety*, contributed to reduced substance use and improved mental health conditions among women heavily using stimulant drugs; the integrated treatment was not more effective compared to education among women engaging in light use of stimulants (Ruglass, Hien, Hu, & Campbell, 2014). These results suggest that integrated treatment may be most effective for individuals experiencing severe symptoms.

Barriers to integrated treatment

Implementing and sustaining integrated treatment can pose challenges for programs (Mueser et al., 2003). Gil-Rivas and Grella (2005) surveyed staff at mental health and substance use agencies, observing that the level of integration greatly varied. Practitioners may not be trained to treat both disorders or may be resistant to changing practices (Blakey & Bowers, 2014; McKee, 2017; Mueser et al., 2003). Billing and licensure of social workers to treat both the MHD and SUD can be problematic. Agencies offering integrated treatment may have to revise their current program, re-train staff, ensure that staff value co-occurring treatment (embrace the culture shift), and create plans for evaluating treatment. Having a scientist-practitioner on staff to assist with implementation and fidelity is one option for promoting effective integrated treatment in a residential setting (McKee et al., 2013).

Another challenge with integrated treatment is that the research literature is often limited to studies focused on treatment of one disorder (Rizvi & Harned, 2013). Potential participants who experience co-occurring disorders are often excluded from studies because their co-occurring disorder is viewed as a confounding variable, making it more difficult to understand the effects of treatment on the focal disorder (Rizvi & Harned, 2013). Investigators have identified the need for more research that includes individuals with co-occurring disorders and the inclusion of assessments for co-occurring disorders in investigation protocols (Rizvi & Harned, 2013).

Harm reduction

Harm reduction is an important approach to consider in all addictive behaviors work, and is especially important when SUD and MHD co-occur. The concept of harm reduction comes from a public health perspective focused on reducing the harm or negative effects associated with alcohol or drug use (Henwood, Padgett, & Tiderington, 2014; Van Wormer & Davis, 2013). More recently, Substance Abuse and Mental Health Services Administration (2019) has updated the definition of recovery to align with harm reduction values. Appropriate use of psychiatric medication to treat MHDs may be considered a harm reduction strategy, because it can help reduce substance use/misuse (Denning & Little, 2017).

Harm reduction attitudes and policies vary from country to country. While the United States continues to support policies that are more oriented to abstinence, countries in Europe, Australia, and Canada more readily offer harm reduction approaches (Van Wormer & Davis, 2013). As policies and practice approaches continue to allow more harm reduction approaches, this continues to be an important approach to use with clients with co-occurring disorders.

Conclusion

Social workers and other health professionals in all fields of practice commonly encounter clients experiencing co-occurring substance use and mental health disorders. Social workers familiar with the various ways co-occurring disorders might develop and the associated problems encountered by clients experiencing more than one disorder are better prepared to meet clients' needs. Social workers should develop awareness of and skills in delivering promising treatment approaches that incorporate tenets of integrated treatment and harm reduction, and advocate for their clients receiving these interventions.

Acknowledgment

The author would like to thank Anne Howard for her assistance in preparing this manuscript.

References

Abroms, M., & Sher, L. (2016). Dual disorders and suicide. *Journal of Dual Diagnosis, 12*(2), 148–149. doi:10.1080/15504263.2016.1172898

Adan, A., Marquez-Arrico, J. E., & Gilchrist, G. (2017). Comparison of health-related quality of life among men with different co-existing severe mental disorders in treatment for substance use. *Health and Quality of Life Outcomes, 15*, 209–221. doi:10.1186/s12955-017-0781-y

Aharonovich, E., Liu, X., Nunes, E., & Hasin, D. (2002). Suicide attempts in substance abusers: Effects of major depression in relation to substance use disorders. *American Journal of Psychiatry, 159*, 1600–1602. doi:10.1176/appi.ajp.159.9.1600

American Psychiatric Association. (2013). *Diagnostic and statistical manual of mental disorders* (5th ed.). Washington, DC: American Psychiatric Association. doi:10.1176/appi.books.9780890425596

Azorin, J. M., Perret, L. C., Fakra, E., Tassy, S., Simon, N., Adida, M., & Belzeaux, R. (2017). Alcohol use and bipolar disorders: Risk factors associated with their co-occurrence and sequence of onsets. *Drug and Alcohol Dependence, 179*, 205–212. doi:10.1016/j.drugalcdep.2017.07.005

Berenz, E. C., Kevorkian, S., Chowdhury, N., Dick, D. M., Kendler, K. S., & Amstadter, A. B. (2016). Posttraumatic stress disorder symptoms, anxiety sensitivity, and alcohol-use motives in college students with a history of interpersonal trauma. *Psychology of Addictive Behaviors, 30*(7), 755–763.

Bisby, J. A., King, J. A., Sulpizio, V., Degeilh, F., Curran, H. V., & Burgess, N. (2015). Extinction learning is slower, weaker and less context specific after alcohol. *Neurobiology of Learning and Memory, 125*, 55–62. doi:10.1037/adb0000193

Bizzarri, J. V., Sbrana, A., Rucci, P., Ravani, L., Massei, G. J., Gonnelli, D., . . . Cassano, G. B. (2007). The spectrum of substance abuse in bipolar disorder: Reasons for use, sensation seeking and substance sensitivity. *Bipolar Disorders, 9*, 213–220. doi:10.1111/j.1399-5618.2007.00383.x

Blakey, J. M., & Bowers, P. H. (2014). Barriers to integrated treatment of substance abuse and trauma among women. *Journal of Social Work Practice in the Addictions, 14*(3), 250–272. doi:10.1080/1533256X.2014.933731

Blanco, C., Xu, Y., Brady, K., Perez-Fuentes, G., Okuda, M., & Wang, S. (2013). Comorbidity of posttraumatic stress disorder with alcohol dependence among US adults: Results from national epidemiological survey on alcohol and related conditions. *Drug and Alcohol Dependence, 123*(3), 630–638. doi:10.1016/j.drugalcdep.2013.04.016

Bland, R. C., Newman, S. C., & Orn, H. (1988). Period prevalence of psychiatric disorders in Edmonton. *Acta Psychiatry Scandinavica, 338*, 33–42. doi:10.1111/j.1600-0447.1988.tb08545.x

Bland, R. C., Orn, H., & Newman, S. C. (1988). Lifetime prevalence of psychiatric disorders in Edmonton. *Acta Psychiatry Scandinavica, 338*, 24–42. doi:10.1111/j.1600-0447.1988.tb08544.x

Bolton, E. E., Litz, B. T., Britt, T. W., Adler, A., & Roemer, L. (2001). Reports of prior exposure to potentially traumatic events and PTSD in troops poised for deployment. *Journal of Traumatic Stress, 14*(1), 249–256. doi:10.1023/A:1007864305207

Boschloo, L., Vogelzangs, N., Smit, J. H., van den Brink, W., Veltman, D. J., Beekman, A. T. F., & Penninx, B. W. J. H. (2011). Comorbidity and risk indicators for alcohol use disorders among persons with anxiety and/or depressive disorders: Findings from the Netherlands study of depression and anxiety (NESDA). *Journal of Affective Disorders, 131*(1–3), 233–242. doi:10.1016/j.jad.2010.12.014

Bountress, K. E., Cusack, S. E., Sheerin, C. M., Hawn, S., Dick, D. M., Kendler, K. S., & Amstadter, A. B. (2019). Alcohol consumption, interpersonal trauma, and drinking to cope with trauma-related distress: An auto-regressive, cross-lagged model. *Psychology of Addictive Behaviors, 33*(3), 221–231. doi:10.1037/adb0000457

Bradizza, C. M., Stasiewicz, P. R., & Paas, N. D. (2005). Relapse to alcohol and drug use among individuals diagnosed with co-occurring mental health and substance use disorders: A review. *Clinical Psychology Review, 26*, 162–178. doi:10.1016/j.cpr.2005.11.005

Canino, G. J., Bird, H. R., Shrout, P. E., Bravo, M., Martinez, R., Sesman, M., & Guevara, L. M. (1987). The prevalence of specific psychiatric disorders in Puerto Rico. *Archives of General Psychiatry, 44*, 727–735. doi:10.1001/archpsyc.1987.01800200053008

Chow, C. M., Wieman, D., Cichocki, B., Qvicklund, H., & Hiersteiner, D. (2013). Mission impossible: Treating serious mental illness and substance use co-occurring disorder with integrated treatment: A meta-analysis. *Mental Health and Substance Use, 6*(2), 150–168. doi:10.1080/1752328 1.2012.693130

Cobb, N. H. (2016). Cognitive behavioral theory and treatment. In N. Coady & P. Lehman (Eds.), *Theoretical perspectives for direct social work practice: A generalist-eclectic approach* (3rd ed., pp. 223–248). New York, NY: Springer Publishing Company, LLC. doi:10.1891/9780826119483.0010

Cohen-Gilbert, J. E., Jensen, J. E., & Silveri, M. M. (2014). Contributions of magnetic resonance spectroscopy to understanding development: Potential applications in the study of adolescent alcohol use and abuse. *Developmental and Psychopathology, 26*, 405–423. doi:10.1017/S0954579414000030

Conrod, P. J., Pihl, R. O., Stewart, S. H., & Dongier, M. (2000). Validation of a system of classifying female substance abusers on the basis of personality and motivational risk factors for substance abuse. *Psychology of Addictive Behaviors, 14*(3), 243–256. doi:10.1037/0893-164X.14.3.243

Conway, K. P., Compton, W., Stinson, F., & Grant, B. F. (2006). Lifetime comorbidity of DSM-IV mood and anxiety disorders and specific drug use disorders: Results from the national epidemiologic survey on alcohol and related conditions. *Journal of Clinical Psychiatry, 67*(2), 247–257. doi:10.4088/JCP.v67n0211

Cooper, L. M., Frone, M. R., Russell, M., & Mudar, P. (1995). Drinking to regulate positive and negative emotions: A motivational model of alcohol use. *Journal of Personality and Social Psychology, 69*(5), 990–1005. doi:10.1037/0022–3514.69.5.990

Dauber, H., Braun, B., Pfeiffer-Gerschel, T., Kraus, L., & Pogarell, O. (2018). Co-occurring mental disorders in substance abuse treatment: The current health care situation in Germany. *International Journal of Mental Health and Addiction, 16*(1), 66–80. doi:10.1007/s11469-017-9784-5

DeHass, R. A., Calamari, J. E., Bair, J. P. (2002). Anxiety sensitivity and the situational antecedents to drug and alcohol use: An evaluation of anxiety patients with substance use disorders. *Cognitive Therapy Research, 26*(3), 335–353. doi:10.1023/A:1016076911164

DeHass, R. A., Clalamari, J. E., Bair, J. P., & Martin, E. D. (2001). Anxiety sensitivity and drug or alcohol use in individuals with anxiety and substance use disorders. *Addictive Behaviors, 26*(6), 787–801. doi:10.1016/S0306-4603(01)00237-4

Denning, P., & Little, J. (2017). *Over the influence: The harm reduction guide to controlling your drug and alcohol use* (2nd ed.). New York, NY: The Guilford Press.

de Waal, M. M., Dekker, J., J., M., & Goudriaan, A. E. (2017). Prevalence of victimization in patients with dual diagnosis. *Journal of Dual Diagnosis, 13*(2), 119–123. doi:10.1080/15504263.2016.1274067

Donoghue, K., Doody, G. A., Murray, R. M., Jones, P. B., Morgan, C., Dazzan, P., . . . MacCabe, H. (2014). Cannabis use, gender and age of onset of schizophrenia: Data from the AESOP Study. *Psychiatry Research, 215*, 528–532. doi:10.1016/j.psychres.2013.12.038

Farrugia, P. L., Mills, K. L., Barrett, E., Back, S. E., Teesson, M., Baker, A., . . . Brady, K. T. (2011). Childhood trauma among individuals with co-morbid substance use and post-traumatic stress disorder. *Mental Health and Substance Use, 4*(4), 314–326. doi:10.1080/17523281.2011.598462

Frank, E., Boland, E., Novick, D. M., Bizzarri, J. V., & Rucci, P. (2007). Association between illicit drug and alcohol use and first manic episode. *Pharmacology, Biochemistry and Behavior, 86*, 395–400. doi:10.1016/j.pbb.2006.11.009

Forsyth, J. P., Parker, J. D., & Finlay, C. G. (2003). Anxiety sensitivity, controllability and experiential avoidance and their relation to drug of choice and addiction severity in a residential sample of substance-abusing veterans. *Addictive Behaviors, 28*(5), 851–870. doi:10.1016/S0306–4603(02)00216-2

Gamble, S. A., Conner, K. R., Talbot, N. L., Yu, Q., Tu, X. M., & Connors, G. J. (2010). Effects of pretreatment and posttreatment depressive symptoms on alcohol consumption following treatment in Project MATCH. *Journal of Studies on Alcohol and Drugs, 71*(1), 71–77. doi:10.15288/jsad.2010.71.71

Gearon, J. S., Kaltman, S. I., Brown, C., & Bellack, A. S. (2003). Traumatic life events and PTSD among women with substance use disorders and schizophrenia. *Psychiatric Services, 54*(4), 523–528. doi:10.1176/appi.ps.54.4.523

Giedd, J. N. (2015). Adolescent neuroscience of addiction: A new era. *Developmental Cognitive Neuroscience, 16*, 192–193. doi:10.1016/j.dcn.2015.11.002

Gil-Rivas, V., & Grella, C. E. (2005). Addictions services: Treatment services and service delivery models for dually diagnosed clients: Variations across mental health and substance abuse providers. *Community Mental Health Journal, 41*(3), 251–266. doi:10.1007/s10597-005-5000-3

Gobbart, S. (2013). 'Changing habits': An evaluation of dual diagnosis focused, integrated, multimodal, psychosocial education and skill building group programme delivered in a community-based setting. *Mental Health and Substance Use, 6*(1), 29–46. doi:10.1080/175323281.2012.660980

Grant, B. F., Goldstein, R. B., Saha, T. D., Chou, S. P., Jung, J., Zhang, H., . . . Hasin, D. S. (2015). Epidemiology of DSM-5 alcohol use: Results from the national epidemiologic survey on alcohol and related conditions (NESARC) III. *JAMA Psychiatry, 72*(8), 757–766. doi:10.1001/jamapsychiatry.2015.0584

Grant, B. F., Saha, T. D., Ruan, W. J., Goldstein, R. B., Chou, S. P., Jung, J., . . . Hasin, D. S. (2016). Epidemiology of DSM-5 drug use disorder: Results from the national epidemiologic survey on alcohol and related conditions-III. *JAMA Psychiatry, 73*(1), 39–47. doi:10.1001/jamapsychiatry.2015.2132

Grant, B. F., Stinson, F. S., Dawson, D. A., Chou, P., Dufour, M. C., Compton, W., . . . Kaplan, K. (2004). Prevalence and co-occurrence of substance use disorders and independent mood and anxiety disorders: Results from the national epidemiologic survey on alcohol and related conditions. *Archives of General Psychiatry, 61*, 807–816. doi:10.1001/archpsyc.61.8.807

Greenfield, S. F., Weiss, R. D., Muenz, L. R., Vagge, L. M., Kelly, J. F., Bello, L. R., & Michael, J. (1998). The effect of depression on return to drinking. *Archives of General Psychiatry, 55*, 259–265. doi:10.1001/archpsyc.55.3.259

Greig, R. L., Baker, A., Lewin, T. L., Webster, R. A., & Carr, V. J. (2006). Long-term follow-up of people with co-existing psychiatric and substance use disorders: Patterns of use and outcomes. *Drug and Alcohol Review, 25*, 249–258. doi:10.1080/09595230600657741

Grella, C. E., & Stein, J. A. (2006). Impact of program services on treatment outcomes of patients with comorbid mental and substance use disorders. *Psychiatric Services, 57*, 1007–1015. doi:10.1176/appi.ps.57.7.1007

Grunebaum, M. F., Galfalvy, H. C., Nichols, C. M., Caldeira, N. A., Sher, L., Dervic, K., . . . Oquendo, M. A. (2006). Aggression and substance abuse in bipolar disorders. *Bipolar Disorders, 8*(5pt1), 496–502. doi:10.1111/j.1399-5618.2006.00349.x

Gurillo, P., Jauhar, S., Murray, R. M., & MacCabe, J. H. (2015). Does tobacco use cause psychosis? Systematic review and meta-analysis. *Lancet Psychiatry, 2*, 718–725.

Hall, J. A., Vaughan-Sarrazin, M., Reedy, A. R., & Huber, D. L. (2008). Comprehensive case management for substance abuse clients who have mood or anxiety disorders. *Mental Health and Substance Use: Dual Diagnosis, 1*(2), 143–157. doi:10.1080/17523280802019935

Hartz, S. M., Pato, C. N., Medeiros, H., Cavazos-Rehg, P., Sobell, J. L., Knowles, J. A., . . . Pato, M. T. (2014). Comorbidity of severe psychotic disorders with substance use. *JAMA Psychiatry, 71*(3), 248–254. doi:10.1001/jamapsychiatry.2013.3726

Hasin, D., Liu, X., Nunes, E., McCloud, S., Samet, S., & Endicott, J. (2002). Effects of major depression on remission and relapse of substance dependence. *Archives of General Psychiatry, 59*, 375–380. doi:10.1001/archpsyc.59.4.375

Henwood, B. F., Padgett, D. K., & Tiderington, E. (2014). Provider views of harm reduction versus abstinence policies within homeless services for dually diagnoses adults. *The Journal of Behavioral Health Services & Research, 41*(1), 80–89. doi:10.1007/s11414-013-9318-2

Kaysen, D., Atkins, D. C., Simpson, T. L., Stappenbeck, C. A., Blayney, J. A., Lee, C. M., & Larimer, M. E. (2014). Proximal relationships between PTSD symptoms and drinking among female college students: Results from a daily monitoring study. *Psychology of Addictive Behaviors, 28*(1), 62–73. doi:10.1037/a0033588

Kessler, R. C., Chiu, W. T., Jin, R., Ruscio, A. M., Shear, K., & Walters, E. E. (2006). The epidemiology of panic attacks, panic disorder, and agoraphobia in the national comorbidity survey replication. *Archives of General Psychiatry, 63*, 415–424. doi:10.1001/archpsyc.63.4.415

Kessler, R. C., Chiu, W. T., Demler, O., & Walters, E. E. (2005). Prevalence, severity, and comorbidity of 12-month DSM-IV disorders in the national comorbidity survey replication. *Archives of General Psychiatry, 62*, 617–705. doi:10.1001/archpsyc.62.6.617

Kessler, R. C., Crum, R. M., Warner, L. A., Nelson, C. B., Schulenberg, J., & Anthony, J. C. (1997). Lifetime co-occurrence of DSM-III-R alcohol abuse and dependence with other psychiatric disorders in the national comorbidity survey. *Archives of General Psychiatry, 54*, 313–321. doi:10.1001/archpsyc.1997.01830160031005

Khantzian, E. J. (1974). Opiate addiction: A critique of theory and some implications for treatment. *American Journal of Psychotherapy, 28*, 59–70. doi:10.1176/appi.psychotherapy.1974.28.1.59

Khantzian, E. J. (1985). The self-medication hypothesis of addictive disorders: Focus on heroin and cocaine dependence. *The American Journal of Psychiatry, 142*(11), 1259–1264. doi:10.1176/ajp.142.11.1259

Khantzian, E. J. (1997). The self-medication hypothesis of substance use disorders: A reconsideration and recent applications. *Harvard Review of Psychiatry, 4*(5), 231–244. doi:10.3109/10673229709030550

Kingston, R. E. F., Marel, C., & Mills, K. L. (2017). A systematic review of the prevalence of comorbid mental health disorders in people presenting for substance use treatment in Australia. *Drug and Alcohol Review, 36*, 527–539. doi:10.1111/dar.12448

Kushner, M. G. (2014). Seventy-five years of comorbidity research. *Journal of Studies of Alcohol and Drug Studies, 75*(S17), 50–58. doi:10.15288/jsads.2014.s17.50

Kushner, M. G., Abrams, K., & Borchardt, C. (2000). The relationship between anxiety disorders and alcohol use disorders: A review of major perspectives and findings. *Clinical Psychology Review, 20*(2), 149–171. doi:10.1016/S0272-7358(99)00027-6

Lacagnina, A. F., Brockway, E. T., Crovetti, C. R., Shue, F., McCarty, M. J., Sattler, K. P., . . . Drew, M. (2019). Distinct hippocampal engrams control extinction and relapse of fear memory. *Nature Neuroscience, 22*, 753–761. doi:10.1038/s41593-019-0361-z

Large, M., Sharma, S., Compton, M. T., Slade, T., & Nielssen, O. (2011). Cannabis use and earlier onset of psychosis: A systematic meta-analysis. *Archives of General Psychiatry, 68*(6), 555–561. doi:10.1001/archgenpsychiatry.2011.5

Leeson, V. C., Harrison, I., Ron, M. A., Barnes, T. R. E., & Joyce, E. M. (2012). The effect of cannabis use and cognitive reserve on age at onset and psychosis outcomes in first-episode schizophrenia. *Schizophrenia Bulletin, 38*(4), 873–880. doi:10.1093/schbul/sbq153

Mangrum, L. F., Spence, R. T., & Lopez, M. (2006). Integrated versus parallel treatment of co-occurring psychiatric and substance use disorders. *Journal of Substance Abuse Treatment, 30*(1), 79–84. doi:10.1016/j.jsat.2005.10.004

Mangrum, L. F., Spence, R. T., & Steinley-Bumgarner, M. D. (2006). Gender differences in substance-abuse treatment clients with co-occurring psychiatric and substance use disorders. *Brief Treatment and Crisis Intervention, 6*(3), 255–267. doi:10.1093/brief-treatment/mhl006

McCauley, J. L., Killen, T., Gros, D. F., Brady, K. T., & Back, S. E. (2012). Posttraumatic stress disorder and co-occurring substance use disorders: Advances in assessment and treatment. *Clinical Psychology: Science and Practice, 19*(3), 283–304. doi:10.1111/cpsp.12006

McHugh, R. K. (2015). Treatment of co-occurring anxiety disorders and substance use disorders. *Harvard Review of Psychiatry, 23*(2), 99–111. doi:10.1097/HRP.0000000000000058

McKee, S. A. (2017). Concurrent substance use disorders and mental illness: Bridging the gap between research and treatment. *Canadian Psychology/Psychologie Canadienne, 58*(1), 50–57. doi:10.1037/cap0000093

McKee, S. A., Harris, G. T., & Cormier, C. A. (2013). Implementing residential integrated treatment for co-occurring disorders. *Journal of Dual Diagnosis, 9*(3), 249–259. doi:10.1080/15504263.2013.807073

Metrik, J., Jackson, K., Bassett, S. S., Zvolensky, M. J., Seal, K., & Borsari, B. (2016). The mediating roles of coping, sleep, and anxiety motives in cannabis use and problems among returning veterans with PTSD and MDD. *Psychology of Addictive Behaviors, 30*(7), 743–754. doi:10.1037/adb0000210

Meyer, H. C., & Lee, F. S. (2019). Translating developmental neuroscience to understand risk for psychiatric disorders. *American Journal of Psychiatry, 176*(3), 179–185. doi:10.1176/appi.ajp.2019.19010091

Miller, M. W., Vogt, D. S., Mozley, S. L., Kaloupek, D. G., & Keane, T. M. (2006). PTSD and substance-related problems: The mediating roles of disconstraint and negative emotionality. *Journal of Abnormal Psychology, 115*(2), 369–379. doi:10.1037/0021-843X.115.2.369

Morisano, D., Babor, T. F., & Robaina, K. A. (2014). Co-occurrence of substance use disorders with other psychiatric disorders: Implications for treatment services. *Nordic Studies on Alcohol and Drugs, 21*, 5–25. doi:10.2478/nsad-2014-0002

Mueser, K. T., Noordsy, D. L., Drake, R. E., & Fox, L. (2003). *Integrated treatment for dual disorders: A guide to effective practice.* New York, NY: The Guilford Press.

Nery, F. B., Hatch, J. P., Monkul, S. E., Matuso, K., Zunta-Soares, G. B., Bowden, C. L., & Soares, J. C. (2013). Trait impulsivity is increased in bipolar disorder patients with comorbid alcohol use disorders. *Psychopathology, 46*, 145–152. doi:10.1159/000336730

Norman, S. B., Haller, M., Hamblen, J. L., Southwick, S. M., & Pietrzak, R. H. (2018). The burden of co-occurring alcohol use disorder and PTSD in US Military veterans: Comorbidities, functioning, and suicidality. *Psychology of Addictive Behaviors, 32*(2), 224–229. doi:10.1037/adb0000348

Norman, S. B., Tate, S. R., Anderson, K. G., & Brown, S. A. (2007). Do trauma history and PTSD symptoms influence addiction relapse context? *Drug and Alcohol Dependence, 90*, 89–96. doi:10.1016/j.drugalcdep.2007.03.002

Nunes, E. V., Liu, X., Samet, S., Matseone, K., & Hasin, D. (2006). Independent versus substance-induced major depressive disorder in substance-dependent patients: Observational study of course during follow-up. *Journal of Clinical Psychiatry, 67*(10), 1561–1567. doi:10.4088/JCP.v67n1010

Ogloff, J. R. P., Talevski, D. Lempher, A., Wood, M., & Simmons, M. (2015). Co-occurring mental illness, substance use disorders, and antisocial personality disorder among clients of forensic mental health services. *Psychiatric Rehabilitation Journal, 38*(1), 16–23. doi:10.1037/prj0000088

Oliva, F., Nibbio, G., Vizzuso, P., Jaretti Sodano, A., Ostacoli, L., Carletto, S., & Picci, R. L. (2018). Gender differences in anxiety and depression before and after alcohol detoxification: Anxiety and depression as gender-related predictors of relapse. *European Addiction Research, 24*(4), 163–172. doi:10.1159/000490046

Oquendo, M. A., Currier, D., Liu, S. M., Hasin, D. S., Grant, B. F., & Blanco, C. (2010). Increased risk for suicidal behavior in comorbid bipolar disorder and alcohol use disorders: Results from the national epidemiologic survey on alcohol and related conditions (NESARC). *The Journal of Clinical Psychiatry, 71*(7), 902–909. doi:10.4088/JCP.09m05198gry

Ouimette, P. C., Coolhart, D., Funderburk, J. S., Wade, M., & Brown, P. J. (2007). Precipitants of first substance use in recently abstinent substance use disorder patients with PTSD. *Addictive Behaviors, 32*(8), 1719–1727. doi:10.1016/j.addbeh.2006.11.020

Painter, J. M., Malte, C. A., Rubinsky, A. D., Campellone, T. R., Gilmore, A. K., Baer, J. S., & Hawkins, E. J. (2018). High inpatient utilization among veterans health administration patients with substance-use disorders and co-occurring mental health conditions. *American Journal of Drug & Alcohol Abuse, 44*(3), 386–394. doi:10.1080/00952990.2017.1381701

Paulus, D. J., Hogan, J. B. D., & Zvolensky, M. J. (2018). Examining emotion dysregulation as an underlying factor explaining relations of anxiety sensitivity and cannabis use severity. *Translational Issues in Psychological Science, 4*(1), 21–32. doi:10.1037/tps0000143

Petrakis, I. L., Rosenheck, R., & Desai, R. (2011). Substance use comorbidity among veterans with posttraumatic stress disorder and other psychiatric illnesses. *The American Journal on Addictions, 20*, 185–189. doi:10.1111/j.1521-0391.2011.00126.x

Price, R. K., Risk, N. K., Haden, A. H., Lewis, C. E., & Spitznagel, E. L. (2004). Post-traumatic stress disorder, drug dependence, and suicidality among male Vietnam veterans with a history of heavy drug use. *Drug and Alcohol Dependence, 76S*, S31–S43. doi:10.1016/j.drugalcdep.2004.08.005

Reedy, A. R., & Kobayashi, R. (2012). Substance use and mental health disorders: Why do some people suffer from both? *Social Work in Mental Health, 10*, 496–517. doi:10.1080/15332985.2012.709480

Regier, D. A., Farmer, M. E., Rae, D. S., Locke, B. Z., Keith, S. J., Judd, L. L., & Goodwin, F. K. (1990). Comorbidity of mental disorders with alcohol and other drug abuse: Results from the epidemiologic catchment area (ECA) study. *Journal of the American Medical Association, 264*, 2511–2518. doi:10.1001/jama.1990.03450190043026

Ritsher, J. B., Moos, R. H., & Finney, J. W. (2002). Relationship of treatment orientation and continuing care to remission among substance abuse patients. *Psychiatric Services, 53*(5), 595–601. doi:10.1176/appi.ps.53.5.595

Rizvi, S. L., & Harned, M. (2013). Increasing the treatment efficiency and effectiveness: Rethinking approaches to assessing and treating comorbid disorders. *Clinical Psychology: Science and Practice, 20*(3), 285–290. doi:10.111/cpsp.12040

Rosenthal, R. N., Nunes, E. V., & Le Fauve, C. E. (2012). Implications of epidemiological data for identifying persons with substance use and other mental disorders. *The American Journal on Addictions, 21*, 97–103. doi:10.1111/j.1521-0391.2011.00198.x

Ruglass, L. M., Hien, D. A., Hu, M., & Campbell, A. N. C. (2014). Associations between post-traumatic stress symptoms, stimulant use, and treatment outcomes: A secondary analysis of NIDA's women and trauma study. *The American Journal on Addictions, 23*(1), 90–95. doi:10.1111/j.1521-0391.2013.12068.x

Shipherd, J. C., Stafford, J., & Tanner, L. R. (2005). Predicting alcohol and drug abuse in Persian Gulf War veterans: What role do PTSD symptoms play? *Addictive Behaviors, 30*, 595–599. doi:10.1016/j.addbeh.2004.07.004

Smith, K. Z., Smith, P. H., Cercone, S. A., McKee, S. A., & Homish, G. G. (2016). Past year non-medical opioid use and abuse and PTSD diagnosis: Interactions with sex and associations with symptoms clusters. *Addictive Behaviors, 58*, 167–174. doi:10.1016/j.addbeh.2016.02.019

Amanda R. Reedy

Sommers-Flanagan, J. S., & Sommers-Flanagan, R. (2004). *Counseling and psychotherapy theories in context and practice: Skills, strategies, and practice.* Hoboken, NJ: John Wiley & Sons, Inc.

Stappenbeck, C. A., Luterek, J. A., Kaysen, D., Rosenthal, C. F., Gurrad, B., & Simpson, T. L. (2015). A controlled examination of two coping skills for daily alcohol use and PTSD symptom severity among dually diagnosed individuals. *Behavior Research and Therapy, 66,* 8–17. doi:10.1016/j.brat.2014.12.013

Stefanis, N. C., Dragovic, M., Power, B. D., Jablensy, A., Castle, & Morgan, V. A. (2013). Age at initiation of cannabis use predicts age at onset of psychosis: The 7-to 8-year trend. *Schizophrenia Bulletin, 39*(2), 251–254. doi:10.1093/schbul/sbs188

Substance Abuse and Mental Health Services Administration. (2017). *Key substance use and mental health indicators in the United States: Results from the 2016 National Survey on Drug Use and Health* (HHS Publication No. SMA 17-5044, NSDUH Series H-52). Retrieved from https://www. samhsa.gov/data/

Substance Abuse and Mental Health Services Administration. (2019). *Recovery and recovery support.* Washington, DC: U.S. Department of Health and Human Services. Retrieved from https://www.samhsa.gov/find-help/recovery

Substance Abuse and Mental Health Services Administration.. (2009). *Integrated treatment for co-occurring disorders (evidence based practices kit).* Washington, DC: U.S. Department of Health and Human Services. Retrieved from https://store.samhsa.gov/system/files/brochure-itc.pdf

Swann, A. C., Moeller, F. G., Steinberg, J. L., Schneider, L., Barratt, E. S., & Dougherty, D. M. (2007). Manic symptoms and impulsivity during bipolar depressive episodes. *Bipolar Disorders, 9,* 206–212. doi:10.1111/j.1399-5618.2007.00357.x

Taft, C. T., Kaloupek, D. G., Schumm, J. A., Marshall, A. D., Panuzio, J., King, D. W., & Keane, T. M. (2007). Posttraumatic stress disorder symptoms, physiological reactivity, alcohol problems, and aggression among military veterans. *Journal of Abnormal Psychology, 116*(3), 489–507. doi:10.1037/0021-843X.116.3.498

Tipps, M. E., Raybuck, J. D., & Lattal, K. M. (2014). Substance abuse, memory, and post-traumatic stress disorder. *Neurobiology of Learning and Memory, 112,* 87–100. doi:10.1016/j.nlm.2013.12.002

Tull, M. T., Gratz, K. L., Aklin, W. M., & Lejuez, C. W. (2010). A preliminary examination of the relationships between posttraumatic stress symptoms and crack/cocaine, heroin, and alcohol dependence. *Journal of Anxiety Disorders, 24,* 55–62. doi:10.1016/j.janxdis.2009.08.006

Ullman, S. E., Filipas, H. H., Townsend, S. M., & Starznski, L. L. (2005). Trauma exposure, posttraumatic stress disorder and problem drinking in sexual assault survivors. *Journal of Studies on Alcohol, 66,* 610–619. doi:10.15288/jsa.2005.66.610

Van Wormer, K., & Davis, D. R. (2013). Strengths and evidence based helping strategies. In K. Van Wormer & D. R. Davis, *Addiction treatment: A strengths perspective* (pp. 405–451). Belmont, CAL: Brooks/Cole.

Velleman, R., & Baker, A. (2008). Moving away from medicalised and partisan terminology: A contribution to the debate. *Mental Health and Substance Use: Dual Diagnosis, 1*(1), 2–9. doi:10.1080/17523280701712366

Washburn, M., Carr, C. L., & Dettlaff, A. J. (2018). The moderating effects of ethnicity on key predictors of trauma in child welfare involved adolescents. *Journal of Adolescence, 67,* 179–157. doi:10.016/j.adolescence.2018.06.008

Wells, J. E., Bushnell, J. A., Hornblow, A. R., Joyce, P. R., & Oakley-Browne, M. A. (1989). Christchurch psychiatric epidemiology study, Part I: Methodology and lifetime prevalence for specific psychiatric disorders. *Australia and New Zealand Journal of Psychiatry, 23,* 315–323. doi:10.3109/00048678909068289

World Health Organization. (2018). *International statistical classification of diseases and related health problems* (11th revision). Retrieved from https://icd.who.int/browse11/l-m/en

Wu, L. T., Woody, G. E., Yang, C., Pan, J. J., & Blazer, D. G. (2011) Abused and dependence on prescription opioids in adults: A mixture categorical and dimensional approach to diagnostic classification. *Psychological Medicine, 41,* 653–664. doi:10.1017/S0033291710000954

34

Substance misuse and intimate partner violence

Cecilia Mengo and Kenneth Leonard

Background

Violence against women has been accepted and even condoned throughout history. Violence against women is broadly defined and includes different types of violence. This chapter focuses on intimate partner violence (IPV): "behavior by an intimate partner or ex-partner that causes physical, sexual or psychological harm, including physical aggression, sexual coercion, and psychological abuse and controlling behaviors" (World Health Organization [WHO], 2010, p. 6). According to the U.S. Centers for Disease Control (CDC, 2012), physical violence is the use of physical force with the intention of harming a person, sexual violence is the exertion of force to coerce a person to engage in sexual activity against her/his will, and psychological or emotional violence is the act of intimidating or humiliating a person, exerting control over her/his life, or isolating the person. Some studies focus on IPV as only physical actions, others include sexual assault and coercion, and still others include emotional or psychological abuse (Basile & Smith, 2011; Romans, Forte, Cohen, Du Mont, & Hyman, 2007). There is no universally agreed-upon definition of IPV (Hamberger, 2005); in fact, some authors argue that it is impossible to form a universal definition of IPV that captures the sentiments of different groups (e.g. Hamby, 2017). In this chapter, the term intimate partner violence (IPV) refers to the use or threat of violence (in any of the forms previously described) between individuals who are, or have been, in an intimate relationship—married, divorced, separated, cohabiting, non-cohabiting, or dating.

The topic of IPV is included in this book concerning addictive behaviors because the two types of problems so frequently co-occur. This chapter begins with an introduction to perspectives and typologies of IPV as a global public health problem. Following this introduction is an analysis of the intersection between substance misuse and IPV, presenting evidence concerning both IPV perpetrators and survivors. The chapter concludes with recommendations for integrated prevention and intervention approaches and research addressing IPV and substance use in social work and other disciplines.

Intimate partner violence as a global public health concern

IPV is an important human rights and public health concern around the world. Although statistics clearly show that men and women are both victimized by IPV, national and international surveys sponsored by the U.S. National Institute of Justice's Bureau of Justice Statistics and the World Health Organization (WHO) conclusively stated that, globally, men are much more likely to perpetrate IPV and women to be victimized through IPV. Moreover, women are more likely to experience injurious and potentially fatal forms of IPV. However, distinguishing between "high intensity" and "low intensity" IPV (Archer, 2018), the more severe form is more often perpetrated by men, and the less severe form appears equally prevalent among men and women. Nevertheless, the potential importance of even "low intensity" aggressive behaviors should not be ignored. These behaviors can be consequential and potentially lead to increased aggression (Leonard, Smith, & Homish, 2014; Schumacher, Homish, Leonard, Quigley, & Kearns-Bodkin, 2008).

IPV has a significant adverse effect on women's physical, emotional, mental, sexual, and reproductive health (Breiding, Chen, & Black, 2010; Golding, 1999; Mechanic, Weaver, & Resick, 2008). Survivors of IPV are more likely to report mental health disorders including post-traumatic stress disorder, depression, anxiety, and substance use disorders (CDC, 2018; Coker, Weston, Creson, Justice, & Blakeney, 2005; Devries, Mak et al., 2013; Johnson, Zlotinick, & Perez, 2008). Experiencing IPV can lead to a variety of cognitive problems as well as traumatic brain injury (Wong, Fong, Lai, & Tiwari, 2014). Women surviving IPV also experience increased risks for physical injury, gynecological problems associated with forced sex, unintended pregnancy, sexually transmitted infections (including HIV/AIDS), and miscarriages (Campbell, Garcia-Moreno, & Sharps, 2004). IPV has also been linked to lower initiation and/or early termination of breast-feeding (Lau & Chan, 2007). Children who witness IPV are predisposed to numerous social and physical problems, including an increased risk of later perpetrating IPV (WHO, 2010).

IPV prevalence

There exist many difficulties associated with accurately estimating the prevalence of IPV, arising from definitional issues, the many different manifestations of IPV, stigma, and fear of legal sanctions for reporting IPV. Regardless of these factors, estimates are tragically high for sexual, psychological, and physical forms of IPV.

Sexual violence

Estimates of lifetime "contact sexual violence" (rape, attempted rape, sexual coercion, and unwanted sexual contact) approach 20% (Smith et al., 2018). These rates reflect *intimate partners*; rates of contact sexual violence by any perpetrator are approximately twice those rates for an intimate partner (see Chapter 35).

Psychological violence

Estimates of psychological violence are very problematic as definitions vary from one study to another. Early research by Stets (1990) and Stets and Straus (1990) reported that 75% of men and 80% of women acknowledged psychological aggression. Follingstad and Rogers (2014) asked a large national sample whether they had experienced 42 psychological abuse items in their worst relationship and found that 84% endorsed at least one item. Smith et al. (2018) reported lifetime rates of experiencing expressive psychological aggression (e.g. insults, made fun of in front of others) of 26% for women and 17% for men. Lifetime rates of experiencing coercive control (e.g. threats of physical harm, demanded to know where you were and what you were doing, tried to keep you from seeing or talking to friends or family) were 31% for women and 30% for men.

Physical violence

Physical aggression was the focus of the earliest national estimates of the prevalence of IPV and has been the most common form of IPV examined over the years. Straus, Gelles, and Steinmetz (1980) reported that over the course of their relationships, 28% of married couples reported either husband or wife violence. Other estimates range from 22% to 31% of women and 7% to 31% of men (Smith et al., 2018; Tjaden & Thoennes, 2000). In terms of annual prevalence, Esquivel-Santoveña and Dixon (2012) reported perpetration rates of 8.0–12.1% for men and 8.0–16.9% for women across numerous of national surveys. Much lower annual rates of physical assault were reported in the U.S. National Violence Against Women Survey (1.3% of men—0.9% of women). The U.S. National Intimate Partner and Sexual Violence Survey conducted by the CDC reported rates of partner violence of 3.8% by women and 2.9% by men. Annual rates of IPV are substantially higher in the early years of marriage, with reports of any physical aggression in the 30–40% range (e.g. O'Leary et al., 1989; Schumacher & Leonard, 2005), although rates of serious or repeated violence tend to be in the 15% range for both women and men.

Alcohol, substance use, and IPV

The role of excessive alcohol and substance use in IPV is both controversial and complex. Meta-analyses of several hundred studies showed that alcohol and substance use are related both to IPV perpetration and IPV victimization (e.g. Cafferky, Mendez, Anderson, & Stith, 2018), as well as violence more generally (Duke, Smith, Oberleitner, Westphal, & McKee, 2018). In fact, excessive men's alcohol use has been shown, both in large-scale international studies (e.g. Greene, Kane, & Tol, 2017) and more focused national and local studies, to be one of the most consistent risk factors for IPV.

Although meta-analyses support a relationship between substance use and IPV, the findings are more complex when specific substances are examined. For instance, meta-analysis identified significant associations between physical IPV and both cocaine and opiate use, but no significant association with marijuana, stimulants, sedatives, or hallucinogens (Moore et al., 2008). In a more recent meta-analysis, Cafferky et al. (2018) identified associations of IPV with amphetamine, cocaine, and marijuana use, but no significant relationship with opiates.

From the perspective of perpetration, there are three broad explanations for these relationships: (1) alcohol and drug use are associated with other factors that facilitate IPV; (2) alcohol and drug use have an indirect effect on IPV, usually through relationship satisfaction and conflict, which lead to IPV; and (3) acute alcohol consumption, in predisposed individuals under certain circumstances, facilitates the occurrence or severity of IPV. For studies of victimization, we would add a fourth explanation: (4) alcohol and drug use reflect efforts at coping with IPV. These four explanations are not mutually exclusive, and the explanations may differ for alcohol and specific other drugs. The large-scale meta-analyses do not provide information that addresses these four explanations.

Alcohol and drugs as spurious factors

There is little doubt that alcohol and drug use are associated with other factors predictive of IPV. For example, Krueger, McGue, and Iacono (2001) presented evidence for an "externalizing" disorder comprised on adult antisocial behavior, and alcohol and drug dependence; antisocial behavior is strongly linked to IPV. This externalizing factor also related to parent-child conflict (Burt, Krueger, McGue, & Iacono, 2003). These and other studies suggest that both substance use disorders and the propensity for violence share common roots.

Alcohol and drugs as indirect causes

Patterns of alcohol and drug use predict relationship deterioration and conflict. One emerging finding is that the discrepancy between partners' alcohol use patterns is often more predictive of IPV than whether one partner or the other engages in heavy use. Discrepant patterns of heavy drinking were longitudinally predictive of reductions in marital satisfaction (Homish & Leonard, 2007) and divorce (Leonard et al., 2014, Ostermann, Sloan, & Taylor, 2005). Although these studies focus on discrepant use, evidence concerning alcohol use disorders appears to be more complex (e.g. Cranford, Floyd, Schulenberg & Zucker, 2011; Mattson, Lofgreen, & O'Farrell, 2017). Furthermore, discrepant marijuana use was not associated with relationship satisfaction (Testa, Wang, Derrick, & Leonard, 2018) or divorce (Leonard et al., 2014).

Alcohol and drugs as acute contributors to IPV

Substantial research has focused on the proximal influence of alcohol or other drugs, both experimentally and in studying IPV episodes. Crane, Godleski, Pryzbyla, Schlauch, and Testa (2016) examined six studies involving responses to both vignettes and verbal cognitive behaviors in the context of conflict or disagreements. They concluded that alcohol significantly increased measures of aggressive behavior. In a subsequent meta-analysis of female aggression, Crane, Licata, Schlauch, Testa, and Easton (2017) concluded that alcohol facilitated female aggression, but the effect size was small. Consistent with the broader literature, these studies suggest a stronger impact of alcohol on IPV among men than among women.

Early studies comparing the presence of alcohol during an aggressive and a non-aggressive conflict support a link between alcohol use and the occurrence of physical aggression (Chermack & Blow, 2002; Leonard & Quigley, 1999). More recent studies have collected daily data about drinking and conflict/IPV for weeks or months. A review of this literature concluded that drinking by men and women "increases the likelihood of perpetrating physical violence on the same day" (de Bruijn & de Graff, 2016, p. 150). Recent studies have assessed the actual time that drinking and IPV occurred. For example, Testa and Derrick (2014) assessed the time of drinking and any aggressive interactions and were able to link alcohol consumption with the perpetration of both verbal (psychological) and physical aggression within four hours of the drinking initiation. This effect was observed for both men and women.

Considerably less research addresses either the experimental impact or the same-day relationship between other drugs and IPV. Experimental studies of marijuana and aggression have yielded contradictory results, and there are very few experimental studies of other drugs in humans. The review by de Bruijn and de Graff (2016) identified six studies addressing cannabis use and partner violence, concluding that the limited evidence did not suggest a relationship. Testa et al. (2018) detected small but significant increases in conflict and verbal aggression within two hours of marijuana use, but no increases in physical aggression. With fewer than five studies addressing same-day cocaine or opioid use, it is difficult to draw definitive conclusions.

Alcohol and drugs as conditional contributors to IPV

Researchers have long known that alcohol (or drugs) do not directly lead to violence but facilitate aggression among certain individuals under certain circumstances (Leonard &

Quigley, 2017). Recent research has sought to understand the interplay of the multiple factors that lead to aggression. One approach reflects a multiple thresholds theory (Fals-Stewart, Leonard, & Birchler, 2005), focused on the interplay between alcohol, provocation, inhibitions, and aggressive motivations. A similar framing, I3 (I-cubed) developed by Finkel (2007), describes three sets of factors that lead to aggression: instigating, impelling, and inhibiting. From both perspectives, intoxication is viewed as disrupting cognitive processes and reducing inhibitions. These approaches suggest that the greatest likelihood of violence, as well as the most severe violence, occurs when intoxicated individuals with high levels of impelling factors (e.g. hostility) and low levels of inhibition are faced with aggressive instigation.

Survey and experimental research strongly support these basic tenets with respect to both general and intimate partner violence. From the perspective of impelling characteristics, excessive alcohol consumption is more strongly associated with IPV among individuals high in anger (e.g. Schumacher et al., 2008), jealousy (Foran & O'Leary, 2008), stressful life events (Margolin, John, & Foo, 1998), and relationship dissatisfaction (Foran, Snarr, Heyman, & Slep, 2012). From the perspective of inhibiting factors, alcohol was more strongly related to IPV among individuals with low/poor impulse control (Watkins, Maldonado, & DiLillo, 2014), emotion regulation (Halmos, Leone, Parrott, & Eckhardt, 2018), and executive functioning (Easton, Sacco, Neavins, Wupperman, & George, 2008). In fact, it is rare to find a study reporting that alcohol leads to aggression among non-aggressive individuals in non-threatening circumstances.

The multiple thresholds model provides some potential clinical guidance with respect to the relative importance of addressing the alcohol use of an individual who engages in IPV. First, alcohol is not likely to result in violence in the absence of aggressive motivations. In other words, it is never just the alcohol; clinical work also needs to address other potential factors. Second, among individuals with high aggressive motivations and low inhibitions (i.e. highly violent individuals), alcohol intoxication is likely to increase IPV frequency and severity. In these individuals, successfully treating excessive drinking is not likely by itself to eliminate violence, but it may reduce very severe violence. Finally, alcohol is likely to have its strongest influence among individuals with moderate levels of aggressive motivations and moderate levels of inhibition fundamentally. Although alcohol is viewed as a contributing cause, clinical work should always include other known causes of IPV at the same time as excessive drinking is being addressed.

Theoretical perspectives on IPV and substance use

Because of the extensive research with respect to alcohol and aggression, most theoretical accounts of IPV perpetration and substance use have grown out of this literature. Two approaches dominate this discussion: alcohol expectancy and alcohol myopia theories.

Alcohol expectancy theory

Alcohol expectancy theory (see Chapter 6) argues that alcohol consumption activates memories (learned expectancies) regarding the expected behaviors and consequences of aggression, leading a person to aggress under specific conditions. The psychopharmacological impact of alcohol is minimized in this theory. One process, deviance disavowal, proposes that individuals learn that, under the influence of alcohol, they can behave in a disinhibited and aggressive fashion with less likelihood of punishment. As a result, when motivated to aggress, the usual restraining impact of anticipated punishment is lessened through the alcohol-related expectancies. Another process, aggressive-cue priming, suggests that consuming alcohol facilitates aggression by leading a person to frame the situation as appropriate for aggression.

Research is not generally supportive of the deviance disavowal position. Studies have presented IPV vignettes with either intoxicated or sober characters and asked men and women to make judgments of causality or blame. Most reported that intoxicated and sober characters received comparable attributions of blame. Similarly, in studies of real-world perpetration, intoxication was not an accepted excuse for the perpetration of violence (Quigley & Leonard, 2006). Moreover, prospective studies examining whether beliefs about alcohol and aggression predict subsequent IPV have been contradictory. Overall, there exists little evidence for deviance disavowal as a factor facilitating the occurrence of IPV. However, individuals perpetrating IPV often *attempt* to excuse their behavior in a variety of ways, including intoxication, and this may have intervention implications.

In contrast, consistent evidence supports alcohol cues as primes, eliciting aggression-promoting cognitions. For example, Bartholow and Heinz (2006) observed that alcohol cues facilitated the recognition of aggressive words. Exposure to alcohol advertising resulted in attributing more hostile motivations to another individual than did exposing them to a neutral advertisement; this effect was more pronounced among participants with stronger alcohol-related expectancies. A subsequent study reported that alcohol cues led to increased aggression but only in response to a provocation with ambiguous intent (Pedersen, Vasquez, Bartholow, Grosvenor, & Truong, 2014).

Alcohol myopia theory

Specifying the psychopharmacological disruption of cognitive processes, this theory argues that intoxication leads to behavior guided by the most salient cues in a situation (Steele & Josephs, 1990; Taylor & Leonard 1983). Taylor and Leonard (1983) hypothesized that because of cognitive disruption, an intoxicated person "will tend to be more responsive to immediate, dominant cues, and less responsive to nonsalient, subtle cues" (p. 97). From this perspective, intoxication may facilitate a variety of behaviors, depending on the most salient cues. Steele and Josephs (1990) demonstrated that alcohol could increase helping behaviors. Similarly, Leonard (1989) reported that level of intoxication was correlated with less aggression in the presence of a non-aggressive partner, and with more aggression in the presence of a threatening partner.

Evidence regarding alcohol myopia is quite strong, although most has focused on basic tenets of the theory, and not specifically on its application to IPV. Various basic studies of alcohol and attentional processes supported the limited ability to process information and the focus on central tasks while drinking (see Chapter 6). More pertinent are studies supporting the hypothesis that alcohol increases aggression when aggressive cues are most salient, either because of individual characteristics (e.g. high anger) or characteristics of the situation (e.g. highly threatening).

Research has also sought to address key elements of myopia theory more directly. For example, the theory suggests that it would be possible to alter the relationship between intoxication and aggression by changing or disrupting attentional processes. Bailey, Leonard, Cranston, and Taylor (1983) reduced intoxicated aggression by providing cues to self-awareness (e.g. mirror, video camera). Giancola and Corman (2007) reduced intoxicated aggression by distracting participants from aggression with a working memory task. Massa, Subramani, Eckhardt, and Parrot (2019) observed that alcohol led to an attentional bias toward anger among individuals engaged in heavy drinking with a recent history of partner violence. This bias was particularly strong for individuals engaged in problematic alcohol use.

In summary, the evidence regarding deviance disavowal as a cause of the alcohol-violence relationship is weak. However, there exists growing evidence that the act of consuming alcohol, as well as the specific environmental and interpersonal contexts of alcohol consumption, may facilitate the perceptual of a situation as hostile. At the same time, alcohol intoxication appears to limit a person's attentional and information processing abilities to salient cues.

Substance misuse and the risk of experiencing IPV

Experiencing IPV is associated with mental health challenges, including substance use problems (e.g. El-Bassel, Gilbert, Wu, Go, & Hill, 2005; Martino, Collins, & Ellickson, 2005; Warshaw, Sullivan, & Rivera, 2013). These problems are complex and highly correlated with each other, and in a potentially bidirectional manner. Some studies report increased substance use following IPV (Martino et al., 2005), whereas others reported that using substances may lead to increased vulnerability to IPV (El-Bassel et al., 2005; Greene et al., 2017). Thus, substance use may be a response to the effects of IPV and/or render individuals more vulnerable to ongoing abuse (Warshaw et al., 2013).

Although it is not clear whether substance use increases vulnerability to IPV, it seems quite clear that the experience of IPV can lead to increased substance use. Research strongly supports the position that alcohol and substance use are often used to manage negative emotions, including anger, depression, anxiety, and distress (Cooper, Kuntsche, Levitt, Barber, & Wolf, 2016), common sequelae of IPV (Stewart, Vigod, & Riazantseva, 2016). Indeed, a meta-analysis (Devries, Child et al., 2013) concluded that IPV significantly predicted subsequent alcohol use, although the effect was not large and was based on a small number of studies. While the evidence is clear that IPV can impact subsequent alcohol and substance use, other factors clearly can increase or mitigate this effect including social support (Suvak, Taft, Goodman, & Dutton, 2013), and resources (Beeble, Bybee, & Sullivan, 2010). More research is warranted in this area.

Intervention and research implications related to substance misuse and IPV

There exists a dire need to develop and evaluate innovative approaches that can address substance misuse and IPV, in terms of both perpetrating and experiencing violence. These interventions need to consider strategies for the different contexts and types of intimate partner relationships where IPV occurs, as well as implications for diverse populations. The majority of IPV intervention efforts come from Western societies and these might not be applicable to other contexts such as Africa, Asia, and South America. In addition, prevention and intervention efforts for ethnic minority women and same sex partners might be different. Furthermore, intervening in substance misuse and perpetration would differ from interventions delivered to individuals experiencing IPV and substance-related problems.

Intervening around substance misuse and IPV perpetration

One of the most prominent contexts for addressing IPV has been the criminal justice system. Men represent 90% of individuals who come before the courts on charges of perpetrating IPV (Feder & Wilson, 2005). One typical outcome is referral to a mandatory IPV/batterer intervention program. Currently, there is wide variation in content, style, and length of batterer intervention programs, from small group weekend treatment programs to 52-week prevention efforts, many of which have demonstrated modest and reasonably enduring effects (Edleson, 2012). Other studies present more questionable or inconsistently positive outcomes (Babcock, Green, & Robie, 2004; Jackson et al., 2003). Notably, most of these programs do not directly address substance use. In a study of 840 men in batterers' programs in four U.S. cities, substance abuse *during the batterers' program* was the best predictor of future partner abuse (Gondolf, 2002). A key recommendation for social workers and other professionals is to screen and evaluate substance abuse by participants in batterers' programs during intake and throughout their time in the program. This would also provide an opportunity for professionals to discuss how substance misuse impacts a person's life. Screening for substance use during intake would also be a first step in establishing that an alcohol or drug problem exists, leading when appropriate to referral for formal assessment by a qualified specialist who could then help develop a treatment plan. Effective treatment programs for service providers to deal with this issue within the batterer intervention programs are still emerging.

A second potential venue of IPV and substance abuse treatment has been addiction treatment centers. Studies conducted over the last decade have consistently revealed that about 44–84% of men in substance use treatment also report a past year history of IPV perpetration (Murphy, Winters, O'Farrell, Fals-Stewart, & Murphy, 2005; Timko et al., 2012). Men receiving substance use treatment who perpetrate IPV are rarely referred to batterer intervention programs (Timko et al., 2012) because most are court mandated and referred by the criminal justice system. Although there exists some empirical support for intervening with men who perpetrate violence and experience coexisting substance use problems, such as motivational enhancement therapy (MET) (Easton, Swan, & Sinha, 2002), new models are also being developed to incorporate an alcohol component into batterer intervention programs. It is important to recognize that violent men presenting for substance use treatment voluntarily are likely to be very different from violent men in the criminal justice system. Moreover, for these men, successful treatment of their substance use, particularly alcohol, can lead to significant reductions in IPV.

Some studies examining the impact of integrating IPV and substance use treatment observed that IPV may be reduced when addressed in the context of substance abuse treatment and supplemented by behavioral couples therapy (e.g. O'Farrell, Murphy, Stephan, Fals-Stewart, & Murphy, 2004). This model of concurrently addressing IPV and substance misuse remains a challenge, especially among IPV service providers, given barriers such as limited trained professionals, lack of drug and alcohol programming, fear and lack of knowledge on the part of staff to handle severe cases of substance use (Warshaw et al., 2013). More trainings are needed around basics of the co-occurring problem of IPV and substance use. Nevertheless, there have been promising results related to reducing both victimization and perpetration of IPV by integrating partner violence treatment with substance use and mental health treatment, especially among couples (Crane & Easton, 2017).

An emerging potential venue for intervention is the health care setting. Overall, the relationship between substance misuse and IPV is apparent in primary health care settings, family practice clinics, prenatal clinics, and rural health clinics (Mason & O'Rinn, 2014). In these settings, the co-occurring problems can be identified through routine screening and addressed through intervention by properly trained professionals. Ideally, these individuals would be referred to systems of care where both problems (IPV and substance misuse) can be concurrently addressed rather than sequentially, although few such programs currently exist. There are, of course, notable challenges to bringing IPV and substance use treatment expertise to the health care setting (see Chapter 27). Nevertheless, the need for health services, and the obvious health implications of IPV and substance use are factors which should foster further exploration of this approach.

Intervening around substance misuse and the experience of IPV

In the United States, much of our current knowledge about these interventions comes from research involving participants from battered women's shelters, batterer intervention programs (BIP) and emergency rooms (or other medical clinics). Much of this research focused on the impact of outreach advocacy on victims' revictimization, quality of life, depression, and social support (e.g. Breiding et al., 2010; Ramsay et al., 2009). Research suggests many positive outcomes especially for individuals who use IPV shelter services For instance, women who sought shelter services reported less revictimization by their partners (Bybee & Sullivan, 2002, 2005), a better quality of life (Sullivan, Bybee, & Allen, 2002), fewer psychological distress/mental health symptoms (Constantino, Kim, & Crane, 2005), more social support (Bybee & Sullivan, 2005), greater safety and emotional support for themselves and their children and more effectiveness in accessing resources (Constantino et al., 2005) than women who did not use shelters.

The critical issue here is that women engaged in alcohol or other drug misuse are seldom permitted to enter shelter care. Despite clear relationships among IPV, mental health, and substance use problems, many prevention and intervention efforts are faced with numerous challenges to addressing these highly correlated issues among IPV survivors (Arroyo, Lundahl, Butters, Vanderloo, & Wood, 2017). Mental health and substance use problems may increase the chances that a person will remain in an abusive partner relationship and, in turn, potentially endure continued abuse (Bell & Goodman, 2001).

Clinicians and frontline providers who work in IPV, health care, mental health, or addiction treatment settings need to routinely screen for these frequently co-occurring problems and recognize how to respond when detected. As discussed in terms of concurrently addressing these in interventions around perpetration, concurrent solutions need to be offered to individuals experiencing IPV, as well. Social work practitioners and other professionals should have access to the most current evidence-supported screening tools for IPV victimization and substance misuse. These screening tools should be comprehensive so that they are appropriate for use with diverse populations. These screening tools should be included in the intake process in both the substance use treatment centers and IPV service agencies for all individuals seeking help within these agencies so as to provide the needed support (Rhodes, 2012).

Research

Researching IPV and substance use problems is challenging because the sensitive, potentially threatening, and traumatic nature of the subject matter presents numerous practical and ethical challenges: the safety and even lives of research participants may be at risk. Innovative strategies are needed to engage these difficult to identify, recruit, and retain populations in studies (Begun, Berger, & Otto-Salaj, 2018). In addition to ethical challenges, Murray and Graybeal (2007) stated that methodological challenges are common. These include varying definitions of key constructs (both in IPV and substance misuse) and measurement issues (e.g. long-term follow-up and validity). Because resources to support extensive research are very limited, use of pre-existing data becomes extremely important as a research strategy. Furthermore, secondary data analysis reduces risks of imposing secondary trauma on study participants. However, use of such data poses different challenges, especially when data were not designed/collected for research purposes. Investigators must collaborate more closely with advocates, providers, and intervention recipient populations to ensure that they frame meaningful questions and produce useful knowledge. For example, use of community based participatory research may help identify and prioritize needs and interventions that align with those needs, as well as enhance intervention fidelity and sustainability.

Overall, past research efforts focused on individual interventions. The CDC urges prevention and intervention efforts beyond individual level factors, addressing macro level factors in communities and society to build sustainable interventions for addressing and preventing IPV. Success is dependent on intervention designers and decision makers understanding that these would be long-term community based participatory approaches requiring a considerable amount of planning and funding (Contreras-Urbina et al., 2016).

Conclusions

IPV has major impacts on individual and family long-term health and well-being. This chapter presented evidence of the various complex relationships between substance misuse (alcohol and other drugs) and both the perpetration and experiencing of IPV. For years, there has been a siloed approach, with IPV and substance use professionals, as well as mental health professionals, addressing only their area of expertise. However, the overlap and complexity of these problems calls for integrating services to address these concurrent problems. Moreover, there are important implications for training. Social workers and other professionals should be trained to routinely engage in substance misuse and IPV screening efforts and know how to respond when these problems arise individually or in a co-occurring manner. Intimate partner violence has many contributing factors including substance use, and our treatment models can no longer justify focusing on only one contributing cause and ignoring other potential contributors (Babcock et al., 2016).

References

Archer, J. (2018). Violence to partners: Gender symmetry revisited. In J. L. Ireland, P. Birch, & C. A. Ireland (Eds.), *International handbook on aggression*. New York, NY: Routledge. doi:10.4324/9781315618777-13

Arroyo, K., Lundahl, B., Butters, R., Vanderloo, M., & Wood, D. S. (2017). Short-term interventions for survivors of intimate partner violence: A systematic review and meta-analysis. *Trauma, Violence, & Abuse, 18*(2), 155–171. doi:10.1177/1524838015602736.

Babcock, J., Armenti, N., Cannon, C., Lauve-Moon, K., Buttell, F., Ferreira, R., . . . Solano, I. (2016). Domestic violence perpetrator programs: A proposal for evidence-based standards in the United States. *Partner Abuse, 7*(4), 355–460. doi:10.1891/1946-6560.7.4.355

Babcock, J., Green, J., & Robie, C. (2004). Does batterers' treatment work? A meta-analytic review of domestic violence treatment outcome research. *Clinical Psychology Review, 23*, 1023–1153. doi:10.1016/j.cpr.2002.07.00

Bailey, D. S., Leonard, K. E., Cranston, J. W., & Taylor, S. P. (1983). Effects of alcohol and self-awareness on human physical aggression. *Personality and Social Psychology Bulletin, 9*, 289–295. doi:10.1177/0146167283092014

Bartholow, B. D., & Heinz, A. (2006). Alcohol and aggression without consumption: Alcohol cues, aggressive thoughts, and hostile perception bias. *Psychological Science, 17*(1), 30–37. doi:10.1111/j.1467-9280.2005.01661.x

Basile, K. C., & Smith, S. G. (2011). Sexual violence victimization of women: Prevalence, characteristics, and the role of public health and prevention. *American Journal of Lifestyle Medicine, 5*, 407–417. doi:10.1177/1559827611409512

Bell, M. E., & Goodman, L. (2001). Supporting battered women involved with the court system: An evaluation of a law-based advocacy intervention. *Violence Against Women, 7*(12), 1377–1404. doi:10.1177/10778010122183919

Beeble, M. L., Bybee, D., & Sullivan, C. M. (2010). The impact of resource constraints on the psychological well-being of survivors of intimate partner violence over time. *Journal of Community Psychology, 38*(8), 943–959. doi:10.1002/jcop.20407

Begun, A. L., Berger, L. K., & Otto-Salaj, L. L. (2018). *Participant recruitment and retention in intervention and evaluation research.* New York, NY: Oxford University Press.

Breiding, M. J., Chen, J., & Black, M. C. (2010). *Intimate partner violence in the United States—2010.* Atlanta, GA: US Department of Health and Human Services, CDC, National Center for Injury Prevention and Control.

Burt, S. A., Krueger, R. F., McGue, M., & Iacono, W. (2003). Parent-child conflict and the comorbidity among childhood externalizing disorders. *Archives of General Psychiatry, 60*(5), 505–513. doi:10.1001/archpsyc.60.5.505

Bybee, D. I., & Sullivan, C. M. (2002). The process through which an advocacy intervention resulted in positive change for battered women over time. *American Journal of Community Psychology, 30*(1), 103–132. doi:10.1023/A:1014376202459.

Bybee, D. I., & Sullivan, C. M. (2005). Predicting re-victimization of battered women 3 years after exiting s shelter program. *American Journal of Community Psychology, 36*(1–2), 85–96. doi:10.1007/s10464-005-6234-5

Cafferky, B. M., Mendez, M., Anderson, J. R., & Stith, S. M. (2018). Substance use and intimate partner violence: A meta-analytic review. *Psychology of Violence, 8*(1), 110–131. doi:10.1037/vio0000074

Campbell, J., Garcia-Moreno, C., & Sharps, P. (2004). Abuse during pregnancy in industrialized and developing countries. *Violence Against Women, 10*(7), 770–789. doi:10.1177/1077201204265551

Centers for Disease Control and Prevention. (2018). *Preventing intimate Partner Violence.* Retrieved from https://www.cdc.gov/violenceprevention/intimatepartnerviolence/fastfact.html

Centers for Disease Control and Prevention. (2012). *Promoting respectful, nonviolent intimate partner relationships through individual, community and societal change: Strategic direction for intimate partner violence prevention.* Atlanta, GA: Centers for Disease Control and Prevention. Retrieved from https://www.cdc.gov/violenceprevention/pdf/IPV_Strategic_Direction_Full-Doc-a.pdf

Chermack, S. T., & Blow, F. C. (2002). Violence among individuals in substance abuse treatment: The role of alcohol and cocaine consumption. *Drug and Alcohol Dependence, 66*(1), 29–37. doi:10.1016/S0376-8716(01)00180-6

Coker, A. L., Weston, R., Creson, D. L., Justice, B., & Blakeney, P. (2005). PTSD symptoms among men and women survivors of intimate partner violence: The role of risk and protective factors. *Violence and Victims, 20*(6), 625–643. doi:10.1891/vivi.20.6.625

Constantino, R., Kim, Y., & Crane, P. A. (2005). Effects of a social support intervention on health outcomes in residents of a domestic violence shelter: A pilot study. *Issues in Mental Health Nursing, 26*, 575–590. doi:10.1080/01612840590959416

Contreras-Urbina, M., Heilman, B., Von Au, A. K., Hill, A., Puerto-Gómez, M., Zelaya, J., & Arango, D. J. (2016). *Community-based approaches to intimate partner violence: A review of evidence and essential steps to adaptation (English).* Washington, DC: World Bank Group.

Cooper, M. L., Kuntsche, E., Levitt, A., Barber, L. L., & Wolf, S. (2016). Motivational models of substance use: A review of theory and research on motives for using alcohol, marijuana, and tobacco. In. K. J. Sher (Ed.), *The Oxford handbook of substance use and substance use disorders* (Vol. 1, pp. 375–421). New York, NY: Oxford University Press. doi:10.1093/oxfordhb/9780199381678.013.017

Crane, C. A., & Easton, C. J. (2017). Integrated treatment options for male perpetrators of intimate partner violence. *Drug and Alcohol Review, 36*, 24–33. doi:10.1111/dar.12496

Crane, C. A., Godleski, S. A., Przybyla, S. M, Schlauch, R. C., & Testa, M. (2016). The proximal effects of acute alcohol consumption on male-to-female aggression: A meta-analytic review of the experimental literature. *Trauma, Violence, & Abuse, 17*(5), 520–531. doi:10.1177/1524838015584374

Crane, C. A., Licata, M. L., Schlauch, R. C., Testa, M., & Easton, C. J. (2017). The proximal effects of acute alcohol use on female aggression: A meta-analytic review of the experimental literature. *Psychology of Addictive Behaviors, 31*(1), 21–26. doi:10.1037/adb0000244

Cranford, J. A., Floyd, F. J., Schulenberg, J. E., & Zucker, R. A. (2011). Husbands' and wives' alcohol use disorders and marital interactions as longitudinal predictors of marital adjustment. *Journal of Abnormal Psychology, 120*(1), 210–222. doi:10.1037/a0021349

de Bruijn, D. M., & de Graaf, I. M. (2016). The role of substance use in same-day intimate partner violence: A review of the literature. *Aggression and Violent Behavior, 27*, 142–151. doi:10.1016/j.avb.2016.02.010

Devries, K. M., Child, J. C., Bacchus, L. J., Mak, J. Y., Falder, G., Graham, K., . . . Heise, L. (2013). Intimate partner violence victimization and alcohol consumption in women: A systematic review and meta-analysis. *Addiction, 109*, 379–391. doi:10.1111/add.12393

Devries, K. M., Mak, J. Y., Bacchus, L. J., Child, J. C. , Falder, G., Petzold, M., . . .Watts, C. H. (2013). Intimate partner violence and incident depressive symptoms and suicide attempts: A systematic review of longitudinal studies, *PLoS Medicine, 10*(5), a1001439. doi:10.1371/journal.pmed.1001439

Duke, A. A., Smith, K. M. Z., Oberleitner, L. M. S., Westphal, A., & McKee, S. A. (2018). Alcohol, drugs, and violence: A meta-meta-analysis. *Psychology of Violence, 8*(2), 238–249. doi:10.1037/vio0000106

Easton, C. J., Sacco, K. A., Neavins, T. M., Wupperman, P, & George, T. P. (2008). Neurocognitive performance among alcohol dependent men with and without physical violence toward their partners: A preliminary report. *American Journal of Drug and Alcohol Abuse, 34*(1), 29–37. doi:10.1080/00952990701764326

Easton, C., Swan, S., & Sinha, R. (2002). Motivation to change substance use among offenders of domestic violence. *Journal of Substance Abuse Treatment, 19*(1), 1–5. doi:10.1016/S0740-5472(99)00098-7

Edleson, J. L. (2012). *Groupwork with men who batter: What the research literature indicates*. Harrisburg, PA: VAWnet, a project of the National Resource Center on Domestic Violence. Retrieved June 19, 2019, from http://www.vawnet.org

El-Bassel, N., Gilbert, L., Wu, E., Go, H., & Hill, J. (2005). Relationship between drug abuse and intimate partner violence: A longitudinal study among women receiving methadone. *American Journal of Public Health, 95*, 3, 465–470. doi:10.2105/AJPH.2003.023200

Esquivel-Santoveña, E. E., & Dixon, L. (2012). Investigating the true rate of physical intimate partner violence: A review of nationally representative surveys. *Aggression and Violent Behavior, 17*(3), 208–219. doi:10.1016/j.avb.2012.02.002

Fals-Stewart, W., Leonard, K. E., & Birchler, G. R. (2005). The occurrence of male-to-female intimate partner violence on days of men's drinking: The moderating effects of antisocial personality disorder. *Journal of Consulting and Clinical Psychology, 73*(2), 239–248. doi:10.1037/0022-006X.73.2.239

Feder, F., & Wilson, D. (2005). A meta-analytic review of court-mandated batterer intervention. Can courts affect abusers' behavior? *Journal of Experimental Criminology, 1*, 239–262. doi:10.1007/s11292-005-1179-0.

Finkel, E. J. (2007). Impelling and inhibiting forces in the perpetration of intimate partner violence. *Review of General Psychology, 11*(2), 193–207. doi:10.1037/1089-2680.11.2.193

Follingstad, D. R., & Rogers, M. J. (2014). The nature and prevalence of partner psychological abuse in a national sample of adults. *Violence and Victims, 29*(1), 3–23. doi:10.1891/0886-6708.09-160

Foran, H. M., & O'Leary, K. D., (2008). Problem drinking, jealousy, and anger control: Variables predicting physical aggression against a partner. *Journal of Family Violence, 23*, 141–148. doi:10.1037/a0027688

Foran, H. M., Snarr, J. D., Heyman, R. E., & Slep, A. M. S. (2012). Hazardous alcohol use and intimate partner violence in the military: Understanding protective factors. *Psychology of Addictive Behaviors, 26*, 471–483. doi:10.1037/a0027688

Giancola, P. R., & Corman, M. D. (2007). Alcohol and aggression: A test of the attention-allocation model. *Psychology Science, 18*, 649–655. doi:10.1111/j.1467-9280.2007.01953.x

Golding, J. M. (1999). Intimate partner violence as a risk factor for mental disorders: A Meta-analysis. *Journal of Family Violence, 14*, 99–130. doi:10.1023/A:1022079418229

Gondolf, E. (2002). *Batterer intervention systems: Issues, outcomes, and recommendations*. Thousand Oaks, CA: Sage Publications, Inc.

Greene, M. C., Kane, J. C., & Tol, W. A. (2017). Alcohol use and intimate partner violence among women and their partners in sub-Saharan Africa. *Global Mental Health, 4*. doi:10.1017/gmh.2017.9

Halmos, M. B., Leone, R. M., Parrott, D. J., & Eckhardt, C. I. (2018). Relationship dissatisfaction, emotion regulation, and physical intimate partner aggression in heavy-drinking, conflict-prone couples: A dyadic analysis. *Journal of Interpersonal Violence*. doi:10.1177/0886260518801019 [Epub ahead of print].

Hamby, S. (2017). On defining violence, and why it matters. *Psychology of Violence, 7*, 167–180. doi:10.1037/vio0000117

Hamberger, L. (2005). Men's and women's use of intimate partner violence in clinical samples: Toward a gender-sensitive analysis. *Violence and Victims, 20*, 131–151. doi:10.1891/vivi.2005.20.2.131

Homish, G. G., & Leonard, K. E. (2007). The drinking partnership and marital satisfaction: The longitudinal influence of discrepant drinking behavior. *Journal of Consulting and Clinical Psychology, 75*(1), 43–51. doi:10.1037/0022-006X.75.1.43

Jackson, S., Feder, D., Forde, D., Davis, R., Maxwell, C., & Taylor, B. (2003). *Batterer intervention programs: Where do we go from here?* Washington, DC: National Institute of Justice. Retrieved from https://www.researchgate.net/publication/265100951_Batterer_intervention_programs_Where_do_we_go_from_here

Johnson, D. M., Zlotnick, C., & Perez, S. (2008). The relative contribution of abuse severity and PTSD severity on the psychiatric and social morbidity of battered women in shelters. *Behavior Therapy, 39*(3), 232–241. doi:10.1016/j.beth.2007.08.003

Krueger, R. F., McGue, M., & Iacono, W. G. (2001). The higher-order structure of common DSM mental disorders: Internalization, externalization, and their connections to personality. *Personality and Individual Differences, 30*, 1245–1259. doi:10.1016/S0191-8869(00)00106-9

Lau, Y., & Chan, K. S. (2007). Influence of intimate partner violence during pregnancy and early postpartum depressive symptoms on breastfeeding among Chinese women in Hong Kong. *Journal of Midwifery & Women's Health, 52*(2), 15–20. doi:10.1016/j.jmwh.2006.09.001

Leonard, K. E. (1989). The impact of explicit aggressive and implicit nonaggressive cues on aggression in intoxicated and sober males. *Personality and Social Psychology Bulletin, 15*(3), 390–400. doi:10.1177/0146167289153009

Leonard, K. E., & Quigley, B. M. (1999). Drinking and marital aggression in newlyweds: An event-based analysis of drinking and the occurrence of husband marital aggression. *Journal of Studies on Alcohol, 60*(4), 537–545. doi:10.15288/jsa.1999.60.537

Leonard, K. E., & Quigley, B. M. (2017). Thirty years of research show alcohol to be a cause of intimate partner violence: Future research needs to identify who to treat and how to treat them. *Drug and Alcohol Review, 36*(1), 7–9. doi:10.1111/dar.12434

Leonard, K. E., Smith, P. H., & Homish, G. G. (2014). Concordant and discordant alcohol, tobacco, and marijuana use as predictors of marital dissolution. *Psychology of Addictive Behaviors, 28*(3), 780–790. doi:10.1037/a0034053

Margolin, G., John, R. S., & Foo, L. (1998). Interactive and unique risk factors for husbands: Emotional and physical abuse of their wives. *Journal of Family Violence, 13*, 315–344. doi:10.1023/A:1022880518367

Martino, S., Collins, R. L., Ellickson, P. L. (2005). Cross-lagged relationships between substance use and intimate partner violence among a sample of young adult women. *Journal of Studies on Alcohol, 66*, 139–148. doi:10.15288/jsa.2005.66.139

Massa, A. A., Subramani, O. S., Eckhardt, C. I., & Parrott, D. J. (2019). Problematic alcohol use and acute intoxication predict anger-related attentional biases: A test of the alcohol myopia theory. *Psychology of Addictive Behaviors, 33*(2), 139–143. doi:10.1037/adb0000426

Mason, R. A., & O'Rinn, S. E. (2014). Co-occurring intimate partner violence, mental health, and substance use problems: A scoping review. *Global Health Action, 7*. doi:10.3402/gha.v7.24815

Mattson, R. E., Lofgreen, A. M., & O'Farrell, T. J. (2017). Dyadic alcohol use, alcohol-specific conflict, and relationship dissatisfaction in treatment-seeking men and their female partners. *Journal of Social and Personal Relationships, 34*(8), 1206–1226. doi:10.1177/0265407516670759

Mechanic, M. B., Weaver, T. L., & Resick, P. A. (2008). Mental health consequences of intimate partner abuse: A multidimensional assessment of four different forms of abuse. *Violence Against Women, 14*(6), 634–654. doi:10.1177/1077801208319283

Moore, T. M., Stuart, G. L., Meehan, J. C., Rhatigan, D. L., Hellmuth, J. C., & Keen, S. M. (2008). Drug abuse and aggression between intimate partners: A meta-analytic review. *Clinical Psychology Review, 28*(2), 247–274. doi:10.1016/j.cpr.2007.05.003

Murphy, C. M., Winters, J., O'Farrell, T. J., Fals-Stewart, W., & Murphy, M. (2005). Alcohol consumption and intimate partner violence by alcoholic men: Comparing violent and nonviolent conflicts. *Psychology of Addictive Behaviors, 19*(1), 35–42. doi:10.1037/0893-164X.19.1.35

Murray, C. E., & Graybeal, J. (2007). Methodological review of intimate partner violence prevention research. *Journal of Interpersonal Violence, 22*, 1250–1269. doi:10.1177/0886260507304293

O'Farrell, T. J., Murphy, C. M., Stephan, S. H., Fals-Stewart, W., & Murphy, M. (2004). Partner violence before and after couples-based alcoholism treatment for male alcoholic patients: The role of treatment involvement and abstinence. *Journal of Consulting and Clinical Psychology, 72*(2), 202–217. doi:10.1037/0022-006X.72.2.202

O'Leary, K. D., Barling, J., Arias, I., Rosenbaum, A., Malone, J., & Tyree, A. (1989). Prevalence and stability of physical aggression between spouses: A longitudinal analysis. *Journal of Consulting and Clinical Psychology, 57*(2), 263–268. doi:10.1037/0022-006X.57.2.263

Ostermann, J., Sloan, F. A., & Taylor, D. H. (2005). Heavy alcohol use and marital dissolution in the USA. *Social Science and Medicine, 61*, 2304–2316. doi:10.1016/j.socscimed.2005.07.021

Pedersen, W. C., Vasquez, E. A., Bartholow, B. D., Grosvenor, M., & Truong, A. (2014). Are you insulting me? Exposure to alcohol primes increases aggression following ambiguous provocation. *Personality and Social Psychology Bulletin, 40*, 1037–1049. doi:10.1177/0146167214534993

Quigley, B. M., & Leonard, K. E. (2006). Alcohol expectancies and intoxicated aggression. *Aggression and Violent Behavior, 11*, 484–496. doi:10.1016/j.avb.2006.01.008

Ramsay, J., Cater, Y., Davidson, L., Dunne, D., Eldridge, S., Feder, G., . . . Warburton, A. (2009). Advocacy interventions to reduce or eliminate violence and promote the physical and psychosocial well-being of women who experience intimate partner abuse (review). *Cochrane Database of Systematic Reviews, Article No. CD005043*(3). doi:10.1002/14651858.CD005043.pub2

Rhodes, K. V. (2012). Taking a fresh look at routine screening for intimate partner violence: What can we do about what we know? *Mayo Clinic Proceedings, 87*(5), 419–423. doi:10.1016/j.mayocp.2012.02.006

Romans, S., Forte, T., Cohen, M. M., Du Mont, J., & Hyman, I. (2007). Who is most at risk for intimate partner violence? A Canadian population-based study. *Journal of Interpersonal Violence, 22*(12), 1495–1514. doi:10.1177/0886260507306566

Schumacher, J. A., Homish, G. G., Leonard, K. E., Quigley, B. M., & Kearns-Bodkin, J. N. (2008). Longitudinal moderators of the relationship between excessive drinking and intimate partner violence in the early years of marriage. *Journal of Family Psychology, 22*(6), 894–904. doi:10.1037/a0013250

Schumacher, J. A., & Leonard, K. E. (2005). Husbands' and wives' marital adjustment, verbal aggression, and physical aggression as longitudinal predictors of physical aggression in early marriage. *Journal of Consulting and Clinical Psychology, 73*, 28–37. doi:10.1037/0022-006X.73.1.28

Smith, S. G., Zhang, X., Basile, K. C., Merrick, M. T., Wang, J., Kresnow, M., & Chen, J. (2018). *The national intimate partner and sexual violence survey (NISVS): 2015 data brief—Updated release.* Atlanta, GA: National Center for Injury Prevention and Control, Centers for Disease Control and Prevention.Steele, C. M., & Josephs, R. A. (1990). Alcohol myopia: Its prized and dangerous effects. *American Psychologist, 45*, 921–933. doi:10.1037/0003-066X.45.8.921

Stets, J. E. (1990). Verbal and physical aggression in marriage. *Journal of Marriage and the Family, 52*, 501–514. doi:10.2307/353043

Stets, J. E., & Straus, M. A. (1990). The marriage license as a hitting license: A comparison of assaults in dating, cohabiting, and married couples. In M. A., Straus & R. J. Gelles (Eds.), *Physical violence in American families: Risk factors and adaptations to violence in 8,145 families* (pp. 227–244). New Brunswick, NJ: Transaction Publishers. doi:10.4324/9781315126401-17

Stewart, D. E., Vigod, S., & Riazantseva, E. (2016). New developments in intimate partner violence and management of its mental health sequelae. *Current Psychiatry Reports, 18*(1). doi:10.1007/s11920-015-0644-3

Straus, M. A., Gelles, R. J., & Steinmetz, S. K. (1980). *Behind closed doors: Violence in the American family.* Garden City, NY: Anchor Press.

Sullivan, C. M., Bybee, D. I., & Allen, N. E. (2002). Findings from a community-based program for battered women and their children. *Journal of Interpersonal Violence, 17*(9), 915–936. doi:10.1177/0886260502017009001

Suvak, M. K., Taft, C. T., Goodman, L. A., & Dutton, M. A. (2013). Dimensions of functional social support and depressive symptoms: A longitudinal investigation of women seeking help for intimate partner violence. *Journal of Consulting and Clinical Psychology 81*(3), 455–466. doi:10.1037/a0031787

Taylor, S. P., & Leonard, K. E. (1983). Alcohol and human physical aggression. In R. Geen & E. I. Donnerstein (Eds.), *Aggression: Theoretical and empirical reviews* (pp.77–101). New York, NY: Academic Press.

Testa, M., & Derrick, J. L. (2014). A daily process examination of the temporal association between alcohol use and verbal and physical aggression in community couples. *Psychology of Addictive Behaviors, 28*(1), 127–138. doi:10.1037/a0032988

Testa, M., Wang, W. J., Derrick, J. L., & Leonard, K. E. (2018). Marijuana use by intimate partners: Does discrepant use impair relationship functioning? *Psychology of Addictive Behaviors, 32*(4), 475–484. doi:10.1037/adb0000357

Timko, C., Valenstein, H., Lin, P. Y., Moos, R. H., Stuart, G. L., & Cronkite, R. C. (2012). Addressing substance abuse and violence in substance use disorder treatment and batterer intervention programs. *Substance Abuse Treatment, Prevention, and Policy, 7*, 37. doi:10.1186/1747-597X-7-37

Tjaden, P., & Thoennes, N. (2000). *Full report of the prevalence, incidence, and consequences of violence against women: Findings from the national violence against women survey* (NCJ Publication No. 183781). Washington, DC: U.S Department of Justice. doi:10.1037/e514172006-001

Warshaw, C., Sullivan, C. M., & Rivera, E. A. (2013). *A systematic review of trauma-focused interventions for domestic violence survivors.* National Center on Domestic Violence, Trauma & Mental Health. Retrieved December 10, 2016 from http://www.nationalcenterdvtraumamh.org/wp, doi:10.1037/e566602013-001

Watkins, L. E., Maldonado, R. C., & DiLillo, D. (2014). Hazardous alcohol use and intimate partner aggression among dating couples: The role of impulse control difficulties. *Aggressive Behavior, 40*, 369–381. doi:10.1002/ab.21528

Wong, J. Y., Fong, D. Y., Lai, V., & Tiwari, A. (2014). Bridging intimate partner violence and the human brain: A literature review. *Trauma, Violence, & Abuse, 15*(1), 22–33. doi:10.1177/1524838013496333

World Health Organization. (2010). *Preventing intimate partner and sexual violence against women: Taking action and generating evidence.* Geneva, Switzerland/London, UK: World Health Organization/London School of Hygiene and Tropical Medicine.

35

Substance-involved sexual assault

Kelly Cue Davis, Mitchell Kirwan, Elizabeth C. Neilson
and Cynthia A. Stappenbeck

Background

Sexual assault is a worldwide, centuries-old problem. In recent decades, there has been a global resurgence of attention directed to sexual assault, which involves nonconsensual sexual activity ranging from unwanted sexual touching to rape. For example, the 1994 passage of the Violence Against Women Act (VAWA) in the United States resulted in sexual assault prevention and education efforts receiving increased federal funding. Originally passed in 1972, Title IX, a U.S. federal civil rights law, more recently has been revised to include sexual assault and sexual harassment as forms of sex discrimination prohibited in education. The application of this law to sexual assault was clarified in 2011 by the Obama administration; however, federal Title IX guidance pertaining to sexual assault is currently in a state of flux as new revisions have been proposed by the Trump administration (U.S. Department of Education, 2018). This increased U.S. legislative focus has occurred concomitantly with grassroots efforts to raise sexual assault awareness through social media efforts such as the #MeToo movement that have taken hold worldwide. Since the #MeToo movement went viral in October 2017, there has been an increase in funds available for victim legal assistance, surges in numbers of victims seeking support and services, and increased efforts to improve relevant cultural norms (Searles, 2018). Indeed, the #MeToo movement has become a global phenomenon involving almost every country in the world (Burke, 2018).

In this chapter, we review the research on sexual assault, with a specific focus on empirical evidence pertaining to associations between substance misuse (alcohol and other drugs) and sexual violence victimization and perpetration. We present research regarding the prevalence of alcohol and drug use during sexual assault events, characteristics of substance-involved assaults, the associations of substance misuse with both sexual assault perpetration and victimization, and prevention and intervention efforts targeting substance-involved sexual assaults. Research on substance-involved sexual assault primarily investigates the role of alcohol in assaults involving male perpetrators and female victims; thus, this is the chapter focus. Additionally, most research on substance-involved sexual assault pertains to assaults that occurred after age 14; thus, childhood sexual abuse is not covered in this chapter. Finally, both domestic research and international research on substance-involved sexual assault are presented where available.

Prevalence

Sexual assault occurs at alarming rates across the globe. The World Health Organization (WHO, 2012) reported that, among women aged 15–49 years, rates of sexual violence by intimate partners ranged from 6% to 59% across 15 settings in 10 countries. When considering non-partner sexual assaults, rates ranged from 0.3% to 12% (WHO, 2012). In Western countries, sexual victimization prevalence rates vary. For example, 36.3% of American women and 20.3% of women in England and Wales report lifetime sexual victimization (Office for National Statistics, 2018; Smith et al., 2017).

Although men do experience sexual violence victimization, women are exposed at much higher rates. The Centers for Disease Control (CDC; Smith et al., 2017) reported that one in three women and one in six men experienced contact sexual violence during their lifetime, with 23 million women and 1.7 million men experiencing rape over the course of their lives. Among female victims, the vast majority of perpetrators were men known to them (i.e. current or former intimate partners, acquaintances, etc.). Male victims are also most likely to have known their perpetrators, but perpetrator gender varied depending on the nature of the sexual assault. For example, male rape victims were most likely to have been raped by a man, while men who experienced sexual coercion were more likely to have a female perpetrator (Smith et al., 2017).

Regarding the prevalence of substance-involved sexual assault, research evidence consistently demonstrates widespread involvement of immoderate alcohol consumption in sexual assault, whereas fewer studies have examined the role of other drugs. Research demonstrates that at least 50% of sexual assaults involved alcohol consumption by the victim, perpetrator, or both (Abbey, Wegner, Woerner, Pegram, & Pierce, 2014). The CDC (Smith et al., 2017) reported that 9% of U.S. women experience alcohol or drug-involved rape over their lifetime.

The use of alcohol and drugs preceding or during sexual assaults varies widely in both the nature and the amount of consumption. For example, victims may become intoxicated or high due to a perpetrator deliberately giving them drugs or alcohol to facilitate sexual assault (alcohol/drug-facilitated sexual assault). Alternatively, a victim may have consumed alcohol or drugs voluntarily to the point of severe intoxication (incapacitated rape). Regardless of whether substances were consumed voluntarily or involuntarily, both types of sexual assault involve the victim being either unconscious or conscious but unable to consent (Kilpatrick, Resnick, Ruggiero, Conoscenti, & McCauley, 2007).

A nationally representative study of U.S. women aged 18–86 reported that 18% of participants experienced rape during their lifetimes; 2.2% reported alcohol-facilitated rape, 0.5% reported drug-facilitated rape, 2.8% reported incapacitated rape due to alcohol, and 0.7% reported incapacitated rape due to drugs (Kilpatrick et al., 2007). Similarly, a U.S. national sample of college women reported that most incapacitated (76%) and alcohol/drug-facilitated rapes (72%) involved alcohol, 25% of both incapacitated and alcohol/drug-facilitated rapes involved drugs and alcohol, and 3% of incapacitated and 7% of alcohol/drug-facilitated rapes involved drugs only, with marijuana being the most commonly reported drug (McCauley et al., 2009). Because alcohol is the substance most commonly involved in sexual assaults, most research has specifically focused on the role of alcohol in these events. The present review reflects this state of the research—primarily focusing on the relationship between alcohol and sexual assault.

Characteristics of alcohol-involved assaults

Victim-perpetrator relationship

Alcohol-involved sexual assault typically occurs among acquaintances (Abbey et al., 2002; Testa & Livingston, 2009), and acquaintance sexual assault is more likely to involve drinking than sexual assault among intimate partners (Davis, Danube, Stappenbeck, Norris, & George, 2015). Acquaintance assaults are especially prevalent on college campuses (Lorenz & Ullman, 2016) where most penetrative assaults occur while "hooking up," in which a woman consents to one casual sexual activity (e.g. kissing), but is later pressured or forced into additional non-consensual activities (Flack et al., 2007). Furthermore, hooking up with an acquaintance is more likely to lead to a sexual assault than hooking up with a stranger, and sexual assaults occur more commonly in hookups following heavy drinking (Tyler, Schmitz, & Adams, 2017).

Although most studies show that drinking is less common during sexual assaults perpetrated within intimate relationships, one recent study reported that heavy drinking contributed more to sexual assault perpetration among intimate partners than among casual partners (Pegram et al., 2018), indicating that alcohol is also an important factor in relationship violence. Notably, an international study by the WHO reported that heavy drinking by one or both partners increased the likelihood of sexual assault perpetration within an intimate relationship (Abramsky et al., 2011). This assertion is supported by a meta-analysis which concluded that women who drink heavily or have an alcohol use disorder are at increased risk of being sexually assaulted by their intimate partner (Devries et al., 2014). However, because these findings are both correlational and inconsistent, more research is needed to better understand the nuances of alcohol-involved sexual assaults perpetrated by casual and intimate partners.

Setting

Most alcohol-involved sexual assaults occur in the context of bars or parties, especially assaults involving college students hooking up (Abbey et al., 2002; Flack et al., 2007). Indeed, a recent longitudinal study of college men demonstrated that frequenting drinking venues such as bars and parties was predictive of greater sexual assault perpetration (Cleveland, Testa, & Hone, 2019). In such drinking-related social contexts, multiple potential perpetrators are often present, and perpetrators are more likely to take advantage of an intoxicated woman whose judgment and awareness are impaired than of a sober woman (Flack et al., 2007; Lorenz & Ullman, 2016; Testa & Livingston, 2009). Frequently, these assaults either begin as consensual hookups, which escalate to nonconsensual sexual activities, or involve a perpetrator taking advantage of an incapacitated victim unable to consent to sexual activity (Testa & Livingston, 2009). For instance, an analysis of 232 male-to-female sexual aggression incidents in Canadian bars reported that 61% involved unwanted physical contact, 57% involved persistent advances after the target refused, 18% involved sexually suggestive or threatening acts, and 9% involved sexual harassment (Graham et al., 2014). Similarly, social norms in South African bar culture encourage men to drink heavily, sexually objectify women, target intoxicated women for sexual assault, engage in transactional sex (i.e. expecting a woman to have sex if he buys her drinks), and support rape myths (Letsela, Weiner, Gafos, & Fritz, 2019; Rich, Nkosi, & Morojele, 2015). In contrast, sexual assaults perpetrated by intimate partners are more likely to occur in the home and involve drinking by the perpetrator only (Abbey et al., 2002). However, further research examining sexual assault among intimate partners is needed to establish more information about the setting of these assaults.

Level of force

Alcohol-involved sexual assaults usually involve greater physical force than assaults not involving alcohol (Kirwan, Parkhill, Schuetz, & Cox, 2016). Similarly, consuming more alcohol is associated with using greater physical force during sexual assaults and perpetrating more severe forms of sexual assault (Kingree & Thompson, 2015). Thus, alcohol-involved sexual assaults often have more severe outcomes than those in which both parties are sober.

Perpetration of alcohol-involved sexual assault

Perpetrator characteristics

Perpetrators of alcohol-involved assaults are more likely to hold negative stereotypes about women who drink, misperceive a woman's sexual intentions, drink in sexual situations, be impulsive, hold sexually dominant attitudes, hold positive attitudes about casual sex, and possess more sex-related alcohol expectancies (i.e. beliefs about how they think alcohol will affect their behaviors), compared to sober perpetrators (Pegram et al., 2018). In laboratory simulations, intoxicated perpetrators provided women with more alcohol and perceived them as being more intoxicated relative to sober perpetrators (Pegram et al., 2018). In contrast, research assessing men who perpetrate sexual assault both with and without alcohol reported that during alcohol-involved assaults, perpetrators had more positive emotions toward their victim, were more attracted to her, had more cognitions about having sex with her, and used more isolating and controlling behaviors to ensure that they were able to assault her than during their sober assaults (Kirwan et al., 2016).

Consistency of perpetrators' alcohol use during perpetration

Most sexual assault perpetrators (61–70%) have perpetrated at least one alcohol-involved assault, and for 17%, all their assaults involved alcohol. Furthermore, 56% of all acts of forced sexual contact were perpetrated following drinking, along with 56% of all instances of verbal coercion, 88% of all incapacitated rapes, 48% of all attempted rapes, and 53% of all completed rapes (Davis et al., 2012; Kirwan et al., 2016). Additionally, alcohol-involved sexual assault perpetrators consumed an average of eight drinks and had an estimated average peak blood alcohol concentration of 0.07% when they perpetrate the assault (Davis et al., 2015). As noted, although the severity of a sexual assault usually increased as perpetrator alcohol consumption increased (Kingree & Thompson, 2015), this may not be true when high levels of intoxication are reached (Brecklin & Ullman, 2001).

Cognitive impairment and misperceptions of sexual intentions

Cognitive impairments associated with acute alcohol intoxication are well documented. These include slowed information processing, reduced multitasking ability, decreased inhibitory control, increased impulsivity, impaired decision-making, increased distractibility, reduced attentional control, and increases in inappropriate behaviors (Fillmore, 2007). Within the context of sexual assault, a meta-analysis of studies examining male-to-female sexual assault perpetration revealed that acute alcohol intoxication caused increases in general, sexual, and intimate partner aggression (Crane, Godleski, Przybyla, Schlauch, & Testa, 2016). This increase in aggression is partially explained by alcohol myopia theory, which states that cognitive impairments associated with alcohol intoxication result in a perpetrator becoming more focused on personally salient cues (e.g. his desire to have sex) than on other salient cues (e.g. a woman's resistance to his advances; Steele & Josephs, 1990). This may lead intoxicated men to misperceive a woman's friendliness as sexual interest, increasing his likelihood of pursuing sex with her, or even sexually assaulting her (Abbey, Jacques-Tiura, & LeBreton, 2011). Similarly, alcohol expectancies may affect alcohol-involved sexual assaults, in that intoxicated men with stronger alcohol expectancies regarding aggression report more motivations and emotions related to sexual aggression than intoxicated men with weaker aggression-related alcohol expectancies (Davis, 2010).

Emotion regulation and impulse control difficulties

Emotion regulation, or the processes which influence what, when, and how individuals experience emotions, may also play a role in sexual assault perpetration (Kirwan, Lanni, Warnke, Pickett, & Parkhill, 2018; Shorey, Brasfield, Febres, & Stuart, 2011), especially following alcohol use, which exacerbates emotion regulation difficulties due to impairment of cognitive processes (Dvorak et al., 2014). For example, emotion regulation difficulties moderate the relationship between drinking and sexual assault perpetration, such that individuals who frequently drink heavily and have greater emotion regulation difficulties are more likely to perpetrate sexual assault than those who have fewer emotion regulation difficulties or who do not often drink heavily—possibly because these individuals are less able to properly regulate a strong, negative emotion, like anger, when they are intoxicated (Kirwan et al., 2018).

Alcohol may interact with emotion regulation to increase an individual's likelihood of perpetrating sexual aggression through its effect on impulse control, a component of emotion regulation (Gratz & Roemer, 2004). Impulse control difficulties are associated with both aggression and violence against women (Gildner, Kirwan, Pickett, & Parkhill, 2018), as well as sexual assault perpetration (Abbey et al., 2011; Kirwan et al., 2018; Shorey et al., 2011). This likely occurs because the cognitive effects of alcohol cause a reduction in self-control, especially among men (Fillmore & Weafer, 2004). Thus, heavy drinking may increase impulse control difficulties, which subsequently increases the risk of sexual assault perpetration by individuals who would not perpetrate when sober due to recognizing legal, social, or moral repercussions of their actions (Abbey, 2002).

Sexual arousal

Sexual arousal increases sexual assault perpetration, in that sexually aroused men are more likely to perpetrate than men who are not sexually aroused (Ariely & Loewenstein, 2006). Furthermore, due to the myopic effects of alcohol, intoxication can lead individuals to focus more strongly on their sexual arousal, pursue sex when less salient cues suggest that they should stop, project their own arousal onto a woman, and ignore cues indicating that she does not want to have sex (Gross, Bennett, Sloan, Marx, & Juergens, 2001; Steele & Josephs, 1990). Additionally, sexual arousal also increases one's desire to drink, which further increases the alcohol myopia effect, and leads to situations which foster sexual arousal, creating a cycle culminating in both high intoxication and high sexual arousal (Spelman & Simons, 2018). These situations are especially problematic because drinking and sexual arousal each independently increases the risk of sexual assault perpetration.

Alcohol-involved sexual assault victimization

Victim drinking factors

Frequent, heavy drinking has been consistently associated with increased risk for sexual assault generally (Lorenz & Ullman, 2016), and alcohol-related sexual assault specifically (Testa & Livingston, 2018). This association may be partly explained by routine activities and lifestyle theories, which posit that exposure to risk factors in drinking-related social contexts increases one's risk for sexual assault (see, Settings; Mustaine & Tewksbury, 2002). Additionally, alcohol expectancies may help explain the link between heavy drinking and sexual assault victimization. For instance, women who drink heavily and experienced sexual assault (Corbin, Bernat, Calhoun, McNair, & Seals, 2001) and alcohol-involved sexual assaults (Bedard-Gilligan, Kaysen, Desai, & Lee, 2011) held greater positive alcohol expectancies, including enhanced tension-reduction, sociability, liquid courage, and sexuality. However, these observations were based on cross-sectional studies, meaning it is unknown whether alcohol expectancies served as risk factors for or consequences of sexual assault.

Victim intoxication during sexual assault

Being intoxicated can impair a victim's ability to mitigate or thwart an attempted sexual assault. Compared to sober victims, intoxicated victims are less likely to perceive sexual assault risk indicators, perhaps due to cognitive impairment and alcohol myopia processes (Melkonian & Ham, 2018). Intoxicated victims are also less likely to forcefully resist and more likely to respond passively to an assault (Davis, George, & Norris, 2004). This lowered resistance may be due to uncertainty and conflict about how to respond and greater self-blame for the assault (Norris, Zawacki, Davis, & George, 2018). Finally, these concerns only apply to situations in which a victim is impaired but not completely incapacitated. In situations of incapacitation (i.e. passed out), victim risk perception and resistance become impossible.

Sequelae of alcohol-involved sexual assault

Sexual assault is associated with significant personal and societal costs. Following a sexual assault, women are significantly more likely to abuse alcohol or other drugs (Kilpatrick, Acierno, Resnick, Saunders, & Best, 1997). Among college women, a history of sexual assault is associated with poor academic performance, dropout, and transfer from the university (Baker et al., 2016). More generally, a history of sexual assault, particularly alcohol-involved assault, is associated with poor psychological functioning, including post-traumatic stress disorder (PTSD), depression, obsessive-compulsive disorder (OCD), disordered eating, and suicidality (Dworkin, in press; Dworkin, Menon, Bystrynski, & Allen, 2017; Peter-Hagene & Ullman, 2015); physical health problems (Stein & Barrett-Connor, 2000); and problems with sexual and relationship functioning (Kelley & Gidycz, 2017; Neilson, Norris, Bryan, & Stappenbeck, 2017). Additionally, the economic burden of sexual assault in the United States is substantial: the estimated lifetime cost per rape victim is $122,278, which includes costs associated with medical care and lost productivity (Peterson, DeGue, Florence, & Lokey, 2017).

Up to 80% of women disclose their sexual assault experience either formally (e.g. police, health care provider, counselor) or informally (e.g. friends, relatives; Lorenz & Ullman, 2016). Disclosures most often are made to peers, with fewer women indicating that they made a formal sexual assault disclosure (Ullman, 1996). Victims who consumed alcohol before the assault were less likely to acknowledge it as an assault compared to victims who were sober (Littleton, Grills-Taquechel, & Axsom, 2009). This is consistent with a low level of formal support seeking following sexual assault: only 7% of sexual assault survivors sought mental health care (Ullman, 1996), and only 5–10% sought rape crisis center services (Golding, Siegel, Sorenson, Burnam, & Stein, 1989). Victims' alcohol use at the time of assault was associated with greater disclosure (Lorenz & Ullman, 2016); however, that may be due to increased informal disclosure and less formal disclosure (Littleton, Grills-Taquechel, & Axsom, 2009).

Despite a majority of women disclosing their sexual assaults, many survivors report that their disclosure experiences were hurtful (Campbell, Wasco, Ahrens, Sefl, & Barnes, 2001), and 20% regretted their disclosure (Jacques-Tiura, Tkatch, Abbey, & Wegner, 2010). Victim intoxication during the assault was associated with increased self-blame (Koss, Figueredo, & Prince, 2002; Peter-Hagene & Ullman, 2018), perhaps because they believe being intoxicated facilitated the assault or because of others' perceptions regarding their alcohol use. Women who were intoxicated during the assault were more likely to be perceived as less credible and more blameworthy than victims who were not drinking (Sims, Noel, & Maisto, 2007). These perceptions may help explain why victims who were drinking at the time of the assault received more negative reactions following disclosure, including blame and disbelief, than victims who were not drinking (Ullman & Najdowski, 2011). Perhaps not surprisingly, victims who blame themselves generally report poorer post-assault functioning (Koss et al., 2002; Peter-Hagene & Ullman, 2015).

The theoretical and empirical literature suggests that sexual assault during childhood interferes with the development of adaptive emotion regulation strategies (Ford, 2017). Childhood sexual assault survivors may not learn how to effectively regulate their emotional arousal and tolerate emotional distress and may easily exhibit high-intensity emotional reactions that continue into adulthood (Cloitre, Miranda, Stovall-McClough, & Han, 2005). Moreover, emotion regulation difficulties can result from sexual assault experienced in adulthood, as these experiences often lead to strong feelings of fear and physiological arousal that may be difficult to regulate (Marx, Heidt, & Gold, 2005).

Sexual assault may be linked to heavy drinking as a result of emotion regulation difficulties. The self-medication hypothesis (Khantzian, 2003) asserts that alcohol consumption reduces the experience of distress in the short-term, which increases a person's likelihood of using alcohol in the future to manage distress. Women with sexual assault histories may consume alcohol in part to regulate emotional distress and cope with negative affective states (Miranda, Meyerson, Long, Marx, & Simpson, 2002). However, this pattern of drinking to cope eventually interferes with recovery following trauma and can result in continued heavy drinking (Kaysen et al., 2007) and development of alcohol use disorders (Fossos, Kaysen, Neighbors, Lindgren, & Hove, 2011). Thus, emotion regulation difficulties may lead to increased motivation to drink to cope with distress and heavy alcohol use for women who have experienced sexual assault (Lindgren, Neighbors, Blayney, Mullins, & Kaysen, 2012), increasing women's risk for revictimization (Messman-Moore, Ward, Zerubavel, Chandley, & Barton, 2015).

Sexual assault interventions

The propensity for sexual assault to occur within the context of alcohol intoxication calls for interventions focused on alcohol-related sexual assault (Orchowski, Barnett et al., 2018; Testa & Livingston, 2009). Such interventions are less common than general sexual assault interventions; however, they include building awareness of alcohol's role in increasing vulnerability to experiencing or perpetrating sexual violence and decreasing alcohol use as a means of intervention. Sexual assault prevention programming should utilize an integrative approach that increases awareness, acknowledges barriers to change, and increases action through skills practice (Orchowski, Edwards et al., 2018). Historically, however, risk reduction and perpetration prevention interventions have been delivered as separate interventions (for review, Orchowski, Edwards et al., 2018). Recently, college campuses have established initiatives to address sexual assault perpetration and victimization, change the culture regarding consent, and share resources (HECAOD, 2019; Thomas, Sorenson, & Joshi, 2016). Further, violence and HIV prevention and intervention programs implemented in communities in South Africa, Zimbabwe, and Uganda have utilized a gender transformative approach with both women and men, such that these approaches address expectations about male and female roles and behavior through reflection, discussion, and practice (Ellsberg et al., 2015).

Risk reduction interventions

Risk reduction programs aim to decrease women's vulnerability to sexual victimization by altering behaviors that enhance their risk. These programs primarily draw from the cognitive ecological model, describing the psychological and environmental factors that contribute to women's responses to sexual assault (Nurius & Norris, 1996) while incorporating situational awareness and self-defense strategies (for review, see Orchowski, Edwards et al., 2018). The foundation of these programs is not to place the responsibility of sexual violence on women but empower them with knowledge and skills to decrease their susceptibility to sexual violence. Contemporary sexual assault risk resistance programs utilize the "Assess, Acknowledge, Act" model of rape resistance (Rozee & Koss, 2001) to increase awareness of the frequency of sexual assault, improve one's ability to perceive and acknowledge a risky situation, teach a continuum of resistance strategies, often called protective behavioral strategies (PBS), to respond to varying levels of risk, and address barriers to resistance strategies. Some of these programs expand the PBS women may already employ to reduce their sexual assault vulnerability, such as walking home with a trusted friend (Moore & Waterman, 1999).

Sexual assault risk reduction programs using a gender transformative approach also include protective behavior strategies within programs while also fostering community mobilization to fight cultural factors that promote or maintain violence against women, such as economic inequality. Prevention programs such as the IMAGE study, *Empowerment and Livelihood for Adolescents*, the *SHAZ!* program, and *Stepping Stones and Creating Futures*, integrate skills to reduce vulnerability to sexual and/or physical intimate partner violence (IPV) and HIV, with microfinance and economic attainment programming, and are associated with decreased sexual and/or physical IPV victimization at follow-up (Bandiera et al., 2012; Dunbar et al., 2014; Jewkes et al., 2014; Pronyk et al., 2006).

Sexual assault risk-reduction programs vary in the degree of inclusion of knowledge about alcohol in the program, with some including psychoeducation regarding alcohol consumption as a sexual assault risk factor (Senn et al., 2015). Alcohol-focused sexual assault risk reduction programs integrate education regarding alcohol and alcohol-involved sexual assault and provide PBS to resist sexual assault and reduce alcohol use, strategies such as identifying a designated friend who does not drink when a group of friends is out for the evening, alternating alcoholic and nonalcoholic beverages, and not attempting to outdrink others (Gilmore, Lewis, & George, 2015; Sell, Turrisi, Scaglione, Cleveland, & Mallett, 2018). Randomized controlled trials of alcohol-focused risk reduction programs indicate that women who receive them report lower sexual victimization at follow-up than women who do not (Senn et al., 2015, 2017; Gilmore et al., 2015). Notably, women at high risk for victimization, such as those with prior sexual victimization, those who drink heavily, those who drink in sexualized drinking contexts (e.g. parties, bars), and/or those who drink to cope, benefit from alcohol-focused risk reduction programs (Gilmore et al., 2015; Gilmore & Bountress, 2016; Senn et al., 2015).

Perpetration prevention programs

The vast majority of interventions have focused on reducing women's vulnerability to assault, with fewer evidence-based interventions focused on decreasing men's perpetration (DeGue et al., 2014). Less than one-third of existing sexual assault prevention programming is directed to male audiences (DeGue et al., 2014). Currently two programs implemented in the United States, *Safe Dates* (Foshee et al., 2005) and *Shifting Boundaries* (Taylor, Stein, Mumford, & Woods, 2013), an anti-sexual coercion program in Spain (Fuertes Martín, Orgaz Baz, Vicario-Molina, Martínez Alvarez, Fernández Fuertes, & Carcedo González, 2012), and a gender transformative prevention program in South Africa, *Stepping Stones* (Jewkes et al., 2008), have demonstrated efficacy in decreasing the perpetration of sexual violence. Furthermore, even fewer explicitly target the role of alcohol as a risk factor for perpetration (for review, Orchowski, Edwards et al., 2018).

Sexual assault perpetration prevention programs are diverse in their foci. Different components include building victim empathy and awareness of sexual assault, correcting misperceptions of the acceptability and frequency of sexual assault, challenging men's socialization to traditional masculine norms, and increasing victims' use of strategies to intervene in sexual assault (for review, Orchowski, Barnett et al., 2018). Some programs, primarily implemented within college-aged samples in the United States, draw from literature that suggests sexually aggressive men underestimate their peers' prosocial attitudes and behaviors and overestimate their peers' conformity to hypermasculine attitudes and behaviors (Gidycz, Orchowski, & Berkowitz, 2011). After assessing men's attitudes and beliefs, these programs provide feedback regarding the frequency and acceptability of sexual assault while challenging adherence to traditional gender norms. Prevention programs may provide skill-building exercises for anger management, negotiating consent, and communication strategies (Choate, 2003; O'Donohue, Yeater, & Fantetti, 2003). Programs also seek to increase men's ability to identify and intervene in sexual assault as bystanders (Salazar, Vivolo-Kantor, Hardin, & Berkowitz, 2014).

The bulk of prevention programs typically include universal interventions, in which all group members receive the same intervention, such as through social marketing campaigns or during college orientations (Potter, 2012). Universal sexual assault prevention programs directed at middle- and high-school students have demonstrated the greatest effect within the United States and Spain (Foshee et al., 2005; Taylor et al., 2013; Fuertes Martín, Baz, Vicario-Molina, Álvarez, Fuertes, & González, 2012). These programs emphasize building healthy relationships, the social construction of gender roles, and the consequences of dating violence and sexual harassment. A gender transformative approach with male and female adolescents and young adults in rural areas of South Africa has also demonstrated efficacy in reducing sexual and/or physical IPV perpetration at a two-year follow-up (*Stepping Stones*; Jewkes et al., 2008). This program emphasizes violence against women and sexual health, gender roles, and peer influences. The *Stepping Stones* program has been expanded and amended to include curriculum to improve economic attainment; however, pilot testing has not demonstrated a decrease in sexual IPV perpetration by men (*Stepping Stones and Creating Futures*; Jewkes et al., 2014). Of these programs, three included discussion of alcohol (Fuertes Martín et al., 2012; Jewkes et al., 2008, 2014), suggesting an ongoing need to develop and evaluate universal interventions integrating alcohol and sexual assault.

Men at high risk for perpetrating sexual assault, such as those who drink heavily or have previously perpetrated sexual assault, do not typically respond to universal interventions (Malamuth, Huppin, & Linz, 2018). Because men who have perpetrated sexual assault in the past are more likely to overuse alcohol and may be particularly defensive in sexual assault interventions, it is recommended that researchers develop and evaluate programs that directly focus on alcohol to more effectively address men's perpetration (Orchowski, Barnett et al., 2018). Integrated alcohol and sexual assault prevention programs have demonstrated feasibility, although their effectiveness has yet to be assessed (Orchowski, Barnett et al., 2018).

Conclusions

Despite the recent social and political gains regarding sexual assault awareness and changing social norms, continued and increased efforts are needed to maintain and capitalize on these advances. Greater research attention to drug-involved sexual assaults globally and alcohol-involved sexual assaults in non-Western countries is needed to advance the field. Moreover, research acknowledging diversity in sexual assault events by moving beyond a singular focus on male perpetrators and female victims is critically warranted. Additionally, although a few risk reduction and perpetration prevention programs have demonstrated promise, increased research is critical for developing evidence-based programs effective at reducing the occurrence of substance-involved sexual assault. Moving beyond research, social workers are well-poised to engage in sexual assault prevention and response efforts that are critical to reducing the incidence and impact of sexual assault. Through clinical practices that support survivors in their recovery and advocacy work that demands policies and legislation which challenge violence-supportive cultural norms, social workers can play an important role in global efforts to abolish sexual violence.

References

Abbey, A. (2002). Alcohol-related sexual assault: A common problem among college students. *Journal of Studies on Alcohol Supplement,* (14), 118–128. doi:10.15288/jsas.2002.s14.118

Abbey, A., Jacques-Tiura, A. J., & LeBreton, J. M. (2011). Risk factors for sexual aggression in young men: An expansion of the confluence model. *Aggressive Behavior, 37*(5), 450–464. doi:10.1002/ab.20399

Abbey, A., Wegner, R., Woerner, J., Pegram, S. E., & Pierce, J. (2014). Review of survey and experimental research that examines the relationship between alcohol consumption and men's sexual aggression perpetration. *Trauma, Violence & Abuse, 15*(4), 265–282. doi:10.1177/1524838014521031

Abbey, A., Zawacki, T., Buck, P. O., Testa, M., Parks, K., Norris, J., . . . Martell, J. (2002). How does alcohol contribute to sexual assault? Explanations from laboratory and survey data. *Alcoholism: Clinical and Experimental Research, 26*(4), 575–581. doi:10.1111/j.1530-0277.2002.tb02576.x

Abramsky, T., Watts, C. H., Garcia-Moreno, C., Devries, K., Kiss, L., Ellsberg, M., . . . Heise, L. (2011). What factors are associated with recent intimate partner violence? Findings from the

WHO multi-country study on women's health and domestic violence. *BMC Public Health, 11*, 109. doi:10.1186/1471-2458-11-109

Ariely, D., & Loewenstein, G. (2006). The heat of the moment: The effect of sexual arousal on sexual decision making. *Journal of Behavioral Decision Making, 19*(2), 87–98. doi:10.1002/bdm.501

Baker, M. R., Frazier, P. A., Greer, C., Paulsen, J. A., Howard, K., Meredith, L. N., . . . Shallcross, S. L. (2016). Sexual victimization history predicts academic performance in college women. *Journal of Counseling Psychology, 63*, 685–692. doi:10.1037/cou0000146

Bandiera, O., Buehren, N., Burgess, R., Goldstein, M., Gulesci, S., Rasul, I., & Sulaiman, M. (2012). *Empowering adolescent girls: Evidence from a randomized control trial in Uganda.* World Bank. doi:10.1596/25529

Bedard-Gilligan, M., Kaysen, D., Desai, S., & Lee, C. M. (2011). Alcohol-involved assault: Associations with posttrauma alcohol use, consequences, and expectancies. *Addictive Behaviors, 36*(11), 1076–1082. doi:10.1016/j.addbeh.2011.07.001

Brecklin, L. R., & Ullman, S. E. (2001). The role of offender alcohol use in rape attacks: An analysis of national crime victimization survey data. *Journal of Interpersonal Violence, 16*(1), 3–21. doi:10.1177/088626001016001001

Burke, L. (2018). *The #MeToo shockwave: How the movement has reverberated around the world.* Retrieved from https://www.telegraph.co.uk/news/world/metoo-shockwave/ (Accessed on February 3, 2019).

Campbell, R., Wasco, S. M., Ahrens, C. E., Sefl, T., & Barnes, H. E. (2001). Preventing the "second rape": Rape survivors' experiences with community service providers. *Journal of Interpersonal Violence, 16*, 1239–1259.

Choate, L. H. (2003). Sexual assault prevention programs for college men: An exploratory evaluation of the men against violence model. *Journal of College Counseling, 6*, 166–176. doi:10.1002/j.2161-1882.2003.tb00237.x

Cleveland, M. J., Testa. M., & Hone, L. S. (2019). Examining the roles of heavy episodic drinking, drinking venues, and sociosexuality in college men's sexual aggression. *Journal of Studies on Alcohol and Drugs, 80*, 177–185. doi:10.15288/jsad.2019.80.177

Cloitre, M., Miranda, R., Stovall-McClough, C., & Han, H. (2005). Beyond PTSD: Emotion regulation and interpersonal problems as predictors of functional impairment in survivors of childhood abuse. *Behavior Therapy, 36*, 119–124. doi:10.1016/S0005-7894(05)80060-7

Corbin, W. R., Bernat, J. A., Calhoun, K. S., McNair, L. D., & Seals, K. L. (2001). The role of alcohol expectancies and alcohol consumption among sexually victimized and nonvictimized college women. *Journal of Interpersonal Violence, 16*(4), 297–311. doi:10.1177/088626001016004002

Crane, C. A., Godleski, S. A., Przybyla, S. M., Schlauch, R. C., & Testa, M. (2016). The proximal effects of acute alcohol consumption on male-to-female aggression: A meta-analytic review of the experimental literature. *Trauma, Violence & Abuse, 17*(5), 520–531. doi:10.1177/1524838015584374

Davis, K. C. (2010). The influence of alcohol expectancies and intoxication on men's aggressive unprotected sexual intentions. *Experimental and Clinical Psychopharmacology, 18*(5), 418–428. doi:10.1037/a0020510

Davis, K. C., Danube, C. L., Stappenbeck, C. A., Norris, J., & George, W. H. (2015). Background predictors and event-specific characteristics of sexual aggression incidents: The roles of alcohol and other factors. *Violence against Women, 21*(8), 997–1017. doi:10.1177/1077801215589379

Davis, K. C., Kiekel, P. A., Schraufnagel, T. J., Norris, J., George, W. H., & Kajumulo, K. F. (2012). Men's alcohol intoxication and condom use during sexual assault perpetration. *Journal of Interpersonal Violence, 27*(14), 2790–2806. doi:10.1177/0886260512438277

Davis, K. C., George, W. H., & Norris, J. (2004). Women's responses to unwanted sexual advances: The role of alcohol and inhibition conflict. *Psychology of Women Quarterly, 28*(4), 333–343. doi:10.1111/j.1471-6402.2004.00150.x

DeGue, S., Valle, L. A., Holt, M. K., Massetti, G. M., Matjasko, J. L., & Tharp, A. T. (2014). A systematic review of primary prevention strategies for sexual violence perpetration. *Aggression and Violent Behavior, 19*, 346–362. doi:10.1016/j.avb.2014.05.004

Devries, K. M., Child, J. C., Bacchus, L. J., Mak, J., Falder, G., Graham, K., . . . Heise, L. (2014). Intimate partner violence victimization and alcohol consumption in women: A systematic review and meta-analysis. *Addiction, 109*(3), 379–391. doi:10.1111/add.12393

Dunbar, M. S., Kang Dufour, M. S., Lambdin, B., Mudekunye-Mahaka, I., Nhamo, D., & Padian, N. S. (2014). The SHAZ! project: Results from a pilot randomized trial of a structural intervention to prevent HIV among adolescent women in Zimbabwe. *PloS One, 9*(11), e113621. doi:10.1371/journal.pone.0113621

Dvorak, R. D., Sargent, E. M., Kilwein, T. M., Stevenson, B. L., Kuvaas, N. J., & Williams, T. J. (2014). Alcohol use and alcohol-related consequences: Associations with emotion regulation difficulties. *American Journal of Drug and Alcohol Abuse, 40*(2), 125–130. doi:10.3109/00952990.2013.877920

Dworkin, E. R. (in press). Risk for mental disorders associated with sexual assault: A meta-analysis. *Trauma, Violence, and Abuse.* doi: 10.1177/1524838018813198

Dworkin, E. R., Menon, S. V., Bystrynski, J., & Allen, N. E. (2017). Sexual assault victimization and psychopathology: A review and meta-analysis. *Clinical Psychology Review, 56,* 65–81. https://doi.org/10.1016/j.cpr.2017.06.002

Ellsberg, M., Arango, D. J., Morton, M., Gennari, F., Kiplesund, S., Contreras, M., & Watts, C. (2015). Prevention of violence against women and girls: What does the evidence say?. *The Lancet, 385*(9977), 1555–1566. doi:10.1016/S0140-6736(14)61703-7

Fillmore, M. T. (2007). Acute alcohol-induced impairment of cognitive functions: Past and present findings. *International Journal on Disability and Human Development, 6*(2), 115–125. doi:10.1515/IJDHD.2007.6.2.115

Fillmore, M. T., & Weafer, J. (2004). Alcohol impairment of behavior in men and women. *Addiction, 99*(10), 1237–1246. doi:10.1111/j.1360-0443.2004.00805.x

Flack, W. F., Jr., Daubman, K. A., Caron, M. L., Asadorian, J. A., D'Aureli, N. R., Gigliotti, S. N., . . . Stine, E. R. (2007). Risk factors and consequences of unwanted sex among university students: Hooking up, alcohol, and stress response. *Journal of Interpersonal Violence, 22*(2), 139–157. doi:10.1177/0886260506295354

Ford, J. D. (2017). Treatment implications of altered affect regulation and information processing following child maltreatment. *Psychiatric Annals, 35*(5), 410–419. doi:10.3928/00485713-20050501-07

Foshee, V. A., Bauman, K. E., Ennett, S. T., Suchindran, C., Benefield, T., & Linder, G. F. (2005). Assessing the effects of the dating violence prevention program "safe dates" using random coefficient regression modeling. *Prevention Science, 6*(3), 245–258. doi:10.1007/s11121-005-0007-0

Fossos, N., Kaysen, D., Neighbors, C., Lindgren, K. P., & Hove, C. M. (2011). Coping motives and a mediator of the relationship between sexual coercion and problem drinking in college students. *Addictive Behaviors, 36,* 1001–1007. doi:10.1016/j.addbeh.2011.06.001

Fuertes Martín, A., Orgaz Baz, M. B, Vicario-Molina, I., Martínez Alvarez, J. L, Fernández Fuertes, A., & Carcedo González, R. J. (2012). Assessment of a sexual coercion prevention program for adolescents. *The Spanish Journal of Psychology, 15*(2), 560–570. doi:10.5209/rev_SJOP.2012.v15.n2.38867

Gidycz, C. A., Orchowski, L. M., & Berkowitz, A. D. (2011). Preventing sexual aggression among college men: An evaluation of a social norms and bystander intervention program. *Violence Against Women, 17,* 720–742. doi:10.1177/1077801211409727

Gildner, D. J., Kirwan, M., Pickett, S. M., & Parkhill, M. R. (2018). Impulse control difficulties and hostility toward women as predictors of relationship violence perpetration in an undergraduate male sample. *Journal of Interpersonal Violence,* Advance online publication. doi:10.1177/0886260518792972

Gilmore, A. K., & Bountress, K. E. (2016). Reducing drinking to cope among heavy episodic drinking college women: Secondary outcomes of a web-based combined alcohol use and sexual assault risk reduction intervention. *Addictive Behaviors, 61,* 104–111. doi:10.1016/j.addbeh.2016.05.007

Gilmore, A. K., Lewis, M. A., & George, W. H. (2015). A randomized controlled trial targeting alcohol use and sexual assault risk among college women at high risk for victimization. *Behaviour Research and Therapy, 74,* 38–49. doi: 10.1016/j.brat.2015.08.007

Golding, J. M., Siegel, J. M., Sorenson, S. B., Burnam, M. A., & Stein, J. A. (1989). Social support sources following sexual assault. *Journal of Community Psychology, 17*(1), 92-107.Graham, K., Bernards, S., Wayne Osgood, D., Abbey, A., Parks, M., Flynn, A., . . . Wells, S. (2014). "Blurred lines?" Sexual aggression and barroom culture. *Alcoholism: Clinical and Experimental Research, 38*(5), 1416–1424. doi:10.1111/acer.12356

Gratz, K. L., & Roemer, L. (2004). Multidimensional assessment of emotion regulation and dysregulation: Development, factor structure, and initial validation of the difficulties in emotion regulation scale. *Journal of Psychopathology and Behavioral Assessment, 26*(1), 41–54. doi:10.1023/B:JOBA.0000007455.08539.94

Gross, A. M., Bennett, T., Sloan, L., Marx, B. P., & Juergens, J. (2001). The impact of alcohol and alcohol expectancies on male perception of female sexual arousal in a date rape analog. *Experimental and Clinical Psychopharmacology, 9*(4), 380–388. doi:10.1037/1064-1297.9.4.380

Higher Education Center for Alcohol and Drug Misuse Prevention and Recovery. (2019). Retrieved from https://hecaod.osu.edu/

Jacques-Tiura, A. J., Tkatch, R., Abbey, A., & Wegner, R. (2010). Disclosure of sexual assault: Characteristics and implications for posttraumatic stress symptoms among African American and Caucasian survivors. *Journal of Trauma & Dissociation, 11*(2), 174–192. doi:10.1080/15299730903502938

Jewkes, R., Gibbs, A., Jama-Shai, N., Willan, S., Misselhorn, A., Mushinga, M., . . . Skiweyiya, Y. (2014). Stepping stones and creating futures intervention: Shortened interrupted time series evaluation of a behavioural and structural health promotion and violence prevention intervention for young people in informal settlements in Durban, South Africa. *BMC Public Health, 14*(1), 1325–1335. doi:10.1186/1471-2458-14-1325

Jewkes, R., Nduna, M., Levin, J., Jama, N., Dunkle, K., Puren, A., & Duvvury, N. (2008). Impact of stepping stones on incidence of HIV and HSV-2 and sexual behaviour in rural South Africa: Cluster randomised controlled trial. *BMJ, 337*, Online. doi:10.1136/bmj.a506

Kaysen, D., Dillworth, T. M., Simpson, T., Waldrop, A., Larimer, M. E., & Resick, P. A. (2007). Domestic violence and alcohol use: Trauma-related symptoms and motives for drinking. *Addictive Behaviors, 32*, 1272–1283. doi:10.1016/j.addbeh.2006.09.007

Kelley, E. L., & Gidycz, C. A. (2017). Mediators of the relationship between sexual assault and sexual functioning difficulties among college women. *Psychology of Violence, 7*(4), 574–582. doi:10.1037/vio0000073

Khantzian, E. J. (2003). The self-medication hypothesis revisited: The dually diagnosed patient. *Primary Psychiatry, 10*(9), 47–54.

Kilpatrick, D. G., Acierno, R., Resnick, H. S., Saunders, B. E., & Best, C. L. (1997). A 2-year longitudinal analysis of the relationships between violent assault and substance use in women. *Journal of Consulting and Clinical Psychology, 65*, 834–947. doi:10.1037/0022-006X.65.5.834

Kilpatrick, D. G., Resnick, H. S., Ruggiero, K. J., Conoscenti, L. M., & McCauley, J. (2007). Drug-facilitated, incapacitated, and forcible rape: A national study. Charleston, SC: Medical University of South Carolina, National Crime Victims Research and Treatment Center. Retrieved from https://www.ncjrs.gov/pdffiles1/nij/grants/219181.pdf

Kingree, J. B., & Thompson, M. (2015). A comparison of risk factors for alcohol-involved and alcohol-uninvolved sexual aggression perpetration. *Journal of Interpersonal Violence, 30*(9), 1478–1492. doi:10.1177/0886260514540806

Kirwan, M., Lanni, D. J., Warnke, A., Pickett, S. M., & Parkhill, M. R. (2018). Emotion regulation moderates the relationship between alcohol consumption and the perpetration of sexual aggression. *Violence Against Women*, Advance online publication. doi:10.1177/1077801218808396

Kirwan, M., Parkhill, M. R., Schuetz, B. A., & Cox, A. (2016). A within-subjects analysis of men's alcohol-involved and nonalcohol-involved sexual assaults. *Journal of Interpersonal Violence*, Advance online publication. doi:10.1177/0886260516670179

Koss, M. P., Figueredo, A. J., & Prince, R. J. (2002). Cognitive mediation of rape's mental, physical and social health impact: Tests of four models in cross-sectional data. *Journal of Consulting and Clinical Psychology, 70*(4), 926–941. doi:10.1037/0022-006X.70.4.926

Letsela, L., Weiner, R., Gafos, M., & Fritz, K. (2019). Alcohol availability, marketing, and sexual health risk amongst urban and rural youth in South Africa. *AIDS and Behavior, 23*(1), 175–189. doi:10.1007/s10461-018-2250-y

Lindgren, K. P., Neighbors, C., Blayney, J. A., Mullins, P. M., & Kaysen, D. (2012). Do drinking motives mediate the association between sexual assault and problem drinking? *Addictive Behaviors, 37*, 323–326. doi:10.1016/j.addbeh.2011.10.009

Littleton, H., Grills-Taquechel, A., & Axsom, D. (2009). Impaired and incapacitated rape victims: Assault characteristics and post-assault experiences. *Violence and Victims, 24*(4), 439–457. doi:10.1891/0886-6708.24.4.439

Lorenz, K., & Ullman, S. E. (2016). Alcohol and sexual assault victimization: Research findings and future directions. *Aggression and Violent Behavior, 31*, 82–94. doi:10.1016/j.avb.2016.08.001

Malamuth, N., Huppin, M., & Linz, D. (2018). Sexual assault interventions may be doing more harm than good with high-risk males. *Aggression and Violent Behavior*. Online. doi:10.1016/j.avb.2018.05.010

Marx, B. P., Heidt, J. M., & Gold, S. D. (2005). Perceived uncontrollability and unpredictability, self-regulation, and sexual revictimization. *Review of General Psychology, 9*, 67–90. doi:10.1037/1089-2680.9.1.67

Mccauley, J. L., Ruggiero, K. J., Resnick, H. S., Conoscenti, L. M., & Kilpatrick, D. G. (2009). Forcible, drug-facilitated, and incapacitated rape in relation to substance use problems: Results from a national sample of college women. *Addictive Behaviors, 34*(5), 458–462. doi:10.1016/j.addb.2008.12.004

Melkonian, A. J., & Ham, L. S. (2018). The effects of alcohol intoxication on young adult women's identification of risk for sexual assault: A systematic review. *Psychology of Addictive Behaviors, 32*(2), 162. doi:10.1037/adb0000349

Messman-Moore, T., Ward, R. M., Zerubavel, N., Chandley, R. B., & Barton, S. N. (2015). Emotion dysregulation and drinking to cope as predictors and consequences of alcohol-involved sexual assault: Examination of short-term and long-term risk. *Journal of Interpersonal Violence, 30*(4), 601–621. doi:10.1177/0886260514535259

Miranda, R., Meyerson, L. A., Long, P. J., Marx, B. P., & Simpson, S. M. (2002). Sexual assault and alcohol use: Exploring the self-medication hypothesis. *Violence and Victims, 17*(2), 205–217. doi:10.1891/vivi.17.2.205.33650

Moore, C., & Waterman, C. K. (1999). Predicting self-protection against sexual assault in dating relationships among heterosexual men and women, gay men, lesbians, and bisexuals. *Journal of College Student Development, 40*, 132–140.

Mustaine, E. E., & Tewksbury, R. (2002). Sexual assault of college women: A feminist interpretation of a routine activities analysis. *Criminal Justice Review, 27*(1), 89–123. doi:10.1177/073401680202700106

Neilson, E. C., Norris, J., Bryan, A. E., & Stappenbeck, C. A. (2017). Sexual assault severity and depressive symptoms as longitudinal predictors of the quality of women's sexual experiences. *Journal of Sex & Marital Therapy, 43*(5), 463–478. doi:10.1080/0092623X.2016.1208127

Norris, J., Zawacki, T., Davis, K. C., & George, W. H. (2018). The role of psychological barriers in women's resistance to sexual assault by acquaintances. In L. M. Orchowski & C. A. Gidycz (Eds.), *Sexual assault risk reduction and resistance* (pp. 87–110). San Diego, CA: Elsevier. doi:10.1016/B978-0-12-805389-8.00005-0

Nurius, P. S., & Norris, J. (1996). A cognitive ecological model of women's response to male sexual coercion in dating. *Journal of Psychology and Human Sexuality, 8*(1–2), 117–139. doi: 10. 1300/J056v08n01_09

O'Donohue, W., Yeater, E. A., & Fanetti, M. (2003). Rape prevention with college males: The roles of rape myth acceptance, victim empathy, and outcome expectancies. *Journal of Interpersonal Violence, 18*, 513–531. doi:10.1177/0886260503251070

Office for National Statistics. (2018). Any sexual assault (including attempts) on women since age 16. Extracted from Table 1. Retrieved from https://www.ons.gov.uk/peoplepopulationandcommunity/crimeandjustice/datasets/sexualoffencesappendixtables

Orchowski, L. M., Barnett, N., Berkowitz, A., Borsari, B., Oesterle, D., & Zlotnick, C. (2018). Sexual assault prevention for heavy drinking college men: Development and feasibility of an integrated approach. *Violence Against Women.* Online. doi:10.1177/1077801218787928

Orchowski, L. M., Edwards, K. M., Hollander, J. A., Banyard, V. L., Senn, C. Y., & Gidycz, C. A. (2018). Integrating sexual assault resistance, bystander, and men's social norms strategies to prevent sexual violence on college campuses: A call to action. *Trauma, Violence, & Abuse.* Online. doi:10.1177/1524838018789153

Pegram, S. E., Abbey, A., Helmers, B. R., Benbouriche, M., Jilani, Z., & Woerner, J. (2018). Men who sexually assault drinking women: Similarities and differences with men who sexually assault sober women and nonperpetrators. *Violence Against Women, 24*(11), 1327–1348. doi:10.1177/1077801218787927

Peter-Hagene, L. C., & Ullman, S. E. (2015). Sexual assault-characteristics effects on PTSD and psychosocial mediators: A cluster-analysis approach to sexual assault types. *Psychological Trauma: Theory, Research, Practice, and Policy, 7*(2), 162–170. doi:10.1037/a0037304

Peter-Hagene, L. C., & Ullman, S. E. (2018). Longitudinal effects of sexual assault victims' drinking and self-blame on posttraumatic stress disorder. *Journal of interpersonal violence, 33*(1), 83–93. doi:10.1177/0886260516636394

Peterson, C., DeGue, S., Florence, C., & Lokey, C. N. (2017). Lifetime economic burden of rape among U.S. adults. *American Journal of Preventive Medicine, 52*, 691–701. doi:10.1016/j.amepre.2016.11.014

Potter, S. (2012). Using a multimedia social marketing campaign to increase active bystanders on the college campus. *Journal of American College Health, 60*, 282–295. doi:10.1080/07448481.2011.599350

Pronyk, P. M., Hargreaves, J. R., Kim, J. C., Morrison, L. A., Phetla, G., Watts, C., . . . Porter, J. D. H. (2006). Effect of a structural intervention for the prevention of intimate-partner violence and HIV in rural South Africa: A cluster randomized trial. *Lancet, 368,* 1973–1983. doi:10.1016/S0140-6736(06)69744-4

Rich, E. P., Nkosi, S., & Morojele, N. K. (2015). Masculinities, alcohol consumption, and sexual risk behavior among male tavern attendees: A qualitative study in North West Province, South Africa. *Psychology of Men & Masculinity, 16*(4), 382–392.

Rozee, P. D., & Koss, M. P. (2001). Rape: A century of resistance. *Psychology of Women Quarterly, 25,* 295–311. doi:10.1037/a0038871

Salazar, L. F., Vivolo-Kantor, A., Hardin, J., & Berkowitz, A. (2014). A web-based sexual violence bystander intervention for male college students: Randomized controlled trial. *Journal of Medical Internet Research, 16,* e203. doi:10.2196/jmir.3426

Searles, R. (2018). *What has #MeToo actually changed?* Retrieved from https://www.bbc.com/news/world-44045291. Accessed February 3, 2109.

Sell, N. M., Turrisi, R., Scaglione, N. M., Cleveland, M. J., & Mallett, K. A. (2018). Alcohol consumptions and use of sexual assault and drinking protective behavioral strategies: A diary study. *Psychology of Women Quarterly, 42*(1), 62–71. doi:10.1177/0361684317744198

Senn, C. Y., Eliasziw, M., Barata, P. C., Thurston, W. E., Newby-Clark, I. R., Radtke, H. L., & Hobden, K. L. (2015). Efficacy of a sexual assault resistance program for university women. *New England Journal of Medicine, 372,* 2326–2335. doi:10.1056/NEJMsa1411131

Senn, C. Y., Eliasziw, M., Hobden, K. L., Newby-Clark, I. R., Barata, P. C., Radtke, H. L., & Thurston, W. E. (2017). Secondary and 2-year outcomes of a sexual assault resistance program for university women. *Psychology of Women Quarterly, 41*(2), 147–162. doi:10.1177/0361684317690119

Shorey, R. C., Brasfield, H., Febres, J., & Stuart, G. L. (2011). An examination of the association between difficulties with emotion regulation and dating violence perpetration. *Journal of Aggression, Maltreatment & Trauma, 20*(8), 870–885. doi:10.1080/10926771.2011.629342

Sims, C. M., Noel, N. E., & Maisto, S. A. (2007). Rape blame as a function of alcohol presence and resistance type. *Addictive Behaviors, 32*(12), 2766–2775. doi:10.1016/j.addbeh.2007.04.013

Smith, S. G., Chen, J., Basile, K.C., Gilbert, L.K., Merrick, M.T., Patel, N., Walling, M., & Jain, A. (2017). *The national intimate partner and sexual violence survey (NISVS): 2010–2012 state report.* Atlanta, GA: National Center for Injury Prevention and Control, Centers for Disease Control and Prevention. Retrieved from https://www.cdc.gov/violenceprevention/pdf/NISVS-StateReportBook.pdf

Spelman, P. J., & Simons, J. S. (2018). Effects of sexual arousal and alcohol cues on acute motivation for alcohol. *Archives of Sexual Behavior, 47*(6), 1577–1589. doi:10.1007/s10508-018-1195-6

Steele, C. M., & Josephs, R. A. (1990). Alcohol myopia. Its prized and dangerous effects. *American Psychologist, 45*(8), 921–933. doi:10.1037//0003-066X.45.8.921

Stein, M. B., & Barrett-Connor, E. (2000). Sexual assault and physical health: Findings from a population-based study of older adults. *Psychosomatic Medicine, 62,* 838–843. doi:10.1097/00006842-200011000-00014

Taylor, B. G., Stein, N. D., Mumford, E. A., & Woods, D. (2013). Shifting boundaries: An experimental evaluation of a dating violence prevention program in middle schools. *Prevention Science, 14*(1), 64–76. doi:10.1007/s11121-012-0293-2

Testa, M., & Livingston, J. A. (2009). Alcohol consumption and women's vulnerability to sexual victimization: Can reducing women's drinking prevent rape? *Substance Use & Misuse, 44*(9–10), 1349–1376. doi:10.1080/10826080902961468

Testa, M., & Livingston, J. A. (2018). Women's alcohol use and risk of sexual victimization: Implications for prevention. In L. M. Orchowski & C. A. Gidycz (Eds.), *Sexual assault risk reduction and resistance* (pp. 135–172). San Diego, CA: Elsevier. doi:10.1016/B978-0-12-805389-8.00007-4

Thomas, K. A., Sorenson, S. B., & Joshi, M. (2016). "Consent is good, joyous, sexy": A banner campaign to market consent to college students. *Journal of American College Health, 64*(8), 639–650. doi:10.1080/07448481.2016.1217869

Tyler, K. A., Schmitz, R. M., & Adams, S. A. (2017). Alcohol expectancy, drinking behavior, and sexual victimization among female and male college students. *Journal of Interpersonal Violence, 32*(15), 2298–2322. doi:10.1177/0886260515591280

Ullman, S. E. (1996). Correlates and consequences of adult sexual assault disclosure. *Journal of Interpersonal Violence, 11*(4), 554–571. doi:10.1177/088626096011004007

Ullman, S. E., & Najdowski, C. J. (2011). Prospective changes in attributions of self-blame and social reactions to women's disclosures of adult sexual assault. *Journal of Interpersonal Violence, 26*(10), 1934–1962. doi:10.1177/0886260510372940

United States Department of Education. (2018). *Secretary DeVos: Proposed Title IX rule provides clarity for schools, support for survivors, and due process rights for all.* Retrieved from https://www.ed.gov/news/press-releases/secretary-devos-proposed-title-ix-rule-provides-clarity-schools-support-survivors-and-due-process-rights-all. Accessed February 1, 2019.

World Health Organization (WHO). (2012). Understanding and addressing violence against women. Geneva: Author. Retrieved from https://apps.who.int/iris/bitstream/handle/10665/77434/WHO_RHR_12.37_eng.pdf;jsessionid=735865601EC819910FADF357F5FE5FCE?sequence=1

Introduction to Section V
Moving forward

Four major issues are addressed in this *Routledge Handbook of Social Work and Addictive Behaviors* concluding section. First, Chapter 36 introduces key principles of implementation science and what this means for social workers and other professionals adopting evidence-supported interventions. Second, curriculum issues related to developing a workforce prepared to guide change around addictive behavior (substance misuse in particular) are explored in Chapter 37. Third, Chapter 38 presents an introduction to new/emerging strategies for social workers and other professionals to integrate data about environmental contexts into our understanding and community-level interventions concerning substance misuse and related/co-occurring problems. Finally, readers are provided with concluding analyses in Chapter 39 discussing (1) a framework for integrating the many disparate theories and evidence concerning addictive behaviors in intervention and policy planning, (2) the relevance of intervention mechanisms of change, common elements, and common factors to practice and science, and (3) emerging priorities and future directions.

36

Implementation of evidence-based substance misuse prevention and treatment interventions

Alicia Bunger, Jim Lange and Erica Magier

Background

Although a range of effective approaches exist, evidence-based interventions (EBIs) for preventing and treating substance misuse can be very challenging to adopt and implement. The ecological model helps explain why alcohol and other drug (AOD) misuse stems from multiple levels ranging from the individual and peer networks to institutions, communities, and ultimately societal norms. Many EBIs involve action within the broader community. And, within communities and real-world treatment settings, EBI selection and training alone often is insufficient. As a result, EBIs are not widely used, slow to be adopted, or not used as intended, raising questions about the quality and impact of existing prevention and treatment efforts (Backer, Kiser, Gillham, & Smith, 2015; Ducharme, Mello, Roman, Knudsen, & Johnson, 2007; Garner, 2009; Griffin & Botvin, 2010). The field of implementation science (IS) (also referred to as dissemination and implementation science, or knowledge translation) offers a structured approach to understanding and addressing implementation challenges to expedite the movement of EBIs into routine practice and policy for widespread public health benefit. This chapter introduces implementation science, describes unique challenges to implementing EBIs for preventing and treating substance misuse, and considers key approaches and tools for practitioners and scholars. In particular, we highlight distinctions between prevention and treatment EBIs, and the implications for implementation research and practice.

Introduction to implementation science

Implementation science is a critical phase in the translational science pipeline, which traces the journey of research evidence from laboratory to practice. While intervention development and testing is intended to translate basic research results into new methods, practices, and treatments—the first area of research translation—*implementation research* aims to translate the results of intervention testing into routine care—the second area of research translation (Westfall, Mold, & Fagnan, 2007; Woolf, 2008). Implementation is "the process of putting to use or integrating evidence-based interventions within a setting" (Rabin & Brownson, 2018, p. 22). By extension, implementation science is the study of methods or strategies for integrating EBIs into practice and policy, and is intended to address critical quality gaps that limit population health and well-being (Brownson, Colditz, & Proctor, 2018; Eccles & Mittman, 2006).

Implementation research includes *pre-implementation studies* that document quality gaps and implementation barriers, *observational studies* examining factors associated with implementation or strategies used in naturally occurring experiments, and controlled *trials* that test effects of implementation strategies on implementation, system, and/or client outcomes. This interdisciplinary field draws from a range of theoretical and research traditions: public health, social work, psychology, organizational science, public policy, economics, and sociology. In this chapter, we introduce key concepts related to the types and nature of effective interventions that represent the focus of implementation science, the multi-level contexts that shape their use, strategies for promoting implementation, and key implementation outcomes.

Effective interventions

Since the focus of implementation science is quality improvement, implementation efforts and research center around efficacious and effective (i.e. evidence-based) interventions. Although there are no clear criteria for determining whether an intervention is "ready" for broad-scale implementation (and this would likely vary across fields), generally an intervention should be supported by strong evidence generated through multiple controlled studies, such as randomized controlled trials and time-series designs. However, beyond the best available research evidence, practitioners, leaders, and other stakeholders might also consider other factors when selecting an intervention to implement: fit with the environment and organizational contexts, the target population's needs and preferences, and available resources and expertise (Satterfield et al., 2009). Ideally, there should also be manuals, toolkits, training, or other supports available to help stakeholders implement an EBI. A variety of online clearinghouses catalog EBIs and other resources might be useful, including the *What Works Clearinghouse* (https://ies.ed.gov/ncee/wwc/) and the *California Evidence Based Clearinghouse for Child Welfare* (https://www.cebc4cw.org/).

Context for implementation

When EBI implementation is discussed, it is often within a multi-level practice context as highlighted by several common frameworks in the field (e.g. Aarons, Hurlburt, & Horwitz, 2011; Damschroder et al., 2009). Successful and sustained use of EBIs often is contingent on front-line practitioners' skills, knowledge, attitudes, and beliefs. For example, communication, norms, and supervision directly influence practice within practitioner teams. Practitioners and their teams are also embedded within organizations, where leadership, structure, supports, incentives, culture, climate, and internal work place rules/policies shape practice. Finally, the organizations responsible for delivering EBIs do so within larger political, funding, and professional environments that influence norms, resources, and broad support for prevention and treatment EBIs. These external, organizational, team, and practitioner-level factors interact to influence implementation, and are a key consideration in the selection and effectiveness of implementation strategies.

Implementation strategies

Proctor and colleagues (2009) conceptualized implementation in terms of two interventions: (1) the EBI to be implemented (interventions with demonstrated effectiveness), and (2) the

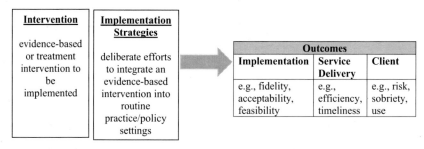

Figure 36.1 Conceptual model of implementation research (as adapted from Proctor et al, 2009)

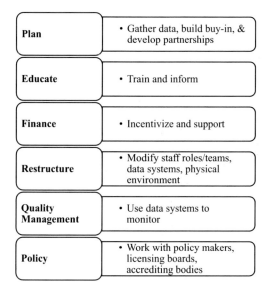

Figure 36.2 Major types of implementation strategies (as adapted from Powell et al, 2012)

implementation strategy (see Figure 36.1). Implementation strategies are deliberate methods, actions, or techniques to integrate and scale up EBIs into routine care (Powell et al., 2012).

A variety of strategies are often necessary for implementation, including specific planning, education, restructuring, financing, quality management, and policy-related activities (see Figure 36.2). Strategies for implementing EBIs might be complex and multifaceted, involving multiple components (e.g. a combination of didactic provider training, coaching, and fidelity monitoring), or straightforward involving only a single component (e.g. clinical reminders). Implementation strategies should be selected and tailored to meet the unique needs of the project, and to overcome anticipated contextual barriers (Baker et al., 2015; Powell et al., 2015; Wensing et al., 2011). Thus, the specific strategies selected may vary based on the specific intervention being implemented, the community/organizational/system context, and stakeholder preferences.

Strategies needed to promote implementation can vary over time (Aarons et al., 2011; Bunger et al., 2017; Chamberlain, Brown, & Saldana, 2011; Saldana, 2014). Before implementation, thorough assessment of the context, including an organization or system's readiness, existing partnerships, and existing resources and needs may be important for informing a specific implementation plan developed to overcome the unique barriers in each setting. Because implementation often requires collaboration across organizations, communities, and systems, selecting and engaging key partners builds buy-in for implementation, and gathers a variety of perspectives for developing the implementation plan. These perspectives are also important for understanding how EBIs might need to be adapted to address the needs of the target population and fit within the community setting.

As implementation planning gets underway, targeted individuals might need to be educated or trained. Professionals may also need to consider methods for altering financing, infrastructure, or policies to support EBIs. Once an EBI launches, there often exists a need for extensive problem solving and adjustments to both the intervention and implementation plan based on early lessons learned, highlighting the importance of a quality management system. Ongoing monitoring, evaluation, and adjustments are important for bringing the EBI to full implementation. Finally, the sustainment phase often includes additional monitoring, evaluation of impact, and plans for continuing or expanding the intervention.

Implementation outcomes

Effective use of implementation strategies is expected to lead to better implementation outcomes, which are indicators of implementation success. A common implementation outcome is fidelity: the degree to which an EBI has been implemented or delivered as intended (Carroll et al., 2007). Implementing EBIs with fidelity helps ensure that an intervention generates the same improvement in client outcomes in the field, as were demonstrated in efficacy and effectiveness trials. However, fidelity is not the only indicator of successful implementation. Practitioners and researchers may also be interested in improving the acceptability, adoption, perceived appropriateness, cost, feasibility, penetration, and sustainability of an EBI (Proctor et al., 2011). These implementation outcomes are distinct but important precursors to other service and client outcomes related to the prevention and treatment of substance misuse.

Implementation challenges in substance misuse prevention and treatment interventions

Both prevention and treatment EBIs focus on a range of factors known to influence substance misuse and its consequences, including access, attitudes, risks, relative attractiveness, and beliefs about AOD. EBIs might target these factors among individuals, groups, or higher levels and structures within the community. For instance, individuals convicted of Driving Under the Influence (DUI) may be required to install an alcohol-detecting ignition interlock device on their vehicles, limiting their ability to drive after drinking (an individual-level intervention). However, to implement an interlock mandate, laws must be in place at the community or societal level, and courts must actually mandate it, and police must enforce it. There must also be available devices and support for their installation and maintenance. Therefore, implementing interventions often requires simultaneous action on multiple social–ecological levels.

Prevention interventions

Prevention interventions intended to inhibit substance misuse and substance use disorders are implemented in a variety of contexts, settings, and populations (Spoth, Guyll, & Day, 2002).

Prevention EBIs often employ environmental approaches to address system-level factors and situations that drive substance misuse, like availability, access, norms, and perceived risks (Clapp et al., 2003; Gorman et al., 2004; Holder, 2000). Examples of these prevention interventions include policy changes regarding alcohol-sales licenses, minimum drinking age laws, responsible beverage service training, reducing hours of alcohol sales, and DUI checkpoints (Holder et al., 1997).

Alcohol and other drug misuse prevention programming that focuses on individual knowledge and attitudes is also common, yet not always an EBI. For instance, in use within primary school settings, Kumar and colleagues identified over 200 commercial prevention programs (Kumar, O'Malley, Johnston, & Laetz, 2013), further noting that those represented a fraction of deployed school-based programs, which were far more likely to be locally developed. With the sea of competing choices, successful implementation of prevention EBIs requires coordinated action and productive working relationships among community stakeholders, as well as well-trained staff knowledgeable in EBI approaches and productive working relationships among stakeholders (Dusenbury & Falco, 1995; Nation et al., 2003). Lack of buy-in from necessary stakeholders and poor partnerships (Winstanley, Clark, Feinberg, & Wilder, 2016), and lack of EBI awareness are often the primary barriers to selection and implementation.

Treatment interventions

Substance use disorder (SUD) treatments address already existing and diagnosed SUDs. Treatments might include Medication-Assisted Treatments (MAT) or brief interventions such as Screening, Brief Intervention, and Referral to Treatment (SBIRT). Treatments can be targeted to specific populations at high risk for SUD. For instance, Brief Alcohol Screening and Intervention for College Students (BASICS) targets college students at risk of substance misuse, as identified by violations of campus alcohol policies (DiFulvio, Linowski, Mazziotti, & Puleo, 2012). Treatment interventions are often implemented within a variety of formal settings, such as mental health clinics, emergency medicine departments, and specialty care venues, and the field has seen a rise in the delivery of SUD treatment through technology-assisted platforms (e.g. eHealth interventions) (Smit et al., 2011). Because the treatment delivery often relies on professional staff employed by treatment organizations, lack of staff and funding, staff skepticism, insufficient staff training, client resistance, and lack of insurance coverage for SUD treatment are often the primary barriers to implementation (Amodeo et al., 2011; Knudsen, Abraham, & Oser, 2011; Nilsen, 2010; Rieckmann, Kovas, Fussell, & Stettler, 2009).

Considerations and tools for implementation

Prevention and treatment EBIs vary in terms of their complexity and settings in which they are implemented. Prevention approaches, especially environmental interventions, are often multi-component interventions implemented within communities and institutions. Treatment interventions are implemented by clinicians within service delivery organizations. Below, we review considerations for implementation and continued implementation research in this area.

Engaging stakeholders

A range of stakeholders from clients to alcohol industry partners may all have an interest in adopting a specific EBI and the strategies used in bringing it to scale within and across communities. Identifying local stakeholders and engaging them in meaningful ways in implementation initiatives or studies can generate broad support for EBIs and inform implementation plans tailored to the local need and context. Teams implementing treatment interventions might engage local practitioners, clients and their families, agency leaders, and addiction treatment service funders (e.g. public or private insurance providers).

For many prevention initiatives, a broad community-based group of stakeholders that includes community coalitions, advocacy groups, and institutions outside of traditional behavioral health service delivery systems (e.g. schools or law enforcement) likely will be needed. For example, consider the role of community stakeholders for implementing a drunk-driving prevention strategy such as High Visibility Enforcement (HVE). Often this is operationalized as a sobriety check point accompanied by intentional publicity through news coverage to increase public perception of the risk for arrest, leading to reduced rates of driving under the influence. While a relatively simple theoretical mechanism, the operational complexity can be daunting: resources to pay for police involvement and publicity coordination require community support. Thus, it is not uncommon to see communities fail to maintain such an effort, drift to easier enforcement styles, or have difficulty maintaining local media attention. Advocacy groups might help sustain community attention, and community support can help sustain the program and justify its cost. However, police departments may resist sustainment because sobriety checkpoints may not fit naturally within their current performance metrics since they often result in few arrests per office-hour worked. Therefore, police need to believe this activity has inherent value within their department and their professional goals. So, the relative simplicity of the operation, once placed in the complexity of the community, institutional, and normative beliefs, exposes the implementation challenges and the necessity of broad stakeholder engagement for community EBIs.

Approaches for understanding the context and capacity for change

Understanding the context, and its capacity is important for informing the EBIs selected and the strategies used to implement them. Existing literature highlights a range of contextual factors relevant to implementation success in communities, schools, and organizations. Local assessments of community needs (e.g. incidence and prevalence statistics) and existing resources and supports are critical for informing these decisions. But those leading local implementation efforts will also want to draw on stakeholders' perceptions of a system's readiness and capacity for change through focus groups, town hall meetings, or even informal conversations. In situations where an event or identified crisis (e.g. the opioid overdose epidemic or a high-profile tragedy) precipitates a community-wide call to action, it is especially important to triangulate these insights with more objective assessments. There exists a variety of quantitative and qualitative tools developed to assess context that might be useful to both practitioners and researchers. For instance, the Consolidated Framework for Implementation Research (CFIR) developers maintain a helpful website (https://cfirguide.org) that defines contextual implementation determinants, and provides a suite of tools for data collection, including interview guides, observation templates, and meeting minute templates.

Tracking and documenting implementation strategies

As communities and providers continue to implement prevention and treatment EBIs, monitoring and documenting the specific implementation strategies used are important for helping others scale up and adapt EBIs across other settings (Powell et al., 2019). Several tools are available for monitoring strategies. For instance, the Stages of Implementation

Completion (SIC) is a tool for monitoring implementation process milestones, and pacing across eight stages (Chamberlain et al., 2011; Saldana, Chamberlain, Wang, & Hendricks Brown, 2012). The SIC is especially useful for understanding implementation pacing as implementers select, adopt, implement, and sustain an EBI. To explore or document specific strategies used to implement EBIs, other approaches including activity logs (e.g. Bunger et al., 2017) and observations (e.g. Boyd, Powell, Endicott, & Lewis, 2018) can be employed to track the types, frequency, and timing of strategies used during implementation. These approaches can be useful for reporting implementation strategies consistent with Proctor, Powell, and McMillen's (2013) recommendations for operationalizing the actor, specific actions, target, timing, dosage, expected outcome, and theoretical justification.

Managing fidelity-adaptation tension

Implementing EBIs with a high degree of fidelity is essential for ensuring that interventions can achieve the same effectiveness in the field as demonstrated in the lab. However, in real-world contexts, EBIs are often adapted. Indeed, many AOD prevention EBIs were initially developed and tested, not in a controlled lab environment, but within real-world trials. EBIs may need to be culturally adapted to fit a different target population than the population on which it was initially tested (Cabassa & Baumann, 2013). Similarly, stakeholders may adapt EBIs to enhance fit within local systems which often have fewer resources and more competing demands than was true in initial trials. Within the college-drinking setting, for instance, SBIRT may be adapted for use in college health centers by increasing the thresholds that trigger brief interventions and referrals for alcohol treatment, since the drinking quantities that were flags for a general population were relatively normative among college students. Higher thresholds allow for fewer referrals in the college setting and help to keep a SBIRT from overwhelming other departments. Thoughtful adaptation requires a firm understanding of an EBI's theoretical underpinnings: the theory that explains the specific behavior change. This requires identification of the core components responsible for producing outcomes and other peripheral intervention features which theoretically can be modified (Damschroder et al., 2009).

For instance, in brief interventions for risky alcohol use, clinicians deliver information about normative drinking behavior and personal risks during in-person discussions. Theoretically, individuals change their drinking behavior when they understand how their alcohol use diverges from the norm. These in-person discussions ensure that individuals receive core content about typical drinking norms, and begin to contemplate how their own risky drinking behavior departs from these norms. Computerized versions of brief interventions may be less costly and have potential to reach larger numbers of individuals, but alter the core components since there is no way to confirm that an individual received and considered information about drinking norms. In fact, computerized adaptations have been demonstrated as less effective than brief interventions delivered in-person (Cadigan et al., 2015; Carey, Scott-Sheldon, Elliott, Bolles, & Carey, 2009).

Theory also plays a role when determining whether a particular intervention might be adapted for a different population or problem. Continuing with our brief intervention example, these approaches have been adapted to address drug use. Yet, brief intervention for drug use has been ineffective, arguably because individuals are often already aware that their drug use is risky (Saitz, 2014): the theory underlying the adapted brief intervention does not align with the theory that explains drug use. Although, a recent trial of the online Marijuana eCheckUpToGo, which provides an intervention featuring personalized feedback did demonstrate significant reductions in cannabis use among college students engaged in heavy use (Riggs et al., 2018). Again, the particular program, setting, and population may dictate an EBI's success.

Sustainability

Many organizations and communities experience difficulty continuing to deliver EBIs as they are intended once initial start-up supports are withdrawn (Wiltsey Stirman et al., 2012). Changes in the external or internal organizational environment might cause leaders to discontinue an EBI. Or, problems maintaining supports for an EBI might cause a gradual drift from fidelity to core components leading to a diminution of the EBI's impact. Financial resources play a strong role in sustainment as do political support, organizational capacity, evidence of impact, strong community partnerships, and planning (Schell et al., 2013). Continued training is also important (Gloppen et al., 2016). However, the factors that influence sustainability vary depending on the nature of the intervention (Scheirer, 2013). EBIs implemented by providers are likely to be shaped by individual motivations and financing, thus staffing changes and new financial priorities threaten their sustainability. However, EBIs that require extensive collaboration across stakeholders are often shaped by administrative supports, fit with organizational contexts, technical assistance, and commitment to working together. Often times, once fully institutionalized, these interventions tend to continue. Policy or automated technology interventions (e.g. eCheck Up to Go and ScreenU) are especially difficult to "undo" because they require an affirmative action to discontinue them. Although more research in this area is needed, those wishing to sustain EBIs for preventing or treating substance misuse likely need to continue their collaborative implementation efforts to ensure maintained impact in the community.

De-implementation

De-implementation involves replacing or removing practices that fail to improve prevention or treatment goals; this includes de-implementing harmful practices. For instance, every 15 minutes programming involved an intense mock funeral, where an actual student was removed from the school and declared deceased because of drunk driving. Although the model was intended to highlight risks, the trauma and distress that many students experienced likely outweighed preventive effects. No easily located studies assess its impact. Stakeholders might also target practices for de-implementation if they are ineffective. For instance, Drug Abuse Resistance Education (D.A.R.E.) is widely used in school settings to prevent drug use among adolescents, yet lacks evidence of effectiveness across multiple rigorous trials (Rosenbaum, 2010). Thus, de-implementing practices that are ineffective, low-value, or harmful is equally important to improving quality, value, and population health impact.

Designing trials to understand impact on clients and communities

Continued research is needed to understand the most effective strategies for implementing and sustaining EBIs, and their long-term impact. Given the strength of the evidence for a particular EBI's effectiveness, or the extent to which it was adapted, researchers might consider designing hybrid implementation trials. Hybrid trials examine effects of implementation initiatives on both implementation and client outcomes (Curran, Bauer, Mittman, Pyne, & Stetler, 2012). Randomized controlled trials (RCTs) are rigorous designs for examining intervention, and implementation strategy effectiveness and generating strong evidence about what works. However, researchers may not always have control over who may be exposed to the intervention or the implementation strategy (e.g. when implementing new policies and environmental prevention strategies). A range of quasi-experimental and other design variations (e.g. cluster RCTs, stepped wedge, interrupted time-series designs), that account for the realities of the context, have promise for generating strong evidence about implementation strategies and interventions (Brown et al., 2017; Mazzucca et al., 2018). The Dissemination and Implementation Research Core at Washington University in St. Louis developed a toolkit that further describes these research designs, and the conditions under which they are appropriate (Lewis et al., 2017).

Conclusions

New insights about implementation of EBIs have strong potential to improve the public health impact of interventions that prevent and treat substance misuse. However, the strategies needed to implement EBIs will likely differ for prevention and treatment since these interventions tend to target different levels of the service ecology. Both practitioners and researchers will need to work together to understand the distinct contexts in which EBIs are implemented, engage a range of stakeholders to plan for implementation, and adapt interventions in thoughtful ways that respond to community needs while preserving core intervention elements. Continued research, evaluation, and documentation of implementation processes will generate evidence to inform implementation and scale up efforts across communities.

References

Aarons, G. A., Hurlburt, M., & Horwitz, S. M. (2011). Advancing a conceptual model of evidence-based practice implementation in public service sectors. *Administration and Policy in Mental Health, 38*(1), 4–23. doi:10.1007/s10488-010-0327-7

Amodeo, M., Lundgren, L., Cohen, A., Rose, D., Chassler, D., Beltrame, C., & D'Ippolito, M. (2011). Barriers to implementing evidence-based practices in addiction treatment programs: Comparing staff reports on motivational interviewing, adolescent community reinforcement approach, assertive community treatment, and cognitive-behavioral therapy. *Evaluation and Program Planning, 34*(4), 382–389. doi:10.1016/J.EVALPROGPLAN.2011.02.005

Backer, P. M., Kiser, L. J., Gillham, J. E., & Smith, J. (2015). The Maryland resilience breakthrough series collaborative: A quality improvement initiative for children's mental health services providers. *Psychiatric Services, 66*(8), 778–780. doi:10.1176/appi.ps.201500036

Baker, R., Camosso-Stefinovic, J., Gillies, C., Shaw, E. J., Cheater, F., Flottorp, S., . . . Jäger, C. (2015, April 29). Tailored interventions to address determinants of practice. In R. Baker, (Ed.), *Cochrane database of systematic reviews*. Chichester, UK: John Wiley & Sons, Ltd. doi:10.1002/14651858. CD005470.pub3

Boyd, M. R., Powell, B. J., Endicott, D., & Lewis, C. C. (2018). A method for tracking implementation strategies: An exemplar implementing measurement-based care in community behavioral health clinics. *Behavior Therapy, 49*(4), 525–537. doi:10.1016/j.beth.2017.11.012

Brown, C. H., Curran, G., Palinkas, L. A., Aarons, G. A., Wells, K. B., Jones, L., . . . Cruden, G. (2017). An overview of research and evaluation designs for dissemination and implementation. *Annual Review of Public Health, 38*, 1–22. doi:10.1146/annurev-publhealth-031816-044215

Brownson, R. C., Colditz, G. A., & Proctor, E. K. (2018). *Dissemination and implementation research in health* (2nd ed.). New York, NY: Oxford University Press. doi:10.1093/oso/9780190683214.001.0001

Bunger, A. C., Powell, B. J., Robertson, H. A., MacDowell, H., Birken, S. A., & Shea, C. (2017). Tracking implementation strategies: A description of a practical approach and early findings. *Health Research Policy and Systems, 15*(1), 15. doi:10.1186/s12961-017-0175-y

Cabassa, L. J., & Baumann, A. A. (2013). A two-way street: Bridging implementation science and cultural adaptations of mental health treatments. *Implementation Science : IS, 8*(1), 90. doi:10.1186/1748-5908-8-90

Cadigan, J. M., Haeny, A. M., Martens, M. P., Weaver, C. C., Takamatsu, S. K., & Arterberry, B. J. (2015). Personalized drinking feedback: A meta-analysis of in-person versus computer-delivered interventions. *Journal of Consulting and Clinical Psychology, 83*(2), 430–437. doi:10.1037/a0038394

Carey, K. B., Scott-Sheldon, L. A. J., Elliott, J. C., Bolles, J. R., & Carey, M. P. (2009). Computer-delivered interventions to reduce college student drinking: A meta-analysis. *Addiction, 104*(11), 1807–1819. doi:10.1111/j.1360-0443.2009.02691.x

Carroll, C., Patterson, M., Wood, S., Booth, A., Rick, J., & Balain, S. (2007). A conceptual framework for implementation fidelity. *Implementation Science, 2*(1), 1–9. doi:10.1186/1748-5908-2-40

Chamberlain, P., Brown, C. H., & Saldana, L. (2011). Observational measure of implementation progress in community based settings: The stages of implementation completion (SIC). *Implementation Science : IS, 6*, 116. doi:10.1186/1748-5908-6-116

Clapp, J. D., Lange, J., Jon, W. M., Shillington, A., Johnson, M., & Voas, R. (2003). Two studies examining environmental predictors of heavy drinking by college students. *Prevention Science, 4*(2), 99–108. doi:10.1023/A:1022974215675

Curran, G. M., Bauer, M., Mittman, B., Pyne, J. M., & Stetler, C. (2012). Effectiveness–implementation hybrid designs: Combining elements of clinical effectiveness and implementation research to enhance public health impact. *Medical Care, 50*(3), 217–226. https://doi.org/10.1097/MLR.0b013e3182408812

Damschroder, L. J., Aron, D. C., Keith, R. E., Kirsh, S. R., Alexander, J. A., & Lowery, J. C. (2009). Fostering implementation of health services research findings into practice: A consolidated framework for advancing implementation science. *Implementation Science: IS, 4*, 50. doi:10.1186/1748-5908-4-50

DiFulvio, G. T., Linowski, S. A., Mazziotti, J. S., & Puleo, E. (2012). Effectiveness of the brief alcohol and screening intervention for college students (BASICS) program with a mandated population. *Journal of American College Health, 60*(4), 269–280. doi:10.1080/07448481.2011.599352

Ducharme, L. J., Mello, H. L., Roman, P. M., Knudsen, H. K., & Johnson, J. A. (2007). Service delivery in substance abuse treatment: Reexamining "comprehensive" care. *Journal of Behavioral Health Services and Research*. doi:10.1007/s11414-007-9061-7

Dusenbury, L., & Falco, M. (1995). Eleven components of effective drug abuse prevention curricula. *Journal of School Health, 65*(10), 420–425. doi:10.1111/j.1746-1561.1995.tb08205.x

Eccles, M. P., & Mittman, B. S. (2006). Welcome to implementation science. *Implementation Science, 1*(1), 1. doi:10.1186/1748-5908-1-1

Garner, B. R. (2009). Research on the diffusion of evidence-based treatments within substance abuse treatment: A systematic review. *Journal of Substance Abuse Treatment, 36*(4), 376–399. doi:10.1016/j.jsat.2008.08.004

Gloppen, K. M., Brown, E. C., Wagenaar, B. H., Hawkins, J. D., Rhew, I. C., & Oesterle, S. (2016). Sustaining adoption of science-based prevention through communities that care. *Journal of Community Psychology, 44*(1), 78–89. doi:10.1002/jcop.21743

Gorman, D. M., Gruenewald, P. J., Hanlon, P. J., Mezic, I., Waller, L. A., Castillo-Chavez, C., . . . Mezic, J. (2004). Implications of systems dynamic models and control theory for environmental approaches to the prevention of alcohol- and other drug use-related problems. *Substance Use and Misuse, 39*(10–12), 1713–1750. doi:10.1081/JA-200033215

Griffin, K. W., & Botvin, G. J. (2010). Evidence-based interventions for preventing substance use disorders in adolescents. *Child and Adolescent Psychiatric Clinics of North America, 19*(3), 505–526. doi:10.1016/j.chc.2010.03.005

Holder, H. D. (2000). Community prevention of alcohol problems. *Addictive Behaviors, 25*(6), 843–859. doi:10.1016/S0306-4603(00)00121-0

Holder, H. D., Saltz, R. F., Grube, J. W., Voas, R. B., Gruenewald, P. J., & Treno, A. J. (1997). A community prevention trial to reduce alcohol-involved accidental injury and death: Overview. *Addiction, 92*(Suppl 2), S155–S171. doi:10.1111/j.1360-0443.1997.tb02989.x

Knudsen, H. K., Abraham, A. J., & Oser, C. B. (2011). Barriers to the implementation of medication-assisted treatment for substance use disorders: The importance of funding policies and medical infrastructure. *Evaluation and Program Planning, 34*(4), 375–381. doi:10.1016/j.evalprogplan.2011.02.004

Kumar, R., O'Malley, P. M., Johnston, L. D., & Laetz, V. B. (2013). Alcohol, tobacco, and other drug use prevention programs in U.S. Schools: A descriptive summary. *Prevention Science, 14*(6), 581–592. doi:10.1007/s11121-012-0340-z

Lewis, E., Baumann, A., Gerke, D., Tabak, R., Ramsey, A., Small, S., & Proctor, E. (2017). *D&I research designs*. St. Louis, MO. Retrieved from https://sites.wustl.edu/wudandi

Mazzucca, S., Tabak, R. G., Pilar, M., Ramsey, A. T., Baumann, A. A., Kryzer, E., . . . Brownson, R. C. (2018, February). Variation in research designs used to test the effectiveness of dissemination and implementation strategies: A review. *Frontiers in Public Health, 6*, 1–10. doi:10.3389/fpubh.2018.00032

Nation, M., Crusto, C., Wandersman, A., Kumpfer, K. L., Seybolt, D., Morrissey-Kane, E., & Davino, K. (2003). What works in prevention: Principles of effective prevention programs. *American Psychologist, 58*(6–7), 449–456. doi:10.1037/0003-066X.58.6-7.449

Nilsen, P. (2010). Brief alcohol intervention-where to from here? Challenges remain for research and practice. *Addiction, 105*(6), 954–959. doi:10.1111/j.1360-0443.2009.02779.x

Powell, B. J., Beidas, R. S., Lewis, C. C., Aarons, G. A., McMillen, J. C., Proctor, E. K., & Mandell, D. S. (2015). Methods to improve the selection and tailoring of implementation strategies. *The Journal of Behavioral Health Services & Research*, 1–18. doi:10.1007/s11414-015-9475-6

Powell, B. J., Fernandez, M. E., Williams, N. J., Aarons, G. A., Beidas, R. S., Lewis, C. C., . . . Weiner, B. J. (2019). Enhancing the impact of implementation strategies in healthcare: A research agenda. *Frontiers in Public Health, 7*, 3. doi:10.3389/fpubh.2019.00003

Powell, B. J., McMillen, J. C., Proctor, E. K., Carpenter, C. R., Griffey, R. T., Bunger, A. C., . . . York, J. L. (2012). A compilation of strategies for implementing clinical innovations in health and mental health. *Medical Care Research and Review: MCRR, 69*(2), 123–157. doi:10.1177/1077558711430690

Proctor, E. K., Landsverk, J., Aarons, G., Chambers, D., Glisson, C., & Mittman, B. (2009). Implementation research in mental health services: An emerging science with conceptual, methodological, and training challenges. *Administration and Policy in Mental Health, 36*(1), 24–34. doi:10.1007/s10488-008-0197-4

Proctor, E. K., Powell, B. J., & McMillen, J. C. (2013). Implementation strategies: Recommendations for specifying and reporting. *Implementation Science: IS, 8*(1), 139. doi:10.1186/1748-5908-8-139

Proctor, E. K., Silmere, H., Raghavan, R., Hovmand, P., Aarons, G. A., Bunger, A., . . . Hensley, M. (2011). Outcomes for implementation research: Conceptual distinctions, measurement challenges, and research agenda. *Administration and Policy in Mental Health, 38*(2), 65–76. doi:10.1007/s10488-010-0319-7

Rabin, B. A., & Brownson, R. C. (2018). Developing the terminology for dissemination and implementation research. In R. C. Brownson, G. A. Colditz, & E. K. Proctor (Eds.), *Dissemination and implementation research in health: Translating science to practice* (2nd ed., pp. 19–46). New York, NY: Oxford University Press.

Rieckmann, T. R., Kovas, A. E., Fussell, H. E., & Stettler, N. M. (2009). Implementation of evidence-based practices for treatment of alcohol and drug disorders: The role of the state authority. *The Journal of Behavioral Health Services & Research, 36*(4), 407–419. doi:10.1007/s11414-008-9122-6

Rosenbaum, D. P. (2010). Just say no to D.A.R.E. *Criminology & Public Policy, 6*(4), 815–824. doi:10.1111/j.1745-9133.2007.00474.x

Saitz, R. (2014). Screening and brief intervention for unhealthy drug use: Little or no efficacy. *Frontiers in Psychiatry, 5*, 121. doi:10.3389/fpsyt.2014.00121

Saldana, L. (2014). The stages of implementation completion for evidence-based practice: Protocol for a mixed methods study. *Implementation Science: IS, 9*(1), 43. doi:10.1186/1748-5908-9-43

Saldana, L., Chamberlain, P., Wang, W., & Hendricks Brown, C. (2012). Predicting program start-up using the stages of implementation measure. *Administration and Policy in Mental Health and Mental Health Services Research, 39*(6), 419–425. doi:10.1007/s10488-011-0363-y

Satterfield, J. M., Spring, B., Brownson, R. C., Mullen, E. J., Newhouse, R. P., Walker, B. B., & Whitlock, E. P. (2009, June 1). Toward a transdisciplinary model of evidence-based practice. *Milbank Quarterly*. doi:10.1111/j.1468-0009.2009.00561.x

Scheirer, M. A. (2013). Linking sustainability research to intervention types. *American Journal of Public Health, 103*(4), e73–e80. Retrieved from http://www.scopus.com/inward/record.url?eid=2-s2.0-84875148564&partnerID=tZOtx3y1, doi:10.1093/oso/9780190683214.001.0001

Schell, S. F., Luke, D. A., Schooley, M. W., Elliott, M. B., Herbers, S. H., Mueller, N. B., & Bunger, A. C. (2013). Public health program capacity for sustainability: A new framework. *Implementation Science: IS, 8*(1), 15. doi:10.1186/1748-5908-8-15

Smit, F., Lokkerbol, J., Riper, H., Majo, M. C., Boon, B., & Blankers, M. (2011). Modeling the cost-effectiveness of health care systems for alcohol use disorders: How implementation of eHealth interventions improves cost-effectiveness. *Journal of Medical Internet Research, 13*(3), e56. doi:10.2196/jmir.1694

Spoth, R. L., Guyll, M., & Day, S. X. (2002). Universal family-focused interventions in alcohol-use disorder prevention: Cost-effectiveness and cost-benefit analyses of two interventions. *Journal of Studies on Alcohol, 63*(2), 219–228. doi:10.15288/jsa.2002.63.219

Wensing, M., Oxman, A., Baker, R., Godycki-Cwirko, M., Flottorp, S., Szecsenyi, J., . . . Eccles, M. (2011). Tailored implementation for chronic diseases (TICD): A project protocol. *Implementation Science, 6*(103). doi:10.1186/1748-5908-6-103

Westfall, J. M., Mold, J., & Fagnan, L. (2007). Practice-based research—"Blue Highways" on the NIH roadmap. *Journal of the American Medical Association: JAMA, 297*(4), 403. doi:10.1001/jama.297.4.403

Wiltsey Stirman, S., Kimberly, J., Cook, N., Calloway, A., Castro, F., & Charns, M. (2012). The sustainability of new programs and innovations: A review of the empirical literature and recommendations for future research. *Implementation Science: IS, 7*(1), 17. doi:10.1186/1748-5908-7-17

Winstanley, E. L., Clark, A., Feinberg, J., & Wilder, C. M. (2016). Barriers to implementation of opioid overdose prevention programs in Ohio. *Substance Abuse, 37*(1), 42–46. doi:10.1080/08897077.2015.1132294

Woolf, S. H. (2008). The meaning of translational research and why it matters. *Journal of the American Medical Association: JAMA, 299*(2), 211–213. doi:10.1001/jama.2007.26

37

Core health professional education curriculum for risky substance use and substance use disorder

Lena Lundgren, Meredith Silverstein and Siv Nyström

Background

Substance Use Disorder (SUD) prevalence rates have steadily increased since the 1990s in many countries of the world, and these rates are now higher than those of diabetes for most countries (GBD 2016 Alcohol and Drug Use Collaborators, 2018). Globally, a lack of knowledge among health professionals and social workers about causes and consequences of alcohol and other drug (AOD) misuse, as well as evidence-based practices (EBPs) in SUD screening, assessment, and treatment, presents barriers to improved treatment access, use, and outcomes. This chapter first provides a rationale for why a core curriculum for social workers and other health professionals concerning alcohol and other drugs is needed. Second, the chapter discusses past and current barriers to implementing AOD knowledge and evidence into the overall social work curriculum. Third, the chapter provides an example of how neglect of AOD content and practice skills in social work education occurs internationally, resulting in institutions other than higher education assuming this responsibility. Fourth, the chapter describes evaluation results from a U.S. National Institute on Alcohol Abuse and Alcoholism (NIAAA)-funded educational training program, Alcohol and Other Drugs Education Program (ADEP), preparing social work faculty to deliver an empirically supported AOD curriculum. Implications from the ADEP project can inform development of an AOD core curriculum for the social work profession. Finally, this chapter presents the authors' recommendations concerning AOD core curriculum for social work and other professional education.

Why an AOD core-curriculum for social work

Social workers practice in a range of organizational settings where use of evidence-based AOD screening and brief intervention skills play an important role in early identification of risky substance use and SUD. These include schools, community health centers (Duong, O'Sullivan, Satre, Soskin, & Satterfield, 2016; Roy-Byrne et al., 2014), inpatient settings, and outpatient mental health centers (Senreich, Ogden, & Greenberg, 2017). Social workers also practice as mental health clinicians and clinical supervisors in psychosocial SUD treatment settings, conducting and/or supervising screening and assessment, and providing a range of psycho-educational and therapeutic interventions.

Approximately 50% of individuals with a mental health disorder (MHD) have, at some time in their life, also experienced a SUD and vice versa (Kelly & Daley, 2013; Ross & Peselow, 2012; see Chapter 33). In the United States, 3.4% of the adult population over the age of 18 has a co-occurring mental health and substance use disorder (Substance Abuse and Mental Health Services Administration [SAMHSA], 2017). Social work practice settings, whether specifically designed or not for addressing AOD problems, engage with large percentages of individuals at risk of or experiencing problems related to their own or someone else's substance misuse. This was demonstrated in a service-user alcohol screening study across many types of community-based agencies in one U.S. community (Rose, Brondino, & Barnack, 2009). While 83.7% of persons seen in substance abuse services had positive screening results, this was true among mental health (53.6%), health care (58.6%), homeless (25.7%), social (22.1%), child welfare (12.8%), and welfare-to-work (9.5%) service agencies.

Given the high percentage of individuals at risk of or experiencing SUDs in many different social work settings, all social workers need familiarity with evidence-based AOD screening, as well as basic knowledge of assessment, treatment, causes, consequences, and epidemiology of AODs. Although integrated care is sometimes considered a relatively new concept, the social work profession is historically based on an integrated care model (Block, Wheeland, & Rosenberg, 2014; Lundblad, 1995; Peterson, 1965). Specifically, social workers trained in case management skills from the profession's conception: promoting ongoing, long-term contact with clients; responding to a range of client biopsychosocial needs; and working with other health professionals in a range of health care institutions.

Additional arguments exist regarding the need for social workers to develop evidence-based AOD skills. For example, many clinical social workers receive training in Motivational Interviewing (MI) (Hohman, Pierce, & Barnett, 2015; Wahab, 2005). Although MI represents a core skill set for professional practice in the AOD/SUD arena (Babor et al., 2007; Duong et al., 2016), critical to screening, brief intervention, and referral to treatment (SBIRT) practices and relapse prevention efforts, the education social workers receive often fails to address how to use these skills with a client experiencing a SUD. Social workers can be critical to implementing EBPs for SUD treatment, since social workers in clinical practice are trained to deliver a range of cognitive behavioral approaches, and these have been established as effective in treating alcohol and other drug use disorders; unfortunately, many social workers are not trained in this.

As health care systems increasingly move toward integrated behavioral health models in primary care (see Chapter 27), increased opportunities emerge for behavioral health specialists, including social workers, trained in assessment, screening, and treatment of SUDs (McLellan & Woodworth, 2014). In the United States, the National Institute on Drug Abuse (NIDA), the National Institute on Alcohol Abuse and Alcoholism (NIAAA), Health Resources Services Administration (HRSA), and the Substance Abuse and Mental Health Services Administration (SAMHSA) have funded portions of behavioral health training in social work programs (Salas-Wright, Lundgren, & Amodeo, 2018), but more training is needed. Finally, many social workers provide services to vulnerable and diverse populations. They train to provide linguistically and culturally appropriate services, and to communicate effectively with clients who have low literacy (Andrews, Darnell, McBride, & Gehlert, 2013; Boulware et al., 2013; Leach & Segal, 2011). Cultural responsiveness skills are especially valuable when working in under-served communities and can increase the efficacy of AOD prevention, identification, and treatment. In short, "Counseling and social work programs educate future practitioners who are likely to be engaged in direct practice with individuals impacted by substance use disorders" (Russett & Williams, 2015, p. 51). Thus, they need to be adequately prepared to do so responsibly.

Barriers to implementing an AOD core curriculum

In general, barriers to university's adopting AOD curricula reflect what is known from implementation science and may parallel barriers to organizations implementing evidence-based treatment practices: organizational capacity, readiness to change, perceived need, and stress (Lundgren, Chassler, Amodeo, D'Ippolito, & Sullivan, 2012; Lundgren, Amodeo, Chassler, Krull, & Sullivan, 2013). Training, supervision, and ultimate use by social work students of an evidence-based practice (EBP) were influenced by school-level factors and their interactions with field placement and student-specific factors (Ogden, Vinjamuri, & Kahn, 2016). How an evidence-based practice is taught, learned, and delivered across four different professions was influenced by components of the intervention itself, encouragement by professional organizations (Wamsley, Satterfield, Curtis, Lundgren, & Sartre, 2018). One key barrier to implementing an alcohol and other drug core curriculum for the social work profession is that many health professionals, including social workers, do not envision themselves or are not drawn to working with clients experiencing SUDs. Whereas the majority of professional social workers report that they do not primarily work with clients experiencing SUDs, large numbers work in organizational settings where they have ongoing interactions with clients engaged in risky substance use or experiencing a SUD (CSWE, 2018), and too many times the social worker may not be aware of this.

Other major barriers to social workers' training in and subsequent use of AOD EBPs include: lack of faculty knowledge about causes and consequences of substance use (including the biomedical aspects) and lack of skills training in SBIRT (Lundgren & Krull, 2018; Wilkey et al., 2013). In the NIAAA-funded program to increase social work faculty SUD knowledge, faculty participants showed statistically significant improvement in AOD-related knowledge in the domains of screening/assessment, brief intervention, medication-assisted treatment, relapse prevention, and recovery. Faculty participants' initial knowledge scores were surprisingly low, and 66% believed that lack of social work faculty knowledge and expertise in AOD content and AOD-related clinical practice skills were barriers to effectively teaching social work students nationwide about SUDs (Krull et al., 2018; Lundgren & Krull, 2018). When re-tested with a second 48-person cohort a year later, lack of faculty expertise was again the highest rated barrier, with lack of space in the current curriculum ranked as the second highest barrier to implementing an AOD curriculum (Lundgren et al., 2012).

University provided AOD education lacking internationally

Many social work programs either do not systematically provide education about AOD or provide this content only through elective courses, often taught by instructors outside of the program's core faculty (Wilkey et al., 2013). This situation at times results in other societal institutions assuming responsibility for educating the behavioral health and social work workforce on AOD content and evidence-based SUD practices. This sends a message that AOD content is "outside" of the profession's scope, or not important for all health professionals and social workers to know.

Currently, the United States has no national-level core AOD content requirement for educational programs in social work. In a review of 97 U.S. master's-level social work programs, investigators identified only about two-third requiring a specific substance abuse course and 12 offering this as an elective; at the bachelor's level, this type of course was required by only 3 of 89 programs reviewed and fewer than half offered a specific elective on this topic (Russett & Williams, 2015). The Council on Social Work Education (CSWE) developed a substance misuse curriculum guide built around its nine Core Competencies (CSWE, in press); however, this provides resources for guiding curriculum development, not a curriculum requirement or mandate.

One international example of systematic change outside of university-based training is Sweden's government response to the lack of university-educated social workers in AOD assessment. They developed a national education and implementation program using the Addiction Severity Index (ASI), an evidence-supported SUD and risky substance use assessment protocol, across Swedish national health and welfare systems. Prior evaluation studies identified significant limitations in the information collected through the nation's social services SUD care system: client information was documented in an unsystematic manner and the information, contained in hand-written client journals, was difficult to use, even by social workers who provided the written descriptions. This necessitated the development of mechanisms for training workers in the National Board of Health and Welfare (NBHW) system to identify and intervene around risky substance use or SUD (Tengvald, 1996). Training and use of this evidence-based assessment instrument began in Sweden during the 1990s.

The ASI as used today in Sweden, based on the fifth version (McLellan et al., 1992) collects relevant and reliable assessment information for use in treatment planning, client follow-up, and evaluation and implementation studies. The NBHW, which manages conduct of the ASI, assumed a coordinating role and supported the nationwide education activities of ASI trainers and methodologists, local and regional experts, R&D departments, regional coordinators, experts, researchers, and IT companies. Results from the first user study showed that both the social workers who used the ASI and their clients viewed the implementation favorably: 90% of clients were very satisfied (Engström, 2005) and approximately 90% of counties in Sweden now use the ASI in assessment. The ASI educational program became a cornerstone in implementing nationwide SUD screening and assessment in Sweden. The NBHW assumed responsibility for the education and training of both new and experienced trainers, an important part of the quality assurance in ASI use. Above all, ASI education contributed to an increase in social workers using empirically based methods in their substance-related work with clients.

In the United States, professional and government organizations actively encouraged educators in health and helping professions to develop AOD curricula and expertise. Examples include the NIAAA's online curriculum for the prevention and treatment of alcohol use disorders, the National Association of Social Workers' AOD specialist certification criteria, and the Association for Multidisciplinary Education and Research in Substance Use and Addiction's (AMERSA) ProjectMainstream curriculum. At the NIH, both the National Institute on Alcohol Abuse and Alcoholism and the National Institute on Drug Abuse have a long history of supporting health professions education initiatives and research on alcohol and drug curricula development for physicians, nurses, psychologists, and social workers. The National Association for Children of Alcoholics (NACoA) sponsored development of a training curriculum for faith leaders, as well.

The Alcohol and Other Drugs Education Program (ADEP)

The Alcohol and Other Drugs Education Program (ADEP) was developed and implemented by Lundgren and colleagues, funded by the NIAAA, and began in 2017. The specific

Table 37.1 Faculty integration of alcohol and other drug use content into social work instruction, by topic

In your teaching about the following topics, how often do you cover alcohol and other drug use/addiction?

2018 cohort: N and % of sample reported they always cover AOD content in detail

	N	%
Life course		
Pregnancy and childbirth	5	11.1
Adolescence and youth development	8	16.7
Aging and older adults	5	10.9
Social environment		
Poverty/inequality	10	20.8
Intimate partner violence	3	6.3
Crime/criminal justice system	9	18.8
Homelessness	2	4.3
Health outcomes	0	0
Mental health disorders	12	25.0
Trauma and posttraumatic stress	9	18.8
HIV/AIDS	2	4.3

aim of ADAP was to train social work faculty to educate social work graduate students in empirically supported AOD identification and treatment methods and evaluate the outcomes. Ultimately, ADEP aims to see AOD content incorporated into social work curricula throughout the United States. Fifty faculty members from 29 MSW programs across 18 states participated in the first ADEP immersion training (2017); 48 from 30 MSW programs across 27 states participated in ADEP 2018.

Most of the faculty participants were not previously incorporating AOD content in their courses despite these courses covering subjects directly associated with substance use: topics such as mental health disorders, adolescent development, trauma, and HIV/AIDS. Fewer than 40% of training participants initially reported having ever taken a course in AOD/substance use or addiction during their own graduate social work training. Compared to their peers, faculty members who had completed AOD coursework were significantly more likely to cover alcohol and other drug abuse/addiction in their teaching (Table 37.1).

The year 1 ADEP program evaluation demonstrated efficacy, significantly increasing faculty members' knowledge and confidence about teaching AOD content and skills (Lundgren et al., 2018). Participants gained in knowledge across all four data collection time points: pretest, posttest, and 6- and 12-month follow-up (see Figure 37.1), although the sample decreased from 50 at pre- and immediate posttest to 31 at 12-month follow-up. The mean number of correct responses to AOD knowledge questions increased from 8.8 at pretest to 13.8 at posttest.

The greatest improvements in trainees' knowledge concerned SBIRT, Medication-Assisted Treatment (MAT), and the biological-genetic causes and consequences of SUD. Trainees followed for one year also demonstrated gains in teaching confidence around

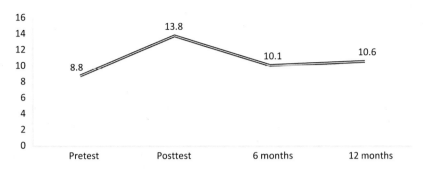

Figure 37.1 Baseline and follow-up correct knowledge scores for ADEP faculty fellows 2017 cohort

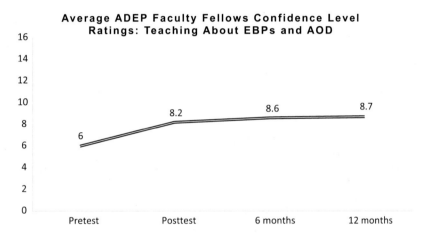

Figure 37.2 Baseline and follow-up confidence scores for ADEP faculty fellows 2017 cohort

evidence-based practices across the four data collection time points (see Figure 37.2), based on means from a 10-point confidence scale (F (3, 30) = 17.51, $p < 0.001$).

AOD knowledge among the faculty participants' students was compared to knowledge among a control group not taught by these faculty participants. At the beginning of the semester (baseline), no significant knowledge difference was detected between the two student groups: $t(133) = 1.09$, $p = 0.28$. Lowest student baseline knowledge scores concerned: (1) evidence-based practices (EBPs)—11.9% had correct answers; (2) screening, brief intervention, and referral to treatment (SBIRT)—12.6% answered correctly; and (3) medication-assisted treatment (MAT)—11.9% answered correctly. Both student groups had the highest baseline knowledge score on alcohol use, with little more than half in each group providing correct answers. At the end of the semester (follow-up), students of ADEP-trained faculty demonstrated significantly greater AOD knowledge (F (1, 126) = 4.22, $p = 0.04$), specifically in areas of MAT and SBIRT. Additionally, students of ADEP participants, compared to control group students, demonstrated significantly higher knowledge of AOD DSM-5 diagnostic severity (t (151.941) = −2.5010, $p = 0.013$), as well as increased knowledge about alcohol.

It is both important and concerning that the lowest levels of faculty and student knowledge with the first ADEP cohort reflected two areas promoted by SAMHSA, NIH, and the World Health Organization as critical in the identification, treatment, and prevention of risky substance use and SUD—SBIRT and MAT)—and treatment of opioid use disorder—MAT. Hence, it is critical that any AOD core curriculum include this content. In addition, 12-month results from cohort 1 indicated not only that ADEP increased faculty participants' AOD knowledge and confidence in teaching AOD content, but also that this knowledge and confidence was transmitted to their students who completed the student survey. Together these results suggest that if faculty members' knowledge and confidence about teaching AOD content improves, student learning benefits.

As the United States and Swedish examples suggest, there need to be significant efforts and investment in promoting AOD curriculum development and implementation, including around empirically supported screening, assessment, and treatment for risky substance use and SUD. Even though a country may lack systematic national AOD education requirements for health professionals, a range of continuing education institutions provide training around MI, SBIRT, and other AOD topics. However, many university programs where social workers and other health professionals receive their core professional education have no core-curriculum in AOD content. Given that there exists significant empirically supported knowledge about AOD and evidence-supported AOD practices, as well as emerging empirical knowledge from studies testing AOD educational programs, it is key that that professional education curricula informed by this significant knowledge base be developed and disseminated.

AOD core curricula for social work education

What currently characterizes many social work and other professional training programs currently is the lack of a systematic, explicit AOD curriculum. Curriculum recommendations provided here are suited to generalist programs around the world; some content is more suited to specialized AOD clinical practice. These curriculum recommendations were developed based on: (1) evaluation results from the ADEP program; (2) consistent themes described by the first two ADEP cohorts; (3) the authors' experiences with implementing ASI as a national assessment instrument in Sweden; (3) recommendations from the United Nations Office on Drugs and Crime (UNODC), National Association of Social Workers (NASW), and CSWE; and (4) authors' experiences reviewing and implementing social work education internationally. The ADEP curriculum is available at https://socialwork.du.edu/about/gssw-directory/lena-lundgren, and the UNODC training materials are available at https://www.unodc.org/unodc/en/treatment-and-care/treatnet-training-package.html. Skill domains recommended for NASW specialist AOD training are presented at https://www.socialworkers.org/LinkClick.aspx?fileticket=BUoelgdF-yQ%3d&portalid=0. The CSWE curriculum guide on substance misuse (in press) represents another resource to direct curriculum development and many topics are developed in the evidence-based practices book by Lundgren and Krull (2018), as well as other chapters in this *Routledge Handbook of Social Work and Addictive Behavior.*

Introductory content

- Why training in AOD matters (global, national, local prevalence/epidemiology evidence;
- Social work or other professional roles where AOD issues are encountered;
- Need for expanded AOD-trained professional workforce); professional responsibility for AOD education;

- Perceptions about individuals engaged in AOD misuse or experiencing SUDs;
- Societal responses to AOD misuse/SUD in different societies/nations;
- International (World Health Organization and United Nations) and national recommendations for AOD education.

Etiology and consequences of AOD misuse and substance use disorders

- AOD/substance misuse as biopsychosocial and transdisciplinary phenomena;
- Biological (genetic, neurobiology), psychological, and social context/social norms influences on AOD use, misuse, and use disorders (see Chapters 4, 5, 6, and 7);
- Biological, psychological, and social consequences of AOD misuse and SUDs, including relationships, finances, housing security, physical and mental health, premature death/disability, disease exposure, accidental injury, fetal exposure, incarceration, child maltreatment, intimate partner violence, and sexual assault (see Chapters 3, 11, 12, 23, 27, 34, and 35);
- Social determinants of AOD-related health parity/disparities; two-way relationships between trauma/stress and AOD misuse (including experiences of war, community violence, interpersonal/family violence, sexual violence, and adverse childhood events).

History and philosophies underlying responses to AOD misuse

- Historical trends and traditions in responding to AOD misuse;
- Harm reduction;
- Treatment versus punishment or incarceration;
- Defining recovery;
- Defining "addiction";
- Evidence and practice (evidence-based practice/EBP, evidence-based practices/EBPs, evidence-supported practice, evidence-informed practice);
- Roles of formal treatment versus informal help (e.g. mutual help/12-step programs, peer support, natural/significant others);
- "Natural" recovery.

AOD screening

- Screening principles, practices, and evidence-supported tools;
- Screening for AOD misuse in non-specialist settings;
- The screening, brief intervention and referral to treatment (SBIRT) model and its supporting evidence (see Chapter 20);
- How to respond to positive and negative screening results;
- How motivational interviewing (MI) skills facilitate screening.

SUD diagnosis and assessment

- Diagnostic and Statistical Manual version 5 (DSM-5) and/or International Classification of Disease version 11 (ICD-11) criteria for diagnosing alcohol and other substance use disorders, withdrawal, and related problems (see Chapter 1 and Appendix A);
- Dynamic nature of diagnostic criteria;
- How diagnosis informs treatment planning (see Chapter 18);

- Evidence-supported tools for AOD/SUD assessment (e.g. Addiction Severity Index/ ASI, Addiction Science for American Medicine (ASAM) criteria, Global Assessment of Individual Needs/GAIN).

Intervening around AOD problems

- Case management and navigator models, treatment modalities, and relapse prevention (evidence-supported practices in these areas; see Chapter 18);
- When and how to refer individuals or families for treatment;
- Medication-assisted treatment (MAT), evidence supporting combined medication and behavioral therapies, resistance to MAT, and social work roles in supporting MAT (see Chapters 18 and 19);
- Other recovery supporting practices, including peer-to-peer, peer recovery specialist models (see Chapter 29), and mindfulness/meditation (see Chapter 21);
- Motivational interviewing in engagement, retention, and relapse prevention; continuity of care.

Co-occurring mental health problems

- Epidemiology of co-occurring mental health disorders (MHDs) and AOD misuse/SUD;
- Impact of MHDs and AOD misuse/SUD on each other and on treatment for each;
- Need and evidence support for integrated care approach;
- Examples of integrated care approach (e.g. Seeking Safety; Integrated Dual Diagnosis Treatment/IDDT).

Conclusions

This chapter began with an acknowledgment that in most countries, social workers and other health professionals do not receive adequate empirically supported AOD education and skills training that enables them to work effectively with clients and patients who engage in risky substance use or experience SUDs. Globally many social workers do not receive sufficient evidence-informed education about AOD misuse and SUDs from a bio-psychosocial framework. Neither do they receive education in the significant amount of empirical knowledge available with respect to causes and consequences of SUDs or treating and preventing SUDs.

This lack of education represents a major barrier to more effective responses to globally increased rates of AOD misuse and SUDs. The lack of university supported education regarding AOD use and SUD leads to a range of funders and institutions having to assume responsibility for educating and training professionals to work with individuals around AOD and SUD concerns. This has resulted in non-systematic, erratically provided education and skills training that is poorly integrated into the conceptual framework of the profession. Thus, developing and implementing standards, guidelines, and examples of evidence-informed and evidence-supported AOD curricula is critically important. This means AOD curricula based on empirical knowledge describing social work and cross-disciplinary approaches that: (1) have been tested and summarized through meta-analysis and systematic review, (2) are implemented in different countries; and (3) can be applied in a range of organizational settings. Finally, curriculum guidelines, such as those suggested in this chapter, can be included in both generalist and more specialized training globally.

Acknowledgments

We acknowledge and thank the National Institute on Alcohol Abuse and Alcoholism for funding grant number 1H79TI025951, the ADEP Program. Results presented in this chapter were developed based on work completed with support from this grant.

References

Andrews, C. M., Darnell, J. S., McBride, T. D., & Gehlert, S. (2013). Social work and implementation of the affordable care act. *Health and Social Work, 38*(2), 67–71. doi:10.1093/hsw/hlt002

Babor, T. F., McRee, B. G., Kassebaum, P. A., Grimaldi, P. L., Ahmed, K., & Bray, J. (2007). Screening, brief intervention, and referral to treatment (SBIRT): Toward a public health approach to the management of substance abuse. *Substance Abuse, 28*(3), 7–30. doi:10.1300/J465v28n03_03

Block, S. R., Wheeland, L., & Rosenberg, S. (2014). Improving human service effectiveness through the deconstruction of case management: A case study on the emergence of a team-based model of service coordination. *Human Service Organizations Management Leadership and Governance, 38*(1), 16–28. doi:10.1080/03643107.2013.853007

Boulware, L. E., Hill-Briggs, F., Kraus, E. S., Melancon, J. K., Falcone, B., Ephraim, P. L., . . . Powe, N. R. (2013). Effectiveness of educational and social worker interventions to activate patients' discussion and pursuit of preemptive living donor kidney transplantation: A randomized controlled trial. *American Journal of Kidney Disease, 61*(3), 476–486. doi:10.1053/j.ajkd.2012.08.039

Council on Social Work Education (CSWE). (2018). *Results of the nationwide survey of 2017 social work graduates. The national workforce study.* Alexandria, VA: CSWE Press.

Council on Social Work Education (CSWE). (in press). *Curricular guide on substance misuse.* Alexandria, VA: CSWE Press.

Duong, D. K., O'Sullivan, P. S., Satre, D. D., Soskin, P., & Satterfield, J. (2016). Social workers as workplace-based instructors of alcohol and drug screening, brief intervention, and referral to treatment (SBIRT) for emergency medicine residents. *Teaching and Learning in Medicine, 28*(3), 303–313. doi:10.1080/10401334.2016.1164049

Engström, C. (2005). *Implementering och utvärdering av addiction severity index (ASI) i socialtjänsten* (Doctoral Dissertation). Institutionen för psykologi, Umeå universitet.

GBD 2016 Alcohol and Drug Use Collaborators. (2018). The global burden of disease attributable to alcohol and drug use in 195 countries and territories, 1990–2016: A systematic analysis for the global burden of disease study 2016. *Lancet Psychiatry, 5*(12), 987–1012.

Hohman, M., Pierce, P., & Barnett, E. (2015). Motivational interviewing: An evidence-based practice for improving student practice skills. *Journal of Social Work Education, 51*(2), 287–97. doi:10.1080/10437797.2015.1012925

Kelly, T. M., & Daley, D. C. (2013). Integrated treatment of substance use and psychiatric disorders. *Social Work and Public Health, 28,* 388–406. doi:10.1080/19371918.2013.774673

Krull, I., Salas-Wright, C., Amodeo, M., Hall, T., Alford, D., & Lundgren, L. (2018). Integrating alcohol and other drug content in the social work curriculum: Practices and perceived barriers. *Journal of Social Work Practice in the Addictions, 18*(1), 30–40. doi:10.1080/1533256X.2017.1412978

Leach, M. J., & Segal, L. (2011). Patient attributes warranting consideration in clinical practice guidelines, health workforce planning and policy. *BMC Health Services Research, 11,* 221. doi:10.1186/1472-6963-11-221

Lundblad, K. S. (1995). Jane Addams and social reform: A role model for the 1990s. *Social Work, 40*(5), 661–669.

Lundgren, L., Amodeo, M., Chassler, D., Krull, I., & Sullivan, L. (2013). Organizational readiness for change in community-based addiction treatment programs and adherence in implementing evidence-based practices: A national study. *Journal of Substance Abuse Treatment, 45*(5), 457–65. doi:10.1016/j.jsat.2013.06.007

Lundgren, L., Chassler, D., Amodeo, M., D'Ippolito, M., & Sullivan, L. (2012). Barriers to implementation of evidence-based addiction treatment: A national study. *Journal of Substance Abuse Treament, 42*(3), 231–238. doi:10.1016/j.jsat.2011.08.003

Lundgren, L., & Krull, I. (2018). *Screening, assessment and treatment for substance use disorder in the era of integrated care.* New York, NY: Oxford University Press.

Lundgren, L., Salas-Wright, C., Amodeo, M., Krull, I., Hall, T., & Alford, D. (2018). Advancing alcohol and other drug education among social work faculty: An evaluation of social work faculty immersion training. *Journal of Social Work Practice in the Addictions*. doi:10.1080/1533256X.2017.1412977

McLellan, A. T., & Woodworth, A. M. (2014). The affordable care act and treatment for "substance use disorders": Implications of ending segregated behavioral healthcare. *Journal of Substance Abuse Treatment, 46*(5), 541–545. doi:10.1016/j.jsat.2014.02.001

McLellan, T. M., Kushner, H., Metzger, D., Peters, R., Smith, I., Grissom, G., . . . Argeriou, M. (1992). The fifth edition of the addiction severity index. *Journal of Substance Abuse Treatment, 9*, 199–213. doi:10.1016/0740-5472(92)90062-S

Ogden, L. P., Vinjamuri, M., & Kahn, J. M. (2016). A model for implementing an evidence-based practice in student fieldwork placements: Barriers and facilitators to the use of "SBIRT". *Journal of Social Service Research, 42*(4), 425–441. doi:10.1080/01488376.2016.1182097

Peterson, J. A. (1965). From social settlement to social agency: Settlement work in Columbus, Ohio, 1898–1958. *Social Service Review, 39*(2), 191–208. doi:10.1086/641739

Rose, S. J., Brondino, M. J., & Barnack, J. L. (2009). Screening for problem substance use in community-based agencies. *Journal of Social Work Practice in the Addictions, 9*(1), 41–54. doi:10.1080/15332560802664938

Ross, S., & Peselow, E. (2012). Co-occurring psychotic and addictive disorders: Neurobiology and diagnosis. *Clinical Neuropharmacology, 35*(5), 235–243. doi:10.1097/WNF.0b013e318261e193

Roy-Byrne, P., Bumgardner, K., Krupski A., Dunn, C., Ries, R., Donovan, D., . . . Zarkin, G. A. (2014). Brief intervention for problem drug use in safety-net primary care settings: A randomized clinical trial. *Journal of American Medical Association, 312*(5), 492–501. doi:10.1001/jama.2014.7860

Russett, J. L., & Williams, A. (2015). An exploration of substance abuse course offerings for students in counseling and social work programs. *Substance Abuse, 36*(1), 51–58. doi:10.1080/08897077.2014.933153

Salas-Wright, C., Lundgren, L., & Amodeo, M. (2018). Introduction to the special issue: Educating social workers about alcohol and other drug use disorders. *Journal of Social Work Practice in the Addictions, 18*(1), 1–7. doi:10.1080/1533256X.2018.1412663

Senreich, E., Ogden, L. P., & Greenberg, J. P. (2017). A postgraduation follow-up of social work students trained in "SBIRT": Rates of usage and perceptions of effectiveness. *Social Work and Health Care, 56*(5), 412–34. doi:10.1080/00981389.2017.1290010

Substance Abuse Mental Health Services Administration (SAMHSA). (2017). *Key substance use and mental health indicators in the United States: Results from the 2016 national survey on drug use and health* (HHS Publication No. SMA 17-5044, NSDUH Series H-52). Rockville, MD: Center for Behavioral Health Statistics and Quality, SAMHSA. Retrieved from https://www.samhsa.gov/data/report/key-substance-use-and-mental-health-indicators-united-states-results-2016-national-survey

Tengvald, K. (1996). *Krav och problem med systematiserad klientinformation. I: Berglund m.fl. Dokumentation i missbrukarvården. Behandlingsarbete Metodutveckling Utvärdering*. Stockholm, Sweden: Liber/CUS.

Wahab, S. (2005). Motivational interviewing and social work practice. *Journal of Social Work, 5*(1), 45–60. doi:10.1177/1468017305051365

Wamsley, M., Satterfield, J., Curtis, A., Lundgren, L., & Sartre, D. (2018). Alcohol and drug screening, brief intervention and referral to treatment (SBIRT) training and implementation: Perspectives from four health professions. *Journal of Addiction Medicine, 12*(4), 262–272. doi:10.1097/ADM.0000000000000410

Wilkey, C., Lundgren, L., & Amodeo, M. (2013). Addiction training in social work schools: A nationwide analysis. *Journal of Social Work Practice in the Addictions, 13*(2), 192–210. doi:10.1081/1533256X.2013.785872

38

Using GIS and spatial analysis to better integrate context into our understanding of addictive behaviors

Bridget Freisthler and Nancy Jo Kepple

Background

Geographic information systems—or GIS—is the process of creating, organizing, and managing geographic data. Essentially, GIS is the process of creating maps from addresses and displaying data by geographic location or areas. Mapping the local environment helps point out areas where alcohol and drug problems appear to cluster. This information can help practitioners identify areas with high densities of substance-related problems or substance availability, and open dialog with neighborhood residents about resources and risks located within their neighborhood or other areas where they spend time.

Creating maps in GIS software is a visual way to depict neighborhood conditions that can motivate neighborhood residents to organize and take action. For example, providing a community member with a list of alcohol outlets may not be as impactful as showing them a map of the locations of alcohol outlets within their neighborhood and surrounding areas. We first explore how GIS can enhance community practice before introducing the benefits of spatial analysis and its application to evaluating place-based drug policies.

Case study: Sacramento Neighborhood Alcohol Prevention Project

The Sacramento Neighborhood Alcohol Prevention Project (SNAPP) applied environmental interventions within a quasi-experimental research design to reduce alcohol-related problems in two California neighborhoods from 1999 to 2003 (see Figure 38.1).

SNAPP included five intervention components: (1) community mobilization; (2) community awareness; (3) responsible beverage service; (4) enforcement of sales to underage minors; and (5) enforcement of sales to intoxicated patrons (Treno, Lee, Freisthler, Remer, & Gruenewald, 2005).

- *Community mobilization* efforts were designed to provide support for all the interventions by reaching out to community gatekeepers and influential community leaders. The mobilization team included business owners, local police, leads of non-profit agencies, and members of the research team. These individuals provided support within the community and guidance for the remaining interventions.

601

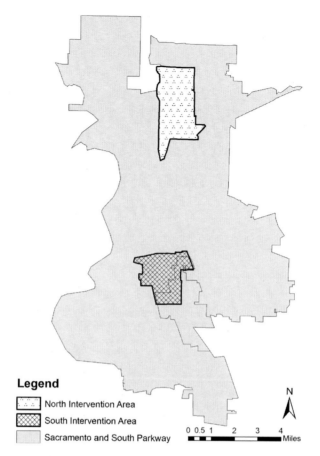

Figure 38.1 Location of North and South intervention areas in Sacramento, CA

- *Community awareness* was designed to inform neighborhood residents about the problems related to youth and young adult drinking, laws about underage possession and sales to intoxicated patrons, and inform them of the remaining interventions. A key focus of this intervention discussing the harms that can occur when alcohol is provided informally to minors. This was implemented through a variety of home meetings where information was shared about the extent of alcohol-related problems within each of the neighborhood areas.
- *Responsible beverage service training* provided two different types of trainings. In the first, training targeted to bars and restaurants focused on strategies that prevent over serving alcohol. This included keeping glasses on the table in order to identify how many alcoholic drinks have been consumed. The second type of training was primarily targeted to off-premise outlets (i.e. those places where alcohol is purchased to be consumed at another location, such as liquor store) and provided specialized training in how to spot fake IDs and ensuring that store clerks do not sell alcohol to individuals without IDs. We collaborated with local police to implement the final two interventions.
- *Enforcement of sales to underage minors* involved police sending underage decoys (referred to as a "sting") into off-premise outlets to determine if the outlet would sell alcohol

illegally to someone who was underage. Businesses that did sell alcohol to underage decoys were given a citation.

• *Enforcement of sales to intoxicated patrons* involved police entering on-premise outlets (bars and restaurants) to watch for sales of alcohol to already intoxicated patrons and provide citations to outlets engaging in those business practices.

A framework for using maps in communities

Elwood (2006) provides one useful framework for thinking about how maps can help communities understand their local environments and enact change to improve their conditions. Specifically, we explain the core tenets of mapping community needs, community assets, injustices, accomplishments, and reinterpretation (Elwood, 2006). As we discuss the core tenets of this framework, we use SNAPP as one illustration of how this appears in practice.

Mapping community needs

Using maps to illustrate community needs shows potential problems with neighborhood spaces and structures, or ills experienced by those living in those areas (Elwood, 2006). Showing community needs via maps provides a powerful depiction of where a neighborhood may need resources or supports (Hillier, 2007). In Sacramento, we used maps in the South intervention area to determine the extent to which off-premise alcohol outlets sold alcohol to underage minors. Figure 38.2 shows the locations of off-premise alcohol outlets and whether they sold to an apparent minor during our baseline survey. An apparent minor is a person who was over 21 but deemed by a panel of individuals who work with youth to look less than 21.

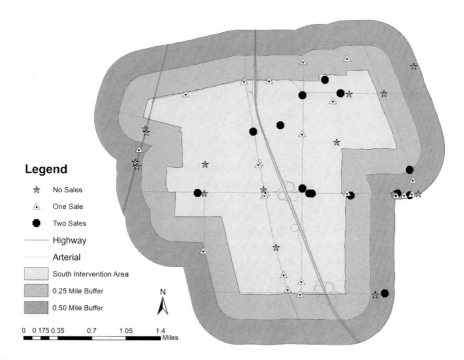

Figure 38.2 Underage alcohol purchases by apparent minors in South intervention area in Sacramento, CA during Wave 1

There are two ways to define "need" based on this map. The first is that 49% of purchase attempts resulted in a successful purchase (two attempts per establishment). In this map, you can see the number of establishments that sold alcohol zero, one, or two times. When looking at the map's legend that includes depictions for number of times each outlet sold alcohol, almost half of the attempts resulted in the sale of alcohol. A second way to understand this map is to look at the number of establishments that sold alcohol. With that orientation to the data, you can see that 67% of all outlets sold to the apparent minors at least once. For underage youth living in that community, the likelihood they could obtain alcohol was fairly high.

Community assets

While needs can begin to reveal problematic locations, assets provide information on what resources already exist to make change in the same areas (Elwood, 2006). The SNAPP interventions for community mobilization needed to know the locations of agencies and individuals that could be mobilized to help create change. A map illustrating community assets may show locations of local community agencies and businesses that provide services to the intervention areas to target with mobilization efforts.

Injustices

Maps can also show inequalities between neighborhoods or other places (Elwood, 2006). By using maps in this way, neighborhood residents can see places—some with similar demographic and economic characteristics—which do not have the same level of problems or have different types of needs. Figure 38.3 shows differences in rates of sales to apparent minors across the entire SNAPP study area. In the South intervention area, 49% of attempts resulted in a successful purchase; however, only 20% of the attempts in the North intervention area resulted in a successful purchase of alcohol, while that number was 38% in the rest of Sacramento (Treno et al., 2005). These disparities become very clear in this map. In fact, the North area had no alcohol establishments that sold alcohol during more than one of the two attempts.

Accomplishments

As an intervention unfolds in an area or as a neighborhood's residents and community organizations begin working together for change, recognizing accomplishments, regardless of size, is important. Sharing accomplishments is one way to show the successes that have already occurred (Elwood, 2006). For SNAPP, these accomplishments initially took the form of assessing process outcomes. First, we measured the number of off-premise establishments taking part in training for Responsible Beverage Service (RBS) (see Figure 38.4a). Just about half (49%) received the RBS training. Off-premise establishments received a letter from the police notifying them that apparent underage youth purchase attempts would be occurring in order to encourage establishments to offer the training to their workers. In the second community accomplishment (Figure 38.4b), we show the locations of police stings, which were conducted in more than half of the outlets in the South intervention area; out of those locations, only seven received citations. The question remains: were these accomplishments enough to reduce sales of alcohol to underage minors?

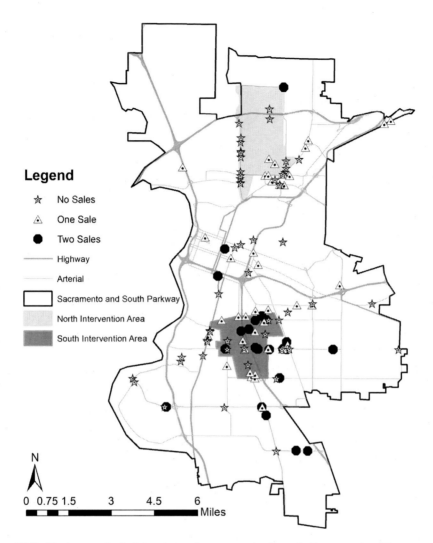

Figure 38.3 Underage alcohol purchases by apparent minors in Sacramento, CA

Reinterpretation

Through reinterpretation, official data can be presented through a new lens that helps advance neighborhood priorities or agendas (Elwood, 2006). In the SNAPP intervention, we conducted another survey of sales to apparent minors two years after the baseline survey was completed. At that point, apparent minors were only able to purchase alcohol 32% of the time (Figure 38.5), representing a 34% decrease. The reinterpretation process occurred on two levels. First, it demonstrated to residents that they could make positive changes in their communities by working together and with local business owners and police. Second, residents more quickly organized around issues related to alcohol outlet density and sales to minors after seeing successful results.

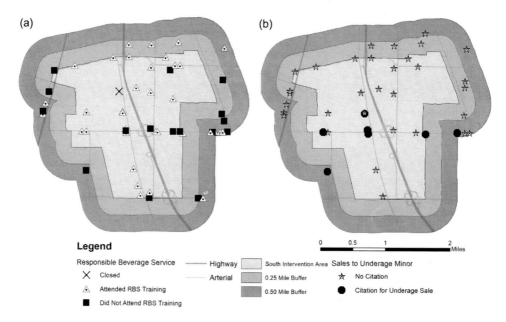

Figure 38.4 Depiction of accomplishments in South intervention area, Sacramento, CA. (a) Locations of off-premise alcohol outlets trained in responsible beverage service in South intervention area. (b) Location of Sacramento Police Stings at off-premise alcohol outlets in South intervention area

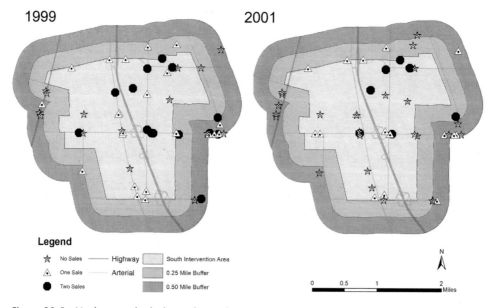

Figure 38.5 Underage alcohol purchases by apparent minors in South intervention area in Sacramento, CA during Wave 1 (1999) and Wave 2 (2001)

Pitfalls of relying on maps alone

What mapping alone cannot do is to indicate whether the observed spatial patterns are artifacts of the data or statistically important relationships. Additionally, how the information in the map is presented can also lead to different interpretations. Information in maps can be presented via points, polygons (i.e. areas, shapes), or lines. Many points (e.g. locations of all people) may clutter the map or make some spatial feature appear overwhelming. However, those same points aggregated to a polygon unit (e.g. count of people per zip codes) ease the interpretation or ability to make sense of the map.

Counts versus rates

Depending on how data are displayed, interpretation may vary. Counts show the exact number of some characteristic or phenomenon (e.g. number of people). For example, Census data are often used to display the demographic and socioeconomic status of areas. These administrative units from the Census are based on population and designed to represent about the same number of people per each unit; the larger the unit, the greater the likelihood the population is distributed across a larger area. While these places visually dominate a map, that visual does not correlate with a larger population size than smaller units.

Alternatively, rates themselves can be misleading. Rates are often based on the underlying population at risk. Despite having a really low population, if everyone engages in substance misuse, the rate will be large. In this case, what looks like a huge problem is really just an artifact of the way the data were presented.

As one example, a map displaying resource counts such as locations of Alcoholics Anonymous (AA) or Narcotics Anonymous (NA) meetings is helpful in assessing where most meetings occur. However, a rate may be a better indicator of whether or not meetings occur in places needed by populations engaged in substance misuse. In order to calculate, you first need to identify the population at risk; in this case, those engaged in substance misuse. Identifying the size of this population is difficult, so we often use proxies like the number of people seeking treatment per zip code or county. This approach standardizes the availability of meetings and allows you to more easily compare across areas. A county may have high numbers of meetings, but a relatively low rate of meetings per person engaged in substance misuse. Thus, depending on the question of interest, data may need to be presented in multiple formats in order to better assess the needs and resources of a community.

Visual versus statistical relationships

Human eyes assess visual patterns and visual anomalies. However, noticing a pattern on a map does not mean that a statistical relationship exists. A map of child abuse and neglect rates by Census tract is presented in Figure 38.6. This figure also overlays the locations of incidents from drug sales. Together, it appears that locations of drug sales are correlated to rates of child maltreatment. However, using spatial analysis techniques, Freisthler, Gruenewald, Johnson, Treno and Lascala (2005) showed they are in fact not related. A map showing two variables is not likely to show other cofounding variables (e.g. poverty) that might be more influential to the problem at hand. To assess the statistical significance of the visual relationship between two variables, we conduct spatial analyses.

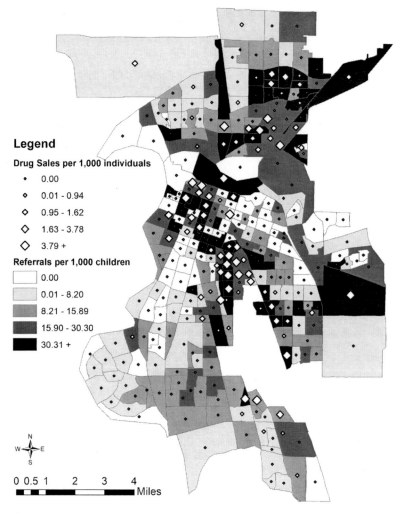

Figure 38.6   Rates of incidents of drug sales overlaid on rates of child abuse and neglect in Sacramento, CA

Spatial analysis

Spatial analysis is the process by which spatial data can be assessed statistically to determine if places share characteristics with other spatial phenomena, how characteristics of places may be related to various outcomes, and how movement across the environment may affect risk of exposure to certain social problems (Waller & Gotway, 2004). Every event occurs in some location; the goal of spatial analysis is to determine if that location was important in understanding that event. Spatial analysis provides techniques to assess the unique role of physical location, density (defined by a measure of locations or events occurring within a specified area), and distance (from a related location or event) in understanding substance misuse and related problems (Bailey & Gatrell, 1995; Waller & Gotway, 2004). The use of spatial analysis, even descriptive, can help provide greater context for the numbers that might otherwise be displayed in a table or reduced to some basic level statistics (e.g. average rate of problems across an area). Seeing in a table a high rate of violence in the zip code where you live might not be as impactful as seeing the same rate on a map showing the rate of violence for your neighborhood to be in the highest quartile. To illustrate this, we use descriptive spatial analyses to explore how to use the maps discussed in the prior section on the Elwood (2006) framework.

While spatial analyses take different forms, we only discuss a few basics here.

Exploratory spatial data analysis

The purpose of exploratory data analysis is similar to exploratory analyses with traditional statistical data (Waller & Gotway, 2004). It provides a feel for the data in order to identify nuances of the information related to place. One concern in mapping data, particularly when looking at rates or counts across areas, is that areas adjacent to each other may have similar values. This can result in spatial autocorrelation (Bailey & Gatrell, 1995), meaning that each areal unit is not independent of another. For example, the density of dispensaries in one neighborhood is dependent, in some way, on the density of dispensaries in its adjacent neighborhoods. From a practical perspective, this might mean that any neighborhood intervention or assessment of needs or resources may have to be assessed in adjacent areas as well. The subsequent sections discuss procedures that can help assess spatial autocorrelation and provide greater context about local areas that may be useful while working with community members to identify how best to represent information using maps.

Local indicators of spatial autocorrelation (LISA)

In the course of studying maps, one is likely to observe that alcohol-related problems (e.g. location of assaults, motor vehicle accidents) appear to cluster across areas (e.g. Gruenewald & Johnson, 2010; Lipton & Gruenewald, 2002). This clustering over geographic areas can identify spatial clusters or spatial outliers (Waller & Gotway, 2004). Spatial clusters show neighborhoods (or local areas) that have statistically significant similarities with adjacent areas. This might include areas where rates of problems or densities of dispensaries cluster in concentrated high rates or in concentrated low rates. Put differently, which areas of high density of dispensaries are located next to areas of similar high density of dispensaries? In contrast, spatial outliers seek to identify areas having high or low density of dispensaries, but that are adjacent to areas with the opposite type of density. In this case, while a local neighborhood may have a high density of dispensaries, the adjacent neighborhoods may have no dispensaries. Thus, the density of dispensaries in one neighborhood is a local outlier when compared with those neighborhoods next to it.

Returning to the Elwood (2006) framework for using maps, the spatial outlier of dispensaries could be used to depict injustice. But what if that was an artifact of how the measure was created? Instead, the neighborhood looking like an outlier was because the neighborhood had six dispensaries and neighboring areas had zero or one dispensary. However, a density measure that standardizes the number of dispensaries by some denominator (e.g. area, per capita) might be a better measure, and show the neighborhood is not an outlier.

The exploratory statistics used to identify spatial clustering and spatial outliers are called local indicators of spatial association (LISA). LISA values are considered to be largely descriptive in nature, but they help interpret the univariate data at hand (Anselin, 1995). LISA values cannot tell whether clusters or outliers are there artificially or are due to specific characteristics of the populations or places found in those areas. Multivariate spatial statistics are needed to understand the complexity of the underlying spatial structure of the data.

Global association of spatial autocorrelation

LISA values provide information about spatial data at a local level. Global associations of spatial autocorrelation—such as Moran's I—provide information about the level of spatial dependence across the entire study area (Waller & Gotway, 2004). Thus, while a local neighborhood may not be a spatial outlier or be in a spatial cluster, the larger area (e.g. city or county) may exhibit either positive or negative spatial autocorrelation. Positive spatial auto-correlation reflects the extent to which adjacent neighborhoods share similarly high values on the measure of interest. Negative spatial autocorrelation appears when a local neighborhood has high values on some variable, but adjacent neighborhoods have a low value, or vice versa. The map of negative spatial autocorrelation would appear more like a checkerboard. Assessing spatial autocorrelation at this level may provide information about how one might frame the overall approach of a place-based intervention. As one example, if a significant overall value of positive spatial autocorrelation is found for rates of alcohol-involved violent crimes, then an intervention to reduce bar density might be implemented at larger than the neighborhood level in order to reduce violent crime rates (Livingston et al., 2007).

Turning again to the Elwood (2006) framework, maps of community needs and assets could be slightly misleading if they are not shown in context. For example, social workers can use a map to show the locations of all alcohol-related violent crime in a local neighborhood and use that map to work with neighborhood residents around intervening to reduce or prevent those types of crime. However, if all surrounding neighborhoods have the same problem, such interventions may not be successful in the one neighborhood. Here, one risks having neighborhood residents withdraw from participating in neighborhood initiatives, as they may feel nothing will reduce the problem. If the larger context is provided, however, neighborhood residents may seek to mobilize adjacent neighborhoods in efforts to coordinate an intervention approach on a larger geographic scale.

Integrating context into community practice

In summary, maps are essential tools for community practices related to organizing residents and stakeholders, planning interventions that address needs and leverage assets, and evaluating intervention progress. However, mapping alone has limitations that we can address with the use of spatial analyses to identify underlying relationships that cannot be determined visually. In the next section, we extend how GIS and spatial analyses are useful tools for social workers to examine consequences of place-based policies related to the distribution of psychoactive substances.

Using maps to understand place-based drug policies

Although not allowing assessment of statistical relationships, GIS can be a crucial step in understanding whether place-based policies may have the desired effect of increasing well-being or reducing social problems. Often, local jurisdictions will include place-based provisions to limit densities of dispensaries, primarily through local zoning laws or policies. This can affect the access to resources or increase risks in certain areas within a city or other jurisdiction. To show how place-based policies can be studied, we consider the example of medical marijuana dispensaries in Los Angeles.

Mapping compliance of medical marijuana dispensaries with place-based ordinances

Medical marijuana dispensaries have been the primary venue for obtaining medical marijuana in California since the mid-2000s (California Police Chief's Association, 2009). The first known dispensary in the Los Angeles area was the Los Angeles Cannabis Resource Center in 1996 (Simmons, 2001). In 2007, Los Angeles placed a moratorium on the opening of new dispensaries. The policy—Medical Marijuana Interim Control Ordinance—stated that those currently in operation were grandfathered in, but no new dispensaries would be allowed. In 2009, a California court ruled the moratorium was illegal. From 2007 to 2009, several hundred new dispensaries began operating; actual counts ranged from about 550 to about 650. In 2010, Los Angeles passed a new ordinance limiting the density of dispensaries based on population, with a cap in the city of 70 dispensaries. The original 186 dispensaries were grandfathered in as long as there had not been a change in ownership (although that was later softened). The new ordinance also provided guidelines about location, zoning, hours of operation, and security. Later that year, parts of the ordinance were ruled illegal. In early 2011, the City Council amended the ordinance to state that the 70 dispensaries would be

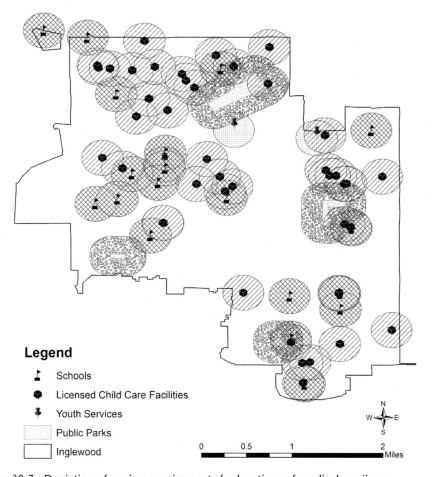

Figure 38.7 Depiction of zoning requirements for locations of medical marijuana

chosen via a lottery process for dispensaries that could prove they were operating in LA in September of 2007 (when the moratorium was passed).

Dispensaries not chosen through the lottery process were to remain closed. Several more policies were enacted after 2011, but for this example, we focus on the guidelines related to location and zoning passed in 2010.

Related to place, the 2010 Los Angeles ordinance provided a list of child and youth organizations, public institutions, and substance abuse facilities from which dispensaries needed to be at least a 1,000-foot radius away. The ordinance also stated that dispensaries may not be located next to residentially zoned property. Where then, could dispensaries be located? We created a map of the City of Inglewood (see Figure 38.7), a much smaller city adjacent to Los Angeles. This map shows only some locations from which a dispensary must be 1,000 feet away. Also shown are locations of the Hollywood Park casino, the Forum stadium, and a local cemetery. This severely limited where dispensaries could be located, even without including the location of residential properties. The concern, then, becomes dispensaries disproportionately locating in areas where already vulnerable populations live. Implicitly (and sometimes even explicitly) the point of these policies is to reduce risk or future problems for residents living in areas of these "undesirable" businesses (e.g. reducing crime, reducing access to illicit use of marijuana, preventing drug abuse). To adequately evaluate the effectiveness of such policies, specific methodological challenges arise and need to be addressed.

Challenges to studying place-based policies using GIS

The first challenge involves understanding the best metric to use when analyzing these data and identifying how the policy operationalizes this metric. For example, one could create a policy that limits dispensary density in an area or per capita, the actual number of those dispensaries, or distances of those places from other types of business or environments. In the example of the Los Angeles policy, the ordinance specifically sought to limit the density per capita (e.g. population). What happens when population changes in those areas? How often will the ordinance assess population changes in relation to where dispensaries are located? The policy does not address these issues but may cause problems over time if locations of dispensaries are related to population loss or zoning changes allow residential areas to emerge. Concerning buffers around locations, what evidence is there that 1,000 feet is the correct distance? In a previous study for the City of Sacramento, we examined the relationship of violent crime at various distances with regard to specific security features dispensaries employed to see if those features were related to lower counts of crime (Freisthler, Kepple, Sims, & Martin, 2013). We found statistically significant differences for buffers at 500 feet or less. While there is only one study with a small sample size, it illustrates that we need more research to understand how place-based policies may actually prevent or reduce substance misuse.

A related problem that occurs when using underlying geographic areas to create place-based policies is that area boundaries may change. Zip codes used by the post office to deliver mail change regularly, largely due to changes in underlying populations and changes in postal carrier routes (Ginsberg, 2011). This results in misalignment of the underlying shape boundaries.

Without attention to this misalignment and changes in population size, the density of dispensaries may look very different over time, even if their locations stay the same (Waller & Gotway, 2004).

Another challenge in understanding effects of place-based policies is that they generally apply to very specific geographic locales. In our previous example, buffers extend into locations beyond the geographic boundaries of the City of Inglewood and into areas not under the jurisdiction of Inglewood policies. In other words, spatial locations end. Thus, nothing prevents dispensaries from opening in areas immediately adjacent to Inglewood. These are known as edge effects (Waller & Gotway, 2004). Examining place-based policies means understanding how these policies are implemented across the areas near the specific area identified for the intervention.

Similar to edge effects, geographic spillover or contamination can also occur. In some instances, this could be good. An intervention in a neighborhood designed to reduce supply of alcohol, for example, could reduce alcohol access in neighboring areas if populations from those adjacent areas purchase alcohol in the intervention neighborhood. However, these effects can be negative for a couple of reasons. First, using our dispensary example, any negative effects of dispensaries (e.g. increases in crime) may not be contained to just the geographic area immediately surrounding the dispensaries. As people move in and out of these areas, problems can increase along the routes these individuals take, or with respect to problematic substance use, in the areas where these individuals spend time. Second, spillover makes it difficult to assess the efficacy of interventions unless they are explicitly modeled. Thus, an understanding of place-based policies requires consideration of areas adjacent to where the policies are implemented. This has significant implications for national policies and borders.

We illustrated only one example of how place-based policies can be assessed by looking at the location of medical marijuana dispensaries. Place-based policies are popular ways for jurisdictions to regulate availability of alcohol and drug supply and their consequences. For example, these approaches can be used to assess locations of alcohol outlets, access to treatment facilities, locations of illicit drug available, or availability of licit drugs (e.g. pharmacies), which have been the focus of thefts during the opioid crisis.

How spatial analysis addresses limitations of GIS to examine place-based policies

In the previous section, we discussed how GIS can help assess the efficacy of place-based policies in achieving desirable outcomes. As noted, this process becomes ripe for misunderstanding or misclassification of results if various challenges are not addressed. The good news is that spatial analysis procedures can address the limitations of mapping to assess policy and provide sound evidence for the effects of policy changes, even at a local level. Spatial regression models can assess and control for spatial autocorrelation so that estimates of the intervention's effects will be less biased (Waller & Gotway, 2004). We describe additional methods, how they address the challenges of mapping to assess place-based policies, and results from work employing some of these statistical techniques.

Addressing misalignment

The success of a place-based policy is dependent on whether these policies independently contribute to a reduction of problems that the policy was designed to address. We previously noted that geographic boundaries are often arbitrary (e.g. zip codes) and change over time. Thus, the provisions in place-based policy around density or per capita numbers of undesirable land features (e.g. dispensaries, alcohol outlets) may not be consistent over time. To identify whether misalignment has occurred, you must assess whether the geographic units in the study stay the same over time, or whether the boundaries can and do shift. Every ten years, when the U.S. Census is conducted, changes to Census geographic areas (e.g. tracts, block groups) will adjust for the underlying size of the population living in these areas. The Census provides a crosswalk that matches old Census areas to the new areas (U.S. Census Bureau, 2015). Not all boundary changes are as easily identified. Statistically, we can address this area instability (or misalignment) by computing and adjusting for the level of misalignment in the model. This was demonstrated by Mair, Freisthler, Ponicki and Gaidus (2015) when they looked at neighborhood features (operationalized as zip codes) related to rates of substance abuse and dependence over time. Their study directly measured zip code instability, adjusting the model coefficients to account for changes in zip code areas. Having a higher density of retail establishments was related to higher rates of marijuana abuse and dependence over time (Mair et al., 2015). These results may have differed had zip code instability not been assessed.

Addressing spillover

We have multiple methods to address the issue of spatial spillover. Since we know geographic boundaries of most neighborhood areas are permeable (i.e. people can move in and out of places), we need to incorporate possible spillover effects into how we assess the efficacy of place-based policies. In Figure 38.2, the South intervention area has a 500- and a 1,000-foot buffer surrounding the entire intervention area. Any alcohol outlets included in that buffer zone were expected to have some effect on youth and young adult access to alcohol. Thus, we included them as part of our intervention activities.

Another alternative involves creating spatial lags to assess similar effects. Although spatial lags can be constructed in a variety of ways, the most common is to average the characteristics of adjacent neighborhoods. Adjacencies can be defined as contiguous areas that share a boundary with a local neighborhood. Spatial lags allow you to control for how rates of problems or density of resources in adjacent neighborhoods may impact the effectiveness of a place-based intervention in a target neighborhood. In some cases, resources or risks in adjacent neighborhoods may be a bigger risk. For example, in Long Beach, California, Freisthler, Ponicki, Gaidus and Gruenewald (2016) were interested in how crime rates changed when Long Beach police made a concerted effort to close illegally operating medical marijuana dispensaries. They observed that dispensary density in adjacent Census block groups (measured using spatial lags) were related to higher rates of violent and property crimes in the local block group. Earlier, we mentioned that dispensaries often employ a variety of security measures to reduce crime in the immediate vicinity of the dispensary. This may push crime or other problems to adjacent areas. In contrast, in the study of marijuana abuse and dependence, spatially lagged dispensary density in adjacent zip codes was not related to higher rates of abuse and dependence in the local zip code (Mair et al., 2015). Thus, different types of problems may have different spatial signatures.

Addressing edge effects

Finally, geographic boundaries end which may affect the likelihood that a place-based policy will successfully reduce problems or increase capacity in local areas. In the prior Inglewood example, some of the limitations of place-based policies arose when they occurred in only one jurisdiction. It is often not feasible or practical to extend the study area to include all adjacent areas. Spatial lags can address some issues resulting from permeable boundaries, but another way is to assess the number of adjacencies for each place.

Spatial lags are created through assessing areas that share boundaries (Waller & Gotway, 2004). If most areas in the study share fewer connections, it may indicate that much of the area is on a spatial edge. In contrast, areas with more connections are less likely to be on the edge of a boundary. Assessing the average number of connections and the percentage of connections with fewer connections provides some context concerning whether edge effects may be an intervention concern. Further, buffers around intervention areas can also be used to address edge effects in intervention areas.

Advances in the study of context

We have described the most common ways GIS and spatial analysis have been used in the field of substance misuse. Now we showcase ways GIS and spatial analysis are combined to better assess and identify contexts that may enhance or reduce substance use and related problems.

Advances in technology and statistical techniques allow us to more easily examine substance use and related problems across spatial areas, time periods, and different levels of geography. Doing so may help uncover previously unrecognized relationships. As one example, Kepple and Freisthler (2012) examined how the location of medical marijuana dispensaries was related to crime for one year. The study detected no relationship between dispensaries and crime. Yet, the space-time analysis showed that dispensaries were related to crime over time, but this relationship occurred in spatially lagged areas, not local areas (Freisthler et al., 2016). As we move forward with prevention and intervention efforts, we should strive to assess these effects in multiple ways, including over multiple geographic areas and time periods.

The permeability of neighborhood areas can be better measured if, instead of focusing on administrative geographic boundaries, we focus on those spaces where people actually spend time during daily living—called activity spaces (Rai et al., 2007). Activity spaces provide detailed information on an individual's risks or resources for substance misuse or related problems. They can be constructed using survey measures or global positioning system (GPS) data to identify the common locations individuals visited (Freisthler, Lipperman-Kreda, Bersamin, & Gruenewald, 2014). Morrison and colleagues (2019) showed that the relationship of alcohol outlets to alcohol use among young adults differed when applying a measure that represents a person's neighborhood versus activity space. Thus, as we move forward and better refine our understanding of how environmental contexts shape behaviors, activity spaces will be an important component.

Studying these contexts can go even further as we combine GPS movement data to ecological momentary assessments (EMA; Shiffman, 2009). EMA "pings" an individual's cell phone at various times during a defined period (e.g. a week, a day) to collect brief survey data regarding what that person is doing and their activity space right at that moment (e.g. present at a party or bar, who else is there, and whether alcohol is being consumed). This can be combined with the GPS data of where the EMA survey is completed. This method is called geographic ecological momentary assessment (GEMA) and has promise in identifying the riskiest contexts for different individuals, and possibly intervening by sending messages to prevent or address problematic behaviors.

One limiting factor in our ability to continue to expand studies of how context affects substance use and related problems is the lack of training in GIS and spatial analysis across many disciplines that study substance use. Very few social work or health services programs include formal training in using GIS or spatial analysis (Hillier, 2007). Although these training opportunities are more prevalent in geography and public health programs, they are not always considered core learning activities. Professional programs (e.g. master's degree in social work or public health) may teach students how to develop interventions or intervene in problems, but the majority focus on preventing or reducing problems experienced by individuals. As we continue to move the research forward in this area, we need to pay special attention to developing community development skills among the next generation of scholars and practitioners, including GIS and spatial analysis skills.

Conclusions

Advances in our ability to capture locations of events and visualize social phenomenon over space have created new opportunities for social workers interested in the community impact of substance availability and use. Mapping these relationships using GIS and analyzing relationships using spatial analysis can enhance current community practice and policy analysis related to intervening at the community level to reduce substance-related harms. These tools can be leveraged by both social workers and community members to better understand how the larger context may contribute to alcohol and other drug problems, and to encourage creative solutions for prevention and intervention in the development of addictive behaviors.

References

Anselin, L. (1995). Local indicators of spatial association—LISA. *Geographical Analysis, 27*(2), 93–115. doi:10.1111/j.1538-4632.1995.tb00338.x

Bailey, T. C., & Gatrell, A. C. (1995). *Interactive spatial data analysis.* Essex, UK: Pearson Education Limited.

California Police Chief's Association. (2009). *White paper on marijuana dispensaries.* Sacramento, CA: Author. Retrieved from http://www.procon.org/sourcefi les/CAPCAWhitePaperonMarijuana-Diepensaries.pdf

Elwood, S. (2006). Critical issues in participatory GIS: Deconstructions, reconstructions, and new research directions. *Transactions in GIS, 10*(5), 693–708. doi:10.1111/j.1467-9671.2006.01023.x

Freisthler, B., Gruenewald, P. J., Johnson, F. W., Treno, A. J., & Lascala, E. A. (2005). An exploratory study examining the spatial dynamics of illicit drug availability and rates of drug use. *Journal of Drug Education, 35*(1), 15–27. doi:10.2190/25QY-PBC3-B1EB-JB5Y

Freisthler, B., Kepple, N. J., Sims, R., & Martin, S. E. (2013). Evaluating medical marijuana dispensary policies: Spatial methods for the study of environmentally-based interventions. *American Journal of Community Psychology, 51*(1–2), 278–288. doi:10.1007/s10464-012-9542-6

Freisthler, B., Lipperman-Kreda, S., Bersamin, M., & Gruenewald, P. J. (2014). Tracking the when, where, and with whom of alcohol use: Integrating ecological momentary assessment and geospatial data to examine risk for alcohol-related problems. *Alcohol Research: Current Reviews, 36*(1), 29–38.

Freisthler, B., Ponicki, W. R., Gaidus, A., & Gruenewald, P. J. (2016). A micro-temporal geospatial analysis of medical marijuana dispensaries and crime in Long Beach, California. *Addiction, 111*(6), 1027–1035. doi:10.1111/add.13301

Ginsberg, W. R. (2011). Changing postal ZIP code boundaries [CRS Report RL33488]. Retrieved from https://www.everycrsreport.com/reports/RL33488.html

Gruenewald, P. J., & Johnson, F. W. (2010). Drinking, driving, and crashing: A traffic-flow model of alcohol-related motor vehicle accidents. *Journal of Studies on Alcohol and Drugs, 71*(2), 237–248.

Hillier, A. (2007). Why social work needs mapping. *Journal of Social Work Education, 43*(2), 205–222. doi:10.5175/JSWE.2007.200500524

Kepple, N. J., & Freisthler, B. (2012). Exploring the ecological association between crime and medical marijuana dispensaries. *Journal of Studies on Alcohol and Drugs, 73*(4), 523–530. doi:10.15288/jsad.2012.73.523

Lipton, R., & Gruenewald, P. (2002). The spatial dynamics of violence and alcohol outlets. *Journal of Studies on Alcohol, 63*(2), 187–195. doi:10.15288/jsa.2002.63.187

Livingston, M., Livingston, M., Chikritzhs, T., Livingston, M., Chikritzhs, T., Room, R., . . . Room, R. (2007). Changing the density of alcohol outlets to reduce alcohol-related problems. *Drug and Alcohol Review, 26*(5), 557–566. doi:10.1080/09595230701499191

Mair, C., Freisthler, B., Ponicki, W. R., & Gaidus, A. (2015). The impacts of marijuana dispensary density and neighborhood ecology on marijuana abuse and dependence. *Drug and Alcohol Dependence, 154*, 111–116. doi:10.1016/j.drugalcdep.2015.06.019

Morrison, C. N., Byrnes, H. F., Miller, B. A., Kaner, E., Wiehe, S. E., Ponicki, W. R., & Wiebe, D. J. (2019). Assessing individuals' exposure to environmental conditions using residence-based measures, activity location-based measures, and activity path-based measures. *Epidemiology, 30*(2), 166–176. doi:10.1097/EDE.0000000000000940

Rai, R. K., Balmer, M., Rieser, M., Vaze, V. S., Schönfelder, S., & Axhausen, K. W. (2007). Capturing human activity spaces: New geometries. *Transportation Research Record, 2021*(1), 70–80. doi:10.3141/2021-09

Shiffman, S. (2009). Ecological momentary assessment (EMA) in studies of substance use. *Psychological Assessment, 21*(4), 486. doi:10.1037/a0017074

Simmons, M. (2001, July 4). One toke over the line. *LA Weekly*. Accessed online: https://www.laweekly.com/arts/one-toke-over-the-line-2133553

Treno, A. J., Lee, J. P., Freisthler, B., Remer, L. G., & Gruenewald, P. J. (2005). 4.4 Application of evidence-based approaches to community interventions. In T. Stockwell, P. J. Gruenewald, J. W. Toumbourou, & W. Loxley (Eds.), *Preventing harmful substance use: The evidence base for policy and practice* (pp. 177–189). New York, NY: John Wiley. doi:10.1002/9780470713624.ch15

U.S. Census Bureau. (2015, May). Geographic boundary change notes [Webpage]. Retrieved from https://www.census.gov/geo/reference/boundary-changes.html

Waller, L. A., & Gotway, C. A. (2004). *Applied spatial statistics for public health data.* Hoboken, NJ: John Wiley & Sons, Inc. doi:10.1002/0471662682

Emerging priorities for practice and research

Audrey L. Begun and Margaret M. Murray

Background

The Routledge Handbook of Social Work and Addictive Behaviors examines a wide array of topics critical to understanding and intervening around substance misuse, substance use disorders, gambling, problematic internet gaming, and problems commonly related to these addictive behaviors. While many chapters identify future directions for the field, this concluding chapter discusses the future in a more general, "umbrella" manner. First, we present a framework for integrating diverse theoretical models into an overall strategic plan for addressing specific problems based on what is known about vulnerability, risk, resilience, and protective factors. Second, we explore implications of research into mechanisms of change. Third, we discuss the relevance of common elements and common factors with the aim of improving future interventions. Fourth, we discuss future directions of global and U.S. National Institutes of Health (NIH) research, policy, and strategic goals. The chapter offers concluding observations related to the book in its entirety.

Integrating diverse theoretical models

A wide range of biological, psychological, and social context theories and models concerning the development and maintenance of addictive behaviors were examined in Section I of this book—for the most part, these theories and domains were discussed independently of one another. At this point, it is important to re-integrate them to more fully reflect a true biopsychosocial perspective. The vulnerability/resilience and risk/protective factors framework for integrating multiple theories offered here helps inform intervention and policy logic models for prevention, treatment, and continuing care (Begun, 1993). This integrative framework reflects both a biopsychosocial and social work strengths perspective. Thus, it can inform interventions and policies that help change individuals, their environments, and the interface between individuals and their environments. The framework seeks to integrate what is known about a specific topic and was derived from E. James Anthony's early work concerning the etiology of schizophrenia. The framework is applied at the group or population level for purposes of planning intervention strategies based on logic models and existing evidence.

The state of evidence, at this time, is not sufficiently honed to predict individual outcomes, so the framework is not used to assess or predict what will happen for an individual person or family. Here, the framework's four steps are outlined.

Specify the problem

The more specific the problem definition, the easier the task of identifying and integrating varied theoretical models becomes (see Begun, 1999). For example, "preventing adolescent initiation of alcohol misuse" is reasonably specific, whereas "preventing substance use disorders" is overly general. Specificity might include specifics of an addictive behavior (e.g. a specific substance, type of technology, or form of gambling) and/or a target population (e.g. a specified age or developmental phase, racial/ethnic group, self-defined gender identity, sexual orientation, co-occurring problems, or problem severity level). It is important, as well, to be specific as to the system level being addressed: individuals, family subsystems, family systems, neighborhoods/communities, institutions, or geographical regions. Processes for building practice questions are well suited to specifying the topic in this framework, as well (see Begun, 2018; Kloda & Bartlett, 2013):

- COPES (Client Oriented Practical Evidence Search),
- ECLIPSE (Expectation, Client Group, Location, Impact, Professionals, Service),
- PECODR (Problem, Exposure, Comparison, Outcome, Duration, Results),
- PESICO (Person, Environments, Stakeholders, Intervention, Comparison, Outcome),
- PICO (Patient, Intervention, Comparison, Outcome),
- PICO+ (Patient, Intervention, Comparison, Outcome, Context, Patient Values and Preferences), and
- PIPOH (Population, Interventions, Professionals/Patients, Outcome, Health Care Setting).

Define the vulnerability/resilience continuum

Once a practice question/problem is clearly specified, evidence concerning known vulnerability and resilience factors can be located and critically analyzed. The vulnerability/resilience continuum refers to factors *intrinsic* to individuals (or other system level specified in the first step). In other words, factors that individuals bring with them to any new situation or experience. These include the factors like: genetics, neurobiology, and other biological processes; temperament and personality characteristics; abilities and disabilities; co-occurring problems; past experiences and learning; and current attitudes, beliefs, knowledge, and behavior patterns. Some factors reflect individuals' vulnerability to the specified problem, and other factors reflect aspects of their resilience. Together evidence concerning these intrinsic factors helps determine where along a vulnerability/resilience continuum a group of individuals might be situated.

Risk/protective factors continuum

As with the vulnerability/resilience continuum, evidence concerning known risk and protective factors is also identified and analyzed. The risk/protective continuum refers to *extrinsic* factors. In other words, factors residing in the current social and environmental contexts. According to a social-ecological model, this includes individuals' interplay with relationships, communities, and societal level factors (CDC, 2019). The relevant science examines

	Vulnerability/Resilience	
	low vulnerability/ high resilience	*high vulnerability/ low resilience*
low risk/ high protection	I low probability	II moderate probability
high risk/ low protection	III moderate probability	IV high probability

Figure 39.1   Integrating vulnerability/resilience and risk/protective factors

social determinants of the (health) behaviors identified in the first step. The risk/protective factors continuum relates to "here and now" contexts and experiences; past interactions with the social context become a part of the vulnerability and resilience continuum—historical experiences of the environment become part of what is brought to new situations. For example, a history of adverse childhood events (ACES) becomes a vulnerability factor related to substance misuse; currently living in a traumatizing environment is a risk factor.

Integration

Consider now how the two continua intersect: bringing together the vulnerability/resilience continuum with the risk/protection continuum. This is conceptually diagrammed as a 2 × 2 grid specifying the general probability (low, moderate, high) for developing the specified problem under these complex circumstances (see Figure 39.1).

The result is an integration of theory and evidence to inform the development of intervention and policy strategies and logic models. For example, the low probability group (I) needs little attention beyond universal preventive efforts to maintain healthful status—maintaining both resilience and protective factors and minimizing new vulnerability and risk exposure. However, the high probability group (IV) warrants a great deal of immediate attention with efforts designed to reduce both vulnerability and risk, as well as promote both resilience and protective factors. The two moderate probability groups (II and III) warrant attention in the form of selective or indicated prevention efforts to prevent their shifting into the high probability group (IV). Ideally, group II and group III populations can also be helped to more closely come to resemble the low probability population (group I).

This is where theoretical models and empirical evidence inform both specific interventions (including policy) and planning broader combined intervention strategies, whether the aim is prevention, treatment, or maintenance of gains achieved. A great deal of literature across many disciplines presents detailed and nuanced evidence related to vulnerability, risk, resilience, and protective factors surrounding different addictive behaviors. This framework provides a logical system for organizing the massive literature, only some of which appears in this handbook.

Mechanisms of change

Numerous approaches to intervening around addictive behaviors have been developed and empirically tested for efficacy and effectiveness in producing healthful outcomes; this type of intervention outcome evidence is woven throughout this handbook's many chapters. A branch of current and future science addresses a somewhat different type of question: rather than asking *if* and intervention works, mechanisms of change science asks *how* interventions produce their observed outcomes (Hayes, Hope, & Hayes, 2007). This knowledge, in turn, helps develop more nuanced interventions and strategies for intervening with more diverse populations, under more diverse circumstances, and where prior intervention attempts have failed.

Studies in the psychotherapy, cognitive behavioral therapy (CBT), and pharmacotherapy areas provide multiple examples of mechanisms of change science, often referred to as studies of mediation. Testing mediation (conceptually) involves examining the relationships that exist in data around the intervention (input), outcomes, and factors believed to fill an intervening role (mediators). For example, coping skills mediated the relationship between CBT and treatment outcomes related to substance misuse; "counter change" and "sustain" talk mediated poor outcomes of motivational interviewing; and strong social support mediated abstinence with 12-step programs (Magill, Kiluk, McCrady, Tonigan, & Longabaugh, 2015). In summary, learning about mechanisms of change regarding addictive behaviors is an important future aim for practitioners, investigators, and students to pursue, and may help inform the development of practice standards in social work and other professions.

Common elements, common factors

Aligned with efforts to understand mechanisms of change are efforts to identify the critical or active "ingredients" of behavioral interventions. Active ingredients research examines the impact of specific intervention components, practices, and processes on outcomes (Barth et al., 2012; Magill et al., 2015), much like over-the-counter product labeling identifies active versus inactive ingredients. Not only does this kind of evidence support the process of refining individual intervention protocols, it contributes to a broader understanding of shared, common elements across different kinds of intervention approaches. This knowledge, in turn, supports intervention development and refinement, as well as helping practitioners select from among evidence-supported psychosocial intervention options (Barth et al., 2012). Examples of common elements include frequency and duration of intervention contacts (e.g. 12 two-hour weekly sessions), curriculum elements (e.g. different forms of cognitive skill building training), or who is engaged in the intervention (e.g. parent involvement in different community-based prevention programs). Ideally, with sufficiently nuanced understanding of the match between specific elements and client circumstances, practitioners can make well-informed decisions about adapting evidence-based intervention protocols to best meet diverse and changing needs. Common elements research of the future needs to analyze effect size associated with specific elements to better inform practice decisions (Barth et al., 2012).

Common factors research questions follow a similar logic to common elements research, the main difference being that common factors science is concerned with factors that may have been unrecognized or unspecified as intervention elements. For example, therapeutic alliance (nature of the client-practitioner working relationship) accounts for as much as 30% of variance in intervention outcomes, more than techniques specified in the intervention model (Fife, Whiting, Bradford, & Davis, 2014), but is not a factor specified in intervention protocols. Or, for instance, studies of client treatment preferences and clients' expectations that an intervention will work for them (treatment credibility) produced mixed results in terms of treatment retention and outcomes (Adamson, Sellman, & Dore, 2005; Serafini et al., 2015), making a difference in some but not in others; treatment expectancies are also not a specified intervention component. "In this view, models become the vehicle through which common curative factors are delivered" (Fife et al., 2014, p. 20). Common elements and common factors thinking has significant implications for practice, establishing practice standards ("best practices"), and future research, as well as how social workers and other professionals are trained to intervene around addictive behaviors.

Future global health policy and NIH research goals

In addition to the above, issues regarding addictive disorders currently receive national attention in many parts of the world (i.e. the opioid epidemic, legalization of marijuana, fetal alcohol exposure), as well as global attention from groups such as the World Health Organization (WHO). WHO began a global tobacco initiative in 1998 in order to call international attention to the global epidemic of tobacco addiction (https://www.who.int/tobacco/en/). This was an important step led by the directing and coordinating body for health at the United Nations (UN). Every year, on May 31, WHO uses a World No Tobacco Day (WNTD) as "… an opportunity to raise awareness on the harmful and deadly effects of tobacco use and second-hand smoke exposure, and to discourage the use of tobacco in any form" (https://www.who.int/news-room/events/detail/2019/05/31/default-calendar/world-no-tobacco-day).

The Organization of Economic Cooperation and Development (OECD) is a post-WWII organization comprised of the world's wealthiest countries and whose mission is to stimulate economic development and world trade. The organization adopted the task of developing a simulation model to determine the most effective policies for reducing harmful alcohol use. Among findings from their model which should be of interest to social workers are that:

- rates of hazardous and heavy drinking (defined as more than 140 grams for women, more than 210 grams for men, and more than 5–8 drinks in one sitting, depending on the country) are growing in many OECD countries;
- in general, individuals from minority ethnic groups drink less alcohol than the majority population;
- brief interventions in primary care settings have the potential to reduce health burdens on life expectancy in three countries studied (Germany, Czech Republic, and Canada); and
- combining alcohol policies in a unified approach can substantially increase impact (Organization on Economic Cooperation and Development, 2015).

Additionally, the United Nations in 2012 argued for reduction in prevalence of tobacco smoking by 30% among persons over 15 years old and 10% relative reduction in the harmful use of alcohol as targets for the WHO non-communicable disease initiative (Ho, & Bethniji, 2013). Non-communicable diseases (NCDs) are the largest contributors to deaths globally, especially premature death (before age 70), and are largely preventable https://www.who.int/nmh/events/ncd_action_plan/en/). Alcohol and tobacco use not only present health risks of their own but also contribute to many other non-communicable diseases of concern (e.g. diabetes, cancer, lung, and heart disease). Many groups are working together on the Sustainable Development Goals 2015–2030, where goal 3.5 is "… strengthen prevention and treatment of substance abuse, including narcotic drug abuse and harmful use of alcohol" (https://www.un.org/sustainabledevelopment/sustainable-development-goals/).

With its sizeable budget (greater than $2 billion in U.S. dollars) directed to research on alcohol, tobacco, and other drugs, the National Institutes of Health (NIH) in the United States currently funds the most research on addiction in the world. It is important to note the strategic plans of three key NIH institutes, the National Institute on Alcohol Abuse and Alcoholism (NIAAA), the National Cancer Institute (NCI), and the National Institute on Drug Abuse (NIDA), as well as the Collaborative Research on Addictions (CRAN) initiative, in identifying the NIH's addictions research priorities (https://www.addictionresearch. nih.gov/cran-strategic-plan-2016-2021; https://www.niaaa.nih.gov/strategic-plan; https:// www.cancer.gov/about-nci/overview/strategic-planning; https://www.drugabuse.gov/ about-nida/2016-2020-nida-strategic-plan). For example, the CRAN strategic plan highlights the ten-year longitudinal Adolescent Brain Cognitive Development (ABCD) Study exploring, among various topics, how exposure to different substances, individually or in combination, affects developmental outcomes and vice versa, how different developmental trajectories might affect substance use/misuse. Another highlighted CRAN initiative concerns the use of social media as tools to address and assess problems related to substance use, misuse, and use disorders. The NIAAA strategic plan includes goals related to basic science, diagnostics and epidemiology, prevention, treatment, and public health; similarly, the NIDA strategic plan includes goals related to basic science, prevention, treatment, and public health. In addition, NIH has recently announced a new $1 billion initiative (U.S. dollars) on opioid addiction and pain research, called Helping to End Addiction Long-Term (HEAL) that covers "… a wide variety of projects: creating a more potent overdose-reversing medicine, studying what helps people stay sober, even developing a vaccine against opioid addiction" (https://www.drugabuse.gov/about-nida/noras-blog/2019/09/nida-announces-new-nih-heal-initiative-awards-to-address-opioid-crisis). As the NIH's priorities evolve over time, it will be important to check for updates to their strategic plans.

Conclusions

Addictive behaviors and their related issues remain a challenge for individuals, families, communities, and societies world-wide. While long standing substances of abuse (alcohol, marijuana, illicit narcotics, and prescription pain medications) are an important piece of the puzzle, behaviors associated with gambling, internet gaming, and related activities are an important emerging focus of some populations, especially in certain parts of the world. Furthermore, these problematic addictive behaviors often co-occur with each other and with other physical health, behavioral health, and social problems, with this added complexity contributing to the challenges of successfully intervening.

In recent decades, medical, behavioral, and social research has expanded our ideas about who engages in addictive behavior, whose addictive behaviors develop into disorders and who remains resilient, as well as how can we best help, not punish, individuals who fall prey to addictive substances and disorders. Organizations focused on health at the highest level are noting the importance of addressing addiction in order to achieve global health, and it is indeed time. The challenges of achieving both mental and physical health and global well-being depend on collective efforts of nations, including scientific, health professions education, clinical and preventive work forces, health and lifestyle policy makers, among others, to meet these challenges. As the increase in the amount of research and advances in research techniques move the field forward, it must be remembered that our goals evolve, change, and priorities re-order.

The preceding 38 chapters in this Handbook of Social Work and Addictive Behavior provide readers with a great deal of information concerning the scope and nature of addictive behaviors and related problems, including the use/misuse of psychoactive substances, gambling, and problematic technology use. The biopsychosocial framework is represented throughout the book and reflects a strong, central social work perspective. Also from the social work perspective, the book presents addictive behavior from a lifespan developmental and human diversity perspective, as well: from prenatal exposure to alcohol and other substances through late adulthood and as experienced among diverse populations. Theory and evidence related to a host of intervention strategies concerning prevention, treatment, and recovery are explored both in general and as related to specific populations. The interventions explored reflect the social work profession's commitment to intervening at the levels of individual, family, community, and policy. Furthermore, the chapters address implementation science and workforce development issues as we move the field forward. It is our hope that the book presents a useful resource chapter-by-chapter and as an integrated whole, that it adequately documents where we are today in prevention, treatment, and recovery service interventions related to addictive behavior, and provides a road map by which to travel into the near future and guide developments in a systematic and practical manner, while taking the field the best way forward.

References

Adamson, S. J., Sellman, J. D., & Dore, G. M. (2005). Therapy preference and treatment outcome in clients with mild to moderate alcohol dependence. *Drug and Alcohol Review, 24,* 209–216. doi:10.1080/09595230500167502

Barth, R. P., Lee, B. R., Linsey, M. A., Collins, K. S., Streider, F., Chorpita, B. F., … Sparks, J. A. (2012). Evidence-based practice at a crossroads: The timely emergence of common elements and common factors. *Research on Social Work Practice, 22*(1), 108–119. doi:10.1177/1049731511408440

Begun, A. L. (1993). Human behavior and the social environment: The vulnerability, risk, and resilience model. *Journal of Social Work Education, 29,* 26–35. doi:10.1080/10437797.1993.10778796

Begun, A. L. (1999). Intimate partner violence: An HBSE perspective. *Journal of Social Work Education, 35*(2), 239–252. doi:10.1080/10437797.1999.10778963

Begun, A. L. (2018). Module 2, chapter 2: Formulating practice evidence questions. In *Coursebook for SWK 3402: Research and statistics for understanding social work interventions.* The Ohio State University: Pressbooks, Open Educational Resources. Retrieved from https://ohiostate.pressbooks.pub/swk3402/chapter/module-2-chapter-2/

Centers for Disease Control and Prevention (CDC). (2019). The social-ecological model: A framework for prevention. Retrieved from https://www.cdc.gov/violenceprevention/publichealthissue/social-ecologicalmodel.html

Fife, S. T., Whiting, J. B., Bradford, K., & Davis, S. (2014). The therapeutic pyramid: A common factors synthesis of techniques, alliance, and way of being. *Journal of Marital and Family Therapy, 40*(1), 20–33. doi:10.1111/jmft.12041

Hayes, A., Hope, D. A., & Hayes, S. (2007). Towards an understanding of the process and mechanisms of change in cognitive behavioral therapy: Linking innovative methodology with fundamental questions. *Clinical Psychology Review, 27*(6), 679–681. doi:10.1016/j.cpr.2007.01.006

Ho, J. K., & Bethniji, R. (2013). Targets for non-communicable disease: What has happened since the UN summit? *British Medical Journal, 346,* f3300. doi:10.1136/bmj.f3300

Kloda, L. A., & Bartlett, J. C. (2013). Formulating answerable questions: Question negotiation in evidence-based practice. *Journal of the Canadian Health Libraries Association/Journal de l'Association des Bibliothèques de la Santé du Canada, 34,* 56–60. doi:10.5596/c13-019

Magill, M., Kiluk, B. D., McCrady, B., Tonigan, J. S., & Longabaugh, R. (2015). Active ingredients of treatment and client mechanisms of change in behavioral treatments for alcohol use disorders: Progress 10 years later. *Alcohol: Clinical and Experimental Research, 39*(10), 1852–1862. doi:10.1111/acer.12848

Organization on Economic Cooperation and Development. (2015). *Tackling the Harmful Use of Alcohol.* Retrieved from OECD, https://www.iogt.org/wp-content/uploads/2015/03/OECD-report-2015.pdf

Serafini, K., Decker, S., Killuk, B. D., Anez, L., Paris, M., Frankforter, T., & Carroll, K. M. (2015). Abstract: Patient pre-treatment expectations and substance use treatment outcomes. *Drug and Alcohol Dependence, 156,* e183–e245. doi:10.1016/j.drugalcdep.2015.07.541

Appendix A
Diagnostic criteria for alcohol use disorder (AUD) and substance use disorders (SUD) in DSM-5® and ICD-11 protocols

Background

One premise underlying the development of major diagnostic systems such as the Diagnostic and Statistical Manual (DSM) and the International Classification of Disease (ICD) is that practitioners (and researchers) benefit from applying standardized guidelines and language to communicate about their diagnoses. Identifying "addiction" is complicated by there being no specific physiological or behavioral test that can be relied on to make such a diagnosis (Peele, 1985). Instead, practitioners rely on systems informed by research evidence to direct the diagnostic process.

The DSM-5®

The DSM guides much of the assessment and treatment planning for mental/psychiatric conditions in the United States and some other nations. The most current version is the fifth edition (DSM-5®), first implemented in 2013. According to the DSM-5® Handbook of Differential Diagnosis symptoms related to substance use and observed in practice may result from direct effects of acute substance intoxication (recent use), chronic substance use (over time), and/or substance withdrawal from one or more psychoactive substances; other possibilities include that substance use is an attempt to self-medicate symptoms of a primary disorder/physical condition, or that the substance use and other symptoms/disorders co-occur independently of each other (First, 2014). Substance-induced disorders include intoxication, withdrawal, and other disorders induced by the use of substances/medications; substance use disorders, on the other hand, relate to symptom patterns specific to the use of certain types of substances (APA, 2013). The DSM-5® substance-related diagnoses relate to ten categories of substances and gambling:

- alcohol
- caffeine
- cannabis
- hallucinogens

- inhalants
- opioids
- sedatives, hypnotics, and anxiolytics
- stimulants (including cocaine)
- tobacco
- other or unknown substances.

Concurrent use of multiple substances (polydrug use) is also considered in the system.

DSM-5® criteria for substance use disorders

"The essential feature of a substance use disorder is a cluster of cognitive, behavioral, and physiological symptoms indicating that the individual continues using the substance despite significant substance-related problems" (APA, 2013). Eleven diagnostic symptoms specified in DSM-5® cluster into four general categories: impaired control, social impairment, risky use, and pharmacological criteria. Substance use disorder severity is determined by the total number of symptoms experienced.

Impaired control

First are the four criteria related to impaired control over one's substance use: (1) larger amounts or longer period of use than originally intended; (2) persistent desire to cut down/ regulate use with or without unsuccessful attempts to decrease/discontinue use; (3) great deal of time spent obtaining or using the substance; and (4) recovering from its effects; experience of craving to use the substance.

Social impairment

Second are the three criteria related to social impairment: (5) use resulting in failure to fulfill major work, school, and/or home role obligations; (6) continued substance use despite persistent/recurrent social or interpersonal problems caused or made worse by effects of the substance used; and (7) giving up or reducing engagement in important social, occupational, or recreational activities because of substance use.

Risky use

Third are two criteria related to risky use patterns: (8) recurrent substance use in physically hazardous situations; and (9) continued use despite knowing a persistent/recurring physical or psychological problem is caused or made worse by the substance.

Pharmacological criteria

The final two criteria reflect changes in a person's physiological/psychology response to use of the substance: developing tolerance (10) manifested by requiring increased doses of the substance to achieve the desired effects and/or a reduced effect of the substance when the usual dose is consumed; and (11) experiencing withdrawal syndrome with reduced dose or eliminating the substance after a period of prolonged heavy use (and renewed use alleviating withdrawal symptoms).

Severity

The continuum of substance use disorder severity specified in the DSM-5® is from mild to severe. Mild substance use disorder is assessed when two or three of the 11 symptoms are present; four or five symptoms reflect a moderate substance use disorder; and six or more symptoms are classified as a severe substance use disorder. Note that severity of an individual's substance use disorder may fluctuate over time as specific symptoms may appear, disappear, and reappear.

The ICD-11

The World Health Organization (WHO) directs the establishment of the International Classification of Diseases (ICD), which is currently being adopted in the 11th version (ICD-11). Similarities between the DSM-5® and ICD-11 diagnostic systems are extensive. For example, the two systems specify many of the same or similar substances, although differentiation in specific substances exists. For example, the ICD-11 not only includes disorders due to cannabis, it also includes synthetic cannabinoids. Cocaine is in a category of its own in the ICD-11, not under the category of stimulants, MDMA as well as dissociative "club" drugs (ketamine, PCP) are specified, and nicotine is specified rather than tobacco in the ICD-11. As in the DSM-5®, multiple substances used concurrently (polydrug use) are also considered in the diagnostic system.

Similar to the DSM-5®, the ICD-11 includes gambling disorder. However, rather than placing gambling disorder alongside substance use disorders, the ICD-11 places gambling disorder in the category of impulse control disorders, which are characterized by repeated failure to resist an impulse, drive, or urge to engage in actions which are experienced by the person as rewarding despite harm to self or others (Grant & Chamberlain, 2016). Compulsive sexual behavior is included, but problematic Internet use was not; how addictive behaviors other than those involving substances is a major dimension along which the two diagnostic systems differ (Grant & Chamberlain, 2016).

The ICD-11, which is generally organized around diseases of human systems, classifies addictive behaviors under the larger umbrella of mental, behavioral, or neurodevelopmental disorders (category 06): disorders due to substance use or addictive behaviors. They are described as "mental and behavioural disorders that develop as a result of the use of predominantly psychoactive substances, including medications, or specific repetitive rewarding and reinforcing behaviours" (retrieved from ICD-11 Coding tool, https://icd.who.int/browse11). Unlike the DSM-5® single continuum of substance use disorder with different degrees of severity, the ICD-11 describes three general categories: single episodes of harmful substance use, substance use disorders, and substance-induced disorders.

Single episodes of harmful substance use

The types of harms included in this category include harm to one's own physical or mental health or behavior causing harm to the health of others. Of note also is attention paid to harms associated with a substance's route of administration, not only to its pharmacological action.

Substance use disorders

This category includes the two sub-categories of harmful patterns of substance use and substance dependence. Harmful patterns of use include the harms previously identified concerning single episodes of use, but they occur with repeated use. Dependence is specified when three or more diagnostic criteria co-occur for at least one month or occur together repeatedly within a single 12-month period (per the ICD-10 definition from WHO https://www.who.int/substance_abuse/terminology/definition1/en/):

- strong desire or sense of compulsion to use the substance;
- difficulty in controlling onset, termination, or levels of substance use;
- physiological withdrawal syndrome with reduced or terminated use of a substance;
- developing tolerance to a substance (increased doses required);
- progressive neglect of alternative pleasures or interests due to substance use, increased amounts of time involved in obtaining or using a substance or recovering from its effects (preoccupation); and
- persisting in use of substance despite evidence of harmful physical or psychological consequences.

Substance-induced disorders

Intoxication and substance withdrawal are two sub-categories of substance-induced disorders. Others are mental disorders, sexual dysfunctions, and sleep-wake disorders identified as being substance-induced.

References

American Psychiatric Association (APA). (2013). *Diagnostic and statistical manual of mental disorders, fifth edition (DSM-5®)*. Arlington, VA: American Psychiatric Association.

First, M. B. (2014). *DSM-5® handbook of differential diagnosis*. Arlington, VA: American Psychiatric Association.

Grant, J. E., & Chamberlain, S. R. (2016). Expanding the definition of addictions: DSM-5 vs. ICD-11. *CNS Spectrums, 21*(4), 300–303.

Peele, S. (1985). *The meaning of addiction: An unconventional view*. San Francisco, CA: Jossey-Bass.

Index

Note: **Bold** page numbers refer to tables and *italic* page numbers refer to figures.

AA *see* Alcoholics Anonymous (AA)
ABCD Study *see* Adolescent Brain Cognitive Development (ABCD) Study
Abrams, K. 536
abstinence 10–11, 307, 309
acamprosate 73, 252–253, **323**; clinical safety 325; drug indications and duration 325; efficacy 325; mechanism of action 324–325
acceptance and commitment therapy (ACT) 359
ACES *see* adverse childhood experiences (ACES)
ACEs *see* adverse childhood events (ACEs)
acetaldehyde 25
ACOAs *see* adult children of alcoholics (ACOAs)
ACOG *see* American College of Obstetrics and Gynecology (ACOG)
ACT *see* acceptance and commitment therapy (ACT)
ACTH *see* adrenocorticotropin-releasing hormone (ACTH)
activity spaces 615
acute alcohol intoxication 384, 387
acute/chronic pancreatitis 439
addiction: allostasis 69; allostatic load 69; anxiety symptoms 70; behavioral responses 62; brain areas 68; brain function 60–61, *61–62*; chronic alcohol consumption 70; compulsive behavior 67; contemporary disease models 78; CRF 70; defined 8, 12, 59; dopamine 70; dynorphin-kappa system 70; goal-directed substance use 66; habit circuits 66–68; hedonic homeostasis 69; homeostasis 68, 69; impulsive behavior 67; KOR 70; maladaptive learning 59; mesocorticolimbic reward pathway 69–70; motivational process 69; negative reinforcement 65–66; neurobiology 60; opponent process theory 69; original disease model 9; positive reinforcement 63–65, *64*, 67; preoccupation/anticipation stage 71–72; recovery 470–471; stimulus-response relationships 60; stress-related neurotransmitters 70; thermoregulation 68;

treatment and recovery 72–73; *see also* substance use disorder (SUD)
Addiction Severity Index (ASI) 300
addictive personality 100
ADEP *see* Alcohol and Other Drugs Education Program (ADEP)
ADH *see* alcohol dehydrogenase (ADH)
adjunct therapy 166
adolescence: COSAPs 370–373; externalizing disorders 80; LGBTQ+ individuals 286–287; MBIs 358
adolescent brain: alcohol consumption 217; BOLD signal 220; cannabis 217; cognitive control circuitry 217; developmental perspective 218; differential brain activation 220; dose-dependent effects 225; electronic cigarettes 217–218, 224; fMRI 220; functional neuroimaging studies 223; functions 216; longitudinal studies 222; MRS 225; neural predictors 218–219; neuroimaging studies 222; neuroplasticity 225; neuropsychological alterations 222–223; neuropsychological predictors 219–220; resilience 225; risk factors 218, 221–222; self-report measures 225; structural brain precursors 220–221, 223–224; THC concentration 217; World Drug Report (2018) 217
Adolescent Brain Cognitive Development (ABCD) Study 218
adrenocorticotropin-releasing hormone (ACTH) 65
adult children of alcoholics (ACOAs) 367
adverse childhood events (ACEs) 112
adverse childhood experiences (ACES) 5, 368
Affordable Care Act 448
Agrawal, A. 86
agreeableness (A) 234
Al-Anon Family Groups 373, 404
alcohol: AA deaths (*see* alcohol-attributable (AA) deaths); acetaldehyde 25; acute contributors 548; ADH 25; adult per capita

consumption 40, **41**; alcohol expectancy theory 549–550; alcohol myopia theory 550–551; ALDH 25; APC 40, 42; AUDs 39 (*see also* alcohol use disorders (AUDs)); child maltreatment 387; cigarette 80; CNS 26; communicable diseases 51; concentration, liquid beverage 25; conditional contributors 548–549; consumption 25–26, 39, 217, 296; cost 58; density 84; ethyl alcohol 25; HED 42; heritability 84; impaired attention and disinhibition 387; indirect causes 548; injury 52; low-risk alcohol consumption, public health guidelines 53; low-risk drinking limits 26, **26**; metabolism 24, 264; metabolizing enzyme 25; noncommunicable diseases 51–52; older adults, substance misuse (*see* older adults, substance misuse); political factors 39; prevalence 40, 235; risk of experience 551; societal factors 39; socio-economic status 53; spurious factors 547–548; statistics 27; substance-specific effects 384, 387; theoretical perspectives 549; tolerance 26; usage 25; WHO 39; withdrawal symptoms 26

alcohol and other drug (AOD) core curriculum 100; ASI 593; barriers 592; co-occurring mental health problems 598; diagnosis and assessment 597–598; education programs 592–593, 593–596, **594**, *595*; etiology 597; history 597; interventions 598; screening 597; social workers 590–592

alcohol and other drugs education program (ADEP) 593–596, **594**, *595*

alcohol-attributable (AA) deaths: causes 46, **47**; GSRAH 46; Levin-based methodology 46; public health policies 46; relative risk 46; women 46–47, **48**, 49, *49–50*

alcohol dehydrogenase (ADH) 25

alcohol expectancy theory 549–550

Alcoholics Anonymous (AA) 9, 98, 308, 473–474

alcohol-induced peripheral neuropathy 440

alcoholism 99

alcohol myopia theory 550–551

alcohol per capita consumption (APC): childbearing age 42; measurement 40; women 40, 42

alcohol-related birth defects (ARBD) 176, 194

alcohol-related cues 72

alcohol-related neurodevelopmental disorder (ARND) 176, 194

Alcohol, Smoking and Substance Involvement Screening Test (ASSIST) 345

alcohol use disorders (AUDs) 6, 20–21, 249, 252, 311, 387; APA clinical practice guidelines 322; characteristics 42; first-line treatments 322–325, **323**; pregnancy **43**, 43–46, *45;* prevalence 42–43; public health policies 42;

racial/ethnic disparities 263–264; second-line treatments 325–326

Alcohol Use Disorders Identification Test (AUDIT) 345

aldehyde dehydrogenase (ALDH) 25

Aldridge, A. 347

Allem, J. 233

allostasis 69

allostatic load 69

American Academy of Pediatrics 162

American Association of Social Work and Social Welfare 2

American College of Obstetrics and Gynecology (ACOG) 161

American Psychiatric Association (APA) 130, 142, 144, 322

American Society for Addiction Medicine (ASAM) 8, 443, 445

Americans with Disabilities Act (ADA) 265, 273

amphetamine 30–31

amphetamine-induced psychosis 30–31

Anslinger, Harry Jacob 501–502

Antabuse®, 252

Anti-Drug Abuse Act 453, 486

anti-harm reduction 13

antihypertensive clonidine 330

antisocial personality 100

anxiety 30

anxiety disorders 531

APA *see* American Psychiatric Association (APA)

APC *see* alcohol per capita consumption (APC)

appendicitis 209

ARBD *see* alcohol-related birth defects (ARBD)

ARND *see* alcohol-related neurodevelopmental disorder (ARND)

Arndt, S. 348

Arnett, J. J. 232–234

ASAM *see* American Society for Addiction Medicine (ASAM)

Ashford, K. 238

ASSIST *see* Alcohol, Smoking and Substance Involvement Screening Test (ASSIST)

AUDIT *see* Alcohol Use Disorders Identification Test (AUDIT)

AUDs *see* alcohol use disorders (AUDs)

Australia Association of Social Work 136

autism spectrum disorder (ASD) 194

autoimmune disorders 195–196, **197**

"average trend" model 9

Ayers, J. 516

BAC *see* blood alcohol concentrations (BAC)

baclofen 253

Baezconde-Garbanati, L. 233

Baggio, S. 232–234

Bailey, D. S. 550

BAL *see* blood alcohol levels (BAL)

Balogh, D. 410
Baltimore City Drug Treatment Court (BCDTC) 459
Bandura, A. 103
barbiturates 27
Barbosa, C. 347
Barbour, R. S. 401
Bartholow, B. D. 550
BCT *see* behavioral couples therapy (BCT)
Begun, A. L. 348
behavioral addictions 5
behavioral couples therapy (BCT) 307, 401
behavioral economics theory 105–106
behavioral genetic studies: additive gene × environment effects 81–82, **83**; genetic control 80; interactive gene × environment effects 82, 84; non-twin adoption studies 81; sibling type 80, **81**; twin study design 80, 81
behavioral health disparities 282
behavioral health interventions 12
behavior change: COM 309–310; MI 305–306; network support 308–309; SOs 307–308
benzodiazepines 27
Bergman, B. G. 238
Berridge, K. C. 72
Bersamira, C. 469–479
BI *see* brief intervention (BI)
biological vulnerability 110
biopsychosocial assessment, dimensions 445
biopsychosocial emphasis 1
biopsychosocial framework 110
Blanco, C. 529
blood alcohol concentrations (BAC) 22
blood alcohol levels (BAL) 22
blood-oxygen-level-dependent (BOLD) signal 220
Bloom, B. 519
Bogenschutz, M. P. 347, 348
Boggs Act 484
Bonnano, G. 414
Borchardt, C. 536
Bowen, S. 358
brain–behavior process 12
brain function: action potential 60; addiction cycle 61, *62*; astrocytes 61; cell types 60; glial cells 61; microglia 61; myelination 61; neurons 60, *61*; neurotransmitter signals 60
brain stress systems 73
Bray, J. 347
Breitenbucher, P. 462
Brendryen, H. 432
brief intervention (BI) 251, 345–346, 426–427; CBI 302; effectiveness 346–347; MI 301, 302; SAMHSA 301; substance-related problems 301
Briley, D. A. 234, 348
Brook, J. 391
Buckley, J. 239

buprenorphine 34, 165, 167, 311–312, **332**; drug indications and duration 333; efficacy and clinical safety 331, 333, 334; mechanism of action 333; naloxone 333–334
bupropion hydrochloride **328**; drug indications and duration 328–329; efficacy and clinical safety 329; mechanism of action 328

caffeine 30, 33
Cafferky, B. M. 547
Campbell, N. D. 497, 502
Campral®, 252
Canadian Prevention Network Action Team on FASD (CanFASD) Prevention 427
Cancer 439; smoking 32; types 207, **208**
cannabinoid receptors 28
cannabis 28–29, 98, 223, 274; acute intoxication and withdrawal 388; adolescent brain 217; cannabis use epidemiology 506–508; child maltreatment 387–388; commercialization and equity 506; Commonwealth 500; decriminalization 503–504; effects 499–500; epidemiology 498–499; history 497–498; implications 508–509; medical 249–250; medicalization 504–505; nonmedical usage 247; penalties 505; prevalence 498; prevention and treatment 505–506; Rasta experience 502–503; social history 501–502; substance-specific effects 387–388
cannabis use disorder 336–337
cardiac arrhythmias 439
cardiomyopathy 439
cardiovascular system 197, **198**
Card, N. A. 285
Caribbean: cannabis use epidemiology 506–508; Commonwealth 500; implications 508–509; Rasta experience 502–503; social history 501–502
case management (CM) 254, 415; client advocacy 303; managers, roles and functions 302–303; medical care team 303; MI strategies 303; services 303; substance-related problems 303
CASIG *see* Client Assessment of Strengths, Interest, and Goals (CASIG)
Cavaiola, A. A. 100
CBCST *see* cognitive behavioral therapy/coping skills training (CBCST)
CBI *see* computer-delivered brief intervention (CBI)
CBT *see* cognitive behavioral therapy (CBT)
CDC *see* Centers for Disease Control and Prevention (CDC)
Center for Substance Abuse Treatment (CSAT) 397
Centers for Disease Control and Prevention (CDC) 28

central nervous system (CNS) 26, 27–28
change strategies 1
CHD *see* congenital heart defect (CHD)
child and family welfare 2
childhood externalizing behaviors 80
child maltreatment 381
children of addicted parents 367
children of alcoholics (COAs) 367
children of substance abusing parents
    (COSAPs): adolescents 370–373;
    Celebrating Families!, 374; child welfare
    system 371; CRAFT 375–376; dysfunctional
    patterns 367; emotional reactions 376;
    family-system dynamics 368; family trauma
    368–369; family treatment 374; FASD 372;
    FOF 374; infants 369–370; MDFT 374–375;
    mentalization-based therapy 375; NAS 372;
    newborns 369–370; parental marijuana 368;
    parent-child relationships 369; parenting skills
    372; school-aged children 370, 372;
    self-supporting adults 368; SFP 374
child welfare system 371
Chow, C. M. 537
chronic alcohol consumption 70
chronic substance use 65
Cichocki, B. 537
cigarette 80
cisgender 285
Client Assessment of Strengths, Interest,
    and Goals (CASIG) 300
clonidine 166
CM *see* case management (CM)
COAs *see* children of alcoholics (COAs)
cocaine 3, 31–32, 335–336, 482
codependency theory 400
cognitive-behavioral interventions 417
cognitive behavioral therapy 96, *96*, 101, 134,
    148–149, 253, 258
cognitive behavioral therapy/coping skills
    training (CBCST) 304–305
cognitive control circuitry 217
cognitive process 105
cognitive social learning theory 237
COM *see* contingency management (COM)
communicable diseases 51
community coethnic density 273
community development 2
community-level determinants 272–273
community reinforcement and family training
    (CRAFT) 307, 375–376, 403–404
community variables 84
community violence 2, 5
Comprehensive Drug Abuse Prevention and
    Control Act 453, 484
Compton, M. T. 535
compulsive behavior 130, 142
computer-delivered brief intervention (CBI) 302

concerned/supportive significant others (CSOs)
    see member's addictive behavior
confrontational interventions 404
congenital disorders 193, **194**
congenital heart defect (CHD) 197
Congruence Couple Therapy (CCT) 402
conscientiousness (C) 234
contemporary brain disease model,
    biopsychosocial framework 12–13
contingency management (COM) 103;
    benefits 310; negative drug screen 309–310
controlled substances 19
Corbit, J. D. 69
Corman, M. D. 550
corticotropin-releasing factor (CRF) 65, 66,
    70, 73
COSAPs *see* children of substance abusing
    parents (COSAPs)
cost-benefit ratio 105
Cowell, A. 347
CRAFT *see* community reinforcement and
    family training (CRAFT)
Crandall, C. 347
Crane, C. A. 548
Cranston, J. W. 550
CRF *see* corticotropin-releasing factor (CRF)
CSAT *see* Center for Substance Abuse
    Treatment (CSAT)
cue-induced response 101, *102*
cultural awareness 1, 275
cultural competence 271
cultural diversity 275
cultural identity 119–120
cytisine 330

Daley, D. C. 410
DALYs *see* disability-adjusted life years (DALYs)
Dannerbeck, A. 461
Dauber, H. 531
Davis, J. P. 234, 235, 348, 360
Davis, T. S. 443
DEA *see* Drug Enforcement Agency (DEA)
de Bruijn, D. M. 548
decisional balance 106, *106*
de Graaf, I. M. 548
de Guglielmo, G. 70
Delfabbro, P. H. 135
dental and oral health 200, **200**
depression 30
detoxification (detox) process 23
develecology model 113
developmental theory, emerging adults:
    acute awareness 233; dimensions of 233;
    experimentation 233; identity exploration
    233; life transitions 234; personality change
    234–235; self-focused 233; *Theory of Emerging
    Adulthood* (Arnett) 232

Diagnostic and Statistical Manual (DSM-5®) 4, 8, 130, 144, 183, 249; impaired control 626; pharmacological criteria 626; risky use patterns 626; severity 627; social impairment 626; substance use disorder 626

Diaz, R. M. 285

DiClemete, Carlo 106

disability-adjusted life years (DALYs): causes 46, **47**; epilepsy 52; GSRAH 46; Levin-based methodology 46; public health policies 46; relative risk 46; women 46–47, **48**, 49, *49–50*

dissociative substances 29–30

distal stressors 286

disulfiram 103, 252, 311, **323**; clinical safety 323; drug indications and duration 323; efficacy 323; mechanism of action 322

diverse theoretical models integration: integration 620, *620*; problem specification 619; risk/protective factors continuum 619–620; vulnerability/resilience continuum 619

Dixon, L. 547

DNA sequence 87

D'Onofrio, G. 348

dopamine 70; VTA 63

drinking behavior patterns 98

drug addiction 59

Drug Enforcement Agency (DEA) 19, 28

drug-related activities 6

drug-related cues 72

drug-related habits 71

Drug trafficking networks 3

drug treatment courts: family drug court 460–461; global reach 454–455; implications 464–465; juvenile and family drug court 455; juvenile drug court 459–460; medication-assisted treatment 462–463; race disparities 461–462; short and long- term 458; similarities and differences 456, **457**, 458; social justice concerns 463–464; ten key components 455–456, **456**; therapeutic jurisprudence 463

drug use disorders 3, 133

Duckert, F. 432

Dumas, T. M. 234

Dutch Ministry of Health Welfare and Sport 425

dynorphin-kappa system 70

dysphoria 71

EAGLES trial 329

early adulthood, MBIs 358

Easton, C. J. 548

eating disorders 439

e-cigarettes 32, 217–218, 224, 330

Edenberg, H. J. 86

education 2

Egan, S. K. 285

Eggers, A. 458

Egizio, L. L. 350

electronic health records (EHR) 448

Eliason, M. J. 291

Elliott, L. 401

Elswick, A. 238

Elwood, S. 603, 609–610

emerging adults: alcohol, prevalence 235; biopsychosocial domains 232; developmental theory (*see* developmental theory, emerging adults); homeless 239–240; LGBTQ+ individuals 288–289; mental health comorbidities 236–237; subgroup variation 236; SUD, prevalence 235–236

emerging priorities, practice and research: common elements and factors 621–622; global health policy 622–623; integration 620, *620*; mechanisms of change 620–621; NIH research goals 622–623; problem specification 619; risk/protective factors continuum 619–620; vulnerability/resilience continuum 619

emotionality (E) 234

endocrine diseases 203–204, **204**

energy drink 33

energy shots 33

environmental hazards 381

epileptic seizures 51–52

epinephrine 65

Esquivel-Santoveña, E. E. 547

ethyl alcohol 25

evidence-informed interventions: CBT 148–149; family-based therapy 150; harm reduction 148; MI 149; mindfulness-based intervention 149–150; multi-level and multi-modality intervention 150; RCT 148

evidence-supported interventions 312

evidence-supported measures 299

exosystem 113

expectancies 104

explicit bias 115

externalizing behavior problems 370

extraversion (X) 234

Fair Sentencing Act 486

Fallin-Bennett, A. 238

family-centered interventions 397, 415; BCT 401; confrontational interventions 404; conjoint treatment 401, 402; CRAFT 403–404; CSO skills 403; evidence-informed interventions 401; family psychoeducation 402–403; family systems interventions 402; healthcare system 400; macro-level barriers 401; mutual aid groups 404–405; services 402, 403; 5-Step Method 402–403

family drinking environment 117

family drug court 455

family-involved treatment approach 308

family psychoeducation 402–403

family system 368 characteristics 117–118; genetic influences 117; human development and behavior 116; interventions 402, 417; maturing pattern 116; parental substance misuse 116; role theory 118
family systems theory 117–118, 398–399
family trauma 368–369
Farrugia, P. L. 534
FAS *see* fetal alcohol syndrome (FAS)
FASD *see* fetal alcohol spectrum disorder (FASD)
FDA *see* Food and Drug Administration (FDA)
Federal Drug and Alcohol Administration 120
federal Uniform State Narcotic Drug Act 484
Fendrich, M. 453–465
Ferdik, F.V. 458
fetal alcohol exposure 439
fetal alcohol spectrum disorder (FASD) 372; ACEs 186; adversity 179; ARBD 176; ARND 176; binge drinking 44; clinical features 176; clinical outcome 176; community factors 178; components 181; costs 177–178; diagnostic categories 176, **177**; diagnostic criteria, elements 181–182, **182**; drinking guidelines 180; DSM-V criteria 183, **183**; epidemiology 177–178; executive function issues **210**, 210–211; facial features 177; FAS 176, 180; functional consequences 174; functional needs 184–185; functional neurodevelopmental domains **182**, 182–183; health care providers 211; health issues, survey (*see* health issues, survey); healthy public policy 186; medical diagnosis 174; multidisciplinary approach 187; PAE (*see* prenatal alcohol exposure (PAE)); pain tolerance 209; pFAS 176; prevalence 44–45, *45*; prevention 423–425, 427–428; RICH approach 185; risk 174; screening 180–181; SDOH 174; secondary adverse outcomes 184, **184**; secondary disabilities 212; sensory issues 209, **209–210**; social determinants 179; social systems 186; social work interventions 46; social work screening 181; TES medicine wheel 185
fetal alcohol syndrome (FAS) 44, 176, 180
fetal neurodevelopment 159
Finkel, E. J. 549
fMRI *see* functional magnetic resonance imaging (fMRI)
focus on families (FOF) 374
Follingstad, D. R. 546
Food and Drug Administration (FDA) 321, 331
Forcehimes, A. 347
Foster, A. 239
France, K. E. 431
Freisthler, B. 388, 607, 614
French, M. T. 347
Freud, S. 130
Friedmann, P. D. 441

Friedman, S. 463
Fuleihan, B.K. 458
functional magnetic resonance imaging (fMRI) 220

GABA *see* gamma-aminobutyric acid (GABA)
Gable, J. 239
Gaidus, A. 614
Gallagher, J.R. 461, 465
gambling disorder 4, 398; bankruptcy 129; characteristics 130; clinical criteria 131; comorbidity 133; compulsive behavior 130; criminality 129; defined 129; desperation phase 130; diagnosis 133–134; emerging issue 135; etiological models 132–133; loot boxes 135; losing phase 130; pathological gambling 130; prevalence 131–132; problem gambling 130; screening instruments 134; "skin" betting 135; social casino games 135; social work programs 136; stress-induced health problems 129; tension 130; treatment outcomes 134–135; WHO 130; winning phase 130; *see also* Internet gaming disorder
Gambling Pathways Questionnaire (GPQ) 132, 134
gaming-related maladaptive cognitions 147
gamma-aminobutyric acid (GABA) 27
gang activities 6
gastrointestinal/digestive system 203, **203**
gastrointestinal problems 439
Gelernter, J. 86
gender identity: LGBTQ+ individuals 283, 285–286; SBIRT models 348
gender non-conformity 285
gene-by-environment (G×E) research 120–121 candidate examples 86; genetic traits 86; polygenic scores 86–87
genome-wide association studies (GWAS) 85–87
geographic ecological momentary assessment (GEMA) 615
geographic information systems (GIS): accomplishments 604, *605*; community assets 604; counts *versus* rates 607; edge effects 614–615; injustices 604, *605*; limitations 613; mapping community needs *603*, 603–604; misalignment 613–614; North and South intervention areas 601, *602*; place-based policies 612–613; reinterpretation 605, *606*; Sacramento Neighborhood Alcohol Prevention Project 601–603; spatial spillover 614; visual *versus* statistical relationships 607, *608*
Giancola, P. R. 550
Gil-Rivas, V. 538
Giroux, I. 134
GIS *see* geographic information systems (GIS)
Glass, J. E. 347, 348

Global Burden of Disease study 53
Global Information System on Alcohol and Health 39
Global Status Report on Alcohol and Health (GSRAH) 40, 42, 46, 52, 53
Gmel, G. 232–234
goal-directed substance use 66
Gobbart, S. 537
Godleski, S. A. 548
GPQ *see* Gambling Pathways Questionnaire (GPQ)
grandfamilies: Black/African American and Latino caregivers 411; case management 415; cognitive-behavioral interventions 417; community programs 415; diversity 411; family-based interventions 415; family system interventions 417; grandchildren 412–413; grandparents 411–412; psychoeducation 416–417; resilience 413–415; social interactions 417; structured interventions 415; SUDs 410; support groups 416
Graybiel, A. M. 67
Grella, C. E. 538
growth and development alterations 193, **194**
Gruenewald, P. J. 388, 607, 614
Grunebaum, M. F. 529
GSRAH *see* Global Status Report on Alcohol and Health (GSRAH)
GWAS *see* genome-wide association studies (GWAS)

habit circuits 66–68
Hajek, P. 330
hallucinogens 29–30
Han, B. 249
Hargrove, Emily Travis 191–192
harm reduction 13–14
Harris, G. 461
Harrison Narcotics Tax Act 484
Hayslip, B. 414
Hazardous/problematic gaming 4
health beliefs model 105
health issues, survey: acute and chronic ear infections 195; appendicitis 209; ARBD 194; ARND 194; ASD 194; autoimmune disorders 195–196, **197**; cancer, types 207, **208**; cardiovascular system 197, **198**; congenital disorders 193, **194**; dental and oral health 200, **200**; endocrine diseases 203–204, **204**; gastrointestinal/digestive system 203, **203**; growth and development alterations 193, **194**; hearing/auditory problem 201, **202**; hernias 207–208; immune disorders 195, **196**; immune system 195; IOM 193, 194; kidney disease 209; mental health disorders 205–206, **206**; metabolic diseases 203–204, **204**; migraine headaches 207, **208**; musculoskeletal system 198, **199**, 200; reproductive health **202**, 202–203; respondent demographics 192, **193**; seizures 207; sleep disorders 204–205, **205**; substance use disorders 206, **207**; Tourette syndrome 209; vision 201, **201**
health-promoting behaviors 106
health promotion programs: alcohol use, during pregnancy 423–425; BI 426–427; FASD 423–425, 427–428; primary prevention activities 425; secondary prevention 425; socio-ecological approach 426, *426*; tertiary prevention 425
hearing/auditory problem 201, **202**
Heath, B. B. 442
Heather, N. 11
heavy episodic drinking (HED) 42
hedonic homeostasis 69
Heinz, A. 550
hemorrhagic stroke 439
hernias 207–208
heroin 34, 35
Heroin Act 484
heroin-related cues 72
HEXACO factors 234, 235
Hiersteiner, D. 537
high visibility enforcement (HVE) 583
Hill, S. C. 436
Himmelreich, Myles 191–192
HIV infection 51
homelessness 6–7
homeostasis 68, 69
homosexuality 288
honesty (H) 234
Horn, B. P. 347
housing/homelessness issues 2
housing vulnerability 7
Huang, H. 460
Hughes, T. 291
human diversity 1, 5; ADA 265; cultural awareness 275; cultural diversity 275; gender roles 264–265; heavy drinking, alcohol-induced disorders 266; intersectionality 263; macro-level practice implications 276–277; micro-level practice implications 275–276; NIMHD 262, 263 (*see also* U.S. National Institute on Minority Health and Health Disparities (NIMHD); physical disabilities 265; racial/ethnic disparities 263–264
Human Genome Project 84, 85
human responsibility 1
human trafficking 2
HVE *see* high visibility enforcement (HVE)
hyperalgesia 73
hyperkatifeia 72–73
hypertension 439
hypohedonia 71

Iacono, W. G. 547

Ialongo, N. S. 86–87

IARC *see* International Agency for Research on Cancer (IARC)

IGD *see* Internet gaming disorder (IGD)

Iglesias, K. 232–234

IHD *see* ischemic heart disease (IHD)

Illes, R. C. 442

illicit drug use 247, 250

IM *see* Intervention Mapping (IM)

IMAGEN Consortium 218

immigrant and refugee populations 6

immune disorders 195, **196**

implementation science: clients and communities 585–586; context and capacity 583; de-implementation 585; effective interventions 579; engaging stakeholders 582–583; fidelity-adaptation tension 584–585; implementation strategies 583–584; multi-level practice context 579; outcomes 581; prevention interventions 581–582; strategies *579*, 579–581; sustainability 585; treatment interventions 582

implicit bias 115–116, 272

Important People and Activities (IPA) instrument 300

impulsive behavior 67

impulsivity 219

incarcerated women: childhood and adult victimization 516; co-occurring disorders 515–516; forever free program 519; Oxford House 519–520; policy and system changes 520–521; prisoner reentry 517–518; promising programs 519; regular and heavy illicit drug use 516; risk factor 517; specialized probation and recovery management checkups 520; treatment barriers 518–519

individual-level determinants 269–270

information processing model: behavior and performance 97, *97*; distortion of 97; information/education intervention 96; short-term memory retention 97

inhalants 35–36

innovative interventions: ASI 300; assessment tasks 298; behavioral treatment (*see* case management (CM)); brief intervention (BI) *see* brief intervention (BI); CASIG 300; CBCST 304–305; COM 309–310; diagnostic process 300; evaluation 299; MAT 310–312; MI 298, 305–306; motivation 300; problem severity 300; SAW 300; screening 299; social support 300

Institute of Medicine (IOM) 193, 194

Integrated and Culturally Relevant Care Curriculum 443

integrated care: behavioral health integration 442; early identification 444; healthcare system 437; PCBH 436; primary healthcare 437 (*see also* primary healthcare settings; skepticism 441); social worker competencies 443; social work practice 442–443; social work profession 442

Intellectual Quotient (IQ) 219

internalized stigma 236

International Agency for Research on Cancer (IARC) 51

International Classification of Disease (ICD)-11, 627–628

International Classification of Disease (ICD-10) 4

Internet gaming disorder (IGD) 4; APA 142, 144; assessment 144, **145**; behavioral addiction 151; comorbid psychopathology 147; compulsive behavior 142; defined 143; etiology 146; evidence-informed interventions (*see* evidence-informed interventions); family environment 148; gaming-related maladaptive cognitions 147; measurement invariance 144; mesolimbic dopaminergic system 142; motivations 147–148; neurological risks 146; personality traits 146–147; prevalence rates 144; psychological distress 144; psychosocial harms 142; risk factors 146; social media addiction 144, **145**; substance use disorders 144; "sunk cost bias," 147; usage and addiction 142; video game genres and titles 143, **143**; virtual online community 147

interpersonal-level determinants 270–272

intervention logic models 95

Intervention Mapping (IM) 433; determinants 430; ethical considerations 430; evaluation plan 432; FASD prevalence 429; implementation 430; logic model 428; maternal behaviors 429; program materials and messages 431; program outcomes and objectives 430; program plan development 430–431; step and tasks 428, *429*; stigma, types 430; sustainability 431; theory-based methods 432

intervention spectrum *297*

intervention studies, older adults 250; acamprosate 252–253; baclofen 253; BI 251; care modalities 254; case and care management models 254; CBT 255; disulfiram 252; individual and group treatments 254; MAT 253; motivational interventions 251–252; naltrexone 253; NRT 253–254; pharmacotherapy 252; psychotherapeutic approaches 254; STMs 255; varenicline 253

intimate partner violence (IPV) 2, 5; acute contributors 548; alcohol expectancy theory 549–550; alcohol myopia theory 550–551; conditional contributors 548–549; externalizing factor 547–548; high *versus*

low intensity 546; indirect causes 548; intervention 551–553; physical violence 547; prevalence 546; psychological violence 546; research implications 553–554; risk of experience 551; sexual violence 546; spurious factors 547–548; theoretical perspectives 549
IOM *see* Institute of Medicine (IOM)
IPA instrument *see* Important People and Activities (IPA) instrument
IPV *see* intimate partner violence (IPV)
IQ *see* Intellectual Quotient (IQ)
ischemic heart disease (IHD) 439
ischemic stroke 439

Jacques, C. 134
Jang, S. A. 431
"J-curve" hypothesis 248
Jellinek Curve 9
Jellinek, E. M. 9–10, 98
Johansen, A. 432
Johnson, F. W. 607
Johnson, J. L. 370
Jones, D. 348
Jones, K. L. 180
Jones-Miller Narcotic Drugs Import and Export Act 484
juvenile drug court 455

Kabat-Zinn, J. 356–357
kappa opioid receptor (KOR) 70
Kaptsis, D. 135
Kennedy, John F. 501
Kennedy, S. C. 516
Kepple, N. J. 615
kidney disease 209
King, D. L. 135
Kingston, R. E. F. 531–532
Kirkpatrick, H. A. 442
Klein, H. 454
Kok, G. 431, 432
Koob, G. 69
Koob, M. L. 67
KOR *see* kappa opioid receptor (KOR)
Kowalchuk, A. 350
Krueger, R. F. 547
Kushner, M. G. 536

Ladouceur, R. 134
Lancianese, D. A. 348
language-use practices 8
Large, M. 535
Lascala, E. A. 607
Laudet, A.B. 471
learning theory: classical conditioning principles 101–102, *102*; operant conditioning functions 102–103, *103*; social learning theory 103–104
Lebel, T. P. 348, 463

legal/criminal justice systems 2
Leonard, K. E. 550
Lesbian, gay, bisexual, transgender, and queer/questioning (LGBTQ+) individuals: adolescence 286–287; behavioral health disparities 282; bisexual individuals 282; community 283; coping process 288; disparities 286; emerging adulthood 288–289; gender identity 283, 285–286; homosexuality 288; identity development 287; identity exploration 289–290; instability 289; intervention research 291–292; middle adulthood 290; minority stress theory (MST) 282, 286; older adulthood 290–291; sexual orientation 283–284, **284**; social climate 288; social environment 287–288
Letarte, H. 134
LGBTQ+ individuals *see* Lesbian, gay, bisexual, transgender, and queer/questioning (LGBTQ+) individuals
Licata, M. L. 548
licensed physical/mental health care 19
life course development, developmental theory 98
life course perspective 1
Lipsey, M. W. 346
Lipton, D. M. 67
Lisha, N. E. 233
Liu, M. 460
liver cirrhosis 52
liver disease 439
Li, Y. 460
Lloyd, K. 461
Lloyd, M. 453–465
local indicators of spatial autocorrelation 609–610
lofexidine 335
"long acting" drug 22
loot boxes 135
loss of control concept 11–12
low-risk alcohol consumption, public health guidelines 53
lung diseases, smoking 32
Lutke, C. J. 191–192

McGue, M. 547
MacKenzie, D.L. 458
macro-level healthcare policy 406
macrosystem 113
magnetic resonance spectroscopy (MRS) 225
Maher, B. 86–87
maladaptive learning 59, 74
Malcore, S. A. 442
Marijuana Tax Act 484
Marlatt, A. 356–357
Marlatt, G. A. 358, 359
Marlowe, D.B. 461

Marmot, M. 186
MAT *see* medication-assisted treatment (MAT)
maternal opioid use 160
May, P. A. 177
MBCT *see* Mindfulness-Based Cognitive Therapy (MBCT)
MBIs *see* mindfulness-based interventions (MBIs)
MBRP *see* Mindfulness-Based Relapse Prevention (MBRP)
MBSR *see* Mindfulness-Based Stress Reduction (MBSR)
McDonald, T. 391
McEwen, B. S. 69
McMillin, H.E. 460
MDFT *see* multidimensional family therapy (MDFT)
mediational mechanisms, acculturation 119
medical costs 159
medical management (MM) approach 312
medication-assisted treatment (MAT) 11, 13, 167, 253, 321, 462–463; abstinence/reduction 311; client-practitioner partnership 313; evidence-supported interventions 312; MM approach 312; OUD 311–312; pharmacotherapies 310–311; social stability 312; social support 312
member's addictive behavior: codependency theory 400; cultural factors 398; family-centered approach 397; family-centered interventions (*see* family-centered interventions); family systems theory 398–399; gambling disorder 398; social work education 405–406; SSCS model 399–400; SUDs 398
mental/behavioral health issues 2
mental health disorders (MHD) 205–206, **206**; anxiety disorders 531; brain development 535; combination models 535–536; gender 529; harm reduction 538; influence models, direction of *532*; integrated treatment barriers 537, 538; intoxication and withdrawal 535; mood disorders 531; parallel treatment 536–537; prevalence 530; PTSD 531–532; sequential treatment 536; severe and persistent 532; shared underlying factors 535; substance-related cognitions 534; substance use disruptions 534; symptom severity 533; trauma 534
mentalization-based therapy 375
mesocorticolimbic dopamine system 63
mesocorticolimbic reward pathway 69–70
mesolimbic dopaminergic system 142
mesosystem 113
MET *see* Motivational Enhancement Therapy (MET)
metabolic diseases 203–204, **204**

methadone 34, 165, 167, 311, **332**; drug indications and duration 331; efficacy and clinical safety 331, 333; mechanism of action 331
methamphetamine 31
Meyers, J. A. 350
MHD *see* mental health disorders (MHD)
MI *see* motivational interviewing (MI)
Michael, K. 98
micro aggression experiences 5
migraine headaches 207, **208**, 440
military members and veteran groups 5
Miller, G. E. 436
Milner, P. M. 63
Mindfulness-Based Cognitive Therapy (MBCT) 355–357, 358–359
mindfulness-based interventions (MBIs) 149–150; ACT 359; adolescence 358; childhood 357; components 356; early adulthood 358; early intervention 357; manualized interventions 357; MBCT 358–359; MBRP 359; MBSR 358; meditation 356; MORE 359; non-manualized approach 359–360; pilot studies 360; prevention 357; psychological issues 356; relapse prevention models 358; SUDs 355; technology-based mindfulness interventions 360; TM 356; treatment 358; TSMP 360; yoga 356
Mindfulness-Based Relapse Prevention (MBRP) 355–357, 359
Mindfulness-Based Stress Reduction (MBSR) 355–357, 358
Mindfulness-oriented recovery enhancement (MORE) 359
minority stress theory (MST) 282, 286, 292
Mitchell, O. 458, 459
Mitchell, S. G. 346
MM approach *see* medical management (MM) approach
Modified Finnegan Neonatal Abstinence Scoring system 162
molecular genomic studies: candidate gene studies 85; genetic variants 85; G×E research 86–87; GWAS 85–86; Human Genome Project 84, 85; human traits and behaviors 84; SNP 84
Mollen, S. 431
mood disorders 531
Moran, E. 130
MORE *see* Mindfulness-oriented recovery enhancement (MORE)
morphine 34, 165
motivation 69, 106
Motivational Enhancement Therapy (MET) 251–252, 552
motivational interviewing (MI) 149, 251–252, 298, 301, 302, 305–306, 313, 346;

affirmations 306; client autonomy 306; clinical utility 305; CM 303; foundational elements 306; open-ended questioning 305–306; optimism 306; practitioner-client relationship 305; reflections 306; SBIRT models 344, 349

MRS *see* magnetic resonance spectroscopy (MRS)

multidimensional family therapy (MDFT) 374–375

Multilateral Evaluation Mechanism (MEM) 506

multi-level and multi-modality intervention 150

Multi-Site Adult Drug Court Evaluation (MADCE) 458

Musci, R. J. 86–87

musculoskeletal system 198, **199**, 200

mutual aid groups 255, 404–405

mutual help networks 309

NA *see* Narcotics Anonymous (NA)

nalmefene 325–326

naloxone, opioid overdose reversal 34, 333–335

naltrexone 253, 311, **323**, 334–335; clinical safety 324; drug indications and duration 324; efficacy 324; mechanism of action 323

Narcotic Drug Control Act 484

Narcotics Anonymous (NA) 308, 473–474

Narcotics Penalties and Enforcement Act 485

NAS *see* neonatal abstinence syndrome (NAS)

nasal inhalation 24

National Association for Children of Alcoholics 373

National Consortium on Alcohol and Neuro Development in Adolescence (NCANDA) 218

National Epidemiologic Survey on Alcohol and Related Conditions (NESARC) 10, 247

National Household Survey by Statistics Canada 410

National Institute of Alcohol Abuse and Alcoholism (NIAAA) 26, 248, 345, 623

National Institute of Drug Abuse (NIDA) 335

National Student Drug Survey (2016) 507–508

National Survey on Drug Use and Health (NSDUH) 247, 366, 436

NCANDA *see* National Consortium on Alcohol and Neuro Development in Adolescence (NCANDA)

ND *see* neurodevelopmental disorder (ND)

neonatal abstinence syndrome (NAS) 372; adjunct therapy 166; brain cell death 159; diagnosis 161; epidemiology 158–159; fetal neurodevelopment 159; fetal opiate levels 161; healthcare team 163; illicit drugs 166; long-term developmental outcomes 159, 166; maternal opioid use 160; medical costs 159; multidisciplinary community 169;

non-pharmacological treatment 163–165; opiate withdrawal 158; pharmacological intervention 164–165; pharmacological treatment 160; prevention 166–168; screening 161; short-acting opiates 161; SNPs 168; social determinants 160–161; social work services 169; societal costs 159; socioeconomic factors 160; standard treatment protocols 163

neonatal meconium testing 161–162

NESARC *see* National Epidemiologic Survey on Alcohol and Related Conditions (NESARC)

Nesvåg, S. 432

neural predictors 218–219

neuroadaptations 74

neurodevelopmental disorder (ND) 175

neuroplasticity 225

neuropsychological assessments, parental cognitive functioning 392

neuropsychological predictors 219–220

New Recovery Advocacy Movement 475–476

NIAAA *see* National Institute of Alcohol Abuse and Alcoholism (NIAAA)

nicotine 32–33

nicotine replacement therapy (NRT) 253–254, **328**; clinical safety 327–328; drug indications and duration 327; efficacy 327–328; mechanism of action 327; pharmacological treatment 326

Nielssen, O. 535

nitrites, inhalants 35

N-methyl-D-aspartate (NMDA) 324

non-benzodiazepine sedative-hypnotics/ sleep aids 27

non-communicable diseases (NCDs) 51–52, 622

non-refugee immigrants 6

NRT *see* nicotine replacement therapy (NRT)

NSDUH *see* National Survey on Drug Use and Health (NSDUH)

observational learning 104

O'Doherty, J. P. 72

OECD *see* Organisation for Economic Co-operation and Development (OECD)

older adults, substance misuse: acamprosate 252–253; aging services 248; alcohol effects 248; baclofen 253; BI 251; cannabis, nonmedical usage 247; care modalities 254; case and care management models 254; CBT 255; disulfiram 252; illicit drug use 247, 250; individual and group treatments 254; "J-curve" hypothesis 248; LGBTQ+ individuals 290–291; MAT 253; medical cannabis 249–250; motivational interventions 251–252; mutual aid groups 255; naltrexone 253; NESARC 247; non-confrontational approach 251; nonmedical prescription 250; NRT 253–254; NSDUH 247, 249;

pharmacotherapy 252; psychotherapeutic approaches 254; risk continuum 249; SAGE 248; STMs 255; tobacco 249; varenicline 253
O'Leary, C. M. 194
OMT *see* opioid maintenance therapy (OMT)
on-demand feeding 163–164
openness to experience (O) 234
opioid maintenance therapy (OMT) 161–162, 167
opioids 24, 34–35, 388–389; PAG 66; receptors 64; substitution drugs 13
opioid use disorder (OUD) 158–159, 311–312; first-line treatments 330–335, **332**; interdisciplinary prenatal substance abuse programs 167; MAT 253; naloxone, overdose reversal 335; during pregnancy 166–167; second-line treatments 325, 335
opium 482
Opium Exclusion Act 482
opponent process theory 69, 74
Orford, J. 399
Organisation for Economic Co-operation and Development (OECD) 40, 622
organized crime 6
original disease model: abstinence 10–11; addiction 9; "average trend" model 9; degree of variability 10; DSM-IV-R criteria 10; loss of control concept 11–12; MAT 11; NESARC data 10; RRD 11; stereotypes 10; treatment 10
Orr, L. C. 401
osteoarthritis 198
osteopenia 198
osteoporosis 198
OUD *see* opioid use disorder (OUD)
over-the-counter (OTC) substances 19

PAE *see* prenatal alcohol exposure (PAE)
PAG *see* periaqueductal gray (PAG)
pain tolerance 209
pancreatitis 52
Papies, E. K. 360
parental substance misuse 116, 121
parent-child relationships 148, 369
parenting behavior **383**; attachment models 384; empathy models 384; individual-level mechanisms 384; parental brain circuits 382; SIP models 382, 384; substance-specific effects **385, 386**
parenting behaviors 112
parenting interventions 392
partial Fetal Alcohol Syndrome (pFAS) 176
pathological gambling 130
pathways model, gambling problems 132
PCBH *see* primary care behavioral health (PCBH)
peer recovery networks 308
periaqueductal gray (PAG) 66
Perry, D. G. 285

personality theory 100–101, 234
PET *see* positron emission tomography (PET)
Pettus-Davis, C. 516
PGS *see* polygenic score (PGS)
pharmacokinetics 21, **22**, *22*; drug half-life 21, *22*; home use urine drug tests 21, **22**; principle 21; therapeutic/effects range 21
pharmacotherapies, addiction treatment 252; AUDs (*see* alcohol use disorders (AUDs)); cannabis use disorder 336–337; cocaine use disorder 335–336; FDA 321; MAT 321; OUD 330–335, **332**; substance use disorder 321; TUD (*see* tobacco use disorder (TUD)); WHO 322
pharmacy computerized networking systems 20
phenotypes 79, 85, 87
physical disabilities 265
physical health issues 2
policy reforms: budget *486*, 486–487; cannabis 484; cocaine 482; criminalization and public health 490–491; decriminalization 492–493; drug policy reform advocacy 491–492; early prohibition 484; harm reduction 492; illicit drug availability 487–488; mass criminalization and racial disparities 488–489; modern war on Drugs 484–486, **485**; notable drug policy reforms 487; opium 482; treatment and criminalization 489–490; in United States 482–483
polydrug use/drug interaction effects 21
polygenic score (PGS) 86, 88
polysubstance use 390–391
Ponicki, W. R. 614
Popova, S. 424
positron emission tomography (PET) 64
post traumatic stress disorder (PTSD) 5, 531–532
pregnancy, alcohol use: clinical guidelines 43; FAS 44; FASD 44–46, *45*; GSRAH 44; OUD treatment 166–167; postpartum mother treatment 168; prevalence 43, **43**, 44; risk factor 43
prenatal alcohol exposure (PAE) 174; alcohol use 178; clinical features 175; community factors 178; costs 177–178; drinking guidelines 180; DSM-V criteria 183, **183**; epidemiology 177–178; prevalence rates 178; screening 180–181; secondary adverse outcomes 184, **184**; WHO 178
prescription drug abuse 19, 20
primary care behavioral health (PCBH) 436
primary healthcare settings: Affordable Care Act 437; alcohol exposure 438–439; cost reimbursement 447; drug screening 440–441; health complications 438; health concerns 438–440; infrastructure issues 447–448; mental health concerns 440; outpatient substance use services 445–446; pain

management 440; stigma 447; substance use assessment 445; SUD 438; team member commitment 447–448; withdrawal management 446; wrap-around services 446

Pringle, J. L. 350

problem gambling 130

Problem Gambling Severity Index 134

Prochaska, J. O. 106

proximal stressors 286

Przybyla, S. M, 548

psychoactive substances 381–382; alcohol (*see* alcohol); AUD 20–21; BAC 22; BAL 22; cannabis 28–29; classification 18–19; CNS depressants 27–28; community level 20; controlled substances 19; dissociative substances 29–30; drug interaction effects 24; dyad level 20; hallucinogens 29–30; individual level 19–20; inhalants 35–36; intended effects 18; licensed physical/mental health care 19; "long acting" drug 22; modes of administration 23–24; opioids 24, 34–35; OTC substances 19; pharmacokinetics 21, **22**, *22*; polydrug use/drug interaction effects 21; prescription drug abuse 19, 20; sedative-hypnotics 27–28; "short acting" drug 22; stimulants (*see* stimulants); SUD 18; tolerance 23; unintended effects 18; withdrawal 23

psychodynamic theory 100

psychoeducation 416–417; interventions, grandfamilies 416psychological models: behavioral economics theory 105–106; cognitive theory 96, *96*; decisional balance 106, *106*; developmental theory 98–99, *99*; expectancies 104; health beliefs model 105; health-promoting behaviors 106; information processing (*see* information processing model); integrated biopsychosocial framework 95; internal mental process 95; intervention logic models 95; learning theory (*see* learning theory); motivation 106; personality theory 100–101; psychodynamic theory 100; self-efficacy 106; stages of change 107; substance use 104–105; TMBC 106; types 95

psychological vulnerability 110

psychomotor 52

psychotomimetic—mimicking psychosis 29

PTSD *see* post traumatic stress disorder (PTSD)

Qvicklund, H. 537

race/ethnicity 236, 263–264

randomized controlled trials (RCTs) 148, 322, 323, 325, 350, 361

Reagan-era Anti-Drug Abuse Act 485

recovery community organizations (RCOs) 469

Recovery Courts 454

recovery housing models 7

recovery management checkups (RMCs) 520

recovery-oriented policy and services: addiction recovery 470–471; addiction treatment, history of 473; chronic disease 474; community empowerment 478; disparate approaches 474; mutual aid 473–474; New Recovery Advocacy Movement 475–476; policy advocacy 478; potential barriers and tensions 478–479; recovery movement implications 474–475; recovery-oriented system of care 472–473, **473**; service delivery 478; social work practices *versus*. addiction recovery values 476–477

recovery-oriented system of care (ROSC) 469–470; definitions 472; *versus* treatment-as-usual 472–473

reduced-risk drinking (RRD) 11

relapse 107; prevention models 358; SDOH 111

relaxation techniques 373

religiosity 120

reproductive health **202**, 202–203

responsible beverage service (RBS) 604, *605*

responsiveness 1

resveratrol, antioxidative properties 51

Revia®, 253

Reynolds, K. 442

Rimal, R. N. 431

Roberts, B. W. 235

Rogerian approach 251

Rogers, M. J. 546

Roozen, S. 428

Rose, S. J. 348

RRD *see* reduced-risk drinking (RRD)

Ruiter, R. A. C. 431

Russell, S. T. 285

Ryan, C. 285

Sacco, P. 350

Sacramento Neighborhood Alcohol Prevention Project 601–603

SAGE *see* Study on Global AGEing and Adult Health (SAGE)

Sagvaag, H. 401

Sahker, E. 348

Salvatore, J. E. 86–87

SAMHSA *see* Substance Abuse and Mental Health Services Administration (SAMHSA)

Samson, A. 105

SAW *see* Strengths Assessment Worksheet (SAW)

school-aged children 370, 372

Schlauch, R. C. 548

screening, brief intervention, and referral to treatment (SBIRT) models 391, 444, **444**; brief intervention 345–346; cost effectiveness 347; defined 344; enhancing motivation 346; gender 348; goals 346; healthcare settings 344, 348–349; MI 344; multiple

meta-analyses 346; quality-of-life outcomes 347; SAMHSA 343, 349; screening 344–345; social workers 349–350; socioeconomic status 348; substance misuse 344; substance type 348; substance use treatment system 343; treatment initiation outcome 347
SDOH *see* social determinants of health (SDOH)
Seale, J. P. 350
secondary disabilities 212
sedative-hypnotics 27–28
seizures 207
Selbekk, A. S. 401
self-efficacy 106
Senreich, E. 291
Sentencing Reform Act 453
service delivery systems 2, 5
Sevigny, E.L. 458
sexual assault 2, 6
sexual dysfunction 439
sexual orientation 283–284, **284**
sexual trauma 5
SFP *see* strengthening families program (SFP)
Sharma, S. 535
"short acting" drug 22
SIC *see* stages of implementation completion (SIC)
SIDS *see* sudden infant death syndrome (SIDS)
significant others (SOs) 307–308; BCT 307; CRAFT 307; family-involved treatment 308
single-nucleotide polymorphisms (SNPs) 84, 168
Single State Authorities (SSA) 469
Sing, M. 436
SIP models *see* social information processing (SIP) models
Sjögren's syndrome 195
"skin" betting 135
Slade, T. 535
sleep: disorders 204–205, **205**, 440; SUD 238–239
Smith, D. C. 348, 350
Smith, E. 410
Smith, G. C. 416
Smith, K. S. 67
smoking 32, 104; cessation 252, 326
SNPs *see* single-nucleotide polymorphisms (SNPs)
social casino games 135
social control 111–112
social determinants of health (SDOH) 111, 174
social ecological model 113, *113*
social environmental contexts: biological vulnerability 110; biopsychosocial framework 110; circularity of influence 111; community level 119; culture 119–120; distal factors 112; family drinking environment 117; family system 116–117; Federal Drug and Alcohol Administration 120; gene-environment

interplay 120–121; neighborhood environment conditions 119; parental substance misuse 116; peers 118–119; proximal factors 112; psychological vulnerability 110; religiosity 120; resilience 110; role theory 118; SDOH 111; social control 111–112; social norms 114–115, **115**; social system 112–114, *113*; social triggers 111–112; stigma 115–116
social information processing (SIP) models 382, 384
social learning theory 103–104
social media addiction 144, **145**
social norms 114–115, **115**
social stigma 115–116, 121
social system 112–114, *113*, 121
social triggers 111–112
social work education 7, 405–406
social workers, recovery-oriented policy and services: community empowerment 478; policy advocacy 478; potential barriers and tensions 478–479; service delivery 478
social work interventions 1
social work treatments protocols 392
societal costs 159
societal-level determinants 273–275
socioeconomic status (SES) 264, 348
Solomon, R. L. 69
SOs *see* significant others (SOs)
Soto, D. W. 233
South Oaks Gambling Screen (SOGS) 134
spatial analysis: exploratory spatial data analysis 609; medical marijuana dispensaries *611*, 611–612; place-based drug policies 610; spatial autocorrelation 609–610
SSCS model *see* Stress-Strain-Coping-Support (SSCS) model
Stade, B. 424
stages of implementation completion (SIC) 583–584
Stein, D.M. 459
Stellar, E. 69
stimulants 389–390; amphetamine 30–31; caffeine 30, 33; cocaine 31–32; methamphetamine 31; nicotine 32–33
stimulus-response relationships 60
STMs *see* supportive therapy models (STMs)
strengthening families program (SFP) 374
Strengths Assessment Worksheet (SAW) 300
stress-coping strategy 133
stress-induced health problems 129
stress-related neurotransmitters 65–66, 70
Stress-Strain-Coping-Support (SSCS) model 399–400
structural brain precursors 220–221, 223–224
Studer, J. 232–234
Study on Global AGEing and Adult Health (SAGE) 248

Substance Abuse and Mental Health Services Administration (SAMHSA) 255, 301, 436, 469, 471
substance-free social networks 304
substance-involved sexual assault: characteristics 563; cognitive impairment s 563–564; drinking factors 565; emotion regulation 564; impulse control difficulties 564; intoxication, sexual assault 565; level of force 563; perpetration prevention programs 568–569; perpetrators' alcohol use 563; prevalence 561–562; risk reduction programs 567–568; sequelae of 565–566; setting 562–563; sexual arousal 564–565; victim–perpetrator relationship 562
substance misuse 1, 5–7; adolescence 78; adult 78; behavioral genetic studies (see behavioral genetic studies); developmental perspective 78–80, 79; emphasis 4; gene-environment interactions 78, 80; implications 87–88; interactive model 80; molecular genomic studies (see molecular genomic studies); older adults (see older adults, substance misuse); primary healthcare (see integrated care); SDOH 111; social system 114; social triggers 112
substance use: adolescent brain 217–224; community functioning 272; community norms 272–273; co-occurring disorders 515–516; coping strategies 270; cultural identity 270; distal factors 112; human diversity 265; interpersonal discrimination 271; LGBTQ+ individuals (see Lesbian, gay, bisexual, transgender, and queer/questioning (LGBTQ+) individuals); patient-clinician relationship 271–272; prisoner reentry 517–518; proximal factor 112; regular and heavy illicit drug use 516; risk factor 517; social control 111–112; social system 114; social triggers 111–112; societal structure 273–274; see also intimate partner violence (IPV)
substance use disorders (SUDs) 1, 5, 7, 18; availability of services 273; CNS depressant drugs 27; cocaine 32; community resources 272; COSAPs (see children of substance abusing parents (COSAPs)); emerging adults 237–238 (see also emerging adults); etiology 80; evidence-based treatment 240; family functioning 271; genetic vulnerability 269–270; health issues, survey 206, 207; health promotion programs (see health promotion programs); human diversity 262; IGD 144; income and insurance coverage 270; member's addictive behavior 398; National Surveys on Drug Use and Health 366; peers 118–119; policies and laws 273; prevalence 235–236; prevention 425; quality of care 274–275;

racial/ethnic disparities 263–264; risk factor 79; severity 367; sleep 238–239; social norms 274; social system 114; stigma 116; in United States 58, 58
sudden infant death syndrome (SIDS) 370
Sundet, P. 461
supportive therapy models (STMs) 254–255, 255
Sussman, S. 234
Sylvain, C. 134

Tanner-Smith, E. E. 346, 459
Taylor, S. P. 550
teratogen see alcohol
TES medicine wheel see "two-eyed seeing" (TES) medicine wheel
Testa, M. 548
tetrahydrocannabinol (THC) concentration 217, 497
Theory of Emerging Adulthood (Arnett) 232
thermoregulation 68
Thornberry, T. P. 388
thyroid diseases 196
TM see transcendental meditation (TM)
TMBC see transtheoretical model of behavior change (TMBC)
tobacco 32–33, 79, 112, 120; older adults, substance misuse 249
tobacco use disorder (TUD): first-line treatments 326–330, 327; second-line treatments 330
Toomey, R. B. 285
Toscolani, J. 410
Tourette syndrome 209
Tracy, S. 476
trafficking 20
transcendental meditation (TM) 356
transgender 285, 287
transtheoretical model of behavior change (TMBC) 106, 107
trauma 5
trauma-informed care 5
trauma-sensitive mindfulness practice (TSMP) 360
Treno, A. J. 607
Tripodi, S. J. 516
TUD see tobacco use disorder (TUD)
"two-eyed seeing" (TES) medicine wheel 185
type 1 diabetes 196

Uhl, G. 86–87
Unger, J. B. 233
United Nations Office on Drugs and Crime (UNODC) 28, 35
United Nations Sustainable Development Goals 3
univariate genetic models 82, 84
UNODC see United Nations Office on Drugs and Crime (UNODC)

U.S. drug scheduling system **485**
U.S. Monitoring the Future study 114
U.S. National Institute on Drug Abuse (NIDA) 12, 25
U.S. National Institute on Minority Health and Health Disparities (NIMHD): Asian-American populations **268**, 269; biological determinants 266; influence levels 266, **267**; social determinants 266

varenicline tartrate **328**; drug indications and duration 329; efficacy and clinical safety 329–330; mechanism of action **328**
Velasquez, M. M. 348
ventral tegmental area (VTA) 63, *64*; glutamate 71
video game genres and titles 143, **143**
Violence Against Women Act (VAWA) 560
virtual community of inquiry (vCoI) model 427
Vogel, M. E. 442

Wagner-Goldstein, K. 463
Wahler, E. A 465
Werner, E. E. 370

Werner-Wilson, R. 238
Westbrook, C. 361
White, W. 472
WHO *see* World Health Organization (WHO)
Wieman, D. 537
Wilson, D.B. 458
Wise, R. P. 442
Wolf, J. P. 388
workplace/economic sufficiency 2
World Cancer Research Fund/ American Institute for Cancer Research (WCRF/AICR) 51
World Drug Report (2018) 217
World Health Organization (WHO) 39, 130, 178, 322, 424
Wu, Q. 460

Yakhnich, L. 98
yoga 356
Yuma-Guerrero, P. J. 346

Zhang, S. 460
Zorrilla, E. P. 67
Zwaans, T. 135